FUNDAMENTALS OF HIV MEDICINE

2023 EDITION

FUNDAMENTALS OF HIV MEDICINE

2023 EDITION

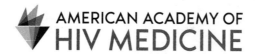

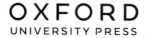

OXFORD
UNIVERSITY PRESS

OXFORD
UNIVERSITY PRESS

ISSN 2752-5767 (Print)
ISSN 2752-5775 (Online)
ISBN 978–0–19–767909–8

DOI: 10.1093/med/9780197679098.001.0001

Printed by Sheridan Books, Inc., United States of America

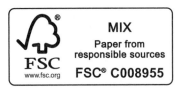

CONTENTS

OVERALL LEARNING OBJECTIVES

After completing these activities, the participant should be better able to:

- Describe the evolving epidemiology of HIV disease in the U.S., with an emphasis on age, gender, sexuality, race/ethnicity, socioeconomic status, emerging subtypes and viral resistance

- Implement appropriate laboratory HIV testing methods for screening and diagnosing HIV

- Adapt pre- and post-testing counseling to best meet individual needs in a variety of situations

- Provide up-to-date HIV care to a broad spectrum of people with HIV, including pediatrics, adolescents, injection-drug users, incarcerated individuals, and an aging population

- Adjust treatment based upon the various co-morbidities that are often found in people with HIV including cardiovascular, renal, and neurologic disease

- Discuss the ethics and legal issues related to caring for people with HIV

FACULTY

LEAD EDITOR

W. David Hardy, MD, AAHIVS
Scientific and Medical Consultant
Attending Physician, Los Angeles General Hospital, Rand Schrader (HIV) Clinic
Adjunct Clinical Professor of Medicine
Keck School of Medicine of USC

CO-EDITORS

Jonathan S. Appelbaum, MD, FACP, AAHIVS
Laurie L. Dozier, Jr. MD Education Director
Professor of Internal Medicine
Department of Clinical Sciences
Florida State University College of Medicine

Roberto C. Arduino, MD
Professor of Medicine
Department of Internal Medicine
Division of Infectious Diseases
McGovern Medical School
The University of Texas Health Science Center at Houston

Philip Bolduc, MD
Associate Professor, Family Medicine and Community Health, University of Massachusetts Chan Medical School
HIV Program and Fellowship Director, Family Health Center of Worcester
Principal Investigator, New England AIDS Education and Training Center

Carolyn Chu, MD, MSc
Associate Professor
Department of Family & Community Medicine
Chief Clinical Officer/PI, National Clinician Consultation Center
University of California, San Francisco

Jarrett K. Sell, MD, FAAFP, AAHIVS
Associate Professor
Department of Family and Community Medicine
Penn State Hershey Medical Center

William R. Short, MD, MPH, FIDSA
Associate Professor of Medicine
Associate Professor of Obstetrics and Gynecology
Perelman School of Medicine
University of Pennsylvania

CONTRIBUTORS

Nancy Aitcheson, MD, MSHP
Assistant Professor of Clinical Medicine
Department of Medicine, Division of Infectious Diseases
Perelman School of Medicine

Saira Ajmal, MD
Clinical Assistant Professor
Division of Infectious Diseases, Advocate Christ Medical Center

Lisa Y. Armitige, MD, PhD
Co-Medical Director, Heartland National TB Center
Professor, Internal Medicine/Pediatrics/Adult ID
University of Texas Health Center at Tyler

Renata Arrington-Sanders, MD, MPH, ScM
Associate Professor
Division of Adolescent and Young Adult Medicine, Department of Pediatrics
Division of Infectious Diseases, Department of Medicine
Johns Hopkins School of Medicine

Olabimpe Asupoto
Research Assistant I
Division of Geographic Medicine and Infectious Diseases
Department of Medicine
Tufts Medicine

Laurel Banach, MD
Instructor
Department of Family Medicine & Community Health
Family Health Center of Worcester
University of Massachusetts Chan Medical School

Jillian T. Baron, MD, MPH
Assistant Professor of Clinical Medicine
Penn Medicine, Division of Infectious Diseases
Medical Director, Penn Community Practice

Katrina Baumgartner, MD, AAHIVS
HIV and Viral Hepatitis Clinical Director
Greater Lawrence Family Health Center

Roger Bedimo, MD
Professor, Department of Internal Medicine
UT Southwestern Medical Center, Division of Infectious
Diseases & Geographic Medicine Infectious Diseases
Section Chief, VA North Texas Health Care System

Christopher M. Bositis, MD, AAHIVS
Associate Clinical Professor, Department of Family and
Community Medicine
Clinical Director, National Clinician Consultation Center
University of California, San Francisco

Christian Brander, PhD
ICREA Senior Research Professor
IrsiCaixa AIDS Research Institute
University of Vic, Spain

Patricia Carr Reese, MD, MPH, AAHIVS
Family Physician, Lancaster General Health Physicians -
Comprehensive Care
Adjunct Faculty, Family Practice - Obstetrics, Lancaster
General Hospital Family Medicine Residency

Ashley Carvalho, MD, MSc
HIV & Viral Hepatitis Fellow
Full Circle Health

Priyanka Chakrabarti, DO
Staff Physician, Family Medicine
Partners in Primary Care

Elizabeth Y. Chiao, MD, MPH
Michael E. DeBakey VA Medical Center

Eva H. Clark, MD, PhD
Assistant Professor
Department of Medicine, Section of Infectious Diseases
Baylor College of Medicine

Jennifer Cocohoba, PharmD, BCPS, AAHIVP
University of California, San Francisco, School of Pharmacy
University of California, San Francisco, Women's HIV
Program

Dagan Coppock, MD, MSCE
Assistant Professor of Medicine
Division of Infectious Diseases
Sidney Kimmel Medical College
Thomas Jefferson University

Elizabeth H. David, MD
Associate Professor, Department of Psychiatry and
Behavioral Sciences
Baylor College of Medicine
Staff Psychiatrist
Thomas Street Clinic

Abby Davids, MD, MPH, AAHIVS
HIV and Viral Hepatitis Fellowship Director
Full Circle Health / Family Medicine Residency of Idaho - Boise

Alejandro Delgado, MD, FACP
Attending Physician, Division of Infectious Diseases
Assistant Program Director, Department of Internal
Medicine
Clinical Assistant Professor of Medicine, Sidney Kimmel
Medical College
Ethics Consultant
Albert Einstein Healthcare Network

Esteban A. DelPilar Morales, MD
Attending Physician, Division of Infectious Diseases
Associate Hospital Epidemiologist
Assistant Professor, UMass Chan Medical School-Baystate
Health

Yash Desai, MD
PGY-1 Categorical IM
University of Maryland Medical Center

Christine M. Durand, MD
Associate Professor
Division of Medicine and Oncology
Johns Hopkins University School of Medicine

Umar Farooq, MD, MS, FASN
Associate Professor of Medicine
Division of Nephrology
Penn State University College of Medicine

Deliana Garcia, MA
Chief Program Officer International and Emerging
Issues
Migrant Clinicians Network

Rajesh T. Gandhi, MD
Director of HIV Clinical Services and Education,
Massachusetts General Hospital (MGH)
Professor of Medicine, Harvard Medical School
Co-Director and Principal Investigator, Harvard University
Center for AIDS Research (CFAR)

Taylor K. Gill, PharmD, BCPS, AAHIVP, FKCHP
Clinical Pharmacist
Ascension Via Christi Hospitals Wichita, Inc.

Zil G. Goldstein, FNP-BC
Associate Medical Director
Callen-Lorde Community Health Center

Meagan Goodier, MSN, APRN, FNP-C
Family Nurse Practitioner
Family Health Center of Worcester

Dennis J. Hartigan-O'Connor, MD, PhD
Associate Professor, Department of Medical Microbiology
and Immunology
Core Scientist, California National Primate Research Center
University of California, Davis

Rodrigo Hasbun, MD, MPH
Professor of Medicine
The University of Texas McGovern Medical School

Emily Heil, PharmD, MS
Associate Professor, Department of Practice, Sciences, and Health-Outcomes Research
University of Maryland School of Pharmacy

Matthew D. Hickey, MD
Assistant Professor
Division of HIV, Infectious Diseases, and Global Medicine
San Francisco General Hospital
University of California, San Francisco

Elizabeth Imbert, MD, MPH
Associate Professor
Clinical Lead, POP-UP Program, Ward 86
Division of HIV, ID and Global Medicine
San Francisco General Hospital
University of California San Francisco

Nikolaus Jilg, MD, PhD
Assistant in Medicine
Division of Infectious Diseases
Massachusetts General Hospital/Harvard Medical School

Boris Juelg, MD, PhD
Associate Professor of Medicine, Harvard Medical School
Division of Infectious Diseases, Massachusetts General Hospital
Ragon Institute of Mass General, MIT and Harvard

Joseph S. Kass, MD, JD, FAAN
Professor
Department of Neurology
Menninger Department of Psychiatry and Behavioral Sciences
Center for Medical Ethics and Health Policy
Baylor College of Medicine

Jeffrey T. Kirchner, DO, FAAFP, AAHIVS
Medical Director - Caring Communities for HIV
Wilkes-Barre, Hazleton, and Bloomsburg, PA

David E. Koren, PharmD, MPH, BCPS, AAHIVP
Clinical Pharmacist Specialist
Temple University Health System

Ramiz Kseri, MD
Assistant Professor, Department of Clinical Sciences
Florida State University College of Medicine

Laszlo Madaras, MD, MPH, FAAFP, SFHM
Chief Medical Officer, Migrant Clinicians Network
Clinical Assistant Professor of Medicine
Penn State College of Medicine

Christina E. Maguire, PharmD, BCIDP
Infectious Diseases Clinical Pharmacist
Penn Presbyterian Medical Center

Poonam Mathur, DO, MPH
Assistant Professor
Institute of Human Virology
University of Maryland School of Medicine

Leslie McGorman, MPPA
Director of Public Policy
American Academy of HIV Medicine

Jessica A. Meisner, MD, MS, MSHP
Assistant Professor
Division of Infectious Diseases
The University of Texas Southwestern Medical Center

Steven Mudroch, MD
Infectious Diseases Fellow, PGY-5
Temple University Hospital

Puja H. Nambiar, MD, MPH
Assistant Attending, Infectious Diseases
Memorial Sloan Kettering Cancer Center
Assistant Professor of Medicine
Weill Cornell Medical College, New York

Peg O'Byrne Nelson, MSN, RN
Infectious Disease Clinic Nurse
Beth Israel Deaconess Medical Center

Karin Nielsen-Saines, MD, MPH
Professor of Pediatrics
Division of Pediatric Infectious Diseases
David Geffen School of Medicine University of California, Los Angeles

Jonathan J. Nunez, MD
Associate Professor of Medicine
Penn State Health, Hershey

Bruce J. Packett II
American Academy of HIV Medicine

Neha Sheth Pandit, PharmD, AAHIVP, BCPS
Professor, Infectious Diseases/Pharmacotherapy
Department of Practice, Sciences, and Health Outcomes Research
University of Maryland Baltimore, School of Pharmacy
Clinical Pharmacist, THRIVE Program

Lealah Pollock, MD, MS
Associate Professor, Department of Family & Community Medicine
University of California, San Francisco

Richard C. Prokesch, MD
Physician
Infectious Diseases Associates

Aroonsiri Sangarlangkarn, MD, MPH
Associate Professor & Lead Geriatrician
Temple University

Claire M. Hutkins Seda, BA
Associate Director of Communications
Migrant Clinicians Network

Rajagopal V. Sekhar, MD
Professor of Medicine
Department of Medicine,
Section of Endocrinology, Diabetes and Metabolism,
Baylor College of Medicine

Robert W. Shafer, MD
Professor of Medicine
Stanford University

Kalpana D. Shere-Wolfe, MD
Assistant Professor of Medicine
University of Maryland

Elizabeth M. Sherman, PharmD
Associate Professor, Barry and Judy Silverman College of
Pharmacy
Nova Southeastern University
Clinical Faculty, Division of Infectious Disease
Memorial Healthcare System

Catherine Silva, MD, MHS
Assistant Professor, Department of Pediatrics, Johns
Hopkins School of Medicine
Clinical Faculty, Johns Hopkins All Children's
Hospital, Adolescent Medicine and Young Adult
Specialty Clinic

Daniel J. Skiest, MD
Vice Chair, Department of Medicine
Professor, Division of Infectious Diseases
Baystate Health/UMass Medical School

Benjamin Sokoloff, DO, AAHIVS
Internal Medicine Physician
Cascade AIDS Project, Prism Health

Gary F. Spinner, DMSc, MPH, PA, AAHIVS
Medical Director, HIV/AIDS Program
Southwest Community Health Center

Zelalem Temesgen, MD, FIDSA
Professor of Medicine
Director, Mayo Clinic Center for Tuberculosis
Division of Public Health, Infectious Diseases, and
Occupational Medicine
Mayo Clinic

Thanh Thuy Truong, MD
Addiction Psychiatry
Assistant Professor, Department of Psychiatry and
Behavioral Sciences
Baylor College of Medicine

Karen J. Vigil, MD, FACP, FIDSA
Associate Professor
Department of Internal Medicine
Division of Infectious Diseases
McGovern Medical School
The University of Texas Health Science Center at Houston

Richa Vijayvargiya, MD
Assistant Clinical Professor
Division of Consultation-Liaison Psychiatry
UF Department of Psychiatry

Craig S. Weeks, MD
Assistant Clinical Professor of Family Medicine
Central Michigan University
Family Physician
Great Lakes Bay Health Centers

Rita Wilson Dib, MD, MPH
Onco-Infectious Diseases Fellow
Division of Infectious Diseases
McGovern Medical School
The University of Texas Health Science Center at Houston

Alysse G. Wurcel, MD, MS
Associate Professor
Tufts Medical Center, Department of Medicine, Division of
Geographic Medicine and Infectious Diseases
Tufts University School of Medicine, Department of Public
Health and Community Medicine

Kruti J. Yagnik, DO
Staff Physician, Division of Infectious Diseases
Director of Antimicrobial Stewardship
Cleveland Clinic Indian River Hospital

DISCLOSURE OF FINANCIAL RELATIONSHIPS

Postgraduate Institute for Medicine (PIM) requires authors, planners, and others in control of educational content to disclose all their financial relationships with ineligible companies. All potential conflicts of interest (COI) are thoroughly mitigated according to PIM policy. PIM is committed to providing its learners with high quality accredited continuing education activities and related materials that promote improvements or quality in healthcare and not a specific proprietary business interest of an ineligible company.

The following financial relationships have all been mitigated:

Jonathan S. Appelbaum reports that he is a consultant for Merck, Theratechnologies, and ViiV Healthcare

Roger Bedimo reports receiving grant support from Merck. He is a consultant for Gilead Sciences, Janssen, Merck, Shionogi, Theratechnologies, and ViiV Healthcare

Jennifer Cocohoba reports receiving grant support from ViiV Healthcare

Christine M. Durrand reports receiving grant support from Gilead Sciences

Umar Farooq reports receiving grant support from Ablative Solutions, Bayer, Genentech, and Remegen. He serves as a speaker for Bayer. He is a consultant for Enochian, Gilead Sciences, GKS Pharmaceuticals, Merck, and ViiV Healthcare

W. David Hardy serves as a consultant for Enochian, Gilead Sciences, GKS Pharmaceuticals, Merck, and ViiV Healthcare. He is a shareholder of Enochian

Dennis J. Hartigan-O'Conner is a speaker for ViiV Healthcare

Rodrigo Hasbun is a speaker for and receives grant support from Biofire. He is a consultant for Melinta

David E. Koren is a speaker for Gilead Sciences. He is a consultant for Gilead Sciences, Janssen, Theratechnologies, and ViiV Healthcare

Poonam Mathur is a consultant for NKG and receives grant support from Merck

Neha Sheth Pandit receives grant support from Gilead Sciences and Theratechnologies

Richard C. Prokesch is a shareholder with Abbot Laboratories, Alnylam Pharmaceuticals, Gilead Sciences, Johnson & Johnson, and Pfizer

Robert W. Shafer is a consultant for Gilead Sciences and GlaxoSmithKline

Bill Short is a speaker for ViiV Healthcare. He is a consultant for Gilead Sciences and ViiV Healthcare

Daniel J. Skiest receives research support from Hoffman-LaRoche

Gary F. Spinner is a consultant for Theratechnologies. He is a speaker and shareholder with Gilead Sciences

Zelalem Temesgen is a consultant for ViiV Healthcare and receives grant support from Gilead Sciences, Merck, and ViiV Healthcare

Karen J. Vigil is a consultant for Theratechnologies and ViiV Healthcare. She receives grant support from Theratechnologies

Alysse G. Wurcel receives grant support from Merck and ViiV Healthcare

The following authors and planners have no relevant financial relationships to disclose:

Nancy Aitcheson

Saira Ajmal

Roberto C. Arduino

Lisa Armitage

Renata Arrington-Sanders

Olabimpe Asupoto

Laurel Banach

Jillian T. Baron

Katrina Baumgartner

Phil Bolduc

Christopher M. Bositis

Christian Brander

Trish Carr Reese

Ashley Carvalho

Priyanka Chakrabarti

Carolyn Chu

Dagan Coppock

Elizabeth H. David

Abby Davids

Alejandro Delgado

Esteban A. DelPilar Morales

Yash Desai

Deliana Garcia

Rakesh T. Ghandi

Taylor K. Gill

Zil G. Goldstein

Meagan Goodier

Emily Heil

Matthew D. Hickey

Aroonsiri Howell

Claire M. Hutkins Seda

Elizabeth Imbert

Nikolaus Jilg

Boris Juelg

Joseph S. Kass

Jeffrey T. Kirchner

Ramiz Kseri

Laszlo Madaras

Christina Maguire

Leslie McGorman

Jessica A. Meisner

Steven Murdoch

Puja H. Nambiar

Peg Nelson

Karin Nielson-Saines

Jonathan Nunez

Lealah Pollock

Clair Seda

Rajagopal V. Sekhar

Jarrett K. Sell

Kalpana D. Shere-Wolfe

Elizabeth M. Sherman

Cathy Silva

Ben Sokoloff

Tri Trang

Richard Vijayvargiya

Craig S. Weeks

Rita Wilson Dib

Kruti J. Yagnik

The planners and reviewers at Postgraduate Institute for Medicine have nothing to disclose. The planners at American Academy of HIV Medicine have nothing to disclose.

DISCLOSURE OF UNLABELED USE

This educational activity may contain discussion of published and/or investigational uses of agents that are not indicated by the FDA. The planners of this activity do not recommend the use of any agent outside of the labeled indications. The opinions expressed in the educational activity are those of the faculty and do not necessarily represent the views of the planners. Please refer to the official prescribing information for each product for discussion of approved indications, contraindications, and warnings.

DISCLAIMER

Participants have an implied responsibility to use the newly acquired information to enhance patient outcomes and their own professional development. The information presented in this activity is not meant to serve as a guideline for patient management. Any procedures, medications, or other courses of diagnosis or treatment discussed or suggested in this activity should not be used by clinicians without evaluation of their patient's conditions and possible contraindications and/or dangers in use, review of any applicable manufacturer's product information, and comparison with recommendations of other authorities.

PREFACE

W. David Hardy, MD, AAHIVS

Welcome to the 2023 edition of *The Fundamentals of HIV Medicine for the HIV Specialist*. First, I want to thank our co-editors, Jonathan Appelbaum, Roberto Arduino, Bill Short, Carolyn Chu, Philip Bolduc and Jarrett Sell whose indefatigable academic fervor and attention to detail make this textbook the success it is, our phenomenal managing editor Amy Keller Thyberg, the "essential ingredient" for overseeing the day-to-day progress of this endeavor culminating in the near-perfection it is and, of course, the AAHIVM staff without whose dedication this textbook would never see the light of day, Scott Brawley, Angela Riley and of course our guiding star Bruce Packett. Second, I want to express our tremendous gratitude to the scores of returning and new authors who shared not only their intellectual prowess and dedicated teaching skills, but also many hours of their time honing their chapters.

This edition marks the 9th edition of this textbook and the 7th for which I have had the distinct honor and pleasure of serving as editor-in-chief.

Since its initial publication in 2007 as a comprehensive, clinically focused textbook detailing the most up-to-date basic science translated to therapeutic and preventative interventions for HIV infection in addition to treatments for and prevention of opportunistic infections and cancers, associated inflammatory co-morbid diseases, substance use disorders, mental health illnesses and diseases associated with social determinants of health, the persistent and overarching goal of this publication has been to keep practitioners of HIV medicine as well-informed as possible to support them in providing optimal patient care.

In my humble opinion, this 9th edition marks a high point for this biennially updated textbook, as it has now reached a persistently elevated quality of regularly reviewed and updated foundational chapters, reviewed, and eliminated or condensed historic chapters and added chapters focused on the ever evolving therapeutic and prophylactic innovations characteristic of HIV medicine along with co-occurring and emerging health events such as the COVID-19 Pandemic and the monkeypox outbreak. In other words, I believe that this is the BEST Fundamentals textbook to date.

I hope that as you use this textbook as your study guide for the AAHIVM Specialist, Pharmacist or Expert credentialing exams, your go-to reference for your clinical practice when making patient care decisions or as a teaching tool for medical and post-graduate medical trainees, you will come to agree with my personal assessment.

Please use this textbook to its fullest extent as it best fits your needs, but don't get too attached to it, as it will be updated again in 2025 to keep abreast with the ever-changing science of HIV medicine.

1.

ENDING OF THE HIV EPIDEMIC
A PLAN FOR AMERICA

Benjamin Sokoloff

LEARNING OBJECTIVES

- Identify the goals of the current nationwide initiative to eliminate new HIV infections in the United States.

- Describe the pillars upon which the initiative is built to achieve these goals.

KEY POINTS

- Ending the HIV epidemic in the United States is possible; the current goal is to reduce the number of new HIV infections by 75% by 2025 and by 90% by 2030.

- The four pillars of the initiative are to increase the diagnosis, treatment, and prevention of HIV infection and the rapid response to new clusters of HIV transmissions. These pillars are based on the most robust evidence-based science, medicine, and public health principles derived from randomized controlled clinical trials.

- The Ending the HIV Epidemic (EHE) Initiative will initially focus on Puerto Rico, Washington, DC, the 48 counties in the United States with the highest rates of new infections, and the seven US states with the highest incidence of HIV in rural communities.

INTRODUCTION

Not only has the medical care of persons with HIV (PWH) evolved significantly over the past 4 decades, so too has the national epidemiological plan for slowing and eventually ending the epidemic. This chapter arrives at an auspicious time. The first edition of this chapter was written within the first 6 months of the SARS-CoV-2 pandemic. This second edition was written within the first 6 months of the hMPXV (human monkeypox virus) pandemic, and we hope that no new pandemics will show themselves at the time of its next writing. However, inevitable pandemics may be, we (i.e., government, healthcare providers, and public health) are not powerless to address them. The US federal government, throughout its

history, has typically responded to emerging epidemics and pandemics with legislative and executive actions with the intent of saving lives and preventing disease.

Unfortunately, new HIV infection rates have remained stubbornly high and static over the last decade, despite many scientific and medical advances. The HIV incidence rate in 2016 was estimated to be 39,972, and the rate only modestly declined to 30,635 in 2020 (Centers for Disease Control and Prevention ((CDC), 2021a). While data from 2020 suggests a more aggressive decline, data from that year must be assessed cautiously given the nationwide lockdowns of testing centers and clinics during the SARS-CoV-2 pandemic. In addition, while the rates of new infections have declined in White men who have sex with men (MSM), they have remained stable in Black MSM and have increased in Hispanic/Latino MSM (CDC, 2021a). The CDC data from the end of 2019 also showed persistent disparities for new infections, with Black/African Americans making up 41% of new infections, while White Americans account for only 25% (CDC, 2021a). The disparities also persist in viral suppression rates between racial groups. Worse still, only 28% of persons with an indication for pre-exposure prophylaxis (PrEP) had a prescription for it in 2020 and still with massive disparities (CDC, 2020).

With our modern antiretroviral therapy (ART) and PrEP regimens, we should be able to suppress HIV in nearly all PWH and prevent most new infections in persons at higher risk for acquiring HIV. Using our tools of Treatment as Prevention (TasP) and PrEP, while expanding HIV screening and focusing on those most at risk, we can see the path to zero new infections. Significant challenges remain that are preventing us from achieving this goal. And so, the EHE initiative was created with the bold goal of eliminating most new infections in the United States by 2030. Mounting evidence has shown how this could be achieved, which is further cemented by the four pillars of this new program. We have come a long way from a time when HIV infection meant certain death, but we have not yet been able to stop the spread of the virus on a broader scale. With this latest initiative, we aspire to use the remarkable tools developed over the last decade to end this 40-year epidemic in the United States.

GOALS AND TIMELINE

The EHE initiative is a 10-year plan with the goal of reducing the number of new HIV infections in the United States by 75% by 2025, and by 90% by 2030, for a total of 250,000 infections averted over this time (USHHS, 2019). This translates to a reduction in the incidence of HIV infections in the United States to fewer than 3,000 annually. The estimated incidence of HIV infections in the United States and dependent areas in 2018 was 34,800 (CDC, 2021a). This goal, set forth by the US government, is in line with the 90-90-90 targets for ending the HIV/AIDS pandemic globally as issued by the United Nations Program for HIV and AIDS (UNAIDS) in 2014. Based on UNAIDS-sponsored modeling, it is predicted that if 90% of persons with HIV/AIDS are diagnosed, 90% of those with a diagnosis are on ART, and 90% of those receiving ART are virally suppressed by 2020, the end of the HIV/AIDS pandemic would be achieved by 2030 (UNAIDS, 2014). Unfortunately, the 90-90-90 goal has only been met by only a handful of countries globally. The EHE initiative represents the US government's ongoing commitment to eliminating HIV/AIDS as a major public health threat.

Over the 10 years of its implementation, the EHE initiative will transition through three phases. The initial phase, slated for the first 5 years, aims to target specific regions in the United States—48 counties along with Puerto Rico and Washington, DC—that constituted more than 50% of all new HIV infections in the United States in 2016 and 2017. It will also focus on seven states where HIV infection remains a large burden in rural areas based on 2016 and 2017 data. Federal agencies will work with and provide support to local facilities already in place to implement the four pillars of diagnosis, treatment, prevention, and response to decreasing new HIV infections by 75%. The second phase of the initiative will seek to expand on the efforts and successes achieved in phase 1 throughout the rest of the country to reach the goal of reducing the infection rate by 90% by 2030. Finally, the third phase of the initiative will focus on improving resources for individuals living with HIV who are connected to care in order to achieve viral suppression and maintain new infection rates at less than 3,000 per year (Giroir, 2020).

THE FOUR PILLARS

DIAGNOSE

According to the latest CDC surveillance report, at the end of 2019, there were an estimated 1.2 million people living with HIV in the United States. Of those, 13.3% remained undiagnosed (CDC, 2021b). These undiagnosed individuals are responsible for a disproportionate share of new HIV transmissions. Thus, expanding HIV testing efforts to diagnose these individuals is vital to initiate treatment for their benefit and halt further forward transmission of HIV. The first pillar of the EHE's key strategies—diagnosis—seeks to address this goal by mobilizing federal and local resources to achieve early diagnosis of all people with HIV. Several agencies within the Department of Health and Human Services (DHHS), including the CDC, Health Resources and Services Administration (HRSA), National Institutes of Health, Indian Health Service, and Substance Abuse and Mental Health Services Administration (SAMHSA), will support community structures already in place to increase testing capabilities in both traditional settings, such as health facilities providing medical and substance abuse services, and nontraditional venues where people congregate, such as festivals, public spaces, and businesses. The overarching goal of this effort is to make HIV testing a noncontroversial, routine screen for all persons in the United States at least once in their lifetime and repeated depending on risk factors.

TREAT

Advances in the treatment of HIV have allowed PWH to live with a well-managed chronic condition rather than a progressive terminal illness. Results from the HPTN 052, PARTNER 1, PARTNER 2, and Opposites Attract trials have demonstrated that PWH who have consistently suppressed viral loads will not transmit the virus to their sexual partners by condomless sex (Bavinton et al., 2018; Cohen et al., 2011; Cohen et al., 2016; Rodger et al., 2019). These studies provide strong support for the role of treatment as prevention (TasP). Yet, as reported by the CDC in 2016, six in ten transmissions were from PWH who knew about their infection but either were not in care or not virally suppressed despite representing only 37% of the HIV community (CDC, 2019). This represents a large failure of the healthcare system and an area for significant improvement. The goal of this pillar of the EHE initiative is to increase the proportion of persons with known HIV infection with suppressed viral loads from where it is now at 65.5% to 95% by 2030. The secondary outcome of this is to reduce new transmissions—what is otherwise known as TasP. Building on the successes of clinics funded by the Ryan White HIV/AIDS Program, DHHS agencies seek to strengthen and expand local infrastructures while tailoring the roll-out of HIV care to the individual needs of each community.

PREVENT

The third pillar of the EHE initiative aims to prevent HIV transmission using PrEP and syringe service programs (SSP). PrEP in its various forms substantially reduces the risk for HIV acquisition, which will be discussed in subsequent chapters. In 2020 it was estimated that there were 1,216,210 people in the United States that had an indication for PrEP. That same year only 301,033 patients received a prescription for PrEP, representing less than a quarter of candidates. While this is a slight improvement from 22.5% of candidates receiving a prescription in 2019, there remains another large gap in medical care (CDC, 2021c).

Ready, Set, PrEP is a program created by DHHS in 2019 to address one of the barriers causing this discrepancy. Thanks to public-private partnerships, this program makes Truvada ((TDF/FTC) one form of PrEP) available to those without prescription drug insurance coverage. The criteria to be funded as a patient are: (1) no prescription drug insurance coverage, (2) a recent negative HIV test, (3) have a prescription for oral PrEP, and (4) live in the United States or its tribal lands or territories. Both patients and healthcare providers can enroll at readysetprep.hiv.gov. It should be noted that Ready, Set, PrEP is not limited to the jurisdictions of the first phase of the EHE and is available to anyone nationwide. It does not cover the cost of medical visits and lab tests, nor does it cover those who are insured, regardless of out-of-pocket cost.

SSPs are community-based prevention programs aimed at providing comprehensive resources to persons who inject drugs (PWID), including access to substance use disorder treatment, needle-exchange programs, and infectious diseases screening with linkage-to-care. A recent meta-analysis of studies in North America and Europe (Aspinal et al., 2014) showed that SSPs contribute to an estimated 58% reduction in incidence of HIV. Unfortunately, congressional funds cannot be used to purchase needles directly for exchange. The CDC and SAMHSA instead will use appropriated funds to support increased access to SSPs and help local communities implement SSPs.

RESPOND

The final pillar of the EHE initiative aims to strengthen communities' ability to respond quickly to new outbreaks through collaboration between the CDC and local health departments via epidemiologic trends and lab surveillance. This partnership endeavors to quickly identify clusters of HIV transmission, otherwise known as outbreaks, using real-time molecular techniques with epidemiologic tracing. The end goal is to offer diagnostic, therapeutic, and prophylactic interventions, as appropriate, and guide the distribution of resources where they are most needed. This partnership is not limited to health departments and can include local physicians, patients, and HIV advocates.

THE TARGETED JURISDICTIONS IN PHASE ONE

COUNTIES

Arizona
- Maricopa County

California
- Alameda County
- Los Angeles County
- Orange County
- Riverside County
- Sacramento County
- San Bernadino County
- San Diego County
- San Francisco County

Florida
- Broward County
- Duval County
- Hillsborough County
- Miami-Dade County
- Orange County

- Palm Beach County
- Pinellas County

Georgia
- Cobb County
- Dekalb County
- Fulton County
- Gwinnett County

Illinois
- Cook County

Indiana
- Marion County

Louisiana
- East Baton Rouge Parish
- Orleans Parish

Maryland
- Baltimore City
- Montgomery County
- Prince George's County

Massachusetts
- Suffolk County

Michigan
- Wayne County

Nevada
- Clark County

New Jersey
- Essex County
- Hudson County

New York
- Bronx County
- Kings County
- New York County
- Queens County

North Carolina
- Mecklenburg County

Ohio
- Cuyahoga County
- Franklin County
- Hamilton County

Pennsylvania
- Philadelphia County

Puerto Rico
- San Juan Municipio

Tennessee
- Shelby County

Texas
- Bexar County
- Dallas County
- Harris County
- Tarrant County
- Travis County

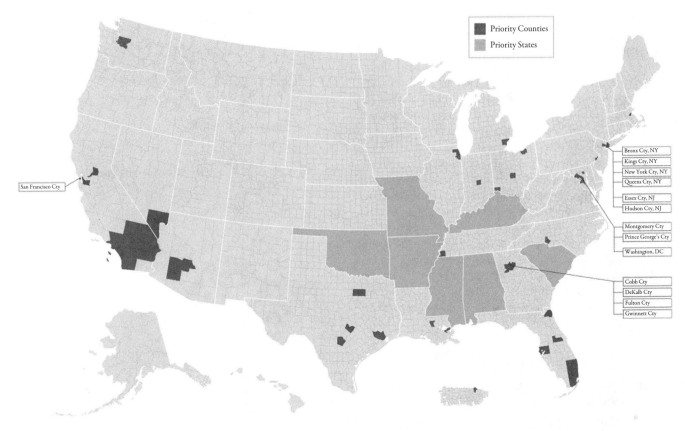

Figure 1.1 Priority jurisdictions for ending the HIV epidemic   SOURCE: https//www.hiv.gov/federal-response/ending-the-hiv-epidemic/jurisdictions/phase-one. Published 2020. Accessed August 15, 2022.

Washington
- King County

Washington, DC.

STATES

- Alabama
- Arkansas
- Kentucky
- Mississippi
- Missouri
- Oklahoma
- South Carolina

This initiative will target resources to the 47 highest burden counties; Washington, DC; San Juan, Puerto Rico; and seven states with a substantial rural HIV burden—with over 75 cases and 10% or more of their diagnoses in rural areas. Programs receiving funding through the EHE for these targeted jurisdictions are the Minority HIV/AIDS Fund, Public Health Service Commissioned Corps, Ryan White HIV/AIDS Programs, AIDS Education and Training Centers, HRSA's Primary Care HIV Prevention fund, the CDC's Division of HIV/AIDS Prevention, and the Indian Health Service (Figure 1.1).

ASSESSMENT OF INTERVENTION

DHHS has assembled a website where progress can be visualized through graphs of data, which you are encouraged to view here: ahead.hiv.gov. It should be noted that because CDC incidence data lags by 1–2 years, there are few comparative years to assess the effects of the EHE. Further, because of disruptions from the SARS-CoV-2 pandemic, data from the first few years should be evaluated cautiously.

REFERENCES

Aspinal EJ, Nambiar D, Goldberg DJ, et al. Are needle and syringe programmes associated with a reduction in HIV transmission among people who inject drugs: a systematic review and meta-analysis. *Int J Epidemiol.* 2014;43(1):235–248. https://academic.oup.com/ije/article/43/1/235/734951

Bavinton BR, Prestage GP, Jin F, et al. Strategies used by gay male HIV serodiscordant couples to reduce the risk of HIV transmission from anal intercourse in three countries. *Journal of the International AIDS Society.* 2019;22(4);e25277. http://doi: 10.1002/jia2.25277

Centers for Disease Control and Prevention (CDC). Ending HIV transmission. *Vital Signs.* https://www.cdc.gov/vitalsigns/test-treat-prevent/index.html. Published December 2019. Accessed August 2022.

CDC. Core indicators for monitoring the Ending the HIV Epidemic Initiative (preliminary data): National HIV Surveillance System data reported through June 2021; and preexposure prophylaxis (PrEP) data reported through March 2021. *HIV Surveillance Data Tables.* 2021;2(4): 10–33. http://www.cdc.gov/hiv/library/reports/hiv-surveillance.html. Published October 2021c. Accessed August 2022.

CDC. Estimated HIV incidence and prevalence in the United States, 2015–2019. *HIV Surveillance Supplemental Report*. 2021;26(1). http://www.cdc.gov/hiv/library/reports/hiv-surveillance.html. Published May 2021a. Accessed August 2022.

CDC. Estimated HIV incidence and prevalence in the United States 2014–2018. *HIV Surveillance Supplemental Report*. 2020;25(1). https://www.cdc.gov/hiv/pdf/library/reports/surveillance/cdc-hiv-surveillance-supplemental-report-vol-25-1.pdf. Published May 2020. Accessed August 2022.

CDC. Monitoring selected national HIV prevention and care objectives by using HIV surveillance data—United States and 6 dependent areas, 2019. *HIV Surveillance Supplemental Report*. 2021;26(2). http://www.cdc.gov/hiv/library/reports/hiv-surveillance.html. Published May 2021b. Accessed August 2022.

Cohen MS, Chen YQ, McCauley M, et al. Antiretroviral therapy for the prevention of HIV-1 transmission. *New England Journal of Medicine*. 2016;375(9):830–839. https://doi.org/10.1056/NEJMoa1600693

Cohen MS, Chen YQ, McCauley M, et al. Prevention of HIV-1 infection with early antiretroviral therapy. *New England Journal of Medicine*. 2011;365(6):493–505. https://doi.org/10.1056/NEJMoa1105243

Giroir BP. The time is now to end the HIV epidemic. *American Journal of Public Health*. 2020;110(1):22–24. https://doi.org/10.2105/AJPH.2019.305380

Rodger AJ, Cambiano V, Bruun T, et al. Risk of HIV transmission through condomless sex in serodifferent gay couples with the HIV-positive partner taking suppressive antiretroviral therapy (PARTNER): final results of a multicentre, prospective, observational study. *Lancet (London, England)*. 2019;393(10189):2428–2438. https://doi.org/10.1016/S0140-6736(19)30418-0

UNAIDS. *90-90-90 An ambitious treatment target to help end the HIV epidemic*. https://www.unaids.org/sites/default/files/media_asset/90-90-90_en.pdf. Published October 2014. Accessed August 15, 2022.

United States Department of Health and Human Services. Office of Infectious Disease and HIV/AIDS Policy. *Ending the HIV epidemic: a plan for America* [blog post]. https://www.hhs.gov/blog/2019/02/05/ending-the-hiv-epidemic-a-plan-for-america.html. Published February 19, 2019. Accessed August 15, 2022.

2.

EPIDEMIOLOGY AND THE SPREAD OF HIV

Laurel Banach, Meagan Goodier, and Philip Bolduc

OVERVIEW OF WORLDWIDE PANDEMIC

LEARNING OBJECTIVE

Discuss the global prevalence, as well as the geographic distribution, of human immunodeficiency syndrome (HIV)-1 and HIV-2 infections, and updates on recent shared global initiatives.

WHAT'S NEW?

The World Health Organization and Joint United Nations Program on HIV and AIDS (WHO/UNAIDS) estimates that in 2021, 38.4 million persons worldwide were living with HIV (UNAIDS, 2022). Although the numbers of new HIV infections and AIDS-related deaths continue to decline in many regions of the world, including Sub-Saharan Africa, there are still certain regions where the incidence of HIV is rising, most notably in the Eastern European and Eastern Mediterranean areas. In 2021, 94% of the new HIV infections outside of Sub-Saharan Africa were in the key populations of sex workers and their clients, gay men and other men who have sex with men, persons who inject drugs, and transgender persons (UNAIDS, 2022). In comparison, these populations comprised only 51% of new HIV infections in Sub-Saharan Africa. While the incidence of HIV has been reduced by 40% since its peak in 1998, the UNAIDS Global AIDS Update of 2022 urges caution when examining data from the COVID-19 pandemic. With the number of infections dropping only 3.6% between 2020 and 2021, UNAIDS Executive Director Winnie Byanyima remarks, "these data show that the global AIDS response is in severe danger. If we are not making rapid progress then we are losing ground, as the [HIV/AIDS] pandemic thrives amidst COVID-19, mass displacement, and other crises" (UNAIDS, 2022). The 95-95-95 initiative, which is described below, highlights both critical improvements and enduring deficits alike.

KEY POINTS

- UNAIDS identified several demographic subgroups at high risk for HIV infection and in danger of being left behind by the global AIDS response, including adolescent girls and young women, men who have sex with men (MSM), transgender persons, persons who inject drugs, prisoners, and sex workers.

- The COVID-19 pandemic most certainly impacted access to HIV testing, but its true toll on HIV/AIDS globally is yet to be known.

OVERVIEW OF THE GLOBAL PANDEMIC

Since the onset of the global epidemic, the WHO estimates that 84.2 million (64–113 million) persons have acquired HIV infection, and 40.1 million have died of AIDS-related illnesses (UNAIDS, 2022). At the end of 2021, an estimated 38.4 million (33.9–43.8 million) persons were living with HIV, while 1.5 million (1.1–2.0 million) persons acquired HIV infection that year. An estimated 0.7% (0.6%–0.9%) of adults aged 15–49 years worldwide are living with HIV, although the burden of the epidemic continues to vary considerably between countries and regions. Africa remains the most heavily burdened, with nearly 1 in every 25 adults (3.7%) living with HIV, representing more than two-thirds of the persons with HIV (PWH) globally.

Across all countries, several key demographic subgroups continue to be most impacted by the HIV/AIDS epidemic. UNAIDS has identified six populations at higher risk of acquiring HIV that are in danger of being left behind by the global AIDS response: adolescent girls and young women, MSM, transgender persons, persons who inject drugs, persons who are incarcerated, and sex workers and their clients. The risk of acquiring HIV is 35-times higher among persons who inject drugs, 28-times higher among MSM of any age, 30-times higher for female sex workers, and 14-times higher for transgender women compared to other adults in the general population (UNAIDS, 2022).

The importance of each of these populations varies by region and within countries. For example, in southern Africa, age-disparate intergenerational sexual relationships and transactional sex place adolescent girls and young women at extremely high risk for HIV; in Eastern Europe and Central Asia, most new HIV acquisitions are associated with persons who inject drugs; and in Latin America, the Caribbean, Western Europe, and North America, the largest proportion of new HIV diagnoses is among MSM. These six key populations and their sexual partners account for 47% of new HIV acquisitions globally, but with wide geographic differences:

just 16% in eastern and southern Africa, but 95% in Eastern Europe, Central Asia, the Middle East, and North Africa (UNAIDS, 2018).

In 2014, the Joint United Nations Program on HIV/AIDS launched the 90-90-90 initiative. Briefly outlined, it sought to assure that 90% of persons with HIV will be diagnosed, 90% of whom will be started and maintained on antiretroviral therapy (ART), among whom 90% will be virally suppressed (or an overall viral suppression rate of 73%). At the end of 2019, 81% of persons living with HIV knew their HIV status; more than two-thirds (67%) were on ART; and 59% of persons living with HIV globally had suppressed viral loads (UNAIDS, 2020).

In 2021, these numbers improved considerably: 85% (75%–97%) of the 38.4 million PWH across the world knew their status. Among them, 88% (78% to >98%) were linked to ART, and of those, 92% (81% to >98%) had suppressed viral loads. Looked at another way, of all persons living with HIV, 85% (75%–97%) knew their status; 75% (66%–85%) were accessing treatment; and 68% (60%–78%) were virally suppressed (UNAIDS, 2022). The next phase of this initiative aims to achieve the even more ambitious targets of 95-95-95 by 2030.

These data show that we continue to close global gaps in treatment coverage, with 20.9 million more PWH on treatment in 2021 than in 2020. AIDS-related deaths dropped by 68% since its peak in 2004, and since 2010, AIDS-related mortality declined by 57% among women and girls and by 47% among men and boys (UNAIDS, 2022). However, global leaders are urging caution about the interpretation of our most recent data given the unprecedented impact of the COVID-19 pandemic on access to HIV testing and medical care and accurate data collection.

HIV & COVID GLOBALLY

With the number of infections only dropping 3.6% between 2020 and 2021, UNAIDS Executive Director Winnie Byanyima remarked, "these data show that the global AIDS response is in severe danger. If we are not making rapid progress then we are losing ground, as the [HIV/AIDS] pandemic thrives amidst COVID-19, mass displacement, and other crises" (UNAIDS, 2022). Given shipping and delivery barriers, the WHO reported 34 countries across the world, predominantly in Africa, and noted disruptions in antiretroviral access (Figure 2.1a June 2020). Fortunately, between June and November 2020, many countries adopted multi-month dispensing of ART and a number of innovative home delivery models, which ultimately resulted in an improvement of global antiretroviral (ARV) access (Figure 2.1b, November 2020).

HIV DIVERSITY

There are two major types of HIV, designated HIV-1 and HIV-2. Each has a similar but distinct genome with a genetic difference of approximately 60%. The vast majority of human infections are caused by HIV-1, with HIV-2 comprising only 1–2 million globally (Campbell-Yesufu & Gandhi, 2011). HIV-2 is found almost exclusively in persons from or living in West Africa, and it is transmitted at lower rates than HIV-1. It appears to have a longer incubation period, produce lower plasma viral load, and lead to AIDS in fewer patients (Apetrei & Marx, 2004). HIV-1 is classified into three genetically related subtypes based on the coding sequence of the envelope gene. Group M (Main) is the most common, and groups O (Outlier) and N (Not-M, Not-O or New) remain rare (Apetrei & Marx, 2004). Group M has at least 11 subtypes, or clades, designated A–K.

There is limited clinical trial information on ART for HIV-2; however, data show that HIV-2 is naturally resistant to nonnucleoside reverse transcriptase inhibitors and enfurvitide (US Department of Health and Human Services (USDHHS), 2020; Witvrouw et al., 2004). HIV-1 subtype (i.e., group) variability may eventually influence how ART is used, but at this point, no data have shown any subtypes to be less sensitive to or to have a greater propensity to develop resistance to current antiretroviral drugs (Gomes et al., 2002; Spira et al., 2003; Wainberg, 2004).

RECOMMENDED READING

UNAIDS. Global HIV & AIDS statistics—2020 fact sheet. unaids.org. http://www.unaids.org/en/resources/fact-sheet. Published 2020. Accessed September 11, 2022.
WHO. HIV/AIDS data and statistics. unaids.org. http://www.who.int/hiv/data/en/. Published 2022. Accessed August September 11, 2022.

OVERVIEW OF THE US EPIDEMIC

LEARNING OBJECTIVE

Describe current demographic trends in HIV in the United States, especially regarding gender, sexuality, race/ethnicity, age, injection-drug use, socioeconomic status, and recent initiatives.

WHAT'S NEW?

The COVID-19 pandemic has had a profound impact on clinical care services. The reduction in HIV incidence is thought to be an underestimate of PWH in the United States. The CDC is still recommending caution when examining statistics of PWH from the COVID-19 pandemic.

KEY POINTS

- HIV incidence among MSM continues to increase, with 50% of new diagnoses being located in the South.

- The leading mode of HIV transmission continues to be male same-sex sexual contact.

- Slowly declining incidence and more rapidly diminishing death rates continue to drive up HIV prevalence and, therefore, workforce demands.

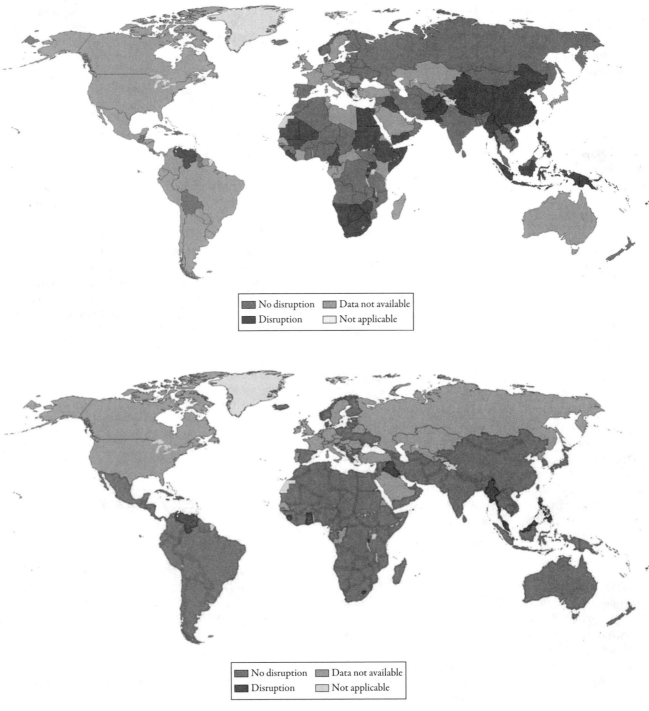

Figure 2.1 Countries reporting on ARV disruption owing to COVID-19, 2020 from June 2022 through November 2022   (A) Results compiled from a survey conducted by WHO between April and June 2020 (*n* = 127); 34 countries reported ARV disruptions; (B) Results compiled from a survey conducted by WHO in November 2020 (*n* = 152); nine countries reported ARV disruptions   **SOURCE:** WHO HIV/HEP/STI COVID-19 Questionnaire, June 2020 and November 2020. https://www.who.int/docs/default-source/hq-hiv-hepatitis-and-stis-library/hhs-service-disruption-slides-dec-2020.pdf?sfvrsn=be10f39d12. Published 2020. Accessed August 15, 2020.

OVERALL US HIV PREVALENCE, INCIDENCE, AND DEATHS

EMPHASIS ON KEY POPULATIONS & PROGRAMS

According to the CDC reports on prevalence and incidence data on HIV and AIDS in the 50 US states and six dependent areas, from 2015 to 2019, the prevalence of PWH increased, while new HIV diagnoses decreased 9%. At year-end 2019, over one million (1,189,700) persons aged 13 years and older were living with a diagnosis of HIV infection (Figure 2.2). The number of new HIV diagnoses in the United States in 2020 (30,403) was 17% lower than in 2019 (36,585), which is thought to be due to disruption in clinical services and decreased testing during the COVID-19 pandemic. At year-end 2020, prevalence remained highest in the Northeast (420.7 per 100,000), followed by 377.4 in the South, 264.9 in the West, and 182.7 in the Midwest. Figure 2.2, however, showing 2020 HIV incidence rates, demonstrates how the southeastern United States suffered the highest rates of new infections.

Pivoting from HIV to AIDS-specific data, despite CDC and US Preventive Task Force recommendations for routine, opt-out, non–risk factor-based HIV screening since 2006, AIDS remains disappointingly common, with 16,990 persons receiving a new AIDS diagnosis in 2020. AIDS diagnoses follow a geographic trend similar to new HIV diagnoses, with the heaviest impact in the South (40%), followed by the Northeast (27%), West (19%), and Midwest (11%). The high rate of AIDS despite widespread availability of effective, tolerable antiretroviral treatment highlights the need for improved HIV screening as well as care linkage,

retention, and treatment for those already diagnosed with HIV (CDC, 2020).

Death rates related to HIV continue on a low, slow decline following the sharp drop-off with the advent of effective antiretroviral treatments in 1996. As expected, with new infections outpacing deaths by approximately 25,000 cases each year, HIV prevalence continues to rise. Two important implications of this are that more clinicians will be needed to care for the burgeoning aging HIV population, and more must be done to prevent HIV transmission by targeting high-risk populations with interventions of proven efficacy, such as pre-exposure prophylaxis (PrEP) and treatment-as-prevention.

THE US HIV CARE CONTINUUM

Since the USDHHS HIV/AIDS Bureau's National HIV/AIDS Strategy (NHAS) release in 2010, the HIV treatment community has focused on what is known as the HIV care continuum as the leading quality indicator in our healthcare system's response to HIV (White House Office of National AIDS Policy, 2015). The care continuum comprises rates of HIV diagnoses among persons estimated to have acquired HIV, care linkage, retention, and viral suppression (Figure 2.3). Although the NHAS goals (i.e., reducing new HIV diagnoses; increasing access to care, and improving health outcomes for persons living with HIV; and reducing HIV-related health disparities) go beyond the care continuum, it nonetheless remains a fundamental indicator of progress not only for the NHAS but also for the newer Ending the HIV Epidemic Initiative (see Chapter 1).

As ART has become increasingly potent, less toxic, and easier to take, the greatest challenges in suppressing what is commonly referred to as "community viral load" (i.e., the

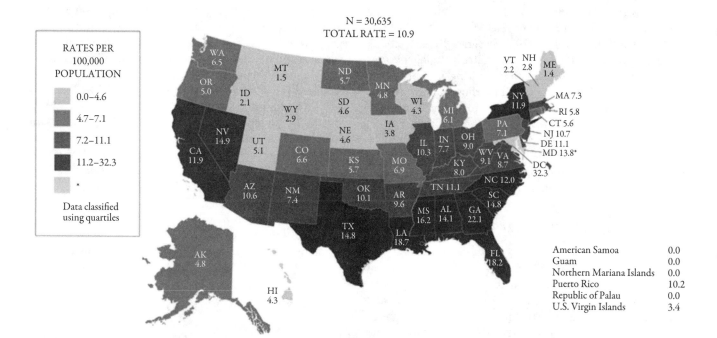

Figure 2.2 Rates of diagnosis of HIV infection among persons aged ≥13 years, 2020 (COVID-19 pandemic)—United States and six dependent areas   SOURCE: CDC. HIV surveillance report, 2020; vol. 33. http://www.cdc.gov/hiv/library/reports/hiv-surveillance.html. Published May 2022.

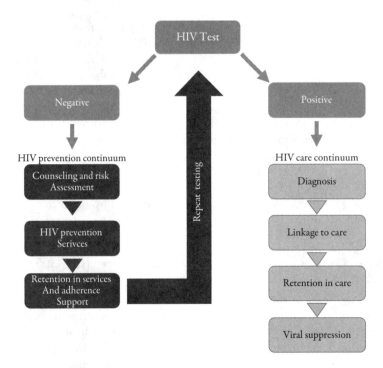

Figure 2.3 HIV testing and care continuum.   SOURCE: Adapted from Horn T, et al. Towards an integrated primary and secondary HIV prevention continuum for the United States: a cyclical process mode. *J Int AIDS Soc.* 2016;19(1):21263.

sum of detectable viral loads among PWH in a community) now exists primarily in the first three steps of the continuum. Unfortunately, little progress was made from 2010 to 2012 in these measures, and in 2012, fewer than one-third of persons with HIV in the United States were virally suppressed. However, by 2018, 86% of persons with HIV knew their status; 65% were engaged in care; and although only 50% were retained in care, 56% had viral suppression (CDC, 2018a). On the prevention side, the number of adults prescribed PrEP increased by more than 300% from 7,972 in 2014 to 33,273 in 2015 (NHAS: 2020 Progress Report, 2020), although even by 2018, only 18.1% of PrEP-eligible persons were prescribed it, including a disappointing 5.9% of eligible Black persons (CDC, 2018a). While those data show real progress, we still have significant work to do for the most at-risk groups and regions. Providing HIV prevention, testing, and care across a variety of settings, particularly community health centers and other medical homes that serve affected populations with cultural competence, is critical to further improving outcomes along the care continuum.

TRANSMISSION GROUP SPECIAL CONSIDERATIONS

Though any person may acquire HIV, it is well-known that the US epidemic disproportionately impacts key populations and geographic areas. As an example, Black gay and bisexual men comprised 39% of new HIV diagnoses among all gay and bisexual men in 2020, more than three times their percentage of the total population (Figure 2.4). From a geographic perspective, the CDC identifies impoverished urban areas as settings of generalized epidemics. By definition, a concentrated epidemic exists when the prevalence rate is <1% in the general population but >5% in at least one high-risk subpopulation, such as is seen with HIV among MSM, persons who inject drugs (PWID), and persons who exchange sex for money (sometimes referred to as commercial sex workers or CSWs) in these areas (Denning & DiNenno, 2019).

Regrettably, we lack population-level data on CSWs, given the frequently criminalized status of commercial sex work, presenting a barrier to understanding transmission dynamics and developing solutions. Similarly important to ending the HIV epidemic is reaching out to PWID, who accounted for 1 in 15 HIV diagnoses in 2020. A focus on these high-risk groups will continue to be critical to HIV work in impoverished urban areas, not all of which are located in major cities, and to continue to appreciate the intersectionality of these high-risk groups in HIV transmission. More HIV clinicians are needed in new locations to reach underserved populations. In addition, in order to end the HIV epidemic, HIV prevention and education must expand beyond historically high-prevalence areas to newer high-incidence states and counties to reduce new infections in a way that we have not been able to do thus far.

RECOMMENDED READING

CDC. CDC HIV/AIDS Resource Library sets. HIV surveillance report 2020. cdc.gov. http://www.cdc.gov/hiv/library/slidesets/index.html. Published 2020a. Accessed September 9, 2022.

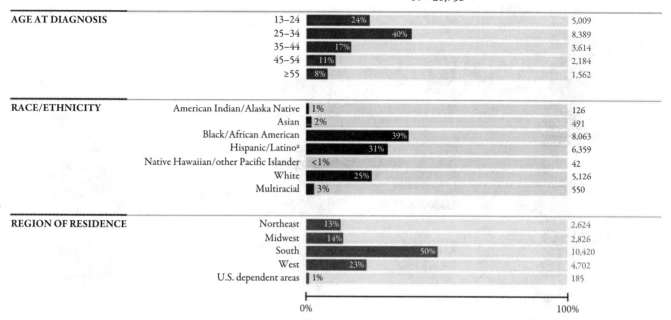

Figure 2.4 Percentages of diagnoses of HIV infection among men who have sex with men, by selected characteristics, 2020 (COVID-19 pandemic)—United States and six dependent areas   NOTE: Data have been statistically adjusted to account for missing transmission category. Data for 2020 should be interpreted with caution due to the COVID-19 pandemic on access to HIV testing, care-related services, and case surveillance activities in state/local jurisdictions[a].
[a]Hispanic/Latino persons can be of any race.
SOURCE: CDC. HIV surveillance report, 2020; vol. 33. http://www.cdc.gov/hiv/library/reports/hiv-surveillance.html. Published May 2022.

HIV AMONG COMMUNITIES OF COLOR

WHAT'S NEW?

HIV infection among Native Hawaiians and other Pacific Islanders (NHOPI) in the United States has increased but young, Black or African American MSM persist at the highest risk for new HIV infection.

KEY POINTS

- The prevalence of HIV among Black persons is more than three times higher than their percentage of the US population, with rates highest in the southeastern United States.

- Young Black MSM have the highest risk for HIV acquisition of any demographic group in the United States.

- AIDS and AIDS-related deaths among Black and Hispanic persons are higher than population norms.

UNEQUAL BURDENS

While the annual number and rate of diagnoses of HIV infection in the United States decreased overall from 2014–2018, this varied widely among different subgroup populations. Among NHOPI, new HIV diagnoses increased 51% during this time frame, with the majority of new cases among NHOPI MSM (although absolute numbers remain relatively low). In contrast, the rates of new HIV diagnoses among Asian, Black, Hispanic/Latinx, White, and persons of multiple races decreased slightly, and the rate for Native American and Alaska Native persons remained stable (Figure 2.5). Although NHOPI make up <1% of new HIV diagnoses in the United States, HIV may affect this group in ways that are not readily apparent because of their small population size (only 0.2% of the US population in 2018) and a lack of representation in clinical trials or epidemiologic analyses. In addition to societal disadvantages, including poverty and limited access to health care, NHOPI cultural customs, such as not discussing sex across generations, may stigmatize sexuality, especially homosexuality, and prevent NHOPI from accessing HIV prevention and care services.

However, the most critical feature to note about US epidemiologic HIV data is that Black persons continue to be the group hardest hit by HIV infections and deaths. Black persons were vastly overrepresented among PWH compared to their percentage of the general population in 2018 (41% vs. 13%). This is also true, but to a lesser extent, for Hispanic persons (22% vs. 18%). These numbers for White persons, by comparison, are 29% and 60%, respectively. The CDC denotes the rate of difference as absolute disparity; if Black/African American adults and adolescents had the same rate as White persons of the same age group, then 33 cases of HIV per 100,000 population would have been prevented (Figure 2.5). Additionally, the largest number of new HIV diagnoses exists in Black/African American MSM living in the US South (Figure 2.5). Figure 2.6 shows how this group increased its percentage among AIDS diagnoses early in the epidemic while cases among White persons declined, overtaking them in 1995 before leveling off in 2000, and continue to far exceed all other racial/ethnic groups.

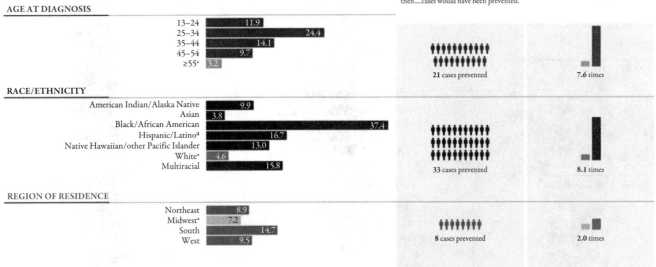

Figure 2.5 Rates and disparities of diagnosis of HIV infection among persons aged ≥13 years, by selected characteristics, 2020 (COVID-19 pandemic)—United States   NOTE: Rates are per 100,000 population. Data for 2020 should be interpreted with caution because of the impact of the COVID-19 pandemic on access to HIV testing, care-related services, and case surveillance activities in state/local jurisdictions. *Absolute disparity* measures the difference between rates in groups with the highest rates and a reference group[s].
[a] Hispanic/Latino persons can be of any race.
SOURCE: CDC. HIV surveillance report, 2020; vol. 33. http://www.cdc.gov/hiv/library/reports/hiv-surveillance.html. Published May 2022.

The current highest-risk demographic in the United States is young Black MSM who live in the South, driving the epidemic in this subgroup across the United States to the extent that the CDC announced in 2016 that if current demographic trends continue, fully one half of Black MSM (and one-quarter of Latino MSM) will be HIV-infected in their lifetime. Death rates are also heavily skewed against Black persons with HIV, with a sevenfold higher death rate than that of White PWH. Death rates among Hispanic persons is almost twice that of White persons, whereas other groups fare the same or better.

Regardless of how these data are examined—whether considering HIV diagnoses, AIDS, or deaths—there is a strikingly excessive burden of HIV shouldered in the United States by Black persons, and, to a lesser extent, by Hispanic persons. The 2016 NHAS recognized this in its call to reduce racial disparities in HIV care, which should be incorporated into the mission of all local, regional, and national HIV programs.

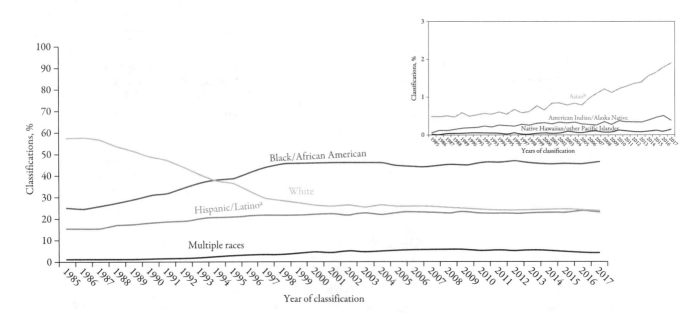

Figure 2.6 Percentages of stage 3 (AIDS) classifications among adults and adolescents with diagnosed HIV Infection, by race/ethnicity, 1985–2017—United States and six dependent areas   SOURCE: CDC HIV/AIDS Resource Library slide sets. http://www.cdc.gov/hiv/library/slidesets/index.html. Accessed September 22, 2022.

Such efforts must address the stigma, fear, discrimination, homophobia, distrust, and socioeconomic issues associated with poor access to care in these at-risk populations (White House Office of National AIDS Policy, 2015). The CDC and its partners are pursuing a high-impact prevention approach, increasing awareness about testing, prevention (including PrEP), and retention in care among populations disproportionately affected by HIV, particularly gay or bisexual men of color (CDC, 2022a).

HIV AMONG IMMIGRANT POPULATIONS

KEY POINTS

- The percentage of new AIDS diagnoses in the United States comprised by minority races/ethnicities continues to climb.

- HIV-2 infection, while still uncommon in the United States, may rise as more persons emigrate from West Africa.

- Different immigrant populations have widely varying rates of HIV infection, and differences within foreign and US-born racial/ethnic minorities are not fully understood.

- Immigrants, legal or not, face many barriers to engagement with the healthcare system.

For several years, the CDC has published data on the incidence and prevalence of HIV, AIDS, and HIV-related deaths among Black, Latinos/Hispanic, Asian, Native American, and Pacific Islander persons. These data are summarized in Tables 2.1 and 2.2 (CDC, 2022a), showing the wide range of impact of HIV in these different groups and the overrepresentation of racial and ethnic minorities as a whole among AIDS diagnoses (72%) (Figure 2.7). However, in these data, the CDC does not separate African-born from US-born Black persons, or foreign-born versus US-born Latinos/Hispanic persons, making it difficult to track the HIV epidemic among these different immigrant populations. Despite this, a 2013 review found HIV incidence among African-born versus US-born Black persons to be two-thirds higher, presentation with AIDS more frequent (30% vs. 22%), and progression to AIDS within 12 months of an HIV diagnosis more likely (45% vs. 37%), this despite the already high rates of these indicators among Black persons as a whole. Paradoxically, survival was better among African-born versus US-born Black persons (7.1 deaths vs. 19.5 deaths per 1,000 per year), possibly because of better engagement in care (Blanas et al., 2013).

Since January 4, 2010, refugees are no longer tested for HIV infection upon arrival to the United States. However, since 2006, CDC guidelines have recommended universal screening for all persons aged 13–64 years regardless of risk factors or country of origin (Branson, 2006). Given

Table 2.1 ADULTS AND ADOLESCENTS LIVING WITH DIAGNOSED HIV INFECTION BY RACE/ETHNICITY, YEAR-END 2020 (COVID-19 PANDEMIC)—UNITED STATES

RACE/ETHNICITY	NUMBER	RATE	%
American Indian/Alaskan Native	3,248	133.5	0.3
Asian	16,198	83.6	1.5
Black/African American	430,015	1,038.0	40.8
Hispanic/Latino	246,097	401.4	23.3
Native Hawaiian/other Pacific Islander	936	152.6	0.1
White	305,956	155.5	29.0
Multiple races	52,423	693.7	5.0
Total	1,054,873	320.4	100

SOURCE: CDC Surveillance Report 2020. https://www.cdc.gov/hiv/pdf/library/reports/surveillance/cdc-hiv-surveillance-report-2020-updated-vol-33.pdf. Published 2022. Accessed August 15, 2022.

that the chaotic and vulnerable conditions of refugee flight and refugee camps create high risk for HIV transmission, HIV screening of all refugees is encouraged. The CDC-recommended fourth-generation testing algorithm differentiates between HIV-1 and HIV-2, whereas older-generation HIV antibody screening tests generally do not. Therefore, if fourth-generation testing is not available, refugees or immigrants native to or who transited through

Table 2.2 DEATHS OF PERSONS WITH DIAGNOSED HIV INFECTION EVER CLASSIFIED AS STAGE 3 (AIDS) BY RACE/ETHNICITY, YEAR-END 2020—UNITED STATES AND SIX DEPENDENT AREAS

RACE/ETHNICITY	NUMBER	RATE	%
American Indian/Alaskan Native	78	3.2	0.4
Asian	97	0.5	0.5
Black/African American	7930	17.4	43.7
Hispanic/Latino	3245	5.3	17.9
Native Hawaiian/other Pacific Islander	10	1.6	<0.1
White	5514	2.8	30.3
Multiple races	1290	17.1	7.1
Total	18,164	5.5	100

SOURCE: CDC HIV/AIDS Resource Library Slide Sets. HIV surveillance Report 2020 (cdc.gov) http://www.cdc.gov/hiv/library/slidesets/index.html. Published 2020. Accessed August 15, 2022.

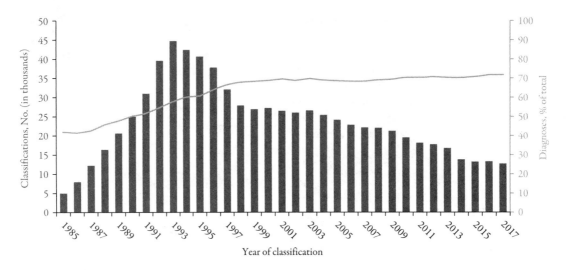

Figure 2.7 Diagnosed HIV infections classified as stage 3 (AIDS) among racial/ethnic minorities, 1985–2017—United States and six dependent areas   SOURCE: CDC HIV/AIDS Resource Library slide sets. http://www.cdc.gov/hiv/library/slidesets/index.html. Accessed September 22, 2022.

countries with high HIV-2 prevalence should have specific testing for HIV-2.

The CDC's 2014 surveillance case definition for HIV and AIDS applies to both variants of HIV and has specified criteria for defining HIV-2 infection. From 1988 to June 2010, 242 HIV-2 cases were reported to the CDC, but, of these, only 166 met the case definition for HIV-2. These cases were concentrated in the Northeast (66%), including 46% in New York City, occurring primarily among persons born in West Africa (81%) (CDC, 2011). During 2010–2017, use of the HIV-1/HIV-2 differentiation test increased, but the number of confirmed HIV-2 diagnoses in the United States remained <0.1%, consistent with previously reported findings (Peruski et al., 2020).

Data from King County, Washington, show the percentage of new HIV cases that were foreign born rising from 23% to 34% from 2006 to 2015. The leading areas of origin were Africa (34%), Latin America (32%), and Asia (22%). Africans with HIV were more likely to be female and heterosexual, while Latin American and Asian persons were similar to US-born individuals by HIV risk factor and gender (male MSM) (Kerani et al., 2018).

Multiple factors contribute to HIV infection among immigrants. Migration within and across national borders in search of work may contribute to increased HIV risk situations. In addition, change in residence can result in loneliness, isolation, and disruption of social, familial, and sexual relationships that can lead to risk-taking behavior (Organista et al., 2004). In another study, the authors found lack of knowledge regarding HIV risk, social stigma, secrecy, and symptom-driven health-seeking behavior (as opposed to routine preventive care) as factors in delayed HIV presentation in immigrants. Further, compared to US-born patients, immigrants were significantly younger; more likely to present with indicators of more advanced HIV disease, including opportunistic infections; had lower CD4 counts; and were more likely to be hospitalized at the time of HIV diagnosis, consistent with findings specific to African-born HIV patients, as mentioned earlier (Levy et al., 2007).

RECOMMENDED READING

CDC. CDC HIV/AIDS Resource Library slide sets. HIV surveillance report 2020. cdc.gov. http://www.cdc.gov/hiv/library/slidesets/index.html. Published 2020. Accessed August 15 2022.

Blanas DA, Nichols K, Bekele M, et al. HIV/AIDS among African-born residents in the United States. *J Immigr Minor Health.* August 2013;15(4):718–724.

HIV AMONG WOMEN, CHILDREN, AND ADOLESCENTS

WHAT'S NEW?

In 2020, in the United States, 18% of HIV diagnoses were among women, and this has remained stable since 2015. With widespread utilization of ART, transmission of HIV from mother to child has decreased to less than 1% in the United States.

KEY POINTS

- High-risk heterosexual contact remains the most common risk factor for HIV acquisition among adult women.

- The CDC recommends opt-out testing for all pregnant women in the first trimester and repeat testing in the third trimester for women at risk for infection. Adolescent HIV transmission mirrors adult patterns, with large majorities of males infected via same-sex contact and females via heterosexual contact.

WOMEN

Worldwide in 2021, women continue to account for more than half of all HIV-infected persons and 43% of new infections largely through heterosexual transmission (World Health Organization (WHO), 2022). In Sub-Saharan Africa, six in seven new infections are among adolescents young women aged 15–19 years, and young women aged 15–24 years are twice as likely as men in this cohort to be living with HIV (UNAIDS, 2022). Conversely, in the United States, women represented only 18% of HIV diagnoses in 2020, comprising an estimated 5,000 new infections. This disparity is due to the preponderance of male-to-male HIV transmission in the United States. This was down from 7,190 new infections among women in 2018, a drop felt to be due to decreased testing during the Covid-19 pandemic. Of the new diagnoses, approximately one-quarter already had AIDS, highlighting the need to improve early detection and prevent ongoing transmission. HIV incidence among US women continues to be highest in the South, followed by the industrial states of the Northeast.

From 2014 through 2020, Black women accounted for the majority of new HIV diagnoses in US females, although the number decreased from 4,573 in 2014 to 4,097 in 2018, and then to 2,970 in 2020 (again, 2020 data reflect decreased testing rates because of COVID-19). The seropositivity rate of these women (23 per 100,000 persons) was nearly 14-times higher than that of White females (1.7/100k) and more than 4-times higher than that of Hispanic females (5.2/100k). Although Black women comprised only 13% of the female population, they accounted for 54% of diagnoses of HIV infection among women, which is 4.5 times the expected population-adjusted rate. Hispanic/Latina women made up 17% of the female population and accounted for 17% of diagnoses. White women were 62% of the US female population and yet accounted for only 24% of HIV diagnoses among women (CDC, 2022a).

Factors that increase a woman's risk of acquiring HIV include not knowing her partner's risk factors for HIV infection, having a lack of HIV knowledge, and having a decreased awareness of risk (CDC, 2022a). Women's relationships with their partners play a pivotal role as well: in relationships in which women are physically abused, vulnerability to HIV is increased because they may not insist on condom use out of fear of being harmed. Women with a history of sexual abuse are more likely to engage in high-risk sexual activity and use drugs compared to women without such behaviors. This includes exchanging sexual activities for drugs and money as well as having difficulty refusing unwanted sex.

Results from CDC's Young Men's Survey (1994–2000) found that many young Black and Latino MSM outwardly identify as heterosexual, with female spouses or partners, but also engage in same-sex encounters with other men, and that this high-risk group represents a bridge for transmitting HIV to women (Fitzpatrick et al., 2004; Millett, 2004; Valleroy et al., 2004). In addition, many poor and/or minority women lack the agency—whether economic, cultural, or otherwise—to use condoms with or separate from abusive or unfaithful men who engage in high-risk sex with other partners or commercial sex workers. HIV prevention efforts must account for such factors to make inroads against HIV transmission in these groups.

The most common mode of transmission for women is high-risk heterosexual contact (64%–92% across various groups), followed by injection-drug use. These rates, current through 2020, may change with the deepening national opioid crisis and outbreaks of HIV transmission among needle-sharing networks (CDC, 2022a).

Sexual HIV transmission occurs through unprotected vaginal or anal sex, with receptive anal sex posing the highest risk, and insertive vaginal sex the lowest. Oral sex is a theoretical risk if there are breaks in the oral and genital mucosa through which blood or genital secretions may pass. Similarly, sexually transmitted infections that disrupt genital mucosa and stimulate a local immune response will increase the likelihood of acquiring or transmitting HIV. Because gonorrhea and syphilis in particular have a higher rate in women of color compared to White women, this heightens their risk of HIV acquisition. Socioeconomic status also plays a role in HIV risk. In states with higher rates of poverty and limited access to healthcare, women are more likely to use drugs and exchange sex for drugs or money, factors shown to increase risk of HIV, directly or indirectly (CDC, 2022a).

CHILDREN

The reduction of perinatal HIV transmission in the United States is a major success of the antiretroviral era. Although the CDC has not published a similar graph showing perinatal HIV transmission rates since the beginning of the epidemic, Figure 2.8 shows the dramatic rise and fall in perinatal AIDS diagnoses since 1985 until 2017. In 1992, an estimated 952 pediatric HIV transmissions were reported in the United States. By 2004, the number declined to 177, and in 2019, a total of 32 children received a diagnosis of HIV through perinatal transmission. The overall rate of perinatal HIV infections reported by the CDC decreased from 1.5 per 100,000 live births in 2014 to 0.9 in 2018, which met the CDC's goal of less than 1 perinatal transmission per 100,000 live births (CDC, 2020).

Despite the powerful role of ART in preventing vertical HIV transmission, its persistence is tied to an increasing number of pregnancies among HIV-positive women, a lack of HIV testing in some pregnant women, and inadequate viral suppression in mothers known to have HIV. Among all perinatal HIV transmissions from 2016–2019, 64% of mothers tested HIV+ before or during pregnancy, representing gaps in linkage and retention in care and viral suppression. An additional 21% did not test positive until at or after delivery, representing missed opportunities to screen and prevent vertical transmission (Figure 2.9). This highlights the importance of screening all pregnant women for HIV at least once during pregnancy and higher-risk women again in the third trimester.

As with adults, HIV disproportionately affects Black children. While accounting for 56% of diagnoses, they comprised only 14% of the population of US children in 2020, whereas Hispanic (16% of HIV diagnoses, 26% of population) and White (21% of HIV diagnoses, 49% of population) children are infected far less often than their population percentages (CDC, 2022a).

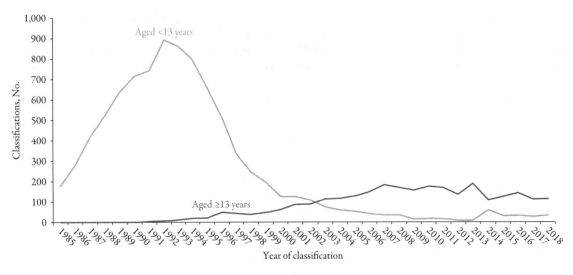

Figure 2.8 Stage 3 (AIDS) classifications among persons with perinatally acquired HIV infection, 1985–2018—United States and six dependent areas   SOURCE: CDC HIV/AIDS Resource Library slide sets. http://www.cdc.gov/hiv/library/slidesets/index.html. Accessed September 22, 2022.

ADOLESCENTS AND YOUNG ADULTS

According to 2020 CDC data, persons aged 13–34 years account for over half of newly diagnosed HIV in the United States. In particular, persons aged 13–24 and young adults aged 25–34 represented 20% and 37% of incident diagnoses, respectively, the majority being MSM. The annual number of HIV infections in 2020 among persons aged 13–24 decreased compared with 2018, but this was likely due to decreased testing because of COVID-19. Young persons with HIV are particularly vulnerable, as they are least likely to be retained in care and to have a suppressed viral load (CDC,2022).

Transmissions remain disproportionately high among Black and Latino MSM youth. In 2020, of all adolescents and young adults aged 13–24 years diagnosed with HIV infection, the CDC reported that 54% were Black, far outpacing their percentage of the general population. Hispanic/Latino persons represented an additional 26% of adolescent HIV diagnoses in the same year (CDC, 2022a).

Male same-sex contact remains the predominant mode of HIV transmission in the adolescent and young adult population, accounting for 92% of new diagnoses. Heterosexual contact accounts for approximately 3%. Transmissions from injection-drug use remain stable at approximately 2% (CDC, 2018b).

In 2020, female sex at birth comprised 15% of the HIV diagnoses in adolescents (13–19 years) and 12% in young adults (20–24 years) compared to 17% of adults older than 24 years. The mode of HIV transmission varies between sexes in this age group, as it does in adults: whereas 84% of adolescent and young adult females are infected through heterosexual contact, more than 90% of males contract HIV through male-to-male sexual contact (CDC, 2022a). Racial disparities persist among Black, Hispanic/Latino, and White adolescent and young adult females, with prevalence rates of 47%, 13%, and 4%, respectively. If African Americans had the same rate of prevalence as White persons among ages 13–24 years, 43 cases per 100,000 would

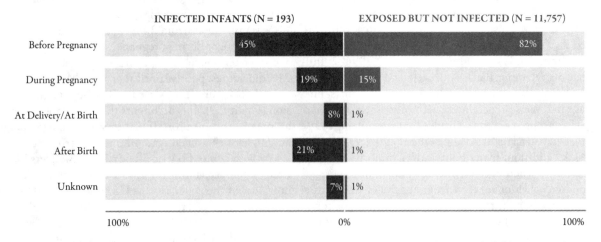

Figure 2.9 Time of maternal HIV testing among children with diagnosed perinatally acquired HIV infection and children exposed to HIV, birth years 2016 to 2019—United States and Puerto Rico   SOURCE: CDC HIV/AIDS Resource Library slide sets. http://www.cdc.gov/hiv/library/slidesets/index.html. Accessed September 22, 2022.

have been prevented (CDC, 2022a). Perinatal transmission accounted for 41% of adolescent and young adult females living with HIV, while only 10% of males with HIV were perinatally acquired, reflecting a higher rate of behavioral transmission among young MSM (as opposed to vertical transmission). However, unstable housing and employment may lead young women to engage in survival sex, leading to disproportionately HIV infection.

RECOMMENDED READING

CDC. HIV surveillance report: diagnoses of HIV infection and AIDS in the United States and dependent areas, vol. 31. cdc.gov. https://www.cdc.gov/hiv/pdf/library/reports/surveillance/cdc-hiv-surveillance-report-2018-updated-vol-31.pdf. Published 2018. Accessed August 15, 2022.

CDC. Adolescents and young adult surveillance. cdc.gov. https://www.cdc.gov/hiv/pdf/library/slidesets/cdc-hiv-surveillance-adolescents-young-adults-2018.pdf. Published 2018. Accessed August 15 2022.

HIV IN THE MSM AND TRANSGENDER COMMUNITIES

WHAT'S NEW?

The CDC estimated in February 2016 that, based on current trends, one in two gay Black MSM would become HIV-positive in their lifetime and that one half of Black transgender women are already living with HIV.

KEY POINTS

- Individuals who identify as gay, bisexual, or as other MSM are the only population group in the United States in which new HIV infections have steadily increased since the 1990s, with young Black MSM being disproportionally affected.

- Transgender women account for the vast majority of HIV diagnoses among transgender individuals. Expanded access to PrEP is essential to help curb the spread in this at-risk population.

Since the beginning of the HIV/AIDS epidemic in the United States, MSM have constituted the largest percentage of persons diagnosed with HIV/AIDS, whereas HIV transmission among women who have sex with women has been exceedingly rare. Since 2015, infection rates have remained stubbornly high in the Black American MSM population (CDC, 2022a). In 2020, 81% of all HIV infections among males were attributed to male-to-male sexual contact, whereas heterosexual, Injection Drug Use (IDU), and MSM with IDU transmissions among men remained stable at about 10%, 5%, and 4%, respectively (CDC, 2022b). In 2020, approximately 71% of all HIV infections were attributed to MSM transmission (Figure 2.10).

The percentage of HIV cases diagnosed in the gay community differs based on race/ethnicity and age. In 2020, the estimated percentage of MSM diagnosed with HIV infection who were Black, Latino, White and Asian were 34%, 32%, 28%, and 3%, respectively (CDC, 2022a) (Figure 2.11). NHOPI MSM each accounted for less than 1% of new infections, and persons of mixed race, 3%. Similar but more pronounced racial disparities exist in the adolescent and young adult population, with incidence rates of 54%, 27%, and 14%, respectively, among Black, Latino, and White MSM.

Looking at HIV transmissions among MSM as a function of age, in 2020 the largest percentage of diagnoses were in those aged 25–34 years (40%), followed by those aged 13–24 (24%), 35–44 (17%), 45–54 (11%), and >55 (8%). With the high prevalence of HIV in the MSM community, the cumulative risk of contracting or transmitting the virus becomes greater as these individuals age. Being unaware of one's HIV status, especially common among MSM of color and young MSM, increases the risk of transmitting HIV infection as well. According to CDC guidelines, MSM who are high risk for HIV infection should be screened at least annually; this

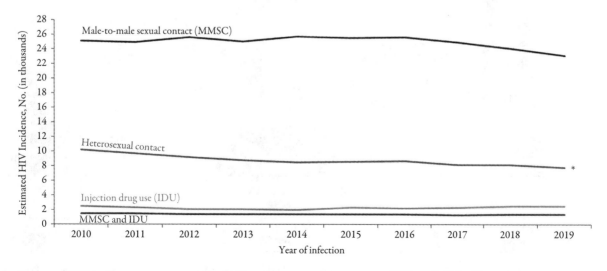

Figure 2.10 Estimated HIV incidence among persons aged >13 years, by transmission category, 2010–2019, United States   SOURCE: CDC. https://www.cdc.gov/hiv/pdf/library/slidesets/cdc-hiv-linley-HIV-Incidence-Prevalence-2010-2019.

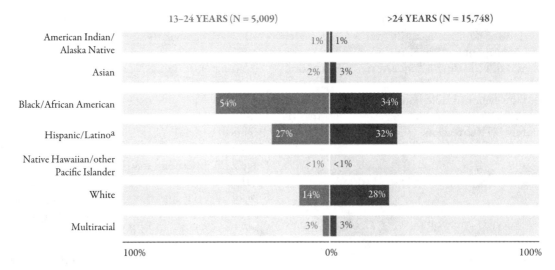

Figure 2.11 Percentages of diagnoses of HIV infection among men who have sex with men, by group and race/ethnicity, 2020, United States and six dependent areas   SOURCE: https://www.cdc.gov/hiv/pdf/library/reports/surveillance/cdc-hiv-surveillance-report-2020-updated-vol-33.pdf.

includes those with more than one sex partner since their last HIV test and MSM who are injection-drug users. Data are insufficient to recommend more frequent screening, but "each clinician can consider the benefits of offering more frequent screening (e.g., once every 3 or 6 months) to individual MSM at increased risk for acquiring HIV infection, weighing their patients' individual risk factors, local HIV epidemiology, and local testing policies" (CDC, 2017).

Transgender individuals are one of the highest-risk groups in the United States for acquiring HIV infection, and epidemiological data on this group are now available from the CDC. In 2020 alone, 697 new cases of HIV infection were documented in the United States; 92% were transgender women; 7% were transgender men; less than 1% had another gender identity; and half of these infected persons lived in the South. One-quarter of transgender women are estimated to have HIV; among Black persons, this figure rises to one half (Figure 2.12).

Despite these worrisome trends, nearly two-thirds of transgender men and women in the Behavioral Risk Factor Surveillance System from 2014 to 2015 were never tested for HIV. The stigma and social rejection faced by transgender persons leads to significant disparities in housing, education, employment, and access to healthcare and preventive services. While studies and firm data are lacking, it is generally observed that transgender females are often forced into survival sex, putting them at heightened risk for HIV acquisition. Social interventions such as advocating for safer sexual practices and condom use, limiting the number of sexual partners, using barrier protection, advocating for stable housing and employment, and pharmacologic PrEP hold promise in helping to stem the tide of transmissions in this at-risk population. This represents an opportunity for improved outreach, education, and testing, as well as for addressing the many factors that put transgender persons at risk for HIV infection (i.e., multiple sexual partners, condomless sex, commercial

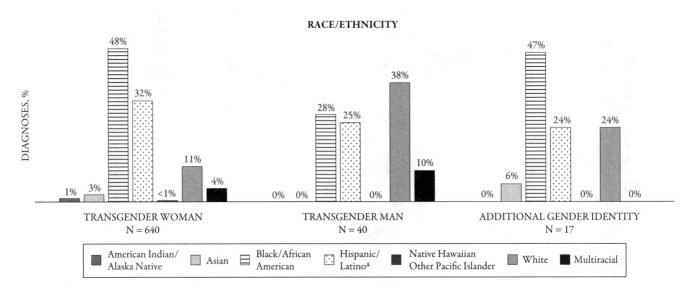

Figure 2.12 Percentages of diagnoses of HIV infection among transgender and additional gender identity persons aged >13 years, by gender and race/ethnicity, 2020, United States and six dependent areas   SOURCE: https://www.cdc.gov/hiv/pdf/library/reports/surveillance/cdc-hiv-surveillance-report-2020-updated-vol-33.pdf.

sex work, mental illness and substance abuse, homelessness, unemployment, targeted violence, and lack of family support) (CDC, 2022a).

HIV AMONG OLDER ADULTS

PWH enjoy increased quality of life for longer periods of time as a result of well-tolerated and highly effective ART regimens. As such, there is a steadily increasing prevalence of HIV among all age groups (CDC, 2022a). While incidence rates among adults are generally stable, those aged 55 years and older (the conventional definition of "older adult" with respect to HIV) still accounted for 10% of new HIV infections in 2020. Of these 3,202 transmissions in 2020, 2,322 (73%) were in men, mainly through male-to-male sexual contact, and 880 (27%) were in women, the majority of which were the result of heterosexual contact. This is a decreased rate of new infection among this population in comparison to 2018 where there were 6,640 new HIV infections, although data from 2020 is likely to be significantly incomplete because of the COVID-19 pandemic. It is critical to remember that this older age group remains at significant risk of HIV acquisition and is less likely to receive guideline-based screening (USPSTF, 2019). A study examining National Health Interview Survey data from 2009 demonstrated that the rate of HIV screening of individuals aged 50 years and older was approximately 25%, with only half of the tests being suggested by a clinician during the encounter (Adekeye et al., 2012). This is an obvious area of opportunity for improved screening, earlier detection, linkage to care, and decreased transmission.

RECOMMENDED READING

Centers for Disease Control and Prevention (CDC). HIV surveillance report, 2020, vol. 33. cdc.gov. https://www.cdc.gov/hiv/library/reports/hiv-surveillance.html. Published May 2022. Accessed August 12, 2022.

CDC. HIV among transgender people in the United States 2018. cdc.gov. https://www.cdc.gov/hiv/group/gender/transgender/index.html. Published 2018a. Accessed August 12, 2022.

CDC. HIV and older Americans. cdc.gov. https://www.cdc.gov/hiv/group/age/olderamericans/index.html. Published November 12, 2019. Accessed August 17, 2020.

REFERENCES

Adekeye OA, Heiman HJ, Onyeabor OS, Hyacinth HI. The new invincibles: HIV screening among older adults in the U.S. *PLoS One.* 2012;7(8):e43618. http://doi/10.1371/journal.pone.0043618

Apetrei C, Marx PA. Simian retroviral infections in human beings. *Lancet.* 2004;364(9429):137–138.

Blanas DA, Nichols K, Bekele M, et al. HIV/AIDS among African-born residents in the United States. *J Immigr Minor Health.* 2013;15(4):718-724. https://doi.org/10.1007/s10903-012-9691-6

Branson BM. To screen or not to screen: is that really the question? *Ann Intern Med.* 2006;145(11):857–859.

Campbell-Yesufu OT, Gandhi RT. Update on human immunodeficiency virus (HIV)-2 infection. *Clin Infect Dis.* 2011;52:780–787. https://doi:10.1093/cid/ciq248

Centers for Disease Control and Prevention (CDC). CDC HIV/AIDS Resource Library slide sets. HIV surveillance report 2020. cdc.gov. http://www.cdc.gov/hiv/library/slidesets/index.html. Published 2020.

CDC. HIV and people who inject drugs. cdc.gov. https://www.cdc.gov/hiv/group/hiv-idu.html. Published February 6, 2020. Accessed August 12, 2022.

CDC. HIV-2 infection surveillance—United States, 1987–2009. *MMWR Morb Mortal Wkly Rep.* 2011;60:985–988.

CDC. HIV surveillance—adolescents and young adults—2018b. cdc.gov. httpss://www.cdc.gov/hiv/pdf/library/slidesets/cdc-hiv-surveillance-adolescents-young-adults-2018.pdf. Published 2018b. Accessed August 15, 2022.

CDC. HIV surveillance report, 2020, vol. 33. cdc.gov. http://www.cdc.gov/hiv/library/reports/hiv-surveillance.html. Published May 2022a. Accessed August 14, 2022.

CDC. MMWR recommendations for HIV screening of gay, bisexual, and other men who have sex with men—United States, 2017. cdc.gov. https://www.cdc.gov/mmwr/volumes/66/wr/mm6631a3.htm. Published 2017. Accessed August 15, 2022.

CDC. Selected national HIV prevention and control outcomes. cdc.gov. https:// www.cdc.gov/hiv/pdf/library/slidesets/cdc-hiv-prevention-and-careoutcomes-2018.pd. Published 2018a. Accessed August 15, 2022.

Denning P, DiNenno E. Communities in crisis: is there a generalized HIV epidemic in impoverished urban areas of the United States? cdc.gov. https://www.cdc.gov/hiv/group/poverty.html. Published December 11, 2019. Accessed August 15, 2022.

Fitzpatrick LK, Grant L, Eure C, et al. Investigation of HIV transmission among young Black men who have sex with men (MSM) in North Carolina: implications for prevention. In: *Program and abstracts of the XV International AIDS Conference.* [Abstract C10746]. Bangkok, Thailand; July 11–16, 2004. Accessed on August 12, 2022.

Gomes P, Diogo I, Gonca Ives MF, et al. Different pathways to nelfinavir genotypic resistance in HIV-1 subtypes B and C. In: *Program and abstracts of the 9th Conference on Retroviruses and Opportunistic Infections.* [Abstract 46]. Seattle, WA; February 24–28, 2002. Accessed August 15, 2022.

Kerani R, Bennett AB, Golden M, Castillo J, et al. Foreign-born individuals with HIV in King County, WA: a glimpse of the future of HIV? *AIDS Behav.* 2018;22(7):2181–2188. http://doi:10.1007/s10461-017-1914-3

Levy V, Prentiss D, Balmas G, et al. Factors in the delayed HIV presentation of immigrants in Northern California: implications for voluntary counseling and testing programs. *J Immigr Minor Health.* 2007;9(1):49–54. http://doi:10.1007/s10903-006-9015-9

Millet G. Men on the "down low": more questions than answers. In: *Program and abstracts of the 11th Conference on Retroviruses and Opportunistic Infections.* [Abstract 83]. San Francisco, CA; February 8–11, 2004. https://www.natap.org/2004/CROI/croi_6.htm

National HIV/AIDS Strategy for the United States. Update to 2020. 2017 Progress report. https://files.hiv.gov/s3fs-public/NHAS_Progress_Report_2017.pdf. Published 2020. Accessed August 12, 2022.

Organista KC, Carillo H, Avala G. HIV prevention with Mexican migrants: review, critique, and recommendations. *J AIDS.* 2004;37 (Suppl 4):S227–S239.

Peruski AH, Wesolowski LG, Delaney KP, et al. Trends in HIV-2 diagnoses and use of the HIV-1/HIV-2 differentiation test—United States, 2010–2017. *MMWR Morb Mortal Wkly Rep.* 2020;69:63–66.

Spira S, Wainberg MA, Loemba H, et al. Impact of clade diversity on HIV-1 virulence, antiretroviral drug sensitivity and drug resistance. *J Antimicrob Chemother.* 2003;51:229–240.

UNAIDS. UNAIDS data 2018. unaids.org. https://www.aidsdatahub.org/sites/default/files/resource/unaids-data-2018.pdf. Published 2018. Accessed August 15, 2022.

UNAIDS. UNAIDS data 2020. Unaids.org. http://www.unaids.org/en/resources/documents/2020/unaids-data. Published 2020. Accessed March 3, 2022.

UNAIDS. Fact sheet 2022. unaids.org. https://www.unaids.org/en/resources/fact-sheet. Published 2022. Accessed August 15, 2022.

UNAIDS. Update. 90-90-90-: good progress, but the world is off-track for hitting the 2020 targets. unaids.org. https://www.unaids.org/en/resources/presscentre/featurestories/2020/september/20200921_90-90-90. 21 September 2020. Published 2020. Accessed August 15, 2022.

USDHHS. HIV clinical guidelines for adults and adolescents. Guidelines for the use of antiretroviral agents in adults and adolescents living with HIV. https://clinicalinfo.hiv.gov/en/guidelines/hiv-clinical-guidelines-adult-and-adolescent-arv/. Published 2022. Accessed September 22, 2022

US Preventive Services Task Force. Screening for HIV Infection. US Preventive Services Task Force recommendation statement. *JAMA*. 2019;321(23):2326–2336. http://doi:10.1001/jama.2019.6587

Valleroy LA, MacKellar D, Behel S, Secura G. The bridge for HIV transmission to women from 15- to 29-year-old men who have sex with men in 7 US cities. In: *Program and Abstracts of the XV International AIDS Conference*. [Abstract 1367]. Bangkok, Thailand; July 11–16, 2004;

Wainberg MA. HIV-1 subtype distribution and the problem of drug resistance. *AIDS*. 2004;18(Suppl 3):S63–S68.

White House Office of National AIDS Policy. National HIV/AIDS strategy for the United States: updated to 2020. https://files.hiv.gov/s3fs-public/nhas-update.pdf. Published July 2015.

Witvrouw M, Pannecouque C, Switzer VM, et al. Susceptibility of HIV-2, SIV and SHIV to various anti-HIV-1 compounds: implications for treatment and postexposure prophylaxis. *Antivir Ther*. 2004;9:57–65.

WHO. Disruption in HIV, hepatitis and STI services due to COVID-19. https://www.who.int/docs/default-source/hq-hiv-hepatitis-and-stis-library/hhs-service-disruption-slides-dec-2020.pdf?sfvrsn=be10f39d12. Published 2020. Accessed August 15, 2022.

WHO. HIV. https://www.who.int/data/gho/data/themes/hiv-aids. Published 2022. Accessed August 15, 2022.

3.

ORIGIN, EVOLUTION, AND SPREAD OF HIV1 & HIV2

Jeffrey T. Kirchner

LEARNING OBJECTIVES

- Discuss the distinct origins of HIV-1 and HIV-2 from SIVs and the multiple cross-transmission events from apes to humans.

- Describe the origin of the initial HIV infections in South-Central Africa, the key reasons for viral dissemination to other areas of Sub-Saharan Africa, and the ultimate global spread of HIV.

- Discuss the diversity of HIV, including viral groups, viral clades, and recombinant forms and their implications for future transmission of HIV, as well as treatments and vaccine developments.

WHAT IS NEW?

- Researchers recently identified a new HIV-1 group M subtype called subtype L. This was based on complete genomic sequencing of non-transmission linked cases (Yamaguchi et al., 2020).

- Additional strains are likely circulating in the Democratic Republic of Congo (DRC). three non-transmission-linked cases (Yamaguchi et al., 2020).

- Recombination between different HIV strains continues to lead to further diversification of the pandemic, and there now have been at least 118 distinct circulating recombinant forms (CRFs) identified, and this number is increasing (Bacque et al., 2021; Elangovan et al., 2021; Mori et al., 2022).

KEY POINTS

- All strains of HIV-1 and HIV-2 are genetic descendants of SIVs. Initial cross-species transmission of the virus occurred from the butchering and eating of bush meat.

- HIV-1 group M ("Major") and 12 associated viral subtypes (A–L) account for approximately 95% of infections globally, with a much smaller number caused by groups N, O, and P.

- HIV-2 and its nine groups (A–I) are mainly limited to West Africa, but since the discovery of HIV-2 in 1986, cases have been reported in Europe and the United States. US. Globally, HIV-2 represents approximately 3% of all HIV infections, although its prevalence appears to be declining. There are data showing a small number of persons are dually infected with HIV-1 and HIV-2.

- Genetic diversity of HIV, including recombination between subtypes, may continue to present challenges to the development of a globally effective vaccine.

ORIGIN OF HIV AND ENTRY INTO HUMANS

The origin of HIV-1 can be traced to the early 1920s from southern Cameroon and then to Kinshasa in what is now the DRC. The combination of rapid population growth, changes in sexual behaviors, and the use of unsterilized needles likely contributed to the rapid spread of HIV, especially groups M and O. Very strong evidence indicated that the first cross-species transmission of HIV to humans that predates the emergence of group M occurred in southeast Cameroon (Sharp & Hahn, 2011). It is not known how humans acquired the zoonotic precursors of HIV-1. However, based on the recognized biology of these viruses, transmission likely arose from cutaneous or mucous membrane exposure to infected chimpanzee blood or body fluid. Such exposures likely occur in the context of the hunting, butchering, and eating of bush meat (Sharp & Hahn, 2011).

HIV, a retrovirus and member of the lentivirus family, was identified as the cause of AIDS 2 years after the first cases were reported in the United States in June 1981 (Gottlieb et al., 1981). Dr. Luc Montaigner in France and Dr. Robert Gallo in the United States are both credited with identifying HIV-1 (Gallo & Montaigner, 2003). The pandemic form of HIV, also referred to as group M (for "Major"), is responsible for most infections globally, and it is currently estimated to be approximately 84 million from the start of the epidemic (UNAIDS, 2022). Since the discovery of HIV-1, followed by HIV-2 in 1986, the reasons for its emergence during the twentieth century, its transmission to humans, its genetic diversity, and the pathogenesis of the virus have been the subjects of extensive research.

It was first noted in 1999, via genetic sequencing, that the chimpanzee *Pan troglodytes troglodytes* infected with the simian immunodeficiency virus (SIV_{cpz}) was likely the primary natural reservoir for HIV-1 (Gao et al., 1999). Later work determined that HIV-1 in humans began with cross-species transmission and recombination of two SIVs (from red-capped mangabeys (*Cercocebus torquatus*) and greater spot-nosed monkeys (*Cercopithecus nictitans*) to chimpanzees that preyed on these animals (Keele et al., 2006). Keele and his group analyzed mitochondrial DNA and viral-specific antibody from 599 fecal samples from chimpanzees. These samples exhibited a strong and broad cross-reactive western blot profile indistinguishable from that of HIV-1 human controls. To date, serologic evidence for SIV infection has been identified in more than 45 nonhuman primate species (NHPS) (Peeters et al., 2014; Sharp & Hahn, 2011). The genetic diversity of these viral species is complex and includes coevolution of virus–host, cross-species transmission, and viral recombination.

Like HIV, SIV is sexually transmitted in NHPS and can be transmitted vertically. In deference to previous thinking, SIV is indeed pathogenic in most NHPS, causing CD4 [+] T-cell depletion (Keele et al., 2009). Chimpanzees infected with SIV have a 10- to 16-fold increased risk of death compared to those that are uninfected. Fertility and survival of offspring are also decreased in SIV-positive female chimpanzees.

THE SPREAD OF HIV THROUGHOUT AFRICA AND THE WORLD

A 2014 study by Faria and colleagues using phylogenetic analysis and "molecular clocks" (based on the assumption that retroviruses mutate over time at a constant rate) confirmed previous work by Hahn and others regarding the dissemination routes of HIV-1 in West Africa (Cohen, 2014; Faria et al., 2014; Sharp & Hahn, 2011). They have also largely determined how group M became the driver of the AIDS pandemic. It is well established that the first-known infections with HIV-1 emerged from Kinshasa (formerly called Leopoldville) in the DRC in approximately 1920. Many refer to Leopoldville/ Kinshasa as the cradle of the AIDS pandemic. From this area, the virus spread eastward to other communities via railway lines that carried up to 1 million passengers yearly to other areas of Africa, including the three largest population centers—Brazzaville, Mbuji-Mayi, and Lubumbashi (Cohen, 2014; Faria, et al. 2014). Rivers were major travel and commerce routes and are believed to have enabled the spread of HIV geographically (Figure 3.1).

Sexual transmission is the primary mode and driver of new HIV transmissions and resultant dissemination of the virus. However, unsterilized injections at clinics in the area

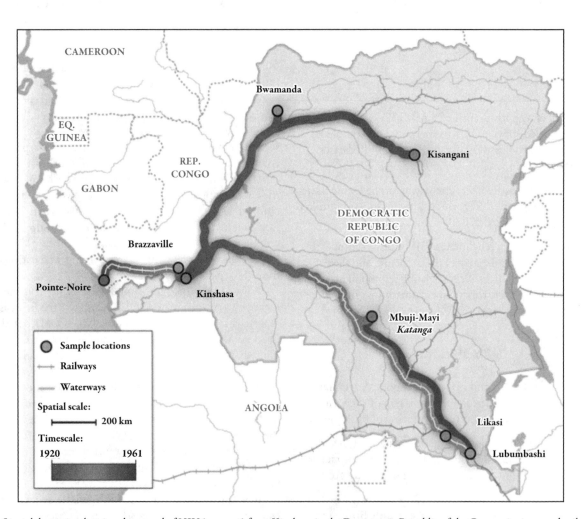

Figure 3.1 Spatial dynamics showing the spread of HIV-1 group, 1 from Kinshasa in the Democratic Republic of the Congo via rivers and railways, which were operational until about 1960 SOURCE: Faria NR, et al. *Science.* 2014;346(6205):56–61.

may have greatly contributed to the spread of HIV. According to Jaques Pepin (2011), well-intended public health interventions by authorities in the Belgian Congo from 1921 to 1959 to treat trypanosomiasis, syphilis, yaws, malaria, and leprosy resulted in the administration of millions of injections to residents of these communities. The majority of injections were intravenous and administered with syringes that clinicians used repeatedly without sterilization of the needles (Pepin, 2011). Consequently, thousands of these individuals may have acquired HIV iatrogenically. Data suggest similar transmission of hepatitis B and C viruses globally through iatrogenic spread during public health campaigns.

The epidemic histories of HIV-1 groups M and O were similar until approximately 1960, when group M infections underwent an epidemiologic transition and exponential increase, outpacing regional population growth (Faria et al., 2014). It is unknown why the growth rate of infections with HIV group M nearly tripled at approximately this time, but likely explanations include virus-specific factors, population growth factors, and the widespread use of injections (Pepin, 2011; Sharp & Hahn, 2011).

Tissues samples collected from two patients in Kinshasa in 1959 and 1960 showed that HIV-1 had diversified into different subtypes much earlier than previously believed. Viral sequencing done on plasma from a sailor who died in 1959 is the oldest case of documented HIV-1 infection (Zhu et al., 1998). Worobey and colleagues (2008) (amplified and identified HIV-1 from a lymph node specimen obtained in 1960 from a female in Kinshasa. The sizable genetic difference between these two HIV specimens demonstrated that diversification of HIV-1 occurred in Kinshasa at least 20 years before the first AIDS cases were observed in the United States. As HIV-1 group M spread globally, its dissemination led to population bottlenecks (founder events) that resulted in different lineages, viral subtypes or clades, and CRFs (Peeters et al., 2014).

How and when HIV first arrived in the United States remains debatable. The virus first appeared in Haiti between 1960 and 1966. The probable source was Haitian professionals who returned from working in the newly independent Congo. It is estimated that during the 1960s, approximately 4,500 skilled Haitian workers were employed by the Congolese government. However, Pepin states that "a single technical assistant infected with HIV-1 subtype B went back to Haiti and stayed long enough to start a local chain of sexual transmission" (2011). Some authorities believe that the selling of sex to American tourists in Haiti led to HIV infection in individuals who in turn brought the virus back to the United States. US. Although perhaps still controversial, Pepin also states, "American gay and bisexual men infected Haitian male sex workers."

Work done by Gilbert and colleagues (2007) using HIV-1 *gag* gene sequences from five Haitians with AIDS, determined that HIV-1 subtype B definitely arrived in Haiti before it spread to the United States and other Western countries. The same group of researchers noted that the most recent common ancestor of HIV-1 subtype B virus appeared in Haiti in 1966, but not in the United States until at least 1969. Consequently, these data suggest that HIV-1 was circulating cryptically in the United States for approximately 12 years before the 1981 cases of AIDS were recognized and reported (Gottlieb et al., 1981). Based on a phylogenetic analyses by Worobey and colleagues (2016), it is likely that HIV was in the United States, specifically New York City, "around 1970." The virus was likely spreading slowly among the heterosexual population before entering the population of men who have sex with men (MSM), in which it spread much more extensively and began to be recognized clinically. The actual scientific facts may never be known; however, Pepin (2011) believes that the blood trade in Port-au-Prince exponentially amplified the number of HIV infections in Haiti and possibly other countries in which blood products were sold, including the United States.

HIV-1 AND HIV-2 GROUPS AND SUBTYPES AND THEIR GEOGRAPHIC DISTRIBUTIONS

HIV-1 comprises four distinct lineages that are termed groups M, N, O, and P. Each has resulted from a distinct and independent cross-species transmission event of SIVs infecting African apes. Using molecular clocks, the most recent common ancestor of group M has been dated to approximately 1920 (Sharp & Hahn, 2011). The four known HIV-1 groups share approximately 50%–60% homology in their nucleotide sequences.

GROUP M

HIV-1 group M (M for "Major") was the first lineage discovered and represents the pandemic form of HIV-1. It has a widespread global distribution and accounts for 90%–95% of HIV-1 transmissions (Sharp & Hahn, 2011). The genetic diversity within HIV-1 group M is the result of subsequent evolution and spread in humans. Based on phylogenic analysis, HIV-1 group M can be further divided into several pure subtypes or clades (A–D, F–H, J, K, and L) and additional sub-subtypes (A1–A4 and F1–F2). The subtypes share 80% homology in their genetic sequences, meaning they differ genetically by approximately 20%. Subtypes and sub-subtypes can form additional mosaic forms through recombination of different strains inside dually or multiply infected individuals. Some CRFs, which are viruses derived from recombination of different viral subtypes and found in more than one person, may further achieve epidemic relevance. To date, researchers have identified 118 distinct CRFs and unique recombinant strains (Mori et al., 2022). This number appears to be increasing over time.

Globally, subtype C, found mainly in Sub-Saharan Africa, represents approximately 50% of HIV-1 infections, although recent data suggest this may be as high as 75% (Faria et al., 2019). This is followed by subtype A (12%), found mainly in Central and East Africa and Russia. Viral subtype B (11%) is the predominant subtype in Europe, the United States, and Oceania and is the most geographically dispersed subtype worldwide (Bbosa et al., 2019). CRFs, most commonly CRF02_AG and CRF01_AE, now account for about 17% of HIV-1 infections

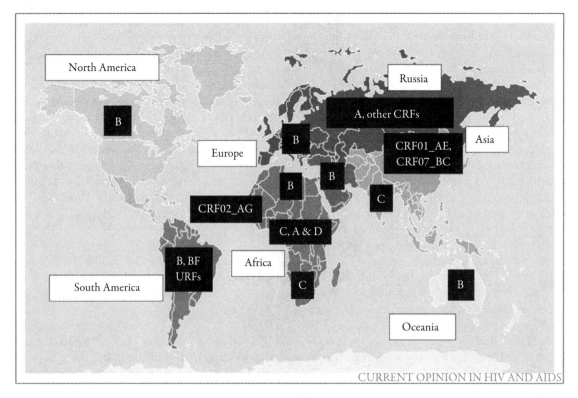

Figure 3.2 HIV subtype diversity worldwide   SOURCE: Bbosa N, et al. *Curr Opin HIV AIDS*. 2019;14:153–60.

worldwide, (Elangovan et al., 2021). Subtypes G and D respectively account for 5% and 2% of infections worldwide (Peeters et al., 2014) (Figure 3.2 and Box 3.1).

HIV-1

GROUP N

Group N ("N" for "non-M, non-O," or "new") was isolated in 1995 from a woman in Cameroon who had AIDS (Pepin,

---

Box 3.1 DISTRIBUTION OF HIV-1 SUBTYPES

Historically, the distribution of subtypes followed the geographic patterns listed here:

- *Subtype A*: Central and East Africa as well as Eastern European countries that were formerly part of the Soviet Union

- *Subtype B*: West and Central Europe, the Americas, Australia, South America, and several Southeast Asian countries (Thailand and Japan), as well as Africa and the Middle East

- *Subtype C*: Sub-Saharan Africa, India, and Brazil

- *Subtype D*: North Africa and the Middle East

- *Subtype F*: South and Southeast Asia

- *Subtype G*: West and Central Africa

- *Subtypes H, J, and K*: Africa and the Middle East

2011). To date, fewer than 20 cases of group N infection have been identified, and all except one were from Cameroon. Like group M, it is the result of chimpanzee-to-human transmission. The small number of infections resulting from this group and limited genetic diversity suggest that its introduction into humans did not occur until approximately 1963 (Peeters et al., 2014).

GROUP O

Group O ("O" for "outlier") was first discovered in 1990 in two Cameroonians living in Belgium (De Leys, 1990) and is thought to represent only approximately 1% of all HIV transmissions. Recent studies have determined that group O originated by cross-species transmission from western lowland gorillas (*Gorilla gorilla*) instead of chimpanzees (D'arc et al., 2015). Like the other groups, it underwent adaptations to the human hosts. Another study found the prevalence of HIV-1 group O in Cameroon to be approximately 0.6%, indicating that the frequency of group O has been stable during the past few decades. The current distribution of the circulating viral strains still does not allow classification as subtypes (Villabona-Arenas et al., 2015). There are also some reports of dual infections with HIV-1 group M and group O but no recombinant forms in coinfected patients (DeOliveira et al., 2017; Ngoupo et al., 2016). Natural resistance to HIV medications, including integrase inhibitors, has not been identified. This suggests that infection with HIV-1 group O can be adequately treated with antiretroviral therapy in countries in which the virus circulates, but this group remains challenging regarding diagnostic and monitoring strategies.

GROUP P

Group P was discovered in 2009, isolated from a Cameroonian woman living in France (Plantier et al., 2009). Despite subsequent screening for more infections caused by this group, only two cases have been identified. It is uncertain when group P virus entered the human population; it is estimated to be any time from 1845 to 1989 (Peeters et al., 2014). In addition, it remains unclear if the source was a chimpanzee or gorilla. The inability to antagonize tetherin protein (human restriction factor) may explain the limited spread of HIV-1 group P in the human population (Sauter et al., 2011).

HIV-2

In 1986, a morphologically similar but antigenically distinct virus was found to cause AIDS in persons living in West Africa and was termed HIV-2 (Clavel et al., 1986, 1987). It was isolated from healthy commercial sex workers in Senegal (Boswell & Rowland-Jones, 2019). This virus only shares approximately 30% (Clavel et al., 1986, 1987). It was isolated from healthy commercial sex workers in Senegal (Boswell & Rowland-Jones, 2019). This virus only shares approximately 30–40% genetic homology with HIV-1; thus, it is considered a different virus and not another HIV-1 group (Pepin, 2011). It was determined that HIV-2 originated in sooty mangabeys (*Cercocebus atys*) with blood-borne transmission to humans, similar to HIV-1 (Chen et al., 1997; Gao et al., 1992). Molecular clock research has determined that the most common recent ancestor for HIV-2 dates to 1940 and 1945 for the first two groups—A and B, respectively (Pepin, 2011).

HIV-2 had been initially found mainly in West Africa, including Guinea-Bissau, Gambia, Cote d'Ivoire, Mali, Nigeria, Senegal, and Sierra Leone. With widespread immigration, cases have been reported throughout other parts of Africa, India, Europe (especially Portugal), and the United States (Campbell-Yesufu & Gandhi, 2011; Kapoor & Padival, 2022; Peruski et al., 2020). However, more recent data suggest that HIV-2 prevalence may be declining, at least in West Africa, because of lower transmission efficacy, decreasing HIV-2 fitness, and competitive exclusion of HIV-1 (Boswell & Rowland-Jones, 2019; Ceccarelli et al., 2021). Importantly, in parts of West Africa, HIV-1 and HIV-2 mixed or dual infections have been found in about 5%–10% of persons diagnosed (Fumarola et al., 2022). Of the approximately 38 million people across the globe living with HIV, about 2 million are infected with HIV-2, although this likely is an underestimation (Ceccarelli et al., 2021).

Since its initial discovery, phylogenic analysis has identified nine different lineages of HIV-2 (groups A–I) (Fumarola et al., 2022). As with HIV-1, each group represents a different host transfer of SIV from nonprimate species (mangabeys) to humans. However, unlike HIV-1, only types A and B have spread to humans to any significant degree. The other groups only represent individual human cases. Also, unlike HIV-1, only one recombinant form has been described for HIV-2, known as CRF01_AB (Ceccarelli et al., 2021).

Of note clinically, persons infected with HIV-2 often have lower viral loads compared to those with HIV-1 (Boswell & Rowland-Jones, 2019). There is also less genital shedding in semen and cervical secretions. This likely accounts for decreased infectivity. It has also been observed that persons infected with HIV-2 have a longer asymptomatic phase and slower progression to AIDS than those with HIV-1. However, in the absence of treatment with antiretroviral agents, the progressive, albeit slower decline in immune function and resultant disease complications will occur (Boswell & Rowland-Jones, 2019; Kapoor & Padival, 2022; Tzou et al., 2020).

THE FUTURE OF HIV REGIONAL AND GLOBAL GENETIC DIVERSITY

By combining historical, phylogenetic, molecular evolutionary, and epidemiological findings researchers have been able to reconstruct the history of the AIDS pandemic and many unique aspects of HIV-1 and HIV-2. This information will be of continued value for HIV vaccine research and development that considers the genetic diversity of the virus as discussed above. It may also determine how strains of HIV, including CRFs, may continue to spread and colonize new geographic regions and host populations. It also raises numerous questions: Given the fact that there are many other nonhuman primates infected with SIV, should there be concern for future zoonotic infections from cross-species transmissions? Will the growing prevalence of sexually transmitted infections continue to facilitate the dissemination and adaptation of HIV-1 and HIV-2? May there be a therapeutic role for host-restriction factors? Will it be possible to develop a single HIV vaccine that will be effective against all HIV groups and subtypes? For any HIV vaccine, it will remain necessary to have up-to-date knowledge of the genetic diversity of the virus to allow prioritization to develop one or more vaccines to provide the greatest benefit to specific countries and regions of the world.

RECOMMENDED READING

Pepin J. *The origins of AIDS*. Cambridge: Cambridge University Press; 2021.

Quammen D. *The chimp and the river: how AIDS emerged from an African forest*. New York: Norton; 2015.

REFERENCES

Bacque J, Delgado E, Benito S, et al. Identification of CRF66_BF, a new HIV-1 circulating recombinant form of South American origin. *Front Microbiol*. 2021;12:774386.

Bbosa N, Kaleebu P, Ssemwanga D. HIV subtype diversity worldwide. *Curr Opin HIV AIDS*. 2019;14:153–60.

Boswell MT, Rowland-Jones SL. Delayed disease progression in HIV-2: the importance of TRIM5a and the retroviral capsid. *Clin Exp Immunol*. June 2019;196(3):305–317. http://doi:10.1111/cei.13280

Campbell-Yesufu OT, Gandhi RT. Update on human immunodeficiency virus (HIV)-2 infection. *Clin Infect Dis*. 2011;52(6):780–787. https://doi.org/10.1093/cid/ciq248

Ceccarelli G, Giovanetti M, Sagnelli C, et al. Human immunodeficiency virus type 2: the neglected threat. *Pathogens.* 2021;10:1377.

Chen Z, Lucky A, Sodora DL, et al. Human immunodeficiency virus type 2 (HIV-2) seroprevalence and characterization of a distinct subtype within the range of SIV-infected sooty mangabeys. *J Virol.* 1997;71:3953–3960.

Clavel F, Guétard D, Brun-Vézinet F. Isolation of a new human retrovirus from West African patients with AIDS. *Science.* 1986;233(4761):343–346.

Clavel F, Mansinho K, Chamaret S. Human immunodeficiency virus type 2 infection associated with AIDS in West Africa. *N Engl J Med.* 1987;316:1180–1185.

Cohen J. Early AIDS virus may have ridden Africa's rails. *Science.* 2014;346:21–22.

D'arc, M, Ayouba A, Esteban A, et al. Origin of the HIV-1 group O epidemic in western lowland gorillas. *Proc Natl Acad Sci USA.* 2015;112(11):E1343–E1352.

De Leys R. Isolation and partial characterization of an unusual HIV retrovirus from two persons of West-Central Africa origin. *J Virol.* 1990;64:1207–1216.

De Oliveira F, Mourez T, Vessiere A, et al. Multiple HIV-1/M + HIV-1/O dual infections and new HIV-1/MO inter-group recombinant forms detected in Cameroon. *Retrovirology.* 2017;14(1):1. https://doi:10.1186/s12977-016-0324-3

Elangovan R, Jenks M, Yun J, et al. Global and regional estimates for subtype-specific therapeutic and prophylactic HIV-1 vaccines: a modeling study. *Front Microbiol.* 2021;12:690647.

Faria, NR, Rambaut A, Suchard MA, et al. The early spread and epidemic ignition of HIV-1 in human populations. *Science.* 2014;346(6205):56–61.

Faria, NR, Vidal N, Lourencio J, et al. Distinct rates and patterns of spread of the major HIV-1 subtypes in Central and East Africa. *PLoS Pathog.* December 2019;15(12):e1007976.

Fumarola B, Calza S, Renzetti S, et al. Immunological evolution of a cohort of HIV-2 infected patients: peculiarities of an underestimated infection. *Mediterr J Hematol Infect Dis.* 2022;14(1):e2022016.

Gallo RC, Montagnier L. The discovery of HIV as the cause of AIDS. *N Engl J Med.* 2003;349:2282–2285.

Gao F, Bailes E, Robertson DL, et al. Origin of HIV-1 in the chimpanzee *Pan troglodytes troglodytes. Nature.* 1999;397:436–441.

Gao F, Yue L, White AT, et al. Human infection by genetically diverse SIVsm-related HIV-2 in West Africa. *Nature.* 1992;358:495–499.

Gilbert MTP, Rambaut A, Wlasiuk G, et al. The emergence of HIV/AIDS in the Americas and beyond. *Proc Natl Assoc Sci USA.* 2007;104(47):18566–18570.

Gottlieb MS, Schanker HM, Fan PT, et al. *Pneumocystis* pneumonia–Los Angeles. *MMWR.* 1981;30(21):1–3.

Kapoor AK, Padival S. *HIV-2.* Treasure Island, FL: StatPearls Publishing; January 2022.

Keele BF, Jones JH, Terio KA, et al. Increased mortality and AIDS-like immunopathology in wild chimpanzees infected with SIV$_{cpz}$. *Nature.* 2009;460:515–519.

Keele BF, Van Heuverswyn F, Li Y, et al. Chimpanzee reservoirs for pandemic and nonpandemic HIV-1. *Science.* 2006;313(5786):523–526.

Mori M, Ode H, Kubota M, et al. Nanopore sequencing for characterization of HIV-1 recombinant forms. *Microbiol Spectr.* 2022;10(4):e0150722.

Ngoupo PA, Sadeu, MB, Alain S, et al. First evidence of transmission of an HIV-1 M/O intergroup recombinant virus. *AIDS.* 2016;30(1):1–8.

Peeters M, D'Arc M, Delaporta E. The origin and diversity of human retroviruses. *AIDS Rev.* 2014;16(1):23–34.

Pepin J. *The origins of AIDS.* Cambridge: Cambridge University Press; 2021.

Peruski AH, Wesolowski LG, Delaney KP, et al. Trends in HIV-2 diagnosis and use of HIV-1/HIV-2 differentiation test—United States, 2010–2017. *Morb Mortal Wkly Rep.* 2020;69(3):63–66.

Plantier JC, Leoz, M, Dickerson JE. A new immunodeficiency virus derived from gorillas designated group "P." *Nature Med.* 2009;15:871–872.

Sauter D, Hué S, Petit S, et al. HIV-1 group P is unable to antagonize human tetherin by Vpu, Env or Nef. *Retrovirology.* 2011;8:103.

Sharp PM, Hahn BH. Origins of HIV and the AIDS pandemic. *Cold Spring Harbor Perspect Med.* 2011;1:1–22.

Tzou PL, Descamps D, Rhee SY, et al. Expanded spectrum of antiretroviral-selected mutations in human immunodeficiency virus type-2. *J Infect Dis.* 2020;211:1962–1972.

UNAIDS. UNAIDS fact sheet. www.unaids.org. Published 2022. Accessed August 10, 2022.

Villabona-Arenas CJ, Domyeum J, Mouacha F, et al. HIV-1 group O infection in Cameroon from 2006–2013: prevalence, genetic diversity, evolution, and public health challenges. *Infect Gener Evo.* 2015;36:210–216. Epub September 11, 2015.

Worobey M, Gemmel M, Teuwen DE, et al. Direct evidence of extensive diversity of HIV-1 in Kinshasa by 1960. *Nature.* 2008;455(7213):661–664.

Worobey, M., Watts, T., McKay, R. et al. 1970s and "Patient 0" HIV-1 genomes illuminate early HIV/AIDS history in North America. *Nature.* 2016;539:98–101.

Yamaguchi J, Vallari A, McArthur C, et al. Complete genome sequencing of GC-0018a-01 establishes HIV-1 Subtype L. *J Acquir Immune Defic Syndr.* 2020;83(3):319–322.

Zhu T, Korber BT, Nahmias AJ, et al. An African HIV-1 sequence from 1959 and implications for the origin of the epidemic. *Nature.* 1998;391(6667):594–597.

4.

MECHANISMS OF HIV TRANSMISSION

Nancy Aitcheson and Puja H. Nambiar

LEARNING OBJECTIVES

Upon completion of this chapter, the reader should be able to:

- Describe the relative risk of HIV transmission based on various types of sexual activity, occupational exposures, drug use, and perinatal transmission.

- Discuss the significance of viral load quantity and its relationship to transmission risk.

- Explain the impact of co-occurring sexually transmitted diseases on HIV transmission.

INTRODUCTION

With over 25 years of experience demonstrating that antiretroviral therapy (ART) is highly effective in reducing the transmission of HIV, there is now clear evidence that individuals living with HIV with an undetectable viral load cannot transmit HIV sexually.

WHAT'S NEW?

- U = U campaign: undetectable viral load equals untransmittable.

- Clinical trial data demonstrate that treatment of HIV is also prevention.

- It has been shown that occupational transmission is extremely rare in the United States.

KEY POINTS

- The risk of HIV transmission to a receptive partner remains higher than that to an insertive one; however, both carry risk.

- Anything that compromises the integrity of mucous membranes, such as sexually transmitted infections, may increase the risk of HIV transmission.

- Keeping a partner with HIV's viral load persistently suppressed to an undetectable level significantly reduces the risk of transmission to an HIV-negative partner.

- Perinatal transmission is a larger concern in developing countries because of the lack of access to perinatal treatment with antiretroviral drugs.

SEXUAL TRANSMISSION

HIV can be transmitted through infected body fluids—blood, seminal fluid, vaginal fluid, rectal fluid, and breast milk. Sexual contact is the most common mode of HIV transmission worldwide. In the United States, HIV is mainly transmitted by anal or vaginal sex and less commonly by other modes such as oral sex, perinatal transmission (during pregnancy, birth, or breastfeeding), needle injury, blood transfusion, or organ transplants. In 2019, of the 36,801 new HIV diagnoses, 69% were accounted for by men who have sex with men (MSM); 23% to high-risk heterosexual activity; and 7% to people who inject drugs (Centers for Disease Control and Prevention and (CDC), 2022).

Acutely infected individuals, often with very high viral loads, are at the highest risk of transmitting the virus. HIV can be readily found in semen and in vaginal fluid from a person with HIV. There is a strong correlation between high plasma viral load and the amount of virus in genital secretions (Zhang et al., 1998). However, discordance, although rare, can exist between levels of HIV in the plasma and genital secretions. Men with HIV on ART with undetectable virus in plasma can infrequently have detectable HIV in their seminal fluid (Zhang et al., 1998).

Condomless anal sex has the highest risk for HIV transmission, with the receptive partner being at higher risk than the insertive partner. The person receiving the semen with HIV is believed to be at highest risk because of the single cell layer of epithelium lining the rectum, which can be easily disrupted and permit entry of the virus across the rectal mucosa. The insertive partner is also at significant risk because HIV can enter the penis through the urethra, the mucosa of the nonkeratinized portions of foreskin, or through cuts, abrasions, or open sores on the penis. Circumcision has been demonstrated to significantly reduce the risk of HIV acquisition but not of transmission (Dosekun & Fox, 2010).

Worldwide, the AIDS epidemic is being driven by new infections occurring in women of childbearing age. During condomless vaginal intercourse, both partners are at risk of contracting HIV, although there is a higher risk of a woman contracting HIV from a man with HIV than a man contracting HIV from a woman with HIV. HIV can enter the body through the vaginal and cervical mucous membrane linings. HIV-1 replicates and persists in the vaginal epithelial dendritic cells (Pena-Cruz et al., 2018), which provides a readily understandable mechanism for transmission via the vaginal mucosa. Although the risk of men acquiring HIV through heterosexual vaginal or anal intercourse is lower, HIV is abundantly present in vaginal secretions, and the anatomic sites of potential infection in the penis are the same as those described previously for anal intercourse (Dosekun & Fox, 2010).

Sexually transmitted infections (STIs) have a significant role in HIV transmission. Genital ulcer disease (i.e., syphilis, chancroid, and herpes simplex infections) and diseases causing mucosal inflammation (i.e., gonorrhea and chlamydia) have been shown to increase HIV transmission threefold. Trichomonas has been shown to increase risk of HIV acquisition among women by 50% (McClelland et al., 2007). This increase is most likely due to both heightened infectivity and susceptibility. Open ulcers aid HIV entry, and inflammation recruits increased numbers of CD4 $^{+}$ cells that serve as targets for HIV. Early diagnosis of STIs has the potential to significantly reduce HIV incidence in general, especially for high-risk populations. Another potential factor is the use of hormonal contraception in women because it may thin the vaginal mucosa, making it more susceptible to tears and trauma. However, large randomized clinical trials have provided conflicting results, and currently, it is not clear whether hormonal contraception has any effect on HIV transmission.

Limiting viral replication in genital secretions is a logical approach to preventing HIV acquisition. Data from the pivotal HPTN 052 study showed dramatic reductions in HIV transmissions in serodifferent couples in which the seropositive partner was virally suppressed with ART along with monthly HIV prevention counseling and regular STI testing and treatment. This unique clinical trial showed that men and women living with HIV had a 96% reduced risk of transmitting the virus to their original linked, HIV-negative sexual partners through early initiation of ART (Cohen et al., 2011). Longer term follow-up of the study showed a sustained, overall, 93% reduction of HIV transmission among linked couples when the HIV-positive partner was taking ART and had a suppressed viral load (Cohen et al., 2016). The results of this historic study provided the initial data to support treatment as prevention (TasP).

Taking evaluation of TasP even further, the prospective, observational PARTNER-1 (Partners of People on ART: A New Evaluation of the Risks) study, although of limited follow-up time (median = 1.3 years per couple) showed no linked HIV transmissions with condomless anal and vaginal sex among serodifferent heterosexual and homosexual couples in which the HIV-positive partner was virologically suppressed on ART (Rodger et al., 2016). The subsequent PARTNER-2 study reported no phylogenetically linked HIV transmission in 415 couple-years of follow-up in male homosexual couples reporting condomless anal intercourse, in which the HIV-positive partners were virally suppressed and HIV-negative partners reported no use of pre-exposure prophylaxis

(Rodger, 2019). An international, prospective, observation cohort study (The Opposites Attract study) examining the association between ART and viral load and HIV transmission in serodifferent male homosexual couples in Australia, Brazil, and Thailand also reported similar results (Bavinton et al., 2018). Together, the PARTNER and Opposites Attract studies have reported no linked transmissions despite nearly 35,000 acts of condomless anal intercourse in HIV serodifferent male homosexual couples not using daily pre-exposure prophylaxis.

Developing novel approaches for the rapid detection and diagnosis of HIV infection and increasing ART coverage are the next important steps in realizing the potential public benefits of these discoveries.

TRANSMISSION IN THE HEALTHCARE SETTING

All persons working in a healthcare setting with potential for exposure to infected blood and body fluids and contaminated medical equipment or surroundings are at risk for HIV acquisition. The risk of occupational HIV transmission is low and occurs when a healthcare worker has a percutaneous injury or contact of mucous membrane or nonintact skin with HIV-infected blood, tissue, or other body fluids. The risk of HIV transmission following percutaneous and mucous membrane exposure to HIV-infected blood has been roughly estimated to be 0.2% and 0.09%, respectively. There is virtually no risk of HIV transmission via contact of HIV-infected body fluids with intact skin (CDC, 2020).

In addition to blood, other bodily fluids, such as cerebrospinal, synovial, amniotic, pleural, peritoneal, and pericardial fluids, are considered potentially infectious. The risk from these fluids remains unknown, owing to the lack of epidemiologic studies in healthcare settings to assess the risk of HIV transmission to healthcare workers from exposure to these fluids. Although semen and cervicovaginal secretions have been shown to contain virus-infected cells, they have not been implicated in occupational transmission from patients to HCP. Feces, urine, nasal secretions, sweat, tears, sputum, vomitus, and saliva are not considered potentially infectious unless visibly bloody (Bell, 1997). The major factors influencing the possibility of transmission include type and severity of exposure and magnitude of viremia. Greater risk of transmission was seen with exposure to large quantity of blood from infected source person, deep injuries, and hollow bore needle injuries. Higher titers of HIV in blood (inoculum)—as seen in persons with acute HIV infection or uncontrolled HIV—increase the transmission risk (CDC, 2020).

Although not common, there have been several documented transmission events from healthcare workers to patients during routine medical or dental care, mostly likely caused by poor adherence to infection control procedures. Further, although increasingly less frequent, there have been documented cases of patient-to-patient transmission, most of which involved the use of contaminated instruments or syringes. Use of universal precautions during all healthcare procedures and encounters cannot be overemphasized. Since 1991, CDC has investigated all cases of HIV infection reported as acquired occupationally by healthcare workers. Until now, the National HIV surveillance system recorded 58 confirmed and 150 possible cases of occupationally acquired HIV transmission among HCPs. Among the 58 confirmed cases, the primary route of exposure resulting in infection was percutaneous puncture or cut (49/58 cases), followed by mucocutaneous exposure (5), both percutaneous and mucocutaneous exposure (2), and unknown (2). The majority were in nurses (41%), followed by laboratory clinicians (35%), physicians (10%), and other health-related workers (14%). Since 1999, there has been only one case of occupationally acquired HIV (a laboratory technician who sustained a needle puncture while working with high-titer HIV cultures in 2008) (Joyce et al., 2015).

For cases in which risk of HIV transmission can be determined, specific guidelines exist for the use of antivirals for postexposure prophylaxis (PEP). Occupational exposures require urgent medical evaluation and initiation of PEP, ideally within 2–6 hours after exposure. Prospective, well-controlled clinical data supporting PEP do not exist. By extrapolation from well-controlled animal model studies, it has been estimated that PEP reduces the risk of infection by approximately 80%, and that it becomes less effective as time lapses (>72 hours). The preferred initial PEP regimen (three or more antiretroviral drugs) is tenofovir disoproxil fumarate/emtricitabine plus raltegravir (TDF/FTC + RAL) or dolutegravir (TDF/FTC + DTG) because of its ease of administration, proven potency against established HIV, and good tolerability. It is recommended to start PEP with this regimen following exposure to a source patient who is known to have HIV or for whom there is a reasonably high suspicion of having HIV. If the source person is determined to be HIV-negative, PEP can be discontinued. The recommended duration of PEP is 28 days.

PEP is also recommended for nonoccupational exposures, referred to as n-PEP. CDC recommendations indicate that n-PEP should be used when the source person is known to be living with HIV, and case-by-case determinations should be in made in instances when the source person has an unknown HIV status. CDC also recommends evaluating patients requiring n-PEP for transition to pre-exposure prophylaxis (PrEP) in the future (CDC, 2016). For both occupational and nonoccupational indications for PEP, administration should not be delayed for HIV test results but rather should be started empirically and discontinued later if tests are negative (Kuhar et al., 2013).

TRANSMISSION THROUGH THE USE OF INJECTION DRUGS

Persons who inject drugs (PWID) are at high risk of acquiring HIV if they use and share needles, syringes, or other drug injection equipment previously used by someone with HIV. Sharing syringes is the second riskiest behavior for acquiring HIV. HIV survival in syringes was associated with volume of blood remaining and the temperature of storage. Viable HIV was isolated from 50% of all syringes stored at 4 °C for up to 42 days (Abdala et al., 2000).

In 2019, PWID accounted for 7% of new HIV diagnosis. In all regions of the United States, the largest percentage of diagnosed HIV infections among PWID was among White persons, followed by African American and Hispanic persons. The prevalence of HIV remains highest among Black/African Americans (46%). Among women, injection-drug use accounts for more than 20% of all infections.

The high-risk practices of sharing needles and syringes, engaging in risky sexual behavior, drug use, and socioeconomic factors limiting access to HIV prevention and care as well as to substance abuse programs are some of the prevention challenges currently identified by the CDC.

The CDC is pursuing a prevention approach by distributing funds to health departments for surveillance and by supporting intervention programs such as community PROMISE (Peers Reaching Out and Modeling Intervention Strategies), syringe service programs that provide access to sterile syringes and needles and thereby reduce transmission of HIV, hepatitis C, hepatitis B virus, and other blood-borne infections, and PrEP and PEP programs, to name a few. Providing comprehensive prevention services and medical and/or addiction treatment referrals for PWID can help increase access to healthcare and substance use treatment (CDC, 2008).

Individuals who use recreational crystal methamphetamine are at increased risk of contracting HIV. However, there is no clear evidence that methamphetamine itself increases HIV transmission or acquisition. Amphetamine users, in general, report several behaviors known to be risk factors for HIV transmission, including greater numbers of sex partners, reduced use of condoms, exchange of sex for money or drugs, sex with PWID, and/or a history of STIs. Further, they are more likely to have unprotected anal or vaginal sex with partners of unknown HIV status. Individuals using other mind-altering drugs, such as alcohol, can also be at increased risk for HIV infection (CDC, 2021).

PERINATAL TRANSMISSION

Perinatal transmission of HIV is a unique setting as the infant exposure to HIV occurs despite the presence of HIV specific antibodies that were passively transferred from the mother while in utero. Several factors have been identified to influence the risk of perinatal HIV infection. High maternal viral load (in blood and genital tract) at the time of delivery, lower $CD4^+$ T-cell count, and advanced disease have been associated with higher risk of perinatal HIV (Yah & Tambo, 2019).

Universal perinatal HIV counseling and testing, ART for all pregnant women with HIV, scheduled cesarean delivery for women with viremia (HIV RNA >1,000 copies/mL), infant ART, and avoidance of breastfeeding have contributed to the remarkable decline in annual rate of perinatal transmission of HIV to less than 1% in the United States. In the absence of any intervention, transmission rates can vary from 15%–45%, and despite scaled-up prevention programs, perinatal HIV infection continues to escalate in regions of Sub-Saharan Africa (Yah & Tambo, 2019). The most common barriers and challenges were nondisclosure of HIV status to partners and family, late initiation of ART treatment or adherence, limited STI screening, long clinic wait times, and infant feeding methods.

Pediatric HIV infection is associated with an accelerated course of disease and high mortality. In the absence of ART, only 65% of children with HIV survive until their first birthday, and less than half will reach 2 years of age. In the absence of breastfeeding and with no ART, the risk of perinatal transmission is estimated at 25%. Up to 20% more children can acquire HIV through breastfeeding. Despite the presence of innate factors in human breast milk that display strong HIV inhibitory activity in vitro, up to 44% of HIV infections in children can be attributed to breastfeeding. The risk of acquiring HIV after a single day of breastfeeding is extremely low: 0.00028 per day of breastfeeding (Richardson et al, 2003). However, after ingesting liters of breast milk over a span of several months to years (~250 liters per year), 5%–20% of infants born to women living with HIV will eventually become infected with HIV in the absence of any preventive measures (WHO, UNICEF, UNFPA, and UNAIDS, 2008). Elevated levels of HIV particles (cell-free virus) and HIV-infected cells (cell-associated virus) in the breast milk of women living with HIV are associated with an increased risk of HIV transmission during breastfeeding. Although it has been reported that a tenfold increase in cell-free or cell-associated HIV in breast milk is associated with a threefold increase in transmission, it is still unclear whether cell-free virus and/or cell-associated virus are transmitted during breastfeeding. Further, it is not known if the frequency of cell-free and cell-associated HIV transmission varies at different stages of lactation (i.e., colostrum, early breast milk, and mature breast milk).

Recent results from the PROMISE study, a randomized control trial of infant nevirapine prophylaxis versus maternal ART comprised of 2,431 mother-child pairs, showed both strategies were safe and associated very low HIV transmission to infants and high rates of infant HIV-free survival (Flynn et al., 2018). Given continued interest on the part of women living with HIV in breastfeeding their infants, further study of HIV transmission through breastfeeding among mothers with viral suppression is warranted.

REFERENCES

Abdala N, Reyes R, Carney JM, Heimer R. Survival of HIV-1 in syringes: effects of temperature during storage external icon. *Subst Use Misuse.* 2000;35(10):1369–1383.

Bavinton BR, Pinto AN, Phanuphak N, et al. Viral suppression and HIV transmission in serodiscordant male couples: an international, prospective, observational, cohort study. *Lancet HIV.* 2018;5(8):e438–e447. http://doi:10.1016/S2352-3018(18)30132-2

Bell DM. Occupational risk of human immunodeficiency virus infection in healthcare workers: an overview. *Am J Med.* 1997;102(5B):9–15.

Centers for Disease Control and Prevention (CDC). HIV and injection drug use. HIV transmission. cdc.gov. https://www.cdc.gov/hiv/bas ics/hiv-transmission/injection-drug-use.html. Published April 2021. Accessed August 16, 2022.

CDC. HIV surveillance report, 2019 (updated), vol. 31. cdc.gov. http://www.cdc.gov/hiv/library/reports/hiv-surveillance.html. Published May 2022. Accessed July 2022.

CDC. HIV transmission. cdc.gov. https://www.cdc.gov/hiv/basics/transmission.html. Published 2020. Accessed August 2022.

CDC. Recommendations for post-exposure interventions to prevent infection with hepatitis B virus, hepatitis C virus, or human immunodeficiency virus, and tetanus in persons wounded during bombings and other mass-casualty events—United States, 2008. *MMWR.* August 1, 2008;57(RR06):1–19.

CDC. Updated guidelines for antiretroviral postexposure prophylaxis after sexual, injection drug use, or other nonoccupational exposure to HIV—United States, 2016. https:// www.cdc.gov/hiv/pdf/progr amresources/cdc-hiv-npep-guidelines.pdf. Published 2016. Accessed August 16, 2022.

Cohen MS, Chen YQ, McCauley M, et al. Prevention of HIV-1 infection with early antiretroviral therapy. *N Engl J Med.* 2011;365:493–505.

Cohen MS, Chen YQ, McCauley M, et al. Final results of the HPTN 052 randomized controlled trial: antiretroviral therapy prevents HIV transmission. *N Engl J Med.* 2016;375:830–839.

Dosekun O, Fox J. An overview of the relative risks of different sexual behaviours on HIV transmission. *Curr Opin HIV AIDS.* 2010;5:291–297.

Flynn PM, Taha TE, Cababasay M, et al. Association of maternal viral load and CD4 count with perinatal HIV-1 transmission risk during breastfeeding in the PROMISE postpartum component. *J Acquir Immune Defic Syndr.* 2021;88(2):206–213. https://www.ncbi.nlm.nih.gov/pubmed/34108383

Joyce MP, Kuhar D, Brooks JT. Occupationally acquired HIV infection by healthcare personnel—United States, 1985–2013. *MMWR.* January 9, 2015;63(53):1245–1246

Kuhar DT, Henderson DK, Struble KA, et al. Updated US Public Health Service guidelines for the management of occupational exposures to human immunodeficiency virus and recommendations for postexposure prophylaxis. *Infect Control Hosp Epidemiol.* November 2013;34(11):1238.

McClelland RS, Sangare L, Hassan WM, et al. Infection with Trichomonas vaginalis increases the risk of HIV-1 acquisition. *J Infect Dis.* 2007;195(5):698–702.

Pena-Cruz V, Agosto, Akiyama et al. HIV replicates and persists in vaginal epithelial dendritic cells. *J Clin Invest.* 2018;128(8):3439–3444. https://doi.org/10.1172/JCI98943

Richardson BA, John-Stewart GC, Hughes JP, et al. Breast-milk infectivity in human immunodeficiency virus type 1-infected mothers. *J Infect Dis.* 2003;187:736–740.

Rodger AJ, Cambiano V, Bruun T, et al. Risk of HIV transmission through condomless sex in serodifferent gay couples with the HIV-positive partner taking suppressive antiretroviral therapy (PARTNER): final results of a multicentre, prospective, observational study. *Lancet.* 2019;393(10189):2428–2438.

Rodger AJ, Cambiano V, Bruun T, et al. Sexual activity without condoms and risk of HIV transmission in serodifferent couples when the HIV-positive partner is using suppressive antiretroviral therapy. *JAMA.* 2016;316(2):171–181. http://doi:10.1001/jama.2016.5148

WHO, UNICEF, UNFPA, and UNAIDS. *HIV transmission through breastfeeding: a review of available evidence: 2007 update.* Geneva: World Health Organization; 2008.

Yah CS, Tambo E. Why is mother to child transmission (MTCT) of HIV a continual threat to new-borns in sub-Saharan Africa (SSA). *J Infect Public Health.* 2019;12(2):213–223. http://doi:10.1016/j.jiph.2018.10.008

Zhang H, Dornadula G, Beumont M, et al. Human immunodeficiency virus type 1 in the semen of men receiving highly active antiretroviral therapy. *N Engl J Med.* December 17, 1998;339(25):1803–1809.

5.

TRANSMISSION PREVENTION STRATEGIES

Carolyn Chu, Katrina Baumgartner, and Christopher M. Bositis

INTRODUCTION

HIV prevention encompasses a vast range of approaches and tools across biomedical, behavioral, social, and structural dimensions. Multiple highly efficacious biomedical options for HIV pre-exposure prophylaxis (PrEP) are now available, including long-acting therapies. HIV "treatment as prevention" (TasP) through rapid antiretroviral therapy (ART) initiation and "U = U" remains impactful. HIV-associated behavioral and social factors continue to be a focus of inquiry, particularly for communities with limited access to and/or utilization of biomedically oriented interventions. Implementation science highlights opportunities to improve uptake and application of evidence-based interventions into "real-world" practices across varied settings. Peer-based service delivery may be especially critical for some communities, such as people who inject drugs, Black and Latinx people, transgender people, and sex workers.

BEHAVIORAL INTERVENTIONS

LEARNING OBJECTIVE

- Describe behavioral and structural factors, as well as biomedical opportunities, surrounding HIV prevention.

- Identify considerations for unique circumstances and populations.

WHAT'S NEW?

Behavioral interventions targeting the individual, dyadic, and organizational levels continue to be refined to optimize not only their acceptability and feasibility, but also their effectiveness in preventing HIV. Digital health, which encompasses both online and mobile technologies, remains a highly active area of interest and investigation—these platforms are able to deliver general, as well as tailored, prevention messaging and promote HIV and sexually transmitted infection (STI) testing and support engagement in care.

KEY POINTS

- Providers should elicit comprehensive sociobehavioral histories in a person-centered, respectful manner to identify the most acceptable and effective HIV prevention opportunities for an individual.

Behavioral interventions to prevent HIV transmission include general informational campaigns about sexual health, including information on condom education, substance use, and specific risk-reduction techniques as well as individually tailored messages. Some gay, bisexual, and other men who have sex with men (MSM) adopt "sero-adaptive" strategies to utilize knowledge of an individual's HIV and virologic suppression status (self-reported or confirmed) when identifying potential sex partners or engaging in specific practices (Malekinejad et al., 2022; Mann et al., 2022). "PrEP-sorting" has also emerged whereby partners are selected based on current PrEP use, although less is currently known about how PrEP is discussed within broader conversations of HIV/STIs among partners and networks (Maloney, 2022).

Adolescents, younger adults, and cis-gender women remain a focus of HIV prevention efforts globally because of multiple socioeconomic and cultural factors (e.g., trafficking and violence, sexual coercion, and economic inequalities), as well as physiologic considerations including in the perinatal, postpartum, and postmenopausal periods that lead to elevated HIV risk (Bhushan et al., 2022; Eastment & McClelland, 2018; Thompson et al., 2018). Behavioral interventions targeted to younger individuals—especially younger cis-gender women and adolescents—have involved delaying sexual debut, promoting or incentivizing condom use, ensuring routine HIV and STI screening, increasing HIV-related knowledge and self-esteem and self-efficacy, addressing unmet mental health needs, preventing substance use, and reducing partner concurrency and/or changes (Chang et al., 2020; Fu et al., 2022; Hoseck & Pettifor, 2019; Opara et al., 2022; Wilkins et al, 2022). Interventions developed for youth and women have utilized group-based knowledge transfer and skills training to support healthy decision-making, sexual negotiation capacity development, relationship building including through couples-based approaches, and overall wellness promotion.

Transgender communities continue to experience some of the highest rates of HIV infection globally, and many individuals face social and legal exclusion and marginalization, sexual and physical violence, economic susceptibility, high levels of stigma and bias, and transphobia. Unsafe injection practices for gender-affirming therapy administration and soft-tissue fillers, as well as substance use and transactional or exchange sex, may also increase risk (Poteat et al., 2017; Reback & Fletcher, 2014). Despite such disproportionate impact, HIV testing rates and PrEP use among transgender people remain low (Malone et al., 2021; Sevelius et al., 2020). Recent studies affirm that factors such as having a usual, trusted health care source and/or provider who offers a welcoming, comfortable space to discuss gender-related health issues, as well as availability of peer support and navigation, may be associated with improved HIV prevention outcomes such as engagement in care and adherence (Ayala et al., 2021; Lee et al., 2022).

Because of ongoing sustainability and dissemination and implementation challenges related to in-person programming, as well as the near-ubiquitous availability of mobile devices with internet access, web-based and mobile health technologies continue to receive much attention. These interventions appear to be particularly acceptable to younger audiences and MSM, and many incorporate design flexibility such that dynamic messages of varying content and structure can be deployed. Some can also be integrated with external social media platforms and/or online peer education and navigation services. Digital health interventions have demonstrated efficacy with regard to delaying sexual initiation and reducing other HIV-associated risk behaviors, increasing HIV/STI knowledge and condom self-efficacy, and increasing HIV testing and PrEP awareness (Biello et al., 2022; Cruess et al., 2018; Melendez-Torres, 2022; Schnall et al., 2018; Veronese, 2020). Importantly, as noted in one exploratory analysis, "technology can be used to engage users in novel and innovative ways that are less dependent on existing institutional structures and may use democratizing approaches to promote community engagement and ownership" (Jones et al., 2022).

Regular HIV and STI screening remains an important cornerstone of prevention. Among other things, universal testing aims to: (1) ensure that people with HIV (PWH) know their status, (2) identify early HIV infections reliably, and (3) assist with timely linkage to HIV care and treatment. The Centers for Disease Control and Prevention (CDC) encourages consideration of HIV self-testing, since some individuals may prefer testing be done outside of traditional, clinic-based channels (CDC, 2021a). The COVID-19 pandemic may have also helped accelerate and expand home-based HIV/STI testing: for example, opt-out HIV screening coupled with SARS-CoV-2 testing led to increased detection of acute HIV for some programs (Spears et al., 2022).

RECOMMENDED READING

Ayala G, Sprague L, van der Merwe LL, et al. Peer- and community-led responses to HIV: a scoping review. *PLoS One*. 2021;16(12): e0260555.

Gamarel KE, King WM, Operario D. Behavioral and social interventions to promote optimal HIV prevention and care continua outcomes in the United States. *Curr Opin HIV AIDS*. 2022;17(2):65–71.

Girometti N, Delpech V, McCormack S, et al. The success of HIV combination prevention: the Dean Street model. *HIV Med*. 2021;22(10):892–897.

STRUCTURAL AND SYSTEMS-LEVEL INTERVENTIONS

LEARNING OBJECTIVES

- Briefly describe safety of the US blood supply and transfusion medicine considerations related to early ART initiation for PWH as well as PrEP use among donors.

- Discuss structural and systems-level considerations that influence HIV transmission, including substance use–related intervention opportunities.

WHAT'S NEW?

Overdose deaths and HIV infection rates among people who inject drugs (PWID) remain high, especially in regions where people are increasingly reliant on an unregulated drug supply and have limited access to effective harm reduction interventions and substance use disorder treatment. HIV outbreaks continue to occur among PWID networks and have largely affected regions experiencing high poverty, unemployment, and homelessness. Effective medications for opioid use disorder are available although underutilized; treatment of stimulant use disorder remains challenging given limited evidence for pharmacotherapy options and poor availability of psychosocial interventions such as contingency management and cognitive behavioral therapy services.

KEY POINTS

- The US blood supply remains extremely safe, and policy changes regarding donor deferral practices among MSM have not been associated with increased incidence of HIV seropositivity among donors.

- Expanded harm reduction services, increased access to (and use of) medications for substance use disorder treatment, integrated substance use and HIV care programs, and large-scale public health and policy efforts are critical for addressing substance use associated HIV transmission.

SAFETY OF THE US BLOOD SUPPLY

With incorporation of nucleic acid testing, the risk of transfusion-transmitted HIV is now approximately one infectious unit per 2–10 million transfusions in the United States and other developed countries (Busch, 2022). Ongoing research has supported a progressive reduction in donor deferral periods such that the FDA revised its guidance for MSM donors in 2015, changing its recommendations from indefinite deferral to a 12-month deferral since last sex. In April 2020, the FDA further reduced the recommended deferral period to 3 months as part of a broader response to the COVID-19 pandemic (FDA, 2020). Early ART initiation and PrEP both continue to pose potential challenges for transfusion-related screening and testing practices, since ART can alter biomarkers of HIV infection progression and may (in rare cases) result in antibody "sero-reversion"; additionally, PrEP use—particularly with long-acting injectable agents—may lead to ambiguous testing results and/or delayed HIV diagnosis among potential donors (Donnell et al., 2017; Lee et al., 2020; Marzinke et al., 2021).

SUBSTANCE USE, HARM REDUCTION, AND HIV PREVENTION

Injection-drug use has long been linked to HIV transmission, with risk estimates ranging from 0.63% to 2.4% per act (Baggaley et al., 2006). Although HIV risk has been demonstrated most clearly for intravenous drug use, any parenteral exposure—including subcutaneous and intramuscular use—to virus-containing material can potentially lead to transmission. Additionally, alcohol, stimulant, and sedative or hypnotic use have all been associated with HIV transmission by affecting decision-making and negotiation around condom use and other sex practices (Berry & Johnson, 2018; Hoenigl et al., 2016; Ickowicz et al., 2015). *Chemsex* is a term that has been used to describe the planned use of one or more psychoactive substances such as methamphetamine and GHB to enhance sexual experiences among gay, bisexual, and other MSM communities. Rather than viewing participation in chemsex as a binary (either/or) phenomenon, an integrated harm reduction framework can help identify opportunities for behavioral, social, as well as biomedical, HIV prevention interventions along a continuum (Strong et al., 2022). Although numerous pharmacotherapy options have been evaluated for methamphetamine use, evidence remains modest regarding medication efficacy, and, therefore, structured behavioral interventions remain the mainstay of treatment for methamphetamine use disorders.

The intersections between substance use, overdose, and HIV encompass a broad array of micro- and macroenvironmental and structural factors, and, therefore, a cross-sector, coordinated response should include: (1) increased access to naloxone and harm reduction services including syringe exchange and supervised consumption spaces; (2) improved recognition of substance use and widespread HIV/viral hepatitis education and screening for all people who use drugs (including through peer-based programs); (3) "low-threshold" provision of medications for substance use disorder treatment and HIV prevention (e.g., PrEP and PEP); (4) flexible, integrated, trauma-informed care that upholds autonomy and supports health promotion; and (5) policy and structural changes to overcome provider-based stigma, as well as ongoing disparities in housing and economic opportunity, racist policing practices, mass incarceration of BIPOC communities, and prohibitive legislation such as the criminalization of HIV and drug possession and use (Bazzi et al., 2018; Biello et al., 2018; Broz et al., 2021; Perlman & Jordan, 2018; Rich et al., 2018; Touesnard et al., 2022).

ADDITIONAL STRUCTURAL AND SYSTEMS-LEVEL CONSIDERATIONS

Several other structural factors influence HIV risk and delivery of evidence-based HIV prevention services: these represent an extensive landscape of physical, sociocultural, organizational, economic, and policy-related dynamics. Physical factors such as proximity to—and convenience of—HIV services can affect motivation to seek care and testing. Stigma, structural racism, sexism and gender-based violence, and intersectional discrimination often influence decision-making related to accessing health care systems, screening/testing and engagement, disclosure to others (including health care providers), sexual and substance use/mental health, and PrEP uptake (Bowleg et al., 2022; Decker et al., 2022; Harrison et al., 2022). Care settings that discreetly offer co-located services and expanded access can help facilitate engagement in care; emergency department-based HIV testing and/or PrEP initiatives may also be a promising strategy in some communities (Carlisle et al., 2022; Simmons, 2022). Inadequate housing, racial residential segregation, and inequitable urban housing policies are also significant barriers to care and increase HIV transmission risk (Aidala et al., 2015; Brawner et al., 2022; Garcia et al., 2015).

Economic factors are closely intertwined with HIV: resource-limited settings are disproportionately affected by high rates of HIV, often related to deindustrialization and unemployment. These disparities involve inequalities in poverty, gender, race, and education; economic instability; labor migration patterns; access to health resources and health literacy; local health care system infrastructure and funding; unmet substance use and mental health needs; drug policies and enforcement; and other factors (Zanakis et al., 2007). Despite efforts to expand testing and prevention broadly across the United States, HIV continues to disproportionately affect communities of color: the COVID-19 pandemic further exacerbated preexisting inequities in testing, and diagnosis rates remain higher among individuals in lower socioeconomic positions including women (DiNenno et al., 2022; Rimmler et al., 2022). Cash transfer programs, although not universally available, have been associated with lower probability of STIs and higher probability of HIV testing among cis-gender women, and reduction in new HIV infections (Richterman & Thirumurthy, 2022; Stoner et al., 2021). Of note, health insurance status is a major determinant affecting access to primary care and preventive services. Lack of uniform access to health care remains a fundamental driver of health inequity and is a critical barrier to ending the US HIV epidemic (Del Rio, 2020).

The epidemiology of incarceration closely reflects that of HIV, and the complex interplay of racial and economic disparities in arrest and incarceration rates, substance use, and HIV is well described (Csete et al., 2016; Iroh et al., 2015; Wirtz et al., 2018). Incarcerated and recently released individuals generally have low rates of HIV awareness, testing, and engagement in care. Incarceration itself could be an important contributor to HIV transmission among networks of PWID, and the period following release represents a unique and potentially high-impact opportunity for reducing HIV transmission and adverse health outcomes including fatal overdose (Khan et al., 2019; Stone et al., 2018).There is considerable variation in HIV prevention, testing, and treatment services across correctional health programs (Valera et al.,

2017). Interventions to address such challenges have included formation of "local change teams," telemedicine and tele-consultation, and transitions programs or care navigators to facilitate engagement in postrelease care (Belenko et al., 2017; Dong et al., 2017).

TREATMENT AS PREVENTION: "UNDETECTABLE = UNTRANSMITTABLE"

In 2016, the Prevention Access Campaign launched the "Undetectable = Untransmittable (U = U)" health equity and antistigma initiative, based on several multinational trials (e.g., HPTN 052, PARTNER, and PARTNER2, Opposites Attract) demonstrating no cases of linked sexual transmission of HIV when the seropositive partner was durably suppressed on ART. Prior to 2016, the paradigm of HIV "treatment as prevention" had been accepted such that most clinical guidelines had removed specific $CD4^+$ thresholds for ART initiation, signaling a universal movement favoring early ART for all PWH. In September 2017, the CDC officially endorsed the campaign, and in 2022 at the International AIDS Conference, the United States federal government joined Canada in formally supporting the "U = U" message.

RECOMMENDED READING

Bowleg L, Malekzadeh AN, Mbaba M, Boone CA. Ending the HIV epidemic for all, not just some: structural racism as a fundamental but overlooked social-structural determinant of the US HIV epidemic. *Curr Opin HIV AIDS*. 2022;17(2):40–45.
Perlman D, Jordan AE. The syndemic of opioid misuse, overdose, HCV, and HIV: structural-level causes and interventions. *Current HIV/AIDS Reports*. 2018;15:96–112.

BIOMEDICAL INTERVENTIONS FOR HIV TRANSMISSION PREVENTION

LEARNING OBJECTIVES

- Describe the recommended baseline and follow-up assessments for oral and injectable PrEP, occupational postexposure prophylaxis (oPEP), and nonoccupational postexposure prophylaxis (nPEP), as well as common side-effects, toxicities, and other potential risks associated with their use.

- Discuss current inequities in PrEP use in the United States, and review potential strategies to close these gaps.

- Describe new or investigational biomedical interventions for HIV prevention and how they complement existing interventions.

WHAT'S NEW

- Injectable cabotegravir (CAB) has been FDA approved for PrEP use in adults and adolescents weighing at least 35 kg to reduce the risk of sexually acquired HIV-1 infection.

- The CDC has updated its PrEP guidelines to include injectable CAB and "on-demand" dosing of emtricitabine/tenofovir disoproxil (F/TDF); other key updates include the recommendation to discuss PrEP with all sexually active adults and adolescents, and offer it to anyone who requests it (CDC, 2021b).

KEY POINTS

- Both oral and injectable PrEP are safe and highly effective for preventing HIV acquisition.

- Despite its effectiveness, significant disparities in PrEP use based on race, gender, geography, and risk behavior exist, threatening to exacerbate existing and similar disparities in HIV incidence.

- Postexposure prophylaxis, when taken within 72 hours of exposure, is also safe and effective for preventing HIV; PEP may be considered as a bridge to PrEP in individuals with anticipated ongoing exposures.

- Continued development and evaluation of novel biomedical prevention approaches are key to an effective, sustainable reduction in the number of new HIV transmissions globally.

INTRODUCTION

Biomedical interventions used to prevent HIV transmission and acquisition among individuals at risk include PrEP, oPEP, and nPEP; STI screening and treatment; voluntary medical male circumcision; prevention of perinatal HIV transmission; and TasP.

PRE-EXPOSUREPREEXPOSURE PROPHYLAXIS

PrEP refers to the use of antiretroviral medications before HIV exposure as a means to prevent HIV acquisition in people who are HIV-negative.

DATA: CLINICAL TRIALS AND REAL-WORLD EFFECTIVENESS

The FDA first approved daily use of fixed-dose FTC 200 mg/TDF 300 mg to reduce the risk of HIV through sexual acquisition in 2012. This was based on multiple studies showing that, when taken consistently, TDF-based PrEP is highly effective at reducing the rate of HIV acquisition in those at highest risk, including MSM, transgender women who have sex with men, persons who inject drugs, and heterosexual women and men (Table 5.1).

"Real-world" data have been encouraging, with the CDC estimating an overall efficacy for preventing

TRIAL	N, STUDY POPULATION; SETTING	INTERVENTION	EFFECT–HAZARD RATIO [ESTIMATED REDUCTION IN HIV ACQUISITION] (95% CI)	REFERENCE
iPrEX	2499 MSM, transgender women; United States, South America, Thailand, South Africa	TDF/FTC	0.56 [44%] (15–63)	Grant, 2010
Partners PrEP	4,747 heterosexual women and men; Kenya and Uganda	TDF TDF/FTC	0.33 [67%] (0.19–0.56) 0.25 [75%] (0.13–0.45)	Baeten, 2012
TDF 2	1,219 heterosexual women and men; Botswana	TDF/FTC	0.38 [62%] (0.22–0.83)	Thigpen, 2012
Thai IDU	2,413 PWIDs; Thailand	TDF	0.51 [49%] (0.1–0.72)	Choopanya, 2013
FemPrEP	2,120 heterosexual women; Africa	TDF/FTC	0.94 [6%] (0.59–1.52)	Van Damme, 2012
VOICE	5,029 heterosexual women; Africa	TDF TDF/FTC	1.49 [-49%] (0.97–2.29) 1.04 [-4%] (0.73–1.49)	Marrazzo, 2015
DISCOVER	2,694 (F/TAF); 2,693 (F/TDF) MSM, TGW; Europe and North America	F/TAF v F/TDF	0.47 [-53%] (0.19–1.15)	Ogbuagu, 2022
HPTN 083	2,282 (LA-CAB), 2,284 (F/TDF) MSM, TGW; United States, Latin America, Asia, Africa	LA-CAB v daily F/TDF	0.34 (0.18–0.62)	Landovitz, 2020
HPTN 084	1,613 (LA-CAB), 1,610 (F/TDF) cis-gender WSM; Africa	LA-CAB v daily F/TDF	0.11 (0.04–0.32)	Delany-Moretlwe S, 2022
MTN020/ASPIRE	2,629 Cis-gender WSM; Africa	DPV ring	0.73 (0.54–1.0)	Baeten, 2016

sexual transmission of 99% with "optimal or consistent use" (CDC, 2022a), based in part on data from the US Kaiser Cohort and UK PROUD studies which showed substantial reductions in incident HIV infections among PrEP users compared to historical or actual controls (McCormack et al., 2015; Volk et al., 2015).

Although daily F/TDF had been the only initially approved strategy, there is now good evidence to support "on-demand" or "event-driven" PrEP (also known as "2-1-1" dosing): two pills of F/TDF taken together 2–24 hours prior to sexual exposure, one pill 24 hours after the initial two pill dose, and one pill 48 hours after that exposure (or one pill daily until 2 sex-free days). The IPERGAY and PRÉVENIR studies showed high rates of protection for MSM with this strategy (Molina et al., 2015, 2017, and 2022), including among participants who reported infrequent sex (Antoni et al., 2017). Moreover, PRÉVENIR demonstrated the high level of interest in event-driven PrEP, with almost 50% of participants choosing this option over daily F/TDF: discontinuations because of side-effects were rare, demonstrating its tolerability as well (Molina et al., 2022). As with daily PrEP, adherence is important: this was demonstrated by HPTN067/ ADAPT, where differences in adherence between daily and event-driven PrEP led to an estimated 18% efficacy reduction

with the latter (Dimitrov et al., 2020). Based on these data, the CDC now includes 2-1-1 dosing of F/TDF as an option for adult MSM who request it and who report infrequent sex (< once/week) and who can anticipate or delay sex to ensure the first dose is taken correctly (CDC, 2021b).

In 2019, the DISCOVER trial comparing F/TAF to F/ TDF was the first to lead to FDA approval of an alternative medication (F/TAF) for PrEP (Mayer et al., 2020). DISCOVER showed noninferiority of daily F/TAF compared to F/TDF among HIV-negative MSM and transgender women who have sex with men. While multiple ongoing studies are evaluating safety and efficacy of F/TAF for prevention in cis-gender women, including those who are pregnant and breastfeeding (ClinicalTrials.gov.NCT05140954; ClinicalTrials.gov.NCT04994509; Joseph Davey et al., 2022), it is not yet recommended for use to prevent HIV acquisition via vaginal sex. Similarly, F/TAF is not approved for on demand dosing, although preliminary data from macaques are promising (Bekerman et al., 2021).

Injectable CAB is also now a recommended PrEP option for all sexually active adults and adolescents with an indication for PrEP use (CDC, 2021b). This is based on safety and efficacy data from HPTN 083 and 084, which found that long-acting CAB given via intramuscular injection every 8 weeks was superior to FTC/TDF in reducing incident HIV in MSM, transgender women, and cis-gender women at risk for sexual acquisition of HIV (Delany-Moretlwe et al., 2022a; Landovitz, 2021). driven primarily by lower adherence for participants receiving F/TDF, LA-CAB was found to be 66% more effective at preventing HIV in MSM and transgender women, and 88% more effective in cis-gender women. There are no data on use of LA-CAB in persons whose primary risk for HIV acquisition is via injection-drug use, although updated CDC PrEP guidelines do endorse its use in persons who inject drugs if they also have sexual risk (CDC, 2021b).

The FDA has controversially decided not to review the dapavirine ring application for approval, in spite of evidence demonstrating that women often prefer this option, as well as its inclusion in the 2021 WHO guidelines as an option for cis-gender women (Ngure et al., 2022; WHO, 2021).

ELIGIBILITY

Multiple guidelines on PrEP eligibility and use have been released. For the purposes of this chapter, specific recommendations are taken from the 2021 CDC/USPHS guidelines. Other guidelines of interest include those from the World Health Organization (WHO, 2021); International Antiviral Society–USA (Saag, 2020); and New York State Department of Health AIDS Institute (New York State Department of Health, 2022). It should also be noted that the US Preventive Services Task Force also now recommends PrEP for individuals with risk factors for HIV acquisition (Grade A) (USPSTF, 2019).

According to CDC guidelines, PrEP is recommended as a prevention option for adults and adolescents with an increased likelihood of acquiring HIV (CDC, 2021b). Importantly, updated guidelines recommend that clinicians discuss PrEP with all sexually active adults and adolescents and offer it to anyone who requests in, as some people may be hesitant to disclose certain behaviors. One simple, non-stigmatizing and nonjudgmental question that can be used is, "Are you interested in learning more about medications that can prevent HIV?" Specific PrEP indications are listed in Table 5.2.

PRESCRIBING PREP: INITIATION AND FOLLOW-UP

Prior to initiating PrEP, clinicians should document the following:

- Absence of acute or chronic HIV.

- Renal function (creatinine clearance (CrCl) ≥60 mL/min for F/TDF use; or CrCl ≥30 mL/min for F/TAF use) for people receiving oral PrEP.

- Hepatitis B (HBV) immunity or infection and vaccination status.

Table 5.2 **SPECIFIC PREP INDICATIONS[1]**

SEXUALLY ACTIVE ADULTS AND ADOLESCENTS	PERSONS WHO USE SUBSTANCES
Any adult or adolescent weighing ≥35 kg without HIV who has had vaginal or anal sex in the last 6 months; *AND* within the last 6 months any of the following: • diagnosed with a bacterial STI[2] • having condomless sex with one or more partners whose HIV status is unknown • having sex with a partner with HIV whose viral load is detectable or unknown	Any adult or adolescent weighing ≥35 kg without HIV who has injected substances in the last 6 months; *AND* • shared injection or drug-preparation equipment

[1]PrEP should also be provided to anyone who requests it, even if the above conditions are not met.

[2] Includes gonorrhea, chlamydia, and syphilis (MSM); gonorrhea or syphilis (MSW, WSM).

SOURCE: Adapted from CDC/US Public Health Service 2021 Guidelines.

To document absence of acute or chronic HIV, the CDC recommends following the algorithms shown in Figures 5.1 and 5.2. Oral rapid HIV testing should not be used due to its lower sensitivity for detecting HIV compared to blood-based tests, and a negative test result should be documented within the week before PrEP initiation. For individuals reporting signs or symptoms of acute HIV (or who have had a high-risk exposure) within the previous 4 weeks, both an HIV viral load and a combined HIV antigen/antibody (Ag/Ab) test should be done. Updated guidelines also recommend both viral load and combined Ag/Ab testing for anyone who has received oral PEP or PrEP within the previous 3 months, or injectable PrEP within the last 12 months, to accurately determine baseline HIV status prior to PrEP initiation (CDC, 2021).

The choice between different PrEP options will be determined by multiple factors, including availability of population-specific safety and efficacy data; co-occurring conditions (e.g., hepatitis B, chronic kidney disease, or osteoporosis) and medications, patient preference, availability, and cost. Daily F/TDF is the most commonly prescribed PrEP regimen and can be used by most eligible individuals, including adolescents weighing at least 35 kg and people who inject substances; it is also available as a generic formulation, making it the most cost-effective option available (Marcus et al., 2022). The 2-1-1 dosing of F/TDF, daily F/TAF, and LA-CAB are additional options and may be considered in specific clinical scenarios (CDC, 2021b). Recommended follow-up and testing are detailed in Tables 5.3 and 5.4.

Given ongoing inequities in PrEP access, uptake and persistence (see below), a number of different strategies have been developed including provision of same-day PrEP as well as PrEP via tele-health, both of which have been shown to be effective in certain settings (Goedel et al., 2022; Kamis et al., 2019). Current CDC guidelines include recommendations

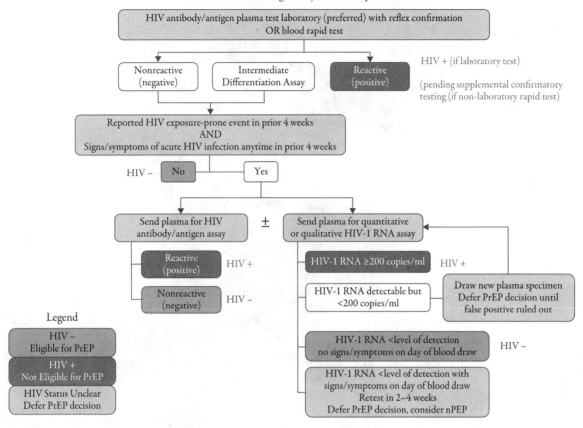

Figure 5.1 Assessment of HIV status prior to PrEP initiation: no recent antiretroviral prophylaxis use SOURCE: https://www.cdc.gov/hiv/pdf/risk/prep/cdc-hiv-prep-guidelines-2021.pdf, Figure 4a.

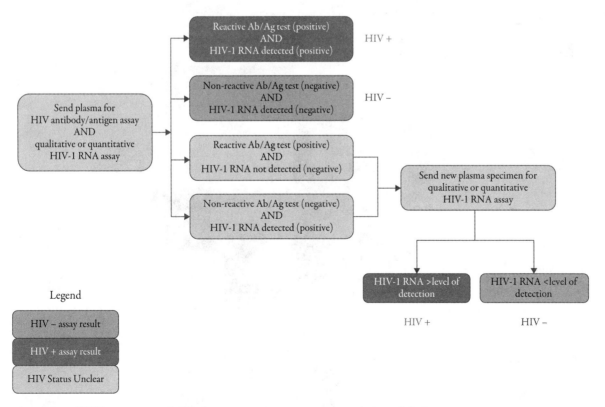

Figure 5.2. Assessment of HIV status prior to PrEP initiation: recent or current antiretroviral prophylaxis use SOURCE: https://www.cdc.gov/hiv/pdf/risk/prep/cdc-hiv-prep-guidelines-2021.pdf, Figure 4b. Published 2021. Accessed September 25, 2022.

Table 5.3 CLINICAL FOLLOW-UP AND MONITORING—ORAL PREP

TEST	BASELINE	EVERY 3 MONTHS	EVERY 6 MONTHS	YEARLY	DISCONTINUATION
HIV Ag/Ab	X	X[1]			X
eCrCl	X		If age >50 y baseline eCrCl< 90 mL/min, or other risk factors for renal disease	X	X
Site-directed STI screening	X	Based on behavior[2]	X		X
Syphilis screening	X	Based on behavior[2]	X		X
Lipid panel (if on F/TAF and age >50 y or risks for CVD)[3]	X			X	
HBV serologies	X				
HCV serology	X			Based on behavior[4]	
Adherence counseling/support	X	X			
Interest in continuing or stopping PrEP	X		X		

[1] CDC guidelines also recommend HIV viral load testing for all people on PrEP.

[2] STI and syphilis screening should be performed periodically; frequency should be based on reported sexual behaviors.

[3] CDC guidelines recommend baseline and yearly lipid testing for all people taking F/TAF.

[4] HCV screening should be repeated in individuals without chronic HCV who are at risk for (re-)infection, including persons who use substances and persons who have anal sex.

SOURCE: Adapted from CDC 2021 Guidelines.

Table 5.4 CLINICAL FOLLOW-UP AND MONITORING—INJECTABLE PREP

TEST	BASELINE	1-MONTH VISIT	EVERY 2 MONTHS	EVERY 4 MONTHS	EVERY 6 MONTHS	YEARLY	DISCONTINUATION
HIV Ag/Ab	X	X	X				X
HIV PCR	X	X	X				X
Site-directed STI screening	X			Based on behavior[1]	X		X
Syphilis screening	X			Based on behavior[1]	X		X
HBV serologies	X						
HCV serology	X					Based on behavior[2]	
Interest in continuing or stopping PrEP	X				X		

[1] STI and syphilis screening should be done periodically; frequency should be based on reported sexual behaviors.

[2] HCV screening should be repeated in individuals without chronic HCV who are at risk for (re-)infection, including persons who use substances and persons who have anal sex.

SOURCE: Adapted from CDC 2021 Guidelines.

for clinicians on required baseline and follow-up care using these models.

CONCERNS RELATED TO PREP USE

Oral PrEP, both as daily F/TDF and F/TAF, is generally very well tolerated, with < 10% of recipients experiencing serious adverse events (CDC, 2021; Ogbuagu, 2021). Common side-effects include nausea, headache, and weight loss. Most symptoms resolve within the first month and can usually be managed supportively.

More serious potential oral PrEP toxicities include acute and/or chronic kidney injury and bone demineralization, both of which appear to be reversible with medication discontinuation (Mulligan et al., 2015; Solomon et al., 2014). Compared to F/TDF, F/TAF as PrEP was associated with favorable and significant differences in bone mineral density and renal marker changes among DISCOVER participants (Ogbuagu et al., 2021). However, participants receiving F/TAF also experienced more weight gain and less favorable lipid changes, the long-term significance of which is not yet clear.

LA-CAB is similarly very well tolerated, with the most commonly reported side effect being local injection site reactions. While frequent (over 80% of HPTN 083 participants experienced injection site reactions), symptoms are typically mild, rarely result in LA-CAB discontinuation, and become less significant over time (Landovitz, 2020). LA-CAB appears to cause more weight gain compared to F/TDF (Delany-Moretlwe et al., 2022a; Landovitz et al., 2021).

Drug–drug interactions between PrEP and other medications are relatively uncommon. Neither F/TAF nor CAB should be administered with antiepileptics such as carbamazepine or with the antituberculous agent rifampicin. Before prescribing PrEP, clinicians should obtain a full list of all prescription and over-the-counter medications and assess for possible interactions. Multiple resources (e.g., University of Liverpool's online HIV drug interaction checker) can be used to assist with this assessment.

Breakthrough HIV acquisition and resistance with oral PrEP is uncommon but has been reported despite optimal dosing and PrEP adherence, primarily because of transmitted drug resistance (Cohen et al., 2018; Colby et al., 2018; Knox et al., 2017; Markowitz et al., 2017; Spinelli et al., 2020; Thaden et al., 2018). Additionally, one individual acquired wild-type HIV while taking oral PrEP; for this case, it is thought that HIV infection progressed systematically only after PrEP discontinuation (Hoorneborg & de Bree, 2017). Most cases in which drug resistance has been observed in people on oral PrEP have occurred in individuals with undiagnosed HIV at the time of PrEP initiation, underscoring the importance of evaluating for possible acute HIV at baseline.

Incident HIV infections in people receiving LA-CAB are extremely uncommon; to date, < 10 breakthrough infections have been reported in people receiving on-time injections despite >4,000 person-years of follow-up (Landovitz et al., 2022). Unlike with oral PrEP, however, HIV drug resistance development has been observed in most of these cases (Landovitz et al., 2022; Marzinke et al., 2021), which is concerning given the central role INSTIs have played in treating most PWH. As with oral PrEP, breakthrough infections without resistance were also observed in HPTN 083 and 084 in the setting of missed or delayed injections (Eshelman et al., 2022; Marzinke et al., 2021).

In addition to breakthrough HIV acquisition and drug resistance, a related concern involves accurate HIV diagnosis. Because antiretroviral exposure can impact viral replication dynamics and the body's immune response to infection, standard HIV testing algorithms may be difficult to interpret. This phenomenon can occur with both oral and injectable PrEP but seems to be more common with the latter. Therefore, the CDC now recommends both a standard HIV Ag/Ab assay and HIV PCR test (e.g., either a qualitative or quantitative RNA test) to assess for incident HIV infection in all PrEP users (CDC, 2021b).

While such issues highlight that PrEP is not infallible, it is notable that there have only been a handful of reported cases of "PrEP failure" among extensive data supporting its efficacy, and the prevalence of multidrug-resistant HIV in individuals with unsuppressed viral load remains low overall in the United States. When used as prescribed, the overwhelming majority of individuals on PrEP will be protected from infection.

STI diagnoses are common among PrEP users. Care must be taken, however, to ensure that concerns about so-called risk compensation are not used to justify withholding PrEP. Rather, the focus should turn toward promoting sexual health using shared decision-making based on individual preferences and priorities, increased STI screening, and engagement in care (Marcus et al., 2019).

For people with chronic HBV as evidenced by a positive/reactive HBV surface antigen (HBsAg) test, the CDC recommends evaluation by an HBV-experienced clinician. Such individuals may be given PrEP but should be counseled on the potential risk of a hepatic flare should they abruptly discontinue tenofovir-containing PrEP, and event-driven PrEP is currently not recommended. While limited data suggest this risk of flares is relatively low (Solomon et al., 2016), many questions about tenofovir-containing PrEP use in people with chronic HBV remain, including what the actual frequency of HBV flares is in this population; whether there could be potential benefit of tenofovir-containing PrEP use by inducing HBsAg loss; what the risk of HBV resistance mutations for those who take event-driven PrEP is; and whether or not it is cost-effective (Mohareb et al., 2022). CAB does not have intrinsic anti-HBV activity; however, there are currently no data on its safety in people with chronic HBV. There are limited data on PrEP use during pregnancy or breastfeeding, and this evidence gap is likely contributing to ongoing inequities in PrEP accessibility and use (Joseph Davey et al., 2022). However, data from the Antiviral Pregnancy Registry demonstrate no evidence of harm to fetuses exposed to F/TDF (Antiretroviral Pregnancy Registry, 2022). Further, it should be emphasized that some HIV-negative women with seropositive partners may be at increased risk for HIV acquisition during pregnancy or peri-conception. Current US guidelines recommend use of F/TDF as PrEP for women trying to conceive or who are pregnant when viral suppression of the seropositive partner is in question (US Department of Health and Human Services, 2022). Although data are limited, use of F/TDF during lactation appears to be safe, and, therefore, breastfeeding is not a contraindication (US Department of Health and Human Services, 2022; CDC, 2021b). While approved for use in pregnant people with HIV, there are currently no data on F/TAF for preventing HIV through vaginal sex, although studies are ongoing (ClinicalTrials.gov. NCT05140954; ClinicalTrials.gov.NCT04994509; Joseph Davey et al., 2022). There are likewise limited data on safety and efficacy of LA-CAB in people who are pregnant or breastfeeding: data from the 49 women in HPTN 084 who became pregnant while receiving LA-CAB suggest it was generally well tolerated (Delany-Moretlwe et al., 2022b). The inclusion of pregnant and breastfeeding persons in the HPTN 084 open label extension should provide additional data.

DISCONTINUING PREP

PrEP should be discontinued in people who experience unacceptable side-effects or toxicities; are unable to adhere to the prescribed regimen or follow-up care; or change their risk status such that PrEP is no longer believed to be indicated. Because LA-CAB levels remain clinically significant for months after last injection, people who discontinue LA-CAB and may have ongoing exposures should be provided with oral PrEP for at least 12 months to reduce the risk of developing drug-resistant HIV during this "tail phase" (CDC, 2021b). Individuals who acquire HIV while taking PrEP should be transitioned to ART as treatment in accordance with current HIV treatment guidelines.

PREP CHALLENGES AND DISPARITIES

Despite established benefits of PrEP, several challenges remain. For example, the role of PrEP for people in serodifferent relationships in which the partner with HIV is on suppressive ART is not clear. It is now established that persons with HIV who maintain an undetectable viral load do not transmit HIV to their sex partners. However, HIV-negative individuals in such relationships may have other partners of unknown status or partners who are positive but not yet on treatment. This possibility was highlighted by the fact that nearly 40% of transmissions in HPTN052 study were unlinked (i.e., they came from someone other than their identified serodifferent partner) (Cohen et al., 2015).

The optimal strategy for initiating PrEP in individuals with frequent, high-risk exposures is unclear and may contribute at least partly to underutilization in persons who inject drugs (Taylor et al., 2019). When a person not on PrEP has a high-risk exposure, current US guidelines recommend PEP initiation within 72 hours and continuation for 28 days (see below) before transitioning to PrEP, after confirming that the exposed person remains HIV-negative (CDC, 2021b). If timing of the last exposure representing significant risk falls outside of the 72-hour window or is uncertain, and HIV cannot be confidently ruled out with immediate testing, providers

should consider consultation with a PEP/PrEP-experienced provider.

Since initial FDA approval of PrEP, the number of at-risk individuals taking PrEP has increased substantially; the CDC now estimates ~25% of eligible adults are now taking it (CDC, 2021d). However, coverage is unequal, with significant differences in rates of PrEP access and uptake along lines of race, gender, and geography: of the ~1.21 million adults at increased risk of HIV who meet indications for PrEP, 39% are Black; 26% Hispanic; and 25% White (CDC, 2021c). This is in stark contrast to 2020 data showing that 66% of people on PrEP are White. Regional differences are also apparent: while about half of all HIV diagnoses are identified in the South, only 27% of PrEP users live in the South (Huang et al., 2018). According to indication, PrEP use is greatest among MSM and substantially lower among cis-gender women and persons who inject drugs (Buchbinder et al., 2018; Kuo et al., 2018; Mayer et al., 2018).

Of particular concern, this unequal distribution of PrEP use could worsen as a result of the US 340B drug pricing system, which (paradoxically) promotes use of more expensive and less accessible PrEP options over less expensive generic ones (Marcus et al., 2022), the end result of which would be perpetuation of already-stark inequities. Individual and population-level efforts must be implemented to close these gaps, while simultaneously addressing the structural racism and internalized biases that have promoted them. Increased training especially for clinicians caring for communities of color, community-level education to promote awareness and reduce stigma, and inclusive public health campaigns all may have an impact, as would ensuring equitable access to health care and health insurance (Kanny et al., 2019).

Providers seeking clinical guidance on PrEP should contact local experts, if available. The National Clinician Consultation Center (nccc.ucsf.edu) also offers free teleconsultation to any US provider through its PrEP line: 1-(855)448-7737 | 1-(855)HIV-PrEP.

PEP

PEP for HIV prevention is a pharmacotherapeutic intervention that takes advantage of the window of time it takes HIV to cross the mucosal barrier and begin viral replication. Established infection ethical considerations preclude PEP trials (for either occupational or nonoccupational exposures), and data supporting its use largely derive from animal models, inference from postnatal prophylaxis studies, observational studies, and one retrospective case-control study showing an 81% reduction in risk of HIV acquisition among health care workers who took zidovudine after exposure (Cardo et al., 1997; Lunding et al., 2015; Otten et al., 2000; Shih et al., 1991; Young et al., 2007). These studies, along with our understanding of HIV viral kinetics, are the foundation for the recommendation to initiate PEP urgently after possible exposure, ideally within 24 hours and at most within 72 hours, and to continue taking it for 28 days. The most recent US-based occupational PEP (oPEP) guidelines were released in 2013 by the CDC/US Public Health Service (Kuhar et al., 2013), and the CDC's nonoccupational PEP (nPEP) guidelines were last updated in 2016 (Dominguez et al., 2016). More recent PEP guidance for both occupational and nonoccupational exposures has been published by the New York State Department of Health AIDS Institute (DeHaan et al., 2022). See Box 5.1.

OCCUPATIONAL EXPOSURES

The use of ART to prevent acquisition of HIV among health care personnel who experience a high-risk occupational exposure was first recommended in 1990. Occupational exposures to HIV encompass penetrating injuries (predominantly sharps or percutaneous needlesticks and mucosal/splash injuries). After exposure in a health care setting, risk of HIV acquisition appears to be related to size of the viral inoculum, which is in turn influenced by the stage of disease of the source individual, and the quantity of blood involved in the exposure (Kuhar et al., 2013).

For occupational exposures (where the source is more often identified and available), timely source person testing is important to guide decisions around whether to initiate and/or continue PEP. If the source's HIV status is unknown, consent should be obtained for testing; if source HIV status is confirmed negative, PEP should be discontinued. If source HIV Ag/Ab testing is negative, but they had an exposure to HIV in the prior 4 weeks, source HIV RNA should also be obtained and PEP should be continued until the RNA returns negative (DeHaan et al., 2022). If the source is known to have HIV or if the source is unavailable, unable, or unwilling to complete HIV testing, oPEP is indicated in the setting of a high-risk exposure. Additionally, when the source is known to have HIV, current viral load, current and prior ART and resistance history, and prescriber information should be obtained.

NONOCCUPATIONAL EXPOSURES

Nonoccupational exposures encompass consensual sex, sexual assault, needle sharing, penetrating injury (sharps or percutaneous needlesticks), bites with blood exposure, and mucosal/splash injuries. Determination of the nature of the exposure is critical, as nPEP is generally only indicated for higher-risk exposures (Table 5.5); when the source is known to be living with HIV; and on a case-by-case basis when source HIV status is unknown (Dominguez et al., 2016). NYS DOH PEP guidance similarly suggests focusing on the nature of the exposure, and recommends PEP for all higher-risk exposures regardless if source person HIV status is unknown or known to be positive; this includes exposures from receptive and insertive vaginal or anal intercourse, needle sharing, penetrating injury, or bites with visible bleeding in the mouth that causes bleeding in the exposed individual (DeHaan et al., 2022).

US-based guidelines recommend against using geographic location of the exposure, residence of the exposed individual, or perceived or assumed source "risk behavior" to guide PEP initiation (DeHaan et al., 2022). Conversely, British 2021 PEP guidelines recommend assessing not only the nature of the exposure, but also the risk of the source having HIV with detectable viremia, ART use, and susceptibility of the exposed individual (i.e., presence of ulcerative genital disease in sexual exposures) (Cresswell et al., 2022). British recommendations to initiate PEP are based on a calculated risk of transmission dependent on known prevalence of HIV viremia in a specific risk-group multiplied by the risk of transmission based on type of exposure (Cresswell et al., 2022). As a result, their most recent guidance varies greatly from US guidelines. It should be noted that British guidelines were developed based on UK-specific population-level data broken down by risk, gender, race, and location and in the context of a largely diagnosed, treated, and virally suppressed national population, which is not broadly generalizable.

While basic principles of PEP initiation and prescribing overlap between nonoccupational and occupational exposures, there are specific considerations for nonoccupational exposures:

- PEP should be discussed with consideration of future and ongoing exposure with attention to PrEP initiation if ongoing HIV vulnerability after PEP completion.

- For consensual sexual exposures, baseline evaluation should include HIV testing, site-specific gonorrhea and chlamydia testing, syphilis screening, and pregnancy testing (if indicated).

- For sexual assault victims, while baseline HIV testing is indicated, other STI testing can be offered but should not be routinely acquired, except in situations of pediatric

Table 5.5 **LEVEL OF RISK BASED ON EXPOSURE TYPE FOR CONSIDERATION OF POSTEXPOSURE PROPHYLAXIS (PEP)**

Higher-risk exposures—PEP should be recommended	Receptive and insertive vaginal or anal intercourse with a source who has HIV and is not known to be virally suppressed on ART with good adherence, or when the source's HIV status is unknown. Needle sharing with a partner who has HIV, or when the partner's HIV status is unknown. Sharps injury[1] with exposure to blood or other potentially infectious fluids (e.g., needlestick or broken glass that has been in a blood vessel, contaminated with blood or is visibly bloody) from a source known to have HIV or with unknown HIV status. Contact of mucosa (mouth, nose, or eyes) or nonintact skin (e.g., open wound, abrasions) with blood, visibly bloody fluid or other potentially infectious material (e.g., semen, vaginal fluid) from a source known to have HIV or with unknown HIV status. Human bites with visibly blood saliva causing bleeding in exposed individual. If history is unreliable or cannot be obtained during sexual assault evaluation (including pediatric cases), PEP is recommended if any physical evidence of sexual abuse.
Lower-risk exposures—require case-by-case evaluation for PEP	Oral–vaginal contact (receptive and insertive). Oral–anal contact (receptive and insertive). Penile–oral contact (receptive and insertive) with or without ejaculation. Factors that increase risk in these situations, and PEP should be offered: • Source is known to have HIV with elevated viral load • Oral mucosa that is not intact (e.g., oral lesions, gingivitis, wounds, or oral trauma as in cases of sexual assault). • Blood exposure. • Presence of genital ulcer disease or other sexually transmitted infections.
Exposures that do not warrant PEP	Kissing. Oral-to-oral contact without mucosal damage (mouth-to-mouth resuscitation). Human bites not involving blood. Exposure to solid-bore needles or sharps[1] not in recent contact with blood (e.g., tattoo needles and lancets). Mutual masturbation without skin breakdown or blood exposure. Exposure to saliva not involving visible blood.

[1] HIV is intolerant to environmental exposure to air and the risk of HIV transmission from community needle stick injury (e.g., discarded needles) extremely low. There have been no documented transmissions through community needlesticks and PEP is generally not recommended in these scenarios.

SOURCE: Adapted from New York State Department of Health AIDS Institute (DeHaan et al., 2022).

assault (as frequently victims are at increased risk of repetitive assault), as these results may subsequently enter bias into court proceedings (DeHaan et al., 2022).

• Other considerations for sexual assault victims include consideration of PEP if there is any mucosal-to-mucosal contact (including oral-penile), or mucosal or broken-skin contact to infectious body fluids, as apparent or occult physical trauma and bleeding are common (DeHaan et al., 2022).

• PEP is not generally indicated for exposed individuals consistently adherent to PrEP: exceptions to this may include recent PrEP initiation, inconsistent adherence, "on-demand" PrEP, or exposure to a source who has HIV resistant to components of a PrEP regimen (DeHaan et al., 2022).

• For consensual sexual exposures, given the evidence behind "U = U," when the source is known to have HIV and is consistently on ART with a confirmed undetectable viral load, PEP is not recommended (Cresswell et al., 2022; DeHaan et al., 2022). British guidelines extrapolate this further, stating PEP "is not generally indicated" in sharps, or needlestick injuries and "is not recommended" in splash injuries (Cresswell et al.,

2022). However, given lack of direct evidence However, given lack of direct evidence for "U = U" in these and other scenarios (i.e., needlestick or needle sharing, breastfeeding) this should not be broadly applied to other exposure types. Current US guidelines continue to recommend PEP in these cases.

RECOMMENDED PEP REGIMENS

To achieve high completion rates, PEP regimens should be convenient with minimal side-effects and drug interactions. Current US-based guidelines recommend FTC/TDF together with DTG or RAL as preferred regimens in most adults and adolescents. Because these medications act prior to HIV integration with cellular DNA, they provide a theoretical advantage over alternative PI-based regimens. PEP updates now include an option for once-daily RAL with FTC–TDF for nonpregnant individuals, which can facilitate adherence (Cresswell et al., 2022; DeHaan et al., 2022). Table 5.6 outlines recommended PEP options.

Newer studies investigating single-tablet regimens (STR) as PEP after sexual exposure show promise toward further regimen simplification (Foster et al., 2015; Gantner et al., 2020; Malinverni et al., 2021; Mayer et al., 2017; Mayer et al.,

Table 5.6 POSTEXPOSURE PROPHYLAXIS (PEP) REGIMENS FOR PERSONS WEIGHING ≥40 KG AND WITH CRCL ≥50 ML/MIN*

PREFERRED REGIMENS	"NRTI BACKBONE"	"ANCHOR ARV"
	Either of the following**:	Emtricitabine 200 mg/tenofovir disoproxil fumarate 300 mg (FTC/TDF) 1 tablet by mouth daily *or* Lamivudine 300 mg/tenofovir disoproxil fumarate 300 mg (3TC/TDF) 1 tablet by mouth daily *Plus* one of the following: Dolutegravir (DTG) 50 mg once daily *or* Raltegravir (RAL) 400 mg twice daily *or* Raltegravir HD 1200 mg once daily (not recommended in pregnancy)
Alternative regimens	Emtricitabine 200 mg/tenofovir disoproxil fumarate 300 mg (FTC/TDF) 1 tablet by mouth daily *or* Lamivudine 300 mg/tenofovir disoproxil fumarate 300 mg (3TC/TDF) 1 tablet by mouth daily	Darunavir (DRV) 800 mg daily + ritonavir (RTV) 100 mg daily 2014 both require dose-adjustment in pregnancy *or* Atazanavir (ATV) 300 mg daily + ritonavir (RTV) 100 mg daily—special considerations exist for use in pregnancy
	Or fixed-dose combination EVG/COBI/FTC/TDF once daily, only if CrCl ≥70mL/min—not recommended in pregnancy)	

NRTI: nucleotide reverse transcriptase inhibitor.

*Majority of ARVs listed are safe during periconception and in pregnancy unless noted. If CrCl< 50mL/min, do not use fixed-dose combinations of NRTIs—should dose adjust components as indicated.

**NYS DOH PEP guidelines recommend NOT to use AZT or TAF.

SOURCE: Adapted from DeHaan et al., 2022; Dominguez et al., 2016; Kuhar et al., 2013.

2022). When compared to historical controls, one study demonstrated that individuals taking co-formulated BIC/FTC/TAF (*n* = 52) experienced fewer side-effects, higher completion rates, and no HIV diagnoses during follow-up (Mayer et al., 2022). When compared to historical controls, one study demonstrated that individuals taking co-formulated BIC/FTC/TAF (*n* = 52) experienced fewer side effects, higher completion rates, and no HIV diagnoses during follow-up (Mayer et al., 2022). Several guidelines now recommend STR PEP options. For example, 2017 French guidelines recommend co-formulated rilpivirine/emtricitabine/tenofovir disoproxil fumarate, although this regimen should only be used in settings with low rates of background transmitted NRTI or NNRTI resistance, as well as low risk of possible HIV-2 exposure, given lack of anticipated NNRTI activity for HIV-2. NYS DOH guidelines state that elvitegravir/cobicistat/emtricitabine/tenofovir disoproxil fumarate can be considered as an alternative regimen (DeHaan et al., 2022).

BASELINE TESTING AND MONITORING

For all exposures, recommended baseline testing of the exposed individual includes laboratory-based HIV Ag/Ab testing, renal and liver function assessment, pregnancy testing (if indicated), and hepatitis B and C serologies. For consensual sexual exposures, additional baseline testing should include syphilis and site-specific STI screening; STI testing can be offered but should not be routine in sexual assault exposures as this may instill bias in future potential court proceedings (DeHaan et al., 2022).

All hepatitis B-susceptible individuals with possible exposure to hepatitis B (source with confirmed hepatitis B infection, or if source status is unknown) should initiate the hepatitis B vaccine series within 24 hours. Individuals exposed to someone with known acute or chronic HBV should receive hepatitis B immune globulin as well. Currently, PEP for HCV is not recommended for occupational exposures (Moorman et al., 2020). In cases of sexual assault, a first dose of HPV vaccine should be administered, and exposed individuals should be offered empiric STI treatment (DeHaan et al., 2022). For sexual exposures, emergency contraceptive should be offered if the exposed individual is of childbearing capacity.

Follow-up testing includes HIV Ag/Ab testing at 4–6 weeks and 3–4 months. While laboratory-based HIV testing is preferred because of improved sensitivity, point-of-care combination HIV Ag/Ab tests may be used for follow-up testing (DeHaan et al., 2022). Newer guidelines emphasize use of more sensitive assays, such as HCV RNA, for earlier detection during the follow-up period (DeHaan et al., 2022; Moorman et al., 2020) as well as consideration for earlier STI testing after sexual exposures (DeHaan et al., 2022). See Table 5.7 for recommended testing and monitoring.

TIME FROM EXPOSURE	RECOMMENDED SERVICES	
	COUNSELING	TESTING AND MANAGEMENT
Baseline	Transmission prevention (condom use; avoidance of blood/tissue donation; avoid breastfeeding) For sexual assault, ensure close follow-up care including support from crisis counselor or outreach worker If prescribing PEP: possible PEP side-effects, drug interactions—counsel on importance of adherence	HIV Ag/Ab testing Hepatitis B surface antigen (HBsAg) and surface Ab (HBsAb); if exposed individual is unvaccinated or non-immune: initiate HBV vaccination, and if source is HBsAg-positive or unknown and high-risk, administer HBIG Hepatitis C antibody (HCV Ab) If sexual exposure: pregnancy test, syphilis, and site-specific testing for gonorrhea and chlamydia (If sexual assault: baseline syphilis, gonorrhea, chlamydia, and trichomonas screening may be offered; offer empiric STI treatment, HPV vaccination, and emergency contraception) If prescribing PEP: pregnancy test, complete blood count, liver function tests, and renal function tests
24-48 hours (may be conducted by telephone)	Transmission prevention Behavioral supports Review additional information about exposure or the source individual if available Assess adherence, drug interactions, and medication tolerance if taking PEP	–
2 weeks (may be conducted by telephone)	Transmission prevention Assess adherence, drug interactions, and medication tolerance if taking PEP	If taking PEP and baseline testing abnormal or adverse effects are reported: complete blood count, liver function tests, and renal function tests If sexual exposure: consider repeat STI screening
4–6 weeks	Transmission prevention Counsel and initiate PrEP if HIV testing negative and ongoing exposures	HIV Ag/Ab testing If source has known HCV or unknown status: HCV RNA and alanine aminotransferase (ALT) testing If childbearing capacity: pregnancy test If taking PEP and baseline testing abnormal or adverse effects are reported: complete blood count, liver function tests, and renal function tests
3–4 months	–	HIV Ag/Ab testing (if negative, HIV is excluded) HBsAg (unless baseline testing HBsAb positive/immune) If source has known HCV or unknown status: HCV RNA and ALT testing (additionally, HCV Ab and ALT should be done at 6 months)

SOURCE: Adapted from DeHaan et al., 2022; Kuhar et al., 2013.

SPECIAL CONSIDERATIONS

- The preferred regimens of DTG or twice daily RAL together with FTC–TDF are safe in pregnancy and in persons of childbearing potential. NYS DOH PEP guidelines have removed the recommendation to discuss teratogenicity and contraception prior to prescribing DTG to pregnant persons or those of childbearing potential (DeHaan et al., 2022). This reflects newer data showing no significant difference in safety outcomes of DTG compared to other antiretrovirals taken during periconception and throughout pregnancy (Zash et al., 2020).

- For individuals who are breastfeeding at the time of potential exposure, person-centered counseling and shared decision-making should be utilized, including considerations of the potential risks and benefits of continued breastfeeding (with or without PEP use) and for surveillance and follow-up testing. Current guidelines recommend that breastfeeding individuals with potential HIV exposure should avoid breastfeeding for 3 months after exposure and until confirmed to be HIV-negative. If the exposed person has a negative HIV Ag/Ab result at 4–6 weeks postexposure, reassessment of breastfeeding plans may be considered.

- If found to have hepatitis B at baseline, exposed individuals should be assessed by a HBV specialist to determine the need to continue HBV therapy post PEP. TDF/FTC should be continued until this assessment occurs, as discontinuation of these medications may lead to inadvertent hepatic flares.

- Antiretroviral (ARV) duration may need to extend beyond 28 days if the exposed individual is found to have an indeterminate HIV test result or is experiencing acute

Table 5.8 SITUATIONS IN WHICH EXPERT CONSULTATION* FOR POSTEXPOSURE PROPHYLAXIS (PEP) IS RECOMMENDED

SCENARIO	CONSIDERATIONS
Delayed (i.e., later than 72 hours) exposure report	If timing of last exposure representing significant risk falls outside of 72 hours or is uncertain, and HIV cannot be confidently ruled out with immediate testing
Unknown source (e.g., needle in sharps disposal container or laundry)	Use of PEP to be decided on a case-by-case basis: consider severity of exposure and epidemiologic likelihood of HIV exposure Do not test needles or other sharp instruments for HIV
Known or possible pregnancy in the exposed individual, or exposed individual is breastfeeding	PEP should not be delayed while awaiting expert consultation
Source has known or suspected ARV-resistant HIV or current or history of ART failure	Selection of a PEP regimen should include ARVs that the source individual's HIV is unlikely to be resistant to Do not delay initiation of PEP while awaiting HIV resistance testing results from source individual
Significant PEP side-effects	Symptoms (e.g., gastrointestinal symptoms, headache) are often manageable without changing PEP regimen—can offer analgesics, antimotility, and antiemetic agents
Limited options for PEP medications owing to potential drug–drug interactions or comorbidities	Significant underlying illness (e.g., renal disease) or multiple medications taken by the exposed individual may increase risk of medication toxicity, drug–drug interactions, and need for ARV dose-adjustment or alternative PEP regimen

*Expert consultation can be sought with local experts or the National Clinician Consultation Center's Post Exposure Prophylaxis Hotline (PEPline) at 1-888-448-4911.

SOURCE: Adapted from DeHaan et al., 2022; Kuhar et al., 2013.

retroviral syndrome during the early follow-up period (i.e., 3–4 weeks after exposure). If the exposed individual is pregnant with a high likelihood of HIV exposure, careful follow-up monitoring and testing and ARV management are warranted.

- Expert consultation is recommended in various scenarios (Table 5.8).

SCREENING AND TREATMENT FOR SEXUALLY TRANSMITTED INFECTIONS

The link between STIs and HIV transmission/acquisition is well established, and supported by both biologic plausibility (e.g., genital tract inflammation leading to increased viral shedding in persons with HIV and increased access of HIV to subepithelial target cells) and epidemiologic synergy (Cohen et al., 2019; Mayer & Venkatesh, 2011). However, multiple confounders have made it difficult to estimate how much these factors contribute to increased risk, and large-scale STI treatment studies have failed to consistently demonstrate a reduction in community-level HIV transmission (Cohen et al., 2019; Mayer & Venkatesh, 2011). The Mwanza study stands out as one notable exception: it demonstrated a 38% reduction in HIV incidence with syndromic STI management (Grosskurth et al., 1995). More recently, data from multiple trials evaluating sexual HIV transmission between serodifferent partnerships as well as from multiple PrEP studies indicate that even with very high STI rates, ART-mediated durable viral suppression of HIV prevents transmission (Cohen et al., 2019).

VOLUNTARY MEDICAL MALE CIRCUMCISION

The presence of penile foreskin may facilitate sexual HIV acquisition as a result of low-grade inflammation and resultant dysbiosis (Cohen et al., 2019). Three large, randomized trials in Sub-Saharan Africa demonstrated that voluntary circumcision led to an approximate risk reduction for heterosexual HIV acquisition of 50% (Auvert et al., 2005; Bailey et al., 2007; Gray et al., 2007; Siegfried et al., 2009). This benefit did not appear to extend to female partners of circumcised men with HIV (Weiss et al., 2009). Based on observational data, circumcision may benefit MSM who practice primarily insertive anal sex, especially in low- and middle-income countries (Yuanet al., 2019). However, data for individuals having receptive anal sex is lacking, and there have been no randomized trials looking at this: thus, a population-level benefit among MSM has not been proven. However, voluntary medical male circumcision (VMMC) remains a critical evidence-based strategy for adolescent boys and men engaging in heterosexual sex in areas of high HIV transmission rates (primarily in Sub-Saharan Africa) as recommended by the WHO and UNAIDS since 2007 (WHO, 2020). The WHO's 2020 guideline update on VVMC continues to not recommend circumcision specifically for MSM, given the paucity of high-quality data, but states MSM should not be excluded in settings where VMMC programs are active for HIV prevention (WHO, 2020). In the United States, VMMC is not recommended broadly for HIV prevention, and decisions around circumcision should be based on individualized discussions incorporating population-specific data, individual behaviors, and potential procedural risks (CDC, 2022b).

NEW AND INVESTIGATIONAL INTERVENTIONS FOR HIV PREVENTION

NOVEL PREP ANTIRETROVIRALS AND DELIVERY METHODS

Active investigation of alternate delivery methods and novel antiretrovirals promise to further expand HIV prevention options. Studies are underway for a once-weekly pill, long-acting injections, and sustained-release implants that may provide long-acting coverage.

Lenacapavir (LEN), a capsid inhibitor that acts across multiple stages of the HIV life cycle, is in phase 3 clinical trials as a 6-month subcutaneous injection for PrEP, hoping to expand options to adolescent girls and young women (PURPOSE 1; Clinicaltrials.gov.NCT04994509) and well as men (cis-gender, transgender, and nonbinary individuals) who have sex with men and transgender women (PURPOSE 2; Clinicaltrials.gov. NCT04925752). Studies of islatravir, a novel nucleoside reverse transcriptase translocation inhibitor, show its promise as a long-acting implantable formulation (Matthews et al., 2019), as well as once-monthly oral PrEP option (IMPOWER-022, Clinicaltrials.gov.NCT04644029; IMPOWER-024, Clinicaltrials.gov.NCT04652700)—of note, these trials are currently on hold by the FDA because of observed decreases in lymphocyte counts. Other antivirals in PrEP studies include LA-RPV, which was found to be safe and effective delivered as two intramuscular injections every 8 weeks in a phase 2 clinical trial (Bekker et al., 2020), as well as a long-acting implant of tenofovir alafenamide (TAF) (Gunawardana et al., 2022) and a long-acting in situ forming implant (ISFI) of CAB (Massud et al., 2022)—the latter two are currently in preclinical studies.

MICROBICIDES

Microbicides are products applied locally to the vaginal or rectal mucosa to reduce risk of STI acquisition. The use of microbicides or other local drug-delivery devices such as vaginal rings have several potential benefits. First, they deliver high concentrations of a drug to the desired tissue with minimal systemic exposure (Hendrix et al., 2013) and can thus potentially provide on-demand protection. Many products are also targeted toward cis-gender women, a group disproportionately excluded from many ART and PrEP trials, but who comprise almost half of new HIV transmissions globally (WHO, 2016). These options may be used discretely, have the potential to be co-formulated with other medications such as contraceptives, and importantly—may be more acceptable to some users compared to other PrEP options. This latter point was illustrated in the REACH trial: after a period of use of each product, 67% of adolescents and young women chose the once-monthly dapivirine vaginal ring over once-daily oral PrEP, with < 5% of visits during the choice period showing no-low adherence (Ngure et al., 2022).

Tenofovir gel as a vaginal microbicide has been extensively studied and found to have mixed efficacy for HIV prevention in cis-gender women, with greatest protection seen in women with high adherence (Abdool Karim et al., 2010). Given poor adherence to this method across multiple trials, as well as concerns that efficacy may be impacted by vaginal dysbiosis or inflammation, it is no longer under active investigation (Abdool Karim et al., 2022). Use of rectal tenofovir gel in MSM and transwomen is under investigation, and has been shown to be safe and acceptable in early stage trials (Cranston et al., 2017). A medicated TDF-based rectal enema (DREAM-01 trial, Clinicaltrials.gov.NCT02750540), tenofovir vaginal ring (CONRAD-128 trial, Clinicaltrials.gov. NCT03762382), and combination topical TAF/EVG as an on-demand vaginal (CONRAD-146 trial, Clinicaltrials.gov. NCT03762772) or rectal (MTN-039 trial, Clinicialtrials. gov.NCT04047420) insert are also under investigation.

MULTIPURPOSE PREVENTION TECHNOLOGIES (MPT)

Options integrating contraception and HIV prevention methods into single combined agents, or MPT, create optimism for expanded choice in women's sexual and reproductive health. Building on already approved and marketed products, the Dual Prevention Pill (a co-formulated combined oral contraceptive once-daily pill with TDF/FTC) may be the first multipurpose prevention technology available in the ensuing years (Friedland et al., 2021). The dapivirine vaginal ring, already approved by the WHO as a stand-alone microbicidal option for HIV prevention for cis-gender women, has been shown to be safe and well tolerated in phase 1 trials as a combined dapivirine-levonorgestrel ring for PrEP and contraception for up to 90 days of continuous use (Achilles et al., 2021). Similarly, the phase 2a CONRAD-128 study showed that 90 days of continuous use of a tenofovir-levonorgestrel ring was safe with adequate protective levels of both medication components for the trial's duration (Mugo et al., 2021). An in situ forming implant injected subcutaneously that may last for ≥3 months combining DTG or CAB for PrEP, with etonogestrel or medroxyprogesterone for pregnancy prevention, is in preclinical investigation (Young et al., 2022). Many other MPTs for HIV prevention, including films, gels, and patches using antiviral, microbicide, and monoclonal antibody platforms, are in varying stages of development (MPT Product Development database).

VACCINES AND BROADLY NEUTRALIZING ANTIBODIES

Multiple challenges, both biomedical and social, have impeded development of an effective HIV vaccine. These include HIV diversity and pathogenesis, difficulty in generating broadly neutralizing antibodies, identification of appropriate immune correlates of protection, community preparedness and concerns about vaccine-induced positivity, and expanded PrEP use (Hammer, 2015). With the exception of the modestly positive Thai vaccine trial RV 144, which demonstrated a 31% reduction in incident HIV among vaccine recipients, clinical trials of HIV vaccines have been disappointing (Table 5.9).

Table 5.9 SUMMARY OF HIV PHASE II/III VACCINE EFFICACY TRIALS

TRIAL	VACCINE PRODUCT	STUDY POPULATION; SITE	RESULTS	REFERENCE
Vax 003	Recombinant gp120 (B/E)	Male and female PWID; Thailand	No efficacy	Pitisuttithum, 2006
Vax 004	Recombinant gp120 (B/B′)	Heterosexual women and MSM; United States and the Netherlands	No efficacy	Flynn, 2005
HVTN 502 (STEP Study)	Recombinant Ad5 (Clade B gag/pol/nef)	MSM, heterosexual women and men; North and South America, Caribbean, Australia	No efficacy	Buchbinder, 2008
HVTN 503 (Phambili Study)	Recombinant Ad5 (Clade B gag/pol/nef)	Heterosexual women and men; South Africa	No efficacy	Gray, 2011
HVTN 505	6-plasmid DNA vaccine and rAd5 vector boost	MSM; United States	No efficacy	Hammer, 2013
RV 144	ALVAC: Canarypox (gag, pol, env) \+ AIDSVAX B/E recombinant gp120	Heterosexual women and men; Thailand	31% reduction in acquisition	Rerks-Ngarm, 2009
HVTN 702 (Uhambo Study)	ALVAC: Canarypox (gag, pol, env) \+ AIDSVAX C recombinant gp120	Adult women and men; South Africa	No efficacy	Gray, 2021
HVTN 705 (Imbokodo Study)	Engineered mosaic Ad26. Mos4.HIV \+ clade C and mosaic gp140	Heterosexual women; Sub-Saharan Africa	No efficacy	Gray, 2022
HVTN 706/ HPX3002 (Mosaico Study)	Engineered mosaic Ad26. Mos4.HIV\ + clade C and mosaic gp140	Cis-gender MSM and transgender women; United States, South America, and Europe	Ongoing, results expected 2023	Clinicaltrials.gov. NCT03964415

SOURCE: Adapted from Rubens et al., 2015; Tieu et al., 2013.

Nevertheless, pursuit of an effective vaccine remains important. Even with widespread ART availability and pharmacologic HIV prevention methods, an effective vaccine is essential to effectively addressing the global HIV epidemic (Fauci, 2017). The ability of a vaccine to elicit broadly neutralizing antibodies (bNAbs, antibodies that can protect against multiple pathogenic HIV strains by binding to highly conserved regions of the virus) is crucial for its success but thus far has been elusive. Recent advances in the identification and understanding of bNAbs have, however, injected new hope into HIV prevention research. While two randomized trials of VRC01, a bNAb targeting the HIV-1 CD4 binding site, did not show broad benefit when administered as infusions, there was a reduction in HIV incidence of HRC01-sensitive HIV-1 isolates, supporting a proof-of-concept that bNAbs can be effective tools for HIV prevention (Corey et al., 2021). Another bNAb, 3BNC117, has shown promise for further development, and in combination with 10-1074, has been shown to be safe and well tolerated (Caskey et al., 2015; Cohen et al., 2019). Such data provide optimism that bNAbs will further development of novel HIV prevention technologies, as well as continue to inform vaccine research. Additionally, the recent initiation of phase I trials looking at mRNA-mediated HIV vaccine delivery, a technology proven successful for SARS-COV-2, provides hope of an accelerated search for a long-awaited highly effective HIV vaccine.

RECOMMENDED READING

Fauci AS. An HIV vaccine is essential for ending the HIV/AIDS pandemic. *JAMA*. October 24, 2017;318(16):1535–1536.

Joseph Davey DL, Bekker LG, Bukusi EA, et al. Where are the pregnant and breastfeeding women in new pre-exposure prophylaxis trials? The imperative to overcome the evidence gap. *Lancet HIV*. March 2022;9(3):e214–e222.

Kanny D, Jeffries WL 4th, Chapin-Bardales J, et al. Racial/ethnic disparities in HIV preexposure prophylaxis among men who have sex with men—23 urban areas, 2017. *MMWR Morb Mortal Wkly Rep.* 2019;68(37):801–806. http://doi:10.15585/mmwr.mm6837a2

Krakower DS, Daskalakis DC, Feinberg J, Marcus JL. Tenofovir alafenamide for HIV preexposure prophylaxis: what can we DISCOVER about its true value? *Ann Intern Med.* 2020;172(4):281–282. http://doi:10.7326/M19-3337

Marcus JL, Killelea A, Krakower DS. Perverse incentives—HIV prevention and the 340B drug pricing program. *N Engl J Med.* June 2022;386(22):2064–2066.

CONCLUSION

Tremendous strides continue to be made in the vast field of HIV prevention. Although much attention has focused on ART-based interventions such as TasP and PrEP, "real-world" application of research findings generates important questions for clinical care delivery across varied resource landscapes, some of which remain unanswered. Ongoing disparities in access, acceptability, and consistent use of these interventions threaten to exacerbate existing disparities in HIV incidence. HIV providers can be important leaders in addressing internal biases and structural factors driving such inequities. Ultimately, a multifaceted approach including behavioral, structural, and established biomedical interventions is needed to make a significant and lasting impact on HIV globally.

REFERENCES

Abdool Karim Q, Abdool Karim SS, Frohlich JA, et al. Effectiveness and safety of tenofovir gel, an antiretroviral microbicide, for the prevention of HIV infection in women. *Science.* 2010;329(5996): 1168–1174.

Abdool Karim SS, Baxter C, Abdool Karim Q. Advancing HIV prevention using tenofovir-based pre-exposure prophylaxis. *Antiviral Therapy.* April 2022;27(2): doi:10.1177/13596535211067589

Achilles S, Kelly CW, Blithe DL, et al. "Pharmacokinetics, safety, and vaginal bleeding associated with continuous versus cyclic 90-day use of dapivirine and levonorgestrel vaginal rings for multipurpose prevention of HIV and pregnancy." Abstract OA06.01 from the 4th HIV Research for Prevention Conference (HIVR4P)// Virtual), 27 & 28 January | 3 & 4 February. 2020 *JIAS.* January 2021;24(S1):15. Accessed September 11, 2022.

Aidala AA, Wilson MG, Shubert V, et al. Housing status, medical care, and health outcomes among people living with HIV/AIDS: a systematic review. *Am J Public Health.* 2015;106:e1–e23.

Antiretroviral Pregnancy Registry Steering Committee. Antiretroviral Pregnancy Registry interim report for 1 January 1989 through 31 January 2022; Wilmington, NC: Registry Coordinating Center. www.APRegistry.com. Published 2022. Accessed September 16, 2022.

Antoni G, Tremblay C, Charreau I, et al. On-demand PrEP with TDF/FTC remains highly effective among MSM with infrequent sexual intercourse: a sub-study of the ANRS IPERGAY trial. [Abstract TUAC102]. In: *Program and abstracts of the 9th International AIDS Society Conference on HIV Science.* Paris, France; July 23–26, 2017.

Auvert B, Taljaard D, Lagarde E, et al. Randomized, controlled intervention trial of male circumcision for reduction of HIV infection risk: the ANRS 1265 trial. *PLoS Med.* 2005;2(11):e298.

Ayala G, Sprague L, van der Merwe LL, et al. Peer- and community-led responses to HIV: a scoping review. *PLoS One.* 2021;16(12):e0260555.

Baeten JM. Donnell D, Ndase P, et al. Antiretroviral prophylaxis for HIV prevention in heterosexual men and women. *N Engl J Med.* 2012;367:399–410.

Baggaley R, Boily M-C, White RG, et al. Risk of HIV-1 transmission for parenteral exposure and blood transfusion: a systematic review and meta-analysis. *AIDS.* 2006;20(6):805–812.

Bailey RC, Moses S, Parker CB, et al. Male circumcision for HIV prevention in young men in Kisumu, Kenya: a randomised controlled trial. *Lancet.* 2007;369:643.

Bazzi AR, Biancarelli DL, Childs E, et al. Limited knowledge and mixed interest in pre-exposure prophylaxis for HIV prevention among people who inject drugs. *AIDS Patient Care STDs.* 2018;32(12):529–537.

Bekerman E, Cox S, Babusis D, et al. Two-dose emtricitabine/tenofovir alafenamide plus bictegravir prophylaxis protects macaques against SHIV infection. *J Antimicrob Chemother.* February 11, 2021;76(3):692–698. https://doi.org/10.1093/jac/dkaa476

Bekker LG, Li S, Pathak S, et al. Safety and tolerability of injectable rilpivirine LA in HPTN 076: a phase 2 HIV pre-exposure prophylaxis study in women. *E Clin Med.* April 1, 2020;21(100303):n. pag. https://doi.org/10.1016/j.eclinm.2020.100303Belenko S, Visher C, Pearson F, et al. Efficacy of structured organizational change intervention on HIV testing in correctional facilities. *AIDS Educ Prev.* 2017;29(3):241–255.

Berry MS, Johnson MW. Does being drunk or high cause HIV sexual risk behavior? A systematic review of drug administration studies. *Pharmacol Biochem Behav.* 2018;164:125–138.

Biello KM, Bazzi AT, Mimiaga MJ, et al. Perspectives on HIV pre-exposure prophylaxis (PrEP) utilization and related intervention needs among people who inject drugs. *Harm Reduction Journal.* 2018;15(1):55.

Biello KB, Daddario SR, Hill-Rorie J, et al. Uptake and acceptability of MyChoices: results of a pilot RCT of a mobile app designed to increase HIV testing and PrEP uptake among young American MSM. *AIDS Behav.* 2022;26:3981–3990. https://doi:10.1007/s10461-022-03724-3. Accessed August 15, 2022.

Bowleg L, Malekzadeh AN, Mbaba M, Boone CA. Ending the HIV epidemic for all, not just some: structural racism as a fundamental but overlooked social-structural determinant of the US HIV epidemic. *Curr Opin HIV AIDS.* 2022;17(2):40–45.

Brawner BM, Kerr J, Castle BF, et al. A systematic review of neighborhood-level influences on HIV vulnerability. *AIDS Behav.* 2022;26(3): 874–934.

Broz D, Carnes N, Chapin-Bardales J, et al. Syringe services programs' role in ending the HIV epidemic in the U.S.: why we cannot do it without them. *Am J Prev Med.* 2021;61(5 Suppl 1):S118–S129.

Buchbinder SP, Mehrotra DV, Duerr A, et al. Efficacy assessment of a cell-mediated immunity HIV-1 vaccine(the Step Study): a double-blind, randomised, placebo-controlled, test-of-concept trial. *Lancet.* 2008;372(9653):1881–1893.

Buchbinder SP, Cohen SE, Hecht J. Getting to zero new diagnoses in San Francisco: what will it take? In: *Program and abstracts of the 2018 Conference on Retroviruses and Opportunistic Infections.* Boston, MA; March 4–7, 2018.

Busch MP. Four decades of HIV and transfusion safety: much accomplished but ongoing challenges. *Transfusion.* 2022;62(7): 1334–1339.

Bhushan NL, Stoner MCD, Groves AK, Kahn K, Pettifor AE. Partnership dynamics and HIV-related sexual behaviors among adolescent mothers in South Africa: a longitudinal analysis of HIV Prevention Trials Network 068 data. *J Adolesc Health.* 2022;71(1):63–69.

Cardo DM, Culver DH, Ciesielski CA, et al.; Centers for Disease Control and Prevention Needlestick Surveillance Group. A case control study of HIV seroconversion in health care workers after percutaneous exposure. *N Engl J Med.* 1997;337(21):1485–1490.

Carlisle NA, Booth JS, Rodgers JB, et al. Utilizing laboratory results to identify emergency department patients with indications for HIV pre-exposure prophylaxis. *AIDS Patient Care STDS.* 2022;36(8):285–290.

Caskey M, Klein F, Lorenzi JC, et al. Viraemia suppressed in HIV-1-infected humans by broadly neutralizing antibody 3BNC117. *Nature.* June 25, 2015;522(7557):487–491. http://doi:10.1038/nature14411. Epub April 8, 2015.

Centers for Disease Control and Prevention (CDC). Core indicators for monitoring the Ending the HIV Epidemic Initiative (preliminary data): National HIV Surveillance System data reported through June 2021; and preexposure prophylaxis (PrEP) data reported through March 2021. *HIV Surveillance Data* Tables 2021;2(No. 4). https://www.cdc.gov/hiv/library/reports/surveillance-data-tables/. Published October 2021c. Accessed September 16, 2022.

CDC. Effectiveness of prevention strategies to reduce the risk of acquiring or transmitting HIV. cdc.gov. https://www.cdc.gov/hiv/risk/estimates/preventionstrategies.html#anchor_1562942347. Published 2022. Accessed September 9, 2022.

CDC). PrEP for HIV prevention in the U.S. cdc.gov. https://www.cdc.gov/nchhstp/newsroom/fact-sheets/hiv/PrEP-for-hiv-prevention-in-the-US-factsheet.html. November 23, 2021d. Accessed September 18, 2022.

CDC. Male circumcision for HIV prevention fact sheet. cdc.gov. https://www.cdc.gov/nchhstp/newsroom/fact-sheets/hiv/male-circumcision-HIV-prevention-factsheet.html. July 12, 2022b. Accessed September 11, 2022.

CDC. Self-testing. cdc.gov. https://www.cdc.gov/hiv/testing/self-testing.html. July 31, 2021a. Accessed August 10, 2022.

CDC. US Public Health Service: preexposure prophylaxis for the prevention of HIV infection in the United States—2021 update: a clinical practice guideline. cdc.gov. https://www.cdc.gov/hiv/pdf/risk/prep/cdc-hiv-prep-guidelines-2021.pdf. Published December 2021b.

Chang JJ, Ashcraft AM. Human immunodeficiency virus in adolescents: risk, prevention, screening, and treatment. *Prim Care*. 2020;47(2):351–365.

Choopanya K, Martin M, Suntharasamai P, et al. Antiretroviral prophylaxis for HIV infection in injecting drug users in Bangkok, Thailand (the Bangkok Tenofovir Study): a randomised, double-blind, placebo-controlled phase 3 trial. *Lancet*. 2013;381:2083–2090.

Clinicaltrials.gov. NCT02750540. 2016. https://clinicaltrials.gov/ct2/show/NCT02750540. Accessed September 17, 2022.

Clinicaltrials.gov. NCT03762382. 2018. https://clinicaltrials.gov/ct2/show/NCT03762382. Accessed September 17, 2022.

Clinicaltrials.gov. NCT03762772. 2018. https://clinicaltrials.gov/ct2/show/NCT03762772. Accessed September 17, 2022.

Clinicaltrials.gov. NCT03964415. 2019. https://clinicaltrials.gov/ct2/show/NCT03964415. Accessed September 17, 2022.

Clinicaltrials.gov. NCT04047420. 2019. https://clinicaltrials.gov/ct2/show/. NCT04047420. Accessed September 17, 2022.

Clinicaltrials.gov. NCT04644029. 2020. https://clinicaltrials.gov/ct2/show/NCT04644029. Accessed September 17, 2022.

Clinicaltrials.gov. NCT04652700. 2020. https://clinicaltrials.gov/ct2/show/NCT04652700. Accessed September 17, 2022.

Clinicaltrials.gov. NCT04994509. 2021. https://clinicaltrials.gov/ct2/show/NCT04994509. Accessed September 17, 2022.

Clinicaltrials.gov. NCT005140954. 2021. https://clinicaltrials.gov/ct2/show/NCT05140954. Accessed September 17, 2022.

Clinicaltrials.gov. NCT04925752. https://clinicaltrials.gov/ct2/show/NCT04925752. Accessed September 17, 2022.

Cohen MS, Council OD, Chen, JS. Sexually transmitted infections and HIV in the era of antiretroviral treatment and prevention: the biologic basis for epidemiologic synergy. *J Int AIDS Soc*. 2019;22(S6):e25355

Cohen MS, Chen Y, McCauley M, t al. Final results of the HPTN 052 randomized controlled trial: antiretroviral therapy prevents HIV transmission. [Abstract MOAC0101LB]. *Program and abstracts of the 8th IAS Conference on HIV Pathogenesis, Treatment & Prevention*. Vancouver, Canada; July 19–22, 2015.

Cohen SE, Sachdev D, Lee SA, et al. Acquisition of tenofovir-susceptible, emtricitabine-resistant HIV despite high adherence to daily preexposure prophylaxis: a case report [published online ahead of print, 2018 Nov 29]. *Lancet HIV*. 2018;S2352–3018(18):30288–1.

Cohen YZ, Butler AL, Millard K, et al. Safety, pharmacokinetics, and immunogenicity of the combination of the broadly neutralizing anti-HIV-1 antibodies 3BNC117 and 10-1074 in healthy adults: a randomized, phase 1 study. *PLoS One*. 2019;14(8):e0219142. http://doi:10.1371/journal.pone.0219142

Colby DJ, Kroon E, Sacdalan C, et al. Acquisition of multidrug-resistant human immunodeficiency virus type 1 infection in a patient taking preexposure prophylaxis. *Clin Infect Dis*. 2018;67(6):962–964.

Corey L, Gilbert P, Juraska M, et al. Two randomized trials of neutralizing antibodies to prevent HIV-1 acquisition. *N Engl J Med*. 2021;18;384(11):1003–1014.

Cranston RD, Lama JR, Richardson BA, et al. MTN-017: A rectal phase 2 extended safety and acceptability study of tenofovir reduced-glycerin 1% gel. *Clin Infect Dis*. 2017;64(5):614–620. http://doi:10.1093/cid/ciw832

Cresswell F, Asanati K, Bhagani S, et al.; British HIV Association. UK guideline for the use of HIV post-exposure prophylaxis 2021. https://www.bhiva.org/file/6183b6aa93a4e/PEP-guidelines.pdf. Published February 14, 2022. Accessed August 22, 2022.

Cruess DG, Burnham KE, Finitsis DJ, et al. A randomized clinical trial of a brief internet-based group intervention to reduce sexual transmission risk behavior among HIV-positive gay and bisexual men. *Ann Behav Med*. 2018;52(2):116–129.

Csete J, Kamarulzaman A, Kazatchkine M, et al. Public health and international drug policy: report of the John Hopkins-Lancet Commission on Drug Policy and Health. *Lancet*. 2016;387(10026):1427–1480.

Decker MR, Lyons C, Guan K, et al. A systematic review of gender-based violence prevention and response interventions for HIV key populations: female sex workers, men who have sex with men, and people who inject drugs. *Trauma Violence Abuse*. 2022;23(2):676–694.

DeHaan E, McGowan JP, Fine SM, et al. *PEP to prevent HIV infection* [Internet]. Baltimore, MD: Johns Hopkins University; August 11, 2022. PMID: 33026756.

Delany-Moretlwe S, Hughes JP, Bock P, et al. Cabotegravir for the prevention of HIV-1 in women: results from HPTN 084, a phase 3, randomized clinical trial. *Lancet*. 2022a;399(10337):1779–1789.

Delany-Moretlwe S, Hughes JP, et al. Evaluation of CAB-LA safety and PK in pregnant women in the blinded phase of HPTN 084. [Abstract 700]. In: *Conference on Retroviruses and Opportunistic Infections*. Virtual; February 12–16, 2022b.

Del Rio C. How do we stop the band from playing on in the US? [Abstract 61]. In: *Conference on Retroviruses and Opportunistic Infections*. Boston, MA; March 8–11, 2020.

DiNenno EA, Delaney KP, Pitasi MA, et al. HIV testing before and during the COVID-19 pandemic—United States, 2019–2020. *MMWR Morb Mortal Wkly Rep*. 2022;71(25):820–824.

Dimitrov D, Moore JR, Wood D, et al. Predicted effectiveness of daily and nondaily preexposure prophylaxis for men who have sex with men based on sex and pill-taking patterns from the Human Immuno Virus Prevention Trials Network 067/ADAPT study. *Clin Infect Dis*. 2020;71(2):249–255. http://doi:10.1093/cid/ciz799

Dominguez K, Smith DK, Vasavi T, et al. Updated guidelines for antiretroviral postexposure prophylaxis after sexual, injection drug use, or other non-occupational exposure to HIV—United States, 2016. US Centers for Disease Control and Prevention. http://stacks.cdc.gov/view/cdc/38856. Published 2018. Accessed September 24, 2020.

Dong BJ, William MR, Bingham JT, et al. Outcomes of challenging HIV case consultations provided via teleconference by the Clinician Consultation Center to the Federal Bureau of Prisons. *J Am Pharm Assoc*. 2017;57(4):516–519.

Donnell D, Ramos E, Celum C, et al. The effect of oral preexposure prophylaxis on the progression of HIV-1 seroconversion. *AIDS*. 2017;31(14):2007–2016.

Eastment MC, McClelland RS. Vaginal microbiota and susceptibility to HIV. *AIDS*. 2018;32(6):687–698.

Esheleman SH, Fogel JM, Piwowar-Manning E, et al. Characterization of human immunodeficiency virus (HIV) infections in women who received injectable cabotegravir or tenofovir disoproxil fumarate/emtricitabine for HIV prevention: HPTN 084. *J Infect Dis*. May 16, 2022;225(10):1741–1749. http://doi:10.1093/infdis/jiab576

Fauci AS. An HIV vaccine is essential for ending the HIV/AIDS pandemic. *JAMA*. October 24, 2017;318(16):1535–1536. http://doi:10.1001/jama.2017.13505. PMID: 29052689.

Foster R, McAllister J, Read TR, et al. Single-tablet emtricitabine-rilpivirine-tenofovir as HIV postexposure prophylaxis in men who have sex with men. *Clin Infect Dis*. October 15, 2015;61(8):1336–1341. http://doi:10.1093/cid/civ511. PMID: 26123937.

Flynn NM, Forthal DN, Harro CD, et al. Placebo-controlled phase 3 trial of a recombinant glycoprotein 120 vaccine to prevent HIV-1 infection. *J Infect Dis*. 2005;191(5):654–665.

Friedland BA, Mathur S, Haddad LB. The promise of the dual prevention pill: a framework for development and introduction. *Front Reprod Health*. 2021;3:682689. http://doi:10.3389/frph.2021.682689.

Fu R, Hou J, Gu Y, Yu NX. Do couple-based interventions show larger effects in promoting HIV preventive behaviors than individualized interventions in couples? A systematic review and meta-analysis of 11 randomized controlled trials. *AIDS Behav*. July 15, 2022. http://doi:10.1007/s10461-022-03768-5. Online ahead of print.

Gantner P, Hessamfar M, Souala MF, et al. E/C/F/TAF PEP Study Group. Elvitegravir-cobicistat-emtricitabine-tenofovir alafenamide single-tablet regimen for human immunodeficiency virus postexposure prophylaxis. *Clin Infect Dis*. February 14, 2020;70(5):943–946. http://doi:10.1093/cid/ciz577. PMID: 31804669.

Garcia J, Parker C, Parker RG, et al. "You're really gonna kick us all out?" Sustaining safe spaces for community-based HIV prevention and control among black men who have sex with men. *PLoS One.* 2015;10(10):e0141326.

Goedel WC, Rogers BG, Li Y, et al. Pre-exposure prophylaxis discontinuation during the COVID-19 pandemic among men who have sex with men in a multisite clinical cohort in the United States. *J Acquir Immune Defic Syndr.* October 1, 2022;91(2):151–156. http://doi:10.1097/QAI.0000000000003042

Grant RM., Lama JR, Anderson PL, et al. Preexposure chemoprophylaxis for HIV prevention in men who have sex with men. *N Engl J Med.* 2010;363:2587–2599.

Gray RH, Kigozi G, Serwadda D, et al. Male circumcision for HIV prevention in men in Rakai, Uganda: a randomised trial. *Lancet.* 2007;369:657–666.

Gray GE, Allen M, Moodie Z, et al. Safety and efficacy of the HVTN 503/Phambili study of a clade-B-based HIV-1 vaccine in South Africa: a double-blind, randomized, placebo-controlled test-of-concept phase 2b study. *Lancet HIV Dis.* 2011;11(7):507–515.

Gray GE, Bekker LG, Laher F, et al; HVTN 702 Study Team. Vaccine efficacy of ALVAC-HIV and bivalent subtype C gp120-MF59 in adults. *N Engl J Med.* 2021;384(12):1089–1100. http://doi: 10.1056/NEJMoa2031499

Gray G, Mngadi K, Lavreys L, et al. Phase IIb efficacy trial of mosaic HIV-1 vaccine regimen in African women: Imbokodo. [Abstract 121.] In: *Program and abstracts of the 2022 Conference on Retroviruses and Opportunistic Infections.* ; February 12–16, 2022. Denver, CO and Virtual.

Grosskurth H, Mosha F, Todd J, et al. Impact of improved treatment of sexually transmitted diseases on HIV infection in rural Tanzania: randomised controlled trial. *Lancet.* 1995;346:530–536.

Gunawardana M, Remedios-Chan M, Sanchez D, et al. Fundamental aspects of long-acting tenofovir alafenamide delivery from subdermal implants for HIV prophylaxis. *Sci Rep.* 2022;12:8224. https://doi.org/10.1038/s41598-022-11020-2

Hammer SM. Advances in preventive HIV vaccines: efficacy trial evolution. [Oral session 0021]. In: *ID Week 2015.* San Diego, CA; October 7–11, 2015.

Hammer SM, Sobieszczyk ME, Janes H, et al. Efficacy trial of a DNA/rAd5 HIV-1 preventive vaccine. *N Engl J Med.* 2013;369:2083–2092.

Harrison SE, Muessig K, Poteat T, et al. Addressing racism's role in the US HIV epidemic: qualitative findings from three Ending the HIV Epidemic prevention projects. *J Acquir Immune Defic Syndr.* 2022;90(S1):S46–S55.

Hendrix CW, Chen BA, Guddera V, et al. MTN-001: randomized pharmacokinetic cross-over study comparing tenofovir vaginal gel and oral tablets in vaginal tissue and other compartments. *PLoS One.* 2013;8(1):e55013. http://doi:10.1371/journal.pone.0055013

Hoenigl M, Chaillon A, Moore DJ, et al. Clear links between starting methamphetamine and increasing sexual risk behavior: a cohort study among men who have sex with men. *J AIDS.* 2016;71(5):551–557.

Hoornenborg E, de Bree GJ. Acute infection with a wild-type HIV-1 virus in PrEP user with high TDF levels. [Abstract 953]. In: *Program and abstracts of the 2017 Conference on Retroviruses and Opportunistic Infections.* Seattle, WA; February 13–16, 2017.

Hosek S, Pettifor A. HIV prevention interventions for adolescents. *Curr HIV/AIDS Rep.* 2019;16(1):120–128.

Huang YA, Zhu W, Smith DK, et al. Preexposure prophylaxis by race and ethnicity—United States, 2014–2016. *MMWR. Morb Mort Wkly Rep.* 2018;67:1147–1150. http://dx.doi.org/10.15585/mmwr.mm6741a3

Ickowicz S, Hayashi K, Dong H, et al. Benzodiazepine use as an independent risk factor for HIV infection in a Canadian setting. *Drug Alcohol Depend.* 2015;155:190–194.

Iroh PA, Mayo H, Nijhawan AE. The HIV care cascade before, during, and after incarceration: a systematic review and data synthesis. *Am J Public Health.* 2015;105(7):e5–e16.

Jones J, Knox J, Meanley S, et al. Explorations of the role of digital technology in HIV-related implementation research: case comparisons of five Ending the HIV Epidemic supplement awards. *J Acquir Immune Defic Syndr.* 2022;90(S1):S226–S234.

Joseph Davey DL, Bekker LG, Bukusi EA, et al. Where are the pregnant and breastfeeding women in new pre-exposure prophylaxis trials? The imperative to overcome the evidence gap. *Lancet HIV.* March 2022;9(3):e214–e222.

Kamis KF, Marx GE, Scott KA, et al. Same-day HIV pre-exposure prophylaxis (PrEP) initiation during drop-in sexually transmitted diseases clinic appointments is a highly acceptable, feasible, and safe model that engages individuals at risk for HIV into PrEP care. *Open Forum Infect Dis.* 2019;6(7):ofz310. http://doi: 10.1093/ofid/ofz310

Kanny D, Jeffries WL IV, Chapin-Bardales J, et al. Racial/ethnic disparities in HIV preexposure prophylaxis among men who have sex with men—23 urban areas, 2017. *MMWR. Morb Mortal Wkly Rep.* 2019;68:801–806. http://dx.doi.org/10.15585/mmwr.mm6837a2

Khan MR, McGinnis KA, Grov C, et al. Past year and prior incarceration and HIV transmission risk among HIV-positive men who have sex with men in the US. *AIDS Care.* 2019;31(3):349–356.

Knox DC, Anderson PL, Harrigan R, et al. Multidrug-resistant HIV-1 infection despite preexposure prophylaxis. *N Engl J Med.* 2017;376:501–502. http://doi:10.1056/NEJMc1611639

Kuhar DT, Henderson DK, Struble KA, et al. Updated USPHS guidelines for the management of occupational exposures to human immunodeficiency virus and recommendations for post-exposure prophylaxis. *Infect Control Hosp Epidemiol.* 2013;34(9):875–892.

Kuo I, Agopian A, Opoku J, et al. Assessing PrEP needs among heterosexuals and people who inject drugs, Washington, DC. [Abstract 1030]. In: *Program and abstracts of the 2018 Conference on Retroviruses and Opportunistic Infection.* Boston, MA; March 4–7, 2018.

Landovitz RJ, Donnell D, Clement ME, et al. Cabotegravir for HIV prevention in cisgender men and transgender women. *N Engl J Med.* 2021;385(7):595–608. http://doi:10.1056/NEJMoa2101016

Landovitz RJ, Donnell D, Tran H, et al. Updated efficacy, safety, and case studies in HPTN 083: CAB-LA vsTDF/FTC for PrEP. [Abstract 96]. *Conference on Retroviruses and Opportunistic Infections.* Virtual; February 12–16, 2022.

Lee K, Trujillo L, Olansky E, et al. Factors associated with use of HIV prevention and health care among transgender women—seven urban areas, 2019–2020. *MMWR Morb Mortal Wkly Rep.* 2022;71(20):673–679.

Lee SS, Anderson PL, Kwan TH, et al. Failure of pre-exposure prophylaxis with daily tenofovir/emtricitabine and the scenario of delayed HIV seroconversion. *Int J. Infect Dis.* 2020;94:41–43.

Lunding S, Katzenstein TL, Kronborg G, et al. The Danish PEP Registry: experience with the use of post-exposure prophylaxis following blood exposure to HIV from 1999–2012. *Infect Dis.* 2016;48(3):195–200. Epub ahead of print.

Malinverni S, Bédoret F, Bartiaux M, et al. Single-tablet regimen of emtricitabine/tenofovir disoproxil fumarate plus cobicistat-boosted elvitegravir increase adherence for HIV postexposure prophylaxis in sexual assault victims. *Sex Transm Infect.* 2021;97(5):329–333. http://doi:10.1136/sextrans-2020-054714. Epub October 26, 2020. PMID: 33106437.

Malone J, Reisner SL, Cooney EE, et al. Perceived HIV acquisition risk and low uptake of PrEP among a cohort of transgender women with PrEP indication in the Eastern and Southern United States. *J Acquir Immune Defic Syndr.* 2021;88(1):10–18.

Maloney KM, Benkeser D, Sullivan PS, et al. Sexual mixing by HIV status and pre-exposure prophylaxis use among men who have sex with men: addressing information bias. *Epidemiology.* 2022;33(6):808–816. http://doi:10.1097/EDE.0000000000001525. Online ahead of print.

Malekinejad M, Jimsheleishvili S, Barker EK, et al. Sexual practice changes post-HIV diagnosis among men who have sex with men in the United States: a systematic review and meta-analysis. *AIDS Behav.* 2023;27(1):257–278. Epub 2022 Jul 12. doi: 10.1007/s10461-022-03761-y.

Mann LM, Kelley CF, Siegler AJ, Stephenson R, Sullivan PS. Seroadaptive strategy patterns of young black gay, bisexual, and other men who have sex with men in Atlanta, Georgia. *J Acquir Immune Defic Syndr.* 2022;89(1):40–48.

Marcus JL, Katz KA, Krakower DS, Calabrese SK. Risk compensation and clinical decision making—the case of HIV preexposure prophylaxis. *N Engl J Med*. 2019;380(6):510–512. http://doi:10.1056/NEJMp1810743

Marcus JL, Killelea A, Krakower DS. Perverse incentives—HIV prevention and the 340B Drug Pricing Program. *N Engl J Med*. 2022;386(22):2064–2066.

Markowitz M, Grossman H, Anderson PL, et al. Newly acquired infection with multidrug-resistant HIV-1 in a patient adherent to preexposure prophylaxis. *J Acquir Immune Defic Syndr*. 2017;76(4):e104–E106. http://doi:10.1097/QAI.0000000000001534

Marrazzo JM, Gita R, Richardson BA, et al. Tenofovir-based preexposure prophylaxis for HIV infection among African women. *N Engl J Med*. 2015;372:509–518.

Marzinke MA, Grinsztejn B, Fogel JM, et al. Characterization of human immunodeficiency virus (HIV) infection in cisgender men and transgender women who have sex with men receiving injectable cabotegravir for HIV prevention: HPTN 083. *J Infect Dis*. 2021;224(9):1581–1592.

Massud I, Kovarova M, Wong-Sam A, et al. In situ forming implants with cabotegravir for ultra long-acting PrEP. [Abstract 855]. In: *Program and abstracts of the 2022 Conference on Retroviruses and Opportunistic Infections*, February 12–16, 2022. Denver, CO and Virtural.

Matthews RP, Barrett SE, Patel M, et al. First-in-human trial of MK-8591-eluting implants demonstrates concentrations suitable for HIV prophylaxis for at least one year. [Late breaker post abstract TUAC0401LB]. *10th IAS Conference on HIV Science (IAS 2019)*. Mexico City; July 21–24, 2019.

Mayer KH, Gelman M, Holmes J, et al. Safety and tolerability of once daily coformulated bictegravir, emtricitabine, and tenofovir alafenamide for postexposure prophylaxis after sexual exposure. *J Acquir Immune Defic Syndr*. 2022;90(1):27–32. http://doi:10.1097/QAI.0000000000002912

Mayer KH, Molina JM, Thompson MA, et al. Emtricitabine and tenofovir alafenamide vs emtricitabine and tenofovir disoproxil fumarate for HIV pre-exposure prophylaxis (DISCOVER): primary results from a randomised, double-blind, multicentre, active-controlled, phase 3, non-inferiority trial. *Lancet*. 2020;396(10246):239–254. http://doi:10.1016/S0140-6736(20)31065-5

Mayer KH, Grasso C, Levine K, et al. Increasing PrEP uptake, persistent disparities in at-risk patients in a Boston Center. [Abstract 101]. In: *Program and abstracts of the 2018 Conference on Retroviruses and Opportunistic Infections*. Boston, MA; March 4–7, 2018.

Mayer KH, Jones D, Oldenburg C, et al. Optimal HIV postexposure prophylaxis regimen completion with single tablet daily elvitegravir/cobicistat/tenofovir disoproxil fumarate/emtricitabine compared with more frequent dosing regimens. *J Acquir Immune Defic Syndr*. 2017;75(5):535–539. http://doi: 10.1097/QAI.0000000000001440. PMID: 28696345; PMCID: PMC5606152.

Mayer KH, Venkatesh KK. Interactions of HIV and other sexually transmitted diseases, and genital tract inflammation facilitating local pathogen transmission and acquisition. *Am J Reprod Immunol*. 2011;65:308–316.

McCormack S, Dunn DT, Desai M, et al. Pre-exposure prophylaxis to prevent the acquisition of HIV-1 infection (PROUD): effectiveness results from the pilot phase of a pragmatic open-label randomised trial. *Lancet*. 2016;387(10013):53–60. doi:10.1016/S0140-6736(15)00056-2.

Melendez-Torres GJ, Meiksin R, Witzel TC, et al. eHealth interventions to address HIV and other sexually transmitted infections, sexual risk behavior, substance use, and mental ill-health in men who have sex with men: systematic review and meta-analysis. *JMIR Public Health Surveill*. 2022;8(4):e27061.

Mohareb AM, Larmarange J, Kim AY, et al. Risks and benefits of oral HIV pre-exposure prophylaxis for people with chronic hepatitis B. *Lancet HIV*. August 2022;9(8):e585–e594. http://doi:10.1016/S2352-3018(22)00123-0

Molina JM, Capitant C, Charreau I, et al. On demand PrEP with oral TDF/FTC in MSM: results of the ANRS Ipergay trial. *N Engl J Med*. 2015;373:2237–2246.

Molina JM, Charreau I, Spire B, Cotte L, Chas J, Capitant C. Efficacy, safety, and effect on sexual behavior of on-demand pre-exposure prophylaxis for HIV in men who have sex with men: an observational cohort study. *Lancet*. 2017;4(9): E402–E410. http://doi:10.1016/S2352-3018(17)30089-9

Molina JM, Ghosn J, Assoumou L, et al. Daily and on-demand HIV pre-exposure prophylaxis with emtricitabine and tenofovir disoproxil (ANRS PREVENIR): a prospective observational cohort study. *Lancet HIV*. 2022;9(8):e554–e562. http://doi:10.1016/S2352-3018(22)00133-3. PMID: 35772417.

Moorman AC, de Perio MA, Goldschmidt R, et al. Testing and clinical management of health care personnel potentially exposed to hepatitis C virus—CDC guidance, United States, 2020. *MMWR Recomm Rep*. 2020;69(RR-6):1–8.

Mugo N, Mudhune V, Heffron R, et al. Randomized, placebo-controlled trial of safety, pharmacokinetics, and pharmacodynamics of 90-day intravaginal rings (IVRs) releasing tenofovir (TFV) with and without levonorgestrel (LNG) among women in Western Kenya. [Abstract OA06.02]. *HIV Research for Prevention (HIVR4P)*. Virtual conference; 2021.

Mulligan K, Glidden DV, Anderson PL, et al. Effects of emtricitabine/tenofovir on bone mineral density in HIV-negative persons in a randomized, double-blind, placebo-controlled trial. *Clin Infect Dis*. 2015;61(4):572–580.

New York State Department of Health AIDS Institute. PrEP to prevent HIV and promote sexual health. https://www.hivguidelines.org/prep-for-prevention/. Published 2022. May 2022 revision. Accessed September 15, 2022.

Ngure K, Nair G, Szydlo D, et al. Choice and adherence to dapivirine ring or oral PrEP by young African women in REACH. [Abstract 82.] *Conference on Retroviruses and Opportunistic Infections*. Virtual; February 12–16, 2022.

Ogbuagu O, Ruane PJ, Podzamczer D, et al. Long-term safety and efficacy of emtricitabine and tenofovir alafenamide vs emtricitabine and tenofovir disoproxil fumarate for HIV-1 pre-exposure prophylaxis: week 96 results from a randomised, double-blind, placebo-controlled, phase 3 trial. *Lancet HIV*. 2021;8(7):e397–e407. http://doi:10.1016/S2352-3018(21)00071-0

Opara I, Pierre K, Assan MA, et al. A systematic review on sexual health and drug use prevention interventions for black girls. *Int J Environ Res Public Health*. 2022;19(6):3176.

Otten RA, Smith DK, Adams DR, et al. Efficacy of postexposure prophylaxis after intravaginal exposure of pig-tailed macaques to a human-derived retrovirus (human immunodeficiency virus type 2). *J Virol*. 2000;74(20):9771–9775.

Perlman D, Jordan AE. The syndemic of opioid misuse, overdose, HCV, and HIV: structural-level causes and interventions. *Current HIV/AIDS Reports*. 2018;15:96–112.

Pitisuttithum P, Gilbert P, Gurwith M, et al. Randomized, double-blind, placebo-controlled efficacy trial of a bivalent recombinant glycoprotein 120 HIV-1 vaccine among injection drug users in Bangkok, Thailand. *J Infect Dis*. 2006;194:1661–1671.

Poteat T, Malik M, Scheim A, Elliott A. HIV prevention among transgender populations: knowledge gaps and evidence for action. *Curr HIV/AIDS Rep*. 2017;14(4):141–152.

Reback CJ, Fletcher JB. HIV prevalence, substance use, and sexual risk behaviors among transgender women recruited through outreach. *AIDS Behav*. 2014;18(7):1359–1367.

Rerks-Ngarm S, Pitisuttithum P, Nitayaphan S, et al. Vaccination with ALVAC and AIDSVAX to prevent HIV-1 infection in Thailand. *N Engl J Med*. 2009;361:2209–2220.

Rich KM, Bia J, Altice FL, et al. Integrated models of care for individuals with opioid use disorder: how do we prevent HIV and HCV? *Curr HIV/AIDS Rep*. 2018;15(3):266–275.

Richterman A, Thirumurthy H. The effects of case transfer programmes on HIV-related outcomes in 42 countries from 1996 to 2019. *Nat Hum Behav*. 2022;6(10):1362–1371. http://doi:10.1038/s41562-022-01414-7. Epub 2022 Jul 18. Rimmler S, Golin C, Coleman J, et al. Structural barriers to HIV prevention and services: perspectives of

African American women in low-income communities. *Health Educ Behav.* 2022;10901981221109138.

Rubens M, Ramamoorthy V, Saxena A, et al. HIV vaccine: recent advances, current roadblocks, and future directions. *J Immunol Res.* 2015;2015:560347. http://doi:10.1155/2015/560347.2015

Saag MS, Gandhi RT, Hoy JF, et al. Antiretroviral drugs for treatment and prevention of HIV infection in adults: 2020 recommendations of the International Antiviral Society–USA Panel. *JAMA.* 2020;324(16):1651–1669. http://doi:10.1001/jama.2020.17025

Schnall R, Kuhns LM, Hidalgo MA, et al. Adaptation of a group-based HIV RISK reduction intervention to a mobile app for young sexual minority men. *AIDS Educ Prev.* 2018;30(6):449–462. http://doi:10.1521/aeap.2018.30.6.449

Sevelius JM, Poteat T, Luhur WE, et al. HIV testing and PrEP use in a national probability sample of sexually active transgender people in the United States. *J Acq Imm Def Syndr.* 2020;84(5):437–442.

Shih CC, Kaneshima H, Rabin L, et al. Post exposure prophylaxis with zidovudine suppresses human immunodeficiency virus type 1 infection in SCID-hu mice in a time-dependent manner. *J Infect Dis.* 1991;163(3):625–627.

Siegfried N, Muller M, Deeks JJ, et al. Male circumcision for prevention of heterosexual acquisition of HIV in men. *Cochrane Database Syst Rev.* 2009;2:CD003362. http://doi:10.1002/14651858.CD003362.pub2

Simmons R, Plunkett J, Cieply L, et al. Blood-borne virus testing in emergency departments—a systematic review of seroprevalence, feasibility, acceptability and linkage to care. *HIV Med.* 2023;24(1):6–26. doi: 10.1111/hiv.13328.

Solomon MM, Lama JR, Glidden DV, et al. Change in renal function associated with oral FTC/TDF use for HIV pre-exposure prophylaxis. *AIDS.* 2014;28:851–859.

Solomon MM, Schechter M, Liu AY, et al. The safety of tenofovir-emtricitabine for HIV pre-exposure prophylaxis (PrEP) in individuals with active hepatitis B. *J AIDS.* 2016;71(3):281–286. http://doi:10.1097/QAI.0000000000000857

Spears CE, Taylor BS, Liu AY, Levy SM, Eaton EF. Intersecting epidemics: the impact of COVID-19 on the HIV prevention and care continua in the United States. *AIDS.* 2022;36(13):1749–1759. http://doi:10.1097/QAD.0000000000003305. Epub 2022 Jun 22.

Spinelli MA, Lowery B, Shuford JA, et al. Use of drug-level testing and single-genome sequencing to unravel a case of HIV seroconversion on PrEP. *Clinical Infectious Diseases.* 2021;72(11):2025–2028. doi.org/10.1093/cid/ciaa1011. Epub 2020 Jul.

Stone J, Fraser H, Lim AG, et al. Incarceration history and risk of HIV and hepatitis C virus acquisition among people who inject drugs: a systematic review and meta-analysis. *Lancet Infect Dis.* 2018;18(12):1397–1409.

Stoner MCD, Kilburn K, Godfrey-Faussett P, Ghys P, Pettifor AE. Cash transfers for HIV prevention: a systematic review. *PLoS Med.* 2021;18(11):e1003866.

Strong C, Huang P, Li CW, et al. HIV, chemsex, and the need for harm-reduction interventions to support gay, bisexual, and other men who have sex with men. *Lancet HIV.* 2022;9(10):e717–e725. doi:10.1016/S2352-3018(22)00124-2. Epub 2022 Aug.

Taylor JL, Walley AY, Bazzi AR. Stuck in the window with you: HIV exposure prophylaxis in the highest risk people who inject drugs. *Subst Abus.* 2019;40(4):441–443. http://doi:10.1080/08897077.2019.1675118

Thaden JT, Gandhi M, Okochi H, Hurt CB, McKellar MS. Seroconversion on preexposure prophylaxis: a case report with segmental hair analysis for timed adherence determination. *AIDS.* 2018;32(9):F1–F4. http://doi:10.1097/QAD.0000000000001825

Thigpen MC, Kebaabetswe PM, Paxton LA, et al. Antiretroviral prophylaxis for heterosexual HIV transmission in Botswana. *N Engl J Med.* 2012;367:423–434.

Tieu HV, Rolland M, Hammer SM, et al. Translational research insights from completed HIV vaccine efficacy trials. *J AIDS.* 2013;63:S150–S154.

Thompson KA, Hughes JP, Baeten J, et al. Increased risk of HIV acquisition among women throughout pregnancy and during the postpartum period: a prospective per-coital-act analysis among women with HIV-infected partners. *J Infect Dis.* 2018;218(1):16–25.

Touesnard N, Brothers TD, Bonn M, Edelman EJ. Overdose deaths and HIV infections among people who use drugs: shared determinants and integrated responses. *Expert Rev Anti Infect Ther.* 2022;20(8):1061–1065.

US Department of Health and Human Services. Panel on Antiretroviral Guidelines for Adults and Adolescents. Guidelines for the use of antiretroviral agents in adults and adolescents with HIV. https://clinicalinfo.hiv.gov/en/guidelines/. Published 2022. Accessed September 10, 2022.

US Food and Drug Administration. Coronavirus (COVID-19) update: FDA provides updated guidance to address the urgent need for blood during the pandemic. fda.gov. https://www.fda.gov/news-events/press-announcements/coronavirus-covid-19-update-fda-provides-updated-guidance-address-urgent-need-blood-during-pandemic. Published 2020. Accessed August 9, 2020.

US Preventive Services Task Force. Screening for hepatitis C virus infection in adolescents and adults: US Preventive Services Task Force recommendation statement. *JAMA.* 2020;323(10):970–975. http://doi:10.1001/jama.2020.1123

Valera P, Chang Y, Lian Z. HIV risk inside US prisons: a systematic review of risk reduction interventions conducted in US prisons. *AIDS Care.* 2017;29(8):943–952.

Van Damme L, Corneli A, Ahmed K, et al. Preexposure prophylaxis for HIV infection among African women. *N Engl J Med.* 2012;367:411–422.

Veronese V, Ryan KE, Hughes C, et al. Using digital communication technology to increase HIV testing among men who have sex with men and transgender women: systematic review and meta-analysis. *J Med Internet Res.* 2020;22(7):e14230.

Volk JE, Marcus JL, Phengrasamy T, et al. No new HIV infections with increasing use of HIV preexposure prophylaxis in a clinical practice setting. *Clin Infect Dis.* 2015;61(10):1601–1603.

Weiss HA, Hankins CA, Dickson K. Male circumcision and risk of HIV infection in women: a systematic review and meta-analysis. *Lancet Infect Dis.* 2009;9:669–677.

Wilkins NJ, Rasberry C, Liddon N, et al. Addressing HIV/sexually transmitted diseases and pregnancy prevention through schools: an approach for strengthening education, health services, and school environments that promote adolescent sexual health and well-being. *J Adolesc Health.* 2022;70(4):540–549.

Wirtz AL, Yeh PT, Flath N, et al. HIV and viral hepatitis among imprisoned key populations. *Epidemiologic Rev.* 2018;40(1):12–26.

WHO. *Consolidated guidelines on HIV prevention, testing, treatment, service delivery and monitoring: recommendations for a public health approach.* Geneva: World Health Organization; 2021. License: CC BY-NC-SA 3.0 IGO.

WHO. *Preventing HIV through safe voluntary medical male circumcision for adolescent boys and men in generalized HIV epidemics: recommendations and key considerations.* Geneva: World Health Organization; 2020. License: CC BY-NC-SA 3.0 IGO.

WHO. World Health Organization consolidated guidelines on the use of antiretroviral drugs for treating and preventing HIV infection. Recommendations for a public health approach—second edition, 2016. https://www.who.int/hiv/pub/arv/arv-2016/en/. Published 2016. Accessed August 15, 2022.

Young TN, Arens FJ, Kennedy GE, et al. Antiretroviral post-exposure prophylaxis (PEP) for occupational HIV exposure. *Cochrane Database Sys Rev.* 2007;1:CD002835.

Yuan T, Fitzpatrick T, Ko NY, et al. Circumcision to prevent HIV and other sexually transmitted infections in men who have sex with men: a systematic review and meta-analysis of global data. *Lancet Glob Health.* April 2019;7(4):e436–e447. http://doi:10.1016/S2214-109X(18)30567-9

Zanakis SH, Alvarez C, Li V. Socio-economic determinants of HIV/AIDS pandemic and nations efficiencies. *Eur J Operational Res.* 2007;176:1811–1838.

Zash R. Update on neural tube defects with antiretroviral exposure in the Tsepamo study, Botswana. *23rd International AIDS Conference*; July 6–10, 2020; virtual. https://www.natap.org/2020/IAC/IAC_112.htm

6.

IMMUNOLOGY

Dennis J. Hartigan-O'Connor and Christian Brander

MECHANISMS OF CD4 + T-CELL DECLINE

LEARNING OBJECTIVE

- Describe the processes contributing to CD4 + T-cell decline and immune activation in untreated HIV infection.

WHAT'S NEW

Chronic inflammation in HIV disease may have its origins in translocation of microbial products across a Th17 cell-deficient mucosal barrier. Collagen deposition in lymph nodes contributes to T-cell loss by interrupting homeostasis. Sensing of intracellular pathogens, including HIV in abortively infected cells, contributes to progressive CD4 + T-cell loss in chronic HIV infection.

KEY POINTS

- Cytopathic infection alone is insufficient to explain CD4+ T-cell loss in HIV infection.

- Chronic inflammation is strongly associated with CD4 + T-cell loss in pathogenic lentiviral infections such as HIV but is not seen in nonpathogenic infections.

- Abortive infection of T-cells leads to their elimination.

- Translocation of microbial constituents and lymph node scarring have been recognized as likely contributors to CD4 + T-cell decline.

The prototypic outcomes associated with untreated HIV infection are progressive CD4 + T-cell decline, consequent immunodeficiency, and chronic inflammation. In untreated disease, circulating memory CD4 + T-cells, some of which are virus infected, are both dividing and dying at an accelerated rate (Hellerstein et al., 1999). In addition, CD4 + T-cells that reside in the gastrointestinal mucosa are important early targets of infection and are decimated early in disease (Guadalupe et al., 2003; Heise et al., 1994; Veazey et al., 1998). Although direct cytopathic infection contributes to CD4 + T-cell loss, many *uninfected* CD4 + T-cells are dying in HIV disease; thus, other mechanisms must be invoked

to fully explain CD4 + T-cell decline. The death of infected cells is likely due to exposure to Tat, Gp120, or other toxic proteins (all of which can induce apoptosis) and/or adaptive immune clearance of HIV-infected cells (Lenardo et al., 2002). In addition, abortive infection of T-cells (i.e., cells that become infected with the virus but where the virus can not complete reverse transcription and thus is not productively infected) can lead to massive cell death in tissue. Such abortive infection drives a process known as *pyroptosis*, a form of programmed cell death triggered by danger signals within the abortively infected cell) and which is believed to significantly contribute to the loss of CD4 + T-cells (He et al., 2022; Ke et al., 2017). Pyroptosis is an intensely inflammatory form of cell death attributed to the release of proinflammatory cytokines including IL-1β, and so additionally contributes to the inflammatory processes discussed below. HIV can also impair CD4 + T-cell regeneration by destroying the immunologic niches that are required for T-cell homeostasis, by depleting essential hematopoietic progenitor cells, and by inhibiting the regenerative process through production of immune mediators (Douek et al., 2003; Grossman et al., 2002).

Chronic inflammation and immune activation have been closely linked to CD4 + T-cell decline. For example, pathogenic lentiviral infections (e.g., HIV infection) and nonpathogenic infections (e.g., lentiviral infections of many nonhuman primates) are each associated with robust virus replication. Immune activation, however, is observed only in the pathogenic models, suggesting that this mechanism is directly responsible for CD4 + decline and disease progression (Silvestri et al., 2003). Further, chronic inflammation and CD4 + T-cell decline may be linked in a self-perpetuating cycle involving gut tissue. CD4 + Th17 cells are among those cells lost from the gastrointestinal tract in early HIV and simian immunodeficiency virus (SIV) infection (Brenchley et al., 2008; Favre et al., 2009). Th17 cells are important for maintenance of the "mucosal barrier" between gut luminal contents and circulation; when these cells are depleted, microbial constituents and even whole microbes can migrate from the gut into circulation, a process referred to as microbial translocation (Brenchley et al., 2006; Raffatellu et al., 2008). These proinflammatory microbial products, in particular lipopolysaccharides (LPS) from the outer membrane of Gram-negative bacteria, vigorously activate the immune system, resulting in activation-induced cell death and/or altered homeostasis. This cycle is initiated early in SIV infection

(Hirao et al., 2014) and appears to be an important driver of disease progression, as presence of sufficient Th17 cells before infection can limit viral replication (Hartigan-O'Connor et al., 2012; Ruiz-Riol et al., 2017).

Two reports emphasized the interplay between HIV and gut homing CD4 [+] T-cells. One showed that the frequency of alpha-4 beta-7 integrin[hi] CD4 [+] T-cells in blood was correlated with acquisition risk in a cohort of women participating in a CAPRISA-sponsored HIV prevention study in South Africa (Sivro et al., 2018). In addition, the preinfectional frequency of alpha-4 beta-7 integrin[hi] CD4 [+] T-cells was strongly correlated with the rate of CD4 [+] T-cell decline following HIV infection. A second report elucidated features intrinsic to the process of naive CD4 [+] T-cell trafficking to gut inductive sites that facilitate viral replication in those inductive tissues (Nawaz et al., 2018). Combined stimulation with retinoic acid and the alpha-4 beta-7 integrin ligand, MAdCAM, was shown to induce a distinct differentiation program in naive CD4 [+] T-cells that leads to the generation of cells with an alpha-4 beta-7 integrin[hi] phenotype, which is supportive of viral replication.

Another increasingly recognized self-perpetuating cycle pertains to the impact of HIV-associated inflammation on lymphoid structures. The inflammatory response generated by HIV results in upregulation of certain countervailing "regulatory" responses, including production of TGF-beta, which stimulates collagen deposition (Estes et al., 2008). Such "scarring" of the lymph nodes, which appears to be irreversible, prevents normal T-cell homeostasis and antigen presentation. The immunodeficiency that follows can lead to an excess burden of a variety of microbes, including CMV, gut microbes, and, perhaps, HIV itself. This microbial burden continues to the cycle by causing even more inflammation and scarring (Arthos et al., 2008).

EFFECTS OF HIV ON THE WHOLE IMMUNE SYSTEM

LEARNING OBJECTIVE

Discuss the effects of HIV on immune cells other than CD4 [+] T-cells.

KEY POINTS

- HIV has broad effects on many immune cell types, including many cells that are not infected by the virus.

- HIV disrupts the entire lymphoid system through its effects on secondary lymphoid organs such as lymph nodes

Although HIV is tropic for CD4-expressing cells, many manifestations of HIV infection result from direct or indirect effects on other immune cell types. One example is the high death rate and turnover of CD8 [+] T-cells, as well as numerical depletion of naive CD8 [+] T-cells, even in the asymptomatic phase of infection (Roederer et al., 1995). HIV also has direct or indirect effects on antigen-presenting cells such as dendritic, B, and NK cells (Ruffin et al., 2017). One factor that likely mediates some of the effects of HIV on the broader immune system, particularly in late disease, is the destruction of lymphoid tissue architecture. In early disease, as antigen-presenting cells are activated and initiate immune responses within lymph nodes, CD4 [+] T-cells are retained within the nodes while activated CD8 [+] T-cells migrate into circulation, a process that contributes to CD8 [+] lymphocytosis and inversion of the CD4:CD8 ratio (Bishop et al., 1990; Bujdoso et al., 1989). In later disease, there is structural damage to primary and secondary lymphoid organs resulting from fibrotic scarring (Estes et al., 2008; Samal et al., 2018). However, naive T-cells, including CD8[+] T-cells, require access to lymph node paracortical T-cell zones for access to critical homeostatic signals and growth factors, including IL-7 (Link et al., 2007). Presumably, therefore, lymphoid tissue scarring is one factor that contributes to failure to fully reconstitute CD4[+] and CD8[+] T-cells despite complete virologic suppression.

HIV-1 can also infect myeloid cells, including macrophages and dendritic cells, both of which can express CCR5. However, myeloid cells are relatively resistant to *productive* infection with HIV, as compared to CD4 [+] T-cells (Coleman & Wu, 2009). The relative inability of SIV and HIV-2 to cause productive infection of these cells is mediated by the cellular restriction factor SAMHD1 (Hrecka et al., 2011; Laguette et al., 2011). The viral accessory protein Vpx blocks this cellular response, thus allowing infection. As HIV-1 lacks this accessory protein, it remains unclear as to how this virus might productively infect macrophages (Hrecka et al., 2011; Laguette et al., 2011; Manel et al., 2010). Surprisingly, it is now appreciated that macrophages and memory CD4 [+] T-cells accumulate in adipose tissue during HIV infection (Damouche et al., 2017; Hsu et al., 2017; Koethe et al., 2018). A replicating virus can be recovered from these adipose tissue-resident cells, indicating that the tissue is a reservoir, though probably a minor one compared to lymphoid tissue. Antiviral effector cells, such as CD8 [+] T-cells and NK cells, are also present in large numbers in adipose tissue (Couturier et al., 2015; Couturier et al., 2016; Damouche et al., 2015; Dupin et al., 2002).

Natural Killer T (NKT) cells are also rapidly and selectively depleted in HIV infection (Sandberg et al., 2002; van der Vliet et al., 2002). NKT cells may be broadly divided into those that are CD4 [+] and those that are CD4 [−], with the former population secreting both Th1 and Th2 cytokines and likely providing B cell help or carrying out immunoregulatory functions, while the latter produces mainly Th1 cytokines and has stronger cytolytic activity. The CD4 [+] NKT population is depleted more rapidly in HIV infection than the CD4 [−] population but is restored more slowly after treatment with ART (Li & Xu, 2008). HIV also interferes with the activation of NKT cells by down-regulating expression of CD1d (an MHC-related protein that presents glycolipid antigens to NKT cells) on antigen-presenting cells (Hage et al., 2005). This down-regulation appears to be mediated mainly by the viral Nef protein (Cho et al., 2005).

There is continued interest in the effect of HIV and other agents of chronic infection on NK cells, particularly subsets with expanded functional capacity including "memory" NK cells (Hwang et al., 2012; Lee et al., 2015; Lopez-Verges et al., 2011; Sun et al., 2009; Zhang et al., 2013). Such cells are considered to be innate cells with adaptive features, including more robust and rapid responses to pathogen encounter (Sun et al., 2009). Limited evidence has been presented demonstrating that HIV infection drives expansion of memory NK cells (Zhou et al., 2015). However, NK cells from SIV-infected macaques or those vaccinated with an Ad26-vectored candidate SIV/HIV vaccine can lyse targets pulsed with SIV peptides in an antigen- and NKG2-dependent fashion (Reeves et al., 2015). CMV infection, which is common in PWH, is thought to be the most important driver of memory NK cell expansion (Brodin et al., 2015; Lopez-Verges et al., 2011; Zhang et al., 2013). People co with HIV and CMV may therefore present unique immunologic features.

MECHANISMS OF CHRONIC INFLAMMATION IN HIV DISEASE

LEARNING OBJECTIVE

Discuss the mechanisms that contribute to chronic inflammation and T-cell activation in HIV disease.

KEY POINTS

- Innate immune responses that result in production of type-I interferons are important drivers of inflammation in early infection.

- Early depletion of CD4 + T-cells from the gastrointestinal mucosa likely contributes to chronic, persistent immune activation.

- CMV and other chronic infections are important contributors to T-cell activation in coinfected individuals.

It was first demonstrated more than 20 years ago that T-cell activation was associated with shorter survival in advanced HIV disease (Giorgi et al., 1999). One might imagine that chronic T-cell activation is simply the inevitable consequence of ongoing viral replication, and that more T-cell activation is indicative of more active disease. However, it is clear from studies of nonpathogenic lentiviral infections that chronic, high-level virus replication can occur without eliciting massive immune activation (Silvestri et al., 2003); indeed, in the natural hosts of SIV, rapid reduction of initial immune activation appears to protect against subsequent CD4 + T-cell decline and disease progression. Efforts are underway to test these factors in rare persons living with HIV and high viral loads but remarkable absence of rapid HIV disease progression (Muenchhoff et al., 2016; Palesch et al., 2018). It is now clear that HIV-associated inflammation is associated with a transformation of "immunometabolism" to greater dependence on aerobic glycolysis, which is partly dependent on mTORC1 activation (Sáez-Cirión & Sereti, 2021). This transformation can in fact be imaged using PET scanning to reveal upregulation of the glucose transporter, GLUT1, and resultant accumulation of FDG tracer in PWH ranging from the successfully ART suppressed to late presenters experiencing opportunistic infection (Brust et al., 2006; Hammoud et al., 2019).

The virion itself elicits innate immune responses via activation of toll-like receptors (TLR) 7, 8, and 9 within antigen-presenting cells. TLR engagement results in production of type-I interferons, including IFN-α. Indeed, a spike of IFN-α production is observed in acute HIV and SIV infection (Favre et al., 2009; Stacey et al., 2009), which doubtless shapes the ensuing adaptive immune responses. Viral proteins such as Tat and Nef have been shown to have proinflammatory effects (Decrion et al., 2005) with consequences that can even affect neurogenesis and other brain functions (Fan et al., 2016). After the first 2 weeks of infection, the induction of adaptive immunity contributes to T-cell activation, although many of these activated T-cells are specific for CMV and other chronic pathogens, rather than HIV (Doisne et al., 2004; Papagno et al., 2004). Less appreciated is the fact that host genetics, in addition to controlling the adaptive immune response, may modulate the intensity of inflammation induced by these proinflammatory influences. Subjects in a Zimbabwean cohort having an IL-10 promoter mutation associated with lower inflammation experienced reductions in both mortality and CD4 + T-cell loss (Erikstrup et al., 2007). Finally, lymphopenia itself can lead to T-cell activation; for example, resting T-cells spontaneously become activated and proliferate when introduced into T-cell-deficient hosts (Srinivasula et al., 2011; Surh & Sprent, 2008). Thus, the progressive loss of CD4 + T-cells can be both a consequence and cause of immune activation (Jones et al., 2009; King et al., 2004).

In addition to these general effects of lymphocyte depletion, the field has discovered the implications of early and profound lymphocyte depletion from the gastrointestinal mucosa (Heise et al., 1994; Veazey et al., 1998). Among the lymphocytes lost in early infection are CD4 + Th17 cells (Pandiyan et al., 2016), which have an important structural role in maintenance of the tight junctions between intestinal epithelial cells (Brenchley et al., 2008; Favre et al., 2009). Loss of these cells contributes to a breakdown in the physical barrier separating the gut lumen from general circulation, which allows bioactive microbial products such as LPS into the blood (Brenchley et al., 2006), while maintenance of sufficient Th17 cells is associated with reduced viral replication (Hartigan-O'Connor et al., 2012; Ruiz-Riol et al., 2017). Mucosal barrier breakdown and proinflammatory processes such as tryptophan catabolism, in turn, are associated with disturbance ("dysbiosis") of the gut-resident microbial community (Vujkovic-Cvijin et al., 2013; Vujkovic-Cvijin et al., 2020). Persistent microbial dysbiosis drives further immune dysregulation and inflammation (Guillén et al., 2019) in part via loss of peroxisomal proliferator-activated receptor-α (PPARα) signaling (Crakes et al., 2019). In animal models, partial reversal of dysbiosis with *Lactobacillus plantarum* leads to recovery of the epithelium because of PPARα activation and restoration of mitochondrial structure and fatty acid β-oxidation (Crakes et al., 2019).

Occult and symptomatic opportunistic infections also contribute to chronic inflammation in HIV disease. In particular, the prevalence of CMV co-infection among PWH is at least 90% (Berry et al., 1988; Lang et al., 1989). Further, CMV infection has been associated with T-cell activation in HIV-negative people (Lenkei & Andersson, 1995). Indeed, CMV-specific T-cells can account for more than 10% of the circulating memory T-cell pool in seropositive individuals, suggesting that CMV replication can have a major influence on the immune system even in healthy individuals who are not immunocompromised (Sylwester et al., 2005) as well as in the growing population of elderly PWH (Margolick et al., 2018). CMV appears to have an even stronger effect on T-cell remodeling in untreated and treated HIV infection (Naeger et al., 2010). A pilot study tested the possibility that chronic immune activation in HIV disease could be reduced by treatment of CMV infection, randomly assigning 30 individuals on antiretroviral therapy to treatment with valganciclovir or placebo (Hunt et al., 2011). A significant 20% reduction in the percentage of activated CD8[+] T-cells was demonstrated in the valganciclovir group, suggesting that CMV infection is a significant contributor to T-cell activation in treated HIV- and CMV-coinfected individuals (Maidji et al., 2017).

IMMUNOLOGIC EFFECTS OF ANTIRETROVIRAL THERAPY AND ROLE OF PERSISTENT IMMUNE DYSFUNCTION DURING THERAPY ON CLINICAL OUTCOMES

LEARNING OBJECTIVE

Discuss the effect of antiretroviral therapy (ART) on immune function.

KEY POINTS

- A small but clinically important subset of PWH exhibit suboptimal CD4[+] T-cell gains after treatment with ART.

- Chronic inflammation, lymphoid fibrosis, hematopoietic progenitor cell loss and thymic dysfunction all likely contribute to failure to reinstate normal T-cell homeostasis.

- Chronic inflammation during treated disease has been associated with disease progression.

Combination antiretroviral therapy is highly effective, resulting in complete or near-complete suppression of HIV replication. Consequently, many of the factors that cause progressive immunodeficiency are reversed. Prevention of continued CD4[+] T-cell destruction (via both direct and indirect effects) and homeostatic regeneration results in eventual restoration of CD4[+] T-cell numbers in blood and tissues in the majority of individuals. The increase in peripheral CD4[+] T-cell counts during therapy appears to be biphasic (Pakker et al., 1998). A robust increase of approximately 50–100 cells/mm[3] is often observed in the first several weeks following initiation of ART.

Because memory cells account for most of the increase, it has long been assumed that the redistribution of cells from tissues to the periphery accounts for this rapid increase. After this early phase, CD4[+] T-cell counts increase more slowly (at a rate of approximately 50 cells/mm^3/year) until they achieve a normal range (i.e., greater than 500 cells/mm^3) (Mocroft et al., 2007). The augmented CD4[+] T-cell population includes naive cells and, hence, is thought to reflect true immune reconstitution. Although less well studied, CD4[+] T-cell gains also occur in tissues during effective antiviral therapy.

Although most PWH exhibit some degree of immune reconstitution during therapy, the outcome is highly variable. Some persons achieving median reference CD4[+] T-cell counts nonetheless exhibit a CD4:CD8 ratio below median because of persisting high CD8[+] T-cell counts (Gras et al., 2019). A small but clinically important subset of PWH fail to achieve normal peripheral CD4[+] T-cell counts, even after many years of therapy. These so-called immunologic nonresponders, or immune-discordant individuals, remain at relatively high risk for cancer, heart disease, liver failure, and other non-AIDS complications, but they usually achieve sufficient restoration of immune function to prevent opportunistic infections. Older persons with HIV and who start ART during late-stage disease often exhibit suboptimal gains in CD4[+] T-cells. In one study, approximately 40% of PWH who delayed therapy initiation until their CD4[+] T-cell count was less than 200 cells/mm^3 failed to achieve a normal CD4[+] T-cell count even after several years of viral suppression (Kelley et al., 2009). Other factors that have been associated with blunted CD4[+] T-cell gains include hepatitis C virus co-infection and high levels of T-cell activation.

Given its clinical importance, there is intense interest in determining the pathogenesis of immunologic failure (defined variably). In untreated disease, HIV-mediated destruction of hematopoietic stem cells, thymic tissue, lymphoid tissue, and central memory cells all contribute to progressive CD4[+] T-cell loss. Treatment-mediated suppression of HIV replication partially restores these factors. Persistent lymph node fibrosis, thymic dysfunction, and loss of cells with stem-like properties have all been associated with CD4[+] T-cell regeneration failure and suboptimal gains during therapy (McCune, 2001; Sauce et al., 2011; Schacker et al., 2002; Teixeira et al., 2001). More recently it has been shown that immunologic nonresponders accumulate CD56[bright] NK cells with cytotoxic activity against autologous, activated CD4[+] T-cells (Giuliani et al., 2017). Those data suggest that autoreactive NK cells, possibly linked to decreased homeostatic control by a depleted T-reg compartment, contribute to suboptimal immune reconstitution.

Untreated HIV infection is associated with heightened levels of immune activation. Long-term suppression of HIV replication dramatically reduces most measures of immune activation, but this effect is often incomplete, as inflammatory markers typically remain higher in treated PWH than in age-matched uninfected adults (Neuhaus et al., 2010). Persistent inflammation during therapy is associated with excess risk of non-AIDS complications, including heart disease, cancer, liver disease, kidney disease, bone disease, and neurologic complications (Deeks,

2011; Kuller et al., 2008; Phillips et al., 2008). Persistent CMV replication may be an important cause of continued inflammation while on therapy, as higher anti-CMV IgG antibody levels are associated with increased prevalence of carotid artery lesions among women with HIV who achieve HIV suppression on ART, but not among viremic or untreated women (Gómez-Mora et al., 2017; Parrinello et al., 2012).

Persistent and possibly irreversible damage to the infrastructure that supports T-cell homeostasis may account for much of the persistent immunodeficiency and inflammation often observed during therapy. Theoretically, collagen deposition and scarring of the lymphoid system during untreated disease result in a loss of the regulatory pathways (particularly those involving IL-7 and IL-27) that control T-cell regeneration and global T-cell homeostasis (Ruiz-Riol et al., 2017; Zeng et al., 2012). This disruption can result in persistently low CD4+ T-cell counts and an inability to generate effective memory T-cells in response to acute or chronic infections. Loss of lymphoid structures may also result in loss of immune surveillance and development of cancer, as well as a loss of key anti-inflammatory regulatory responses and, as a result, autoimmune-related clinical syndromes. In a self-perpetuating "vicious" cycle that persists in absence of any HIV replication, persistent immunodeficiency results in a reduced capacity of host responses to clear pathogens. The resulting burden of these pathogens contributes to more inflammation, which in turn continues to damage the lymphoid tissues. The collective outcome is a combination of low CD4+ T-cell counts and chronic inflammation. It is hoped that knowledge about these pathways will lead to novel interventions aimed at preventing or reversing this immunodeficient and proinflammatory environment. Such potential treatment options may also help to increase immunological responses to therapeutic vaccines included in HIV cure strategies.

PATHOGENESIS OF IMMUNE RECONSTITUTION INFLAMMATORY SYNDROMES (IRIS)

LEARNING OBJECTIVE

Discuss the leading hypotheses explaining pathogenesis of IRIS syndromes, including antigen persistence and immune dysregulation.

WHAT'S NEW

Presence of a more inflammatory environment in untreated HIV disease is associated with IRIS episodes after treatment. Data on the role of T-regs in IRIS syndromes have been unclear.

KEY POINTS

- IRIS are seen most in PWH initiating ART with low CD4+ T-cell counts and preexisting opportunistic infections.

- Many IRIS symptoms are localized to sites of previous infection, suggesting the presence of persistent microbial antigens.

- Development of IRIS is associated with increased T-cell activation before initiation of ART.

A subset of PWH who are immune restored with ART develop inflammatory conditions in the early stages of treatment initiation, known collectively as IRIS (Church et al., 2017). A large meta-analysis showed that 16% of PWH starting ART therapy developed an IRIS event (Muller et al., 2010). PWH most likely to be affected are those initiating ART with low CD4+ T-cell counts and preexisting opportunistic infections (Muller et al., 2010; Price et al., 2009). The symptoms of IRIS are often localized to sites of previous infection with certain co-pathogens (Lawn et al., 2007), which led to the suggestion that IRIS is caused by adaptive immune responses to persistent co-pathogen-derived antigens (Muller et al., 2010). For example, IRIS in persons with a history of cytomegalovirus retinitis (CMVR) can manifest as inflammation of the posterior uveal tract of the eye (Nussenblatt & Lane, 1998). The most frequent clinical manifestation of cryptococcal IRIS, by contrast, is aseptic meningitis (Boulware et al., 2010).

The hypothesis that IRIS is caused by the host immune response to persistent antigen (in the form of intact organisms, dead organisms, or debris) has the appeal of simplicity, but there are surprisingly few data to support this idea. One study demonstrated that, among PWH with recent cryptococcal meningitis who were placed on ART, those developing cryptococcal IRIS had fourfold higher titers of cryptococcal antigen in serum (Boulware et al., 2010). However, in a more recent study, low cryptococcal antibody levels were associated with a significantly increased risk of developing C-IRIS (Yoon et al., 2019). Guidelines based on the Cryptococcal Optimal Antiretroviral Timing trial (Scriven et al., 2015), recommend initial antifungal treatment followed by a minimum 5-week delayed initiation of ART (Balasko & Keynan, 2019). The approach aims to decrease fungal burden and allow immune balance restoration prior to ART initiation. In cases of *Mycobacterium tuberculosis* or *Mycobacterium avium* complex-associated IRIS, PWH normally convert to skin test positivity, suggesting that at a minimum the disease is mediated by pathogen-specific T-cells (French et al., 2004). Worth noting is that preexisting infection with *M. tuberculosis* appears to create an immune environment that influences the susceptibility of CD4+ T-cells to HIV-1 replication (He et al., 2020). In the case of CMV immune recovery uveitis, however, the presence of CMV antigens has not been demonstrated in PWH undergoing an IRIS event.

Several studies have suggested that the pretherapy inflammatory environment predicts IRIS. For example, Antonelli and colleagues showed that individuals who presented with an IRIS episode had a higher proportion of activated CD4+ T-cells before starting ART therapy compared with those who did not develop IRIS (Antonelli et al., 2010). These activated T-cells had a Th1/Th17 skewed cytokine profile before therapy began. Further, PWH with IRIS displayed higher serum

IFN-γ levels near the time of their IRIS events. Another study trying to understand the importance of regulatory CD4 [+] T-cells (T-regs) in controlling immune responses to self-antigens suggests that failure to reconstitute these anti-inflammatory cells predisposes to IRIS (Seddiki et al., 2009). However, data on this hypothesis have been inconsistent (Bourgarit et al., 2006; Hartigan-O'Connor et al., 2011). Other groups have argued that poorly regulated innate immune responses may be central to IRIS. Pretherapy and early treatment-mediated changes in various nonspecific inflammatory biomarkers (including CRP, IL-6, TNF-alpha and D-dimers) have been associated with increased risk of IRIS and mortality during the first several months of effective ART (Barber et al., 2012; Boulware et al., 2011). In general, corticosteroids remain the only treatment for paradoxical IRIS whose use is supported by randomized clinical trial data (Meintjes et al., 2010; Walker et al., 2018).

In summary, the pathogenesis of IRIS seems dependent on the presence of both lymphopenia and antigen-specific CD4 [+] T-cells. These T-cells may be responding to persistent pathogen-derived antigens, to self-antigens, or to unrelated foreign antigens. In these latter cases, the opportunistic pathogen may be the trigger rather than the target of the pathogenic T-cell response. The pathogenic response goes hand in hand with marked lymphopenia, which establishes a dysregulated environment in which either the response of the antigen-specific T-cells or the effect of that response on the host is exaggerated, and effective control mechanisms of exuberant immune responses have been impaired throughout the period of untreated HIV infection.

MECHANISMS AND CONSEQUENCES OF VIRUS CONTROL IN "ELITE" CONTROLLERS

LEARNING OBJECTIVE

Discuss how some individuals maintain durable control of HIV in the absence of therapy.

KEY POINTS

- HIV-specific CD8 [+] T-cells contribute to durable control of virus in HIV "elite" controllers.

- Despite the lack of readily detectable HIV RNA in plasma, "elite" controllers have higher than normal levels of immune activation, which may contribute to eventual disease progression.

- Neutralizing antibodies are more likely relevant to post-treatment control, than to elite control.

Fewer than 1% of adults with HIV who are not taking ART have no readily detectable HIV RNA in plasma. These individuals are generally referred to as "elite" controllers, although other terms have been used to define this or similar groups of individuals who are able to suppress viral replication in absence of ART. The term *long-term nonprogressors* refers to a partly overlapping group of PWH who maintain healthy CD4 [+] T-cell counts despite HIV infection. Given that the host mechanisms which might account for virus control in these individuals could inform vaccine and cure research, there has been long-term interest in understanding their mechanisms of viral control, as well as describing the degree to which most elite controllers exhibit any evidence of disease progression.

Researchers interested in determining the mechanisms of virus control in these individuals have assessed specific candidate host factors in controllers and noncontrollers. These studies have generally been cross-sectional, making it difficult to determine if a given host response is a cause or consequence of virus control (Deeks & Walker, 2007; Mothe et al., 2009). Some efforts have been made to follow individuals closely during the pre-HIV infection period, both to capture information about the earliest events after infection as well as to study dynamic changes that may be important for eventual control (Ndhlovu et al., 2015). Confoundingly, there is reason to believe that the immune responses that bring about control of acute HIV infection are distinct from those that maintain long-term viral suppression once control of viremia has been achieved (Goulder & Deeks, 2018).

Although the mechanisms have not been conclusively defined, the collective data support a central role for potent HIV-specific CD8 [+] T-cells and to a lesser degree CD4 [+] T-cells in maintaining virus control. This is also supported by the fact that most genetic predictors of virus control are found on chromosome 6 in the HLA class I region that governs the antigenic specificity of CD8 [+] T-cells (Pereyra et al., 2010). Studies in SIV-infected monkeys further support the importance of virus-specific CTL responses in virus control, although in the RhCMV-vectored vaccine setting, the responding T-cells are MHC class II- and MHC-E-restricted (Hansen et al., 2013a; Hansen et al., 2013b). Similarly, the role of the Th17 cell compartment in sustaining viral replication has been highlighted in recent monkey studies and the important role of IL-17- and IL-27-producing T-cells in humans has been highlighted (Hartigan-O'Connor et al., 2012; Ruiz-Riol et al., 2017). Abrupt breakdown of such control may also involve changes in viral cell tropism (Rosas-Umbert et al., 2019).

The contribution of humoral immunity to elite control is unclear. Most elite controllers have lower antibody titers than viremic individuals (Laeyendecker et al., 2008). Some studies have shown that elite controllers may have the capacity for more antibody-dependent cellular cytotoxicity than viremic people (Lambotte et al., 2013), which may also be linked to more or less functional NK cell compartments. It was recently shown that PWH receiving ART treatment harbor IgG antibodies that can block outgrowth of a substantial fraction of viruses in the latent reservoir (Bertagnolli et al., 2020). Although these data are not relevant to spontaneous elite control, they emphasize the possibility that neutralizing antibodies could frequently contribute to stringent posttreatment control (i.e., reduced viremia after cessation of ART).

Other factors that have been associated with virus control include (1) strong natural killer cell responses (Martin et al., 2007; Sips et al., 2012), (2) prevention of apoptosis/cell death in central memory cells (van Grevenynghe et al., 2008), (3) intrinsic intracellular restriction to HIV replication mediated by p21 (Chen et al., 2011) and other as yet poorly characterized factors (O'Connell et al., 2011; Saez-Cirion et al., 2011), and (4) acquisition of a replication-deficient virus. The importance of the latter is supported by recent studies of transmitted virus in a cluster of elite controllers, showing the presence of envelope sequences with a reduced binding affinity to the CD4 receptor (Casado et al., 2018). However, care must be taken not to confuse causative, functional markers of virus control with simple correlates of controlled infection. For instance, biomarkers such as proliferative capacity of HIV-specific T-cells or specific cytokine profiles may be the consequence of otherwise controlled/uncontrolled HIV infection rather than its physiological cause (Côrtes et al., 2018; Zhang et al., 2018). Longitudinal studies capturing PWH within days of infection and following them in the absence of treatment may be ethically challenging but could prove highly informative in defining true causes of control in vivo. However, even studies in hyperacute infection have not really been able to dissect the cause and effect conundrum and highly targeted, mechanistic studies in NHP models may be required to provide clarity (Muema et al., 2020; Ndhlovu et al., 2015). In addition, epigenetic predisposition to infection and/or virus control need to be further explored as recent studies have indicated an important role of epigenetic signatures on virus containment (Oriol-Tordera et al., 2020; Oriol-Tordera et al., 2022; Ruiz-Riol & Brander, 2019).

Given that controllers are being studied as a potential model for "functional cure," the consequences of long-term, host-mediated virus control on overall health is also of interest (Migueles & Connors, 2010). HIV persists at very low levels in nearly all controllers and appears to be replicating (Hatano et al., 2009; Mens et al., 2010). Persistent virus production generates a sustained inflammatory environment (Hunt et al., 2008), which in turn might cause end-organ damage, including cardiovascular disease (Hsue et al., 2009). In addition, potential alterations in the gut microbiota of chronically infected individuals may contribute to or be the result of ongoing viral replication, even in elite controllers (Williams et al., 2015), and have been shown to impact the efficacy of a therapeutic HIV vaccination (Borgognone et al., 2022). These considerations suggest that even elite controllers might benefit from antiretroviral drugs, and have spurred treatment guidelines and recommendation to treat all HIV-infected individuals immediately at diagnosis.

FUTURE OF IMMUNE-BASED THERAPEUTICS IN HIV DISEASE

LEARNING OBJECTIVE

Discuss experimental approaches to chronic inflammation in antiretroviral-treated disease, as well as recent advances in therapeutic vaccination.

WHAT'S NEW

Many promising immune-based therapeutics are now being tested in small clinical trials.

KEY POINTS

- Proving that HIV-associated inflammation is causally associated with disease progression will ultimately require a clinical endpoint study involving an immune-based therapy that directly affects these pathways.

- There is optimism in the field that a combination of T-cell vaccination and immunomodulation could be therapeutically effective.

Much of the effort of clinical investigators over the past 2 decades has focused on the development and optimization of combination ART for treating HIV disease. Now that most individuals with access to ART can achieve and maintain undetectable HIV RNA levels for years, it is increasingly apparent that in order to fully restore health, other adjunctive therapies may be needed. Given the consistent observation that inflammation remains elevated despite effective therapy and that the degree of inflammation predicts disease progression, there has been a renewed effort to testing existing drugs for potentially beneficial effects on inflammation in conjunction with suppressed viremia or to developing new approaches that will modify the inflammatory process (Fumaz et al., 2012; Perez-Matute et al., 2015).

With increased focus of the field on the possibility of an HIV cure, there has been both increased development and testing of therapeutic HIV vaccines—and increasing attention to the question of how best to combine therapeutic vaccination with immunomodulators. The most successful combinations to date, however, have generally focused on combining therapeutic vaccines with latency reactivating agents (LRAs) that might expose latent virus to immune attack. Yet, no LRA used in clinical trials of therapeutic vaccination has shown noticeable potency to reactivate latent virus and reduce the latent reservoir (Fidler et al., 2020; Rosas-Umbert et al., 2020). Thus, several clinical trials are ongoing that employ for instance Toll-like receptor agonists or other immune checkpoint modulators in combination with therapeutic vaccines and/or passive immunization with BnAb.

Human clinical trials of anti-inflammatory or immunosuppressive therapeutics have largely yielded disappointing results. Prednisone, hydroxyurea, cyclosporine, and mycophenolate acid have been studied in numerous trials with minimal or no clinical benefit. Although there were some promising early results, all these drugs proved to be either too toxic or to lack any clear efficacy, and, hence, there is limited interest in using nonspecific drugs that globally affect immune responses. The only exceptions to this rule are possibly the HMB-CoA reductase inhibitors also known simply as "statins." These agents are known to have broad anti-inflammatory effects (although the mechanism for this effect remains controversial) and are safe and generally well tolerated. Pilot data in adults with HIV infection suggest these drugs might reduce HIV-associated

T-cell activation and, hence, might prove to be beneficial in PWH for reasons independent of their lipid-lowering effects (Ganesan et al., 2011). At least one meta-analysis suggests that statins confer moderate mortality benefits in PWH (Uthman et al., 2018), although the drugs are consistently underprescribed for these individuals when compared to their HIV-uninfected counterparts (De Socio et al., 2016; Ladapo et al., 2017; van Zoest et al., 2017). A large clinical endpoint study known as REPRIEVE was started in 2015 with a current full enrollment of 7,770 PWH (Grinspoon, 2020).

As noted earlier, many factors contribute to persistent immune activation during therapy, including (1) irreversible breakdown of gut mucosa and subsequent microbial translocation, (2) excess CMV burden and/or enhanced immune responses to CMV (and perhaps other herpes viruses), (3) loss of immunoregulatory cells such as T regulatory cells, (4) ART toxicity, including generation of proinflammatory lipids and development of metabolic syndrome, and (5) lymphoid fibrosis, hematopoietic stem cell dysfunction, and thymic dysfunction. Many, if not all of these mechanisms can be addressed therapeutically. For example, a number of drugs including rifaximin (an antibiotic that is not absorbed systemically), sevelamer (which binds LPS/endotoxin in vivo), colostrum-related products (which bind LPS/endotoxin in the gut), chloroquine (which blocks LPS-mediated TLR signaling in myeloid cells), and mesalamine (which is an aspirin-like anti-inflammatory drug used in ulcerative colitis) have been or are being tested as means to reduce the inflammatory consequences of microbial translocation (Byakwaga et al., 2011; Gori et al., 2011; Murray et al., 2010; Piconi et al., 2011). Interventions that aim to restore certain bacterial species to the gut microbiota are also being studied, although a complete characterization of alterations in gut microbiota and related confounders is still needed before such approaches can be effective, either alone (Noguera, 2016; Vujkovic-Cvijin et al., 2020) or in combination with therapeutic vaccination (Borgognone et al., 2022). Valganciclovir-mediated reduction in CMV has been shown to reduce immune activation in HIV disease (Hunt et al., 2011), and there is new optimism that letermovir may have an even greater effect (Acosta et al., 2020). The drug pirfenidone and ACE inhibitors, among other drugs, are being studied in nonhuman primates and humans as a means to prevent and/or reverse fibrosis. Interleukin-7 has shown promise as a means to enhance immune function during treated disease (Levy et al., 2009). Treatment with the interleukin-15 "superagonist" compound, N-803, caused increased HIV transcription and proviral DNA initially, but eventually led to a decrease in the frequency of peripheral blood cells with an inducible HIV provirus (Miller et al., 2022). Although these studies will provide important insights into the relationship between immune activation and control, it remains unclear as to how such drugs could eventually be tested in phase III clinical trials.

Immunomodulatory therapies may also have a contribution to make in developing a regimen that could functionally cure HIV infection, permitting durable suppression of viremia in the absence of ART. There has been considerable interest in the potential of antibodies to $\alpha_4\beta_7$ integrin to block

homing of lymphocytes to gut tissue and thus eliminate the substrate for viral growth in its most important anatomic site (Guzzo et al., 2017). A first-in-human clinical trial (Fauci, 2018) did not confirm early positive signals from SIV models; however, a more recent report demonstrated reduction in both the size and number of lymphoid aggregates in the terminal ileum (Uzzan et al., 2018). This finding is noteworthy because lymphoid aggregates are inductive sites that can support viral replication and possibly contribute to viral reservoirs. Other studies explored or will explore the immunomodulatory effects of interferon-alpha, TLR-7 agonist, TLR-9 agonist, or even vitamin D (Eckard et al., 2017; Martinsen et al., 2020; Perreau et al., 2017) some of which have shown promising results in SIV-infected NHP studies (Lim et al., 2018), and as mentioned above, are being tested in human clinical trials.

Many investigators in the field would now offer cautious optimism that a combination of immunomodulators and therapeutic vaccines could be developed that would allow at least a fraction of treated people to control viremia without ART. Both preclinical and clinical studies of T-cell vaccines alone have generally demonstrated detectable viral rebound in all vaccine recipients following ART interruption (Colby et al., 2020; Okoye et al., 2021; Sneller et al., 2017). Nonetheless, one recent clinical trial of an optimized T-cell vaccine designed to induce functional T-cell responses with particular HIV-specificity, which were associated with better viral control in more than 1,000 HIV-1 clade B- and C-infected individuals, demonstrated a prolonged time off ART in a subgroup of vaccine recipients (Bailon et al., 2021). This success provides hope that combining T-cell vaccination with immunomodulators may achieve more relevant virologic outcomes. For instance, administration of vesatolimod may act to reverse latency and unmask infected cells for attack by vaccine-induced T-cells. Alternatively or in addition, to avoid or partially curtail viral rebound, it has been proposed to combine therapeutic vaccines with bNAbs—which in addition to neutralization may act by enhancing suppressive capacity of vaccine-induced responses through a vaccinal effect (Caskey, 2020; Mendoza et al., 2018; Nishimura et al., 2017).

Given the role of chronic inflammation in heart disease and aging, it is hoped that the management of inflammation in PWH might be informed by what is happening in those other disciplines. Daily exercise; a balanced diet rich in fish, legumes, grains and fresh vegetables (e.g., the Mediterranean diet); prevention of excess weight gain; and aggressive management of traditional risk factors, such as hypertension, hyperlipidemia, as well as lipid levels, can all have anti-inflammatory aspects, and will almost certainly contribute to successful aging in persons with HIV.

REFERENCES

Acosta E., Bowlin T, Brooks J, et al. Advances in the development of therapeutics for cytomegalovirus infections. *J Infect Dis.* 2020;221:S32–S44.

Antonelli LR, Mahnke Y, Hodge JN, et al. Elevated frequencies of highly activated CD4+ T cells in HIV+ patients developing immune reconstitution inflammatory syndrome. *Blood.* 2010;116:3818–3827.

Arthos J, Cicala C, Martinelli E, et al. HIV-1 envelope protein binds to and signals through integrin alpha4beta7, the gut mucosal homing receptor for peripheral T cells. *Nat Immunol.* 2008;9:301–309.

Bailon L, Llano A, Cedeño S, et al. A placebo-controlled ATI trial of HTI vaccines in early treated HIV infection. Abstract O161. In: *Conference on Retroviruses and Opportunistic Infections* (Virtual). San Francisco, CA. 2021. pp. 50.

Balasko A, Keynan Y. Shedding light on IRIS: from pathophysiology to treatment of cryptococcal meningitis and immune reconstitution inflammatory syndrome in HIV-infected individuals. *HIV Med.* 2019;20:1–10.

Barber DL, Andrrade BB, Sereti I, Sher A. Immune reconstitution inflammatory syndrome: the trouble with immunity when you had none. *Nat Rev Microbiol.* 2012;10(2):150–156.

Berry NJ, Burns DM, Wannamethee G, et al. Seroepidemiologic studies on the acquisition of antibodies to cytomegalovirus, herpes simplex virus, and human immunodeficiency virus among general hospital patients and those attending a clinic for sexually transmitted diseases. *J Med Virol.* 1988;24:385–393.

Bertagnolli LN, Varriale J, Sweet S. Autologous IgG antibodies block outgrowth of a substantial but variable fraction of viruses in the latent reservoir for HIV-1. *Proc Natl Acad Sci USA.* 2020;117:32066–32077.

Bishop DK, Ferguson RM, Orosz CG. Differential distribution of antigen- specific helper T cells and cytotoxic T cells after antigenic stimulation in vivo: a functional study using limiting dilution analysis. *J Immunol.* 1990;144:1153–1160.

Borgognone A, Noguera-Julian M, Oriol B, et al. Gut microbiome signatures linked to HIV-1 reservoir size and viremia control. *Microbiome.* 2022;10:59.

Boulware DR, Hupper Hullsiek K, Puronen CE, et al. Higher levels of CRP, d-dimer, IL-6, and hyaluronic acid before initiation of antiretroviral therapy (ART) are associated with increased risk of AIDS or death. *J Infect Dis.* 2011;203(11):1637–1646.

Boulware DR, Meya DB, Bergemann TL, et al. Clinical features and serum biomarkers in HIV immune reconstitution inflammatory syndrome after cryptococcal meningitis: a prospective cohort study. *PLoS Med.* 2010;7:e1000384.

Bourgarit A, Carcelain G, Martinez V. Explosion of tuberculin-specific Th1-responses induces immune restoration syndrome in tuberculosis and HIV co-infected patients. *AIDS.* 2006;20:F1–F17.

Brenchley JM, Paiardini M, Knox KS, et al. Differential Th17 CD4 T-cell depletion in pathogenic and nonpathogenic lentiviral infections. *Blood.* 2008;112:2826–2835.

Brenchley JM, Price DA, Schacker TW, et al. Microbial translocation is a cause of systemic immune activation in chronic HIV infection. *Nat Med.* 2006;12:1365–1371.

Brodin P, Jojic V, Gao T, et al. Variation in the human immune system is largely driven by non- heritable influences. *Cell.* 2015;160:37–47.

Brust D, Polis M, Davey R, et al. Fluorodeoxyglucose imaging in healthy subjects with HIV infection: impact of disease stage and therapy on pattern of nodal activation. *AIDS.* 2006;20:495–503.

Bujdoso R, Young P, Hopkins J, et al. Non-random migration of CD4 and CD8 T cells: changes in the CD4:CD8 ratio and interleukin 2 responsiveness of efferent lymph cells following in vivo antigen challenge. *Eur J Immunol.* 1989;19:1779–1784.

Byakwaga H, Kelly M, Purcell DF, et al. Intensification of antiretroviral therapy with raltegravir or addition of hyperimmune bovine colostrum in HIV-infected patients with suboptimal CD4+ T-cell response: a randomized controlled trial. *J Infect Dis.* 2011;204:1532–1540.

Casado C, Marrero-Hernández S, Márquez-Arce D, et al. Viral characteristics associated with the clinical nonprogressor phenotype are inherited by viruses from a cluster of HIV-1 elite controllers. *mBio.* 2018;9:e02338–17.

Caskey M. Broadly neutralizing antibodies for the treatment and prevention of HIV infection. *Curr Opin HIV AIDS.* 2020;15:49–55.

Chen H, Li C, Huang J, et al. CD4+ T cells from elite controllers resist HIV-1 infection by selective upregulation of p21. *J Clin Invest.* 2011;121:1549–1560.

Cho S, Knox KS, Kohli LM, et al. Impaired cell surface expression of human CD1d by the formation of an HIV- 1 Nef/CD1d complex. *Virology.* 2005;337:242–252.

Church LWP, Chopra A, Judson MA. Paradoxical reactions and the immune reconstitution inflammatory syndrome. *Microbiol Spectr.* 2017;5(2).

Colby DJ, Sarnecki M, Barouch DH, et al. Safety and immunogenicity of Ad26 and MVA vaccines in acutely treated HIV and effect on viral rebound after antiretroviral therapy interruption. *Nat Med.* 2020;26:498–501.

Coleman CM, Wu L. HIV interactions with monocytes and dendritic cells: viral latency and reservoirs. *Retrovirology.* 2009;6:51.

Côrtes FH, de Paula HHS, Bello G, et al. Plasmatic levels of IL-18, IP-10, and activated CD8(+) T cells are potential biomarkers to identify HIV-1 elite controllers with a true functional cure profile. *Front Immunol.* 2018;9:1576.

Couturier J, Agarwal N, Nehete PN, et al. Infectious SIV resides in adipose tissue and induces metabolic defects in chronically infected rhesus macaques. *Retrovirology.* 2016;13:30.

Couturier J, Suliburk JW, Brown JM. Human adipose tissue as a reservoir for memory CD4+ T cells and HIV. *AIDS.* 2015;29:667–674.

Crakes KR, Santos Rocha C, Grishina I. PPARα-targeted mitochondrial bioenergetics mediate repair of intestinal barriers at the host-microbe intersection during SIV infection. *Proc Natl Acad Sci USA.* 2019;116:24819–24829.

Damouche A, Lazure T, Avettand-Fenoel V, et al. Adipose tissue is a neglected viral reservoir and an inflammatory site during chronic HIV and SIV infection. *PLoS Pathog.* 2015;11:e1005153.

Decrion AZ, Dichamp I, Varin A, Herbein G. HIV and inflammation. *Curr HIV Res.* 2005;3:243–259.

Deeks SG. HIV infection, inflammation, immunosenescence, and aging. *Annu Rev Med.* 2011;62:141–155.

Deeks SG. Human immunodeficiency virus controllers: mechanisms of durable virus control in the absence of antiretroviral therapy. *Immunity.* 2007;27:406–416.

De Socio GV, Ricci E, Parruti G. Statins and Aspirin use in HIV-infected people: gap between European AIDS Clinical Society guidelines and clinical practice: the results from HIV-HY study. *Infection.* 2016;44:589–597.

Doisne JM, Urrutia A, Lacabaratz-Porret C, et al. CD8+ T cells specific for EBV, cytomegalovirus, and influenza virus are activated during primary HIV infection. *J Immunol.* 2004;173:2410–2418.

Douek D, Picker LJ, Koup RA. T cell dynamics in HIV-1 infection. *Annu Rev Immunol.* 2003;21:265–304.

Dupin N, Buffet M, Marcelin AG, et al. HIV and antiretroviral drug distribution in plasma and fat tissue of HIV- infected patients with lipodystrophy. *AIDS.* 2002;16:2419–2424.

Eckard AR, O'Riordan MA, Rosebush JC, et al. Vitamin D supplementation decreases immune activation and exhaustion in HIV-1-infected youth. *Antivir Ther.* 2018;23(4):315–324.

Erikstrup C, Kallestrup P, Zinyama-Gutsire RB, et al. Reduced mortality and CD4 cell loss among carriers of the interleukin-10-1082G allele in a Zimbabwean cohort of HIV-1-infected adults. *AIDS.* 2007;21:2283–2291.

Estes JD, Haase AT, Schacker TW. The role of collagen deposition in depleting CD4+ T cells and limiting reconstitution in HIV-1 and SIV infections through damage to the secondary lymphoid organ niche. *Semin Immunol.* 2008;20:181–186.

Fan Y, Gao X, Chen J, et al. HIV Tat impairs neurogenesis through functioning as a notch ligand and activation of notch signaling pathway. *J Neurosci.* 2016;36:11362–11373.

Fauci AS. Durable control of HIV infections in the absence of antiretroviral therapy: opportunities and obstacles. In: 22nd International AIDS Conference, 2018; Amsterdam, The Netherlands. July 22–27, 2018.

Favre D, Lederer S, Kanwar B, et al. Critical loss of the balance between Th17 and T regulatory cell populations in pathogenic SIV infection. *PLoS Pathog.* 2009;5:e1000295.

Fidler S, Stohr W, Pace M, et al. Antiretroviral therapy alone versus antiretroviral therapy with a kick and kill approach, on measures of the

HIV reservoir in participants with recent HIV infection (the RIVER trial): a phase 2, randomised trial. *Lancet.* 2020;395:888–898.

French MA, Price P, Stone SF. Immune restoration disease after antiretroviral therapy. *AIDS.* 2004;18:1615–1627.

Fumaz CR, Gonzalez-Garcia M, Borras X. Psychological stress is associated with high levels of IL-6 in HIV-1 infected individuals on effective combined antiretroviral treatment. *Brain Behav Immun.* 2012;26:568–572.

Ganesan A, Crum-Cianflone N, Higgins J, et al. High dose atorvastatin decreases cellular markers of immune activation without affecting HIV-1 RNA levels: results of a double-blind randomized placebo controlled clinical trial. *J Infect Dis.* 2011;203:756–764.

Giorgi JV, Hultin LE, McKeating JA, et al. Shorter survival in advanced human immunodeficiency virus type 1 infection is more closely associated with T lymphocyte activation than with plasma virus burden or virus chemokine coreceptor usage. *J Infect Dis.* 1999;179:859–870.

Giuliani E, Vassena L, Di Cesare S, et al. NK cells of HIV-1-infected patients with poor CD4(+) T-cell reconstitution despite suppressive HAART show reduced IFN-gamma production and high frequency of autoreactive CD56(bright) cells. *Immunol Lett.* 2017;190:185–193.

Gómez-Mora E, García E, Urrea V, et al. Preserved immune functionality and high CMV-specific T-cell responses in HIV-infected individuals with poor CD4(+) T-cell immune recovery. *Sci Rep.* 2017;7:11711.

Gori A, Rizzardini G, Van't Land B, et al. Specific prebiotics modulate gut microbiota and immune activation in HAART-naive HIV-infected adults: results of the "COPA" pilot randomized trial. *Mucosal Immunol.* 2011;4:554–563.

Goulder P, Deeks SG. HIV control: is getting there the same as staying there? *PLoS Pathog.* 2008;14:e1007222.

Gras L, May M, Ryder LP, et al. Determinants of restoration of CD4 and CD8 cell counts and their ratio in HIV-1-positive individuals with sustained virological suppression on antiretroviral therapy. *J Acquir Immune Defic Syndr.* 2019;80:292–300.

Grinspoon SK, Douglas PS, Hoffman U, Ribaudo HJ. Leveraging a landmark trial of primary cardiovascular disease prevention in human immunodeficiency virus: introduction from the REPRIEVE coprincipal investigators. *J Infect Dis.* 2020;222(Suppl 1):S1–S7.

Grossman Z, Meier- Schellersheim M, Sousa AE. CD4+ T- cell depletion in HIV infection: are we closer to understanding the cause? *Nat Med.* 2002;8:319–323.

Guadalupe M, Reay E, Sankaran S. Severe CD4+ T- cell depletion in gut lymphoid tissue during primary human immunodeficiency virus type 1 infection and substantial delay in restoration following highly active antiretroviral therapy. *J Virol.* 2003;77:11708–11717.

Guillén Y, Noguera-Julian M, Rivera J, et al. Low nadir CD4+ T-cell counts predict gut dysbiosis in HIV-1 infection. *Mucosal Immunol.* 2019;12:232–246.

Guzzo C, Ichikawa D, Park C, et al. Virion incorporation of integrin alpha4beta7 facilitates HIV-1 infection and intestinal homing. *Sci Immunol.* 2017;2(11):eaam7341.

Hage CA, Kohli LL, Cho S, et al. Human immunodeficiency virus gp120 downregulates CD1d cell surface expression. *Immunol Lett.* 2005;98:131–135.

Hammoud DA, Boulougoura A, Papadakis GZ, et al. Increased metabolic activity on 18F-fluorodeoxyglucose positron emission tomography-computed tomography in human immunodeficiency virus-associated immune reconstitution inflammatory syndrome. *Clin Infect Dis.* 2019;68:229–238.

Hansen SG, Piatak M Jr, Ventura AB, et al. Immune clearance of highly pathogenic SIV infection. *Nature.* 2013a;502:100–104.

Hansen SG, Sacha JB, Hughes CM, et al. Cytomegalovirus vectors violate CD8+ T cell epitope recognition paradigms. *Science.* 2013b;340:1237874.

Hartigan-O'Connor DJ, Abel K, Van Rompay KK, et al. SIV replication in the infected rhesus macaque is limited by the size of the preexisting TH17 cell compartment. *Sci Transl Med.* 2012;4:136ra169.

Hartigan-O'Connor DJ, Jacobson MA, Tan QX. Sinclair E development of cytomegalovirus (CMV) immune recovery uveitis is associated with Th17 cell depletion and poor systemic CMV-specific T cell responses. *Clin Infect Dis.* 2011;52:409–417.

Hatano H, Delwart EL, Norris PJ, et al. Evidence for persistent low-level viremia in individuals who control human immunodeficiency virus in the absence of antiretroviral therapy. *J Virol.* 2009;83:329–335.

He X, Eddy JJ, Jacobson KR, et al. Enhanced HIV- 1 replication in CD4+ T cells derived from individuals with latent mycobacterium tuberculosis infection. *J Infect Dis.* 2020;222(9):1550–1560.

Heise C, Miller CJ, Lackner A, Dandekar S. Primary acute simian immunodeficiency virus infection of intestinal lymphoid tissue is associated with gastrointestinal dysfunction. *J Infect Dis.* 1994;169:1116–1120.

Hellerstein M, Hanley MB, Cesar D. Directly measured kinetics of circulating T lymphocytes in normal and HIV-1-infected humans. *Nat Med.* 1999;5:83–89.

Hirao LA, Grishina I, Bourry O. Early mucosal sensing of SIV infection by paneth cells induces IL-1beta production and initiates gut epithelial disruption. *PLoS Pathog.* 2014;10:e1004311.

Hrecka K, Hao C, Gierszewska M, et al. Vpx relieves inhibition of HIV-1 infection of macrophages mediated by the SAMHD1 protein. *Nature.* 2011;474:658–661.

Hsu DC, Wegner MD, Sunyakumthorn P, et al. CD4+ cell infiltration into subcutaneous adipose tissue is not indicative of productively infected cells during acute SHIV infection. *J Med Primatol.* 2017;46:154–157

Hsue PY, Hunt PW, Schnell A, et al. Role of viral replication, antiretroviral therapy, and immunodeficiency in HIV-associated atherosclerosis. *AIDS.* 2009;23:1059–1067.

Hunt PW, Brenchley J, Sinclair E, et al. Relationship between T cell activation and CD4+ T cell count in HIV-seropositive individuals with undetectable plasma HIV RNA levels in the absence of therapy. *J Infect Dis.* 2008;197:126–133.

Hunt PW, Martin JN, Sinclair E. Valganciclovir reduces T cell activation in HIV-infected individuals with incomplete CD4+ T cell recovery on antiretroviral therapy. *J Infect Dis.* 2011;203:1474–1483.

Hwang I, Zhang T, Scott JM, et al. Identification of human NK cells that are deficient for signaling adaptor FcRgamma and specialized for antibody-dependent immune functions. *Int Immunol.* 2012;24:793–802.

Jones JL, Phuah CL, Cox AL, et al. TIL-21 drives secondary autoimmunity in patients with multiple sclerosis, following therapeutic lymphocyte depletion with alemtuzumab (Campath-1H). *J Clin Invest.* 2009;119:2052–2061.

Ke R, Cong ME, Li D, et al. On the death rate of abortively infected cells: estimation from simian-human immunodeficiency virus infection. *J Virol.* 2017;91(18):e00352–17. doi: 10.1128/JVI.00351-17. Print 2017, September 15.

Kelley CF, Kitchen CM, Hunt PW, et al. Incomplete peripheral CD4(+) cell count restoration in HIV-infected patients receiving long-term antiretroviral treatment. *Clin Infect Dis.* 2009;48:787–794.

King C, Ilic A, Koelsch K, Sarvetnick N. Homeostatic expansion of T cells during immune insufficiency generates autoimmunity. *Cell.* 2004;117:265–277.

Koethe JR, McDonnell W, Kennedy A, et al. Adipose tissue is enriched for activated and late- differentiated CD8+ T cells and shows distinct CD8+ receptor usage, compared with blood in HIV-infected persons. *J Acquir Immune Defic Syndr.* 2018;77:e14–e21.

Kuller LH, Tracy R, Belloso W, et al. Inflammatory and coagulation biomarkers and mortality in patients with HIV infection. *PLoS Med.* 2008;5:e203.

Ladapo JA, Richards AK, DeWitt CM, et al. Disparities in the quality of cardiovascular care between HIV-infected versus HIV-uninfected adults in the United States: a cross-sectional study. *J Am Heart Assoc.* 2017;6(11):e007107.

Laeyendecker O, Rothman RE, Henson C. The effect of viral suppression on cross-sectional incidence testing in the Johns Hopkins hospital Emergency Department. *J Acquir Immune Defic Syndr.* 2008;48:211–215.

Laguette MJ, Abrahams Y, Prince S, et al. Sequence variants within the 3'-UTR of the COL5A1 gene alters mRNA stability:

implications for musculoskeletal soft tissue injuries. *Matrix Biol.* 2011;30(5–6):338–345.

Lambotte O, Pollara J, Boufassa F, et al. High antibody-dependent cellular cytotoxicity responses are correlated with strong CD8 T cell viral suppressive activity but not with B57 status in HIV-1 elite controllers. *PLoS One.* 2013;8:e74855.

Lang DJ, Kovacs AA, Zaia JA, et al. Seroepidemiologic studies of cytomegalovirus and Epstein- Barr virus infections in relation to human immunodeficiency virus type 1 infection in selected recipient populations. Transfusion Safety Study Group. *J Acquir Immune Defic Syndr.* 1989;2:540–549.

Lawn SD, Myer L, Bekker LG, Wood R. Tuberculosis-associated immune reconstitution disease: incidence, risk factors and impact in an antiretroviral treatment service in South Africa. *AIDS.* 2007;21:335–341.

Lee J, Zhang T, Hwang I, et al. Epigenetic modification and antibody-dependent expansion of memory- like NK cells in human cytomegalovirus- infected individuals. *Immunity.* 2015;42:431–442.

Lenardo MJ, Angleman SB, Bounkeua C, et al. Cytopathic killing of peripheral blood CD4(+) T lymphocytes by human immunodeficiency virus type 1 appears necrotic rather than apoptotic and does not require env. *J Virol.* 2002;76:5082–5093.

Lenkei R, Andersson B. High correlations of anti-CMV titers with lymphocyte activation status and CD57 antibody-binding capacity as estimated with three-color, quantitative flow cytometry in blood donors. *Clin Immunol Immunopathol.* 1995;77:131–138.

Levy Y, Lacabaratz C, Weiss L, et al. Enhanced T cell recovery in HIV-1-infected adults through IL-7 treatment. *J Clin Invest.* 2009;119:997–1007.

Li D, Xu XN. NKT cells in HIV-1 infection. *Cell Res.* 2008;18:817–822.

Lim SY, Osuna CE, Hraber PT, et al. TLR7 agonists induce transient viremia and reduce the viral reservoir in SIV-infected rhesus macaques on antiretroviral therapy. *Sci Transl Med.* 2018;10(439):eaao4521

Link A, Vogt TK, Favre S, et al. Fibroblastic reticular cells in lymph nodes regulate the homeostasis of naive T cells. *Nat Immunol.* 2007;8:1255–1265.

Lopez- Verges S, Milush JM, Schwartz BS, et al. Expansion of a unique CD57(+)NKG2Chi natural killer cell subset during acute human cytomegalovirus infection. *Proc Natl Acad Sci USA.* 2011;108:14725–14732.

Maidji E, Somsouk M, Rivera JM, et al. Replication of CMV in the gut of HIV-infected individuals and epithelial barrier dysfunction. *PLoS Pathog.* 2017;13:e1006202.

Manel N, Hogstad B, Wang Y, et al. A cryptic sensor for HIV-1 activates antiviral innate immunity in dendritic cells. *Nature.* 2010;467:214–217.

Margolick JB, Bream JH. Nilles TL, et al. Relationship between T-cell responses to CMV, markers of inflammation, and frailty in HIV-uninfected and HIV-infected men in the Multicenter AIDS Cohort Study. *J Infect Dis.* 2018;218:249–258.

Martin MP, Qi Y, Gao X, et al. Innate partnership of HLA-B and KIR3DL1 subtypes against HIV-1. *Nat Genet.* 2007;39;733–740.

Martinsen JT, Gunst JD, Højen JF, et al. The use of toll-like receptor agonists in HIV-1 cure strategies. *FrontImmunol.* 2020;11:1112.

McCune JM. The dynamics of CD4+ T-cell depletion in HIV disease. *Nature.* 2001;410: 974–979.

Meintjes G, Wilkinson RJ, Morroni C, et al. Randomized placebo-controlled trial of prednisone for paradoxical tuberculosis-associated immune reconstitution inflammatory syndrome. *AIDS.* 2010;24:2381–2390.

Mendoza P, Gruell H, Nogueira L, et al. Combination therapy with anti-HIV-1 antibodies maintains viral suppression. *Nature.* 2018;561: 479–484.

Mens H, Kearney M, Wiegand A, et al. HIV-1 Continues to replicate and evolve in patients with natural control of HIV infection. *J Virol.* 2010;84(24):12971–12981.

Migueles SA, Connors M. Long-term nonprogressive disease among untreated HIV-infected individuals: clinical implications of understanding immune control of HIV. *JAMA.* 2010;304:194–201.

Miller JS, Davis ZB, Helgeson E, et al. Safety and virologic impact of the IL-15 superagonist N-803 in people living with HIV: a phase 1 trial. *Nat Med.* 2022;28:392–400.

Mocroft A, Phillips AN, Gatell J. Normalisation of CD4 counts in patients with HIV-1 infection and maximum virological suppression who are taking combination antiretroviral therapy: an observational cohort study. *Lancet.* 2007;370:407–413.

Mothe B, Ibarrondo J, Llano A, Brander C. Virological, immune and host genetic markers in the control of HIV infection. *Dis Markers.* 2009;27:105–120.

Muema DM, Akilimali NA, Ndumnego OC, et al. Association between the cytokine storm, immune cell dynamics, and viral replicative capacity in hyperacute HIV infection. *BMC Med.* 2020;18:81.

Muenchhoff M, Adland E, Karimanzira O, et al. Nonprogressing HIV-infected children share fundamental immunological features of non-pathogenic SIV infection. *Sci Transl Med.* 2016;8:358ra125.

Muller M, Wandel S, Colebunders R, et al. Immune reconstitution inflammatory syndrome in patients starting antiretroviral therapy for HIV infection: a systematic review and meta-analysis. *Lancet Infect Dis.* 2010;10:251–261.

Murray SM, Down CM, Boulware DR, et al. Reduction of immune activation with chloroquine therapy during chronic HIV infection. *J Virol.* 2010.84:12082–12086.

Naeger DM, Martin JN, Sinclair E, et al. Cytomegalovirus-specific T cells persist at very high levels during long-term antiretroviral treatment of HIV disease. *PLoS One.* 2010;5:e8886.

Nawaz F, Goes LR, Ray JC, et al. MAdCAM costimulation through integrin- α(4)β(7) promotes HIV replication. *Mucosal Immunol.* 2018;1:1342–1351.

Ndhlovu ZM, Kamya P, Mewalal N, et al. Magnitude and kinetics of CD8+ T cell activation during hyperacute HIV infection impact viral set point. *Immunity.* 2015;43:591–604.

Neuhaus J, Jacobs DR Jr, Baker JV, et al. Markers of inflammation, coagulation, and renal function are elevated in adults with HIV infection. *J Infect Dis.* 2010;201:1788–1795.

Nishimura Y, Gautam R, Chun T, et al. Early antibody therapy can induce long-lasting immunity to SHIV. *Nature.* 2017;543:559–563.

Noguera- Julian M, Rocafort M, Guillén Y, et al. Gut microbiota linked to sexual preference and HIV infection. *EBioMedicine.* 2016;5:135–146.

Nussenblatt RB, Lane HC. Human immunodeficiency virus disease: changing patterns of intraocular inflammation. *Am J Ophthalmol.* 1998;125:374–382.

O'Connell KA, Rabi SA, Siliciano RF, Blankson JN. CD4+ T cells from elite suppressors are more susceptible to HIV-1 but produce fewer virions than cells from chronic progressors. *Proc Natl Acad Sci USA.* 1998;108:E689–E698.

Okoye AA, Duell DD, Fukazawa Y, et al. CD8+ T cells fail to limit SIV reactivation following ART withdrawal until after viral amplification. *J Clin Invest.* 2021;131(8):e1416777.

Oriol-Tordera B, Berdasco M, Llano A, et al. Methylation regulation of antiviral host factors, interferon stimulated genes (ISGs) and T-cell responses associated with natural HIV control. *PLoS Pathog.* 2020;16:e1008678.

Oriol-Tordera B, Esteve-Codina A, Berdasco M, et al. Epigenetic landscape in the kick-and-kill therapeutic vaccine BCN02 clinical trial is associated with antiretroviral treatment interruption (ATI) outcome. *EBioMed.* 2022;78:103956.

Pakker NG, Notermans DW, de Boer RJ, et al. Biphasic kinetics of peripheral blood T cells after tripe combination therapy in HIV-1 infection: a composite of redistribution and proliferation. *Nat Med.* 1998;4:208–214.

Palesch D, Bosinger SE, Tharp GK, et al. Sooty mangabey genome sequence provides insight into AIDS resistance in a natural SIV host. *Nature.* 2018;553:77–81.

Pandiyan P, Younes SA, Ribeiro SP, et al. Mucosal regulatory T cells and T helper 17 cells in HIV-associated immune activation. *Front Immunol.* 2016;7:228.

Papagno L, Spina CA, Marchant A, et al. Immune activation and CD8(+) T-cell differentiation towards senescence in HIV-1 infection. *PLoS Biol.* 2005;2:E20.

Parrinello CM, Sinclair E, Landay AL, et al. Cytomegalovirus immunoglobulin G antibody is associated with subclinical carotid artery disease among HIV-infected women. *J Infect Dis.* 2012;205:1788–1796.

Pereyra F, Jia X, McLaren PJ, et al. The major genetic determinants of HIV-1 control affect HLA class I peptide presentation. *Science.* 2010;330:1551–1557.

Perez-Matute P, Perez-Martinez L, Aguilera-Lizarraga J, et al. Maraviroc modifies gut microbiota composition in a mouse model of obesity: a plausible therapeutic option to prevent metabolic disorders in HIV-infected patients. *Rev Esp Quimioter.* 2015;28:200–206.

Perreau M, Banga R, Pantaleo G. Targeted immune interventions for an HIV-1 cure. *Trends Mol Med.* 2017;23:945–961.

Phillips AN, Neaton J, Lundgren JD. The role of HIV in serious diseases other than AIDS. *AIDS.* 2008;22:2409–2418.

Piconi S, Parisotto S, Rizzardini G, et al. Hydroxychloroquine drastically reduces immune activation in HIV-infected, antiretroviral therapy-treated immunologic nonresponders. *Blood.* 2011;118:3263–3272.

Price P, Murdoch DM, Agarwal U, et al. Immune restoration diseases reflect diverse immunopathological mechanisms. *Clin Microbiol Rev.* 2009;22:651–663.

Raffatellu M, Santos RL, Verhoeven DE, et al. Simian immunodeficiency virus-induced mucosal interleukin-17 deficiency promotes Salmonella dissemination from the gut. *Nat Med.* 2008;14:421–428.

Reeves RK, Li H, Jost S, et al. Antigen- specific NK cell memory in rhesus macaques. *Nat Immunol.* 2015;16:927–932.

Roederer M, Dubs JG, Anderson MT, et al. CD8 naive T cell counts decrease progressively in HIV-infected adults. *J Clin Invest.* 1995;95:2061–2066.

Rosas-Umbert M, Llano A, Bellido R, et al. Mechanisms of abrupt loss of virus control in a cohort of previous HIV controllers. *J Virol.* 2019;5;93(4):e01436–18. doi: 10.1128/JVI.01436-18. Print 2019 Feb 15.

Rosas-Umbert M, Ruiz-Riol M, Fernandez MA. In vivo effects of romidepsin on T-cell activation, apoptosis and function in the BCN02 HIV-1 Kick&Kill clinical trial. *Front Immunol.* 2020;11:418.

Ruffin N, Hani L, Seddiki N. From dendritic cells to B cells dysfunctions during HIV-1 infection: T follicular helper cells at the crossroads. *Immunology.* 2017;151:137–145.

Ruiz-Riol M, Berdnik D, Llano A, et al. Identification of interleukin-27 (IL-27)/IL-27 receptor subunit alpha as a critical immune axis for in vivo HIV control. *J Virol.* 2017;91(16):e00441–17.

Ruiz-Riol M, Brander C. Can we just kick-and-kill HIV: possible challenges posed by the epigenetically controlled interplay between HIV and host immunity. *Immunother.* 2019;11:931–935.

Saez-Cirion A, Hamimi C, Bergamaschi A, et al. Restriction of HIV-1 replication in macrophages and CD4+ T cells from HIV controllers. *Blood.* 2011;118:955–964.

Sáez-Cirión A, Sereti I. Immunometabolism and HIV-1 pathogenesis: food for thought. *Nat Rev Immunol.* 2021;21(1):5–19.

Samal J, Kelly S, Na- Shatal A, et al. Human immunodeficiency virus infection induces lymphoid fibrosis in the BM-liver-thymus-spleen humanized mouse model. *JCI Insight.* 2018;3(18):e120430.

Sandberg JK, Fast NM, Palacios EH, et al. Selective loss of innate CD4(+) V alpha 24 natural killer T cells in human immunodeficiency virus infection. *J Virol.* 2002;76:7528–7534.

Sauce D, Larsen M, Fastenackels S, et al. HIV disease progression despite suppression of viral replication is associated with exhaustion of lymphopoiesis. *Blood.* 2011;117(19):5142–5151.

Schacker TW, Nguyen PL, Beilman GJ, et al. Collagen deposition in HIV-1 infected lymphatic tissues and T cell homeostasis. *J Clin Invest.* 2002;110:1133–1139.

Scriven JE, Rhein J, Hullsiek KH, et al. Early ART after cryptococcal meningitis is associated with cerebrospinal fluid pleocytosis and macrophage activation in a multisite randomized trial. *J Infect Dis.* 2015;212:769–778.

Seddiki N, Sasson SC, Santner-Nanan B, et al. Proliferation of weakly suppressive regulatory CD4+ T cells is associated with over-active CD4+ T-cell responses in HIV-positive patients with mycobacterial immune restoration disease. *Eur J Immunol.* 2009;39:391–403.

Silvestri G, Sodora DL, Koup RA, et al. Nonpathogenic SIV infection of sooty mangabeys is characterized by limited bystander immunopathology despite chronic high-level viremia. *Immunity.* 2003;18:441–452.

Sips M, Sciaranghella G, Diefenbach T, et al. Altered distribution of mucosal NK cells during HIV infection. *Mucosal Immunol.* 2012;5:30–40.

Sivro A, Schuetz A, Sheward D, et al. Integrin α(4)β(7) expression on peripheral blood CD4(+) T cells predicts HIV acquisition and disease progression outcomes. *Sci Transl Med.* 2018;10(425):eaam6354.

Sneller MC, Justement JS, Gittens KR, et al. A randomized controlled safety/efficacy trial of therapeutic vaccination in HIV-infected individuals who initiated antiretroviral therapy early in infection. *Sci Transl Med.* 2017;9(419):eeaan8848.

Srinivasula S, Lempicki RA, Adelsberger JW, et al. Differential effects of HIV viral load and CD4 count on proliferation of naive and memory CD4 and CD8 T lymphocytes. *Blood.* 2011;118:262–270.

Stacey AR, Norris PJ, Qin L, et al. Induction of a striking systemic cytokine cascade prior to peak viremia in acute human immunodeficiency virus type 1 infection, in contrast to more modest and delayed responses in acute hepatitis B and C virus infections. *J Virol.* 2009;83:3719–3733.

Sun JC, Beilke JN, Lanier LL. Adaptive immune features of natural killer cells. *Nature.* 2009;457:557–561.

Surh CD, Sprent J. Homeostasis of naive and memory T cells. *Immunity.* 2008;29:848–862.

Sylwester AW, Mitchell BL, Edgar JB. Broadly targeted human cytomegalovirus-specific CD4+ and CD8+ T cells dominate the memory compartments of exposed subjects. *J Exp Med.* 2005;202:673–685.

Teixeira L, Valdez H, McCune JM, et al. Poor CD4 T cell restoration after suppression of HIV-1 replication may reflect lower thymic function. *AIDS.* 2001;15:1749–1756.

Uthman OA, Nduka C, Watson SI, et al. Statin use and all-cause mortality in people living with HIV: a systematic review and meta-analysis. *BMC Infect Dis.* 2018;18:258.

Uzzan M, Tokuyama M, Rosenstein AK, et al. Anti-α4β7 therapy targets lymphoid aggregates in the gastrointestinal tract of HIV-1-infected individuals. *Sci Transl Med.* 2018;10(461):eaau4711.

van der Vliet HJ, von Blomberg BM, Hazenberg MD, et al. Selective decrease in circulating V alpha 24+V beta 11+ NKT cells during HIV type 1 infection. *J Immunol.* 2002;168:1490–1495.

van Grevenynghe J, Procopio FA, He Z, et al. Transcription factor FOXO3a controls the persistence of memory CD4(+) T cells during HIV infection. *Nat Med.* 2008;14:266–274.

van Zoest RA, van der Valk M, Wit FW, et al. Suboptimal primary and secondary cardiovascular disease prevention in HIV-positive individuals on antiretroviral therapy. *Eur J Prev Cardiol.* 2017;24:1297–1307.

Veazey RS, DeMaria M, Chalifoux LV, et al. Gastrointestinal tract as a major site of CD4+ T cell depletion and viral replication in SIV infection. *Science.* 1998;280:427–431.

Vujkovic-Cvijin I, Dunham RM, Iwai S, et al. Dysbiosis of the gut microbiota is associated with HIV disease progression and tryptophan catabolism. *Sci Transl Med.* 2013;5(193):193ra191. doi: 10.1126/scitranslmed.3006438.

Vujkovic-Cvijin I, Sortino O, Verheij E, et al. HIV-associated gut dysbiosis is independent of sexual practice and correlates with noncommunicable diseases. *Nat Commun.* 2020;11:2448.

Walker NF, Stek C, Wasserman S, et al. The tuberculosis-associated immune reconstitution inflammatory syndrome: recent advances in clinical and pathogenesis research. *Curr Opin HIV AIDS.* 2018;13:512–521.

Williams WB, Liao HX, Moody MA, et al. HIV-1 VACCINES. Diversion of HIV-1 vaccine-induced immunity by gp41-microbiota cross-reactive antibodies. *Science.* 2015;349:aab1253.

Yoon HA, Nakouzi A, Chang CC, et al. Association between plasma antibody responses and risk for cryptococcus-associated immune reconstitution inflammatory syndrome. *J Infect Dis.* 2019;219:420–428.

Zeng M, Southern PJ, Reilly CS, et al. Lymphoid tissue damage in HIV-1 infection depletes naive T cells and limits T cell reconstitution after antiretroviral therapy. *PLoS Pathog.* 2012;8:e1002437.

Zhang T, Scott JM, Hwang I. Cutting edge: antibody- dependent memory-like NK cells distinguished by FcRgamma deficiency. *J Immunol.* 2013;190:1402–1406.

Zhang W, Ambikan AT, Sperk M, et al. Transcriptomics and targeted proteomics analysis to gain insights into the immune-control mechanisms of HIV-1 infected elite controllers. *EBioMedicine.* 2018;27:40–50.

Zhou J, Amran FS, Kramski M, et al. An NK cell population lacking FcRgamma is expanded in chronically infected HIV patients. *J Immunol.* 2015;194:4688–4697.

7.

HIV TESTING AND COUNSELING

Alejandro Delgado

CHAPTER GOALS

Upon completion of this chapter, the reader should be able to:

- Describe the types of HIV testing.

- Present an overview of HIV counseling, as well as how to adapt counseling to the variety of situations or environments in which these conversations can take place.

- Initiate early HIV therapy.

HIV TESTING: HISTORY AND EVOLUTION

In 1985, when HIV testing first became available, the main goal of testing was for blood banks to screen the US blood supply. When it was discovered that those who simply wished to learn their HIV status were using blood donation testing sites, alternative testing sites were implemented. Because at that time no treatment was available and routes of transmission were still being investigated, opinion was divided about the value of testing. By 1987, the implications of a positive HIV serology were clear, and the US Public Health Service and the Centers for Disease Control and Prevention (CDC) issued the first set of guidelines for HIV testing and counseling (CDC, 1987). Earlier guidelines targeted those in "high-risk groups," but experience taught that a more productive approach focused on behaviors rather than membership in a particular population. Hence, the thrust of the current guidelines is that HIV screening is recommended for all persons aged 13–65 years, regardless of risk factors. Periodic revisions informed by the epidemiology of the pandemic extended the outreach and flexibility of testing, culminating in the "Revised Recommendations for HIV Testing of Adults, Adolescents, and Pregnant Women in Health-Care Settings" (Branson et al., 2006).

LEARNING OBJECTIVES

- Describe the types of HIV testing.

- Prepare an overview of HIV counseling as well as how to adapt counseling to the variety of situations or environments in which these conversations can take place.

WHAT'S NEW?

- During the past decade, the evidence favoring the early institution of therapy for HIV has been steadily growing, showing benefits in virologic control and decreased transmission of HIV. The World Health Organization (WHO) has published data from 2017 showing that the proportion of low- to middle-income countries that have adopted the "Treat All ART initiation" has increased from 33% to 70%.

- The most recent data published by the CDC estimate that approximately 14% of people living with HIV are unaware of their diagnosis. In certain states and among men who have sex with men (MSM), who constitute 82% of new yearly diagnoses, the percentage of people who are unaware of their HIV infection may be as high as 25%, prompting the CDC to update its HIV screening recommendations for the MSM population.

- In June 2014, the CDC revised its testing algorithm favoring the use of fourth-generation assays that are capable of early detection of HIV-1 and HIV-2 antibodies as well as the p24 antigen. This has substantially narrowed the window between initial infection and positive test results. For the first time since 1989, the CDC has eliminated the use of confirmation testing with a first-generation western blot or immunofluorescence assay, now recommending that a nucleic acid amplification test be used (Figure 7.1).

KEY POINTS

- HIV testing should be offered as part of routine medical care to all people. The US Preventive Services Task Force put forth recommendations in 2013 that clinicians screen all people between the ages of 15 and 65 years. Testing in younger and older persons should be offered when special circumstances deem this appropriate.

- The CDC recommends that clinicians screen asymptomatic sexually active MSM at least annually and more frequently (i.e., every 3 or 6 months) for MSM at increased risk for HIV infection.

- All persons screened for HIV should be counseled regarding risk-reduction strategies including pre-exposure

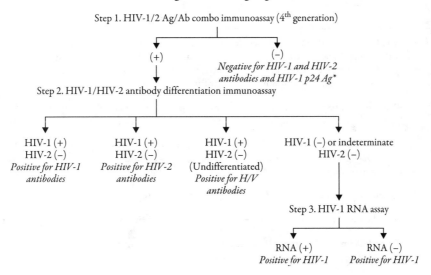

HIV Diagnostic Testing Algorithm

Step 1. HIV-1/2 Ag/Ab combo immunoassay (4th generation)

(+)

(–)
*Negative for HIV-1 and HIV-2
antibodies and HIV-1 p24 Ag**

Step 2. HIV-1/HIV-2 antibody differentiation immunoassay

HIV-1 (+)
HIV-2 (–)
*Positive for HIV-1
antibodies*

HIV-1 (+)
HIV-2 (–)
*Positive for HIV-2
antibodies*

HIV-1 (+)
HIV-2 (–)
(Undifferentiated)
*Positive for H/V
antibodies*

HIV-1 (–) or indeterminate
HIV-2 (–)

Step 3. HIV-1 RNA assay

RNA (+)
Positive for HIV-1

RNA (–)
Positive for HIV-1

(+) = Reactive (or repeatedly reactive) test result, in accordance with manufacturer's instructions
(–) = Nonreactive test result, in accordance with manufacturer's instructions
Italics = Final interpretation; No further testing indicated for the specimen
*For 3rd generation HIV-1/2 immunoassay, interpretation is 'Negative for HIV-1 and HIV-2 antibodies'.

Figure 7.1 Recommended laboratory HIV testing algorithm for serum or plasma specimens   SOURCE: Centers for Disease Control and Prevention and Association of Public Health Laboratories. Laboratory testing for the diagnosis of HIV infection: updated recommendations. http://dx.doi.org/10.15620/cdc.23447. Published June 27, 2014.

prophylaxis (PrEP) and other prevention methods depending on test results.

- All pregnant women should be screened for HIV at the earliest instance possible.

HIV TESTING TERMINOLOGY, TYPES, AND ALGORITHM

Initially, the CDC guidelines focused on the diagnosis of HIV-1 using a sensitive antibody immunoassay with validation of those results by a more specific test such as the western blot or indirect immunofluorescence assay. By 1992, the guidelines also included testing recommendations for the diagnosis of HIV-2. In 2004, protocols for rapid antibody test results were issued with recommendations that all rapid testing be confirmed with either western blot or immunofluorescence assay. With the advent of improved immunoassays and tests, recommendations regarding HIV diagnostic testing have undergone changes.

The CDC's guidelines for laboratory testing for HIV are outlined in an algorithm (Figure 7.1). Initial testing should be done with an antigen/antibody combination immunoassay that detects both HIV-1 and HIV-2 antibodies and HIV-1 p24 antigen. If a positive result is obtained, the specimen should be tested with an antibody immunoassay that differentiates HIV-1 and HIV-2 antibodies. In the situation of a reactive antigen/antibody combination immunoassay with a nonreactive or indeterminate HIV-1/HIV-2 antibody differentiation immunoassay, the specimen should be further tested with an HIV-1 nucleic acid test. If the nucleic acid test is reactive, then it indicates acute HIV infection if the antibody differentiation immunoassay was negative. If the antibody differentiation immunoassay was indeterminate and the nucleic acid test is reactive, this indicates confirmed infection. A negative nucleic acid test indicates a false-positive result of the initial immunoassay.

Table 7.1 enumerates the various types of HIV testing.

LABORATORY MARKERS FOR HIV

There is a brief period immediately after HIV infection where there are no laboratory markers that can be detected in plasma; this is termed the *eclipse period*. After about 5–10 days of infection, HIV RNA can be detected by nucleic acid tests, followed by HIV-1 p24 antigen within 4–10 days after RNA is detected. HIV-1 p24 antigen is detected by fourth-generation immunoassays, but, as antibodies begin developing, the p24 antigens begin forming immune complexes with the antibodies and become no longer detectable. Immunoglobulin M antibodies start to be expressed about 3–5 days after the p24 antigen is detected, which are detected by third- and fourth-generation immunoassays. This is followed by immunoglobulin G antibodies, which will remain throughout the course of the infection (Branson et al., 2014).

WHO SHOULD BE TESTED?

HIV testing should be undertaken in anyone who has symptoms and signs of acute or chronic HIV infection.

In the healthcare setting, every individual between the ages 13 and 65 years should be offered testing once in their lifetime. For higher-risk groups, repeat testing may be indicated.

Table 7.1 HIV TESTING TERMINOLOGY

TEST TYPE	DESCRIPTION
Anonymous testing	No identifying information links the patient to the test sample. At the time of testing, the patient is handed a code number, and a matching code number is affixed to the sample. No institutional record of the code is kept. Results are given only verbally because no medical record is created. Treatment cannot be instituted based on this form of testing. Useful for personal informational purposes.
Confidential testing	Test is linked to patient identifiers, and access to results is available for review only by those identified within "need to know" medical standards, including local, state, and national (e.g., CDC) public health agencies.
Screening	Performing an HIV test for all persons in a defined population. For individual patients, screening is most cost-effective through an antibody-based test, the most common of which is the enzyme-linked immunosorbent assay (ELISA).
Opt-in screening	Patient approaches the provider and requests HIV testing.
Opt-out screening	Healthcare provider offers routine HIV testing to all patients unless refused by patient.
Point-of-care or rapid testing	Simplified antibody- or antibody- and antigen-based testing procedure that can give a screening-level result in approximately 20 minutes or less and that can be implemented by a trained nonhealthcare individual.
Diagnostic testing	Testing prompted by the presence of clinical signs or symptoms. The term may also refer to the antigen-based confirmation of a positive ELISA. In the United States, the validation test formerly used most often was the western blot analysis. New CDC guidelines now recommend using a fourth-generation HIV Ag/Ab enzyme immunoassay test or HIV RNA test for diagnostic confirmation. The validation testing may also be referred to as *confirmatory testing*.
Targeted testing	Performing an HIV test on persons perceived to be at higher risk, as defined by behavioral, clinical, or demographic characteristics. Formerly the main strategy for HIV testing, it has been supplanted by the recommendation to treat HIV screening as a routine part of medical care.

Healthcare providers should offer yearly testing to at-risk groups such as persons who inject drugs, people who engage in sex with an HIV-positive partner, people who exchange money for sex, MSM, or heterosexual persons who have had one more sex partner since their last HIV test. These individuals should be offered annual testing or more frequently if indicated by their risk factors.

Unless recent HIV test results are immediately available, any person whose blood or body fluid is the source of an occupational exposure for a healthcare provider should be informed of the incident and tested for HIV infection at the time the exposure occurs.

Any person seeking testing or having been diagnosed with any sexually transmitted infection (STI) should be offered HIV testing.

PRE- AND POSTTEST COUNSELING ELEMENTS

PRETEST COUNSELING

According to the CDC's 2006 recommendations for HIV testing in the healthcare setting, written consent and prevention counseling is not required. A meta-analysis of 27 published studies saw that HIV counseling and testing was effective in secondary prevention but not an effective strategy for primary prevention (Weinhardt et al., 1999). However, randomized controlled studies suggest that the quality and delivery of the counseling affects its efficacy on primary prevention (Kamb et al., 1998; Koblin et al., 2004). As such, HIV testing in itself can offer the opportunity to refer people for prevention counseling especially in those with high-risk behaviors.

Effective pretest counseling is an interactive process of assessing risk, recognizing specific risk-inducing behaviors, and reviewing risk-reduction strategies. This may be done in a variety of ways—through written material, films, or orally by a variety of trained staff. Of greatest importance is setting a nonjudgmental atmosphere, imparting accurate information in a useful format, offering an opportunity for questions, and maintaining strict confidentiality of personal information.

If deemed to be appropriate, elements of pretest counseling should include the following:

- A functional assessment of the person's decision-making capacity.
- The meaning, sensitivity, and specificity of the test.
- The potential ramifications of a positive test result.
- A discussion about confidentiality and disclosure of test results by the healthcare providers to public health authorities and by the person to sexual and/or drug partners.
- A frank discussion of risk-reduction behaviors.
- Specific instructions about accessing treatment in the event of a positive result.

POSTTEST COUNSELING

Elements of posttest counseling should include the following. For a negative result:

- The validity of the negative result.

- Possible retesting if indicated.

- Reinforcement of transmission reduction behaviors (US Department of Veterans Affairs, 2002).

- Prevention strategies including PrEP, condom use, safer sex practices, and clean needle and syringe services.

For a positive result:

- Optimally given during a face-to-face meeting.

- Review of the availability and effectiveness of treatment.

- Reinforcement of disclosure to spouse and/or sexual and/or drug-using partners.

- Reinforcement of transmission reduction behaviors.

- An assessment of any intent to harm self or others.

SPECIAL POPULATIONS AND ENVIRONMENTS

BLOOD SUPPLY SCREENING

Since 1990, all persons desiring to donate blood or plasma are required to undergo testing, as are those donating sperm for artificial insemination or tissue or organs for transplantation. The donor is notified only if the specimen tests positive. The laboratory assays used for testing blood, blood products, tissues, and organs have evolved along with those used to screen individuals (and often are the same). However, because the volume of testing is larger, pooled testing using nucleic acid tests is commonly done to improve testing and to possibly detect blood or blood products from acutely infected persons.

PERINATAL SCREENING

HIV screening should be a routine component of prenatal testing and should be performed during the first trimester or at entry into care. Retesting in the third trimester (preferably < 36 weeks of gestation) is recommended for women at high risk for HIV exposure, for those who receive healthcare in high-incidence areas, and for those with signs or symptoms consistent with acute HIV infection. Women with undocumented HIV status at the time of labor or delivery should be screened with a point-of-care (POC) HIV test unless they opt out. If a mother's HIV status is unknown postpartum, POC testing of the newborn is recommended (and is legally mandated in many states) as soon as possible so that antiretroviral prophylaxis can be offered to HIV-exposed infants. The mother should be informed that the identification of HIV antibodies in the newborn indicates that the mother is infected (Branson et al., 2006).

MSM

MSM have been identified as a population that is at high risk for HIV infection as well as STIs. Disproportionately higher rates of HIV infection are seen within the Black and Hispanic MSM population compared to White and Asian MSM, with up to 44% being unaware of their serostatus (CDC, 2009). Because of the high-risk nature of the MSM population, the CDC recommends screening for HIV and syphilis at least annually. In addition, it is recommended to screen for urethral and rectal gonorrhea and chlamydia along with pharyngeal gonorrhea in sexually active people.

In the 2021 (most current version), CDC Sexually Transmitted Disease (STD) Screening and Treatment Guidelines, it is now recommended to do more frequent STD screening (i.e., for syphilis, gonorrhea, and chlamydia) at 3- to 6-month intervals with MSM, including those with HIV infection, if risk behaviors persist or if they or their sexual partners have multiple partners. Evaluation for HSV-2 infection with type-specific serologic tests also can be considered if infection status is unknown in persons with previously undiagnosed genital tract infection (Workowski, 2021).

TESTING SETTINGS

There are two primary models of HIV testing as per the CDC: routine testing in a standard medical setting and targeted testing in nonclinical settings. Nonclinical settings are sites where medical services are not routinely provided but select diagnostic services are offered, such as HIV testing. Examples of nonclinical settings include mobile testing units, churches, shelters, syringe services programs, and homes. The essential elements for HIV testing are the same for both a standard medical setting and a nonclinical setting. An important principle with HIV testing in a nonclinical setting is to link any persons living with HIV (PWH) into medical care.

HOME TESTING

Currently, there are only two home HIV tests: the Home Access HIV-1 Test System and the OraQuick In-Home HIV Test. While these tests seek to empower people and allow them to seek testing outside of healthcare settings, the limitations of oral swab testing especially should be emphasized.

The Home Access HIV-1 Test System is a home collection kit that involves pricking the finger to collect a blood sample, sending the sample to a licensed laboratory, and then calling in for results as early as the next business day. This test is anonymous. If the test is positive, a follow-up test is performed by the lab right away, and the results include the follow-up test. The manufacturer provides confidential counseling and referral for treatment. The tests conducted on the blood sample collected at home find infection later after exposure than most lab-based tests using blood from a vein but earlier than tests conducted with oral fluid.

The OraQuick In-Home HIV Test provides rapid results in the home. The testing procedure involves swabbing the gums or mucosal surface for an oral fluid sample and using a kit to test it. Results are available in 20 minutes. Those who test positive need a follow-up test. The manufacturer provides confidential counseling and referral to follow-up testing sites. Because the level of antibody in oral fluid is lower than it is in blood, oral fluid tests detect infection later after exposure than do blood tests. Up to 1 in 12 infected people may test falsely negative with this test.

Data from eSTAMP, a study performed in 2019 where MSM were mailed self-test kits, showed that, compared to control arms, patients were more likely to test themselves frequently and they identified more HIV infections, did not increase sexually risky behavior, and shared their results with their social network.

STRATEGIES TO IMPROVE UPTAKE OF HIV TESTING

HIV screening should be voluntary and undertaken only with the person's knowledge and understanding. Testing is optimally undertaken with the goal of preventing newly acquired infection in those found to be negative and of providing linkage to care in those found to be positive. The knowledge imparted and self-reflection on the part of the person during testing is an essential part of the screening process. Without knowledge of risk reduction for those who are negative and linkage to care for those who are positive, screening is of little benefit to the persons being tested (CDC, 2011). The commonality of concurrent STDs in HIV practices argues against the notion that safer sex practices are promoted through knowledge of one's positive status alone. In the highly structured, technical, reimbursement-driven healthcare environment, a truly successful screening program is not one that is measured by the number of tests performed but, rather, one that takes into account that HIV screening deals with the most elemental and intimate aspects of human existence.

AREAS FOR IMPROVEMENT

Recently published data have demonstrated that, despite current recommendations by various medical organizations including the CDC, an important percentage of at-risk individuals goes untested annually.

In a recent survey, high-risk individuals were interviewed anonymously and tested for HIV infection. Of the MSM population interviewed, 22% had a positive test result, and 8% of people who injected drugs had a positive test result. Of those who were HIV-positive, 8% of MSM and 12% of people who injected drugs were unaware of their infection. Most notably, the majority of people surveyed reported visiting a clinician, but fewer than 50% were offered HIV testing.

Clearly, an opportunity for education and increased testing is still present.

RECOMMENDED READING

Centers for Disease Control and Prevention (CDC). Sexually transmitted diseases treatment guidelines: special populations. cdc.gov. https:// www.cdc.gov/std/default.htm. Published January 25, 2017. Accessed September 30, 2022.

Hall HI, Tang T, Espinoza L. Late diagnosis of HIV infection in metropolitan areas of the United States and Puerto Rico. *AIDS Behav.* 2016;20(5):967–972. http:// www.ncbi.nlm.nih.gov/pub med/26542730

Kelen GD, Hsieh YH, Rothman RE, et al. Improvements in the continuum of HIV care in an inner-city emergency department. *AIDS.* 2016;30(1):113–120. http:// www.ncbi.nlm.nih.gov/pubmed/ 26731757

Truong H. Sentinel surveillance of HIV- 1 transmitted drug resistance, acute infection, and recent infection. PLoS One. October 6, 2011;6:e25281.

Weeks BS, Alcamo EL. *AIDS: the biological basis.* Sudbury, MA: Jones & Bartlett; 2010.

Wejnert P. Prevalence of missed opportunities for HIV testing among persons unaware of their infection. *JAMA.* 2018;319(24):2555.

REFERENCES

Branson BM, Hansfield HH, Lampe MA, et al. Revised recommendations for HIV testing of adults, adolescents, and pregnant women in health-care settings. *CDC MMWR recommendations and reports.* cdc. gov. https://www.cdc.gov/mmwr/ preview/mmwrhtml/rr5514a1.htm. Published September 22, 2006. Accessed September 30, 2022.

Branson BM, Owen SM, Wesolowski LG, et al. Laboratory testing for the diagnosis of HIV infection: updated recommendations. cdc.gov. https://stacks.cdc.gov/view/cdc/23447. Published June 27, 2014. Accessed September 30, 2022.

Centers for Disease Control and Prevention. HIV infection among young black men who have sex with men: Jackson, Mississippi, 2006–2008. cdc.gov. https://www.cdc.gov/mmwr/preview/mmwrhtml/mm580 4a2.htm. Published February 6, 2009. Accessed September 30, 2022.

Centers for Disease Control and Prevention. Perspectives in disease prevention and health promotion public health service guidelines for counseling and antibody testing to prevent HIV infection and AIDS. cdc.gov. https://www.cdc.gov/mmwr/preview/mmwrhtml/00015 088.htm. Published August 14, 1987. Accessed September 30, 2022.

Centers for Disease Control and Prevention. Vital signs: HIV prevention through care and treatment. https:// www.cdc.gov/ mmwr/ preview/ mmwrhtml/ mm6047a4.htm. Published August 29, 2011. Accessed September 30, 2022.

Kamb ML, Fishbein M, Douglas JM, et al. Efficacy of risk-reduction counseling to prevent human immunodeficiency virus and sexually transmitted diseases. *JAMA.* 1998;280:1161–1167.

Koblin B, Chesney M, Coates T, et al. Effects of a behavioural intervention to reduce acquisition of HIV infection among men who have sex with men: the EXPLORE randomised controlled study. *Lancet.* 2004;364 (9428):41–50. https://www.ncbi.nlm.nih.gov/pubmed/15234855

US Department of Veterans Affairs. *The VA prevention handbook: a guide for clinicians.* Washington, DC: Veterans Health Administration; 2002.

Weinhardt LS, Carey MP, Johnson BT, et al. Effects of HIV counseling and testing on sexual risk behavior: a meta-analytic review of published research, 1985–1997. *Am J Public Health.* 1999;89(9):1397–1405. https://www.ncbi.nlm.nih.gov/pmc/articles/PMC1508752

Workowski KA, Bachmann LH, Chan PA, et al. Sexually transmitted infections treatment guidelines, 2021. *MMWR Recomm Rep.* 2021;70(4):1–187. http://doi:10.15585/m

8.

LABORATORY TESTING STRATEGIES, DETECTION, AND DIAGNOSIS

Kruti J. Yagnik and Jessica A. Meisner

CHAPTER GOALS

Upon completion of this chapter, the reader should be able to:

- Discuss the various laboratory and home testing methods used for screening and diagnosis of HIV infections.

- Explain how available immunoassays can be used for screening and diagnosing most early and primary HIV infections.

- Discuss when virologic assays should be considered as complementary diagnostics to immunoassays for screening and confirmation of HIV-1 and HIV-2 infections.

- Explain the rationale behind the HIV testing algorithm.

- Describe how HIV infection can be diagnosed in newborns and children younger than age 18 months.

SEROLOGIC TESTING METHODS

LEARNING OBJECTIVE

- Explain how available immunoassays can be used for screening and diagnosing most early and primary HIV infections.

KEY POINTS

- Laboratory confirmation of HIV infection is primarily through the detection of HIV antibodies and/or the p24 antigen in an individual.

- The western blot is no longer used as a confirmation test.

- The prevalence of HIV-2 is increasing in the United States, so it is important to use immunoassays approved for detecting HIV-2 (as well as other non–group M HIV-1 strains).

- Using the current immunoassays and confirmatory testing, false-positive results are exceedingly rare. However, providers should use clinical judgment when interpreting test results and consider additional follow-up testing when appropriate.

- False-negative immunoassays are exceedingly rare except for individuals who are early in their infection and have yet to produce HIV antibodies that are detectable by current assays.

- Rapid HIV tests can be useful testing options for settings such as health fairs, nonclinical locations, and other situations in which quickly receiving preliminary test results would be beneficial (e.g., pre- and/or postexposure prophylaxis).

IMMUNOLOGY BEHIND TESTING

Following HIV infection there is a seroconversion "window" that includes an "eclipse period" and an acute infection period during which HIV infection may not be detectable by immunological or serologic assays. Although there is no accepted laboratory definition for an acute HIV infection, a current operational definition is the detection of HIV RNA or p24 antigen in the blood before antibodies have formed (Cohen et al., 2010). In these individuals, nonserologic assays should be used or follow-up serological testing should be performed after 2–3 weeks. In addition, it is important to understand that viral kinetics and serologic markers may not always be as accurate with non–clade B subtype infections (Hackett, 2012; Swenson et al., 2014).

HISTORY OF TESTING

The first enzyme immunoassay (EIA) was licensed in 1985 (CDC, 1990). HIV EIAs are typically described as being from particular "generations," which helps to classify them based on technological advancements throughout the years. These advancements have shortened the detection window significantly. The first-generation EIAs used whole HIV lysate as an antigen to capture antibodies present in a blood sample but could only detect HIV-1. However, these had a significant number of false positives because of cellular protein contamination (Houn et al., 1987; Louie et al., 2006). The second-generation EIAs used recombinant viral proteins or peptides, which limited cellular protein contamination (Chappel et al., 2009). This generation was used to screen blood donations in the 1980s. Third-generation EIAs in the 1990s used a technique that was able to bind both immunoglobulin G (IgG) and IgM antibodies and so even further reduced the window period.

The first western blot assay was approved in 1987; thereafter, it was recommended as a confirmatory assay for positive immunoassays (CDC, 1988). A western blot separates the individual proteins of the HIV-1 lysate into bands that allow for capturing antibodies specific to selected HIV antigens in an individual's blood or urine (Healey et al., 1992). Assays are reported positive if the bands present meet an established criterion; assays are reported as indeterminate if bands are detected, but do not meet the criteria for a positive test (CDC, 1989). Western blots are no longer used for confirmation of positive immunoassays.

ENZYME IMMUNOASSAYS

Enzyme immunoassays are currently the most reliable and cost-effective testing method for most individuals in the United States. Screening and testing for HIV-2 infections have become more common in the United States and require the use of assays that are specifically approved to detect this virus type. HIV-2 assays are essential in certain locations outside the United States (Hackett, 2012; Swenson et al., 2014). EIAs are still not completely reliable for screening and diagnostic testing for individuals with acute HIV infections (see the section "Virologic Assays"), self-testing kits (see the section "HIV Self-Testing"), or for screening and diagnostic testing for infants and newborns (see the section "Alternative Algorithms for Screening and Diagnosing HIV Infections").

Antigen/antibody combination assays are also known as *fourth-generation EIAs*. These assays act as both a third-generation assay and a capture immunoassay, directly detecting the p24 antigen (Kabir et al., 2020). Thus, fourth-(Kabir et al., 2020). Thus, fourth generation EIAs reduce the detection window period even further while maintaining the third generation's accuracy (Pandori et al., 2009; Rosenberg et al., 2015; Sickinger et al., 2004). It is important to note that fourth generation EIAs may have a second window period in some patients, but this has not been observed in more recent testing systems that can detect IgM (Gray et al., 2018). The fifth-generation test detects both the p24 antigen and antibodies but can separate results for HIV-1 p24 antigen, HIV-1 antibody, and HIV-2 antibody.

RAPID HIV TESTS

Rapid HIV tests detect HIV antibodies present in an oral fluid, finger-stick blood, or venipuncture whole blood/plasma sample. Fourth- and fifth-generation EIAs have shorter detection windows compared to the currently available rapid tests, but rapid tests are as accurate, and test results are available in less than 30 minutes (Kabir et al., 2020). However, there are data that describe lower sensitivity of HIV rapid tests in high-income countries compared to low-income countries, likely because of the larger proportion of acute infections in targeted populations (Tan, 2016). They show maximum potential utility in resource-limited settings, or to speed up decision-making processes by avoiding turn-around-times (Setty & Hewlett, 2014). Individuals with a potential exposure and those with ongoing high risk for HIV infection who have negative rapid test results should be counseled to be retested or considered for testing that is more sensitive for detecting acute HIV infections in these situations. There are currently more than 15 rapid HIV tests approved by the FDA. Several of these rapid tests have received Clinical Laboratory Improvement Amendment waivers, making them available for point-of-care testing and screening in settings in which transporting specimens to a laboratory is either not possible or not practical.

When determining whether to use an approved rapid HIV test or EIA testing for screening and/or diagnosing HIV infections, one should consider the setting in which testing will occur, the cost, and the population being tested. Rapid tests generally cost more compared to EIA assays, especially if large numbers of tests are being performed. Rapid testing can be particularly useful for public health testing programs outside of clinical settings, such as during health fairs or at social venues where high-risk individuals may be located. Testing women who are in labor is another situation in which rapid HIV testing may be a more suitable choice for compared to EIAs (Setty & Hewlett, 2014). Rapid testing platforms for point-of-care HIV RNA testing are also under development (Agutu et al., 2019; Curtis et al., 2016).

RECOMMENDED READING

Kabir MA, Zilouchian H, Caputi M, et al. Advances in HIV diagnosis and monitoring. *Crit Rev in Biotechnol*. 2020;40(5):623–638.

Tan WS, Chow EPF, Fairley CK, et al. Sensitivity of HIV rapid tests compared with fourth-generation enzyme immunoassays or HIV RNA tests. *AIDS*. 2016;30(12):1951–1960.

Centers for Disease Control and Prevention (CDC). Branson BM, Owen SM, Wesolowski LG, et al. Laboratory testing for the diagnosis of HIV infection. Available at: https:// stacks.cdc.gov/view/cdc/23447. Published 2014. Accessed January 2023.

Masciotra S, Luo W, Westheimer E, et al. Performance evaluation of the FDA-approved determine HIV-1/2 Ag/Ab combo assay using plasma and whole blood specimens. *J Clin Virol*. 2017;91:95–100.

VIROLOGIC ASSAYS

LEARNING OBJECTIVE

Discuss when virologic assays should be considered as complementary diagnostics to immunoassays for screening and confirmation of HIV-1 and HIV-2 infections.

KEY POINTS

- Virologic assays should be used in diagnosing acute HIV infections and infections in newborns and infants younger than age 18 months.

- Compared to immunoassays, virologic assays are more expensive and have an increased rate of false-positive results; virologic assays may also be falsely negative in individuals with chronic infections, undetectable viral loads, and non–clade B infections.

- To improve cost-effectiveness, several public health laboratories in the United States are pooling negative immunoassay samples and testing the pooled samples using a nucleic acid amplification test (NAAT). This method increases a screening program's overall accuracy by detecting individuals with acute infections who would have otherwise received a negative test result.

Virologic assays include qualitative and quantitative DNA and RNA assays as well as p24 antigen assays. Fourth- and fifth-generation antigen/antibody combination immunoassays use the HIV p24 core protein as the antigen component and thus can be considered both a serologic and a virologic assay (Stone et al., 2018). Stand-alone p24 antigen assays are available; however, the p24 antigen rapidly becomes undetectable after antibodies develop, thereby limiting the period during which a p24 antigen assay uniquely provides diagnostic information. Multiple p24-only tests are under investigation for a myriad of roles in HIV management and prevention, but no conclusive data are available yet (Gray et al., 2018).

Virologic assays should be considered for the following:

- Diagnosing HIV infection in newborns and infants younger than age 18 months.

- Diagnosing acute HIV infections in cases in which patients would likely not yet have detectable antibodies.

Because infection transmission risk correlates well with an individual's plasma viral load (Chan, 2012; Rodger et al., 2016), considerable attention has been given to detecting acute HIV infections (Cohen et al., 2010; Henn et al., 2017; Patel et al., 2010; Parekh et al., 2018). Individuals acutely infected will typically have relatively high viral loads before seroconverting and are likely unaware of their infection (Henn et al., 2017). Studies have shown that recently infected individuals are likely the source of transmission for up to 50% of all new infections (Yerly & Hirschel, 2012).

QUANTITATIVE ASSAYS FOR DETECTING HIV-1 RNA (VIRAL LOAD ASSAYS)

There are several commercially available assays reliably quantify HIV-1 RNA in plasma. These tests quantify plasma HIV-1 RNA within variable dynamic range. These assays detect most HIV-1 subtypes, and, although they have become increasingly effective at detecting non–subtype B infections, there is some variability based on clade variations and each assay's performance characteristics. Both kPCR and RT-PCR assays are proficient at quantitation of many non–clade B strains of HIV-1 (Alvarez et al., 2015; Parekh et al., 2018; Karasi et al., 2011).

Because of the rate of false positives, these quantitative assays must be used with caution as a diagnostic test. In an acute HIV infection, plasma HIV-1 RNA levels are typically very high, whereas levels of false positives tend to be very low (Henn et al., 2017).

QUALITATIVE ASSAYS FOR DETECTING HIV-1 RNA

Currently, there is one qualitative virologic assay, frequently referred to as NAAT, which was approved for use in October 2006 by the FDA, as an aid in the diagnosis of HIV-1 (APTIMA; Gen-Probe, San Diego, CA). This assay can be used to assist with diagnosing an acute HIV infection and as an additional test to confirm an HIV-1 infection when an EIA or a rapid test is repeatedly reactive for HIV-1 antibodies. Qualitative assays are not commonly used because quantitative assays are the preferred detection for HIV RNA. The qualitative assays' role in point-of-care HIV management, especially in resource-limited settings, is under investigation. Point-of-care HIV viral load testing shows potential due to its ease of use, quick turnaround time for results, and cost-effectiveness (Ochodo et al., 2022). Despite showing acceptable clinical accuracy, more data are required to assess its clinical utility, quality assurance, and its role in future diagnostic algorithms (Agutu et al., 2019).

HIV-2 VIROLOGIC ASSAYS

Despite increasing use of the HIV-1/HIV-2 differentiation test, few HIV-2 infections are diagnosed in the United States. The US CDC continues to recommend that laboratories follow the laboratory-based algorithm with the HIV-1/HIV-2 differentiation test as the second step (Peruski et al., 2020).

An approved HIV-2 virologic assay is not currently commercially available in the United States. Although some assays may detect a viral load, caution should be exercised when utilizing these results to monitor response to treatment because under quantification is common when viremia is detected and not all HIV-2 infected individuals will have a detectable viral load (Campbell-Yesufu & Gandhi, 2011). A number of international laboratories use in-house (or laboratory-developed) HIV-2 viral load assays. There are two current labs in the United States with HIV-2 quantitative viral loads available (New York State Department of Health and University of Washington, 2020). Reference laboratory resources are available through the CDC for public health laboratories evaluating HIV-2–reactive specimens.

RECOMMENDED READING

Chang M, Gottlieb GS, Dragavon JA, et al. Validation for clinical use of a novel HIV-2 plasma RNA viral load assay using the Abbott m2000 platform. *J Clin Virol*. 2012;55(2):128–133. http://doi:10.1016/j.jcv.2012.06.024

Damond F, Bernard C, Jurg Boni M, et al. An international collaboration to standardize HIV-2 viral load assays: results from the 2009 ACHIEV2E quality control study. *J Clin Microbiol*. 2011;49:3491–3497.

New York State Department of Health. HIV nucleic acid testing. Wadsworth Center Website. https://www.wadsworth.org/programs/id/bloodborne-viruses/clinical-testing/hiv-2-nucleic-acid. Published 2020. Accessed August 14, 2020.

HIV SELF-TESTING

HIV self-testing (HIVST) at home is gaining popularity as a new tool in the diagnosis of HIV, with updated WHO 2019guidelines recommending it be offered as an additional approach to HIV testing services (WHO, 2019). Facility-based testing uses more sensitive assays, can provide onsite counseling, and accelerates linkage to care. However, HIVST has been shown to have high acceptability in high-risk patients from all socioeconomic strata (Figueroa et al., 2015; Krause et al., 2013; Stephenson et al., 2017), and could be very promising in low-to-middle-income countries (Moshoeu et al., 2019). The processes of dissemination, adoption, and implementation continue to remain significant hurdles, mainly because of challenges with cost, testing performance variability, risk of social harm, and linkage to care (Johnson et al., 2014; Hurt & Powers, 2014; Pai et al., 2013; Ruzagira et al., 2017; WHO, 2019).

The OraQuick In-Home HIV Test is the only HIV test approved by the FDA for home use and self-testing in the United States. OraQuick was approved in 2012 for sale in stores and online to anyone aged 17 years and older. It tests for HIV-1/2 antibodies in the oral fluid using a swab and delivers results in 20 to 40 minutes. Main limitations are its lower sensitivity and an extended negative window of at least 3 months after exposure. PrEP or PEP may affect results given its effect on antibody levels (Kabir et al., 2020). If the home test is positive, a follow-up laboratory test will need to be done to confirm the results.

Despite the lower sensitivity in detecting recent HIV infection, owing to the COVID-19 pandemic, CDC guidelines have added HIVST as options for PrEP monitoring when other options are not available or feasible (home specimen collection kits or self-testing via an oral swab-based test) (CDC, 2020).

RECOMMENDED READING

Figueroa C, Johnson C, Verster A, Baggaley R. Attitudes and acceptability on HIV self-testing among key populations: a literature review. *AIDS Behav*. 2015;19(11):1949–1965.

Kabir MA, Zilouchian H, Caputi M, et al. Advances in HIV diagnosis and monitoring. *Crit Rev in Biotechnol*. 2020;40(5):623–638.

Stephenson R, Freeland R, Sullivan SP, et al. Home-based HIV testing and counseling for male couples (Project Nexus): a protocol for a randomized controlled trial. *JMIR Res Protoc*. 2017 May 30;6(5):e101.

World Health Organization (WHO). Consolidated guidelines on HIV testing services for a changing epidemic. November 2019. Available at: https://www.who.int/publications/i/item/WHO-CDS-HIV-19.31. Accessed March 8, 2023.

WHO. Facts about in-home HIV testing. fda.gov. https://www.fda.gov/consumers/consumer-updates/facts-about-home-hiv-testing. Published 2020. Accessed September 26, 2022.

ALGORITHMS FOR SCREENING AND DIAGNOSING HIV INFECTIONS

LEARNING OBJECTIVE

Explain the rationale behind the HIV testing algorithm.

KEY POINTS

- The algorithm no longer recommends the use of the western blot assay because of its limitations, particularly in confirming acute or recent HIV infections.

- The algorithm recommends using the most sensitive immunoassay (fourth-generation EIA) as a screening test, as well as following any repeatedly positive results with a different immunoassay that can discriminate between HIV-1 and HIV-2.

- Samples with a positive screening assay but negative confirmation assay should be tested using a NAAT.

In 2014, an updated testing algorithm was recommended by the CDC and the Association of Public Health Laboratories (APHL) that recommends the use of the most sensitive immunoassays for primary screening along with a confirmatory test that discriminates HIV-1 from HIV-2 after a repeatedly positive screening test (Wesolowski et al., 2014). Figure 8.1 shows the current recommended HIV testing algorithm (CDC, 2018). In this algorithm, if the confirmatory test is negative, HIV NAAT should be performed. A positive NAAT would be confirmatory for an acute HIV infection.

RECOMMENDED READING

CDC and Association of Public Health Laboratories (APHL). Laboratory testing for the diagnosis of HIV infection: updated recommendations. http:// stacks.cdc.gov/view/cdc/23447. Published June 27, 2014. Accessed September 26, 2022.

Delaney KP, Hanson DL, Masciotra S, Ethridge SF, Wesolowski L, Owen SM. Time until emergence of HIV test reactivity following infection with HIV-1: implications for interpreting test results and retesting after exposure. *Clin Infect Dis*. 2017;64(1):53–59. http://doi:10.1093/cid/ciw666

Delaney KP, Wesolowski LG, Owen SM. The evolution of HIV testing continues. *Sex Transm Dis*. 2017;44(12):747–749. http://doi:10.1097/OLQ.0000000000000736

Rosenberg NE, Pilcher CD, Busch MP, et al. How can we better identify early HIV infections? *Curr Opin HIV AIDS*. 2015;10(1):61–68. http://doi:10.1097/COH.0000000000000121

Wesolowski LG, Parker MM, Delaney KP, Owen SM. Highlights from the 2016 HIV diagnostics conference: the new landscape of HIV testing in laboratories, public health programs and clinical practice. *J Clin Virol*. 2017;91:63–68. http://doi:10.1016/j.jcv.2017.01.009

SCREENING AND DETECTING HIV IN NEWBORNS AND CHILDREN

LEARNING OBJECTIVE

Describe how HIV infection can be diagnosed in newborns and children younger than age 18 months.

KEY POINTS

- Maternal antibodies passed in utero are detectable in a newborn's blood using current immunoassays, so combination assays are not recommended.

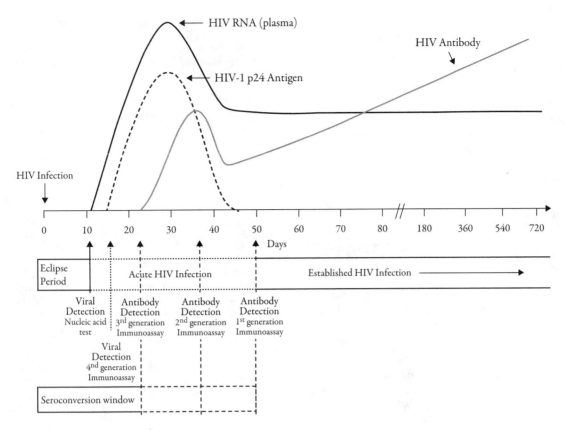

Figure 8.1 Timeline of HIV-1 laboratory markers   SOURCE: Centers for Disease Control and Prevention and Association of Public Health Laboratories. Laboratory testing for the diagnosis of HIV infection: updated recommendations. Available at http://dx.doi.org/10.15620/cdc.23447. Published June 27, 2014. Accessed September 12, 2020.

- Newborn testing requires nucleic acid amplification testing; DNA- and RNA-based assays show similar performance so either can be used.

- HIV testing should be performed for all infants at 14–21 days, at 1 to 2 months of age, and at 4 to 6 months of age in infants who are born of HIV-positive women.

- Laboratory confirmation of HIV infection requires that more than one test be positive; infections typically can be diagnosed by the age of 1 month and definitively in almost all children at age 6 months.

Maternal-to-child transmission of HIV infection can occur in utero, at the time of labor and delivery, and through breastfeeding (Kourtis et al., 2001). Because maternal antibodies passed in utero can be detected in uninfected newborns, immunoassays may be positive in uninfected newborns until 18–24 months of age. Given this, HIV serological testing cannot be used to confirm HIV infection in younger infants because maternal antibodies transferred across the placenta may persist in the newborn up to 18 months (Chantry et al., 1995). Therefore, virologic assays represent the gold standard for diagnostic testing of infants and children younger than 18 months (Read, 2007).

When interpreting immunoassay results for an infant, it is important to consider serological window periods after each of these potential exposure events, as well as the presence of maternal antibodies. Non-breastfed children can be considered presumptively uninfected if there is at least two or more

negative virologic tests (at >2 weeks and >4 weeks) or one negative virologic test and one negative HIV antibody at >6 months, and they can be considered definitively uninfected if there are two negative virologic tests (>1 month and >4 months) or two negative serological tests at >6 months (US DHSS, 2022a).

Virologic assays should be performed at birth on infants born to HIV-infected mothers who meet the following criteria: did not receive prenatal care, did not receive antepartum or intrapartum antiretroviral (ARV) drugs, received intrapartum ARV drugs only, initiated antiretroviral therapy late in pregnancy, were diagnosed with acute HIV during pregnancy, had detectable HIV viral load close to delivery, received ARV combination drugs, and did not have viral suppression (Momplaisir et al., 2015).

Additionally, testing should occur at 14–21 days, at 1 or 2 months of age, and at 4 to 6 months of age. Testing should also be performed for infants with higher risk of perinatal infection 2–4 weeks after cessation of ARV prophylaxis. Some experts also recommend serologic testing to confirm the absence of infection between 12 and 18 months. If any tests are positive, repeat testing is recommended, and the diagnosis of HIV infection can be made based on two separate positive results.

Maternal antibody is present at birth and begins to fade with time, but infant antibody production begins after infant infection occurs (Ciaranello et al., 2011). If an infant is uninfected at birth but becomes infected through breastfeeding, HIV RNA is undetectable while the infant is uninfected but rises rapidly within the first few weeks after infection.

While women living with HIV in the United States are often discouraged from breastfeeding, infants who are breastfed should have standard virologic testing as well as testing every 3 months throughout breastfeeding (WHO, 2010). Many experts also recommend monitoring at 4–6 weeks, 3 months, and 6 months after breastfeeding has stopped (US DHHS, 2022a).

Infants born to HIV-2–infected mothers should be tested with HIV-2–specific virologic assays at time points similar to those used for HIV-1 testing. HIV-2 virologic assays are not commercially available, but the National Perinatal HIV Hotline (1-888-448-8765) can provide a list of sites that perform this testing (US DHHS, 2022b).

TESTING NEWBORNS IN RESOURCE-LIMITED SETTINGS

Access to early infant diagnosis of HIV infection is improving in resource-limited settings (Ciaranello et al., 2011), but key barriers continue to exist. Virologic assays are generally more expensive than immunoassays, and additional barriers, such as accurate specimen collection, transport, and laboratory processing, can limit their use in these settings. However, multiple RNA and DNA PCR assays are currently being used, and the use of dried blood spots has decreased the phlebotomy requirements. Dried blood spots may be obtained through a finger or heel stick, and are heat stable, noninfectious, and can be shipped via mail or courier (Ciaranello et al., 2011).

Breastfeeding may be recommended for children born in resource-limited settings through the age of 12 months, provided the mother and/or child is receiving ARV prophylaxis, so clinical and laboratory monitoring for HIV transmission should take into consideration this ongoing exposure risk (WHO, 2010).

RECOMMENDED READING

Centers for Disease Control and Prevention (CDC) and APHL. Laboratory testing for the diagnosis of HIV infection: updated recommendations. http://stacks.cdc.gov/view/cdc/23447. Published June 27, 2014. Accessed May 22, 2016.

Jourdain G, Mary JY, Coeur SL, et al. Risk factors for in utero or intrapartum mother-to-child transmission of human immunodeficiency virus type 1 in Thailand. *J Infect Dis.* 2007;196(11):1629–1636. http://www.ncbi.nlm.nih.gov/pubmed/18008246

King CC, Kourtis AP, Persaud D, et al. Delayed HIV detection among infants exposed to postnatal antiretroviral prophylaxis during breastfeeding. *AIDS.* 2015;29(15):1953–1961. http://www.ncbi.nlm.nih.gov/pubmed/26153671

US Department of Health and Human Services. Panel on Antiretroviral Therapy and Medical Management of Children Living with HIV. Guidelines for the use of antiretroviral agents in pediatric HIV infection. https://clinicalinfo.hiv.gov/sites/default/files/guidelines/documents/pediatric-arv/guidelines-pediatric-arv.pdf. Published 2022a. Accessed September 26, 2022.

US Department of Health and Human Services. Panel on Treatment of Pregnant Women with HIV Infection and Prevention of Perinatal Transmission. Recommendations for the use of antiretroviral drugs in pregnant women with HIV infection and interventions to reduce perinatal HIV transmission in the United States. https://clinicalinfo.

hiv.gov/sites/default/files/guidelines/documents/Perinatal_GL.pdf. Published 2022b. Accessed September 26, 2022.

Read JS; Committee on Pediatric Aids AAoP. Diagnosis of HIV-1 infection in children younger than 18 months in the United States. *Pediatrics.* 2007;120(6):e1547–1562. http://www.ncbi.nlm.nih.gov/pubmed/18055670

Wessman MJ, Theilgaard Z, Katzenstein TL. Determination of HIV status of infants born to HIV-infected mothers: a review of the diagnostic methods with special focus on the applicability of p24 antigen testing in developing countries. *Scand J Infect Dis.* 2012;44(3):209–215. http://www.ncbi.nlm.nih.gov/pubmed/22074445

REFERENCES

Agutu CA, Ngetsa CJ, Price MA, et al. Systematic review of the performance and clinical utility of point of care HIV-1 RNA testing for diagnosis and care. *PLoS One.* 2019;14(6):e0218369.

Alvarez P, Martin L, Prieto L, et al. HIV-1 variability and viral load technique could lead to false positive HIV-1 detection and to erroneous viral quantification in infected specimens. *J Infect.* 2015;71(3):368–376. http://doi:10.1016/j.jinf.2015.05.011

Campbell-Yesufu OT, Gandhi RT. Update on human immunodeficiency virus (HIV)-2 infection. *Clin Infect Dis.* 2011;52(6):780–787.

Centers for Disease Control and Prevention (CDC). Information from CDC's Division of HIV/AIDS Prevention. https:// stacks.cdc.gov/view/cdc/50872. Published May 2020. Accessed March 8, 2023.

CDC. Interpretation and use of the western blot assay for serodiagnosis of human immunodeficiency virus type 1 infections. *MMWR Morb Mortal Wkly Rep.* 1989;38:1–7.

CDC. Serologic testing for antibody to human immunodeficiency virus. *MMWR Morb Mortal Wkly Rep.* 1988;36:509–515.

CDC. The 2018 quick reference guide: recommended laboratory HIV testing algorithm for serum or plasma specimens. cdc.gov. https:// stacks.cdc.gov/view/cdc/50872. Published January 2018. Accessed September 1, 2018.

CDC. Update: serologic testing for HIV-1 antibody—the United States, 1988 and 1989. *MMWR Morb Mortal Wkly Rep.* 1990;39:380–383.

Chan DJ. Can HIV-1 Incidence be estimated from plasma viral load and sexual behavior. *Int J STD AIDS.* 2012;23(10):724–728.

Chantry CJ, Cooper ER, Pelton SI, et al. Seroreversion in human immunodeficiency virus-exposed but uninfected infants. *Pediatr Infect Dis J.* 1995;14:382–387.

Chappel RJ, Dax EM, Wilson KM. Immunoassays for the diagnosis of HIV: meeting future needs by enhancing quality of testing. *Fut Microbiol.* 2009;48:963–982.

Ciaranello AL, Park JE, Ramirez-Avila L, et al. Early infant HIV-1 diagnosis programs in resource-limited settings: opportunities for improved outcomes and more cost-effective interventions. *BMC Medicine.* 2011;9:1–15.

Cohen MS, Gay CL, Busch MP, et al. The detection of acute HIV infection. *J Infect Dis.* 2010;202:S270–S277.

Curtis KA, Rudolph DL, Morrison D, et al. Single-use, electricity-free amplification device for detection of HIV-1. *J Virol Methods.* 2016;237:132–137.

Figueroa C, Johnson C, Verster A, Baggaley R. Attitudes and acceptability on HIV self-testing among key populations: a literature review. *AIDS Behav.* 2015;19(11):1949–1965.

Gray ER, Bain R, Varsaneux O, et al. p24 revisited: a landscape review of antigen detection for early HIV diagnosis. *AIDS.* 2018;32(15):2089–2102.

Hackett J Jr. Meeting the challenge of HIV diversity: strategies to mitigate the impact of HIV-1 genetic heterogeneity on performance of nucleic acid testing assays. *Clin Lab.* 2012;58(3–4):199–202.

Healey D, Maskill W, Howard T, et al. HIV-1 Western blot: development and assessment of testing to resolve indeterminate reactivity. *AIDS.* 1992;6:629–633.

Hecht F, Wellman R, Busch M, et al. Identifying the early post-HIV antibody seroconversion period. *J Infect Dis.* 2011;204:526–533.

Henn A, Flateau C, Gallien S, et al. Primary HIV infection: clinical presentation, testing, and treatment. *Curr Infect Dis Rep.* 2017;19:7.

Houn HY, Pappas AA, Walter EM. Status of current clinical tests for human immunodeficiency virus (HIV): applications and limitations. *Ann Clin Lab Sci.* 1987;17:279–285.

Hurt CB, Powers KA. Self-testing for HIV and its impact on public health. *Sex Transm Dis.* 2014;41(1):10–12.

Johnson C, Baggaley R, Forsythe S, et al. Realizing the potential for HIV self-testing. *AIDS Behav.* 2014;18(Suppl 4):S391–S395.

Kabir MA, Zilouchian H, Caputi M et al. Advances in HIV diagnosis and monitoring. *Crit Rev in Biotechnol.* 2020;40(5):623–638.

Karasi JC, Dziezuk F, Quennery L, et al. High correlation between the Roche COBAS AmpliPrep/COBAS TaqMan HIV-1, v2.0 and the Abbott m2000 Real Time HIV-1 assays for quantification of viral load in HIV-1 B and non-B subtypes. *J Clin Virol.* 2011;52(3):181–186. http://doi:10.1016/j.jcv.2011.07.002

Kourtis AP, Bulterys M, Nesheim SR, et al. Understanding the timing of HIV transmission from mother to infant. *JAMA.* 2001;285:709–712.

Krause K, Subklew-Sehume F, Kenyon C, et al. Acceptability of HIV self-testing: a systematic literature review. *BMC Public Health.* 2013;13:735.

Louie B, Pandori M, Wong E, et al. Use of an acute seroconversion panel to evaluate a third-generation enzyme-linked immunoassay for detection of human immunodeficiency virus-specific antibodies relative to multiple other assays. *J Clin Microbiol.* 2006;44:1856–1858.

Momplaisir FM, Brady KA, Fekete T, et al. Time of HIV diagnosis and engagement in prenatal care impact virologic outcomes of pregnant women with HIV. *PLoS One.* 2015;10(7):e0132262.

Moshoeu PM, Kuupiel D, Gwala N, et al. The use of home-based HIV testing and counseling in low-and-middle income countries: a scoping review. *BMC Public Health.* 2019;19:132.

New York State Department of Health. HIV nucleic acid testing. Wadsworth Center Website. https://www.wadsworth.org/progr ams/id/bloodborne-viruses/clinical-testing/hiv-2-nucleic-acid. Published 2022. Accessed September 26, 2022.

Ochodo EA, Olwanda EE, Deeks JJ, Mallett S. Point-of-care viral load tests to detect high HIV viral load in people living with HIV/AIDS attending health facilities. *Cochrane Database Syst Rev.* 2022;3(3):CD013208. http://doi:10.1002/14651858.CD013208. pub2. PMID: 35266555; PMCID: PMC8908762.

Pai NP, Sharma J, Shivkumar S, et al. Supervised and unsupervised self-testing for HIV in high-and low-risk populations: a systematic review. *PLoS Med.* 2013;10(4):e1001414.

Pandori MW, Hackett J Jr, Louie B, et al. Assessment of the ability of a fourth-generation immunoassay for human immunodeficiency virus (HIV) antibody and p24 antigen to detect both acute and recent HIV infections in a high-risk setting. *J Clin Microbiol.* 2009;47(8):2639–2642. http://doi:10.1128/JCM.00119-09

Parekh BS, Ou CY, Fonjungo PN, et al. Diagnosis of human immunodeficiency virus infection. *Clin Microbiol Rev.* 2018;32:e00064–18.

Patel P, Mackellar D, Simmons P, et al. Detecting acute human immunodeficiency virus infection using 3 different screening immunoassays and nucleic acid amplification testing for human immunodeficiency virus RNA, 2006–2008. *Arch Int Med.* 2010;170:66–74.

Peruski AH, Wesolowski LG, Delaney KP, et al. Trends in HIV-2 diagnoses and use of the HIV-1/HIV-2 differentiation test United States, 2010–2017. *MMWR Morb Mortal Wkly Rep.* 2020;69:63–66.

Read JS; Committee on Pediatric AIDS, American Academy of Pediatrics. Diagnosis of HIV-1 infection in children younger than 18 months in the United States. *Pediatrics.* 2007;120:e1547–e1562.

Rodger AJ, Cambiano V, Bruun T, et al. Sexual activity without condoms and risk of HIV transmission in serodifferent couples when the HIV-positive partner is using suppressive antiretroviral therapy. *JAMA.* 2016;316(2):171–181.

Rosenberg NE, Pilcher CD, Busch MP, et al. How can we better identify early HIV infections. *Curr Opin HIV AIDS.* 2015;10(1):61–68. http://doi:10.1097/COH.0000000000000121

Ruzagira E, Baisley K, Kamali A, et al. Linkage to HIV care after home-based HIV counselling and testing in sub-Saharan Africa: a systematic review. *Trop Med Int Health.* 2017;22(7):807–821.

Setty MKHG, Hewlett IK. Point of care technologies for HIV. *AIDS Res Treat.* 2014;2014:Article ID 497046. https://doi.org/10.1155/2014/497046

Sickinger E, Steiler M, Kaufman B, et al. Multicenter evaluation of a new, automated enzyme-linked immunoassay for detection of human immunodeficiency virus-specific antibodies and antigen. *J Clin Microbiol.* 2004;42:21–29.

Stephenson R, Freeland R, Sullivan SP, et al. Home-based HIV testing and counseling for male couples (Project Nexus): a protocol for a randomized controlled trial. *JMIR Res Protoc.* 2017;6(5):e101.

Stone M, Bainbridge J, Sanchez AM, et al. Comparison of detection limits of fourth- and fifth-generation combination HIV antigen-antibody, p24 antigen, and viral load assays on diverse HIV isolates. *J Clin Microbiol.* 2018;56(8):e02045–17.

Swenson LC, Cobb B, Geretti AM, et al. Comparative performances of HIV-1 RNA load assays at low viral load levels: results of an international collaboration. *J Clin Microbiol.* 2014;52(2):517–523. http://doi:10.1128/JCM.02461-13

Wesolowski LG, Parker MM, Delaney KP, Owen SM. Highlights from the 2016 HIV diagnostics conference: the new landscape of HIV testing in laboratories, public health programs and clinical practice. *J Clin Virol.* 2017;91:63–68. http://doi:10.1016/j.jcv.2017.01.009

World Health Organization (WHO). Consolidated guidelines on HIV testing services for a changing epidemic. https://www.who.int/publications/i/item/consolidated-guidelines-on-hiv-testing-servi ces-for-a-changing-epidemic. Published November 2019. Accessed September 26, 2022.

WHO. Guidelines on HIV and infant feeding. Principles and recommendations for infant feeding in the context of HIV and a summary of evidence. https://apps.who.int/iris/bitstream/han dle/10665/44345/9789241599535_eng.pdf;jsessionid=15ADE7474 DEDABB0968A7C34F83EF6E9?sequence=1. Published 2010. Accessed: September 26, 2022.

Yerly S, Hirschel B. Diagnosing acute HIV infection. *Expert Rev Ant Infect Ther.* 2012;10:31–41.

9.

INITIAL EVALUATION OF THE PERSON WITH HIV
HISTORY, PHYSICAL EXAMINATION, AND LABORATORY EVALUATION

Esteban A. DelPilar Morales and Daniel J. Skiest

LEARNING OBJECTIVES

- Describe the important details regarding the history and physical examination and appropriate laboratory evaluation for the initial evaluation of the PWH.

- Be familiar with challenges unique to the HIV population.

WHAT'S NEW?

This chapter provides additional insight into gender identity and cultural challenges that can affect the management of some persons living with HIV (PWH). Further, it offers an expanded discussion of the role of telehealth in managing PWH.

KEY POINTS

- A comprehensive history, including a complete sexual and social history, is important in assessing a PWH's risks and possible barriers to treatment.

- A comprehensive physical examination and laboratory evaluation are important to identify any abnormal findings, which may require prompt intervention and to provide a baseline and comparison for future findings.

- Awareness of a person's gender identity and cultural background will allow the health care provider to better understand the person's perception of their condition and is fundamental in caring for PWH.

- PWH presenting for their initial clinic visit may have early infection, asymptomatic chronic infection, or advanced HIV. Recognition of the clinical stage of infection is important, so that appropriate prophylactic medications, prognosis, and counseling can be provided.

THE HIV-ORIENTED MEDICAL HISTORY

The initial office or clinic visit of a PWH, either newly diagnosed or chronically infected, has several objectives. The most obvious purpose is to obtain the necessary information essential for the current and future management. Some PWH may not feel comfortable divulging all relevant medical and social history at the first visit. The hope is that as the patient-provider relationship develops, they will feel more comfortable disclosing more information at subsequent visits. The initial visit also represents an opportunity to establish a trust-based relation between patient and provider. It is important that the provider establish a nonjudgmental tone in a supportive environment. The patient-provider relationship can affect how the patient views the advice received from the provider, including beliefs about the effectiveness of the medications being prescribed (Berghoff et al., 2018). A strong patient-provider relationship has been shown to result in improved retention in care and medication adherence, and is predictive of future therapeutic success (Doshi et al., 2015; Flickinger et al., 2013).

If the PWH is accompanied by another person (e.g., friend, spouse, partner, and family member) the provider should not assume the accompanying person is aware of the patient's HIV diagnosis or other medical history. Prior to proceeding, the provider should determine if the accompanying person is aware of the HIV diagnosis without disclosing the diagnosis. Our practice is to first ask the patient if they want the accompanying person to leave the room or stay during the evaluation. If the patient indicates they want the person to stay, the provider should then ask whether it is okay to discuss "everything" and/ or "Do you know why patient (name) is here today?" In most cases the person will indicate that the patient is here for HIV care; however, if it is still not clear, the provider should consider asking the person to leave the room so they can ask the patient in private, without disclosing the HIV diagnosis.

A comprehensive history and physical examination, as well as past medical history, social, family history, review of all medications and allergies, and review of systems, should be performed at the initial visit (Tables 9.1 and 9.2). The provider should be mindful to identify possible risk factors for progression of illness and potential complications and determine if the patient has sufficient social support.

In addition to the standard history, the following items should be addressed:

- Address the emotional status of the patient.
  - What is the level of anxiety regarding the HIV diagnosis?

Table 9.1 KEY ELEMENTS OF THE MEDICAL HISTORY AT THE INITIAL HIV VISIT

HISTORY COMPONENT	DETAILS	COMMENTS
HIV-specific history:	• Date of seroconversion (if known) • Risk factors for transmission • CD4 count: nadir and pretreatment (if already on treatment) • Detailed history of previous treatment regimens as well as related adverse effects (if any) • Prior HIV resistance testing (if any) and HLA-B5701	Patients previously treated might not recall all of their past treatments, so medical records from previous providers should be obtained
Medical history:	• Viral hepatitis: coinfection with hepatitis B virus (HBV) or hepatitis C virus (HCV)HCV is common, can progress faster in PWH, might need treatment • Cardiovascular risk/disease: hypertension, diabetes mellitus, dyslipidemia can affect choice of ART • Other comorbidities: e.g., CKD, endocrine disorders, cerebrovascular disease • Malignancies: increased incidence in PWH, some might be indicative of AIDS • OB/GYN: prior pregnancies, present contraceptives (if any), previous Pap smears and mammography results, potential plans for future pregnancies • Tuberculosis: risk factors and potential exposures • Previous hospitalizations • Surgeries (including complications, if any) • Childhood infections	Should focus on presence of common comorbidities, particularly those that might affect choice of ART or response to it
Sexual history:	• Gender identity and sexual orientation • Sexual partners: number and gender of partners • Type of sexual activities: oral, vaginal, anal, use of sex toys • Use of condoms: type and frequency • Activities associated with sex: alcohol/drug consumption, exchange for favors (e.g., money, goods) • Sexually transmitted infections (STIs)STIs: any previous diagnosis and treatments • Partners: HIV status and other STIs	Risk of STIs varies greatly if patients are identified by gender identity and sexual orientation rather than just sex (male or female) Can identify patient who might be candidates for cervical/anal Pap smears Can help identify potential sites of testing (e.g., oral testing for chlamydia in patient that perform oral sex)
Psychiatric history:	• Diagnosis and treatments • Sleep patterns: could indicate underlining depression or adverse effects of ART	Depression is frequent in PWH and if not adequately managed can significantly decrease adherence
Medications and allergies:	• List all medications presently taken (including over-the-counter (OTCs and supplements) • Allergies and reactions	Some OTC and supplements may interact with ART Allergies: note reaction as well as date of first/last occurrence if known
Social history:	• Employment and travel: provide insight into potential exposures and risk factors • Alcohol and tobacco use • Substance abuse: details of what type, frequency, and method of administration should be sought • Domestic violence: does the patient feel safe at home? • Hobbies and past times • Animal/pet exposure	Will give the provider insight into the persons safety net and social/home support Can identify potential barriers to treatment
Family history:	• First degree family members • Any family member known to have HIV	May identify potential risk factor for heart disease Can provide information regarding support in the family if other members have HIV
Immunizations:	• All vaccines with dates (if possible)	Will help determine any vaccines the patient may require
Healthcare maintenance:	• Age appropriate as per guidelines • Risk factor-appropriate as per guidelines	Can vary by age, gender, and exposures
Healthcare system information:	• Other healthcare providers managing the PWH • Primary contact information (including emergency contacts) • Healthcare proxy and anyone authorized to access PWH's information • Advance directives • Disclosure information	Patient might want restricted access to his/her information (including spouse occasionally) It is important to reinforce confidential nature of information provided

Table 9.2 KEY ELEMENTS OF THE REVIEW OF SYSTEMS FOR PWH

REVIEW OF SYSTEMS	
Constitutional	Intentional/unintentional weight change, fever, chills, night sweats, fatigue, malaise
Head, eyes, ears, nose, and throat (HEENT)	Hearing changes, ear pain, nasal congestion, sinus pain, hoarseness, sore throat, rhinorrhea, swallowing difficulty, oral lesion, eye pain, swelling, redness, foreign body, discharge, vision changes (floaters or blurred vision)
Cardiovascular	Chest pain, dyspnea, orthopnea, claudication, edema, palpitations
Respiratory	Cough, sputum, bloody sputum, wheezing, shortness of breath
Genitourinary	Dysmenorrhea, bleeding, dyspareunia, dysuria, urinary frequency, hematuria, urinary incontinence, urgency, flank pain, urinary flow changes, hesitancy, genital lesion
Musculoskeletal	Arthralgias, myalgias, joint swelling, joint stiffness, back pain, neck pain, injury history
Skin	Skin lesion, pruritus, hair changes, breast/skin changes, nipple discharge, rash
Neurologic	Weakness, numbness, paresthesia, loss of consciousness, syncope, dizziness, headache, coordination changes, recent falls
Psychiatric	Anxiety/panic, depression, insomnia, personality changes, delusions, rumination, suicidal ideation, homicidal ideation, hallucinations, social issues, memory changes, violence/abuse history, eating concerns
Hematologic	Bruising, bleeding, transfusion history, lymphadenopathy
Endocrine	Polyuria, polydipsia, heat or cold intolerance

- How is he or she coping with the diagnosis of HIV?
- Does the patient have an established social support network?

- Has the patient disclosed his/her HIV status to anyone (e.g., partner, family member(s), or friends)?

- Which sexual partners (or needle-sharing partners) may have been exposed and are potentially at risk for HIV? Have they been notified and tested? If not, would the PWH benefit from assistance in contacting past or recent sexual or needle-sharing partners?

An important aspect of the initial clinic encounter is to determine how the PWH is coping with their HIV diagnosis (particularly if newly diagnosed) and the patient's emotional status following the diagnosis (particularly if newly diagnosed), and ask if they have shared their diagnosis with anyone (e.g., friends, partner, family member, roommate) (Yu et al., 2018). Nondisclosure of HIV status may lead to lower medication adherence and increased anxiety. While some patients are fearful of the reaction of others with whom they disclose their diagnosis, we generally encourage patients to disclose their diagnosis to at least close friends and/or family members. In most cases it leads to more emotional support, less anxiety, and improved patient well-being. The provider should also ask the PWH "What fears do you have?" Often, asking and answering this question can lower the anxiety level of the patient by dispelling myths or misinformation the patient may have heard or read about (Ruffell, 2017).

THE MORE PATIENTS KNOW, THE BETTER THEY CAN CARE FOR THEMSELVES

Assessing PWH's level of understanding of the disease process, medications, and risks is essential in the comprehensive care of the individual with HIV. Studies have demonstrated that PWH with more knowledge of their disease status do better over time. Incomplete medication knowledge has been associated with lower adherence (Miller et al., 2003; Molla et al., 2018), showing the need to ensure patients understand their condition and their medications. The level of sophistication will obviously be different depending on a person's background, level of education, health literacy, years of infection, and other factors. Lower educational level does not correlate with lower adherence (Kim et al., 2018). Any opportunity to emphasize education, understanding, and knowledge of the disease state should be fully embraced.

The provider should not assume that the patient has a thorough understanding of HIV, even in patients with long-standing infection. Open-ended questions such as the following are recommended:

- What do you know about HIV?

- What do you think you can do to maintain your health long term?

- Do you understand the significance of the HIV viral load and T-cell count?

The provider (or team member) should explain (in simple terms, depending on the patient's health literacy) the significance and meaning of CD4 or T-cells, HIV viral load, opportunistic infection, and risks of transmission. The "teach back" method is useful to demonstrate the patient's level of understanding and to improve adherence to treatment in patients with chronic diseases (Ha Dinh et al., 2016).

THE PATIENT-PROVIDER RELATIONSHIP

Medical care for PWH should be patient-centered, with the primary focus on the person's needs and preferences. The care should be sensitive to PWH's educational, cultural, and socioeconomic background. Understanding each person in their unique circumstances, not only helps establish trust, but has been shown to increase adherence to treatment (Ciechanowski et al., 2001). Previous studies have shown that PWH who feel that their HIV provider is providing personalized, patient-centered care were more likely to be adherent to treatment, and to achieve an undetectable viral load (Beach et al., 2006). Ideally the patient-provider relationship will be strengthened with each encounter as PWH gain more confidence and comfort with their provider.

More recent studies indicate that motivational interviewing is an effective, evidence-based, and patient-centered communication strategy that enhances readiness for behavioral changes and can help patients improve motivation as well as treatment adherence for individuals disengaged from HIV care. This typically involves empathic listening, shared decision-making, and a change-focused talk, which should elicit personal motivation for behavioral changes (Sued et al., 2022).

SENSITIVE, RESPECTFUL, AND NONJUDGMENTAL

HIV providers frequently care for patients with a wide variety of sexual practices, patients who have been victims of abuse, people who are/have been commercial sex workers, people who have used intravenous drugs, and individuals in the gay/lesbian/transgender/bisexual/queer communities. Issues of privacy and cultural sensitivity are especially relevant in these encounters. Fostering trust and encouraging truthfulness and openness in the patient-provider relationship requires special attention to cultivating a nonjudgmental and approachable demeanor. It is important to be sensitive to persons' priorities, be respectful of their individuality, and be aware of their self-perception.

CULTURAL COMPETENCY ISSUES

PWH are ethnically and culturally diverse, spanning the spectrum of socioeconomic status. PWH's background may be quite different from that of the clinician providing care. Thus, it is important for the clinician to be aware of the unique cultural background of the person. Evidence shows that noninclusion of cultural norms and values of target populations can act as stumbling blocks in effective communication (Uwah, 2013). The effects of cultural competency in the care of PWH were identified early in the HIV epidemic, and its impacts were notable (O'Connor, 1996). Cultural competency involves not only race identity, but also sexual orientation and gender identity. At times specific groups of people can feel disenfranchised if they feel their cultural identity is not being taken into consideration (Shover et al., 2018). Cultural awareness can identify substantial economic disadvantages, pervasive childhood adversity, limited education, and limited resources that jointly put members of a particular community at risk for the acquisition of HIV, development of depression, and addiction (Le et al., 2016). By practicing cultural competency in medicine, providers can shape patient care and strengthen the patient-provider relationship, leading to increased treatment adherence and health literacy. This highlights the importance of providers being aware of these issues, especially given the disproportionate impact of HIV on historically underserved groups such as people of color (Mogobe et al., 2016). It is important for providers to be aware of the culture surrounding PWH and work to minimize any barriers to treatment. As an example, some communities incorporate their religious beliefs into healthcare (Nyashanu et al., 2022). Being aware of these concepts can help use that faith-based practice to promote health literacy and compliance. Identifying potential gaps in cultural competency, as well as ongoing training sessions, has been shown to significantly improve knowledge, attitudes, self-efficacy, and intentions among providers (Rhoten et al., 2022).

LANGUAGE

PWH in the United States and elsewhere originate from many regions of the world. For many patients English is not their primary language. Thus, an important issue is ensuring effective communication between the patient and the members of the health care team. Language-concordant care reassures that the patient and provider understand each other; it also optimizes health outcomes, advances health equity for diverse populations, and enhances trust between patient and provider (Molina & Kasper, 2019). At times, out of convenience, providers may be tempted to use family members or friends to provide language assistance. These strategies may be associated with a number of problems, including the translator not directly translating the provider or patient's intent, leaving out key details, and it may also result in breaches of confidentiality (Bischoff & Hudelson, 2010). Providing medically trained interpreter services is vital to promoting equitable health care and overcoming misinterpretation and patient-perceived prejudice that can be associated with being a patient who does not speak the local language (Bischoff & Hudelson, 2010; Ngo-Metzger et al., 2009).

THE HIV-ORIENTED PHYSICAL EXAMINATION

Sir William Osler is credited with the saying, "He who knows syphilis knows medicine." The modern-day equivalent of the old adage is "He who knows HIV knows medicine," because indeed HIV infection and its sequelae can affect every organ system and can present in every clinical way possible. The HIV-oriented exam, therefore, needs to be especially comprehensive, both for the assessment of current complaints and for establishing a baseline to compare with future findings (Table 9.3). At times the physical exam can provide clues to the patient's immunological status. As an example, erythematous candidiasis is often present at CD4 $^+$ cell counts between 200 and 500 cells/mm^3, while pseudomembranous candidiasis often indicates more immunosuppression (CD4 counts at or less than 200 CD4 $^+$ cells/mm^3) and oral hairy leukoplakia is usually associated with a CD4 counts< 400 cells/mm^3 (Levy et al., 2012; Nokta et al., 2008). The physical exam can also provide insight to any substance use issues, particularly if noting the person with poor personal hygiene,

Table 9.3 PHYSICAL EXAMINATION OF THE PWH

BODY ORGAN/ SYSTEM	BE ESPECIALLY ATTENTIVE TO:
Vital signs	Weight loss, body mass index, fat distribution, blood pressure, pulse, respiration rate, temperature Pain/tenderness
General	Body habitus, nutritional status, obvious disabilities
Skin	Rash, seborrheic dermatitis, folliculitis, moles, psoriasis, lichen planus, Kaposi sarcoma lesions warts, vesicular lesions, dermatophytes, molluscum contagiosum Needle marks
HEENT	Visual acuity Retinal hemorrhages and exudates (suggestive of CMV) HIV retinopathy (cotton-wool spots) Oral exam: thrush, oral hairy leukoplakia, Kaposi's lesions, gingivitis, aphthous ulcers, chancres, dentition, herpetic lesions, angular cheilitis Thyroid exam
Hemolymphatic	Regional versus generalized lymphadenopathy Splenomegaly
Cardiac	Heart sounds, murmurs, gallop
Pulmonary	Focal or generalized abnormalities
Gastrointestinal	Jaundice, hepatomegaly, splenomegaly Abdominal masses Anorectal exam (ulcers, vesicles, chancres, masses, hemorrhoids, warts) if indicated, anal Pap smear
Genitourinary	Ulcers, warts, chancres, herpetic vesicles Gender-specific exam: For women: pelvic exam, cervical exam, cervical Pap smear For men: testicular exam
Neurologic	Mental status, cognitive function—consider baseline HIV cognitive assessment (e.g., Montreal Cognitive Assessment test) Cranial nerves, motor strength, sensation, gait, vibratory/proprioceptive exam
Psychiatric	Depression screen should be done at baseline (PHQ-2 as a screen or other validated tools) Evidence of self-injury or self-mutilation Evidence of abuse

significant weight loss/gain, scars at injection sites on the skin, or abnormalities in the nasal mucosa associated with inhalations (Mertens et al., 2008). Other findings should be sought on physical exam that might suggest opportunistic infections, such as skin lesions suggestive of Kaposi's sarcoma or cryptococcemia or spider angiomata suggestive of chronic liver disease (hepatitis B and C) (Srivastava et al., 2015; Tappero et al., 1995).

RECOGNITION OF ACUTE AND ADVANCED HIV INFECTION

As the trend toward earlier HIV diagnosis continues (prior to any significant immune dysfunction), the majority of PWH presenting to the clinic for the initial visit will be asymptomatic or have minor nonspecific symptoms that are typically unlikely to be mentioned by the individual outside of a study (Robb et al., 2016). Some of these newly diagnosed patients may still have signs or symptoms of acute infection, a mononucleosis like syndrome, which is characterized by fever, lymphadenopathy, sore throat, rash, muscle aches, diarrhea, and headache (Hoenigl et al., 2016; Niu et al., 1993) (Table 9.4). The symptoms usually resolve within 2 weeks but may go on longer. The presence of prolonged symptomatic illness appears to correlate with more rapid progression to AIDS (Pedersen et al., 1989). Although usually associated with later stages of HIV disease, opportunistic infections can rarely occur during transient CD4 lymphopenia and early HIV infection (Braun et al., 2015). Oral and esophageal candidiasis is the most commonly diagnosed opportunistic infection during acute HIV, but other infections including CMV, *Pneumocystis jirovecii* pneumonia, and cryptosporidiosis have been reported.

Specific symptoms and signs that suggest chronic HIV infection should prompt testing in the hopes of early diagnosis; these include the following:

- Any sexually transmitted infection
- Oral ulcers/aphthous stomatitis

Table 9.4 SIGNS AND SYMPTOMS OF ACUTE RETROVIRAL ILLNESS

SIGNS AND SYMPTOMS	APPROXIMATE INCIDENCE (%)
Fever	48–88
Pharyngitis/sore throat	21–51
Lymphadenopathy	36–45
Rash	12–47
Oral ulcers	12–17
Myalgia/arthralgia	28–46
Diarrhea	17–35
Headache	34–44
Hepatosplenomegaly	10–15
Oral/oropharyngeal or vaginal candidiasis	10
Weight loss	21–39
Neurologic syndromes: Aseptic meningitis Peripheral neuropathy Guillain–Barré syndrome	~10

SOURCE: Hoenigl et al. *Emerg Infect Dis.* 2016;22(3):532–534.

- Oral hairy leukoplakia
- Oral candidiasis
- Unexplained weight loss
- Unexplained chronic fatigue
- Persistent or difficult-to-control seborrheic dermatitis
- Persistent or difficult-to-control vaginal candidiasis
- Unexplained/persistent fevers
- Herpes zoster/shingles (especially if more than one dermatome or recurrent, and especially in young people)
- Chronic diarrhea
- Persistent night sweats
- Persistent generalized lymphadenopathy
- Severe or difficult-to-control psoriasis
- Chronic or persistent herpes simplex infection of the genital tract or perianal region

Likewise, some laboratory findings may clue the clinician to the possibility of chronic HIV infection:

- Any sexually transmitted infection
- Chronic thrombocytopenia
- Leukopenia
- Anemia of chronic inflammation, especially without an alternative explanation
- Low lipid levels (low cholesterol, high-density lipoprotein, and low-density lipoprotein (LDL)), with elevated triglycerides; this has been attributed to chronic inflammatory cytokines (Grunfeld et al., 1992)
- Elevated globulin: albumin ratio, indicating polyclonal gammopathy
- Persistent or intermittent unexplained transaminitis
- Low albumin or prealbumin, especially if wasting is present
- Decreased renal function with proteinuria (HIV nephropathy)

Also, a new diagnosis of certain diseases should prompt an HIV test because their increased incidence in individuals with HIV:

- Active tuberculosis
- Non-Hodgkin's lymphoma or Hodgkin's disease
- Cervical carcinoma in situ
- Listeriosis in an otherwise immunocompetent or pregnant patient

- Extraintestinal salmonellosis
- Recurrent bacterial pneumonia
- Bacteremic pneumococcal pneumonia
- Pelvic inflammatory disease

INITIAL LABORATORY EVALUATION

A comprehensive initial laboratory evaluation should be performed at or before the first clinic visit to establish a baseline of, for example, CD4 count, HIV-1 viral load, and hepatic and renal function (see Table 9.5). Laboratory data should ideally be available prior to the initial interaction, but at times, patients will present for the initial evaluation without any previous records or work-up aside from their positive HIV test (Thompson, et al., 2021). Laboratory testing can be divided into HIV-specific testing, assessing risk factors, and routine medical care labs. The initial laboratory evaluation is fairly extensive but can be simplified thereafter since many of the initial tests need not be repeated.

DISCUSSING INITIATION OF THERAPY

In the last several years, some communities have successfully initiated "rapid initiation of ART" programs, in which antiretroviral therapy is started immediately following diagnosis, a significant shift from previous recommendations. In the early years of the HIV epidemic, limited resources and concerns about suboptimal adherence led to a cautious approach in which PWH underwent multiple counseling sessions that could last several weeks or months before starting ART (World Health Organization (WHO), 2017). More recent data support a rapid initiation (within 1 week and at times even the same day) of ART (Ford et al., 2018b). This strategy improves outcomes across the HIV treatment cascade including reducing loss to care. However, there is also some evidence that indicates that in certain circumstances this approach could lead to an increase in lost to follow-up, because of insufficient time to accept and disclose HIV status and prepare for lifelong treatment (Boyd, et al., 2019; Ford, et al., 2018a). However, when possible, HIV therapy should be started promptly, taking into consideration social and psychological aspects of committing to lifelong therapy. Consideration of contraindications such as co-current infection with tuberculosis or cryptococcus needs to be entertained, and if suspected, therapy should be delayed to lessen the likelihood of the immune reconstitution syndrome (Lawn et al., 2011). Before initiating therapy, obtaining complete and thorough list of all the patient's present medications as well as any natural supplements should be sought. There is still an alarming number of contraindicated drug interactions and high prevalence of potential drug interactions over the time in the treatment of PWH (El Moussaoui et al., 2020). Identifying to prevent and manage any potential interactions should be of paramount importance since experiencing potential

Table 9.5 INITIAL HIV LABORATORY EVALUATION

CATEGORY	TEST	FREQUENCY	COMMENTS
HIV-specific testing	HIV serology (fourth-generation Ab-Ag test)	• At baseline if not available in records	• If no prior results available and viral load expected to be undetectable (patient on treatment), needed to establish diagnosis
	CD4$^+$ count (absolute and percentage)	• At baseline • Monitor every 3 to 6 months initially • If viral load < 20 copies/mL and CD4$^+$ count more than 300–500 cells/mm^3 for 2 years, repeat only every 12 months If CD4 >500 cells/mm^3, CD4$^+$ monitoring is optional	• Establishes clinical stage of HIV • Establishes risk of opportunistic complications and the need for initiation and discontinuation of opportunistic infection prophylaxis • Note: CD4$^+$ percentage, should be noted as it tends to be less variable than the absolute CD4$^+$ cell count and may better assess immune function
	HIV viral load	• At baseline • Repeat 2 to 8 weeks after starting ART, Subsequently, monitor every 3 to 4 months Monitor every 6 months in adherent patients with consistent viral suppression	• May affect selection of antiretroviral regimen (some antiretrovirals should not be used if viral load more than 100,000 copies/mL) Follow-up viral load testing determines response to antiviral therapy
	Resistance testing	• Initially • Repeat if treatment failure noted	• Rate of drug-resistant gene detection in developed countries 5% to 15% • Genotypic testing preferred; phenotypic testing can be helpful in highly treatment-experienced patients with history of multiple resistance mutations • Integrase resistance testing generally not recommended initially—rare at baseline; consider testing for Integrase resistance if patient failing integrase inhibitor-based regimen
	HLA-B5701	• At baseline if abacavir is a consideration	• Establishes risk of abacavir hypersensitivity • If positive, abacavir contraindicated
	Tropism testing	• If CCR5 antagonist being considered	• Only use maraviroc if virus is CCR5 tropic
	G6PD screen	• Baseline or when appropriate	• If deficient increases risk of hemolytic anemia particularly with the use of primaquine and dapsone
General blood work	CBC with differential	• Baseline; as needed thereafter	• Screen for anemia, leukopenia, lymphopenia, thrombocytopenia (incidence 30% to 40% in patients with advanced HIV disease) • Neutropenia: could represent bone marrow suppression because of HIV or other infiltrative infections (e.g., *Mycobacterium avium*) • Anemia: could indicate medication toxicity (e.g., zidovudine) or viral infection (Parvovirus B19) or nutritional deficiencies (iron, B12, folate) • Eosinophilia may be a clue to a parasitic infection, allergy or atopy or eosinophilic folliculitis or drug reaction
	Complete metabolic panel	• Baseline • Every 3 to 6 months thereafter	• Decreased renal function may affect selection of ART may require renal dosing of certain medications • Elevated BUN/creatinine may be a sign of HIV-associated nephropathy • Elevated transaminases and bilirubin levels may provide clues regarding possible liver pathology (e.g., viral hepatitis, drug-induced liver injury, steatohepatitis)

Table 9.5 CONTINUED

CATEGORY	TEST	FREQUENCY	COMMENTS
	Glucose and lipid profile	• Baseline • Every 6 to 12 months thereafter or as indicated by the risk profile	• Will help to identify any baseline metabolic abnormalities and estimate cardiovascular risk • May influence ART choice
	Vitamin D level	• Baseline • As appropriate thereafter	• Consider especially if at risk for risk for osteopenia or osteoporosis
	Urinalysis	• Baseline	• Assess effect of ART on kidney function (especially tenofovir); proteinuria- may be a sign of HIV nephropathy
	Pregnancy test	• Baseline and as appropriate thereafter	• For women of childbearing age
Coinfection/ comorbidity testing	Viral hepatitis serology	• Baseline • Repeat as indicated depending on risk	• May require vaccination against hepatitis A and/or B • Identifies patients requiring further evaluation for hepatitis C infection • May influence ART selection (particularly hepatitis B)
	Tuberculosis	• Baseline and yearly thereafter	Baseline tuberculin skin test (PPD) or IGRA is indicated in all PWH, unless there is a history of prior positive test or treatment for latent TB • Note that a PPD result ≥5 mm induration is considered reactive in PWH • If positive, a chest X-ray should be obtained to rule out active disease along with a careful review of systems and exam to rule out extrapulmonary TB
	STIs: Syphilis Chlamydia/gonorrhea	• Baseline • Annually if sexually active • More frequent testing depending on other risk factors	• Screening for trichomonas indicated in women • Test for latent syphilis • Testing for chlamydia/gonorrhea should include pharyngeal, urine, and rectal samples, depending on sexual practices • If positive testing, treatment and counseling on preventing STIs indicated
	Toxoplasma	• Baseline	• If seronegative, counseling on avoidance of new infection • If seropositive prescribe prophylaxis if CD4 + count≤ 100 cells/mm3
	Varicella and CMV	• Baseline	• To identify PWH who may require primary immunization against varicella or against herpes zoster • If CMV negative, if the patient were to require any blood products that should be CMV negative for leukocyte reduced products, as well as counseling about possibility of sexual transmission of CMV
Other screening	Cervical Pap smear	• Baseline • Repeat every 6–12 months	• Determines if there is human papilloma virus (HPV) infection and risk for neoplastic transfor-mation • Same frequency of testing evaluate more frequently in women PWH
	Anal Pap smear	• Baseline	• Consider if history of receptive anal intercourse or history of genital warts (or abnormal cervical Pap smear in women) • Optimal follow-up not yet established

(continued)

Table 9.5 CONTINUED

CATEGORY	TEST	FREQUENCY	COMMENTS
	Bone density scan		• Baseline screening for osteoporosis in postmenopausal woman and men aged 50 years or older • Could be considered in patients at risk (on tenofovir-based regimens)
	Age-appropriate healthcare maintenance		• Breast and colon cancer screening should follow age-appropriate guidelines • ASCVD score should be considered to evaluate need for statin therapy • Depression screening with repeat PHQ-2 should be considered • Cognitive screening mini-cog/MoCA • Should consider dental care as part of routine healthcare maintenance • Other risk-appropriate screening as per US Preventive Service Task Force Recommendations

drug-drug interactions might be associated with intentional nonadherence to therapy (Castro-Granell et al., 2021).

TELEHEALTH IN HIV

The US Health Resources and Services Administration defines *telehealth* as the use of electronic information and telecommunications technologies to support long-distance clinical healthcare, patient and professional health-related education, public health, and health administration. Many studies have supported the use of telehealth to increase convenience to patients by decreasing travel time, improve patient satisfaction, diminish healthcare disparities, and reduce cost that will ultimately lead to improvement in clinical outcomes and quality of care (Kruse et al., 2017). Guaranteeing confidentiality, educating patients and providers, and obtaining insurance reimbursement are some of the challenges that face the implementation of telehealth programs (Dandachi et al., 2019). In the setting of the recent COVID-19 pandemic the use of telemedicine increased and allowed providers the ability to assess and evaluate patients without exposing patients or healthcare professionals to COVID-19 (Smith et al., 2020). This recent experience allows payors to reimburse for routine telehealth visits including for PWH.

The literature indicates that telehealth programs for PWH can improve retention in care by decreasing travel time, better fitting the patient schedule, and providing more privacy; however, some worry about effective communication and examination as well as personal information safety (Dandachi et al., 2020a). Studies of telehealth indicate that people feel relieved to avoid travel time and physical contact with the clinic itself, and most patients view it positively. Many even prefer to have telehealth visits and rated them better compared to traditional in clinic visits, particularly those patients who have difficulties with travel (more specifically people in rural areas). Providers' concerns with the use of telehealth are usually around inability to perform a physical exam, longer visit times, and technology issues. However, in general, providers feel that with the use of telehealth they are able to communicate well with patients, especially with already established patients. (Dandachi et al., 2020b). Barriers to telehealth include lack of access to high-speed Internet, which is common in remote areas. Technical challenges, such as being comfortable with computers and computer software and new telehealth platforms, can also be challenging (Cole et al., 2019).

Benefits of telemedicine in HIV therapy include ability to reengage patients into care, and the opportunity to engage family as well as other providers. However, the barriers continue to be technical challenges, privacy concerns, and the loss of routine clinical experience and interaction not just with the providers but also with case managers and nursing staff, among others. There is also the concern of limited objective monitoring through physical examination. Despite improved reimbursement, this continues to be a concern as medicine notes beyond the COVID-19 pandemic (Harsono et al., 2022). In general, when used appropriately, telehealth can be a useful tool for managing PWH.

RECOMMENDED READING

Thompson, MA, Horberg MA, Agwu AL, et al. Primary care guidance for persons with human immunodeficiency virus: 2020 update by the HIV Medicine Association of the Infectious Diseases Society of America. *Clin Infect Dis.* 2021;73(11):e3572–e3605.

REFERENCES

Beach MC, Keruly J, Moore RD. Is the quality of the patient-provider relationship associated with better adherence and health outcomes for patients with HIV? *J Gen Intern Med.* 2006;21(6):661–665.

Berghoff CR, Gratz KL, Portz KJ, et al. The role of emotional avoidance, the patient-provider relationship, and other social support in ART adherence for HIV+ individuals. *AIDS Behav.* 2018;22(3): 929–938.

Bischoff A, Hudelson P. Communicating with foreign language-speaking patients: is access to professional interpreters enough? *J Travel Med*. 2010;17(1):15–20.

Boyd MA, Boffito M, Castagna A, Estrada V. Rapid initiation of anti-retroviral therapy at HIV diagnosis: definition, process, knowledge gaps. *HIV Med*. 2019;20(Suppl 1):3–11.

Braun DL, Kouyos RD, Balmer B, Grube C, Weber R, Gunthard HF. Frequency and spectrum of unexpected clinical manifestations of primary HIV-1 infection. *Clin Infect Dis*. 2015;61(6):1013–1021.

Castro-Granell V, Garin N, Jaen A, Cenoz S, Galindo MJ, Fuster-RuizdeApodaca MJ. Prevalence, beliefs and impact of drug-drug interactions between antiretroviral therapy and illicit drugs among people living with HIV in Spain. *PLoS One*. 2021;16(11):e0260334.

Ciechanowski PS, Katon WJ, Russo JE, Walker EA. The patient-provider relationship: attachment theory and adherence to treatment in diabetes. *Am J Psychiatry*. 2001;158(1):29–35.

Cole B, Pickard K, Stredler-Brown A. Report on the use of telehealth in early intervention in Colorado: strengths and challenges with tele-health as a service delivery method. *Int J Telerehabil*. 2019;11(1):33–40.

Dandachi D, Dang BN, Lucari B, Teti M, Giordano TP. Exploring the attitude of patients with HIV about using telehealth for HIV care. *AIDS Patient Care STDS*. 2020a;34(4):166–172.

Dandachi D, Freytag J, Giordano TP, Dang BN. It is time to include tele-health in our measure of patient retention in HIV care. *AIDS Behav*. 2020b;24(9):2463–2465.

Dandachi D, Lee C, Morgan RO, Tavakoli-Tabasi S, Giordano TP, Rodriguez-Barradas MC. Integration of telehealth services in the healthcare system: with emphasis on the experience of patients living with HIV. *J Investig Med*. 2019;67(5):815–820.

Doshi RK, Milberg J, Isenberg D, et al. High rates of retention and viral suppression in the US HIV safety net system: HIV care continuum in the Ryan White HIV/AIDS Program, 2011. *Clin Infect Dis*. 2015;60(1):117–125.

El Moussaoui M, Lambert I, Maes N, et al. Evolution of drug interactions with antiretroviral medication in people with HIV. *Open Forum Infect Dis*. 2020;7(11):ofaa416.

Flickinger TE, Saha S, Moore RD, Beach MC. Higher quality communication and relationships are associated with improved patient engagement in HIV care. *J Acquir Immune Defic Syndr*. 2013;63(3):362–366.

Ford N, Meintjes G, Calmy A, et al. Managing Advanced HIV Disease in a Public Health Approach. *Clin Infect Dis*. 2018a;66(Suppl 2):S106–SS110.

Ford N, Migone C, Calmy A, et al. Benefits and risks of rapid initiation of antiretroviral therapy. *AIDS*. 2018b;32(1):17–23.

Grunfeld C, Pang M, Doerrler W, Shigenaga JK, Jensen P, Feingold KR. Lipids, lipoproteins, triglyceride clearance, and cytokines in human immunodeficiency virus infection and the acquired immunodeficiency syndrome. *J Clin Endocrinol Metab*. 1992;74(5):1045–1052.

Ha Dinh TT, Bonner A, Clark R, Ramsbotham J, Hines S. The effectiveness of the teach-back method on adherence and self-management in health education for people with chronic disease: a systematic review. *JBI Database System Rev Implement Rep*. 2016;14(1):210–247.

Harsono D, Deng Y, Chung S, et al. Experiences with telemedicine for HIV care during the COVID-19 pandemic: a mixed-methods study. *AIDS Behav*. 2022;26(6):2099–2111.

Hoenigl M, Green N, Camacho M, et al. Signs or symptoms of acute HIV infection in a cohort undergoing community-based screening. *Emerg Infect Dis*. 2016;22(3):532–534.

Kim J, Lee E, Park BJ, Bang JH, Lee JY. Adherence to antiretroviral therapy and factors affecting low medication adherence among incident HIV-infected individuals during 2009-2016: a nationwide study. *Sci Rep*. 2018;8(1):3133.

Kruse CS, Krowski N, Rodriguez B, Tran L, Vela J, Brooks M. Telehealth and patient satisfaction: a systematic review and narrative analysis. *BMJ Open*. 2017;7(8):e016242.

Lawn SD, Torok ME, Wood R. Optimum time to start antiretroviral therapy during HIV-associated opportunistic infections. *Curr Opin Infect Dis*. 2011;24(1):34–42.

Le HN, Hipolito MM, Lambert S, et al. Culturally sensitive approaches to identification and treatment of depression among HIV infected African American adults: a qualitative study of primary care providers' perspectives. *J Depress Anxiety*. 2016;5(2):223.

Levy TH, Jacobson DF. Dermatologic manifestations as indicators of immune status in HIV/AIDS. *J Gen Intern Med*. 2012;27(1):124.

Mertens JR, Flisher AJ, Satre DD, Weisner CM. The role of medical conditions and primary care services in 5-year substance use outcomes among chemical dependency treatment patients. *Drug Alcohol Depend*. 2008;98(1–2):45–53.

Miller LG, Liu H, Hays RD, et al. Knowledge of antiretroviral regimen dosing and adherence: a longitudinal study. *Clin Infect Dis*. 2003;36(4):514–518.

Mogobe KD, Shaibu S, Matshediso E, et al. Language and culture in health literacy for people living with HIV: perspectives of health care providers and professional care team members. *AIDS Res Treat*. 2016;2016:5015707.

Molina RL, Kasper J. The power of language-concordant care: a call to action for medical schools. *BMC Med Educ*. 2019;19(1):378.

Molla AA, Gelagay AA, Mekonnen HS, Teshome DF. Adherence to antiretroviral therapy and associated factors among HIV positive adults attending care and treatment in University of Gondar Referral Hospital, Northwest Ethiopia. *BMC Infect Dis*. 2018;18(1):266.

Ngo-Metzger Q, Sorkin DH, Phillips RS. Healthcare experiences of limited English-proficient Asian American patients: a cross-sectional mail survey. *Patient*. 2009;2(2):113–120.

Niu MT, Stein DS, Schnittman SM. Primary human immunodeficiency virus type 1 infection: review of pathogenesis and early treatment intervention in humans and animal retrovirus infections. *J Infect Dis*. 1993;168(6):1490–1501.

Nokta M. Oral manifestations associated with HIV infection. *Curr HIV/AIDS Rep*. 2008;5(1):5–12.

Nyashanu M, Ganga G, Chenneville T. Exploring the impact of religion, superstition, and professional cultural competence on access to HIV and mental health treatment among black Sub-Sahara African Communities in the English city of Birmingham. *J Relig Health*. 2022;61(1):252–268.

O'Connor BB. Promoting cultural competence in HIV/AIDS care. *J Assoc Nurses AIDS Care*. 1996;7(Suppl 1):41–53.

Pedersen C, Lindhardt BO, Jensen BL, et al. Clinical course of primary HIV infection: consequences for subsequent course of infection. *BMJ*. 1989;299(6692):154–157.

Rhoten B, Burkhalter JE, Joo R, et al. Impact of an LGBTQ cultural competence training program for providers on knowledge, attitudes, self-efficacy, and intensions. *Journal of Homosexuality*. 2022;69(6):1030–1041.

Robb ML, Eller LA, Kibuuka H, et al. Prospective study of acute HIV-1 infection in adults in East Africa and Thailand. *N Engl J Med*. 2016;374(22):2120–2130.

Ruffell S. Stigma kills! The psychological effects of emotional abuse and discrimination towards a patient with HIV in Uganda. *BMJ Case Rep*. 2017;2017(Suppl 1):41–53.

Shover CL, DeVost MA, Beymer MR, Gorbach PM, Flynn RP, Bolan RK. Using sexual orientation and gender identity to monitor disparities in HIV, sexually transmitted infections, and viral hepatitis. *Am J Public Health*. 2018;108(S4):S277–S283.

Smith AC, Thomas E, Snoswell CL, et al. Telehealth for global emergencies: Implications for coronavirus disease 2019 (COVID-19). *J Telemed Telecare*. 2020;26(5):309–313.

Srivastava GN, Tilak R, Yadav J, Bansal M. Cutaneous Cryptococcus: marker for disseminated infection. *BMJ Case Rep*. http://doi:10.1136/bcr-2015-210898. Published July 21, 2015. Accessed August 30, 2022. bcr2015210898.

Sued O, Cecchini D, Rolon MJ, et al. A small cluster randomized clinical trial to improve health outcomes among Argentine patients disengaged from HIV care. *The Lancet Regional Health—Americas*. 2022;13:100307. doi: 10.1016/j.lana.2022.100307. Epub 2022 Jun 23.

Uwah C. The role of culture in effective HIV/AIDS communication by theatre in South Africa. *SAHARA J.* 2013;10(3–4):140–149.

Tappero JW, Perkins BA, Wenger JD, Berger TG. Cutaneous manifestations of opportunistic infections in patients infected with human immunodeficiency virus. *Clin Microbiol Rev.* 1995;8(3):440–450.

Thompson, MA, Horberg MA,et al. Primary care guidance for persons with human immunodeficiency virus: 2020 update by the HIV Medicine Association of the Infectious Diseases Society of America. *Clinical Infectious Diseases.* 2021;73(11):e3572–e3605.

Uwah C. The role of culture in effective HIV/AIDS communication by theatre in South Africa. *SAHARA J.* 2013;10(3–4):140–149.

World Health Organization (WHO). Guidelines for managing advanced HIV disease and rapid initiation of antiretroviral therapy. WHO. Geneva. https://www.who.int/publications/i/item/9789241550062. Published July 1, 2017. Accessed January 21, 2023.

Yu Y, Luo D, Chen X, Huang Z, Wang M, Xiao S. Medication adherence to antiretroviral therapy among newly treated people living with HIV. *BMC Public Health.* 2018;18(1):825.

Uwah C. The role of culture in effective HIV/AIDS communication by theatre in South Africa. *SAHARA J.* 2013;10(3–4):140–149.

10.

HEALTH MAINTENANCE

Ramiz Kseri

HIV HEALTHCARE FLOW SHEETS FOR PRIMARY CARE

Most electronic health record (EHR) systems include individually designed disease-specific flow sheets. These flow sheets can be designed to address specific centers' care reporting needs. At minimum, flow sheets should include HIV-specific information such as CD4$^+$ T-cell counts, HIV-1 viral loads, immunization records, and healthcare maintenance reports. HIV drug resistance test results are more difficult to enter into flow sheets. Ideally, the EHR flow sheet is designed to trigger clinical reminders regarding the need for opportunistic infection prophylaxis and vaccinations or health maintenance screening based on patients' current CD4$^+$ T-cell counts, serologies, age, and sex.

RECOMMENDED READING

Thompson MA, Horberg MA, Agwu AL, et al. Primary care guidance for persons with human immunodeficiency virus: 2020 update by the HIV Medicine Association of the Infectious Diseases Society of America. *Clin Infect Dis.* 2021;73(11):E3572–E3605. https://Doi.Org/10.1093/Cid/Ciaa1391

TB SCREENING AND ASSESSMENT

LEARNING OBJECTIVE

Describe TB screening indications (including exposure history) and assessment methods (including selection, interpretation, and limitations of screening tests in PWH).

WHAT'S NEW?

Interferon-gamma release assays (IGRAs) are an alternative to tuberculin skin tests (TSTs) for detection of *Mycobacterium tuberculosis* infection and are preferred for individuals aged 5 years or older who are Bacillus Calmette–Guérin (BCG) vaccinated.

KEY POINTS

- Because of immunodeficiency, PWH are at increased risk for developing active TB disease and thus should be routinely screened for TB.

- PWH also frequently have other indications for TB screening, including contact with persons from areas of the world where there is a high incidence of TB and high-risk exposures in correctional and residential facilities.

- In PWH, TSTs or IGRAs should be performed at the time of initial HIV diagnosis. For persons who are initially TST or IGRA negative when their CD4 + T cells were < 200/mm³, testing should be repeated in those who have experienced an improvement in immune function owing to antiretroviral therapy (ART). Annual testing may be considered in persons with ongoing or repeated exposure to TB.

- TST responses of <u>5 mm or larger induration</u> are considered positive in persons with HIV. However, even negative TST or IGRA results may warrant preventive therapy in the setting of high-risk exposures.

- Chest radiography is indicated regardless of TST or IGRA results in PWH with recent exposure to patients with active TB or with a history of symptoms consistent with TB, as well as in any HIV-infected person with a positive test result.

HIV-associated immune compromise is associated with an increased incidence of TB among HIV-infected individuals, with a relative risk of 10 times that of HIV-negative persons (Horsburgh & Rubin, 2011). As with other opportunistic infections, there has been a substantial decrease in the incidence of TB among persons receiving ART. However, untreated TB is one of the few opportunistic infections transmissible to others and thus has additional public health implications for control and prevention.

PWH are at increased risk for developing active disease by reactivation of untreated latent TB infection (LTBI), at an estimated rate of 3%–16% *per year* compared to 5%–10% *lifetime* risk in HIV-negative persons with no other risk factors. Once infection with *M. tuberculosis* occurs, there can be rapid progression of newly acquired infection to disease—for example, within the first month following exposure to an infectious person. Similarly, reactivation disease may also progress rapidly, particularly in highly immunocompromised individuals. The majority of individuals without HIV and infected with TB who develop active disease in the United States were born, previously lived, or traveled for extended periods in TB endemic areas. Currently, 8% of individuals with active TB have underlying HIV disease. However, prior to the advent of ART, in the United States, the proportion of individuals with TB who had underlying HIV was nearly 50%. TB outbreaks were identified among individuals living with HIV in US institutional settings, including healthcare facilities, correctional facilities, and homeless shelters. Although transmission in institutional settings in the United States is now rare, there is substantial risk in resource-limited settings in which TB is endemic in the general population. PWH who are employees or volunteers in settings identified as high risk by local health authorities should be advised of their risk of exposure to TB and offered alternate sites of work. HIV-positive healthcare workers who intermittently work or volunteer in TB endemic countries should be similarly advised about their risk. The healthcare provider should seek assistance with assessing the level of risk by evaluating factors such as the prevalence of TB in the community, the precautions against transmission that are in place, and the HCP's specific duties in those settings.

HIV-positive individuals, especially those with CD4$^+$ T-cell counts of less than 200/μL, are more likely to present with extrapulmonary TB, miliary pulmonary disease, and disseminated TB compared to HIV-negative persons. Persons with HIV may have active pulmonary TB with normal chest radiographs. Similarly, persons with HIV and TB may present with negative acid-fast bacilli (AFB) sputum in up to 70% of cases (Getahun et al., 2007). In a high-incidence setting and active case-finding study of patients with culture-positive TB, up to 32% had normal chest radiographs; of those who were AFB smear-negative and had normal chest radiographs, 8% had TB, 5% had CD4$^+$ T-cell counts of 350/μL or greater, and 10% had CD4$^+$ T-cell counts of less than 350/μL (Cain et al., 2010). Nucleic acid amplification tests such as Gene Xpert MTB/RIF are more sensitive than AFB smear, and they may identify up to 70% of smear-negative, culture-positive cases (Boehme et al., 2010).

INDICATIONS FOR LTBI SCREENING

Many indications for LTBI screening may be present concurrently in PWH, which represent conditions with higher risk of development of TB than those without these conditions, or in situations that pose high risks of exposure or recent infection with *M. tuberculosis*. Indications for screening include the following:

- Foreign-born persons, or persons in close contact with recent immigrants or refugees, from regions with high rates of TB (i.e., Africa, Asia, Latin America, Russia, and countries of the former Soviet Union).

- Other medical conditions, such as diabetes mellitus, silicosis, chronic renal failure, being underweight (≤ 10% below normal), gastrectomy, injection drug use, malignancies (lymphoma, leukemia, and head and neck cancer), cardiac and renal transplantation, or use of immunosuppressive therapies (especially tumor necrosis factor-α inhibitors).

- Persons from situations with a high risk for person-to-person transmission, such as those working or residing in correctional facilities (3% of TB cases in the United States), homeless shelters (6% of TB cases in the United States), and other congregate settings (American Thoracic Society, Centers for Disease Control and Prevention (CDC), and Infectious Diseases Society of America, 2005).

- Close contacts of person with active TB, 30%–40% of whom will be found to have latent tuberculosis infection (LBTI), and 1% or 2% of whom will have active disease.

- Children born to HIV-positive mothers who have TB or who are at high risk for possible LBTI (e.g., close contacts of persons with active disease).

- Persons previously treated for latent or active TB who are re-exposed to someone with active TB can become reinfected, particularly in hyperendemic settings.

SCREENING TESTS FOR *M. TUBERCULOSIS* INFECTION

TUBERCULIN SKIN TESTING

The time-honored method for diagnosis of *M. tuberculosis* infection is the TST, which measures a polycellular delayed-type hypersensitivity response at the site of injection following the administration of purified protein derivative (PPD), an admixture of mycobacterial antigens. The preferred skin test is the intradermal, or Mantoux, method. It is administered by injecting 0.1 mL of 5 tuberculin units (TU) PPD intradermally into the dorsal or volar surface of the forearm. Tests should be read 48–72 hours after test administration, and the diameter of induration transverse to the long axis of the arm should be recorded in millimeters. Multiple puncture tests (i.e., tine test, Heaf test) and PPD strengths of 1 and 250 TU are not sufficiently accurate and should not be used (American Thoracic Society/Centers for Disease Control and Prevention, 2000). Induration of 5 mm or greater in PWH indicates a positive TST. TSTs require two visits to perform and confirm the results of the test, as well as experience in intradermal placement of the test. There is some subjectivity in its interpretation, and false-positive results may occur from exposure to nontuberculous mycobacteria or prior vaccination with *M. bovis* BCG. A positive TST has been shown to be predictive of progression to active TB in PWH, who benefit from preventive therapy with a reduction in TB incidence.

IGRASS

IGRAs are blood tests that measure interferon-γ (IFN-γ) secreted by sensitized T lymphocytes after exposure to TB-specific antigens ESAT-6 and CFP-10. Two tests are currently approved by the US Food and Drug Administration (FDA) and in use for the detection of *M. tuberculosis* infection: QuantiFERON-TB Gold In-Tube (QFT-GIT) and T-SPOT TB test (T-Spot). QFT measures IFN-γ concentration using an enzyme-linked immunosorbent assay (ELISA), whereas the T-Spot enumerates T cells releasing IFN-γ using an ELISPOT assay. QFT requires fresh blood to be incubated for 18–24 hours with plasma separation, ELISA testing, and comparison to negative and positive mitogen control antigens (phytohemagglutinin). T-Spot assays must be done on fresh blood specimens, processed within 12 hours, and incubated overnight. IGRAs require a single visit, are less subjective in interpretation than TSTs, and are more specific for detection of *M. tuberculosis* infection—that is, less cross-reactivity to nontuberculous mycobacteria (except *M. kansasii*, *M. szulgai*, and *M. marinum*) and BCG (CDC, 2010).

Current evidence suggests that IGRAs have higher specificity (92%–97%) compared to TSTs (56%–95%) (NIH-CDC-HIVMA/IDSA, 2013). TSTs are more likely to identify persons with long-standing cellular immune responses to TB antigens, and IGRAs are more likely to be positive in persons with recent *M. tuberculosis* infection (Horsburgh & Rubin, 2011). For diagnosis of LTBI, the correlation between TSTs and IGRAs is poor to moderate among PWH (Cattamanchi, 2011). For PWH with active TB, in one study, sensitivity was low for both QFT-GIT and TST (63% and 55%, respectively) and was inversely correlated with low CD4 $^+$ T-cell counts (Raby et al., 2008). In PWH at low risk of TB exposure, false-positive tests with QFT have also been reported, suggesting the need to repeat a positive QFT test to confirm the diagnosis of LTBI when patients are at low risk of exposure (Gray et al, 2012). There have been no definitive comparisons of TSTs and IGRAs for LTBI screening of persons with HIV infection in low-incidence settings.

Either TSTs or IGRAs are appropriate for TB screening among PWH in the United States. Some experts have suggested using both the TST and an IGRA to screen for LTBI, but the predictive value of this approach is not clear, and use of this strategy would be more expensive and more difficult to implement. The routine use of both TSTs and IGRAs to screen for LTBI in the same patient is not recommended in the United States (NIH-CDC-HIVMA/IDSA, 2020).

TESTING FREQUENCY

PWH should receive a test for LTBI at the time of initial HIV diagnosis, with repeat testing considered for those who are TST or IGRA negative initially with advanced HIV infection (CD4 $^+$ T-cell counts< 200/μL) and who have improvement in immune function due to ART (CD $^+$ T-cell counts ≥200/μL). Annual testing may also be considered in those who have ongoing or repeated exposure to TB, such as individuals who travel for extended periods of time to hyperendemic TB settings. Intercurrent testing should be done based on recent exposure to a case of active TB, including repeat testing 8 to 12 weeks after the initial negative test for TB infection because it may take this long for the TST or IGRA to become positive following infection.

ANERGY TESTING

PWH are at increased risk to have impaired delayed-type hypersensitivity responses to skin test antigens because of decreased CD4 $^+$ T-cell counts and, therefore, to have a compromised ability to react to tuberculin skin testing (i.e., to have cutaneous anergy). Anergy testing has not been helpful in attempting to distinguish false-negative TST results owing to anergy from true-negative results. Anergy testing is not recommended for routine use in PWH because of problems with test standardization and reproducibility, the variable risk for TB in the setting of anergy, and the lack of demonstrated benefit of preventive therapy in anergic HIV-infected individuals.

CHEST RADIOGRAPHY AND SYMPTOM SCREENING IN HIV-INFECTED PATIENTS

In asymptomatic persons with positive tests for LTBI, chest radiography should be done to exclude active TB. Persons with symptoms of TB, such as cough, fever, and night sweats, should be evaluated for TB regardless of IGRA or skin test results. The absence of these symptoms has a high negative predictive value for excluding active TB (Cain et al., 2010). Chest radiography should also be considered following recent exposure to a person with active TB regardless of skin test or IGRA results. PWH with pulmonary TB are more likely to exhibit atypical radiological presentations, especially those with low CD4 $^+$ T-cell counts and, in some cases, normal chest radiographs (Palmieri et al., 2002).

PREVENTIVE THERAPY

Preventive therapy is recommended following exposure to persons with active TB, regardless of initial or repeat TST results, or in persons with TST of 5 mm or greater and who have not been treated for active or latent TB and have no clinical evidence of active TB. Preventive therapy should be considered in persons with a history of potential exposure in high-risk settings (as listed previously) regardless of results of testing for LTBI.

For further information on evaluation and treatment of active TB disease, see Chapter 28.

RECOMMENDED READING

CDC. Anergy skin testing and preventive therapy for HIV-infected persons: revised recommendations. *MMWR Morb Mortal Wkly Rep.* 1997;46(RR-15):1–12.

ACKNOWLEDGMENTS

This section is an update from the original version authored by David Cohn, MD, in the previous edition.

DENTAL CARE

LEARNING OBJECTIVE

Discuss the importance of routine dental care for PWH and essential information to be included in the treating physician's written referral.

WHAT'S NEW?

A large proportion of PWH do not receive needed dental and oral care despite the high prevalence of such disorders in this population. Referrals for dental care should include information about the patient's risk for secondary infection and bleeding, infectious status, and current medications.

KEY POINTS

- PWH are at increased risk for oral and dental problems because of immunodeficiency, salivary gland dysfunction, substance use, tobacco use, poor oral hygiene, and limited access to dental care.

- Oral cavity problems can undermine the success of ART by exacerbating existing medical, nutritional, and psychosocial problems; compromising adherence to treatment regimens; and diminishing quality of life.

- Providers should include basic oral screening in their routine clinic visits and advocate for routine dental care for patients.

- Referrals for dental care should include information about the patient's risk for secondary infection and bleeding, infectious status, and current medications.

Oral healthcare is an important component of the management of patients with HIV infection. Oral cavity problems can undermine the success of ART by exacerbating existing medical, nutritional, and psychosocial problems; compromising adherence to treatment regimens; and diminishing quality of life (New York State Department of Health AIDS Institute (NYSDOH), 2020).

Oral disease occurs disproportionately in the same individuals most affected by HIV: those of low socioeconomic status, those with limited healthcare access and use of services, and substance users whose attention to personal health and hygiene is often suboptimal (NYSDOH, 2020). They do not receive the dental care they need. In the HIV Cost and Services Utilization Study, which examined a nationally representative sample of persons in HIV care, 35% of patients had no regular source of dental care; 22% had not received dental care in more than 2 years; 25% had not received needed dental care; and 48% had no dental insurance coverage (Freed et al., 2005).

Significant proportions of PWH have HIV-related oral problems such as untreated caries (39%), gum problems (47%), missing teeth (47%), and xerostomia (dry mouth) (37%) (Freed et al., 2005). PWH with advanced immunosuppression are also at risk for serious systemic opportunistic infections and neoplasms, many of which can manifest in the oral cavity. Examples include candidiasis, hairy leukoplakia, Kaposi's sarcoma, and aphthous ulcerations (Bonito, 2001). The presence of oral candidiasis without medical explanation (e.g., recent antibiotics) is most often related to a low $CD4^+$ T- cell number and is considered a marker for cell-mediated immunodeficiency. Deterioration of oral immunologic functions and changes in salivary flow rate and composition also aid in the development of caries and periodontal diseases, including gingivitis, which can progress to serious necrotizing gingivitis and compromise masticatory functions and nutrition (Bonito, 2001). The presence of necrotizing ulcerative periodontitis, a more aggressive form of periodontal disease, should also be considered a sign of severe immune deterioration. It is a rapidly progressing disease, and treatment should be initiated as early as possible.

Thus, oral healthcare should be an integral component of primary healthcare for persons with HIV disease (NYSDOH, 2020). Providers must become familiar with oral conditions that affect HIV-infected persons and include basic oral screening in routine clinic visit exams. Providers also must be aware of and advocate for oral healthcare and dental services in their communities. Finally, providers must educate patients about the importance of good oral hygiene practices and regular dental care (at least twice annually) (NYSDOH, 2020).

When considering referral to a dental specialist, the main issues of concern are the patient's risk for bleeding, risk for infection, and infectiousness. Accordingly, the following information should be provided in dental referrals:

- *Bleeding risk*: platelet count (platelet count< 60,000/mm³ may require platelet transfusion or steroids prior to dental treatment), liver biochemical tests, history of coagulation or other bleeding disorders, history of liver disease, and current hemoglobin (to ascertain risk of anemia should significant bleeding occur).

- *Infection risk*: total white blood cell count, absolute neutrophil count, CD4 + T-cell count, history of valvular or congenital heart disease, and other medical risks for infection (e.g., active intravenous drug use posing a risk for endocarditis).

- *Antibiotic prophylaxis*: Based on the individual need of each patient, antibiotic prophylaxis may be indicated prior to dental care. The need for antibiotic prophylaxis is not based on CD4 + T-counts, viral load, or AIDS diagnosis. Patients with severe neutropenia (neutrophil count< 500/mm³) should be premedicated with antibiotics prior to dental treatment. Otherwise, antibiotic prophylaxis is recommended based on the standard guidelines set forth by the American Heart Association (http://www.aha.org) for the prevention of bacterial endocarditis.

- *Concurrent infections*: current HIV viral load, chronic active hepatitis B or hepatitis C infections, and contagious respiratory diseases such as active/untreated TB.

All medications also should be detailed to prevent drug interactions or adverse effects if medications will be used or prescribed as part of the dental care.

RECOMMENDED READING

Freed JR, Marcus M, Freed BA, et al. Oral health findings for HIV-infected adult medical patients from the HIV Cost and Services Utilization Study. *J Am Dental Assoc.* 2005;136:1396–1405.

Greenspan JS, Greenspan D, Winkler JR. Diagnosis and management of the oral manifestations of HIV infection and AIDS. *Infect Dis Clin North Am.* 1988;2:373–385.

Integrating HIV Innovating Practices. Implementing oral healthcare into HIV primary care settings curriculum. https://careacttarget.org/library/implementing-oral-health-care-hiv-primary-care-settings-curriculum-0. Published December 2013. Accessed November 15, 2015.

Lee KC, Tami TA. Otolaryngologic manifestation of HIV disease. In: Cohen PT, Sande MA, Volberding PA, eds. *The AIDS knowledge base.* 3rd ed. Philadelphia, PA: Lippincott Williams & Wilkins; 1999:559–575.

IMMUNIZATIONS

LEARNING OBJECTIVE

Discuss the immunization schedule for PWH.

WHAT'S NEW?

Information in this section is based on the recommendations from the Advisory Committee on Immunization Practices (ACIP), released in February 2022 (Murthy et al., 2022).

KEY POINTS

- Response to vaccinations is based on the CD4 + T-cell count.

- Response to vaccinations is best as early as possible in the infection or soon after immune reconstitution with ART.

- Vaccinations may need to be repeated when immune reconstitution occurs with ART, as immunosuppression can cause a suboptimal response initially.

- Live-virus vaccinations are not safe in PWH with a CD4+ T-cell count< 200 cells/mm³.

CONCERN WITH IMMUNIZATIONS?

Prior to ART in the 1980s, the concern was that immunizations could inadvertently up-regulate the immune system and cause elevations in HIV replication, ultimately accelerating infection progression. However, it was found the this increase in HIV RNA was only transient. Also, in PWH who are on ART, immunization causes no detectable elevations in the RNA levels. The only contraindication to immunizations is low CD4 + T-cell count (less than 200 cells/mm³) for live vaccinations as they can cause life-threatening disseminated infections.

CORONAVIRUS (SARS-COV-2 OR COVID-19)

In the general population, the individuals who are at the highest risk of severe COVID-19 include those aged >60 years; those who are pregnant; those who have received solid organ transplants; and those with comorbidities, such as cancer, obesity, diabetes mellitus, cardiovascular disease, pulmonary disease, a history of smoking, chronic kidney disease, or chronic liver disease. Many PWH have one or more comorbidities that increase their risk for a more severe course of COVID-19. The COVID-19 Treatment Guidelines Panel (the Panel) recommends that PWH receive COVID-19 vaccines regardless of their CD4 + T-cell count or HIV viral load because the potential benefits outweigh the potential risks. Three vaccines are authorized or approved for use in the United States to prevent COVID-19. For primary and booster vaccinations, the mRNA vaccines (i.e., BNT162b2 (Pfizer-BioNTech) or mRNA-1273 (Moderna)) are preferable. The Ad26.COV2.S (Johnson & Johnson/Janssen) vaccine, because of its risk of serious adverse events, has been limited in use by the FDA. The ACIP recommends that people with advanced or untreated HIV who received a two-dose mRNA COVID-19 vaccine should receive a third dose at least 28 days after the second dose. Advanced HIV is defined as people with CD4 + T-cell counts< 200 cells/mm³, a history of an AIDS-defining illness without immune reconstitution, or clinical manifestations of symptomatic HIV.

- Bottom line:
  - Vaccine:
    - Two-dose series 3–8 weeks apart for BNT162b2 (Pfizer-BioNTech); can be given 21 days apart in high-risk populations.
    - Two-dose series 4–8 weeks apart for mRNA-1273 (Moderna); can be given 28 days apart in high-risk populations.

- One dose of Ad26.COV2.S (Johnson & Johnson/Janssen) is no longer recommended.
- Booster:
  - Most people are recommended to receive one booster, preferably of either Pfizer-BioNTech or Moderna COVID-19 vaccine at least 5 months after the final dose in the primary series.
  - For adults aged 50 years and older, a second booster of either Pfizer-BioNTech or Moderna COVID-19 vaccine at least 4 months after the first booster.
  - Further boosters will likely be recommended in the future.

HAEMOPHILUS INFLUENZA TYPE B (HIB)

Infection caused by *Haemophilus influenzae* is more common in PWH, although the annual incidence remains relatively low. In addition, only about 33% of the cases involve *H. influenzae* type b. Therefore, HIB is not recommended for routine administration to adults with HIV.

- Bottom line: one dose only if there is an indication (e.g., sickle cell disease, leukemia, or anatomic or functional asplenia).

HEPATITIS A VIRUS (HAV)

HAV rates in general have declined with the introduction of the vaccine in 1990s. However, rates are increased in homeless individuals, people who inject drugs, and men who have sex with men. It is recommended to administer a hepatitis A vaccine to all PWH regardless of CD4$^+$ T-cell count.

- Bottom Line: Two doses at least 6 months apart. A three-dose series can be administered with combined hep A-hep B vaccine; minimum intervals are 4 weeks between the first and second dose and 5 months between the second and third dose.

HEPATITIS B VIRUS (HBV)

There is an increased risk for PWH of acquiring HBV from injection drug use and/or condomless sex. It is recommended to administer hepatitis B vaccine to all PWH regardless of CD4$^+$ T-cell count. Screening labs are done pre- and postvaccination to assess the need for the series and adequacy of response if given.

- Screening interpretation:
  - Positive hepatitis surface antigen (HBsAg): Active infection and no indication for vaccination.
  - Positive HBsAg and core antigen may indicate chronic infection and further evaluation would be needed.
  - Positive antibody to hepatitis surface and core antigens (HBsAb, HBcAb): previous infection and no need for vaccination.
  - Positive antibody to hepatitis surface antigen (HBsAb) with a titer >10 mIU/mL; adequately vaccinated.

- Bottom Line: Two- or three-dose series. The two-dose series (Heplisav-B) is given 1 month apart. The three-dose series (PreHevbrio or Engerix-B) is given at 0, 1, and 6 months. If screening reveals a nonresponder, recommendation is to administer a four-dose series double-dose hepatitis B vaccine at 0, 1, 2, and 6 months. Vaccines that contain both hepatitis A and B vaccines are available (Twinrix). If CD4$^+$ T-cell count was below 200 cell/mm^3 with initial series, waiting until immune reconstitution occurs before doing the second series is an option.

HUMAN PAPILLOMAVIRUS VIRUS (HPV)

For PWH, there is a higher incidence of disease associated with HPV. The series is recommended for PWH who are 9 through 26 years of age; some guidelines have recommended extending the age of vaccination up to 45 years.

- Bottom line: Three-dose series given at 0, 1–2, and 6 months. The two-dose series should NOT be used with PLWH. The series should not be given to pregnant women or continued during pregnancy. However, a pregnancy test is not required before administration. Series can be continued after the completion of pregnancy.

INFLUENZA

For PWH, there is higher risk of adverse outcomes with infection when compared with general population. Recommended influenza vaccines include inactivated influenza vaccine (IIV) or recombinant influenza vaccine (RIV). Live attenuated vaccine is contraindicated.

- Bottom line: o: ne dose annually of IIV or RIV.

MEASLES MUMPS RUBELLA (MMR)

As with influenza, for PWH, there is higher risk of adverse outcomes with infection when compared with general population. It is important to remember that the MMR vaccine is a live-virus vaccine.

- Bottom line: Two-dose series if CD4$^+$ T-cell count is 200 cells/mm^3 or greater (for at least 6 months) if born in 1957 or later. The doses administered at least 4 weeks apart. Combination vaccination with varicella is NOT recommended. If the CD4$^+$ T-cell count is less than 200 cells/mm^3, both MMR and MMRV are contraindicated. The vaccine is also contraindicated in pregnancy, which should be avoided for 28 days after vaccination.

VARICELLA VIRUS (VAR)

For PLWH, primary varicella zoster virus infection is uncommon because of immunity from childhood infection. The varicella vaccine is a live-virus vaccine.

- Bottom line: Two doses 3 months apart. Recommended for PLWH with no evidence of immunity and a CD4$^+$ T-cell count of 200 cells/mm^3 or greater. The vaccination is contraindicated with low CD4$^+$ T-cell count (< 200 cells/mm^3).

ZOSTER

For PWH, incidence of zoster is 15-fold higher than among age-matched immunocompetent adults, with highest risk when CD4$^+$ T-cell count is less than 200 cells/mm^3. Vaccination is intended to prevent zoster and reduce the severity of zoster if it does occur.

- Bottom line:
  - **Recombinant zoster vaccine (RZV)**: two doses, given 2 to 6 months apart, for persons aged 50 years and older regardless of CD4$^+$ T-cell count. RZV is preferred over Zoster vaccine live (ZVL) by the ACIP.
  - **ZVL**: Is no longer available. Persons who have previously been vaccinated with this product should be vaccinated with two doses of the RZV.

MENINGOCOCCUS

For PWH there is an increased risk of developing meningococcal disease, with the relative risk estimated at 5- to 13-fold higher than in persons without HIV; the risk in persons with HIV infection appears to be higher with low CD4$^+$ T-cell counts and high HIV RNA levels. Men who have sex with men are particularly at risk for meningococcal meningitis. Recent outbreaks of meningococcal meningitis have been reported in MSMs.

- Bottom Line: For serogroups (A, C, W, Y), two doses (8–12 weeks apart) with a booster in 5 years. Meningococcal B vaccine recommended only if PWH are aged 18 years or older, and they have an indication for receiving meningococcal B vaccine, such as functional or anatomic asplenia, persistent complement component deficiency or receiving complement inhibitor. If given, the two-dose series is given one month apart. If the three-dose series is given, it is at 0, 1–2, and 6 months.

PNEUMOCOCCUS

For PWH there is an increased risk of developing pneumococcal disease, with the relative risk estimated at sevenfold higher than in persons without HIV. In 2022, the ACIP updated its pneumococcal vaccination recommendations. The PCV13 is no longer available.

- Bottom line:
  - **Pneumococcal vaccine-naive**: One dose of PCV20 or PCV15. If PCV15 is used; this should be followed by a dose of PPSV23 given at least 1 year after the PCV15 dose.

A minimum interval of 8 weeks between PCV15 and PPSV23 can be considered for immunocompromised adults to minimize the risk of invasive pneumococcal disease caused by serotypes unique to PPSV23 in these vulnerable groups.

TETANUS, DIPHTHERIA, AND PERTUSSIS (TDAP)

For PWH, an adequate immune response is usually amounted against the toxins produced from these organisms. Therefore, the recommendation for vaccination does not differ from general population.

- Bottom line: One dose of Tdap, followed by a Td or Tdap booster every 10 years. If previously given Td only, give one dose of Tdap. Tdap should be given in every pregnancy regardless of immunization history.

REFERENCES

American Thoracic Society/Centers for Disease Control and Prevention. Targeted tuberculin testing and treatment of latent tuberculosis infection: joint statement of the American Thoracic Society and the Centers for Disease Control and Prevention. *Am J Respir Crit Care Med.* 2000;161:S221–S247.

American Thoracic Society, Centers for Disease Control and Prevention, and Infectious Diseases Society of America. Controlling tuberculosis in the United States. *Am J Respir Crit Care Med.* 2005;172:1169–1227.

Boehme CC, Nabeta P, Hillemann D, et al. Rapid molecular detection of tuberculosis and rifampin resistance. *N Engl J Med.* September 9, 2010;363(11):1005–1015.

Bonito AJ. Management of dental patients who are HIV positive. Summary, evidence report/technology assessment: number 37. AHRQ Publication No. 01-E041. Rockville, MD: Agency for Healthcare Research and Quality. http://www.ncbi.nlm.nih.gov/books/NBK11965. Published March 2001. Accessed November 15, 2015.

Cain KP, McCarthy KD, Heilg CM, et al. An algorithm for tuberculosis screening and diagnosis in people with HIV. *N Engl J Med.* 2010;362:707–716.

Cattamanchi A, Smith R, Steingart KR, et al. Interferon-gamma release assays for the diagnosis of latent tuberculosis infection in HIV-infected individuals: a systematic review and meta-analysis. *J AIDS.* 2011;56:230–238.

Centers for Disease Control and Prevention (CDC). COVID-19 information for specific groups of people. cdc.gov. https://www.cdc.gov/coronavirus/2019-ncov/need-extra-precautions/index.html. Published 2021. Accessed January 24, 2022.

CDC. Updated guidelines for using interferon gamma release assays to detect *Mycobacterium tuberculosis* infection—United States, 2010. *MMWR Morb Mort Wkly Rep.* 2010;59(RR-5):1–26.

COVID-19 Treatment Guidelines Panel. Coronavirus disease 2019 (COVID-19) treatment guidelines. National Institutes of Health. https://www.covid19treatmentguidelines.nih.gov/. Published 2019. Accessed August 11, 2022.

Freed JR, Marcus M, Freed BA, et al. Oral health findings for HIV-infected adult medical patients from the HIV Cost and Services Utilization study. *J Am Dental Assoc.* 2005;136:1396–1405.

Getahun H, Harrington M, O'Brien R, et al. Diagnosis of smear-negative pulmonary tuberculosis in people with HIV infection or AIDS in resource-constrained settings: informing urgent policy changes. *Lancet.* 2007;369(9578):2042–2049.

Gray J, Reves R, Johnson S, et al. Identification of false-positive QuantiFERON-TB Gold In-Tube assays by repeat testing in PLWH at low risk of tuberculosis. *Clin Infect Dis.* 2012;54:e20–e23.

Horsburgh CR, Rubin EJ. Latent tuberculosis infection in the United States. *N Engl J Med.* 2011;364:1441–1448.

New York State Department of Health AIDS Institute (NYSDOH). HIV and oral health: general principles. http://www.hivguidelines.org/clinical-guidelines/hiv-and-oral-health/general-principles. Published 2020. Accessed July 15, 2020.

Murthy N, Wodi AP, Bernstein H, et al. Advisory committee on immunization practices recommended immunization schedule for adults aged 19 years or older—United States, 2022. *MMWR Morb Mortal Wkly Rep.* 2022;71:229–233. http:// www.cdc.gov/mmwr/volumes/71/wr/mm7107a1.htm.

Palmieri F, Girardi E, Pellicelli AM, et al. Pulmonary tuberculosis in HIV-infected patients presenting with normal chest radiograph and negative sputum smear. *Infection.* 2002;30(2):68–74.

Panel on Opportunistic Infections in Adults and Adolescents with HIV. Guidelines for the prevention and treatment of opportunistic infections in adults and adolescents with HIV: recommendations from the Centers for Disease Control and Prevention, the National Institutes of Health, and the HIV Medicine Association of the Infectious Diseases Society of America. https:// clinicalinfo.hiv.gov/sites/default/files/guidelines/documents/adult-adolescent-oi/guidelines-adult-adolescent-oi.pdf. Published January 18, 2023. Accessed March 8, 2023.

Raby E, Moyo M, Devendra A, et al. The effects of HIV on the sensitivity of a whole blood IFN-gamma release assay in Zambian adults with active tuberculosis. *PLoS One.* June 18, 2008;3(6):e2489.

11.

DIVERSITY AWARENESS

Gary F. Spinner

CHAPTER GOALS

Upon completion of this chapter, the reader should be able to:

- Discuss the concepts of social determinants of health and racial/ethnic disparities, and how the failure to address them leads to health inequity in HIV, COVID-19, and other diseases.

- Discuss the meaning of systemic racism, and how it has contributed to, or failed to rectify, the health disparities among many people living with HIV (PWH).

- Understand how clinical trials have generally failed to recruit adequate numbers of women and racial and ethnic minorities into trials and the potential clinical implications from failing to do so.

- Provide an understanding of the diversity of PWH, the complexity of their unique cultures that are shaped by a multitude of factors and the importance of becoming competent in developing a clinician–patient relationship across cultural differences.

- Relate how a patient's values, beliefs, and judgments may create barriers to successful treatment if the HIV provider does not competently navigate the cultural differences between patient and provider and the importance of becoming aware of one's personal biases that may hinder the patient-clinician relationship in caring for a diverse population of PWH.

- Recognize the challenges in addressing racial and ethnic disparities in healthcare and in HIV.

- Discuss the impact that culture, ethnicity, immigration status, sexual orientation, gender identity, religion, gender, and behavioral health problems may have on the care of PWH.

- Equip providers with the knowledge and skill to develop and provide gender-affirming primary and HIV care and prevention for transgender persons.

- Discuss limitations in HIV care and special needs among migrant populations or patients with undocumented citizenship.

DIVERSITY AWARENESS

LEARNING OBJECTIVES

- Discuss how a patient's values, beliefs, and judgments may create barriers to successful treatment if the HIV provider does not competently navigate the cultural differences between the patient and the healthcare provider.

- Recognize the challenges in addressing racial and ethnic disparities in healthcare and in HIV.

- Analyze one's personal (implicit) biases regarding race, ethnicity, sexual and gender diversity, and cultural practices and understand how that bias can hinder the development of an effective patient-clinician relationship.

- Discuss the impact that culture, ethnicity, immigration status, sexual orientation, gender identity, religion, gender, and behavioral health problems may have on the care of PWH.

WHAT'S NEW?

The COVID-19 pandemic, in its third year as of this writing, has impacted Black and Brown communities more severely than White communities. Some recent studies show that the COVID-19 pandemic affects PWH with greater severity than those not living with HIV (Danwang, 2022); Danwang et al., 2022). In addition, the same racial and ethnic disparities that have long persisted in the pandemic of HIV hold true for COVID-19. Black and Latinx populations have significantly higher rates of HIV and COVID-19 infections, along with higher rates of mortality from both pandemics.

Also new in this chapter is how clinical trials have long failed to include adequate numbers of women and racial and ethnic minorities, as well as the clinical implications when therapeutics are approved but unstudied sufficiently in diverse populations.

KEY POINT

- Patients with HIV come from diverse backgrounds and are often mistrustful of healthcare providers.

- Social determinants of health significantly impact persons living with HIV.

INTRODUCTION

This textbook, *Fundamentals of HIV Medicine*, is filled with thousands of scientific facts, evidence-based guidelines, and a compendium of knowledge needed to provide optimal care for patients living with HIV. However, even the most expert health care provider, if lacking adequate understanding of how the health of patients living with HIV is affected by race, ethnicity, gender, and sexual orientation, will be far less effective in helping their patients attain optimal health. This chapter on caring for diverse patients provides insight on how the multitude of living conditions, economic factors, geography, neighborhoods, housing, access to healthcare, employment, education, and economic factors, can be as important to the life of someone living with HIV as the best antiviral therapy. It will also provide insight on how clinical trials that are performed to determine whether medications and other therapeutics are safe and effective, are underrepresented by women and racial and ethnic minorities, and the potential impact that can have on diverse populations that might ultimately use those treatments. In this third year of the COVID-19 pandemic, and the forty-first year of the HIV pandemic, the concept of syndemic theory, first articulated by Singer in 1996, suggests that structural inequalities can interact synergistically to undermine the health of vulnerable populations (Singer, 1996). Syndemic theory helps explain how the interaction of a multitude of social factors impact the pandemics of HIV, and COVID-19, and why populations affected by one pandemic are concurrently and disproportionately impacted by others. A systematic review and meta-analysis of 44 studies of persons with HIV who were co-infected with COVID-19 found them to be at increased risk of hospital admission, and two studies demonstrated an increased risk of mortality (Danwang et al., 2022). One section of this chapter will explore the intersectionality of HIV, COVID-19, and systemic racism, and how they synergistically impact each other, and how ending the HIV epidemic (and perhaps the COVID-19 pandemic) will likely require addressing the mutually reinforcing social systems that precipitate the conditions of inequality.

THE IMPORTANCE OF DIVERSITY IN CLINICAL TRIALS

In 2019, emtricitabine plus tenofovir alafenamide (FTC/TAF) was approved by the Food and Drug Administration (FDA) for the prevention of HIV in cisgender men who have sex with men (MSM), and transgender women. The phase 3 Discover trial was a noninferiority trial comparing emtricitabine plus tenofovir disoproxil fumarate (FTC/TDF) to emtricitabine plus tenofovir alafenamide (FTC/TAF), in about 5,300 MSM and transgender women at high risk of contracting HIV (Mayer et al., 2020). When the trial demonstrated noninferiority of FTC/TAF for pre-exposure prophylaxis (PrEP), Gilead Sciences, the pharmaceutical company which funded the clinical trial, requested FDA approval for FTC/TAF to be used in both cisgender men, transgender women, and cisgender women, in even though the study did not include any cisgender women. When the FDA only approved its use in cisgender men and transgender women, citing the fact that no cisgender women were included in the study to prove noninferiority to FTC/TDF, Gilead explained to critics that they did not find it feasible to study FTC/TAF in cisgender women because the proposed methodology would require too large a study population of women to prove noninferiority. Gilead is now enrolling a study of FTC/TAF in cis-gender women (Gilead, 2020). This example, of exclusion of women in clinical trials, despite biological differences between men and women, is not unusual.

The FDA underscores the importance of testing drugs and medical products in the people they are meant to help (FDA, 2020). This means that people of different races, ages, ethnic groups and genders are included in clinical trials (FDA, 2018). Section 907 of the FDA Safety and Innovation Act directed the FDA to investigate how well demographic subgroups (sex, age, and race and ethnicity) are included in clinical trials and analyze subgroup-specific safety and effectiveness data (FDA, 2012).

It is important to understand that while there are no biologic differences between races, and that genetic differences are more common within races then between them, there is a possibility that missed genetic variants in certain populations excluded from clinical trials can potentially lead to differences in efficacy, adverse effects, or incorrect dosing, all of which may lead to patient harm.

Racial and ethnic minorities and women are significantly underrepresented in clinical trials. For example, a review of enrollment of minorities and women in oncology trials found that over the past 14 years, there has been a decrease in recruitment, with Black and Latinx persons and women less likely to be enrolled in cancer clinical trials as compared with White men (Duma et al., 2018). There is a significant racial disparity in cancer outcomes, yet clinical trials for cancer treatments are overrepresented by White male participants (Guerrero et al., 2018). In 2021, the FDA published the Drug Trials Snapshots that documented the imbalance of study participants. In studies that included almost 5,000 enrollees that led to 18 new cancer treatments approved, 73% of participants were White; half were male; only 5 % were Black; and 6% were Latinx (FDA, 2021).

Cardiovascular disease (CVD) is the number one cause of death in the United States, and although there are significant racial and ethnic disparities in outcomes from CVD, women, Black persons, and Latinx persons are underrepresented in CVD clinical trials (Michos et al., 2021). Lack of participation can undermine how generalizable trial evidence is for populations excluded from the clinical trial.

An analysis by Pro-Publica found that Black and Native American persons are underrepresented in clinical trials for many drugs, even when those groups suffer disproportionately from the condition for which the drug is intended (Chen & Wong, 2018). For example, Bhatnagar and colleagues found that despite Black persons having 2–3 times higher rates of multiple myeloma cases, pivotal trials for multiple myeloma therapeutics enrolled only 1.8% of Black study enrollees (Bhatnagar et al., 2017).

The incidence and rates of mortality from prostate cancer are significantly higher in Black men compared with White men, yet Black men participate significantly less in clinical trials of prostate cancer treatments. In one large clinical trial that *did* include a larger percentage of Black participants, it was found that the particular treatment studied led to better outcomes for survivals in Black participants as compared to White participants in the study (Sartor et al., 2020).

Women absorb, metabolize, distribute, and eliminate drugs differently than men do (Ravindran, 2020). Historically, women have been excluded from clinical trials, exemplified by the FDA, in 1977 recommending the exclusion of women of childbearing years from phase I and phase II clinical trials (Samaei et al., 2022). For many years, this caused clinical trials to almost exclusively recruit White men. However, in 1993, the National Institutes of Health established guidelines for including women and minorities in all government-funded research (US Congress, 1993). There has been improvement in the inclusion of women in clinical trials since then, and the FDA Drug Trials Snapshots of 5-year data between 2015 and 2019 showed that women represented 51% of clinical trial participants globally and 56% of trial participants in the United States (FDA, 2020). Exclusion of pregnant women from clinical trials is based on concern for the fetus, and while well intentioned, it results in more than 80% of pregnant patients being prescribed medications that have not been studied in pregnancy (Heyrana et al., 2018). For women taking antivirals for HIV who become pregnant, HIV specialists can help contribute to the knowledge on the safety of antiviral medications by reporting all cases to the antiretroviral pregnancy registry (Antiviral Pregnancy Registry, 2022).

WHY ARE THERE INSUFFICIENT NUMBERS OF WOMEN AND RACIAL AND ETHNIC MINORITIES PARTICIPATING IN CLINICAL TRIALS?

For racial and ethnic minorities and for women (FDA, 2012), there are multiple reasons for not participating in clinical trials. Mistrust in the healthcare system, discussed elsewhere in this chapter, and in clinical research in particular, has long been a reason why many racial and ethnic minorities have little interest in clinical trials. This mistrust is based on a multitude of historical examples of experimentation on people of color, and on women, including not being informed of needed treatment, and the withholding of syphilis treatment (CDC, 2021) to enable the study of untreated syphilis. There is also a history of forced sterilization of women without consent that occurred from 1973 to 1976 (Torpy, 2007).

Another significant reason for the underrepresentation of racial and ethnic minorities in clinical trials is lack of access to healthcare, an issue also discussed in more depth in this chapter. An draft guidance on Diversity in Clinical Trials (FDA, 2022), cites language and cultural differences, health literacy, lack of transportation, and time and resource constraints among other reasons for low rates of minority participation.

Lack of access to health care (Riner et al., 2022) centers that conduct clinical research programs for new therapies and lack of awareness of clinical trials that are conducted there is another explanation.

Another barrier to recruitment of women and minorities into clinical trials is that many clinicians in the United States are not affiliated with large academic medical centers and may be unaware of trials being conducted in their communities to which to refer eligible patients, or simply do not have the time to discuss and refer patients to clinical trials. In 2019, of the nearly 30 million patients who receive their primary care in Federally Qualified Health Centers (FQHC), 62% were racial and ethnic minorities (National Institutes of Health, 2020). Many FQHCs lack the resources or time to conduct clinical research, and often, the mission-driven need to provide clinical care to a vulnerable population of patients supersedes involvement in clinical research. In addition, eligibility criteria in some clinical trials can perpetuate disparities. Many clinical trials exclude individuals who are unable to read, speak, and/or understand English, or who are not native English speakers (Muthukumar et al., 2021). Other eligibility criteria, such as exclusion for renal dysfunction, are more likely to exclude Black persons in some trials (Riner et al., 2022).

THE POTENTIAL FOR CHANGE

The Medicaid program, in which about 20% of the US population receive health insurance, has not covered the cost of recipient participation in clinical trials, which thus passes costs to low-income people least able to afford it, while private insurers are required to provide reimbursement for clinical trial participation. This disproportionately impacted racial and ethnic minorities. However, the Clinical Treatment Act, passed by the US Congress, went into effect on January 1, 2022, and requires Medicaid to pay the cost of routine care for recipients enrolled in clinical trials who have life-threatening conditions (Raths, 2022). Woodcock and colleagues (2021) argue that it is time for the biomedical industry, policymakers, government agencies, contract research organizations, and patient advocates—to support the development and long-term sustainability of an infrastructure that unites clinical research with clinical care. Academic-community-government partnerships in a community engagement model can help address the lack of diversity in clinical trials, with partnerships between community members, clinicians, scientists, governmental officials, and the pharmaceutical industry (Woodcock et al., 2021).

This chapter explores in more depth the relationship between social determinants of health (SDOH) and health inequity, along with the impact of systemic racism and its impact on health. To further understand the role that SDOH play in clinical outcomes, collecting a uniform data set of demographic and socioeconomic data in clinical trials can facilitate the measurement of care, quality, utilization, and outcomes in vulnerable populations (Kahn et al., 2022).

To alleviate the discrepancy between who participates in clinical trials, and the real-world experience of patients who ultimately are prescribed the treatments studied, more robust efforts are needed to eliminate the barriers of gender, race, and ethnicity in clinical trial participation.

HIV AND COVID-19: TWO PANDEMICS—SAME RACIAL AND ETHNIC DISPARITIES

The dual pandemics of HIV, caused by the RNA virus HIV, and COVID-19, caused by the RNA virus SARS-CoV-2, share much in common beyond their viral etiologies. Both HIV and COVID-19 disproportionately affect Black and Latinx populations far more than White populations. Yet the health disparities in these two pandemics have nothing to do with any biological differences or virus pathology. These disparities are directly related to SDOH, racial and ethnic health inequities, and societal policies that have either created or failed to address these unequal conditions. While PWH do not appear to be at greater risk of becoming infected with SARS-CoV-2 (Park, 2020), nor do they appear to have worse outcomes than people without HIV, people of color are significantly more likely to become infected with SARS-CoV-2 and have higher rates of mortality. To understand the similarities of these two pandemics is to recognize how SDOH create health inequity among people of color, leading to worse outcomes among those with HIV, COVID-19, or many other health conditions. The importance of knowing why racial and ethnic minorities are more likely to acquire HIV can help the HIV specialist become a more culturally competent and ultimately a better health care provider.

According to the World Health Organization (2019), "SDOH (SDH) are the conditions in which people are born, grow, work, live, and age, and the wider set of forces and systems shaping the conditions of daily life. These forces and systems include economic policies and systems, development agendas, social norms, social policies, and political systems."

Blacks, Latinxs, and Native Americans all experience significant health disparities in the United States. A *health disparity* is "a particular type of health difference that is closely linked with social, economic, and/or environmental disadvantage." Health disparities adversely affect groups of people who have systematically experienced greater obstacles to health care based on their racial or ethnic group; religion; socioeconomic status; gender; age; mental health; cognitive, sensory, or physical disability; sexual orientation or gender identity; geographic location; or other characteristics historically linked to discrimination or exclusion (US Department of Health and Human Services, 2020). While unequal access to health care can be one determinant of less-than-equal health outcomes, the disparities go far beyond access to care. For example, even with equal access to health care in the Veterans Health Administration, there were mortality disparities for Black veterans with stage 4 chronic kidney disease, colon cancer, diabetes, HIV, rectal cancer, and stroke; for Native American and Alaska Native veterans undergoing noncardiac major surgery; and for Latinx veterans with HIV (Peterson, 2018).

What follows are examples of the racial and ethnic disparities for HIV and for COVID-19, and why it is important for HIV specialists to have a sound understanding of these disparities and how they affect clinical outcomes. Healthcare provider attitudes, biases, and beliefs will also be addressed, as it is important for the HIV specialist to recognize how racial and ethnic biases, whether conscious or unconscious, can have a profound impact on the health outcomes of patients.

HIV: RACIAL AND ETHNIC DISPARITIES

Black and Latinx populations account for a vastly disproportionate percentage of PWH. According to CDC data (2022c), while Black persons account for only 13.4% of the US population, they comprised 42% of all newly diagnosed PWH in the United States in 2019. Latinxs comprise 18.5 % of the US population but accounted for 29% of HIV incidence in 2019. Black men and women have higher rates of some sexually transmitted diseases than other racial/ethnic groups, increasing risk for HIV acquisition and transmission (CDC, 2022c). The lifetime risk of acquiring HIV is 6 times higher for Black men, and nearly three times higher for Latino men, than for White men. Black women have a 14 times higher lifetime risk of HIV, and Latina women have 3 times higher lifetime risk of acquiring HIV as compared with White women. Among MSM, one of every two Black MSM has a lifetime risk of HIV acquisition, compared with 1 in 6 Latino MSM and 1 in 11 White MSM (CDC, 2016).

In every category, comparing viral suppression between White and Black persons, White persons are more likely to be virally suppressed (Crepaz, 2018; CDC, 2020b). While 56% of White persons were suppressed, only 41% of Black persons were suppressed, and this held true by gender, by age, among MSM, and people-who-inject-drugs.

PrEP is 99% effective in the prevention of HIV when taken optimally, yet while Black and Latino MSM have the highest risk of acquiring HIV, PrEP is far more likely to be offered to White MSM (Kanny, 2019). This disparity between White and Black MSM persisted among those who had health insurance and had a usual source of healthcare. According to data presented at the International AIDS Conference 2022, analysis of the number of PrEP prescriptions from 2012 to 2021 showed that while PrEP prescriptions increased significantly in the United States, in all regions of the country, more significantly, more PrEP prescriptions were written for White people, and least for Black people (Sullivan et al., 2022).

In summary, Black and Latinx persons, compared with White persons, have higher rates of HIV transmission, have higher risk of infection, are less likely to be virally suppressed when on antiviral therapy, and are less likely to be offered HIV prevention with PrEP.

COVID-19: RACIAL AND ETHNIC DISPARITIES

Like HIV, COVID-19 disproportionately affects people of color, who are more likely than White people to become infected with COVID-19, and more likely to have severe disease and death. Although the CDC data in the early days of the COVID-19 pandemic at the time, was incomplete and missing racial and ethnic data for many patients, an early study analyzing county data through mid-April 2020 (Millett, 2020a), in which there are disproportionately more Black persons residing, found that 97% of predominantly Black counties had at least one COVID-19 case, compared to 80% of other counties. They also found that 49% of Black counties had at least one COVID-19 death compared with 28% in all other nonmajority Black counties. The predominantly Black counties tended to have lower rates of insurance, higher rates of unemployment, crowded housing, poor air quality, and reduced ability to practice social distancing. In addition, employed persons in predominantly Black counties were more likely to be classified as essential workers, use public transportation, and have jobs that did not allow working from home. When using the same methodology to look at Latinx majority counties, a similar outcome of disproportionately high COVID-19 cases and deaths was found.

The CDC has tracked the risk for COVID-19 infection, hospitalizations, and death by race and ethnicity for the past several years. As of June 2022, Native American or Alaska Native, Black, and Latinx persons have had 1.5 times higher case rates of COVID-19 as compared with non-Hispanic Whites persons. Rates of hospitalizations for COVID-19, a marker for severity of infection is 3 times higher for Native American/Alaska Native persons;, 2.3 times higher for Black persons; and 2.2 times higher for Latinx persons. The mortality rate from COVID-19 follows similar trends, with 2.2 times higher; 1.7 times higher; and (Cases, data, and surveillance, 2020) 1.8 times higher deaths in Native American/Alaska Native, Black, and Latinx persons, respectively (CDC, 2022f).

Among the social factors most likely contributing to the increased morbidity and mortality of COVID-19 in racial and ethnic minorities are poverty, high-density and crowded housing, and employment that precludes working from home, and the higher likelihood of being employed as essential services workers. Other factors include reliance on public transportation; over-representation in jails, prisons, homeless shelters, and detention centers where social distancing is not possible; living in multigenerational households where it is difficulty to protect older family members; not having sick leave (which increases the likelihood that someone keeps working while ill); lack of health insurance; and distrust of the health care system, along with racism, stigma, and systemic inequities (CDC, 2022d).

COVID-19, HIV, AND THEIR LINK TO SYSTEMIC RACISM

Health equity (US Department of Health and Human Services definition) is the attainment of the highest level of health for all people. It requires valuing everyone equally with focused and ongoing societal efforts to address avoidable inequalities, historical and contemporary injustices, and the elimination of health and health care disparities (DHHS, 2010).

The significant health disparities experienced by people of color are examples of health inequity. The unequal adverse health impact of HIV and COVID-19 holds true for other health conditions as well, including certain cancers, respiratory diseases, diabetes, hypertension, and other conditions, along with worse health care outcomes for most of these conditions. Infant mortality for Black infants is 2.5 times higher than for White infants (CDC, 2022b). A Black man has a nearly 5-year shorter life expectancy than a White man, is 30% more likely to die from heart disease, twice as likely to be diagnosed with diabetes, twice as likely to have a stroke, and 40% more likely to have hypertension but 10% less likely to have it under control (Graham, 2015).

The Black Lives Matter movement taking place at the time of this writing is not only about Black persons being more than 2.5 times as likely to be killed while in the hands of the police (Roper, 2020) or incarcerated at 5.1 times the rate for White persons (Nellis, 2016) but also about these health inequities, among other issues comprising systemic racial injustice.

To truly understand the racial and ethnic disparities of the pandemics of HIV and COVID-19 one must recognize the pandemic of racism. According to Ibram Kendi (2019), a scholar of race and discriminatory policy in America, "Racism is a marriage of racist policies and racist ideas that produces and normalizes racial inequities, and that racial inequity is when two or more racial groups are not standing on approximately equal footing. A racist policy is any measure that produces or sustains racial inequity between racial groups."

The social conditions that lead to adverse health conditions, including poverty, lack of access to health care, lower wage employment, segregated and overcrowded housing, and educational disadvantages among many other inequities, are systemic problems related either to policies that have created these disadvantages or a lack of appropriate policies to address and eliminate these disadvantages.

Systemic racism, also known as *institutional racism*, is a form of racism that is embedded as normal practice within society or an organization that can lead to such issues as discrimination in employment, housing, health care, political power, criminal justice, and education, among other issues.

Systemic racism must be recognized for causing many of the social inequities that people of color experience. Crowded, high-density housing, low-wage essential service jobs that preclude working from home, and reliance on public transportation are linked to COVID-19. There are a multitude of programs and policies that can be traced back to the racial and ethnic discrimination. For example, the practice of banks denying housing loans to Black people or charging them higher rates of interest with stricter repayment terms, has led to fewer Black than White people owning homes. Historically, the Federal Housing Administration's refusal to insure mortgages in Black neighborhoods, and their requirement of developers receiving subsidized loans to build subdivisions that specifically exclude Black people, are systemically racist policies that created segregated and more densely populated housing and denied Black people of one of the most common ways to build personal wealth, home ownership (Rothstein, 2017).

Another example of systemic racism relates to unemployment benefits for workers laid off because of COVID-19. Almost a quarter of Black workers live in the South, where 52% of all new HIV infections currently occur, and where race has long played a role in limiting safety net program. During the COVID-19 pandemic, the US unemployment rate skyrocketed, but the unemployment insurance program is state controlled, and many Southern states have excluded from unemployment programs many of the jobs that are more likely to employ Black and Latinx persons. The average high school–educated White person is twice as likely to receive unemployment benefits as the average high school–educated Black person (Nichols, 2012), and Black persons receive lower rates of compensation than White persons, according to Kathryn Edwards of the Rand Corporation (Badger, 2020).

Despite the significant progress in treating PWH, there continues to be approximately 38,000 new HIV infections each year. While people of color are far more likely to acquire HIV, and PrEP is 99% effective in preventing infection when taken optimally, people of color are less likely to be offered it. "Ending the HIV Epidemic: A Plan for America" is the current administration's effort to address some of the geographic disparities where people are at greatest risk of acquiring HIV. It targets the 48 counties along with seven rural communities with greatest risk for HIV (HRSA, 2020). However, the SDOH faced by people of color threaten to undermine the plan's intended progress. A modeling study of HIV incidence (Nosyk, 2020) suggests the goal of ending the HIV epidemic is unlikely to be met because of many barriers, including lack of access to health care, proposed cutbacks to and/or outright elimination of the Affordable Care Act, and failure to expand Medicaid in many of the Southern states. Millet (2020b) pointed out at the AIDS 2020Millet pointed out at the AIDS 2020 conference that income inequality, poverty, and the degree of Black/White segregation, housing instability, and homelessness are associated with HIV in certain communities where poverty, vacant housing, unemployment, and isolation are most prevalent.

WHAT NEEDS TO BE DONE?

The Ryan White Program has been a hugely successful program with significantly better outcomes in Ryan White–funded clinics compared with other HIV clinics in the United States. Serving over half a million patients with HIV, 73.6% of whom are racial and ethnic minorities, and 69% of whom are living below the federal poverty level, the highest measure of HIV treatment success/viral suppression, was 89.4% for Ryan White–funded clinics compared with the national average of 63% (Cheever et al., 2021; HIV by age: viral suppression, 2022). Ryan White clinics are funded to address barriers many patients face, such as transportation, primary medical care, food bank services, housing, linguistic services, childcare services, emergency financial services, substance use treatment services, case management, and a host of other services. Through the Ryan White clinics efforts to address these barriers, the level of health equity for patients served by this program is raised. The program success can be attributed to

its intent to specifically address the racial and ethnic disparities impacting people of color, as well as other marginalized groups. The high degree of success of the Ryan White model of care, in which SDOH are actively addressed, can serve as a model of health care delivery to all patients.

PROVIDING CULTURALLY COMPETENT CARE

It is not uncommon for health care providers to harbor false beliefs about biological differences between Black and White persons. One study of medical students and residents found that half of those surveyed believed one or more false statements about biological differences between Black and White persons, including the belief that Black persons to not feel pain the same way that Whites persons do, or that Black skin is thicker than White skin (Hoffman, 2016). These prejudices alienate patients who rightfully perceive the racism and implicit bias that their care health care providers harbor.

Provider bias, and sometimes overt racism, can lead to longer waiting times for people of color as compared with White people, taking patient concerns less seriously, doing a less-thorough workup of problems, recommending different treatment options based on a perceived lack of patient adherence, along with many other differences in the treatment of some racial and/or ethnic groups than others. A systematic review of 15 peer-reviewed studies to identify implicit racial and ethnic bias among health care providers found that in 14 of those 15 studies, most health care providers demonstrated implicit bias through more favorable attitudes toward White persons and negative attitudes toward Black and Latinx persons (Hall, 2015). Four studies found that health care providers saw Black persons as less cooperative, less compliant, and less responsive to medical advice. Several studies found health care providers associating poor adherence and noncompliance to Latinx patients, and two studies found moderate amounts of bias against darker-skinned patients than lighter-skinned patients.

Even healthcare providers who sees themselves as providing equitable care may unknowingly be interacting with their patients of color differently and less effectively than with their White patients. Clearly, our system of medical education needs to address issues of race and ethnicity more actively in the training of physicians, nurses, and other healthcare workers. Unless we acknowledge and change our individual racist and ethnic biases, and work to implement health and social policies that eliminate racism and ethnic bias, we will continue to perpetuate the health disparities we see with HIV, COVID-19, and a multitude of other health conditions. What follows in this chapter are further examples of the diversity of patients with HIV, and how we can elevate our awareness and appreciation of those who entrust us with their healthcare.

RETENTION IN CARE

Retaining patients in care requires culturally competent staff at all levels of an organization. It could be easy for the busy

HIV specialist to focus more intensely on the complex medical aspects of HIV medicine and relegate the issues of diversity and cultural competence to "soft areas" that are of lesser importance than learning resistance mutations or developing expertise in the use of the latest antiviral drugs. However, to do so runs the risk of failing to adequately comprehend how patients' behaviors, beliefs, and the characteristics of their unique social, ethnic, racial, religious, gender identity, sexual orientation, or country of origin may affect their engagement with the healthcare system. Failing to understand the important cultural context within which a patient interacts with the healthcare system often leads to poor patient adherence with treatment, misunderstandings about the treatment plan, or worse, loss of retention in care. To successfully treat patients and to achieve the treatment goals, we need to do our best to understand the unique context of our diverse group of patients and to provide care that acknowledges the cultural values that may impact acceptance of treatment.

An analysis (Skarbinski, 2015) estimated that PWH who were out of care were responsible for 61% of new HIV infections in the United States. Further, a statewide study from North Carolina that analyzed patients with acute HIV infection found that most transmission events (77%) were attributable to partners with previously diagnosed infection, of whom only 23% were reportedly in care and taking antiviral medication within the time that transmission was likely to have occurred (Cope, 2015). This is compelling evidence that the system of HIV care in the United States is failing to treat and retain many PWH. There are likely many reasons for lack of success in patient retention, but it underscores the crucial need to improve the ways healthcare providers interact with patients in order to successfully keep them engaged in care and adherent with their antiviral medications. Developing competence in understanding the attributes of a diverse patient population is challenging, but failure to do so will allow greater numbers of PWH to lose contact with care. The greater challenge in becoming culturally competent is for all healthcare providers to develop awareness of their own values, beliefs, and attitudes, and what biases may be inherent in the providers' own culture.

DIVERSITY OF PATIENTS

Medical providers caring for PWHs are likely caring for a population of patients from racial or ethnic groups different from their own. In the United States, PWH are disproportionately Black and Latinx, and, regardless of race or ethnicity, are often affected by poverty, drug or alcohol abuse, mental health problems, lack of employment, lack of permanent housing, histories of incarceration, inadequate education, and sexual preferences different from those of the general population. Some patients may be immigrants or refugees whose language and cultural differences may cause barriers to acceptance of healthcare services from a system of care culturally different from their own. Understanding how patients' spiritual and religious values may impact their healthcare decision-making is important when caring for a diverse group of patients.

However, in our attempt to develop cultural understanding of their diversity, it is critical to avoid stereotyping patients, which also creates barriers to acceptance of treatment. The values, beliefs, and judgments of patients may differ from those of their healthcare provider, and unless the healthcare providers are able to withhold their own judgment of patients' circumstances, trusting relationships may never develop.

THE IMPORTANCE OF TRUST

Trust is a critically important component of a successful patient-clinician relationship. Without trust, a patient is less likely to adhere to a treatment plan. Patients who do not trust their healthcare provider or the healthcare system will be less likely to take prescribed medications, keep scheduled appointments, or accept the advice of their clinician.

Mistrust by certain racial and ethnic minorities in the United States is common. A telephone survey by the Kaiser Family Foundation (James, 1999) found that one-third of Black and one-third of Latinx persons reported experiencing unfair treatment by the healthcare system compared to less than half those numbers of White persons (James, 1999). Black persons were used without their informed consent in medical experimentation by the US Public Health Service from 1932 to 1972 in the notorious Tuskegee syphilis study, which created a legacy of mistrust (Skarbinski, 2015). Mistrust has led to conspiracy theories about the origins of HIV. In 2005, a national telephone survey of 500 Black persons (Bogart, 2005) found that 53% agreed that "there is a cure for AIDS, but it is being withheld from the poor"; 27% agreed that "AIDS was produced in a government laboratory"; and 16% agreed that "AIDS was created by the government to control the Black population."

DISPARITIES IN HEALTHCARE

The HIV epidemic in the United States is characterized by significant racial and ethnic disparities. In 2020, the distribution of new diagnoses of HIV by race/ethnicity was 25% for White; 29% for Latinx/Latino; 42.% for Black; 2% for Asian; 1% for Native Americans/Alaskan Natives; 2% for those of multiple races; and less than 1% for Native Hawaiian/Other Pacific Islander persons (CDC, 2022a). For many patients, the route of HIV transmission carries significant stigma. Among Black men, of whom 80% contracted the disease by male-to-male sexual contact, being gay or bisexual carries a stigma that is prevalent both in the general population and within the Black community. Stigma creates barriers that keep many men from being tested for HIV or connecting to care once identified as being PWH. Understanding the effects of stigma and developing nonjudgmental ways to communicate effectively with patients require that we first acknowledge that patients may enter their relationship with a healthcare provider assuming the healthcare provider harbors the same biases as the general population. Becoming culturally competent requires clinicians to develop strategies with each patient to allay the patient's fear of disapproval by his or her or their healthcare provider as well as to provide reassurance that the patient's personal health information will be protected and kept confidential.

With significant racial and ethnic disparities concerning who is living with HIV, the need to provide culturally appropriate care is evident. Failing to adequately understand a patient's culture—best defined as the unique set of beliefs, characteristics, and behaviors formed by the communities in which a patient resides—can create a barrier between patient and healthcare provider. A lack of trust by the patient may prevent successful treatment. Mistrust of healthcare providers occurs particularly if patients believe they will receive unequal treatment. Many studies across all disease states have documented the unequal treatment provided to Black and Latinx persons. According to the Institute of Medicine (Smedley, 2003), racial and ethnic minorities often receive a lower quality of healthcare services even when insurance status and income are the same as those for nonminorities. Black and Latinx patients have higher risk of acute myocardial infarction, rehospitalization, and death from acute coronary syndrome, yet are less likely than White patients to receive angiography or other coronary interventions (Graham, 2015).

Healthcare clinicians need to understand what objections a patient may have to the recommended treatment in an effort to help the patient understand potential consequences that may occur without treatment. Clinicians need to take the time to ask patients open-ended questions. Asking questions such as What are your concerns about taking this medication? allows the patient to express his or her concerns and gives the healthcare provider the opportunity to address them.

BIAS IN HEALTHCARE

Cultural competence requires taking time to learn what cultural barriers might exist. Ethnocentric healthcare providers only view a patient's culture from the perspective of their own culture and risks losing patient trust. Healthcare providers are not immune to the biases that exist in the general population. Weisse (2001) found that White males were twice as likely as Black males to be prescribed analgesics for pain, whereas female physicians prescribed higher doses for Black than for White patients. A study examining how patient race affects physician perceptions found that physicians rated Black patients as less intelligent, less educated, more likely to abuse drugs and alcohol, and less likely to adhere to treatment even when considering the patient's income and education (van Ryn, 2000). A systematic review of 15 studies that looked at racial and ethnic biases found that in all but one study, racial and ethnic bias by health care providers existed (Hall, 2015). These studies show how racism and personal bias can lead to unequal care.

Bias can be either overt (explicit) or covert (implicit). Derogatory comments made by either providers or office staff about particular "types" of patients are an example of bias. Judgmental comments about how frequently certain patients develop sexually transmitted infections, use the emergency room, look for pain medications, and have too many uncared-for children are examples of overt bias and stereotyping. Such comments, in addition to being highly unprofessional and judgmental, may reinforce among medical staff involved in patient care that bias and judgment are an acceptable form of professional conduct. Negative comments about a patient, especially if overheard by other patients, can transmit to patients that they may be the topic of unwanted conversation. Healthcare organizations need to make certain that staff at all levels and functions within the institution become culturally competent. Recognizing the cultural differences that might exist between a patient and a healthcare provider is an essential step to welcoming each patient with acceptance and understanding. Only by attempting to recognize and to understand these differences can a healthcare provider comprehend what may be needed to best inspire patient trust in the provider, the institution, and the plan of treatment.

WOMEN AND HIV

There are 18 million women worldwide living with HIV, and in the United States, 19% of people with HIV are women (UN AIDS, 2015). Most women diagnosed with HIV (75%) acquire the virus through heterosexual sex (CDC, 2022c). Black women are disproportionately HIV-positive, with 58% of US women living with HIV being Black (CDC, 2022c). Women living with HIV experience intimate partner violence at twice the national average (Gruskin, 2014). The meta-analysis by Gruskin and colleagues (2014) showed that 55% of women with HIV in the United States have experienced trauma and violence. Women and transgender women living with HIV who have experienced trauma and violence had a fourfold higher likelihood of nonadherence to ART (Machinger, 2012). The HIV provider should inquire about a history of violence and abuse and should refer the patient to appropriate crisis and domestic violence services as needed. Healthcare providers should understand that many women who are victims of domestic abuse feel powerless and trapped because of economic dependency, primary responsibility for children, and fear of homelessness. Many women may be slow or unwilling to seek help. A careful mental health and depression screening should be done, and referral to appropriate mental health services should be made when indicated.

SEXUAL AND GENDER MINORITY PATIENTS

Many lesbian, gay, bisexual, transgender and queer (LGBTQ+) patients do not feel welcome by their healthcare providers. Many LGBTQ+ people do not seek medical care because they have had bad experiences with healthcare providers (National LGBT Health Education Center, 2015). One recent study of Black MSM found that 29% experienced racial and sexual stigma from their healthcare providers, and 48% reported mistrust of the healthcare system (Eaton, 2015). If patients feel uncomfortable speaking about their sexual orientation, they are far more likely to withhold important information. Ways to help LGBTQ+ patients feel more welcome include using gender-neutral pronouns, allowing LGBTQ+ patients to be called by their preferred name (even if their legal name may be different), and training staff to have a nonjudgmental attitude. Learning and using the language that patients use may make patients feel more comfortable. For example, patients may use the terms "top" or "bottom" to describe insertive anal sex or receptive anal sex. Asking patients about the gender(s) of their partner(s) is an appropriate way to learn patients' sexual orientation. Avoidance of words that imply a patient has a relationship with someone of the opposite sex is also important. "Do you have a partner?" or "Are you in a relationship?" are more appropriate questions than "Do you have a husband or wife?" A patient who feels accepted by his or her care provider is more likely to return for care. Conversely, a patient who perceives disapproval of his or her lifestyle, sexual orientation, or practices will feel uncomfortable and is much less likely to return.

BEHAVIORAL HEALTH PROBLEMS

The HIV Costs and Services Utilization Study found that nearly 50% of adults treated for HIV have symptoms of a psychiatric disorder—a four-to-eight-times higher prevalence than the general population (Bing, 2001). In the general population, there is a 10- to 20-year reduction in life expectancy in people with severe mental health disorders (Chang, 2011). Mental illness caries a risk of mortality greater than that of smoking (Chesney, 2014).

Identifying patients with mental illness or addiction is crucial in caring for PWH. Carefully acquiring a history, followed by referral to mental health services as needed, is important because patients with mental illness have been reported to have lower levels of adherence (Paterson, 2000). Stigma about mental health diagnoses may keep many patients from accessing mental health services. Onsite behavioral health services increase the likelihood that patients will connect to treatment. Many patients with substance abuse problems may experience a sense of rejection when they reveal that they have chemical dependency or are participating in a substance abuse treatment program. They may assume that mentioning pain will be perceived as drug-seeking by their healthcare provider—a common stereotype of healthcare providers. Cultural competence requires communicating with patients openly and without judgment. It requires efforts to develop trust and to help reduce the stigma that most drug users have about their chemical dependency.

LANGUAGE AND COMMUNICATION

Language comprehension and communication are essential to patient understanding and, ultimately, to good adherence. Many PWH speak languages other than English. Language barriers can interfere with the success of treatment. Exit interviews of emergency room patients found that Spanish-speaking patients were less likely to understand their discharge instructions or carry out follow-up plans (Crane, 1997). Another survey found that one in five Spanish-speaking patients delayed or refused medical treatment because of language barriers, underscoring the need to provide linguistically appropriate services to HIV patients who will need lifelong care (USDHHS, 2020).

Hiring bilingual and bicultural staff is important in a culturally competent organization when there are significant numbers of patients in the local population who speak a particular language. The culturally competent clinical practice needs to make use of professional interpreter services for patients who do not speak the language of the healthcare provider. The use of family members or friends may inhibit patient honesty when asked to discuss personal information. Telephone interpreter services, although costly, are a necessary tool when onsite interpretation is unavailable. This is especially important for immigrant populations, for whom linguistic barriers, often combined with significant cultural differences, may greatly impede the delivery of healthcare. Patients who used the interpreter services received significantly more recommended preventive services, made more office visits, and had more prescriptions written and filled (Jacobs, 2004).

RELIGION AND SPIRITUALITY

A 2014 Gallup survey found that 81% of Americans identify with a particular religion (Newport, 2014). Patients turn to religion in times of illness, and this often influences the way a person perceives and copes with his or her situation. Many PWH have strong religious affiliations (Cotton, 2006). A patient's faith may sometimes conflict with medical advice, which can lead to a lack of adherence to treatment. It is important to ask patients about their spiritual beliefs and how those beliefs may affect their perception of illness and acceptance of treatment.

CREATING A CULTURALLY COMPETENT PATIENT-CENTERED HIV PRACTICE

Racial and ethnic diversity in healthcare leadership and staff is a priority in building culturally competent healthcare organizations. Including community members and consumer representatives on governing boards, as is done at FQHCs, can help hold an organization accountable for providing culturally competent care to a diverse patient population. Providing materials that are linguistically appropriate to the population being served at a literacy level appropriate to the level of most patients is important.

Changing the model of care from the traditional physician-centered practice to a model that places the patient in the center of the relationship—the patient-centered medical home (PCMH) model—can improve the quality of care. This model relies on reorganizing care to ensure that it is comprehensive, with integrated physical and mental health services. Care that is patient-centered supports patients' efforts to manage their own care to whatever degree they may choose. It is coordinated so that there is a smoother transition across levels of care, such as primary care, hospital care, and specialty care. Services are accessible, with after-hours access to a healthcare provider, along with flexible office hours. Last, there is a focus on quality and safety, using evidence-based standards and data for performance improvement (Agency for Healthcare Research and Quality, 2015). Culturally and linguistically appropriate services are offered. In one study, retention in care for PWH was improved with the PCMH model (Sitapati, 2012).

Patients want healthcare providers who communicate with them and who are empathic. Better healthcare outcomes have been associated with providers with whom patients can share their feelings and thoughts. Patients of empathic and communicative healthcare providers are far more likely to comply with their treatment plans (Sitapati, 2012).

The patient-centered approach incorporates cultural competency interventions to better address the racial, ethnic, and cultural differences between provider and patient, and it offers training to providers and to all staff who interact with patients in order to make them more culturally competent (Kim, 2004). Healthcare provider training to improve providers' knowledge and attitudes about diverse populations is essential to creating a culturally competent system of care.

Perhaps most important, aspiring culturally competent healthcare providers must raise their individual self-awareness of their own cultural beliefs, values, and attitudes and any biases that may be inherent in them. Consciousness of one's own cultural biases and an honest attempt to transcend them will allow the HIV provider to communicate effectively, with empathy, and without prejudgment, facilitating an improved and mutually satisfying relationship with each patient.

REFERENCES

Agency for Healthcare Research and Quality. Defining the PCMH. https://www.pcmh.ahrq.gov/page/defining-pcmh. Published 2015. Accessed October 1, 2022.

Agency for Healthcare Research and Quality. Improving cultural competence to reduce health disparities for priority populations. http://content.healthaffairs.org/content/24/2/354.full?firstpage=354. Published 2005. Accessed December 1, 2015.

AIDS 2020. Abstract book. https://www.aids2020.org/wp-content/uploads/2020/09/AIDS2020_Abstracts.pdf. Published 2020. Accessed September 24, 2020.

Antiretroviral Pregnancy Registry. www.apregistry.com. Published 2022. Accessed August 15, 2022.

Badger, E, Parlapiano A, Bui Q. Black workers will hurt the most if congress doesn't extend jobless benefits. New York Times, August 7, 2020. https://www.nytimes.com/2020/08/07/upshot/unemployment-benefits-racial-disparity.html

Baillargeon J, Giordano T, Rich J, et al. Accessing antiretroviral therapy following release from prison. JAMA. 2009;301(8):848–857.

Bass M. Language barriers and illiteracy can affect patient healthcare. Robert Wood Johnson Foundation. http://www.rwjf.org/en/library/research/2000/12/language-barriers-and-illiteracy-can-affect-patient-health-care.html. Published 2000. Accessed December 1, 2015.

Beckwith C, Zaller N, Fu J, et al. Opportunities to diagnose, treat, and prevent HIV in the criminal justice system. J AIDS. 2010;55(Suppl 1):S49–S55.

Bernard K, Sueker J, et al. Provider perspectives about the standard of HIV care in correctional settings and comparison to the community standard of care: how do we measure up? Infect Dis Corrections Rep. March 2006;9(3):1–2, 4–6.

Bhatnagar V, Gormley N, Kazandjian D, et al. FDA analysis of racial demographics in multiple myeloma trials. Blood. 2017;130(Suppl 1):4352–4352. http://doi:10.1182/blood.V130.Suppl_1.4352.4352

Bing EG, Burnam A, Longshore D, et al. Psychiatric disorders and drug use among HIV-infected adults in the US. Arch Gen Psychiatry. 2001;58:721–728.

Bogart LM, Thorburn S. Are HIV/AIDS conspiracy beliefs a barrier to HIV prevention among African Americans? J AIDS. 2005;38(2):213–218.

Boone MR, Cherenack EM, Wilson PA, et al. Self-efficacy for sexual risk reduction and partner HIV status as correlates of sexual beliefs about biological differences between blacks and whites. PNAS. https://doi.org/10.1073/pas. Published April 2016. Accessed August 15, 2022.

Braithwaite R, Hammett T, Mayberry R. Prisons and AIDS: a public health challenge. San Francisco, CA: Jossey-Bass; 1996.

Braverman, P, Arkin Ek, Proctor D, et al. Systemic and structural racism: definitions, examples, health damages, and approaches to dismantling. Health Affairs. 2022;41(2):171–178 2022

Centers for Disease Control and Prevention (CDC). Health equity considerations & racial & ethnic minority groups. cdc.gov. https://www.cdc.gov/coronavirus/2019-ncov/community/health-equity/vaccine-equity.html. Published March 29, 2022a. Accessed August 30, 2022.

CDC. HIV and African American people, 2020. cdc.gov. https://www.cdc.gov/hiv/group/racialethnic/africanamericans/index.html). Published June 28, 2022b. Accessed July 26, 2020.

CDC. HIV by age: viral suppression. cdc.gov. https://www.cdc.gov/hiv/group/age/viral-suppression.html. Published July 1, 2022d. Accessed July 22, 2022.

CDC. HIV in the United States by race/ethnicity: HIV diagnoses. cdc.gov. https://www.cdc.gov/hiv/group/racialethnic/other-races/diagnoses.html. Published July 1, 2022c. Accessed August 4, 2022.

CDC. Reproductive health. Infant mortality. https://www.cdc.gov/reproductivehealth/maternalinfanthealth/infantmortality.htm#:~:text=Infant%20Mortality%20Rates%20by%20Race%20and%20Ethnicity%2C%202016,-*Source%3A%20p.&text=Native%20Hawaiian%20or%20other%20Pacific,Asian%3Abhos203.6. Published June 22, 2022b. Accessed August 30, 2022.

CDC. Risk for COVID-19 infection, hospitalization, and death by race/ethnicity. cdc.gov. https://www.cdc.gov/coronavirus/2019-ncov/covid-data/investigations-discovery/hospitalization-death-by-race-ethnicity.html. Published July 28, 2022f. Accessed August 2022.

CDC. The US Public Health Service Syphilis Study at Tuskegee: timeline. cdc.gov. http://cdc.gov/Tuskegee/timeline.htm. Published April 21, 2021. Accessed July 24, 2022.

Chang CK, Hayes RD, Perera G, et al. Life expectancy at birth for people with serious mental illness and other major disorders from a secondary mental healthcare case register in London. PLoS One. 2011;10:1371.

Chen C, Wong R. Black patients miss out on promising cancer drugs. propublica.org. ww.propublica.org/article/blackw-patients-miss-out-on-promising-cancer-drugs. Published September 19, 2018. Accessed October 1, 2022.

Cheever L. HRSA announces increase in HIV viral suppression rate in new 2020 Ryan White HIV/AIDS program client-level data report. https://www.hiv.gov/blog/hrsa-announces-increase-hiv-viral-suppression-rate-new-2020-ryan-white-hivaids-program-client. Published 2021. Accessed July 22, 2022.

Chesney E, Goodwin GM, Fazel S. Risks all-cause and suicide mortality in mental disorders: a meta-review. World Psychiatry. June 2014;13(2):153–160.

Cope AB, Power KA, Kuruc JD, et al. Ongoing HIV transmission and the HIV care continuum in North Carolina. PLoS One. 2015;10(6):e0127950.

Cotton S. Spirituality and religion in patients with HIV/AIDS. Gen Intern Med. 2006;12;21(Suppl 5):S5–S13.

Crane JA. Patient comprehension of doctor–patient communication on discharge from the emergency department. Emerg Med. January–February 1997;15(1):1–7.

Crepaz N, Dong X, Wang X, et al. Racial and ethnic disparities in sustained viral suppression and transmission risk potential among persons receiving HIV care—United States, 2014. *Mor Mortal Wkly Rep.* February 2, 2018;67(4):113–118.

Duma N, Vera Aguilera J, Paludo J, et al. Representation of minorities and women in oncology clinical trials: review of the past 14 years. *JCO.* 2018;14(1):e1–e10. http://doi:10.1200/JOP.2017.025288

Eaton LA, Driffin DD, Kegler C, et al. The role of stigma and medical mistrust in the routine healthcare engagement of black men who have sex with men. *Am J Public Health.* 2015;105(2):75–82.

US Food & Drug Administration (FDA). 2015–2019 drug trials snapshots summary report: five-year summary and analysis of clinical trial participation and demographics. fda.gov. www.fda.gov/media/143 592/download. February 2020. Accessed July 2022.

FDA. Diversity plans to improve enrollment of participants from underrepresented racial and ethnic populations in clinical trials guidance for industry. fda.gov. www.fda.gov/media/157635/download. Published April 2022. Accessed August 20, 2022.FDA. Drug trials snapshots summary report 2020. fda.gov. www.fda.gov/media/145 718/download. February 2021. Accessed August 15, 2022.

FDA. US Food & Drug Administration Food and Drug Safety and Innovation ACT (FDASIA). www.fda.gov/regulatory-information/selected-amendments-fdc-act/food-and-drug-administration-safety-and-innovation-act-fdasia. Published 2018. Accessed March 9, 2023.

FDA Center for Drug Evaluation and Research. Drug trials snapshots. *Summary Report 2021.* Retrieved from https://www.fda.gov/drugs/drug-approvals-and-databases/drug-trials-snapshots. Published April 2022. Accessed July 2022.

Gilead.com. Gilead announces new arm of HIV women's prevention study. https://www.gilead.com/news-and-press/company-statements/gilead-announces-new-arm-of-hiv-womens-prevention-study. Published 2021. Accessed July 20, 2022.

Gordon MR, Smale A, Lyman R. US will accept more refugees as crisis grows. *New York Times,* September 20, 2015.

Graham G, Disparities in cardiovascular disease risk in the United States. *Curr Cardiol Rev.* 2015;11(3):238–245.

Gruskin S, Safreed-Harmon K, Moore CL, et al. HIV and gender-based violence: welcome policies and programmes, but is the research keeping up? *Reprod Health Matters.* 2014;22(44):174–184.

Guerino P, Harrison P, Sabol W. Prisoners in 2010. US Department of Justice, Bureau of Justice Statistics. http://www.bjs.gov. Published 2011. Accessed August 15, 2023.

Guerrero S, López-Cortés A, Indacochea A, et al. Analysis of racial/ethnic representation in select basic and applied cancer research studies. *Scientific Reports.* 2018;8(1);1–8. http://doi:10.1038/s41 598-018-32264-x

Hall WJ, Chapman MV, Lee KM, et al. Implicit racial/ethnic bias among health care professionals and its influence on health care outcomes: a systematic review. *Am J Public Health.* December 2015;105(12):e60–e76.

Hammet T, Kennedy S, Kuck S. National survey of infectious diseases in correctional facilities: HIV and sexually transmitted diseases. US Department of Justice. https://www.ncjrs.gov/pdffiles1/nij/gra nts/217736.pdf. Published 2007. Accessed October 1, 2022.

Health Resources and Services Administration. Ending the HIV epidemic: a plan for America. https://ahead.hiv.gov. Published February 2021. Accessed March 9, 2023..

HealthyPeople.gov. Healthy People 2030. The Secretary's Advisory Committee on National Health Promotion and Disease Prevention objectives for 2020. Phase I report: recommendations for the framework and format of Healthy People 2020. Section IV: Advisory Committee findings and recommendations. http://www.health ypeople.gov/sites/default/files/PhaseI_0.pdf. Published October 28, 2008. Accessed March 9, 2023.

Heyrana K, Byers HM, Stratton P. Increasing the participation of pregnant women in clinical trials. *Jama.* 2018;320(20):2077–2078. http://doi:10.1001/jama.2018.17716

Hirsch J, Higgins J, Bentley M, Nathanson V. The social constructions of sexuality: marital infidelity and sexually transmitted disease–HIV risk in a Mexican migrant community. *American Journal of Public Health.* August 2002;92(8):1227–1237.

Hirsch J, Meneses S, Thompson B, Negroni M, Pelcastre B, del Rio C. The inevitability of infidelity: sexual reputation, social geographies, and marital HIV risk in rural Mexico. *American Journal of Public Health.* June 2007;97(6):986–996.

International Organization for Migration. Key migration terms. https://www.iom.int/key-migration-terms. Published 2020. Accessed October 1, 2022.

Jacobs EA, Shepard D, Suaya JA, et al. Overcoming language barriers in healthcare: costs and benefits of interpreter services. *Am J Public Health.* 2004;94(5):866–869.

James C. Race ethnicity and medical care: a survey of public perceptions and experiences. Kaiser Family Foundation, September 1999.

Kahn JM, Gray DM, Oliveri JM, Washington CM, DeGraffinreid CR, Paskett ED. Strategies to improve diversity, equity, and inclusion in clinical trials. *Cancer.* 2022;128(2):216–221. http://doi:10.1002/cncr.33905

Kanny D, Jeffries 4th WL, Chapin-Bardales J, et al. Racial/ethnic disparities in HIV preexposure prophylaxis among men who have sex with men—3 urban areas, 2017. *Morb Mortal Wkly Rep.* September 20, 2019;68(37):801–806.

Kendi IX. *How to be antiracist.* New York: Penguin Random House; 2019.

Levy V, Prentiss D, Balmas G, et al. Factors in the delayed HIV presentation of immigrants in Northern California: implications for voluntary counseling and testing programs. *Journal of Immigrant and Minority Health.* 2007;9:49–54. https://doi.org/10.1007/s10 903-006-9015-9

Maruschak L. HIV in prisons, 2007–08. US Department of Justice, Bureau of Justice Statics. http://www.bjs.gov/content/pub/pdf/hiv p08.pdf. Published 2009. Accessed October 1, 2023.

Mayer KH, Agwu A, Malebranche D. Barriers to the wider use of pre-exposure prophylaxis in the United States: a narrative review. *Advances in Therapy.* 2020;37(5):1778–1811. http://doi:10.1007/s12 325-020-01295-0

Mayer KH, Molina J, Thompson MA, et al. Emtricitabine and tenofovir alafenamide vs emtricitabine and tenofovir disoproxil fumarate for HIV pre-exposure prophylaxis (DISCOVER): primary results from a randomized, double-blind, multicenter, active-controlled, phase 3, non-inferiority trial. *Lancet.* 2020;396(10246):239–254. http://doi:10.1016/S0140-6736(20)31065-5

Michos ED, Reddy TK, Gulati M, et al. Improving the enrollment of women and racially/ethnically diverse populations in cardiovascular clinical trials: an ASPC practice statement. *American Journal of Preventive Cardiology.* 2021;8:100250. https://doi.org/10.1016/j.ajpc.2021.100250

Millet G. Casualties on the road to ending HIV: context matters in addressing HIV disparities. Prime session 1. 40 Year HIV pandemic, July 7, 2020. AIDS2020.org. Virtual IAS Conference; July 4–10, 2020.

Millett G, Jones AT, Benkeser D, et al. Assessing differential impacts of COVID-19 on black communities. *Ann Epidemiol.* 2020. PMID: 32419766.

Muthukumar AV, Morrell W, Bierer BE. Evaluating the frequency of English language requirements in clinical trial eligibility criteria: a systematic analysis using ClinicalTrials.gov. *PLOS Medicine.* 2021;18(9):e1003758. http://doi:10.1371/journal.pmed.1003758

National Institutes of Health. National Health Center Program Uniform Data System, Awardee. https://data.hrsa.gov/tools/data-reporting/program-daata/national. Published 2020. Accessed October 1, 2022.

National LGBT Health Education Center. Providing welcoming services and care for LGBT people. http://www.lgbthealtheducation.org/wp-content/uploads/Learning-Guide.pdf. Published 2015. Accessed December 1, 2015.

Nellis A. The color of justice: racial and ethnic disparity in state prisons. The Sentencing Project. https://sentencingproject.org/staff/ashley-nellis/. Published June 14, 2016. Accessed July 26, 2020.

Newport F. Three-quarters of Americans identify as Christian. Gallup.com. http://www.gallup.com/poll/180347/three-quarters-americ

ans-identify-christian.aspx. Published December 2014. Accessed December 1, 2015.

Nichols A, Simms M. Racial and ethnic differences in receipt of unemployment insurance benefits during the great recession, Urban Institute. https://www.urban.org/sites/default/files/publication/25541/412596-Racial-and-Ethnic-Differences-in-Receipt-of-Unemployment-Insurance-Benefits-During-the-Great-Recession.PDF. Published June 2012. Accessed July 26, 2020.

Nosyk B, Zang X, Krebs E, et al. Ending the HIV epidemic in the USA: an economic modeling study in six cities. *Lancet HIV*. July 2020;7(7):e491–e503.

O'Laughlin B. Pragmatism, structural reform and the politics of inequality in global public health. *Development and Change*. 2016;47(4):686–711. http://doi10.1111/dech.12251

Paterson DL, Swindells S. Adherence to protease inhibitor therapy and outcomes in patients with HIV infection. *Ann Intern Med*. 2000;133:21–30.

Peterson K, Anderson J, Boundy E, et al. Mortality disparities in racial/ethnic minority groups in the Veterans Health Administration: an evidence review and map. *Am J P Public Health*. 2018;108(3):e1–e10.

Pew Research Center. Radford J. https://www.pewresearch.org/fact-tank/2019/06/17/key-findings-about-u-s-immigrants/. Published 2019. Accessed October 1, 2022.

Prosser AT, Tang T, Hall HI. HIV in persons born outside the United States 2007–2010. *JAMA*. August 8, 2012;308(6):601–607.

Raths D. New law requires Medicaid coverage of clinical trial participation. /policy-value-based-care/medicare-medicaid/news/21251951/new-law-requires-medicaid-coverage-of-clinical-trial-participation. Published 2022. Accessed October 1, 2022.

Ravindran TK. Making pharmaceutical research and regulation work for women. *BMJ*. 2020;371. https://doi.org/101136/bjm.m3808

Riner AN, Girma S, Vudatha V, et al. Eligibility criteria perpetuate disparities in enrollment and participation of black patients in pancreatic cancer clinical trials. *Journal of Clinical Oncology*. 2022;40(20):2193–2202. http://doi:10.1200/JCO.21.02492

Roper W. Black Americans 2.5X more likely than whites to be killed by police. Stasta.com. https://www.statista.com/chart/21872/map-of-police-violence-against-black-americans/. Published June 2, 2020. Accessed July 26, 2020.

Ross J, Cunningham CO, Hanna DJ. HIV outcomes among migrants from low- and middle-income countries living in high-income countries: a review of recent evidence. *Curr Opin Infect Dis*. 2018 February;31(1):25–32. http://doi:10.1097/QCO.0000000000000415

Rothstein R. *The color of law: a forgotten history of how our government segregated America*. New York: Liveright; 2017.

Samaei M, McGregor AJ, Jenkins MR. Inclusion of women in FDA-regulated premarket clinical trials: a call for innovative and recommended action. *Contemporary Clinical Trials*. 2022;116:106708. http://doi:10.1016/j.cct.2022.106708

Sartor O, Armstrong AJ, Ahaghotu C, et al. Survival of African-American and Caucasian men after sipuleucel-T immunotherapy: outcomes from the PROCEED registry. *Prostate Cancer and Prostatic Diseases*. 2020;23(3):517–526. http://doi:10.1038/s41391-020-0213-7

Singer M. A dose of drugs, a touch of violence, a case of AIDS: a conceptualizing of the SAVA syndemic. *Creative Sociology*. 1996;24(2):99–110.

Sitapati AM, Limneos J, Bonet-Vázquez M, et al. Retention: building a patient-centered medical home in HIV primary care through PUFF (patients unable to follow-up found). *J Health Care Poor Underserved*. 2012;23(3 Suppl):81–95.

Skarbinski J, Rosenberg E, Paz-Bailey G, et al. Human immunodeficiency virus transmission at each step of the care continuum in the United States. *JAMA Intern Med*. 2015;175(4):596–597.

Spaulding A, Stephenson B, Macalino G, et al. Human immunodeficiency virus in correctional facilities. *Clin Infect Dis*. 2002;35:305–312.

Sullivan PS. Trends in PrEP inequity by race and census region, United States, 2012–2021. AIDS 2022, Abstract 12943. https://programme.aids2022.org/Abstract/Abstract/?abstractid=12943. Published 2022. Accessed October 1, 2022.

Torpy SJ. Native American women and coerced sterilization: on the trail of tears in the 1970s. *American Indian Culture and Research Journal*. 2007;24(2):1–22. http://doi:10.17953/aicr.24.2.7646013460646042

UNAIDS. How AIDS changed everything—MDG6: 15 years, 15 lessons of hope from the AIDS response. UNAIDS Secretariat, Geneva, Switzerland. https://issuu.com/unaids/docs/mdg6_executivesummary_en. Published July 2015. Accessed December 1, 2015.

US Congress. United States Congress National Institutes of Health Revitalization Act of 1993: Subtitle B-Clinical Research Equity Regarding Women and Minorities. Public Law 103-43.Congress.gov/bill/103rd-congress/senate-bill/1. Accessed July 24, 2022. Accessed October 1, 2022.

US Department of Health and Human Services (DHHS), Office of Minority Health. HHS action plan to reduce racial and ethnic health disparities. A nation free of disparities in health and health care. https://www.minorityhealth.hhs.gov/npa/files/Plans/HHS/HHS_Plan_complete.pdf. Published 2010. Accessed July 26, 2020.

van Ryn M, Burke J. The effect of patient race and socioeconomic status on physicians' perceptions of patients. *Social Sci Med*. 2000;50:813–828.

Weingbaum C, Sabin K, Santibanez S. Hepatitis B, hepatitis C, and HIV in correctional populations: a review of epidemiology and prevention. *AIDS*. 2005;19(Suppl 3):S41–S46.

Weisse CS, Sorum PC, Sanders KN, et al. Do gender and race affect decisions about pain management? *J Gen Intern Med*. 2001;16(4):211–217.

Woodcock J, Araojo R, Thompson T, Puckrein GA. Integrating research into community practice—toward increased diversity in clinical trials. *New England Journal of Medicine*. 2021;385(15):1351–1353. http://doi:10.1056/NEJMp2107331

WHO. Social determinants of health. https://www.who.int/social_determinants/en/. Published 2020. Accessed July 26, 2020.

Wortham JM, Lee JT, Althomsons S, et al. Characteristics of persons who died with COVID-19—United States, February 12–May 18, 2020. *Morb Mortal Wkly Rep*. July 17, 2020;69(28):923–929.

Yancy CV. COVID-19 and African Americans. *JAMA*. 2020;323(19):1891–1892. PMID:32293639.

12.

SPECIAL POPULATIONS

Catherine Silva, Renata Arrington-Sanders, Zil G. Goldstein, Madeline B. Deutsch,

Olabimpe Asupoto, Alysse G. Wurcel, Elizabeth Imbert, Matthew D. Hickey, Abby Davids,

Ashley Carvalho, Deliana Garcia, Claire M. Hutkins Seda, and Laszlo Madaras

12.1 ADOLESCENT HIV CARE

CATHERINE SILVA AND RENATA ARRINGTON-SANDERS

LEARNING OBJECTIVES

- Describe the developmental, cognitive, social, and environmental factors affecting treatment adherence and secondary prevention in adolescents.

- Identify special populations within adolescents who are at increased risk of acquiring HIV.

- Discuss HIV pre-exposure prophylaxis (PrEP) options with sexually active adolescents.

WHAT'S NEW?

- In the United States, young men who have sex with men (MSM) of color have higher rates of HIV infection compared to White MSM youth.

- Transgender adults and adolescents, especially transgender women of color, have had an increase in HIV infection.

- The COVID-19 pandemic led to a substantial decrease in HIV testing and surveillance activities.

- PrEP should be discussed with all sexually active adolescents.

- In addition to the oral preparation of antiretroviral therapy (ART) and PrEP, long-acting injectable options are approved for use in adolescents who are 12 years of age or older or weigh 35 kg or more.

KEY POINTS

- Adolescents are at risk for HIV through sexual behaviors; most adolescents acquire HIV through condomless sex.

- Adolescents in late puberty per (sexual maturing rating) SMR staging (Stage 4–5) can be managed according

to adult/adolescent guidelines; prepubescent and early pubescent adolescents (per SMR staging Stage 1–3) can be managed according to pediatric guidelines.

- Psychosocial factors that could affect adherence should be addressed before initiating treatment.

- Sexual risk behaviors in adolescents living with HIV should be given special attention.

The period of adolescence (defined as ages 12–24 years) is a critical time of physical, social, emotional, and cognitive growth and development (Sanders, 2013). In the US, the average age at first sexual intercourse for males and females is 17 years (Abma et al., 2017). The American Academy of Pediatrics, and other professional medical organizations, recommend eliciting a thorough sexual history from adolescents to provide appropriate anticipatory guidance, screening, and treatment of sexually transmitted infections including HIV. However, there are multifactorial challenges that adolescents face when accessing appropriate medical care and other services, resulting in a heightened risk for HIV acquisition. Among adolescents, there are significant disparities in HIV infection rates among gender and sexual minority youth, individuals who identify as gay, lesbian, bisexual, or transgender; racial and ethnic minority youth; youth with unstable housing; youth who use injection drugs; individuals who have a mental illness; those who have been sexually or physically abused; and those who are incarcerated or in foster care.

Health disparities occur as a result of an individual's interaction with socioenvironmental factors at the interpersonal (e.g., family and social/sexual networks), intermediate structural (e.g., community, social institutions, culture, social norms, and values), and macrostructural (e.g., socioeconomic conditions) levels that contribute to high rates of HIV. For example, despite the overall drop in new HIV infections, young Black and Hispanic/Latino MSM continue to be disproportionately impacted by HIV in the United States (CDC, 2020a; CDC, 2020b) and account for most new HIV transmissions in their age group (CDC, 2020b). Worldwide, adolescent females disproportionately account for new HIV transmissions (UNAIDS, 2022). Such high rates do not result from increased individual behavior but rather from the complex interrelationship of multiple social identities—such as race, ethnicity, gender, socioeconomic status, and sexual orientation—that intersect at the individual's experience, existence within high HIV prevalent sexual networks, and larger social-structural inequities experienced on the macro level (Raj & Bowleg, 2012). In the United States, approximately 1 million adults and 300,000 youth aged 13 to 17 years identify as transgender (i.e., a person who has a gender identity that differs from the sex they were assigned at birth) (Herman et al., 2022). In 2019, 2% of new HIV diagnoses in the United States were among transgender people, with most occurring among African Americans (CDC, 2020b). One meta-analysis estimates that 14% of transgender women in the United States are living with HIV (Becasen et al., 2019). More than one-third (36.3%) of these women were adolescents and young adults less than 24 years old (Becasen et al., 2019). This represents a 34-fold increased odds of HIV infection compared to that of all reproductive-age adults (Baral et al., 2013) (see Figures 12.1 and 12.2).

Transwomen of color are particularly affected. Some have suggested that rates of HIV among Black transgender women are as high as 44% (Becasen et al., 2019). The CDC's National HIV Behavioral Surveillance system, which collects biobehavioral surveillance data every 3 years among individuals at high risk for HIV infection, found that 62% of Black transgender women and 35% of Hispanic transgender women interviewed are living with HIV (CDC, 2020b). Higher rates of HIV are attributed to experiences of stigma, discrimination, negative healthcare encounters, lack of familial support,

limited healthcare and housing access, and high mental health diagnoses (Eaton et al., 2015). These factors contribute to increased drug and alcohol use, sex work, incarceration, homelessness, and attempted suicide.

Adolescents with HIV (AWH) from perinatal transmission are another group of adolescents and young adults living with HIV. Given there is near universal maternal screening and treatment in most high-income countries, this population is small. The same cannot be said for low-resource countries, in which perinatal transmission continues to be an ongoing concern. AWH from perinatal transmission share many common issues with AWH acquired behaviorally—namely, stigma, sexuality, disclosure, unplanned pregnancy, nonadherence, and substance misuse. However, this population generally is on more complicated ART regimens based on the development of resistance mutations during childhood.

The same socioecologic factors (e.g., discrimination, isolation, microaggressions, and minority stress) that contribute to HIV risk predispose youth to comorbidities (e.g., high rates of mental health and substance use disorders) and medical nonadherence in their HIV treatment and management. Differences in the treatment cascade of care by age have been hypothesized as an explanation for the increase in HIV infections by at-risk youth nationally (Zanoni & Mayer, 2014). Less than half (40%) of those aged 13–29 years are aware of their HIV status, and best estimates suggest that only 62% of those are connected to care within their first year of diagnosis (Zanoni & Mayer, 2014). Other studies have suggested that adolescents have much lower linkage rates, ranging from 29% to 73% successfully linked within the first year of diagnosis (Craw et al., 2008). The CDC and the US Preventive

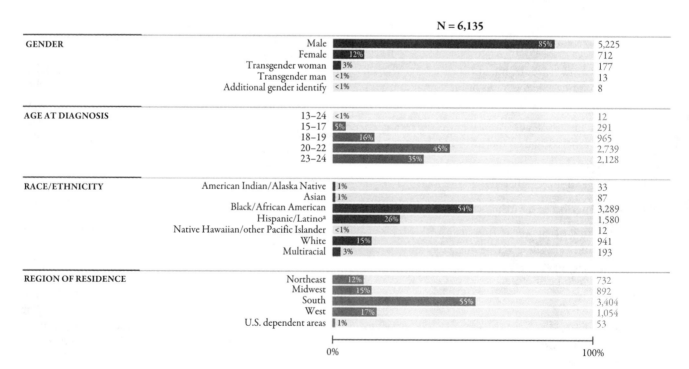

Figure 12.1 Percentage of diagnoses of HIV infection among persons aged 13–24 years, by selected characteristics, 2020—United States and six dependent areas   SOURCE: https://www.cdc.gov/hiv/pdf/library/reports/surveillance/cdc-hiv-surveillance-report-2020-updated-vol-33.pdf. Published 2022. Accessed August 15, 2022.

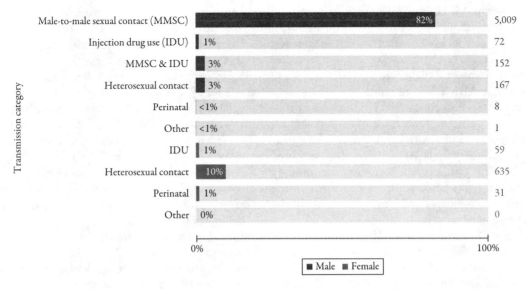

Figure 12.2 Percentage of diagnoses of HIV infection among persons aged 13–24 years, by sex assigned at birth and transmission category, 2020—United States and six dependent areas   SOURCE: https://www.cdc.gov/hiv/pdf/library/reports/surveillance/cdc-hiv-surveillance-report-2020-updated-vol-33.pdf. Published 2022. Accessed August 15, 2022.

Services Task Force recommend routine HIV screening for all youth (Branson et al., 2006; Moyer, 2013). People at risk of HIV acquisition should be screened at least annually. Health care providers should increase frequency of screening every 3–6 months based on sexual risk behavior (e.g., unprotected sex) and other groups (e.g., cisgender young men who report sex with other men, transgender or gender diverse adolescents, who may be at increased risk of HIV infection) (Workowski et al., 2021). Venue-based and social networking testing is another effective strategy to reach high-risk youth and increase the identification and linkage of youth into care (Barnes et al., 2010; Boyer et al., 2013; Straub & Tanner, 2018). Once diagnosed with HIV, special efforts to improve engagement in care are often necessary to maximize youth accessing care.

DEVELOPMENTAL ISSUES

Adolescents face the same barriers to treatment adherence as adults, but they have additional challenges owing to their developmental stage and legal circumstances. Social stigma, fear of alienation from peer groups, medication side effects, lack of transportation, dependence on parents or other caregivers, growing autonomy, and "feeling fine" are major contributors to nonadherence (Ingerski et al., 2021).

MEDICAL MANAGEMENT

The newest guidelines recommend ART for all individuals with HIV, regardless of CD4 + T lymphocyte cell count and age (Department of Health and Human Services (DHHS), 2022). Therapy should be initiated as soon as possible, and treatment deferral should be determined on a case-by-case basis. Recent guidelines for adolescents and young adults include data on the efficacy and feasibility of immediate ART and recommendations for certain populations. Earlier initiation of ART has been associated with reduced morbidity and mortality associated with HIV. Data extrapolated from the START and TEMPRANO trials favor initiating ART in all individuals who are able and willing to commit to treatment, understand the benefits and risks of therapy, and understand the importance of adherence (DHHS, 2022). The course of disease in youth is similar to that in adults, and they generally should be treated according to the same guidelines (DHHS, 2022).

Rapid ART initiation has the potential to improve overall health outcomes and reduce time during which people with newly diagnosed HIV can transmit HIV. Two randomized controlled trials in South Africa and in Haiti have demonstrated that rapid ART initiation resulted in higher sustained viral suppression and retention in care (Koenig et al., 2017; Labhardt et al., 2018; Rosen et al., 2016). There have been no randomized trials in the United States; however, data from a city-wide implementation of the San Francisco RAPID program in the United States suggests that both immediate initiation of ART (on the day of diagnosis) or rapid ART initiation (within days or weeks of diagnosis) were associated with 92% virological suppression at 1 year (Coffey et al., 2019). This study also highlights the intense support required for ART initiation on the same day of HIV diagnosis, clinical evaluation, counseling, laboratory testing, and assessment of insurance coverage (Coffey et al., 2019). Adolescents may also present with high viral loads and multiclass resistance at time of diagnosis (Koay et al., 2021). Review of guidelines to determine best class based on viral load level is critical.

Concerns have been raised about some of the regimens in certain populations of AWH. Initial data from the Tsepamo study raised concerns about dolutegravir (DTG)-based regimens predisposing newborns of women on this medication to neural tube defects (NTDs). However, data presented at AIDS 2020 by Dr. Rebecca Zash, where she reviewed 39,200 births surveyed from March 2019 to April 2020, found that newborns of mothers who were on DTG at the time of conception were not significantly more likely to have NTDs compared with newborns of mothers taking non-dolutegravir ARTs (Davey et al., 2020). In the ADVANCE trial, presented at AIDS 2020, weight gain was more common among study participants on the DTG-based regimens compared to the EFV-based regimen. Providers should be aware of side effects that can occur with regimens (Zash, 2021).

Prevention is a key component of HIV treatment. Most adolescents acquire HIV through sexual transmission and are unaware of their diagnosis, making them excellent candidates for prevention counseling, linkage to and engagement in care, and initiation of ART (DHHS, 2022). All adolescents with HIV should be informed that maintaining a plasma HIV RNA (viral load) of < 200 copies/mL prevents sexual transmission to their partners (Undetectable = Untransmittable). This has been established in a randomized clinical trial and several large observational cohort studies (Cohen et al., 2016). Promoting HIV treatment as a prevention can also promote disclosure of one's HIV status by normalizing HIV and removing some of the stigma, fear, and rejection associated with disclosing to partners and publicly (Bavinton et al., 2018; Rodger et al., 2016, 2019).

SEXUAL RISK

High rates of HIV in adolescents are multifactorial. Data suggest that many adolescents do not experience greater numbers of sexual partners. Instead, sexual risk results from multiple psychosocial factors that predispose youth to HIV. Sexual networks, with a partner who is living with HIV, is more common among adolescents living in higher density, lower income areas, that are characterized by violence and limited access to care. AWH exist in communities with high rates of unintended pregnancy (Nachman et al., 2009), STIs (Trent et al., 2007), and condomless sex (Clum et al., 2009; Weiner et al., 2007). This, combined with low rates of screening for STIs in HIV clinics that lag rates of non-HIV clinics, can promote high rates of STI and transmission of HIV (Berry et al., 2015). Additionally, condom negotiation is often not always a simple task for some AWH. In one sample, females with HIV had lower self-efficacy overall (B = −0.15, P = 0.01), to discuss safe sex with one's partner (B = −0.14, P = 0.01), and to refuse sex without a condom (B = −0.21, P = 0.01), and self-efficacy was related to condomless vaginal and anal intercourse episodes (Boone et al., 2015). In young men, some have suggested that age-discordant partnerships, limited condom negotiation, alcohol and other substances, may be a key contributor to condomless sex with HIV-negative or unknown status partners (Arrington-Sanders et al., 2013; Bruce et al., 2012; Mustanski & Newcomb, 2013). Other studies suggest a complicated relationship with psychological stress, substance use, and mental health that contributes to condomless sex (Arrington-Sanders et al., 2022). Young transgender women and sexual minority men may also exist within social contexts that predispose them to exchange sex (sex for money or a place to stay), substance use, and violence, that may put them at risk for HIV. There is a need to regularly address the risk for pregnancy, acquiring STIs, and the secondary transmission of HIV to sexual partners. The CDC recommends screening for STIs in women younger than age 25 years because of the high rates of STIs in this age range. In young MSM, screening for STIs is recommended from extragenital body sites because oropharyngeal, rectal, and urethral infections are commonly present in this population (Workowski et al., 2021). The CDC provides complete screening guidelines for youth living with HIV. Clinic-based motivational interviewing can improve condom use (Xu et al., 2017). The CDC also recommends PrEP for persons at risk for HIV acquisition. PrEP is recommended for sexually active adolescents who had anal or vaginal sex in the past 6 months and any of the following: having a partner living with HIV (partner with unknown or detectable viral load), a bacterial STI in the past 6 months, history of inconsistent or no condom use with sexual partners, and using injection drugs with a partner living with HIV or sharing injection equipment (Workowski, 2021). As of 2021, the CDC PrEP Clinical Practice Guidelines were updated to recommend that health care providers offer PrEP to all sexually active adolescents even if they do not report high-risk behaviors for HIV infection (CDC, 2021). Normalizing discussions of PrEP with sexually active adolescents will increase knowledge about PrEP among youth. The oral preparation of PrEP is approved for use in adolescents and young adults weighing 35 kg or more. In 2021, the US Food and Drug Administration (FDA) approved the use of extended-release cabotegravir, a long-acting injectable PrEP option, for use by at-risk adolescents who weighed 35 kg or more (FDA, 2021). The long-acting injectable is given first as two injections 1 month apart and then every 2 months.

A client-centered approach that includes culturally grounded risk reduction and addresses not only the client's individual risk but also the complicated contextual factors that impact risk is most helpful. For example, to be effective, providers will also need to also address key social factors that may contribute to risk including discrimination, housing, employment, food insecurity, mental health, and substance use. Personalized cognitive counseling (PCC) and Many Men, Many Voices (MMMV) are two evidence-based interventions that have been suggested to address the needs of vulnerable, at-risk communities. PCC uses an individual approach focusing on last sexual risk behavior, while MMMV attempts to address the intersecting factors and identities impacting adolescents.

SUBSTANCE USE

According to the 2019 National Youth Risk Behavior Survey, approximately 38% of youth described ever having sex, with 27% of high school students reporting that they were currently sexually active. Among youth who described being currently sexually active, 21% drank alcohol or used drugs prior to last sexual intercourse. Substance use predisposes adolescents to other high-risk sexual behaviors like inadequate condom use, and, for AWH, substance use can interfere with clinical care. In a large AIDS Treatment Network (ATN) study of 1,712 youth, 61% of males and 45% of females scored 2 or higher on the CRAFT screening tool (Gamarel et al., 2017). Daily or weekly use of cannabis was 33% for males and 19% for females. Daily or weekly use of alcohol was reported for 27% of males and 12% of females. Substance use prior to and during sex was commonly described. The regular assessment of substance use with appropriate counseling and referral is a key requirement in care.

MENTAL HEALTH

In an ATN study of 1,712 youth, 21% had a positive screen for depression and 15% for anxiety. In the cohort 15% had reported seriously considering suicide, and 14% were prescribed psychotropics. Further, 70% of the cohort recalled seeing a mental health provider while in care, and 38% of men and 42% of women reported currently wanting to receive mental health services (data presented at the October 2011 ATN meeting). These data suggest that regular screening and referral for mental health disorders is crucial. Stigma is another common concern for youth living with and at risk for HIV (Arrington-Sanders et al., 2020; Dowshen et al., 2009) and can relate to HIV status, sexual identity, or racial/ethnic minority. Stigma can lead to feelings of marginalization and mistrust and engagement in risky behaviors including condomless sex, nonadherence to medications, and delay in HIV testing care. Providers will need to approach AWH from an intersectionality lens to be effective—acknowledging all identities (e.g., race/ethnicity, gender identity, and socioeconomic status).

MEDICATION ADHERENCE

Youth living with HIV are at risk for nonadherence because of psychosocial, developmental, and cognitive factors. Several studies have documented nonadherence in youth living with HIV. Rates of adherence to HIV medications during the past 30 days range from 28% to 70% (Reisner et al., 2009). Barriers include medical, psychological, and logistical issues. Medical barriers include an AIDS diagnosis (Johnson et al., 2015), a difficult ART regimen (Buchanan et al., 2012), the absence of symptoms, and an unwelcoming medical environment (Philbin et al., 2014). Psychological barriers include depression, anxiety (Tanney et al., 2012), stigma associated with the diagnosis or transmission history (Rao et al., 2007), and lack of social support (Williams et al., 2022). Positive self-efficacy and outcome expectancy were associated with better adherence, and logistical barriers such as lack of housing, insurance, and transportation were associated with poorer adherence (MacDonell, et al., 2016). A comprehensive, multidisciplinary healthcare team is required to serve the medical, logistical, and psychosocial needs of AWH. Individually tailored interventions that address social and psychological factors (e.g., substance use, lack of insurance despite universal access to care, and lack of social support) and structural barriers (e.g., housing and insurance instability) will need to be developed in order to better meet the needs of youth living with HIV. Attention to potential barriers to adherence prior to treatment initiation is likely to improve outcomes.

Long-acting regimens may simultaneously address psychosocial needs of HIV stigma experienced by adolescents and medication nonadherence. In January 2021, the FDA approved the use of coformulated, extended-release cabotegravir and rilpivirine, a long-acting injectable ART option, for use by adolescents who were 12 years or older or weighed 35 kg or more (US FDA, 2021). In February 2022, the FDA approved it to be administered every 2 months, and the oral lead-in was made optional in March 2022. The long-acting ART is approved to replace the current antiretroviral regimen in adolescents who are virologically suppressed (HIV-1 RNA< 50 copies/mL), on a stable antiretroviral regimen, and have no history of treatment failure or known suspected resistance to either cabotegravir or rilpivirine.

COVID-19

In late 2019, a new pathogen, SARS-CoV2, spread across the globe, killing hundreds of thousands of people. Older adults experienced the highest rates of SARS-CoV2, but adolescents and young adults, aged 15–25 years accounted for up to 20.5% of new COVID-19 infections in some US locales, despite data suggesting that youth had lower COVID-19 testing rates (CDC, 2020c). Black and Latinx adolescents and emerging adults, aged 18–29 years, disproportionately accounted for 35.6% COVID-related age-specific deaths (CDC, 2020a). The same social determinants of health that predisposed communities to COVID-19 illness, contributed to high rates of HIV in adolescents at risk for HIV. These included concomitant comorbidities, adverse social determinants of health, structural racism, access to testing centers, population density, inadequate housing, and poor access to healthy foods.

AWH should follow COVID-19 prevention, testing, treatment, and vaccination guidelines from the Centers for Disease Control and Prevention (CDC). COVID-19 vaccinations are safe for people with HIV and do not interact or interfere with ART or PrEP. The number of doses for the COVID-19 vaccine will depend on the type of vaccine received but overall AWH should receive the primary series followed by boosters. In addition, providers should ensure that adolescents are up to date on all immunizations, including pneumococcal and influenza immunizations, and are provided necessary care for potentially worsening manifestations of mental health and substance use issues that may have increased during the COVID-19 pandemic. These additional comorbidities are prevalent in AWH, so it is vital that providers address these topics and refer them to appropriate mental health and substance use providers when necessary and continue to use a multidisciplinary team to support AWH.

Further guidance suggested that AWH should maintain an adequate supply of medications, 30 days or longer, to prevent barriers to medication access during the pandemic. It is important for providers to consider when an in-person visit including laboratory visits is necessary pending patient's clinical status and needs, and when possible, use telemedicine visits, assist youth in using electronic hardware for appointments (e.g., webcams, virtual platforms), and accommodating schedules to meet the needs of AWH (Armbruster et al., 2020). Care models based on the high rates of psychosocial problems reviewed previously and developmentally based care models that use multidisciplinary care teams are preferable. When a multidisciplinary model is not available, it becomes imperative that the management of complex youth with behavioral problems be facilitated by close communication among physicians, nurses, social workers or case managers, and behavioral health providers. Avoiding potentially catastrophic health outcomes, including rapid HIV progression, multiclass drug resistance, depression and suicide, chronic homelessness, prolonged incarceration, drug addiction, and secondary transmission of HIV, will likely require intensive attention to psychosocial issues. At times, a temporary approach of delaying early ART initiation may improve outcomes by allowing time to focus on developmental and social barriers.

TRANSITION TO ADULT CARE

Finally, clinicians must plan for the transition of AWH into adult care. In a joint statement, the American Academy of Pediatrics, the American Academy of Family Physicians, the American College of Physicians, and the American Society of Internal Medicine affirmed that all adults, including those with special medical needs, benefit from care by doctors who are trained in adult medicine (Cohen, 2002). They recommend that an identified healthcare provider be responsible for the transition, that a portable medical summary be maintained, and that a written transition plan be developed with the patient and family by age 14 years. In addition to these recommendations, Valenzuela and colleagues (2011) recommend the following:

- Optimizing provider communication between adolescent and adult clinics.

- Identifying adult care providers willing to care for adolescents and young adults.

- Addressing patient and family resistance to transition of care caused by lack of information, concerns about stigma or risk of disclosure, and differences in practice styles.

- Helping youth develop life skills, including counseling them on the importance of appropriate use of a primary care provider, managing appointments, symptom recognition and reporting, and self-efficacy.

- Identifying an optimal clinic model based on specific needs.

- Implementing ongoing evaluation to measure the success of a selected model.

- Engaging adult and adolescent care providers in regular multidisciplinary case conferences.

- Implementing interventions that may improve outcomes, such as support groups and mental health consultation.

- Incorporating a family planning component into clinical care.

- Educating HIV care teams and staff about transitioning.

The National Health Alliance also has resources that organize transition into the Six Core Elements. These resources can effectively be used in any clinical setting (see http://www.got-transition.org/providers/index.cfm). Guidance from Straub and Tanner (2018) identifies additional key components of transition including: having a formal, written transition policies, staff training in adolescent development, life skills and self-care plans for AWH, tailored programs that target resources toward AWH, and integrative patient registries that allow for sharing across pediatric and adult clinics.

ADOLESCENT HIV CARE SUMMARY

Adolescents or youth who are living with HIV may have multiple developmental, cognitive, social, contextual, and environmental challenges that impact their identification, linkage, and engagement with care. Attention to the factors noted previously will likely improve the care, treatment, and adherence of youth living with HIV and, potentially, will prevent them from "falling through the cracks."

12.2 HIV AND TRANSGENDER POPULATIONS

ZIL G. GOLDSTEIN AND
MADELINE B. DEUTSCH

LEARNING OBJECTIVE

Equip providers with the knowledge and skill to develop and provide gender-affirming primary care, HIV care, and HIV prevention.

WHAT'S NEW?

- Transgender people suffer from disparities in HIV infection, viral load suppression, and efficacy of tenofovir (TDF)/emtricitabine (FTC) as a PrEP regimen. Biomedical factors are not responsible for these disparities; interactions between antiretrovirals (ARVs) and hormone therapy are rare and should be considered separately from health disparities in this population. Emerging research connects these factors with experiences of trauma and discrimination because of persons' transgender status. New modalities of PrEP medications have shown efficacy in transgender populations.

KEY POINTS

- Transgender people have a range of identities and sexual orientations, as well as transition-related goals; each transgender patient should be approached as an individual.

- Special considerations with transgender populations should focus on minimizing transphobia during the healthcare experience with special attention paid to the documentation and use of the correct name and pronouns in patient documentation.

- Transgender people and programs should not be aggregated with MSM; programs and materials should be developed specifically for transgender populations using a culturally grounded approach.
  - Gender-affirming hormone therapy with estrogens and androgen blockers is generally safe and compatible with ART regimens.
    - Hormone therapy and other gender-affirming interventions improve HIV outcomes and reduce risk.
    - Gender-affirming surgeries are generally safe among transgender PWH, but should not be considered unless the HIV viral load is suppressed
- Transgender patients require ongoing primary and preventive care, as do cisgender patients; it is important to tailor transgender primary care based on the hormonal status and individual organ inventory of each patient.

- Providers should maintain a high index of suspicion for injected silicone and other fillers and related morbidity.

EPIDEMIOLOGY, DEMOGRAPHICS, AND TERMINOLOGY

Transgender is an umbrella term used to describe persons whose gender identity and/or expression of gender is different from the sex they were assigned at birth. Transgender individuals may identify as men, women, nonbinary, or something else. It is important to ask, record, and use the correct pronouns (such as *he*, *she*, or *they*) and the correct name (which may be different from the legal name and/or the name on insurance documentation) to engage and retain transgender patients. It is also important to recognize that there is no set path for transition. Some transgender people may seek only gender-affirming hormone therapy (HT), whereas others may seek surgical interventions such as genital reassignment surgery or other procedures on the face, breast, or body with or without concurrent hormone therapy. Still other transgender persons may present with a more complex gender identity; some may choose to seek HT or surgical treatments but continue to live part- or full-time in their birth gender, whereas others may assume a fluid gender expression that is not categorizable in either polar gender (Deutsch, 2015a). Some transgender people may choose to not pursue any gender-affirming medical or surgical treatments. A 2015 national survey of transgender people found that 30% of respondents identified as genderqueer or nonbinary; that is, neither male nor female (James, 2016). Table 12.1 presents a description of selected terminology and identities.

Table 12.1 DESCRIPTION OF SELECTED TERMINOLOGY AND IDENTITIES

TERM	DESCRIPTION
Transgender	Umbrella term for gender-nonconforming persons; more "modern" and inclusive term, preferred by many
Transsexual	Older, more clinical term, some use to identify those seeking medical or surgical treatment
Trans	Colloquial term increasingly used in place of *transgender*, especially among younger populations
Nonbinary	Describes a range of gender identities that are neither male nor female
Travesti	Term used by some Latina/Spanish speaking transgender women
Gay	Term used by some Latina/Spanish speaking transgender women with complex gender/sexual identities
Transgender woman/ transfeminine person	Person with a female or feminine-spectrum nonbinary gender identity who was assigned male birth sex
Transgender man/ transmasculine person	Person with a male or masculine-spectrum gender identity who was assigned female birth sex
Gender identity	The internal gendered sense of oneself as a man, woman, or something else
Gender expression	Signals that people use to communicate their gender to the outside world including body modification, the way people dress, talk, or walk; there are numerous ways to alter one's expression with and without medica/surgical intervention

Note: People may use pronouns and/or names that differ from those listed on legal identity documents. Some may use *they/them* or other gender-neutral pronouns.

The sexual orientations of transgender persons also lie on a spectrum, with the same 2015 survey 15% identified as heterosexual; 16% as gay or lesbian; 21% as queer; and 32% as bi/pansexual. In most cases, transgender persons define their sexual orientation based on their affirmed gender. For example, a transgender MSM would identify as gay. However, this also varies across cultural and linguistic lines with many transgender women who have sex with men sometimes also identifying as gay. Instead of focusing on identity, the most effective method for determining the sexual history and health of a patient is to ask, "What are the gender(s) of people you have sex with? Are any of them transgender people? What kind of genitals do they have?" or "What kind of genitals are involved in the sex you have?" (Deutsch, 2018). Using the terms *penis* and *vagina* may be alienating to transgender patients who have other words they use to describe their body. Allowing transgender persons to define their own body, identity, and experience will enhance the patient–provider relationship and may serve to improve adherence with ART and other care (Melendez, 2009).

The World Professional Association for Transgender Health's *Standards of Care for the Health of Transgender and Gender Diverse People, Version 8* (SOCv8; Coleman, 2022) states:

> The expression of gender characteristics, including identities that are not stereotypically associated with one's sex assigned at birth is a common and culturally diverse human phenomenon that should not be seen as inherently negative or pathological.
>
> In order to access covered medical and surgical procedures, transgender people are generally given a billable diagnosis. The DSM-V and ICD-10 use "Gender Dysphoria," a state of distress caused by mismatch between gender identity and birth-assigned sex, as the primary diagnosis. The need for a diagnosis to access care, including ongoing routine care when dysphoria is absent after gender transition has occurred has historically forced all transgender people to carry a mental health diagnosis. ICD-11 changed this diagnosis to "gender incongruence" and categorizes this term as a condition rather than a disorder, but slow uptake of ICD-11 in the United States hinders progress in de-pathologizing transgender health. (WHO, 2019)

Epidemiologic surveillance in transgender populations has been limited because of inconsistencies in the collection of gender identity data. Incomplete or inconsistent identification of transgender populations represents a significant structural determinant of the health disparities seen in transgender populations. Best practice for the measurement of gender identity data involves the use of at least two questions, such as gender identity and birth-assigned sex (Cahill, 2013, 2014; Deutsch, 2013), or some other combination of questions that allow differentiation of all transgender and gender nonbinary people, including those who identify as "male" or "female" from cisgender people, which records both the current gender identity and the birth-assigned sex (Cahill, 2013, 2014; Deutsch, 2013). This method has been found to identify twice as many transgender people as a "one-step" method in which a single "sex/gender" question is asked (Tate, 2012). The current estimate of the proportion of the transgender population by the UCLA Williams Institute recently doubled from 0.3% to 0.6% of the US population (Flores, 2016).

A 2019 meta-analysis found an HIV prevalence of 14.3% among transgender women living in the United States (Becasen, 2019). This striking rate is driven by interactions between structural, personal, behavioral, and biological risks unique to transgender women. Structural factors include a lack of legal recognition or protections that often result in survival sex work. Personal factors include the higher rates of mood disorders seen in transgender populations as a result of ongoing discrimination, as well as drive for gender affirmation; the model of gender affirmation describes the relationship between denial of gender affirmation (through lack of access to medical interventions or legal rights such as the ability to change one's name and gender on identity documents) and high-risk sexual behavior (Sevelius, 2013). Increasing gender affirmation through hormone treatment and surgery has been shown to have a positive effect on viral load suppression (Sevelius, 2021). Other behavioral factors include increased rates of condomless sex with primary male partners and anecdotes of increased earnings from sex work when no condom is used. Biological factors have not been explored in depth, but they could include changes to the anal epithelium in the presence of feminizing hormones, reduced erectile function resulting in impaired condom effectiveness, and unknowns such as HIV transmission through receptive vaginal sex in those who have undergone vaginoplasty (Poteat, 2015).

Transgender women have lower rates of virologic suppression (84% vs. 89% among cisgender women, and 90% among cisgender men) in 2020 Ryan White HIV/AIDS Program monitoring data (HRSA, 2021). A study of HIV indicators comparing transgender women to cisgender male and female controls found significant differences between transgender women and cisgender men in rates of ART adherence (78.4% vs. 87.4%, $P = 0.0143$) for 100% last 3-day adherence and virologic suppression (50.8% vs. 61.4%, $P = 0.0127$), but no difference in these measures when compared to cisgender women (Mizuno, 2015). Another study found that a high rate of adherence to hormone regimens was associated with a positive odds ratio of 34.5 ($P = 0.002$) for reported high ART adherence, though there was no effect on the rate of undetectable viral load. Satisfaction with current gender expression was also associated with higher reported adherence (OR 2.56, $P = 0.03$) but not with undetectable viral load (Sevelius, 2014). Other factors associated with viral load suppression are having a primary care provider who manages both HT and HIV, stable housing, employment, longer time since HIV diagnosis, and achieving gender affirmation as desired (Jin, 2019; Bukowski, 2018; Subino, 2020; Sevelius, 2019).

Few data exist on HIV risks and prevalence among transgender men, although some data suggest an increased risk (Green, 2015). A 2010 San Francisco study found that 61% of transgender men engaged in sex with other men, with 51% participating in vaginal receptive sex, and 39% participating in anal receptive sex. Transgender men have reported feeling that HIV testing was less accessible to them than to cisgender male controls (43.5% vs. 56.9%, $P = 0.04$) (Sevelius, 2014).

INITIATING HORMONE THERAPY

Gender-affirming HT has been found to have a number of benefits on quality of life and on symptoms of depression, anxiety, and poor social functioning (Colton, 2011; Gómez-Gil, 2011). SOCv8 defines hormonal and surgical treatment as medically necessary and states that it is unethical to deny surgical care solely on the basis of HIV or hepatitis B or C serostatus. SOCv8 endorses initiating hormone therapy with an assessment from a medical provider. There are no minimums with regard to time spent in psychotherapy prior to HT. This "informed consent" pathway destigmatizes and depathologizes transgender identities, and it overcomes several perceived or actual barriers to accessing HT. While some patients may benefit from additional mental health support to address ambivalence around, social barriers to GAHT, or other issues that come up before and during hormone initiation, a rigorous mental health screening process may neither be available (lack of resources or lack of trained/willing providers) nor culturally applicable (language barriers and cultural differences between Western-oriented psychotherapy and persons of Latinx, African, Aboriginal, or Asian background) (Deutsch, 2013). It is also appropriate to offer physician-supervised HT to those patients who may otherwise turn to unprescribed sources of hormones (internet and street purchase) or who have already fully adjusted and socially transitioned to the affirmed (new) gender. A 2009 study of transgender women in New York City found that 10% receiving physician-supervised HT were also obtaining hormones from other sources and that patients were frequently taking two or three concomitant hormone regimens. This same study reported as barriers to accessing physician-supervised HT a lack of a knowledgeable provider (32%), lack of a transgender-friendly provider (30%), cost (29%), location (18%), and language (13%) (Sanchez, 2009). It is important that transgender persons have reasonable and realistic expectations about what HT and other treatments can and cannot do. Once gender-affirming hormones have begun, there should be continued monitoring for underlying psychosocial factors or mental health conditions, with interventions as indicated.

FEMINIZING HORMONE REGIMENS

Feminizing HT involves testosterone blockade in combination with estrogen replacement and the possible use of a progestogen. The most commonly used testosterone blocker in the United States is spironolactone, a potassium-sparing diuretic taken in divided doses of 50–300 mg twice daily. SOC8 recommends the use of GNRH agonists and progestogens to achieve testosterone blockade as well (Coleman, et al., 2022). In the US context, it is most reasonable to start testosterone blockade with spironolactone because of its cost, efficacy, and common inclusion in drug formularies before progressing to other methods. Caution must be used with patients on angiotensin-converting enzyme (or ACE) inhibitors because of the potential for increases in serum potassium or those with impaired renal function. Concomitant use of ART medications that may affect renal function, such as tenofovir, is a theoretical risk; however, no case reports exist of spironolactone causing or worsening renal function in these patients. If spironolactone, GNRH agonists, and progestogens are not available, failed, or contraindicated, it is reasonable to consider 5-alpha reductase inhibitors, which will lower serum dihydrotestosterone levels, but raise total testosterone. Fosamprenavir and amprenavir are the only ARVs known to have interactions with estrogens that result in lower ARV

drug levels, but these ARVs are rarely used. Side effects of spironolactone are mainly orthostatic hypotension and polyuria, both of which tend to resolve after several weeks. Routine monitoring of potassium and renal function (baseline, every 3 months for the first year, and then every 6–12 months) is reasonable. A 2022 systematic review found a nonsignificant drop in serum creatinine (CI: –0.16 to 0.05 mg/dL) among transgender people on feminizing hormone therapy. While interpretation is still under investigation, it is reasonable to consider the amount of time on GAHT as well as muscle mass changes resulting from GAHT in interpreting serum creatinine. Some transgender women, especially those whose only opportunity for income is sustenance sex work, prefer to retain erectile function and may choose to avoid or use lower doses of testosterone blockers (Hembree, 2017).

Estrogen treatment may be via an oral, transdermal, or injectable route. SOC8 recommends changing to transdermal estrogens at the age of 45 and above because of the lower risk of vascular thrombotic VTE events (VTE) events. Transdermal routes of estradiol (50- to 200-µg patch changed one or two times per week) has been studied extensively and is very safe with respect to risk of thromboembolic disease: a 2008 meta-analysis of VTEs in postmenopausal hormone therapy found a relative risk of VTEs in users of transdermal estradiol of 1.1 versus nonuser controls. This same review found a two- to threefold increased risk of VTEs among users of any type of oral estrogen in the first year of treatment only; however, this increase translates to only an additional 1.5 VTEs per 1,000 woman-years (Canonico, 2008). A subsequent 2019 review found the incidence of VTE to be 2.3 events per 1,0001000 patient years (Khan, 2019). The transdermal route also delivers fairly constant and physiologic serum estradiol levels, which helps minimize common estrogenic symptoms such as migraine, weight gain, or mood swings; however, transdermal preparations tend to be expensive, may irritate the skin, and is not always included in HIV formularies. Oral 17β-estradiol in divided doses of 2–4 mg twice daily also delivers a constant and physiologic dose and is well tolerated. Some providers recommend administering oral estradiol sublingually to minimize first-pass metabolism and effects on clotting factors. Prior studies reporting 20- to 40-fold increases in VTE risk in transgender women involved the use of high-dose, highly thrombogenic synthetic ethinyl estradiol, which is no longer used in cross-sex treatment, and did not control for tobacco use (Asscheman, 1989; van Kesteren, 1997). More recent outcome studies of patients using 17β-estradiol have mixed findings, with one cohort of Dutch transgender women using only transdermal estradiol showing no increased risk of VTE, and a US cohort of transgender enrollees in a managed healthcare plan using estrogen therapy showing a 3.2-fold increased risk (Asscheman, 2011; Nash, 2018).

Many patients may arrive at clinic requesting, or even demanding, injectable estrogens. Although estradiol valerate 5–30 mg intramuscular every 2 weeks or estradiol cypionate 2.5–10 mg weekly are included in SOC8, these routes may deliver supraphysiologic estrogen levels that can vary widely over the injection cycle. Almost no data exist on the short- or long-term effects of this route, although anecdotally it is well tolerated. This route may be useful in a harm-reduction setting in which there is concern that a patient may turn to unprescribed hormone sources if an injected medication is not prescribed, or in settings where transdermal estrogens are not available and drug–drug interactions make avoiding first-pass metabolism a priority. This route may also be useful in patients who have low psychosocial functioning, poor medication adherence, high pill burden, or to provide an opportunity to bundle HIV-related and other care with frequent hormone injection visits (Ickovics, 2008). Fluctuation of levels may be minimized by dividing the dose into weekly injections and, if needed, titrating peak and trough serum estradiol levels to manage any estrogenic side effects. Further, changes in the hormonal milieu can lead to changes in the balance of Th1–Th2 T lymphocyte function and theoretical alterations in cellular immunity, furthering the argument in favor of constant and physiologic dosing of estrogen.

Interactions between estrogen HT and ART medications are complex and inconsistent. Three small studies have investigated possible drug–drug interactions between PrEP and feminizing HT. Tenofovir/emtricitabine (TDF/FTC) does not affect the levels of feminizing HT, and both masculinizing and feminizing hormone therapy reduce serum and target tissue TDF concentrations (Cotrell, 2018; Hiransuthikul, 2018). While a subanalysis of the iPrex study showed that there was no significant increase in risk for HIV transmission among transgender women with serum levels equivalent to taking TDF/FTC five or more times per week, subsequent data suggest that achieving this concentration of serum TDF may require better adherence than was previously thought (Deutsch 2015). These data also suggest the "PrEP On-Demand," requires further study in transgender populations before it can be recommended as an effective prevention strategy to transgender people on hormone therapy.

Data from contraceptive studies are mixed with regard to findings that PI and non-nucleoside reverse transcriptase inhibitor (NNRTI) medications may cause changes in serum estrogen and progesterone levels (Kearney, 2009; Marrazzo, 2015). However, it is important to monitor serum estradiol levels in all transgender patients, particularly before and after concurrent PI or NNRTI use. In addition to the previously mentioned tests, monitoring of transgender women using HT should include baseline fasting glucose and lipid profiles, with subsequent monitoring as clinically indicated.

Many community members claim progestogens may help with breast development; however, a single small ($n = 23$) study found no effects of progesterone on mood or Tanner stage (Nolan et al., 2022). Clinical practice suggests two main uses of progesterone: as an additional antiandrogen with failure of spironolactone alone, or as a first step to increase energy and libido before trying low-dose testosterone after gonadectomy. It is reasonable to attempt a trial of oral micronized progesterone 100–200 mg every night at bedtime or, if unavailable, medroxyprogesterone acetate 5–10 mg orally at bedtime. However, regardless of estrogens used, there is an increase in thrombogenicity with the addition of medroxyprogesterone

acetate, and a lesser increase with the use of other progestogens (Scarabin, 2018).

MASCULINIZING HORMONE REGIMENS

Masculinizing hormone therapy primarily involves testosterone administration. The primary goal of therapy is to keep total testosterone levels in the normal cis male range. Routes include intramuscular or subcutaneous testosterone cypionate or enanthate at 25–100 mg once a week or transdermal routes such as patches (2–8 mg/d) or gels and creams (20–100 mg/d). Testosterone cypionate and enanthate can also be administered in 100–200 mg every 2 weeks, but this dosing may increase peak/trough effects and lead to low energy at trough, often days 10–14 of a 2-week injection cycle. Testosterone undecanoate is available in both an IM injection formulation that is given every 10 weeks after two monthly loading doses or as a twice daily oral regimen. Intranasal testosterone cypionate is also available but must be administered three times daily. Long-acting implantable testosterone pellets are also available: insertion involves a minor in-office procedure, and maintaining cisgender male range testosterone levels often requires placement of new pellets every 2–4 months. Oral testosterone undecanoate preparation requires a dosing up-titration and is administered twice daily; a FDA "black box" warning has been placed on this medication regarding a risk of hypertension; notably, the effect size of the increase in blood pressure when seen is small (Swerdloff, 2020).

Many providers have begun using the subcutaneous route with testosterone cypionate and enanthate, which is less painful and traumatic and has been found to be noninferior (Olson, 2014). This treatment is well tolerated, with a minimum of side effects in most cases. Dose is titrated to cessation of menses and progression of virilization while keeping total testosterone levels in the normal cis male range. Prior concerns about hepatic injury are currently unfounded with the use of nonoral, nonsynthetic androgens. Monitoring should include baseline and periodic (every 6–12 months) fasting serum lipids, glucose, and hematocrit. Because of the lack of menstruation and the hematopoietic influence of testosterone, hematocrit should be compared to cis male normal ranges. Because testosterone administration alone is not a reliable contraceptive, even in the setting of prolonged amenorrhea, transgender men who are sexually active with a partner who has any detectable sperm in their semen should be counseled on contraceptive use and the teratogenic risks of unplanned pregnancy while using testosterone. While some transgender men may be averse to taking estrogen-containing contraceptives, others may prefer it over more invasive methods. It is important to have an individualized discussion with each patient over their contraceptive preferences and consider nonhormonal and progestin-only options (Krempasky et al., 2020). The effects of testosterone on the vagino-cervical mucosa with regards to HIV transmission risk are unknown, though transgender men using testosterone do tend to have higher rates of atrophic vaginitis and inadequate specimens on cervical Pap sampling (Peitzmeier, 2014).

Primary HPV screening via self-swab is a viable alternative for transmasculine patients who are uncomfortable with a pelvic exam, and it has been shown to dramatically increase cervical cancer screening rates in this population (Goldstein et al., 2020). This method of screening is preferred by transmasculine people and increases cervical cancer screening rates in the clinical setting but is less sensitive than traditional provider-collected specimens (Reisner 2017). However, increases in screening rates lead to the detection of more high-risk HPV infection than screening fewer individuals with a more sensitive test (Goldstein, 2020). Conversely, since many high-risk HPV infections do not result in cervical dysplasia requiring intervention, high-risk HPV-only screening may result in over-detection and unnecessary downstream testing such as colposcopy, which can be particularly of concern in those transgender men and transmasculine people for whom pelvic examinations are traumatic (Deutsch, 2020).

SOC8 requires assessment by a licensed professional prior to any gender-affirming surgery. Common surgical procedures and recommendations from SOCv8 for referral to surgery are listed in Table 12.2. While SOC8 suggests that the focus of this assessment should be on verifying the patient's gender identity, it is also important to assess for surgical readiness and psychosocial factors that may influence the course of surgery. Expanded insurance coverage for gender-affirming surgeries is available under the Affordable Care Act. Medicaid coverage is on a state-by-state basis and where available and has made such procedures available to patients with lower levels of psychosocial functioning and health literacy. Providers should consider additional and ongoing assessments of such perioperative essentials as housing, social support, transportation, and ability for postoperative care and self-care, and they should provide resources and support to address identified needs or gaps (Deutsch, 2016). Patients may also present with a history of any number of surgical procedures. In some cases, the surgery may have been performed in another state or even overseas; as such, local primary care providers may be called upon to provide postoperative care. Most surgeons are willing to work with local physicians and when contacted may ask for photographs to be transmitted by email. For those patients with a complex wound care issue and remote surgeon, referral to a local wound care center may be a reasonable alternative approach.

Most vaginoplasties are performed using a penile-inversion technique resulting in a vaginal lined by skin. However, it is important to ask each patient if they know how their vagina was created as different vaginal linings may lead to different bacterial STI susceptibility (Radix et al., 2019). The erectile tissue is removed and a "neovagina" is created by inverting the penile skin into a pocket created in the pelvis in the very narrow space between the urethra and the rectum. A clitoris is created using the glans penis. The creation of labia minora and majora varies based on the surgeon's technique with some using skin in the pelvis, and some using scrotal skin if it was not used to line the neovagina. The neovagina requires lifelong periodic dilation and/or sexual activity to maintain depth and girth, and an artificial lubricant is required for penetration.

Table 12.2 COMMON SURGICAL PROCEDURES

PROCEDURE	DESCRIPTION
FEMINIZING	
Vaginoplasty	Creation of a vagina between the urethra and rectum; vaginal lining may vary based on surgical technique
Orchiectomy	Removal of the testes; commonly referred to as castration
Augmentation mammoplasty	Using implants and/or fat grafting to increase the size of the breasts
Facial feminization	Can involve a variety of procedures including forehead reconstruction, jaw reconstruction, rhinoplasty, tracheal shave, and others to create a more feminine face
Body contouring	Liposuction and fat grafting to create a more feminine figure
MASCULINIZING	
Reduction mammoplasty/ mastectomy	A variety of surgical techniques create a flat, male-appearing chest and remove mammary and ductal tissue
Hysterectomy ± oophorectomy	Removal of the uterus with or without removing the ovaries
Metoidioplasty	Creation of a small phallus out of the clitoris; can be done with or without vaginectomy and/or urethral reconstruction
Phalloplasty	Creation of a phallus using a skin flap from a variety of techniques varying by donor site
Body contouring	Liposuction and fat grafting to create a more masculine figure

Diseases of the neovagina are usually a result of remaining or recurrent granulation tissue or mixed-skin flora or sebum and debris conditions resulting from a deep inverted pocket of keratinized skin. Granulation tissue can be treated with moderate strength topical steroids applied to a dilator and inserted into the vagina. Cauterization with silver nitrate is also an option but is painful and can lead to rectovaginal fistulae if applied to the posterior vaginal wall. Candida infections are uncommon, and the pH would not be expected to be acidic as in a natal vagina (Weyers, 2009). There is no squamocolumnar junction in a neovagina eliminating the need for Pap testing, but providers should maintain a reasonable index of suspicion for occult penile conditions such as Bowen's disease or other internal skin conditions including skin dysplasia. A small minority of transgender patients receive a vaginoplasty in which a self-lubricating vagina is created using a segment of sigmoid colon. These patients must be monitored for possible malignancy or inflammatory bowel disease of the neovagina. The prostate is not removed during the vaginoplasty procedure; examination of the prostate in a patient who has undergone vaginoplasty may be more effective when performed endovaginally as the vagina is most often posterior to the prostate. The risk of transmission of HIV via penile-neovaginal receptive sex in transgender women is unknown. Care of transgender women with a history of silicone or saline implant breast augmentation is identical to that of nontransgender persons.

PRIMARY CARE

Transgender persons require the same general primary and preventive care considerations as do nontransgender persons. However, it is important to take an inventory of organs on a patient-by-patient basis. For example, transgender women will retain their prostate after vaginoplasty, and some transgender men may have a hysterectomy but retain their ovaries or cervix. Additionally, chest exams may still be warranted if there is any remaining mammary or ductal tissue after transmasculine patients undergo removal of their breasts. This surgery is not a radical mastectomy; rather, it is an aesthetic surgery most often completed by plastic surgery to create a male-appearing chest, and some mammary or ductal tissue may be left behind. All organ screening should be based on a combination of age and risk factors, maintaining sensitivity to the patient's anxiety, which may be provoked due to examinations and studies on organs related to the birth sex. Screening for breast cancer in transgender women has not been studied; case series exist showing a possible increased risk above that of nontransgender men but lower risk than that of nontransgender women (Brown, 2015; Gooren, 2013). Some experts recommend that after 5–10 years of HT, patients should be considered for breast cancer screening, as are their age-matched nontransgender peers. Overall, providers should attribute HT as the etiology of any new health condition only after other more common causes have been excluded. Solid, long-term health outcome data are lacking. The largest population-based study on mortality outcomes to date is a retrospective series in the Netherlands of more than 2,000 transgender men and women. In this study, overall mortality among transgender women was increased by 51% in comparison to that of the general Dutch population; however, besides a 64% increase in risk of death as a result of cardiovascular disease, most of this increase was due to HIV, suicide, and substance abuse, and the study did not control for tobacco use. Transgender men did not have an increased overall mortality compared to the general population, but they had a 25-fold increased mortality relating to substance abuse (Asscheman, 2011).

HIV CARE AND PREVENTION CONSIDERATIONS

HIV prevention, care, and research programs have historically grouped transgender women with MSM. This linkage fails to recognize the significant behavioral and social differences between these two groups, not the least of which is that transgender women are not men (Poteat, 2015). Other than the possible negative impact of estrogens on amprenavir

and fosamprenavir, and theoretical renal interaction between tenofovir and spironolactone, there are no clear biomedical differences in the prevention or management of HIV in transgender persons (El-Ibiary, 2008). The most important considerations are ensuring that programs and clinic settings are culturally appropriate; electronic medical record systems should have the capacity to record and display the correct name and pronoun; social marketing and recruitment materials should include imaging and messaging appropriate for transgender populations; waiting rooms should have transgender-oriented pamphlets and wall art; and clinic bathroom policies should allow all patients agency in choosing which bathroom to use without being harassed by clinic staff. Providers and clinic staff should have adequate cultural fluency and sensitivity (Sevelius, 2014).

HIV PrEP in transgender women has not been studied in depth. The only published study to date of PrEP in transgender women is a subgroup analysis of the iPrEx trial that found no efficacy on an intention-to-treat basis. However, none of the transgender women who seroconverted had detectible drug levels at the time of HIV detection. Hormone use was associated with lower drug levels overall, as well as lower likelihood of having therapeutic drug levels, but the relationship between specific drug levels and HIV risk was identical between MSM and transgender women. It remains to be determined if reduced drug levels in transgender women using hormones are due to a direct interaction or to other confounders, such as increased pill burden or personal fear of interaction between hormones and ARVs (Deutsch, 2015b). Trials for cabotegravir and tenofovir alafenamide/emtricitabine as PrEP both included transgender women (Mayer et al., 2020; Landovits et al., 2021). While no subanalyses have been done on these studies examining transgender participants, inclusion was significant enough in these studies to show efficacy among transgender participants for both regimens. No PrEP studies have included transgender men, and only methods approved for cisgender women should be used in this population. Specifically, tenofovir alafenamide/emtricitabine combinations should not be used in transgender men as neither transgender men nor cisgender women were included in clinical trials.

SILICONE

The use of injected silicone and other soft tissue fillers (pumping) has become an increasingly prevalent practice, particularly among transgender women of color and sex workers. Unscrupulous practitioners, medical assistants, or laypersons will inject up to 1 liter or more of medical- or industrial-grade silicone, lubricant oil, insulating caulk, tire sealant, and other chemicals with the intent of bringing drastic and rapid changes to the physique (Silva-Santisteban, 2013). Most patients are unaware of exactly what is being injected, and the colloquial "silicone" may refer to any one of a number of injected fillers. In addition to the risks associated with the injected material, risks of acute bacterial infections and sepsis, as well as transmission of HIV and hepatitis, are high under these uncontrolled operating conditions. Thromboembolic events such as DVT and PE have been observed acutely post-silicone injection; patients should be monitored closely if they disclose that they will be getting silicone injections in the future. Some patients may have a sterile systemic inflammatory response mimicking sepsis or suffer embolization syndromes. The free filler substances could serve as an immunoadjuvant that precipitates an IRIS (Alvarez, 2016). These episodes are often treated with antibiotics as they can mimic cellulitis; however, particularly painful flares should be treated with systemic steroids. Long-term risks include chronic pain and disfigurement as the injected material migrates and calcifies. It is particularly important to assess for injected fillers when using parenteral hormone regimens or long-acting injectable ARVs as the location of fillers may affect available injection sites, and the effects of fillers on transdermal estrogens are unknown.

This procedure is sought because of a variety of factors; in addition to peer pressure and a lack of understanding of the risks, more complex factors of survival are at play. Patients engaging in survival sex work may believe that they need to obtain a hyperfeminine figure to pay for food and rent. Others may place a priority on erectile function and avoid HT, using silicone as their sole method of body feminization. Still others may live in neighborhoods in which they do not feel safe being identified as a transgender person, and they believe that silicone will assist them in blending in as a nontransgender person (Clark, 2008). For many, injected silicone is the only accessible option for body modification beyond hormone therapy.

Treatment of silicone-related morbidities is limited and mostly supportive. Two case reports describe improved symptoms with subcutaneous etanercept 25 mg twice weekly; however, the applicability of etanercept when chemicals other than silicone are used, as well as its safety in PWH, is unclear (Desai, 2006; Pasternack, 2005; Rapaport, 2005). An additional concern is subcutaneous or intramuscular medications used in PWH, such as penicillin and enfuvirtide, and how these injections may be affected by or complicate preexisting soft tissue fillers. One case report described the safe and successful use of subcutaneous enfuvirtide in a patient with extensive migratory silicone material under ultrasound guidance (Gabrielli, 2010).

HIV AND TRANSGENDER POPULATIONS SUMMARY

Most of the special considerations in the care of transgender people living with HIV relate to provider and staff cultural competency, tone and content of messaging, using the correct name and pronoun, and avoiding categorizing transgender women together with MSM. Gender affirmation through hormone and surgical treatment improves quality of life and, when bundled with HIV care or prevention efforts, may have synergistic benefits. More study is needed to evaluate the role of PrEP in transgender communities.

12.3 CARE OF PWH WHO EXPERIENCE HOMELESSNESS OR UNSTABLE HOUSING

ELIZABETH IMBERT AND
MATTHEW D. HICKEY

LEARNING OBJECTIVE

Describe special considerations affecting the medical management of people experiencing homelessness or unstable housing.

WHAT'S NEW?

- Long-acting injectable ART.

- Innovative low-barrier models of care improve care engagement and viral suppression.

KEY POINTS

- Establishing mutual trust is paramount.

- Linkage to care and retention in care require enhanced multidisciplinary teamwork.

- Long-acting injectable antipsychotics are important treatment options for individuals with psychosis who face challenges with adherence.

- Long-acting injectable ART is a new innovative tool that is promising for individuals who face challenges with daily adherence.

INTRODUCTION

PWH who experience homelessness or unstable housing have lower rates of viral suppression and higher mortality than their housed counterparts. While housing is ultimately needed to address disparities in HIV outcomes, navigation and linkage to low-barrier clinic-based and mobile care are promising interventions. Successful linkage to and retention in care is best met through the establishment of a trusting relationship with care teams who can partner with patients to treat HIV and simultaneously address housing, mental health and substance use.

EPIDEMIOLOGY OF HOMELESSNESS AND HIV

Homelessness and unstable housing exist on a spectrum, ranging from unsheltered to living in severely inadequate or insecure accommodation). In the United States, an estimated 580,000 people were unsheltered or in temporary/emergency shelter on a single night in 2020 in the United States Department of Housing and Urban Development (HUD) Continuum of Care Homeless Assistance Program, 2021). These estimates are based on point-in-time homeless counts of individuals living on the street, in emergency shelter, or in transitional housing and likely significantly underestimate the number of people experiencing homelessness over the course of any given year or experiencing other forms of housing instability.

PWH face a high burden of homelessness and unstable housing. In a representative sample of PWH accessing care at outpatient HIV clinics during 2020–2021, 17% reported homelessness or unstable housing, and 8% reported homelessness in the prior year (CDC, 2022). People experiencing homelessness also face a disproportionate burden of new HIV diagnoses. In San Francisco, 18% of new HIV diagnoses occurred in people experiencing homelessness, despite representing less than 1% of the total population (Colfax et al., 2021). Once diagnosed with HIV, people experiencing homelessness experience disparities in treatment outcomes throughout the cascade of HIV care. Greater degree of housing instability is associated with lower rates of HIV viral suppression, even among those engaged in care (Clemenzi-Allen et al., 2018; Griffin et al., 2020), and homelessness at the time of HIV diagnosis is associated with a 27-fold greater odds of mortality (Spinelli et al., 2019). In a large study analyzing the differences in causes of death among housed and unhoused individuals diagnosed with HIV in San Francisco between 2002 and 2016, decedents who were homeless were more likely to be younger, Black, female or transgender, and living below the poverty level; have a history of injection-drug use; and were less likely to have been prescribed ART. Compared to those who were housed, those who were homeless were more likely to die of causes related to mental health or substance use disorders (Hessol et al., 2019).

PWH who experience homelessness also face a disproportionate burden of violence, stigma, mental illness, and substance use and may benefit from a syndemic approach to these related conditions (Jones et al., 2020; Tsai et al., 2015, 2017). Worsening housing instability is associated with more severe mental health symptoms and diagnoses, which are in turn associated with worse HIV treatment outcomes (Aidala et al., 2016). Globally, people who inject drugs have an 18% prevalence of HIV (Degenhardt et al., 2017), and concurrent homelessness further increases HIV prevalence and risk of new infection (Stone et al., 2022) Mental health diagnoses and substance use disorders are both associated with lower rates of retention in HIV care (Rooks-Peck et al., 2018). In an analysis in a Ryan White clinic in Miami, those experiencing a combination of homelessness, mental health symptoms, and a substance use disorders had lower rates of viral suppression than those with any one isolated condition (Dawit et al., 2021), highlighting the importance of a treatment approach that provides integrated care for HIV, substance use, mental health, and social services to support housing needs.

CARE MODELS FOR PEOPLE EXPERIENCING HOMELESSNESS

Traditional HIV primary care models based on scheduled appointments may be difficult to access for people experiencing homeless, resulting in higher utilization of urgent and emergency department care (Clemenzi-Allen et al., 2019). Other barriers to care engagement may include competing sustenance needs, secure location to store medications and belongings, insurance challenges, lack of phone availability to receive appointment reminders, and comorbidities such as substance use and mental health diagnoses (Dombrowski et al., 2015; Holtzman et al., 2015; Yehia et al., 2015). Ultimately, supportive housing is the most-needed and effective intervention to address homelessness and unstable housing (Wiewel et al., 2020). Housing assistance has an independent effect on improving outcomes for inadequately housed PWH (Aidala et al., 2016).

While simultaneously advocating for greater access to permanent supportive housing, local partnership between community-based organizations, departments of public health, health systems, and advocacy groups is essential for addressing current medical and psychosocial needs of PWH and experiencing homelessness. Driven by the UNAIDS "Getting to Zero" campaign and US Ending the HIV Epidemic initiative, many local jurisdictions have developed forums for collaboration between local organizations that can be invaluable for identifying local resources such as legal aid, showers, and harm-reduction services (UNAIDS, 2010; Fauci et al., 2019; Buchbinder & Havlir, 2019). Engagement with "Getting to Zero" coalitions can facilitate both greater local advocacy and important referral networks for community-based services of which clinicians may not otherwise be aware.

For people experiencing homelessness who are not currently engaged in care, navigation services can provide an important link back into clinical care (Mizuno et al., 2018). Navigators are often peers who can meet patients in the community and accompany them to medical appointments. Navigators often develop close relationships with clients that are critical both for ensuring successful linkage to medical care and building client self-efficacy for active participation in their care (Roland et al., 2020). Because of the intensely personal nature of navigator-client relationships, it is important for navigation programs to provide support for boundary setting and burnout prevention (Roland et al., 2022). Navigation is often most successful when eligible patients are identified by a medical or social service provider, and may be less successful when patients are only identified by public health surveillance reports of patients who are out of care (Dombrowski et al., 2018a; Sachdev et al., 2020). Navigation services also help improve linkage to care and prevent declines in viral suppression postincarceration (Cunningham et al., 2018; Myers et al., 2018). Clinic-based programs such as the PHAST team in San Francisco can help ensure that recently diagnosed or newly reengaged patients are immediately started on ART and effectively navigated into routine HIV primary care (Coffey et al., 2019; Bacon et al. 2021a, 2021b). Other peer navigation interventions have not been successful in improving care engagement for people experiencing homelessness, highlighting the challenges of relinking patients to a system that does provide adequate support for them to remain engaged (Cabral et al., 2018).

Multidisciplinary healthcare teams, clinics, and health systems also play an important role in designing HIV and primary care services in a manner that minimizes barriers for people experiencing homelessness. Research among PWH experiencing homelessness demonstrates that this population has strong preferences for a care team that knows them as a person (as opposed to an urgent care model with an unknown provider) and the ability to drop-in for care (vs. a scheduled appointment), with a willingness to trade $32.79 (95% CI: 14.75 to 50.81) and $11.45 (95% CI: 2.95 to 19.95) in gift cards/visit, respectively (Conte et al., 2020). Integration of substance use disorder treatment and mental health services into routine HIV care is also essential for clinics providing care to people experiencing homelessness who face a disproportionate burden of these comorbidities (Garcia & Kushel, 2022; Haldane et al., 2022). The POP-UP low-barrier care model in San Francisco is integrated within the Ward 86 county HIV clinic and provides drop-in comprehensive HIV primary care and social work services for people experiencing homelessness (Imbert et al., 2021; Hickey et al., 2022). The POP-UP model also includes integrated psychiatric and substance use treatment, providing a one-stop-shop for many common patient medical needs. The MAX clinic in Seattle provides similar drop-in services for people experiencing homelessness or other barriers to engagement with routine HIV primary care (Dombrowski et al., 2018b, 2019). Such care models address a key barrier to care by eliminating appointments and providing on-demand access to care, while also routinely reviewing patients who have fallen out of care to conduct outreach when needed.

Mobile care offers another approach to provide care for people whose psychosocial barriers prevent engagement with clinic-based care. Street medicine programs have a long history of providing medical care to people experiencing homelessness outside of traditional clinic settings (Lynch et al., 2022). Street medicine services have successfully delivered mental health care, substance use disorder treatment with low-barrier buprenorphine, and hepatitis C treatment to people living on the streets or in shelters (Carter et al., 2019; Khalili et al. 2022; Lo et al., 2021; Rosecrans et al., 2022). Mobile HIV care programs integrated with medical care and housing navigation services can also improve both health outcomes and successful transition to stable housing (Rajabiun et al., 2020). Other mobile services focus on veterinary care for pets of people experiencing homelessness; this approach can be helpful for engaging patients and for addressing medical needs of their pets that may serve as a barrier to accessing needed healthcare (Geller, 2022). For patients requiring hospitalization but who have a pet, coordination with the local animal care and control to provide temporary boarding for pets can be critical for ensuring the patient can comfortably remain in the hospital to receive needed treatment.

CLINICAL CARE

Clinical care of PWH who experience homelessness and unstable housing should address individual and structural barriers to care. Drop-in access (i.e., no appointments required) to comprehensive primary care with a multidisciplinary care team who can address HIV, mental health diagnoses, substance use disorders, other comorbidities, and housing access is key. Pharmacists and pharmacy technicians can assist with prior authorizations for medications, support clinicians, work with pharmacies, and assist with in-clinic medication distribution. Eligibility workers can assist with insurance issues. Clinic should consider providing gift cards to address immediate sustenance needs, clothing, and hygiene kits; opportunities to pick up medications directly from clinic; and outreach and navigation, including transportation assistance, for patients who have lapses in care engagement (Imbert et al., 2021). Regular case conferences with the multidisciplinary team are helpful to discuss complex cases, review care gaps, and come up with shared care plans (Hickey et al., 2022). The care team should also work closely with emergency rooms, hospitals, psychiatric services, jails, and community-based organizations, including case managers and navigators to coordinate care for patients.

Developing a trusting relationship with patients to partner on their care is key (Conte et al., 2020). The care team should elicit PWH's concerns and priorities, share their concerns, and develop a joint care plan with specific next steps. It is important to listen to PWHs in a nonjudgmental way and try to understand the challenges they are facing and elicit ways in which the clinical team might be able to partner with them to address these challenges, recognizing that it may take time to build trust. The care team should address immediate needs (i.e., reason patient came to the visit) and partner with patient on long-term goals. Care teams should be trained in crisis de-escalation and support for frontline staff should be provided (Audain et al., 2013).

Obtaining information about housing status and stability should be a routine part of obtaining a psychosocial history for PWH. Providers should seek to understand individuals history of homelessness, exploring factors that precipitated homelessness, psychosocial factors that may impact housing, and patient preferences regarding housing. At each visit, it is important to collect living situation and contact information, including location where the patient is staying and a phone number or, email address, or additional contact persons (e.g., family members, friends, case managers) (Audain et al., 2013). For each person, meeting with a social worker to assess source of income, conduct housing assessments, and refer to temporary and long-term housing is important. Compared with unplaced persons not achieving stable housing quickly, persons quickly achieving stable housing were more likely to engage in care, and to be virally suppressed (Wiewel et al., 2020).

In addition to collecting HIV history (diagnosis date, CD4 + nadir, history of opportunistic infections, prior regimens and side effects, and prior genotypes), it is important to explore adherence including pattern and duration of nonadherence as well as individual-identified challenges to adherence. When picking a regimen, it is important to elicit personal preferences including oral (one or more pills) or injectable, side-effects concerns, and medication delivery options (i.e., come to clinic, pharmacy, deliver to location etc.). Having medications in a clinic where PWH can pick up frequently and engage with a medical team and have frequent adherence counseling can be helpful (Imbert et al., 2021).(Imbert et al., 2021). For those dosing at a methadone clinic or engaging in outpatient psychiatric day programs, consider partnering with these programs to deliver oral antiretrovirals as directly observed therapy. For individuals who have faced challenges to engagement in care or adherence to non-HIV medications, consider choosing high genetic barrier to resistance regimens including bictegravir/tenofovir alfenamide/emtricitabine or dolutegravir/tenofovir alfenamide/emtricitabine. Darunavir-based regimens (particularly fixed-dose darunavir, cobisistat, tenofovir alfenamide, and emtricitabine) have a very high barrier to resistance and may be a good treatment option for individuals with inconsistent adherence to oral medications (DHHS, 2022; Lathouwers et al., 2021).

An exciting recent development is the advent of long-acting ART (LA-ART), which is a promising tool for people experiencing homelessness or unstable housing who face barriers to oral medication adherence. Because of its extended dosing interval, LA-ART has the potential to mitigate many barriers to daily oral ART adherence, including lack of safe storage for pills, pills getting lost or stolen, pill fatigue, pills as a reminder of living with HIV, fear of inadvertent disclosure from possessing pills, and inability to take a daily medication (Kanazawa et al., 2021; Scarsi & Swindells, 2021). A demonstration project of LAI-ART in a diverse group of patients with high levels of substance use and marginal housing at the county hospital-based Ward 86 HIV clinic in San Francisco demonstrated promising early treatment outcomes, including in those with detectable viremia because of adherence challenges. LAI-ART was started via a structured process of provider referral, multidisciplinary review by a doctor, nurse, and pharmacist, and monitoring for on-time injections. Inclusion criteria were willingness to receive monthly injections and a reliable contact method; patients with any history of rilpivirine-associated resistance mutations were not considered for LAI-ART; however, the program allowed up to one integrase-associated resistance mutation. The program also allowed patients with hepatitis B infection to enter if they are willing to continue or initiate hepatitis B–directed treatment (Christopoulos et al., 2022).

Addressing severe mental illness and substance use disorders is imperative. Integrated psychiatry consultation in primary care can increase access to needed mental health services and support primary care clinicians to meet the psychiatric needs of the population (Zeidler Schreiter et al., 2013). When treating psychosis, it is important to consider starting an oral antipsychotic that if tolerated can be switched to a long-acting injectable antipsychotic (i.e., risperidone or aripiprazole). Long-acting antipsychotics have demonstrated significant benefit as compared to oral antipsychotics in preventing hospitalization or relapse in schizophrenia (Kishimoto et al., 2021). Methamphetamine-induced psychosis can also be treated with antipsychotics (Glasner-Edwards & Mooney, 2014; Verachai et al., 2014), and in patients with challenges with adherence, long-acting injectable antipsychotics should be considered. Contingency management is an evidence-based intervention to reduce methamphetamine use and should be implemented in outpatient clinics who treat patients with methamphetamine use disorder (Brown & DeFulio, 2020). Assessment for and treatment of opiate use disorder is important during routine HIV care visits, including low-threshold buprenorphine treatment (Jakubowski & Fox, 2020), referral to methadone clinics when indicated, and naloxone distribution "Life-Saving Naloxone from Pharmacies" (CDC, 2019). It is also important to offer harm-reduction services, safe education kits, and education, during clinic encounters (Peckham & Young, 2020). Given the high prevalence of smoking among people experiencing homelessness and its impact on life expectancy for PWH, smoking cessation should also be addressed (Baggett et al., 2013; Reddy et al., 2016). Alcohol use disorder is also high among PWH, and screening and appropriate management is key (Duko et al., 2019).

In addition to partnering with patients on their health goals, it is important to offer standard health care maintenance per United States Preventative Services Task Force (USPSTF) guidelines, including routine vaccinations and age-appropriate cancer screening when patients present for care. Specific attention should be given to test and treat for sexually transmitted infections and hepatitis C and ensure vaccination against hepatitis A/B, COVID-19, meningitis, and pneumococcus. Tuberculosis screening should be offered, and latent tuberculosis infection treated as indicated (see Chapter 10).

CARE OF PWH WHO EXPERIENCE HOMELESSNESS OR UNSTABLE HOUSING SUMMARY CONCLUSION

PWH who experience homelessness or unstable housing face individual and structural barriers that interfere with achieving viral suppression and place patients at increased risk of death. While housing is ultimately needed to address disparities in HIV outcomes, innovative programs that assist with navigation and linkage to low-barrier multidisciplinary care teams who can develop trusting relationships with patients to partner on their care are key.

12.4 HIV IN CRIMINAL-LEGAL INVOLVED PEOPLE

OLABIMPE ASUPOTO AND ALYSSE G. WURCEL

LEARNING OBJECTIVE

Describe the current state of HIV care delivery to people who are criminal-legal involved, with a focus on opportunities for improving care.

WHAT'S NEW?

There is increasing evidence for the feasibility, acceptability, and efficacy of treatment for substance use disorder in PWH. This treatment has been shown to improve rates of retention in HIV care and HIV viral suppression. Although there are challenges to implementation, there are increasing data supporting strategies aimed at broadening access to medication for prevention of HIV (i.e., PrEP) to people who are incarcerated.

KEY POINTS

- Criminal-legal involved people are at increased risk for HIV compared to people who have never been incarcerated or detained.

- Rates of HIV in state and federal carceral facilities are decreasing.

- Similar to healthcare standards in the community, all people who are incarcerated and detained should receive HIV medications with the goal of HIV viral suppression.

- HIV viral suppression is suboptimal in people who are released from jail and prison, signaling the need for intensified linkage to care programs upon release.

- Assessment for and treatment of substance use disorder is necessary to provide quality care to PWH who are incarcerated.

- Implementation of programs supporting the prescription of PrEP to people at risk for HIV should occur in jails and prisons.

INTRODUCTION

As a result of the intersection of criminalization of drug use disorder, poverty, and racism, HIV prevalence in criminal-legal involved populations (CLIP) is higher than in people who have never been incarcerated or detained (Bowleg et al., 2022; Brinkley-Rubinstein et al., 2018; Schneider, 1998). The spectrum of criminal-legal involvement is broad, and includes the experience of being arrested, being incarcerated in jail or prison, and community supervision including parole and probation. In 2020, 1 in every 47 adults in the United States were under some form of carceral supervision across this spectrum, and about 75% of CLIP were under community supervision (Kluckow & Zeng, 2022). People who are marginalized, including but not limited to Black, Hispanic/Latino, and Native American people, are more likely than White people to be incarcerated (Dauria et al., 2021). Similarly, PWH who are impacted by criminal justice system are more likely to be Black, Hispanic/Latino, or Native American than White (Bovell-Ammon et al., 2021).

Although there are several commonalities across the criminal-legal spectrum for HIV care, there are barriers to the operationalization of HIV care that are setting specific. In this review, we will focus on four broad carceral settings (1) prisons and jails, (2) detention centers, (3) resource-limited international carceral settings, and (4) community carceral control and re-entry. Following these site-specific reviews, we discuss the importance of testing and treatment for infectious and noninfectious illnesses that co-occur with HIV, HIV transmission in carceral settings, and best practices for HIV-related care and prevention in carceral settings.

Of note, as the language describing people who are incarcerated has shifted away from use of words like *offender* or *inmate* toward person-first language, we will refer to people with criminal-legal involvement as CLIP, and criminal-legal involved individuals (CLII). The terms *CLIP* and *CLII* include people who are incarcerated as well as people with a history of previous incarceration.

HIV TREATMENT IN PRISONS AND JAILS

Before we discuss HIV in carceral settings, it is important to understand the distinction between prisons and jails. Although the terms *prison* and *jail* are often used interchangeably, there are distinct differences between these facilities, and these differences impact healthcare delivery. Prisons are run at the federal and state level, and incarcerate people for longer periods of time, typically >2 years. Jails are run at the county or city level, and typically have shorter periods of incarceration (average length of jail incarceration in 2020 was 28 days) (Minton, 2021).

HIV infection is three times more prevalent in state and federal prisons than the general population (CDC, 2022). There has been a decrease (14,180 in 2019 to 11,940 in 2020) in the number of people in state prisons with HIV recently (Maruschak, 2022). There are no nationally available estimates of people in jails with HIV, but a range of 1%–9% HIV prevalence has been reported (Javanbakht et al., 2014; Parvez et al., 2013). Approximately 22% of individuals living with HIV who were incarcerated were unaware of their HIV status when they entered prison and jail, and approximately 69% of new infections are spread by those who are diagnosed with HIV infection but who are not receiving treatment (Dauria et al., 2022; Iroh et al., 2015).

Most of the research on HIV treatment for people who are in jail and prison is about barriers to receiving HIV medications. One notable study conducted with CLIP in jails demonstrated that while most individuals received HIV medication and met with healthcare providers during incarceration, access to their medication in a timely manner was inadequate (Blue et al., 2022). In this study, participants reported missing medication for extended periods of time because of delays in obtaining correct medications, unpredictable length of stay, jail staff refusing to provide medication because of the financial burden, and lack of communication between correctional officers. Many CLIP were forced to rely on family members to bring their HIV medication to jail, but correctional officers can even prevent this by citing jail policies (Blue et al., 2022). Despite these challenges, one benefit of this study was that CLIP individuals were able to consult with HIV clinicians (Blue et al., 2022). Individuals involved in the study felt well treated, and clinicians tried to improve their care by utilizing local resources (Blue et al., 2022).

When the barriers to receiving HIV medications are overcome, the methods by which the medications are distributed also pose unique challenges to CLIP living with HIV. The most-common method of distribution of HIV medications in carceral settings is direct-observation therapy (DOT), rather than "keep on person" (KOP). Many jails and prisons prefer

DOT to keep track of medication adherence. However, for the CLIP with HIV, DOT poses a threat to confidentiality because medical staff may state the medication's name or other CLIP may see the medication during distribution (White et al., 2015). Other issues with DOT distribution of HIV medications include inability to take the medication with food and prevention of CLIP with HIV to independently establishing their own medication regimen (White et al., 2015). Prior to release, facilities that use DOT may want to consider introducing a more practical KOP system to help individuals manage their own medications.

It is imperative that PWH have consistent access to their medications and their HIV provider. Unfortunately, qualitative research has revealed major gaps in HIV care delivery in jails and prisons. Justice-involved women in Alabama carceral facilities reported barriers to continuous HIV care owing to unfair limitations, including forced isolation, food rationing, refusal to provide counseling after initial HIV diagnosis, and outright denial of treatment. Disruptions in treatment can also result from transferring between facilities, being segregated, and being in "lockdown," which is when officials restrict individuals from leaving their cells for a period of time (Culbert, 2014).

HIV CARE IN DETENTION SETTINGS

There are over 200 Immigration and Customs Enforcement (ICE) detention facilities in the United States, housing 300,000 people (Terp et al., 2021). Individuals detained in detention settings are subjected to a detention process that is unorganized and complex, which results in gaps in access to appropriate medical care and medications. According to Human Rights Watch, the US immigration detention systems have poor medical care, slow responses to care requests, and inexperienced medical staff, which all contributed to avoidable deaths, including HIV-related deaths (Blunt, 2017). In addition to the poor care offered in detention centers, many people are discouraged from disclosing their HIV status for fear of how it will affect their case or ability to leave the detention facility (Page et al., 2018). Another barrier to the management of HIV in people who are detained in ICE facilities is medication choice because HIV medications vary between countries. Patients with HIV resistance mutations may not benefit from first-line treatment because drug resistance patterns in the United States may differ from those in the patient's home country (Beyrer & Pozniak, 2017).

If persons who are detained are able to overcome all the above barriers to receiving care while in a detention facility, they still face significant barriers to quality HIV care once they are deported. When they are deported, a 30-day supply HIV treatment may be prescribed, but only if they received treatment while in the detention facility (Page et al., 2018). When PWH return to their home countries, returning to the United States often takes precedence over finding HIV clinics for treatment (Grimes et al., 2016). There have been reports of programs aimed at increasing linkage to care for PWH detained in ICE facilities, such as increasing detainees access to infectious diseases consultation during detention (Mishreki et al., 2021). Although some progress has been made in linkage to care, there is still room for improvement in order to encourage continued HIV treatment and viral suppression after deportation.

HIV TREATMENT IN RESOURCE-LIMITED INTERNATIONAL CARCERAL SETTINGS

Although the United States has the highest rates of incarceration, jails and prisons exist globally, including countries that are considered resource-limited settings where HIV prevalence rates are higher. The HIV prevalence in jails and prisons in resource-limited settings is often unknown but is estimated to be quite high, with some countries reporting 25% of CLIP are living with HIV (Dolan et al., 2016). Prisons in Kyrgyzstan found the prevalence of HIV to be 10.3%, making it the third most-common infectious disease they face. More than half of the CLIP living with HIV in these facilities were unaware of their status (Azbel et al., 2016). Twelve of the fifteen people who knew their HIV status were taking antiretroviral medication (Azbel et al., 2016). According to a Malaysian study, less than half of CLIP who qualified for ART received it, and a quarter later developed AIDS (Fuge et al., 2020). Similarly, a cross-sectional retrospective study carried out in South African prisons reported that only half of PWH who were eligible for the initiation of ART treatment were able to do so. Frequently, CLIP were unable to receive HIV care because of a shortage of healthcare workers, disorganized health systems, and facility transfers (Stevenson et al., 2020). An investigation of HIV care access in Malawi's prisons revealed that there is more access to HIV services at entry and throughout incarceration in urban facilities compared to rural ones because of onsite clinics (Gondwe et al., 2021). In contrast, ART was not routinely provided in rural prisons; instead, individuals had to travel to a nearby hospital to receive antiretroviral therapy (Gondwe et al., 2021). Further, many CLII reported significant delays in medical staff providing care for seriously ill patients in urban facilities (Gondwe et al., 2021). Barriers that emerged in resource-limited settings include stigma, unequal access to HIV care for women, shortage of healthcare staff, and insufficient diet (Telisinghe et al., 2016).

Structural interventions that address discrimination, HIV stigma, and human rights violations and make healthcare more accessible are needed in jails and prisons. There is evidence that Sub-Saharan African carceral facilities were more aware of HIV risk after employing structural interventions to reduce HIV-related stigma, and created safer work environments (Lyons et al., 2020). Further, integrating HIV care with gender-affirming care (Maiorana et al., 2021), mental health services (Collins et al., 2021), and harm reduction (Chang et al., 2021) helps to meet the key population's health and wellness needs. In Kenya, the establishment of community clinics and drop-in centers run by key populations resulted in an immediate improvement in HIV care engagement and a significant increase in individuals initiating ART (DiCarlo et al., 2022). PWH from South African carceral facilities were linked to care within 90 days of release and were interviewed by phone or in person to evaluate medication adherence. The study found that there were no lapses in ART medication (Mabuto et al., 2020).

HIV TRANSMISSION IN CARCERAL SETTINGS

The actual transmission of HIV within jails and prisons is thought to be relatively low, and it is believed to be lower than the transmission rates in the general public (Valera et al., 2017). Especially with increased access to well-tolerated HIV treatment efficacious at viral suppression, HIV transmission in jails and prisons is likely a rare occurrence. However, it is challenging to track HIV transmission in carceral settings because CLIP might be reluctant to report potential exposures for fear of punishment. These exposures include tattooing, injection-drug use, and consensual and nonconsensual sexual activity. Despite the need for condoms, only a few carceral facilities provide them. Jails with condoms include Los Angeles, San Francisco, New York City, Philadelphia, and Washington, DC. State prisons in Mississippi and men's prisons in Vermont and California provide condoms (Lucas et al., 2020). Increasing testing, access to HIV prevention medications, and access to harm-reduction tools, like substance use disorder treatment, are strategies to decrease HIV transmission in jails and prisons (Reddon et al., 2019). These measures should be universally implemented in carceral settings globally to prevent HIV transmission.

RELEASE PLANNING: TRANSISION TO COMMUNITY

Release from jail and prison is a time when people may experience barriers to getting HIV care (Masyukova et al., 2018). The majority (3.9 million) of the 5.5 million people who are CLII in the United States are under some sort of community carceral control. HIV infection rates in community supervision programs in New York are 13% in men and 17% in women, which is significantly higher than the rates in carceral facilities (El-Bassel et al., 2019).

Barriers to care for PLWH postrelease include interruptions in health insurance, untreated substance use disorders, and mental health conditions (Campbell et al., 2018). One study in Connecticut found the rates of HIV suppression following release from incarceration were 67% at 1 year and 43% at 3 years (Loeliger et al., 2018b). A study in Illinois compared ART rates between CLII who are incarcerated and CLII who are reincarcerated, and found that the proportion of people on ART decreased from 73% at the time of release to 50% at the time of reincarceration (Badowski & Patel, 2022). Increased linkage to care upon release from prison is critical to maintaining viral suppression. A study conducted in Rhode Island and North Carolina carceral facilities examined the retention of HIV care in CLII postrelease and in those already receiving care in the community. It found HIV care retention in PWH following release was 20% lower than in those already in community (Costa et al., 2018). Within the first 30 days following release from jail in Connecticut, < 20% of people filled their HIV medications or went to an HIV clinic. Less than 50% of those who were released saw an HIV provider within 90 days, and 33% had detectable viremia at the initial appointment (Loeliger et al., 2018a). Conversely, though, a study conducted in a Massachusetts jail to evaluate the transition of care back to the community, 70% of participants met with an HIV care provider in a timely manner (within 30 days) (Dong et al., 2021; Sprague et al., 2017). These findings suggest linkage to care differ by state.

There have been several studies examining the role of a navigator to assist in linkage to care following incarceration (Iryawan et al., 2022; Monroe et al., 2017; Taylor et al., 2018). A case management intervention study was conducted in Baltimore, where justice-involved PWH met with a clinical social worker and an outreach worker to develop treatment plans and attend follow-up visits to assess treatment adherence (Crable et al., 2021). As a result of this intervention, justice-involved PLWH were 5.6 times more likely to receive linkage to HIV clinical services, 5.8 times more likely to be prescribed ART, and 4 times more likely to report medication adherence at follow-up visits (Crable et al., 2021). Data to Care (D2C) is a public health strategy that uses available data from HIV surveillance and other sources to reengage PWH who have fallen out of care in order to improve health outcomes (Villanueva et al., 2022). A recent qualitative review found that applying the D2C strategy to county jails had both potential benefits for public health and risks for PWH (PLWH) (Buchbinder et al., 2020). Implementing D2C had the advantages of increased public trust in state health services, decreased HIV transmission, improved access to HIV care, and continuity of care following release from jail. However, potential drawbacks include invasions of privacy, unintentional or intentional disclosure of HIV status, threats of violence, and coerced HIV treatment (Buchbinder et al., 2020). The implementation of a peer navigator intervention, instead of a D2C intervention, builds trust, reduces stigma, and lessens other discrimination-related barriers to healthcare engagement (Dauria et al., 2022). Once the CLII are released, navigators accompanied them to appointments and aided in patient–provider interactions (Woznica et al., 2021). Prior to release, this intervention should be started, and support can be provided to assist the individuals in setting goals to overcome barriers to HIV care engagement and medication adherence (Taylor et al., 2018).

Untreated substance use disorder is a major reason why people do not engage in HIV care in the community (Dong et al., 2021; Korthuis & Edelman, 2018). Substance use disorder affects 85% of CLII incarcerated in jail (Rubenstein et al., 2016). There is a strong correlation between mental health conditions and substance use disorders (Baranyi et al., 2019, 2022). There is a strong correlation between mental health conditions and substance use disorders (Baranyi et al., 2019; 2022). The presence of a substance use disorder is linked to poor treatment compliance and nonadherence to medication (Hunt et al., 2020). Three treatments for opioid use disorder are buprenorphine, naltrexone, and methadone. A study of 21 state carceral facilities found that all three medications were available in 62% of these facilities. Unfortunately, only 7% of the 538 prisons in these 21 carceral facilities offered all three medications (Scott et al., 2021). This study demonstrates the need for increased access to more types of medications for substance use disorder. A study conducted in Rhode Island carceral facilities found that the use of extended-release buprenorphine, a monthly injectable medication, resulted in minimal side effects and was used for longer than other drugs/formulations postrelease. Buprenorphine will help prevent substance use for longer with prolonged use (Martin et al., 2022). Another study conducted with CLII found extended-release naltrexone reduced opioid use relapse (Lier et al., 2022). Internationally, there are also data that demonstrate the initiation of substance use disorder treatment improves linkage to HIV care (Azbel et al., 2018; Mjaland, 2015; Polonsky et al., 2016). Treatment for substance use disorder is an evidence-based intervention that decreases substance use and, therefore, increases linkage to and adherence to HIV care upon release from jails and prisons.

TESTING AND MANAGEMENT OF COMORBID CONDITIONS WITH HIV

Any discussion about the optimal treatment of HIV in carceral settings needs to highlight the treatment of noninfectious and infectious illnesses that are prevalent in PWH. HIV medications are highly effective and well tolerated, so morbidity and mortality from HIV and opportunistic infections has decreased (Justiz Vaillant & Naik, 2022). Screening for other infections, including hepatitis B and C (HBV, HCV) and sexually transmitted infections like syphilis, are necessary to provide the best care for PWH (Workowski et al., 2021). PWH involved in the justice system who have a history of drug injection have a 78% chance of HIV/HCV coinfection and a 15% chance of HIV/HBV coinfection (Ahmadi et al., 2021). Direct-acting antiviral drugs are the current standard of treatment for HCV and should be offered to all people who are incarcerated and detained. HIV has been linked to premature aging (Aberg, 2020), increased cardiovascular disease (Aberg, 2020), and increased risk of cancer (Castilho et al., 2022). The treatment of PWH should follow national guidelines for preventive care including, for example, cancer screening and blood pressure control (Lakshmi et al., 2018).

HIV TESTING AND PREVENTION

The Centers for Disease Control and Prevention (CDC) recommends that CLII in carceral facilities be routinely screened for HIV through opt-out HIV testing, offered antiretroviral medication, and evaluated by clinicians with experience treating HIV (CDC, 2022). Opt-out testing is not widely employed in US carceral facilities, according to the most recent research (Solomon et al., 2014). Routine opt-out testing is specifically mentioned at 5% of surveyed jail facilities, and 7 % of surveyed jails offered HIV testing for all CLII at intake (Maner et al., 2022). While this is not surprising, routine opt-out testing strategies yield greater numbers of screenings and subsequent HIV diagnoses and, therefore, should be universally employed. Jails, as opposed to prisons, typically have short lengths of stay, high turnover rates, and poor communication with healthcare providers, making routine or opt-out HIV screening and follow-up difficult to implement. The majority of the jails in the nation do not regularly conduct HIV screenings (Hutchinson et al., 2021). Results from studies conducted with individuals who have been incarcerated demonstrated that being African American, having higher education, having been previously incarcerated, and having more HIV knowledge all increased the likelihood of ever receiving HIV screening (Farel et al., 2019). It is critical to promptly diagnose individuals living with HIV in order to overcome the obstacles preventing effective HIV therapy. The US Initiative to End the HIV Epidemic encourages state and local health departments to strengthen their existing programs to increase access to HIV testing (Fauci et al., 2019).

People who inject drugs and people who are incarcerated are not offered PrEP routinely, and this is an area where jails and prisons should focus more resources. Medications that prevent HIV transmission have been available as a daily pill since 2012 (Bolland & Grey, 2013; Mayer & Krakower, 2012). PrEP is approved to prevent HIV infection through sexual contact and intravenous drug use (Choopanya et al., 2013; Grant et al., 2010; Murnane et al., 2013). In the past year, injectable forms have been approved (Garrison & Haberer, 2021). A study on the continuum of PrEP care for men who are incarcerated and at high risk for HIV was conducted in Rhode Island's carceral facilities. The study found that increased PrEP awareness, support from carceral and medical leadership, and linkage to care postrelease contributed to the successful use of PrEP in carceral settings (Murphy et al., 2022). In a comparable study conducted in Thailand, where PrEP was administered through directly observed therapy in prison facilities, 94% of CLIP missed fewer than eight doses of oral medication (Colby et al., 2015). Since the injections are given less frequently, once a month or every two months, missed dosages are significantly reduced. HIV medication is equally effective when taken orally or given intramuscular; therefore, either method of treatment is beneficial. More research is being published about successful implementation of PrEP in carceral settings and during the process of reentry (Brinkley-Rubinstein et al., 2018; Marcus et al., 2016; Murphy et al., 2022).

12.5 RURAL POPULATIONS AND HIV

ABBY DAVIDS AND ASHLEY CARVALHO

LEARNING OBJECTIVE

Describe obstacles to and best practices for optimal HIV care for PWH in rural settings.

WHAT'S NEW?

PWH in rural areas face unique challenges including the need for expanded HIV prevention, testing, and care services.

KEY POINTS

- The HIV epidemic in the United States has begun to shift to more rural areas.

- Rural residence creates barriers for HIV care and is a risk factor for lower HIV testing overall, later HIV diagnosis, and increased HIV-related mortality.

- The increasing rurality of the US opioid epidemic highlights additional challenges and needs for both HIV and HCV care in rural areas.

Although the HIV epidemic in the United States began in large cities, it has since moved to more rural areas (Schafer et al., 2017). The Southern United States currently has the highest incidence and prevalence of HIV in the country; accounting for approximately 46% of all HIV transmissions and 49% of new transmissions, while only 37% of the US population lives in the South (CDC, 2022). Some nonurban counties in the Southern United States now have higher HIV prevalence than many large US cities (Rural Health Information Took Kit, 2022). Racial disparities in the burden of HIV transmissions, particularly among Black populations, are amplified in the South as well (CDC, 2020a).

Rural/nonurban residence creates several barriers to engagement in the HIV continuum of care. HIV testing rates are lower in rural areas; in one study, the rate of lifetime HIV testing was 66% for nonurban participants versus 88% for urban participants (Wallace et al., 2011). MSM in rural areas are less likely to be tested for HIV than those in urban areas, as were undocumented migrant and seasonal farmworkers in rural areas (Fernandez et al., 2005; Goldenberg et al., 2014). Rural providers may not offer HIV testing routinely as well; in one study, primary care providers in North Carolina were only 10% adherent to CDC HIV testing guidelines, despite being aware of the recommendations (White et al., 2015).

Access to care also remains a challenge for PWH in rural areas. Many rural residents travel to urban areas for their medical care, citing lack of local provider expertise as one reason for this. In 2013, 95% of nonurban counties in the United States lacked a Ryan White HIV medical provider, compared to 69% of urban counties (Vyavaharkar, 2013). In 2017, of the 2,000 organizations funded by the Ryan White program, only 6% were located in rural areas (Klein, 2020). Additionally, PWH in rural areas were less likely to have regular outpatient visits with their HIV care provider than PWH in urban areas, and they were less likely to take ART. PWH in rural areas were also less likely to be prescribed newer antiretroviral agents than those living in urban areas (Schafer, 2017). In one study from the US Veteran's Administration, PWH in rural areas had more advanced HIV infection at diagnosis than those in urban areas, and the mortality hazard ratio for rural PWH versus urban PWH was 1.34 (Ohl, 2012). Additional barriers to care for PWH in rural areas include stigma, lack of support services, and transportation difficulties.

Rural areas are also less likely than urban areas to have harm-reduction programs in place to reduce one of the root causes of HIV transmission. The 2014 outbreak of HIV in rural Scott County, Indiana, showcases the potential for rapid progression of HIV and hepatitis C through communities affected by the opioid epidemic. Currently in the United States, new opioid injectors reside primarily in nonurban areas, and opioid users who switch from oral formulations to injection use engage in injection practices with greater risk of HIV and hepatitis C transmission. The CDC estimates that the counties at greatest risk for an IDU-associated HIV outbreak are mostly rural, and this combined with high rates of poverty and lower educational attainment make rural areas particularly vulnerable (CDC, 2021). Hepatitis C similarly affects nonurban populations disproportionately, and many of the areas with highest rates of acute HCV in the United States are in rural Appalachian states (Schranz et al., 2018).

Clearly, to provide state-of-the-art healthcare to the large rural population of PWH, programs are needed to address barriers to care and stigma that PWH in rural areas face. Strategies that keep in mind the social determinants of health and the importance of involving local community members have proven to be most successful (Schafer et al., 2017). These include:

- Community engagement: involving community members in research and programming, such as lay health adviser interventions.

- Leveraging existing data sources: agreement on a universal definition of "rurality" in order to study and understand populations in rural areas more fully.

- Human resource capacity development: addressing the HIV care provider shortage in rural areas and conducting needs assessments of rural primary care providers to better understand knowledge gaps and training needs.

- Innovative service delivery: consideration of non-clinic-based locations to deliver HIV prevention and testing, such as emergency departments (EDs) or pharmacies, use of telehealth to reach remote patients, use of teleconferencing to connect specialists in urban areas with primary care providers in rural areas, and optimizing the use of technology including text messaging and app-based services.

Resources for rural HIV care are available through the National Rural Health Association and the Rural Health Information Hub. The Rural Health Information Hub includes an "HIV/AIDS Prevention and Treatment Toolkit" (available at: https://www.ruralhealthinfo.org/toolkits/hiv-aids). A web resource is available to locate nearby federally funded community health centers (US Department of Health and Human Resources; available at http://findahealthcenter.hrsa.gov/Search_HCC.aspx).

12.6 CARE OF MIGRANT AND IMMIGRANT PERSONS WITH HIV

DELIANA GARCIA, CLAIRE M. HUTKINS SEDA, AND LASZLO MADARAS

LEARNING OBJECTIVE

- Discuss the important distinction between "migrants" and "immigrants."

- Discuss the differences in HIV risk, presentation, and comorbidities among immigrants from different regions of the world.

- Discuss the impact of stigma on healthcare-seeking behavior, treatment adherences, and safe practices.

WHAT'S NEW?

- Migration is recognized as a social determinant of health (SDH) by the International Organization for Migration (IOM, 2009) and requires a careful assessment of the person beyond ethnicity and language preference.

KEY POINTS

- The complex combination of population characteristics and barriers to care requires a careful consideration of each person's circumstances when considering HIV risk, testing, treatment adherence, and perceived or experienced stigma.

- Research in these populations is challenging because of a myriad factors, including absence of accommodations in the study structure, recruitment issues, ethical challenges, and subgroup differentiation.

- A distinction in premigration transmission and intra/postmigration transmission appears when considering migrants from the Americas versus those from the African continent and Eastern Europe.

- Prevalence and incidence of HIV in Black and Indigenous people of color in the United States are higher than those of White people, and these populations have less access to care and treatment than do White populations.

- Among immigrant PWH, the prevalence and presentation of opportunistic infections (OIs) or coinfections differ from those of US-born PWH.

Migrants, those in the United States for a time-limited stay usually to engage in remunerated activity like farm work, and newly arrived immigrants, those who wish to resettle permanently in the United States, are largely from Mexico and Central and South America. A smaller percentage are from Africa and Asia (Radford, 2019). Some migrants and recent immigrants live and work in the United States without authorization, although it is unclear how many. A crucial characteristic of these target populations is its geographic instability and high mobility. Migrants, by definition, move frequently for work purposes, family reunification, or pursuit of safe haven, contributing to an unstable and stressful lifestyle (IOM, 2020).

A natural consequence of such mobility is that migrants face many barriers to accessing care. Migration and immigration—and the federally defined immigration status that migrants and immigrants hold as a result—prevent the acquisition and/or continuation of health insurance. Most people without authorization to live in the United States are not eligible for health insurance or are eligible only for private coverage that is prohibitively expensive. Those with authorization who are migrating within the United States may find it unfeasible to sign up for care after each move as health coverage is geographically fragmented. Mobility is just one negative SDH, a condition in which people are born, raised, work. Some SDHs include employment and working conditions, income and social status, social support and connectedness, environment and housing, access to health care and literacy, and gender issues (O' Laughlin, 2018). The discrepancies attributable to these categories shape individual health status and outcomes through their impact on intermediary determinants such as living conditions, psychosocial circumstances, behavioral and/or biological factors, and the health system itself (WHO, 2019). In addition to mobility, migrants and new immigrants face numerous negative SDHs that overlap and amplify each other. They frequently work in labor-based occupations with high risk for injury and illness (Levy et al., 2007). Low income; a lack of strong networks in the receiving communities; considerable social and cultural isolation, frequently the result of language barriers; economic limitations; cultural differences; and fear over immigration status are common SDHs among migrants and new immigrants. These SDHs limit migrants and new immigrants' access to HIV health education, testing, and treatment. They also reduce migrants and new immigrants' participation in data and surveys.

As a result, developing an accurate picture of the HIV epidemic among migrants and immigrants to the United States has been hampered by a lack of national data. The CDC only recently began tracking country of origin for PWH, and currently there are few national publications on the topic. Most published reports on HIV and immigrant populations are based on studies at the county, city, and state levels. An example is a report from a study conducted through the San Mateo County Health Department in California. Immigrants within the study population presented with lower CD4[+] T-cell counts, were more likely to have an OI and be hospitalized at the time of HIV diagnosis. Immigration status was significantly associated with delayed presentation, although the study did not separate out newly arrived immigrants and long-term immigrants (Levy et al., 2007). A cross-sectional population-based survey conducted in Tijuana, Mexico, found that repeat male migrants returning from their home communities were more likely to have sex with men, not use a condom, and use substances before sex (Zhang et al., 2017). Historically, such local epidemiologic studies have been the predominant method for assessing need and planning services for immigrant populations.

A 2018 review of published literature since 2015 on known HIV outcomes among migrants from low- and middle-income countries living in high-income countries suggests that a high proportion of migrants acquire HIV after migration and are disproportionally affected by HIV (Ross et al., 2018). Migrants from Latin America and the Caribbean have the highest rates of postmigration infection, and migrants from Africa have the lowest.

Research in these populations is challenging, as migrants living with HIV are difficult to identify and monitor. The combination of factors such as stigma, along with increased risk behaviors and reluctance to use condoms or seek testing, increases the risk of migrants acquiring HIV infection (Ross et al., 2018). High levels of mobility are predictive of poor engagement in HIV care and ART disruption (Ross et al., 2018). Reliance on the community for daily survival may negatively affect care seeking and adherence if the migrant living with HIV fears ostracism from the social group. Studies of sexual practices among male migrants note riskier behaviors such as sex with casual female partners and sex workers, condomless anal and vaginal intercourse, and substance use, likely while transiting or in the receiving country. For example, in Mexico, after MSM, the greatest risk for HIV transmission is among those who have migrated to the United States or had a partner who migrated (Hirsch et al., 2002, 2007). Poor HIV outcomes are primarily driven by stigma and limited access to care (Ross et al., 2018). Additionally, there is limited evidence on appropriate interventions for migrants living with HIV.

Among immigrants, the picture is slightly clearer, although the available data do not segment newly arrived immigrants from those who may have lived in the United States for many years. HIV was diagnosed in 191,697 persons in the United States between 2007 and 2010, with 16.2% among those born outside the United States. Nearly half of those diagnosed with HIV for whom a specific country or region of birth outside of the United States was known were from Central America and Mexico. A little more than 20% were from the Caribbean, and approximately 15% were from Africa. California, Florida, New York, and Texas reported the highest numbers of persons born outside the United States diagnosed with HIV. They are also the states with the highest overall case rates. Slightly more than 73% of persons born outside the United States living with HIV were male. The racial breakdown for persons PWH born outside of the United States were: 3.3% White, 10% Black, 42.2% Hispanic, and 64.3% Asian. Thirty-nine percent of persons born outside of the United States were infected through heterosexual contact versus 27.2% for US-born persons (Prosser et al., 2012).

The COVID-19 pandemic widened preexisting health disparities. PWH experienced a reduction of access for HIV services as health systems shifted focus to COVID-related care. Disrupted treatment regimens, stalled or discontinued preventive services and educational opportunities, and overwhelmed health care facilities contributed to an estimated 10 years' loss of advances in HIV/TB care. Additionally, those with the worst outcomes hospitalized with serious COVID-19 infection were often patients with compromised immune systems from poorly controlled HIV or complicated by chemotherapy for cancer, immunosuppressive medications after organ transplant, and taking medications to suppress chronic autoimmune diseases (Trajman et al., 2022).

In 2022 the emergence of monkeypox on a global scale presents new challenges for health care workers treating HIV. While monkeypox thus far has not been as lethal to immunocompetent individuals as historical smallpox, those with poor immune systems, especially in places where HIV medication are not readily available, have increased morbidity and mortality. The US public health system is insufficiently comprehensive to be able to respond to emerging health concerns or crises without diverting resources from HIV care, which compromises the gains that have been achieved over years of HIV focus (CDC, 2022).

Migrants and newly arrived immigrants living with HIV are vulnerable to numerous comorbidities. Tuberculosis (TB) is the most-common presenting comorbidity among migrant and immigrant PWH. In regions of the world where TB is endemic, the *Mycobacterium tuberculosis* (MTB) can persist for years in a person who has been exposed yet has not developed active disease. TB can progress from infection to active disease if the PWH has a suppressed CD4$^+$ count, and it can involve every organ system. Some of the typical medications used in treating MTB must be used with caution in patients also being treated for HIV. For example, when coadministered with the MTB medication rifampin, concentrations of many protease inhibitors are severely diminished compromising HIV treatment efficacy, yet simultaneous treatment of HIV and MTB can greatly improve global survival in vulnerable populations. Extrapulmonary TB should be considered if the person presents with fatigue, weakness, weight loss, and fever, but without an active productive cough. ART may be more toxic in persons with chronic hepatitis and the prevalence of HBV infection in Asian immigrants may complicate attempts to treat HIV. OIs not usually seen in US-born persons may present in immigrant PWH, reflecting the epidemiology of their country of origin. Examples include *Penicillium marnefii* in persons of Southeast Asian origin, and a variety of parasitic diseases in persons of African descent.

Immigrants and migrants face significant barriers to access medical care, including for diagnosis and treatment of HIV and comorbidities. Efforts to reduce these barriers should include legislation that will support and enhance the public health system, improved access to HIV services, better epidemiologic data on immigrants to the United States living with HIV, and enhanced training and support for healthcare providers who serve immigrant populations. Often crucial to success in working with migrant and immigrant populations is the utilization of a team approach involving interpreters, social workers, and case managers, including virtual case management to support immigrants between care sites; hiring of cultural-appropriate staff; inclusion of peer navigators and community health workers; networking with local community-based organizations working with the impacted populations; Ryan White Program and 340B Pharmacy access; and legal services. The CDC has a useful website dedicated to immigrant and refugee health issues (http://www.cdc.gov/immigrantrefugeehealth).

REFERENCES

Aberg JA. Aging and HIV infection: focus on cardiovascular disease risk. *Top Antivir Med.* 2020;27(4):102–105. https://www.ncbi.nlm.nih.gov/pubmed/32224501

Abma JC, Martinez GM. Sexual activity and contraceptive use among teenagers in the United States, 2011–2015. National Health Statistics Reports, Hyattsville, MD; 2017.

Ahmadi GH, Fararouei M, Mirzazadeh A, et al. The global and regional prevalence of hepatitis C and B co-infections among prisoners living with HIV: a systematic review and meta-analysis. *Infect Dis Poverty.* 2021;10(1):93. https://doi.org/10.1186/s40249-021-00876-7

Aidala AA, Wilson MH, Shubert V, et al. Housing status, medical care, and health outcomes among people living with HIV/AIDS: a systematic review. *Am J Pub Health.* 2016;106(1):e1–e23. https://doi.org/10.2105/AJPH.2015.302905

Alvarez H, Marino A, Garcia-Rodriguez JF, et al. Immune reconstitution in inflammatory syndrome in an HIV-infected patient using subcutaneous silicone fillers. *AIDS.* 2016;30(16):2561–2563.

Armbruster M, Fields EL, Campbell N, et al. Addressing health inequities exacerbated by COVID-19 among youth with HIV: expanding our toolkit. *J Adolesc Health.* 2020;67(2):290–295. http://doi:10.1016/j.jadohealth.2020.05.021

Arrington-Sanders R, Leonard L, Brooks D, et al. Older partner selection in young African-American men who have sex with men. *J Adolesc Health.* 2013;52(6):682–688. http://doi:10.1016/j.jadohealth.2012.12.011

Arrington-Sanders R, Alvarenga A, Galai N, et al. Social determinants of transactional sex in a sample of young black and Latinx sexual minority cisgender men and transgender women. *J Adolesc Health.* 2022;70(2):275–281. http://doi:10.1016/j.jadohealth.2021.08.002

Asscheman H, Giltay EJ, Megens JAJ, et al. A long-term follow-up study of mortality in transsexuals receiving treatment with cross-sex hormones. *Eur J Endocrinol.* 2011;164(4):635–642.

Audain G, Bookhardt-Murray LJ, Fogg CJ, et al. (Eds.). *Adapting your practice: treatment and recommendations for unstably housed patients with HIV/AIDS.* Nashville, TN: Health Care for the Homeless Clinicians' Network, National Health Care for the Homeless Council; 2013.

Azbel L, Polonsky M, Wegman M, et al. Intersecting epidemics of HIV, HCV, and syphilis among soon-to-be released prisoners in Kyrgyzstan: Implications for prevention and treatment. *Int J Drug Policy.* 2016;37:9–20. https://doi.org/10.1016/j.drugpo.2016.06.007

Azbel L, Wegman MP, Polonsky M, et al. Drug injection within prison in Kyrgyzstan: elevated HIV risk and implications for scaling up opioid agonist treatments. *Int J Prison Health.* 2018;14(3):175–187. https://doi.org/10.1108/IJPH-03-2017-0016

Bacon O, Chin J, Cohen SE, et al. Decreased time from HIV diagnosis to care, ART initiation, and virologic suppression during the citywide RAPID initiative in San Francisco. *Clin Infect Dis.* 2021;73(1):e122–e128. http://doi.org/10.1093/cid/ciaa620

Bacon OML, Coffey SC, Hsu LC, et al. Development of a citywide rapid antiretroviral therapy initiative in San Francisco. *Am J Prev Med.* 2021;61(5 Suppl 1):S47–S54. https://doi.org/10.1016/j.amepre.2021.06.001

Badowski ME, Patel M. Evaluation of immunologic and virologic function in reincarcerated patients living with HIV or AIDS. *J Correct Health Care.* 2022;28(3):203–206. https://doi.org/10.1089/jchc.20.07.0055

Baggett TP, Lebrun-Harris LA, Rigotti NA. Homelessness, cigarette smoking and desire to quit: results from a US national study. *Addiction.* 2013;108(11):2009–2018. http://doi.10.1111/add.12292

Baranyi G, Fazel S, Langerfeldt SD, Mundt AP. The prevalence of comorbid serious mental illnesses and substance use disorders in prison populations: a systematic review and meta-analysis. *Lancet Public Health.* 2022;7(6):e557–e568. https://doi.org/10.1016/S2468-2667(22)00093-7

Baranyi G, Scholl C, Fazel S, et al. Severe mental illness and substance use disorders in prisoners in low-income and middle-income countries: a systematic review and meta-analysis of prevalence studies. *Lancet Glob Health.* 2019;7(4):e461–e471. https://doi.org/10.1016/S2214-109X(18)30539-4

Barnes W, D'Angelo L, Yamazaki M, et al. Identification of HIV-infected 12–24-year-old men and women in 15 cities through venue-based testing. *Arch Pediatr Adolesc Med.* 2010;164:273–276.

Bavinton BR, Pinto AN, Phanuphak N, et al. Viral suppression and HIV transmission in serodiscordant male couples: an international, prospective, observational, cohort study. *Lancet HIV.* 2018;5(8):e438–e447. http://doi:10.1016/S2352-3018(18)30132-2

Becasen JS, Denard CL, Mullins MM, et al. Estimating the prevalence of HIV and sexual behaviors among the US transgender population: a systematic review and meta-analysis, 2006–2017. *Am J Public Health.* 2019;109(1):e1–e8. http://doi:10.2105/AJPH.2018.304727

Berry SA, Ghanem KG, Mathews WC, et al. Brief report: gonorrhea and chlamydia testing increasing but still lagging in HIV clinics in the United States. *J AIDS.* 2015;70(3):275–279. http://doi:10.1097/QAI.0000000000000711

Beyrer C, Pozniak A. HIV drug resistance—an emerging threat to epidemic control. *N Engl J Med.* 2017;377(17):1605–1607. https://doi.org/10.1056/NEJMp1710608

Blue C, Buchbinder M, Brown ME, et al. Access to HIV care in jails: perspectives from people living with HIV in North Carolina. *PLoS One.* 2022;17(1):e0262882. https://doi.org/10.1371/journal.pone.0262882

Blunt M. US: detention hazardous to immigrants' health. Humans Rights Watch. https://www.hrw.org/report/2017/05/08/systemic-indifference/dangerous-substandard-medical-care-us-immigration-detention. Published 2017. Accessed September 15, 2022.

Bolland MJ, Grey A. Antiretroviral preexposure prophylaxis for HIV prevention. *N Engl J Med.* 2013;368:82.

Boone MR, Cherenack EM, Wilson PA, et al. Self-efficacy for sexual risk reduction and partner HIV status as correlates of sexual beliefs about biological differences between blacks and whites. *AIDS Patient Care STDS.* 2015;29(6):346–353.

Bovell-Ammon BJ, Xuan Z, Paasche-Orlow MK, LaRochelle MR. Association of incarceration with mortality by race from a national longitudinal cohort study. *JAMA Netw Open.* 2021;4(12):e2133083. https://doi.org/10.1001/jamanetworkopen.2021.33083

Bowleg L, Malekzadeh AN, Mbaba M, Boon CA. Ending the HIV epidemic for all, not just some: structural racism as a fundamental but overlooked social-structural determinant of the US HIV epidemic. *Curr Opin HIV AIDS.* 2022;17(2):40–45.

Boyer CB, Hightow-Weidman L, Bether J, et al. An assessment of the feasibility and acceptability of a friendship-based social network recruitment strategy to screen at-risk African American and Hispanic/Latina young women for HIV infection. *JAMA Pediatr.* 2013;3:289–296. http://doi:10.1001/2013.jamapediatrics.398

Branson BM, Handsfield H, Lampe M, et al. Revised recommendations for HIV testing of adults, adolescents, and pregnant women in healthcare settings. *MMWR.* 2006;55(RR-14):1–17.

Brinkley-Rubinstein L, Dauria E, Tolou-Shams M, et al. The path to implementation of HIV pre-exposure prophylaxis for people involved in criminal justice systems. *Curr HIV/AIDS Rep.* 2018;15(2):93–95. https://doi.org/10.1007/s11904-018-0389-9

Brown HD, DeFulio A. Contingency management for the treatment of methamphetamine use disorder: a systematic review. *Drug Alcohol Depend.* 2020;216:108307. http://doi: 10.1016/j.drugalcdep.2020.108307

Brown GR, Jones KT. Incidence of breast cancer in a cohort of 5,135 transgender veterans. *Breast Cancer Res Treat.* 2015;149(1):191–198. http://doi.org/10.1007/ s10549-014-3213-2

Bruce D, Harper GW, Fernandez IM, et al. Age-concordant and age-discordant sexual behavior among gay and bisexual male adolescents. *Arch Sex Behav*. 2012;41(2):441–448. http://doi:10.1007/s10508-011-9730-8

Buchbinder M, Blue C, Juengst E, et al. Expert stakeholders' perspectives on a Data-to-Care strategy for improving care among HIV-positive individuals incarcerated in jails. *AIDS Care*. 2020;32(9):1155–1161. https://doi.org/10.1080/09540121.2020.1737641

Buchbinder SP, Havlir DV. Getting to zero San Francisco: a collective impact approach. *J Acquir Immune Defic Syndr*. 2019;82(Suppl 3):S176–S182. https://doi.org/10.1097/QAI.0000000000002200

Buchanan A, Montepiedra G, Sirois PA, et al. Barriers to medication adherence in HIV-infected children and youth based on self- and caregiver report. *Pediatrics*. 2012;129(5):e1244–e1251. http://doi:10.1542/peds.2011-1740

Bukowski LA, Chandler CJ, Creasy SL, et al. Identifying barriers and facilitators to HIV diagnosis and viral suppression among black transgender women in the United States. *J Acquir Immune Defic Syndr*. 2018;79(4):413–420.

Busch-Geertsema V, Culhane D, Fitzpatrick S. Developing a global framework for conceptualising and measuring homelessness. *Habitat International*. 2016;55:124–132. http://doi:10.1016/j.habitat int.2016.03.004

Cabral HJ, Davis-Plourde K, Sarango M, et al. Peer support and the HIV continuum of care: results from a multi-site randomized clinical trial in three urban clinics in the United States. *AIDS Behav*. 2018;22(8):2627–2639. http://doi:org/10.1007/s10461-017-1999-8

Cahill S, Makadon H. Sexual orientation and gender identity data collection in clinical settings and in electronic health records: a key to ending LGBT health disparities. LGBT Health. http:// online.liebertpub.com/doi/abs/10.1089/lgbt.2013.0001. Published 2013. Accessed September 15, 2022.

Cahill S, Makadon HJ. Sexual orientation and gender identity data collection update: US government takes steps to promote sexual orientation and gender identity data collection through meaningful use guidelines. LGBT Health. http:// doi.org/10.1089/lgbt.2014.0033. Published 2014. Accessed September 15, 2022.

Campbell ANC, Wolff M, Weaver L, et al. "It's never just about the HIV:" HIV primary care providers' perception of substance use in the era of "universal" antiretroviral medication treatment. *AIDS Behav*. 2018;22(3):1006–1017. https://doi.org/10.1007/s10461-017-2007-z

Carter J, Zevin B, Lum PJ. 2019. Low barrier buprenorphine treatment for persons experiencing homelessness and injecting heroin in San Francisco. *Addict Sci Clin Pract*. 2019;14(1):20. http://doi:org/10.1186/s13722-019-0149-1

Castilho JL, Bian A, Jenkins CA, et al. CD4/CD8 ratio and cancer risk among adults with HIV. *J Natl Cancer Inst*. 2022;114(6):854–862. https://doi.org/10.1093/jnci/djac053

Centers for Disease Control and Prevention (CDC). Behavioral and clinical characteristics of persons with diagnosed HIV infection—medical monitoring project, United States, 2020 cycle (June 2020–May 2021). HIV Surveillance Special Report 29. cdc.gov. https://www.cdc.gov/hiv/library/reports/hiv-surveillance.html. Published 2022. Accessed September 15, 2022.

CDC. CDC recommendations for correctional and detention settings. cdc.gov. https://www.cdc.gov/nchhstp/dear_colleague/2022/dcl-041822-correctional-health.html. Published August 19, 2022. Accessed September 15, 2022.

CDC. Health equity considerations and racial and ethnic minority groups. https://www.cdc.gov/coronavirus/2019-ncov/need-extra-precautions/racial-ethnic-minorities.html. Published 2020c. Accessed September 27, 2022.

CDC. HIV and African Americans, 2018. cdc.gov. https://www.cdc.gov/hiv/group/racialethnic/africanamericans/index.html). Published 2020a. Accessed July 26, 2022.

CDC. *HIV surveillance report, 2018 (Updated)*; vol. 31. cdc.gov. http://www.cdc.gov/hiv/library/reports/hiv-surveillance.html. Published May 2020. Accessed July 26, 2020b.

CDC. HIV surveillance report, 2020; vol. 33. cdc.gov. https://www.cdc.gov/hiv/library/reports/hiv-surveillance.html. Published May 2022. Accessed October 22, 2022.

CDC. Life-saving naloxone from pharmacies. cdc.gov. https:// www.cdc.gov/vitalsigns/naloxone/index.html#:~:text=Naloxone%20is%20a%20life-saving%20medication%20that%20can%20reverse,standing%20orders%29%2C%20which%20have%20contributed%20to%20lowering%20deaths. Published 2019. Accessed October 19, 2022.

CDC. Vulnerable counties and jurisdictions experiencing or at-risk of outbreaks. cdc.gov. https://www.cdc.gov/pwid/vulnerable-counties-data.html. August 31, 2021. Accessed August 8, 2022.

CDC and US Public Health Service. Preexposure prophylaxis for the prevention of HIV infection in the United States—2021 update: a clinical practice guideline. https://www.cdc.gov/hiv/pdf/risk/prep/cdc-hiv-prep-guidelines-2021.pdf. Published 2021. Accessed January 24, 2023.

Chang J, Shelly S, Busz M, et al. Peer driven or driven peers? A rapid review of peer involvement of people who use drugs in HIV and harm reduction services in low- and middle-income countries. *Harm Reduct J*. 2021;18(1):15. https://doi.org/10.1186/s12954-021-00461-z

Christopoulos KA, Grochowski J, Mayorga-Munoz F et al. First demonstration project for long-acting injectable antiretroviral therapy for persons with and without detectable HIV viremia in an urban HIV clinic. *Clin Infect Dis*. 2023;76(3):e645–e651. http://doi: 10.1093/cid/ciac631

Choopanya K, Martin M, Suntharasamai P, et al. Antiretroviral prophylaxis for HIV infection in injecting drug users in Bangkok, Thailand (the Bangkok Tenofovir Study): a randomised, double-blind, placebo-controlled phase 3 trial. *Lancet*. 2013;381(9883):2083–2090. https://doi.org/10.1016/s0140-6736(13)61127-7

Clark RF, Cantrell FL, Pacal A, et al. Subcutaneous silicone injection leading to multi-system organ failure. *Clin Toxicol*. 2008;46(9):834–837. http://doi.org/10.1080/15563650701850025

Clemenzi-Allen A, Geng E, Christopoulos K, et al. Degree of housing instability shows independent 'dose-response' with virologic suppression rates among people living with human immunodeficiency virus. *Open Forum Infect Dis*. 2018;5(3):ofy035. http://doi: org/10.1093/ofid/ofy035

Clemenzi-Allen A, Neuhaus J, Geng E, et al. Housing instability results in increased acute care utilization in an urban HIV clinic cohort. *Open Forum Infect Dis*. 2019;6(5):ofz148. http://doi:org/10.1093/ofid/ofz148

Clum G, Chung SE, Ellen JM. Mediators of HIV-related stigma and risk behavior in HIV infected young women. *AIDS Care*. 2009;2(11):1455–1462.

Coffey S, Bacchetti P, Sachdev D, et al. RAPID antiretroviral therapy: high virologic suppression rates with immediate antiretroviral therapy initiation in a vulnerable urban clinic population. *AIDS*. 2019;33(5):825–832. http://doi:10.1097/QAD.0000000000002124

Cohen D, Farley T, Taylor S, et al. When and where do youths have sex? The potential role of adult supervision. *Pediatrics*. 2002;110:1–6.

Cohen MS, Chen YQ, McCauley M, et al. Antiretroviral therapy for the prevention of HIV-1 transmission. *N Engl J Med*. 2016;375(9):830–839. http://doi:10.1056/NEJMoa1600693

Colby D, Srithanaviboonchai K, Vanichseni S, et al. HIV pre-exposure prophylaxis and health and community systems in the Global South: Thailand case study. *J Int AIDS Soc*. 2015;18(4 Suppl 3):19953. https://doi.org/10.7448/IAS.18.4.19953

Coleman E, Bockting W, Botzer M, et al. Standards of care for the health of transsexual, transgender, and gender-nonconforming people, version 7. *Intl J Transgenderism*. 2012;13(4):165–232.

Colfax G, Philip S, Enanoria W, et al. *HIV epidemiology: annual report*, 2020. San Francisco: San Francisco Department of Public Health; 2021.

Collins PY, Velloza J, Concepcion T, et al. Intervening for HIV prevention and mental health: a review of global literature. *J Int AIDS Soc*. 2021;24S2:e25710. https://doi.org/10.1002/jia2.25710

Colton Meier SL, Fitzgerald KM, Pardo ST, et al. The effects of hormonal gender affirmation treatment on mental health in female-to-male transsexuals. *J Gay Lesbian Mental Health.* 2011;15(3):281–299.

Conte M, Eshun-Wilson I, Geng E, et al. Understanding preferences for HIV care among patients experiencing homelessness or unstable housing: a discrete choice experiment. *J Acquir Immune Defic Syndr.* 2020;85(4):444–49. http://doi: 10.1097/QAI.0000000000002476

Costa M, Montague BT, Solomon L, et al. Assessing the effect of recent incarceration in prison on HIV care retention and viral suppression in two states. *J Urban Health.* 2018;95(4):499–507. https://doi.org/10.1007/s11524-018-0255-5

Crable EL, Blue TR, McKenzie M, et al. Effect of case management on HIV outcomes for community corrections population: results of an 18-month randomized controlled trial. *J Acquir Immune Defic Syndr.* 2021;87(1):755–762. https://doi.org/10.1097/QAI.0000000000002624

Craw JA, Gardner LI, Marks G, et al. Brief strengths-based case management promotes entry into HIV medical care: results of the antiretroviral treatment access study-II. *JAIDS.* 2008;(5):597–606. http://doi:10.1097/QAI.0b013e3181684c51

Culbert GJ. Violence and the perceived risks of taking antiretroviral therapy in US jails and prisons. *Int J Prison Health.* 2014;10(2):94–110. https://doi.org/10.1108/IJPH-05-2013-0020

Cunningham WE, Weiss RE, Nakazono T, et al. Effectiveness of a peer navigation intervention to sustain viral suppression among HIV-positive men and transgender women released from jail: the LINK LA randomized clinical trial. *JAMA Intern Med.* 2018;178(4):542–553. http://doi:10.1001/jamainternmed.2018.0150

Dauria EF, Kulkarni P, Clemenzi-Allen A, et al. Interventions designed to improve HIV continuum of care outcomes for persons with HIV in contact with the carceral system in the USA. *Curr HIV/AIDS Rep.* 2022;19(4):281–291. https://doi.org/10.1007/s11904-022-00609-x

Dauria EF, Levine A, Hill SV, et al. Multilevel factors shaping awareness of and attitudes toward pre-exposure prophylaxis for HIV prevention among criminal justice-involved women. *Arch Sex Behav.* 2021;50(4):1743–1754. https://doi.org/10.1007/s10508-020-01834-4

Davey S, Ajibola G, Maswabi K, et al. Mother-to-child HIV transmission with in utero dolutegravir vs. efavirenz in Botswana. *J Acquir Immune Defic Syndr.* 2020;84(3):235–241.

Dawit R, Trepka MJ, Gbadamosi SO, et al. Latent class analysis of syndemic factors associated with sustained viral suppression among Ryan White HIV/AIDS program clients in Miami, 2017. *AIDS Behav.* 2021;25(7):2252–2258. http://doi:10.1007/s10461-020-03153-0

Degenhardt L, Peacock A, Colledge S, et al. Global prevalence of injecting drug use and sociodemographic characteristics and prevalence of HIV, HBV, and HCV in people who inject drugs: a multistage systematic review. *Lancet Glob Health.* 2017;5(12):e1192–e1207. https://doi.org/10.1016/S2214-109X(17)30375-3

Department of Health and Human Services (DHHS). Panel on Antiretroviral Guidelines for Adults and Adolescents: guidelines for the use of antiretroviral agents in adults and adolescents with HIV. Department of Health and Human Services. https://clinicalinfo.hiv.gov/en/guidelines/adult-and-adolescent-arv. Published 2022. Accessed September 26, 2022.

Desai AM, Browning J, Rosen T. Etanercept therapy for silicone granuloma. *J Drugs Dermatol.* 2006;5(9):894–896.

Deutsch MB. Pre-exposure prophylaxis in trans populations: providing gender-affirming prevention for trans people at high risk of acquiring HIV. *LGBT Health.* October 2018;5(7):387–390.

Deutsch MB. Gender-affirming surgeries in the era of insurance coverage: Developing a framework for psychosocial support and care navigation in the perioperative period. *J Health Care Poor Underserved.* 2016;27(2):386–391.

Deutsch MB, Bhakri V, Kubicek K. Effects of cross-sex hormone treatment on transgender women and men. *Obstet Gynecol.* 2015a;125(3):605–610.

Deutsch MB, Glidden DV, Sevelius J, et al. HIV pre-exposure prophylaxis in transgender women: a subgroup analysis of the iPrEx trial. *Lancet HIV.* 2015b;2(12):e512–519. http:// doi.org/10.1016/S2352-3018(15)00206-4

Deutsch MB, Green J, Keatley J, et al. (2013). Electronic medical records and the transgender patient: Recommendations from the World Professional Association for Transgender Health EMR Working Group. *J Am Med Informat Assoc.* 2013;20(4):700–703. http://doi.org/ 10.1136/amiajnl-2012-001472

Deutsch MB, Reisner SL, Peitzmeier S, et al. Recent penile sexual contact is associated with an increased odds of high-risk cervical human papillomavirus infection in transgender men. *Sex Transm Dis.* 2020;47(1):48–53.

DiCarlo MC, Dallabetta GA, Akolo C, et al. Adequate funding of comprehensive community-based programs for key populations needed now more than ever to reach and sustain HIV targets. *J Int AIDS Soc.* 2022;25(7):e25967. https://doi.org/10.1002/jia2.25967

Dolan K, Wirtz AL, Moazen B, Ndeffo-Mbah, M., et al. Global burden of HIV, viral hepatitis, and tuberculosis in prisoners and detainees. *Lancet.* 2016;388(10049):1089–1102. https://doi.org/10.1016/S0140-6736(16)30466-4

Dong KR, Daudelin DH, Koutoujian PJ, et al. Lessons learned from the Pathways to Community Health Study to evaluate the transition of care from jail to community for men with HIV. *AIDS Patient Care STDS.* 2021;35(9):360–369. https://doi.org/10.1089/apc.2021.0060

Dombrowski JC, Galagan SR, Ramchandani M, et al. HIV care for patients with complex needs: a controlled evaluation of a walk-in, incentivized care model. *Open Forum Infect Dis.* 2019;6(7):ofz294. http://doi:10.1093/ofid/ofz294

Dombrowski JC, Hughes JP, Buskin SE, et al. A cluster randomized evaluation of a health department data to care intervention designed to increase engagement in HIV Care and antiretroviral use. *Sex Transm Dis.* 2018a;45 (6):361–367. https://doi.org/10.1097/OLQ.0000000000000760

Dombrowski JC, Ramchandani M, Dhanireddy S, et al. The Max Clinic: medical care designed to engage the hardest-to-reach persons living with HIV in Seattle and King County, Washington. *AIDS Patient Care STDs.* 2018b;32 (4):149–156. https://doi.org/10.1089/apc.2017.031

Dombrowski JC, Simoni JM, Katz DA, et al. Barriers to HIV care and treatment among participants in a public health HIV care relinkage program. *AIDS Patient Care STDs.* 2015;29(5):279–87. http://doi: 10.1089/apc.2014.0346

Dowshen N, Binns HJ, Garofalo R. Experiences of HIV-related stigma among young men who have sex with men. *AIDS Patient Care STDS.* 2009;23(5):371–376. http://doi:10.1089/apc.2008.0256

Duko B, Ayalew M, Ayano G. The prevalence of alcohol use disorders among people living with HIV/AIDS: a systematic review and meta-analysis. *Subst Abuse Treat Prev Policy.* 2019;14(1):52. http://doi:10.1186/s13011-019-0240-3

Eaton LA, Driffin DD, Kegler C, et al. The role of stigma and medical mistrust in the routine healthcare engagement of black men who have sex with men. *Am J Public Health.* 2015;105(2):75–82.

El-Bassel N, Gilbert L, Goddard-Eckrich D, et al. Effectiveness of a couple-based HIV and sexually transmitted infection prevention intervention for men in community supervision programs and their female sexual partners: a randomized clinical trial. *JAMA Netw Open.* 2019;2(3):e191139. https://doi.org/10.1001/jamanetworkopen.2019.1139

El-Ibiary SY, Cocohoba JM. Effects of HIV antiretrovirals on the pharmacokinetics of hormonal contraceptives. *Eur J Contraception Reproduc Health Care.* 2008;13(2):123–132. http:// doi.org/10.1080/13625180701829952

Farel CE, Golin CE, Ochtera RD, et al. Underutilization of HIV testing among men with incarceration histories. *AIDS Behav.* 2019;23(4):883–892. https://doi.org/10.1007/s10461-018-02381-9

Fauci AS, Redfield RR, Sigounas G, et al. Ending the HIV epidemic: a plan for the United States. *JAMA.* 2019;321(9):844–845. http://doi: 10.1001/jama.2019.1343

Fernandez M, Collazo JB, Bowen GS et al. Predictors of HIV testing and intention to test among Hispanic farmworkers in South Florida. *J Rural Health*. 2005;21(1):56–64.

Flores AR, Herman JL, Gates GJ, et al. How many adults identify as transgender in the United States? The Williams Institute. https://williamsinstitute.law.ucla.edu/wp-content/ uploads/How-Many-Adults-Identify-as-Transgender-in-the United-States.pdf. Published June 2016. Accessed January 25, 2023.

Fuge TG, Tsourtos G, Miller ER. A systematic review and meta-analyses on initiation, adherence and outcomes of antiretroviral therapy in incarcerated people. *PLoS One*. 2020;15(5):e0233355. https://doi.org/10.1371/journal.pone.0233355

Gabrielli E, Ferraioli G, Ferraris L, et al. Enfuvirtide administration in HIV-positive transgender patient with soft tissue augmentation: US evaluation. *New Microbiologica*. 2010;33:263–265.

Gamarel KE, Nelson KM, Brown L, et al. The usefulness of the CRAFFT in screening for problematic drug and alcohol use among youth living with HIV. *AIDS Behav*. 2017;21(7):1868–1877. http://doi:10.1007/s10461-016-1640-2

Garcia CM, Kushel MB. Integrating mental health and substance use treatment with HIV care for people experiencing homelessness. *Lancet Psych*. 2022;9(8):606–608. http://doi: 10.1016/S2215-0366(22)00228-0

Garrison LE, Haberer JE. Pre-exposure prophylaxis uptake, adherence, and persistence: a narrative review of interventions in the U.S. *Am J Prev Med*. 2021;61(5 Suppl 1): S73–S86. https://doi.org/10.1016/j.amepre.2021.04.036

Geller JM. Street medicine: caring for the pets of the homeless. *J Am Vet Med Assoc*. 2022;260(2):181–185. http://doi:10.2460/javma.21.05.0249

Glasner-Edwards S, Mooney LJ. Methamphetamine psychosis: epidemiology and management. *CNS Drugs*. 2014;28(12):1115–1126. http://doi: 10.1007/s40263-014-0209-8

Goldenberg T, McDougal S, Sullivan P, et al. Preferences for a mobile HIV prevention app for men who have sex with men. *JMIR Mhealth Uhealth*. 2014;2(4):e47. http://doi: 10.2196/mhealth.3745

Goldstein Z, Martinson T, Ramachandran S, et al. Improved rates of cervical cancer screening among transmasculine patients through self-collected swabs for high-risk human papillomavirus DNA testing. *Transgender Health*. February 28, 2020:trgh.2019.0019. http://doi:10.1089/trgh.2019.0019

Gómez-Gil E, Zubiaurre-Elorza L, Esteva I, et al. Hormone-treated transsexuals report less social distress, anxiety and depression. *Psychoneuroendocrinology*. 2012;37(5):662–670.

Gondwe A, Amberbir A, Singogo E, et al. Prisoners' access to HIV services in southern Malawi: a cross-sectional mixed methods study. *BMC Public Health*. 2021;21(1):813. https://doi.org/10.1186/s12889-021-10870-1

Gooren LJ, van Trotsenburg MAA, Giltay EJ, et al. Breast cancer development in transsexual subjects receiving cross-sex hormone treatment. *J Sexual Med*. 2013;10(12):3129–3134. http:// doi.org/10.1111/ jsm.12319

Grant RM, Lama JR, Anderson PL, et al. Preexposure chemoprophylaxis for HIV prevention in men who have sex with men. *N Eng J Med*. 2010;363(27):2587–2599.

Green, N, Hoenigl, M, Morris, S, et al. Risk behavior and sexually transmitted infections among transgender women and men undergoing community-based screening for acute and early HIV infection in San Diego. *Medicine*. 2015;94(41):e1830.

Griffin A, Dempsey A, Cousino W, et al. Addressing disparities in the health of persons with HIV attributable to unstable housing in the United States: the role of the Ryan White HIV/AIDS program. *PLoS Med*. 2020;17(3) e1003057. http://doi: 10.1371/journal.pmed.1003057

Grimes RM, Hallmark CJ, Watkins KL, et al. Re-engagement in HIV care: a clinical and public health priority. *J AIDS Clin Res*. 2016;7(2):543. https://doi.org/10.4172/2155-6113.1000543

Haldane V, Jung AS, De Foo C, et al. Integrating HIV and substance misuse services: a person-centred approach grounded in human rights. *Lancet Psych*. 2022;9(8):676–688. http://doi:10.1016/S2215-0366(22)00159-6

Health Resources and Services Administration. Ryan White HIV/AIDS program annual client-level data report 2020. www.hab.hrsa.gove/data/data-reports. Published December 2021. Accessed January 25, 2023.

Hembree WC, Cohen-Kettenis P, Gooren L, et al. Endocrine treatment of gender-dysphoric/ gender-incongruent persons: an endocrine society clinical practice guideline. *Endocr Pract*. 2017;23(12):1437.

Herman J, Flores AR, O'Neill KK. How many adults and youth identify as transgender in the US? The Williams Institute. https:// williamsinstitute.law.ucla.edu/wp-content/uploads/Trans-Pop-Update-Jun-2022.pdf. Published 2022. Accessed September 27, 2022.

Hessol NA, Eng M, Vu A, et al. A longitudinal study assessing differences in causes of death among housed and homeless people diagnosed with HIV in San Francisco. *BMC Pub Health*. 2019;19(1):1440. https://doi.org/10.1186/s12889-019-7817-7

Hickey MD, Imbert E, Appa A, J et al. HIV treatment outcomes in POP-UP: drop-in HIV primary care model for people experiencing homelessness. *J Infect Dis*. 2022;jiac267. http://doi: 10.1093/infdis/jiac267

Hiransuthikul A, Himmad K, Kerr S, et al. Drug-drug interactions between the use of feminizing hormone therapy and pre-exposure prophylaxis among transgender women: the iFACT study. TUPDX0107LB. Abstract/13177. http://programme.aids2018.org/Abstract/ 13177. Published 2018. Accessed September 15, 2022.

Hirsch J, Higgins J, Bentley M, Nathanson V. The social constructions of sexuality: marital infidelity and sexually transmitted disease–HIV risk in a Mexican migrant community. *Am J Public Health*. 2002;92(8):1227–1237.

Hirsch J, Meneses S, Thompson B, et al. The inevitability of infidelity: sexual reputation, social geographies, and marital HIV risk in rural Mexico. *Am J Public Health*. 2007;97(6):986–996.

Holtzman CW, Shea JA, Glanz K, et al. Mapping patient-identified barriers and facilitators to retention in HIV care and antiretroviral therapy adherence to Andersen's behavioral model. *AIDS Care*. 2015;27(7):817–828. https://doi.org/10.1080/09540121.2015.1009362

Housing and Urban Development (HUD). Continuum of Care Homeless Assistance Program homeless populations and subpopulations reports. HUD Exchange. https:// files.hudexchange.info/reports/published/CoC_PopSub_NatlTerrDC_2021.pdf. Published 2021. Accessed October 22, 2022.

Hunt GE, Malhi GS, Lai HMX, Cleary M. Prevalence of comorbid substance use in major depressive disorder in community and clinical settings, 1990–2019: systematic review and meta-analysis. *J Affect Disord*. 2020;266:288–304. https://doi.org/10.1016/j.jad.2020.01.141

Hutchinson AB, MacGowan RJ, Margolis AD, et al. Costs and consequences of eliminating a routine, point-of-care HIV screening program in a high-prevalence jail. *Am J Prev Med*. 2021;61(5 Suppl 1):S32–S38. https://doi.org/10.1016/j.amepre.2021.06.006

Ickovics JR. "Bundling" HIV prevention: integrating services to promote synergistic gain. *Prevent Med*. 2008;46(3):222–225. http://doi.org/ 10.1016/ j.ypmed.2007.09.006

Imbert E, Hickey MD, Clemenzi-Allen A, et al. Evaluation of the POP-UP Programme: a multicomponent model of care for people living with HIV with homelessness or unstable housing. *AIDS*. 2021;35(8):1241–1246. http://doi:10.1097/QAD.0000000000002843

Ingerski LM, Means B, Wang F, et al. Preventing medication nonadherence of youth (13–24 years) with HIV initiating antiretroviral therapy. *J Adolesc Health*. 2021;69(4):644–652. https://doi.org/10.1016/j.jadohealth.2021.04.006

International Organization for Migration. Key Migration Terms 2022. Available at https://www.iom.int/key-migration-terms. Published 2022. Accessed September 15, 2022.

Institutional racism—Wikipediaen.wikipedia.org › wiki › Institutional racism. Published 2022. Accessed September 15, 2022.

Iroh PA, Mayo H, Nijhawan AE. The HIV care cascade before, during, and after incarceration: a systematic review and data synthesis. *Am J Public Health.* 2015;105(7):e5–e16. https://doi.org/10.2105/AJPH.2015.302635

Iryawan AR, Stoicescu C, Sjahrial F, et al. The impact of peer support on testing, linkage to and engagement in HIV care for people who inject drugs in Indonesia: qualitative perspectives from a community-led study. *Harm Reduct J.* 2022;19(1):16. https://doi.org/10.1186/s12954-022-00595-8

Jakubowski A, Fox A. Defining low-threshold buprenorphine treatment. *Journal of Addict Med.* 2020;14(2):95–98. http://doi:10.1097/ADM.0000000000000555

James SE, Herman, JL, Rankin, S, et al. *The report of the 2015 U.S. Transgender Survey.* Washington, DC: National Center for Transgender Equality; 2016.

Javanbakht M, Boudov M, Anderson LJ, et al. Sexually transmitted infections among incarcerated women: findings from a decade of screening in a Los Angeles County jail, 2002–2012. *Am J Public Health.* 2014;104(11):e103–e109.

Johnson M, Samarina A, Xi H, et al. Barriers to access to care reported by women living with HIV across 27 countries. *AIDS Care.* 2015;27(10):1220–1230. http://doi:10.1080/09540121.2015.1046416

Jones AA, Gicas KM, Seyedin S, et al. Associations of substance use, psychosis, and mortality among people living in precarious housing or homelessness: a longitudinal, community-based study in Vancouver, Canada. *PLoS Med.* 2020;17(7):e1003172. http://doi: 10.1371/journal.pmed.1003172

Justiz Vaillant AA, Naik R HIV-1 associated opportunistic infections. *StatPearls.* https://www.ncbi.nlm.nih.gov/pubmed/30969609. Published 2022. Accessed September 1, 2022.

Kanazawa JT, Saberi P, Sauceda JA, et al. The LAIs are Coming! implementation science considerations for long-acting injectable antiretroviral Therapy in the United States: a scoping review. *AIDS Res Human Retrovir.* 2021;37(2):75–88. http://doi:10.1089/AID.2020.0126

Kearney BP, Mathias A. Lack of effect of tenofovir disoproxil fumarate on pharmacokinetics of hormonal contraceptives. *Pharmacotherapy.* 2009;29(8):924–929. http://doi.org/10.1592/phco.29.8.924

Khalili M, Powell J, Park HH, Bush D, et al. Shelter-based integrated model is effective in scaling up hepatitis C testing and treatment in persons experiencing homelessness. *Hepatol Comm.* 2022;6(1):50–64. http://doi:10.1002/hep4.1791

Khan J, Schmidt RL, Spittal MJ, et al. Venous thrombotic risk in transgender women undergoing estrogen therapy: a systematic review and meta-analysis. *Clin Chem.* 2019;65(1):57–66.

Kishimoto T, Hagi K, Kurokawa S, et al. Long-acting injectable versus oral antipsychotics for the maintenance treatment of schizophrenia: a systematic review and comparative meta-analysis of randomised, cohort, and pre–post studies. *Lancet Psychiatry.* 2021;8(5):387–404. http://doi:10.1016/S2215-0366(21)00039-0

Klein PW, Psihopaidas D, Xavier J, Cohen SM. HIV-related outcome disparities between transgender women living with HIV and cisgender people living with HIV served by the Health Resources and Services Administration's Ryan White HIV/AIDS program: a retrospective study. *PLoS Med.* 2020:17(5): e1003125. https://doi.org/10.1371/journal.pmed.1003125

Kluckow R, Zeng Z. *Correctional populations in the United States, 2020—statistical tables.* https://bjs.ojp.gov/library/publications/correctional-populations-united-states-2020-statistical-tables. Published 2022. Accessed September 1, 2022

Koay WL, Kose-Otieno J, Rakhmanina N. HIV drug resistance in children and adolescents: always a challenge? *Curr Epidemiol Rep.* 2021;8(3):97–107. http://doi:10.1007/s40471-021-00268-3

Koenig SP, Dorvil N, Devieux JG, et al. Same-day HIV testing with initiation of antiretroviral therapy versus standard care for persons living with HIV: a randomized unblinded trial. *PLoS Med.* 2017;14(7):e1002357. http://doi:10.1371/journal.pmed.1002357

Korthuis PT, Edelman EJ. Substance use and the HIV care continuum: important advances. *Addict Sci Clin Pract.* 2018;13(1):13. https://doi.org/10.1186/s13722-018-0114-4

Labhardt ND, Ringera I, Lejone TI, et al. Effect of offering same-day ART vs usual health facility referral during home-based HIV testing on linkage to care and viral suppression among adults with HIV in Lesotho: the CASCADE randomized clinical trial. *JAMA.* 2018;319(11):1103–1112.

Lakshmi S, Beekmann SE, Polgreen PM, et al. HIV primary care by the infectious disease physician in the United States: extending the continuum of care. *AIDS Care.* 2018;30(5):569–577. https://doi.org/10.1080/09540121.2017.1385720

Landovitz RJ, Donnell D, Clement ME, et al. Cabotegravir for HIV prevention in cisgender men and transgender women. *N Engl J Med.* 2021;385(7):595–608. http://doi:10.1056/NEJMoa2101016

Lathouwers E, Weinsteiger S, Baugh B, et al. Week 96 resistance analyses of the once-daily, single-tablet regimen (STR) darunavir/cobicistat/emtricitabine/tenofovir alafenamide (D/C/F/TAF) in adults living with HIV-1 from the phase 3 randomized AMBER and EMERALD trials. *J Med Virol.* 2021;93(6):3985–3990. https://doi.org/10.1002/jmv.26721

Levy V, Prentiss D, Balmas G, et.al. Factors in the delayed HIV presentation of immigrants in Northern California: implications for voluntary counseling and testing programs. *J Immigrant Minority Health.* 2007;9:49–54. https://doi.org/10.1007/s10903-006-9015-9

Lier AJ, Seval N, Vander Wyk B, et al. Maintenance on extended-release naltrexone is associated with reduced injection opioid use among justice-involved persons with opioid use disorder. *J Subst Abuse Treat.* 2022;142:108852. https://doi.org/10.1016/j.jsat.2022.108852

Lo E, Lifland B, Buelt EC, et al. Implementing the street psychiatry model in New Haven, CT: community-based care for people experiencing unsheltered homelessness. *Community Ment Health J.* 2021;57(8):1427–1434. http://doi:10.1007/s10597-021-00846-1

Loeliger KB, Altice FL, Desai MM, et al. Predictors of linkage to HIV care and viral suppression after release from jails and prisons: a retrospective cohort study. *Lancet HIV.* 2018a;5(2):e96–e106. https://doi.org/10.1016/S2352-3018(17)30209-6

Loeliger KB, Meyer JP, Desai MM, et al. Retention in HIV care during the 3 years following release from incarceration: a cohort study. *PLoS Med.* 2018b:15(10):e1002667. https://doi.org/10.1371/journal.pmed.1002667

Lucas KD, Bick J, Mohle-Boetani JC. California's Prisoner Protections for Family and Community Health Act: Implementing A Mandated Condom Access Program In State Prisons, 2015–2016. *Public Health Rep.* 2020;135(Suppl 1):50S–56S. https://doi.org/10.1177/0033354920920629

Lynch KA, Harris T, Jain SH, et al. The case for mobile "street medicine" for patients experiencing homelessness. *J Gen Intern Med.* June 9, 2022;37:3999–4001. http://doi: 10.1007/s11606-022-07689-w

Lyons CE, Schwartz SR, Murray SM, et al. The role of sex work laws and stigmas in increasing HIV risks among sex workers. *Nat Commun.* 2020;11(1):773. https://doi.org/10.1038/s41467-020-14593-6

Mabuto T, Woznica DM, Lekubu G, et al. Observational study of continuity of HIV care following release from correctional facilities in South Africa. *BMC Public Health.* 2020;20(1):324. https://doi.org/10.1186/s12889-020-8417-2

MacDonell KK, Jacques-Tiura AJ, Naar S, et al. Predictors of self-reported adherence to antiretroviral medication in a multisite study of ethnic and racial minority HIV-positive youth. *J Pediatr Psychol.* 2016;41(4):419–428. http://doi:10.1093/jpepsy/jsv097

Maiorana A, Sevelius J, Keatley J, Rebchook G. "She is like a sister to me." Gender-affirming services and relationships are key to the implementation of HIV care engagement interventions with transgender women of color. *AIDS Behav.* 2021;25(Suppl 1):72–83. https://doi.org/10.1007/s10461-020-02777-6

Maner M, Omori M, Brinkley-Rubinstein L, et al. Infectious disease surveillance in U.S. jails: findings from a national survey. *PLoS*

One. 2022;17(8):e0272374. https://doi.org/10.1371/journal.pone.0272374

Marcus JL, Volk JE, Pinder J, et al. Successful implementation of HIV preexposure prophylaxis: lessons learned from three clinical settings. *Curr HIV/AIDS Rep*. 2016;13(2):116–124. https://doi.org/10.1007/s11904-016-0308-x

Marrazzo JM, Ramjee G, Richardson BA, et al. Tenofovir-based pre-exposure prophylaxis for HIV infection among African women. *N Engl J Med*. 2015;372(6):509–518. http://doi.org/10.1056/NEJMoa1402269

Martin RA, Berk J, Rich JD, et al. Use of long-acting injectable buprenorphine in the correctional setting. *J Subst Abuse Treat*. 2022;142:108851. https://doi.org/10.1016/j.jsat.2022.108851

Maruschak LM. *HIV in prisons, 2020—statistical tables*. ojp.gov. https://www.ojp.gov/library/publications/hiv-prisons-2020-statistical-tables. Published 2022. Accessed August 25, 2022.

Masyukova MI, Hanna DB, Fox AD. HIV treatment outcomes among formerly incarcerated transitions clinic patients in a high prevalence setting. *Health Justice*. 2018;6(1):16. https://doi.org/10.1186/s40352-018-0074-5

Mayer KH, Krakower D. Antiretroviral medication and HIV prevention: new steps forward and new questions. *American College of Physicians*. 2012;156:312–314.

Mayer KH, Molina JM, Thompson MA, et al. Emtricitabine and tenofovir alafenamide vs emtricitabine and tenofovir disoproxil fumarate for HIV pre-exposure prophylaxis (DISCOVER): primary results from a randomised, double-blind, multicentre, active-controlled, phase 3, non-inferiority trial. *Lancet*. 2020;396(10246):239–254. http://doi.org/10.1016/S0140-6736(20)31065-5

Melendez RM, Pinto RM. HIV prevention and primary care for transgender women in a community-based clinic. *J Assoc Nurses AIDS Care*. 2009;20(5):387–397.

Minton DT, Zhen Z, BJS statisticians. *Jail inmates in 2020: statistical tables*. bjs.ojp.gov. https://bjs.ojp.gov/library/publications/jail-inmates-2020-statistical-tables. Published 2021. Accessed September 1, 2021.

Mishreki AM, Boardman NJ, Brodine SK, et al. Predictive factors of facilitating linkage to care for HIV-positive detainees in ICE Health Service Corps-staffed facilities. *J Public Health*. 2021;43(3):611–617. https://doi.org/10.1093/pubmed/fdaa003

Mizuno Y, Frazier EL, Huang P, et al. Characteristics of transgender women living with HIV receiving medical care in the United States. *LGBT Health*. 2015;2(3):228034.

Mjaland K. The paradox of control: an ethnographic analysis of opiate maintenance treatment in a Norwegian prison. *Int J Drug Policy*. 2015;26(8):781–789. https://doi.org/10.1016/j.drugpo.2015.04.020

Monroe A, Nakigozi G, Ddaaki W, et al. Qualitative insights into implementation, processes, and outcomes of a randomized trial on peer support and HIV care engagement in Rakai, Uganda. *BMC Infect Dis*. 2017;17(1):54. https://doi.org/10.1186/s12879-016-2156-0

Moyer VA; US Preventive Services Task Force. Screening for HIV: U.S. Preventive Services Task Force recommendation statement. *Ann Intern Med*. 2013;159(1):51–60. http://doi:10.7326/0003-4819-159-1-201307020-00645

Murnane PM, Celum C, Nelly M, et al. Efficacy of pre-exposure prophylaxis for HIV-1 prevention among high risk heterosexuals: subgroup analyses from the Partners PrEP Study. *AIDS*. 2013;27(13):2155–2160.

Murphy M, Sosnowy C, Rogers B, et al. Defining the pre-exposure prophylaxis care continuum among recently incarcerated men at high risk for HIV infection: protocol for a prospective cohort study. *JMIR Res Protoc*. 2022;11(2):e31928. https://doi.org/10.2196/31928

Mustanski B, Newcomb ME. Older sexual partners may contribute to racial disparities in HIV among young men who have sex with men. *J Adolesc Health*. 2013;52(6):666–667. http://doi.org/10.1016/j.jadohealth.2013.03.019

Myers JJ, Dufour MK, Koester KA, et al. The effect of patient navigation on the likelihood of engagement in clinical care for HIV-infected individuals leaving jail. *Am J Pub Health*. 2018;108(3):385–392. http://doi:10.2105/AJPH.2017.304250

Nachman SA, Cheroff M, Gona P, et al. Incidence of noninfectious conditions in perinatally HIV-infected children and adolescents in the HAART era. *Arch Pediatr Adolesc Med*. 2009;163:164–171.

Nash GD, Flanders WD, Baird TC, et al. Cross-sex hormones and acute cardiovascular events in transgender persons: a cohort study. *Ann Intern Med*. August 21, 2018;169(4):205–213. http://doi:10.7326/M17-2785.

Nolan BJ, Frydman AS, Leemaqz SY, et al. Effects of low-dose oral micronised progesterone on sleep, psychological distress, and breast development in transgender individuals undergoing feminising hormone therapy: a prospective controlled study. *Endocrine Connections*. 2022;11(5):e220170. http://doi:10.1530/EC-22-0170

Ohl M, Perencevich E, McInnes DK, et al. *Antiretroviral adherence among rural compared to urban veterans with HIV infection in the United States [issue brief]*. Veterans Rural Health Resource Center—Central Region. Washington, DC: VHA Office of Rural Health; 2012:W(1). https://www.ruralhealth.va.gov/docs/issue-briefs/antiretroviral-adherence-121812.pdf

O'Laughlin B. Structural reform and the politics of inequality in global public health. *Development and Change*. 2018;47(4):686–711. http://doi:10.1111/dech.12251

Olson J, Schrager SM, Clark LF, et al. Subcutaneous testosterone: an effective delivery mechanism for masculinizing young transgender men. *LGBT Health*. 2014;1(3):165–167. http://doi.org/10.1089/lgbt.2014.0018

Page KR, Grieb SD, Nieves-Lugo K, et al. Enhanced immigration enforcement in the USA and the transnational continuity of HIV care for Latin American immigrants in deportation proceedings. *Lancet HIV*. 2018;5(10):e597–e604. https://doi.org/10.1016/S2352-3018(18)30074-2

Parvez F, Katyal M, Alper H, et al. Female sex workers incarcerated in New York City jails: prevalence of sexually transmitted infections and associated risk behaviors. *Sex Transm Inf*. 2013;89(4):280–284.

Pasternack FR, Fox LP, Engler DE. Silicone granulomas treated with etanercept. *Arch Dermatol*. 2005;141(1):13.

Peckham AM, Young EH. Opportunities to offer harm reduction to people who inject drugs during infectious disease encounters: narrative review. *Open Forum Infect Dis*. 2020;7(11):ofaa503. https://doi.org/10.1093/ofid/ofaa503

Peitzmeier SM, Reisner SL, Harigopal P, et al. Female-to-male patients have high prevalence of unsatisfactory Paps compared to non-transgender females: implications for cervical cancer screening. *J Gen Intern Med*. May 2014;29(5):778–784.

Philbin MM, Tanner AE, Duval A, et al. Linking HIV-positive adolescents to care in 15 different clinics across the United States: creating solutions to address structural barriers for linkage to care. *AIDS Care*. 2014;26(1):12–19. http://doi:10.1080/09540121.2013.808730

Polonsky M, Azbel L, Wickersham JA, et al. Accessing methadone within Moldovan prisons: prejudice and myths amplified by peers. *Int J Drug Policy*. 2016;29:91–95. https://doi.org/10.1016/j.drugpo.2015.12.016

Poteat T, Wirtz AL, Radix A, et al. HIV risk and preventive interventions in transgender women sex workers. *Lancet*. 2015;385(9964):274–286. http://doi.org/10.1016/S0140-6736(14)60833-3

Prosser AT, Tang T, Hall HI. HIV in persons born outside the United States 2007–2010. *JAMA*. 2012:308:(6):601–607.

Radford J. Key findings about U.S. immigrants. Pew Research Center. https://www.pewresearch.org/fact-tank/2019/06/17/key-findings-about-u-s-immigrants/. Published 2019. Accessed January 25, 2023.

Radix AE, Harris AB, Belkind U, Ting J, Goldstein ZG. Chlamydia trachomatis infection of the neovagina in transgender women. *Open Forum Infectious Diseases*. November 11, 2019;6(11):ofz470. http://doi:10.1093/ofid/ofz470

Raj A, Bowleg L. Heterosexual risk for HIV among black men in the United States: a call to action against a neglected crisis in black communities. *Am J Men's Health*. 2012;6(3):178–181. http://doi:10.1177/1557988311416496

Rajabiun S, Davis-Plourde K, Tinsley M, et al. Pathways to housing stability and viral suppression for people living with HIV/AIDS: findings from the building a medical home for multiply diagnosed HIV-positive homeless populations initiative. *PloS One.* 2020;15(10):e0239190. http://doi: 10.1371/journal.pone.0239190

Rao D, Kekwaletswe TC, Hosek S, et al. Stigma and social barriers to medication adherence with urban youth living with HIV. *AIDS Care.* 2007;19(1):28–33. http://doi:10.1080/09540120600652303

Rapaport MJ. Silicone granulomas treated with etanercept. *Arch Dermatol.* 2005;141(9):1171. http:// doi.org/ 10.1001/ archderm.141.9.1171-a

Reddon H, Marshall BDL, Milloy MJ. Elimination of HIV transmission through novel and established prevention strategies among people who inject drugs. *Lancet HIV.* 2019;6(2):e128–e136. https://doi.org/10.1016/S2352-3018(18)30292-3

Reddy KP, Parker RA, Losina E, et al. Impact of cigarette smoking and smoking cessation on life expectancy among people with HIV: a US-based modeling study. *J Infect Dis.* 2016;214(11):1672–1681. http://doi:10.1093/infdis/jiw430

Reisner SL, Deutsch MB, Peitzmeier SM, et al. Comparing self- and provider-collected swabbing for HPV DNA testing in female-to-male transgender adult patients: a mixed-methods biobehavioral study protocol. *BMC Infect Dis.* 2017;17(1):444.

Reisner SL, Mimiaga MJ, Skeer M, et al. A review of HIV antiretroviral adherence and intervention studies among HIV-infected youth. *Top HIV Med.* 2009;17(1):14–25.

Rodger AJ, Cambiano V, Brunn T, et al. Risk of HIV transmission through condomless sex in serodifferent gay couples with the HIV-positive partner taking suppressive antiretroviral therapy (PARTNER): final results of a multicentre, prospective, observational study. *Lancet.* 2019;393(10189):2428–2438. http://doi:10.1016/S0140-6736(19)30418-0

Rodger AJ, Cambiano V, Bruun T, et al. Sexual activity without condoms and risk of HIV transmission in serodifferent couples when the HIV-positive partner is using suppressive antiretroviral therapy. *JAMA.* 2016;316(2):171–181. http://doi:10.1001/jama.2016.5148

Roland KB, Higa DH, Leighton CA, et al. Client perspectives and experiences with HIV patient navigation in the United States: a qualitative meta-synthesis. *Health Promot Pract.* 2020;21(1):25–36. https://doi.org/10.1177/1524839919875727

Roland KB, Higa DH, Leighton CA, et al. HIV patient navigation in the United States: a qualitative meta-synthesis of navigators' experiences. *Health Promot Pract.* 2022;23 (1):74–85. http://doi: 10.1177/15248 39920982603

Rooks-Peck CR, Adegbite AH, Wichser ME, et al. Mental health and retention in HIV care: a systematic review and meta-analysis. *Health Psychol.* 2018;37(6):574–585. http://doi: 10.1037/hea0000606

Rosecrans A, Harris R, Saxton RE, et al. Mobile low-threshold buprenorphine integrated with infectious disease services. *J Subst Abuse Treat.* 2022;133:108553. http://doi: 10.1016/j.jsat.2021.108553

Rosen S, Maskew M, Fox MP, et al. Initiating antiretroviral therapy for HIV at a patient's first clinic visit: the RapIT randomized controlled trial. *PLoS Med.* 2016;13(5):e1002015. http://doi:10.1371/journal.pmed.1002015

Ross J, Cunningham CO, Hanna DJ. HIV outcomes among migrants from low- and middle-income countries living in high-income countries: a review of recent evidence. *Curr Opin Infect Dis.* 2018;31(1):25–32. http://doi:10.1097/QCO.0000000000000415

Rubenstein LS, Amon JJ, McLemore M, et al. HIV, prisoners, and human rights. *Lancet.* 2016;388(10050):1202–1214. https://doi.org/10.1016/S0140-6736(16)30663-8

Rural Health Information Hub. RHI Hub tool kit. https://ww.ruralhealthinfo.org/toolkits/hiv-aids. Published 2022. Accessed October 22, 2022.

Sabino TE, Avelino-Silva VI, Cavalcantte C, et al. Adherence to antiretroviral treatment and quality of life among transgender women living with HIV/AIDS in Sao Paulo, Brazil. *AIDS Care.* 2021;33(1):33–38.

Sachdev DD, Mara E, Hughes AJ, et al. "Is a bird in the hand worth 5 in the bush?": a comparison of 3 data-to-care referral strategies on HIV care continuum outcomes in San Francisco. *Open Forum Infect Dis.* 2020;7(9):ofaa369. http://doi: 10.1093/ofid/ofaa369

Sanchez NF, Sanchez JP, Danoff A. Health care utilization, barriers to care, and hormone usage among male-to-female transgender persons in New York City. *Am J Public Health.* 2009;99(4):713.

Sanders RA. Adolescent psychosocial, social, and cognitive development. *Pediatr Rev.* August 2013;34(8):354–358.

Scarabin PY. Progestogens and venous thromboembolism in menopausal women: an updated oral versus transdermal estrogen meta-analysis. *Climacteric.* 2018;21(4):341–345.

Scarsi KK, Swindells S. The promise of improved adherence with long-acting antiretroviral therapy: what are the data? *J Int Assoc Provid AIDS Care.* 2021;20:232595822110090. https://doi.org/10.1177/23259582211009011

Schafer KR, Albrecht H, Dillingham R, et al. The continuum of HIV Care in rural communities in the United States and Canada: what is known and future research directions. *J Acquir Immune Defic Syndr.* 2017;75(1):35–44. http://doi:10.1097/QAI.0000000000001329. PMID: 28225437; PMCID: PMC6169533.

Schneider, CL. Racism, drug policy, and AIDS. *Polit Sc Q.* 1998;113(3):427–446.

Schranz AJ, Barrett J, Hurt CB, et al. Challenges facing a rural opioid epidemic: treatment and prevention of HIV and hepatitis C. *Curr HIV/AIDS Rep.* 2018;15(3):245–254. http://doi:10.1007/s11904-018-0393-0

Scott CK, Dennis ML, Grella CE, et al. The impact of the opioid crisis on U.S. state prison systems. *Health Justice.* 2021;9(1):17. https://doi.org/10.1186/s40352-021-00143-9

Sevelius JM. Gender affirmation: a framework for conceptualizing risk behavior among transgender women of color. *Sex Roles.* 2013;68(11–12):675–689.

Sevelius J, Chakravarty D, Neilands TB, et al. Evidence for the model of gender affirmation: the role of gender affirmation and health-care empowerment in viral suppression among transgender women of color living with HIV. HRSA SPNS Transgender Women of Color Study Group. *AIDS Behav.* 2021;25(Suppl 1):64–71. http://doi:10.1007/s10461-019-02544-2

Sevelius JM, Patouhas E, Keatley JG, et al. Barriers and facilitators to engagement and retention-in-care among transgender women living with human immunodeficiency virus. *Ann Behav Med.* 2014a;47(1):5–16.

Sevelius JM, Saberi P, Johnson MO. Correlates of antiretroviral adherence and viral load among transgender women living with HIV. *AIDS Care.* August 2014b;26(8):976–982.

Solomon L, Montague BT, Beckwith CG, et al. Survey finds that many prisons and jails have room to improve HIV testing and coordination of postrelease treatment. *Health Affairs.* 2104;33(3):434–442.

Spinelli MA, Hessol NA, Schwarcz S, et al. Homelessness at diagnosis is associated with death among people with HIV in a population-based study of a US city. *AIDS.* 2019;33(11):1789–1794. http://doi:10.1097/QAD.0000000000002287

Sprague C, Scanlon ML, Radhakrishnan B, Pantalone DW. The HIV prison paradox: agency and HIV-positive women's experiences in jail and prison in Alabama. *Qual Health Res.* 2017;27(10):1427–1444. https://doi.org/10.1177/1049732316672640

Stevenson KA, Podewils LJ, Zishiri VK, et al. HIV prevalence and the cascade of care in five South African correctional facilities. *PLoS One.* 2020;15(7):e0235178. https://doi.org/10.1371/journal.pone.0235178

Stone J, Artenie A, Hickman M, et al. The contribution of unstable housing to HIV and hepatitis C virus transmission among people who inject drugs globally, regionally, and at country level: a modelling study. *Lancet Public Health.* 2022;7(2):e136–e145. http://doi: 10.1016/S2468-2667(21)00258-9

Straub DM, Tanner AE. Health-care transition from adolescent to adult services for young people with HIV. *Lancet Child Adolesc Health.* 2018;3:214–222. http://doi:10.1016/S2352-4642(18)30005-1

Swerdloff RS, Wang C, White WB, et al. A new oral testosterone undecanoate formulation restores testosterone to normal concentrations in hypogonadal men. *J Clin Endocrinol Metab.* 2020;105(8):2515–2531.

Tanney MR, Naar-King S, MacDonnel K. Depression and stigma in high-risk youth living with HIV: a multi-site study. *J Pediatr Health Care.* 2012;26(4):300–305. http://doi:10.1016/j.pedhc.2011.02.014

Tate CC, Ledbetter JN, Youssef CP. A two-question method for assessing gender categories in the social and medical sciences. *J Sex Research.* 2012;50:1–10.

Taylor BS, Fornos L, Tarbutton J, et al. Improving HIV care engagement in the South from the patient and provider perspective: the role of stigma, social support, and shared decision-making. *AIDS Patient Care STDS.* 2018;32(9):368–378. https://doi.org/10.1089/apc.2018.0039

Telisinghe L, Charalambous S, Topp SM, et al. HIV and tuberculosis in prisons in sub-Saharan Africa. *Lancet.* 2016;388(10050):1215–1227. https://doi.org/10.1016/S0140-6736(16)30578-5

Terp S, Ahmed S, Burner E, et al. Deaths in Immigration and Customs Enforcement (ICE) detention: FY2018-2020. *AIMS Public Health.* 2021;8(1):81–89. https://doi.org/10.3934/publichealth.2021006

Trent M, Chung SE, Ellen JM, et al. New sexually transmitted infections among adolescent girls infected with HIV. *Sex Transmitted Infect.* 2007;83:468–469

Tsai AC, Mendenhall E, Trostle JA, et al. Co-occurring epidemics, syndemics, and population health. *Lancet.* 2017;389(10072):978–982. http://doi:10.1016/S0140-6736(17)30403-8

Tsai AC, Weiser SD, Dilworth SE, et al. Violent victimization, mental health, and service utilization outcomes in a cohort of homeless and unstably housed women living with or at risk of becoming infected with HIV *Am J Epidemiol.* 2015;181(10):817–826. http://doi: 10.1093/aje/kwu350.

UNAIDS. UNAIDS fact sheet 2022. unaids.org. https: www.unaids.org/en/resources/fact-sheet. Published 2022. Accessed September 26, 2022.

UNAIDS. *Getting to zero: 2011–2015 strategy.* Joint United Nations Programme on HIV/AIDS; 2019. Geneva, Switzerland.

US Food and Drug Administration (FDA). FDA approves first injectable treatment for HIV pre-exposure prevention. fda.gov. https://www.fda.gov/news-events/press-announcements/fda-approves-first-injectable-treatment-hiv-pre-exposure-prevention. Published 2021. Accessed September 4, 2022.

Valenzuela JM, Buchanan CL, Radcliffe J, et al. Transition to adult services among behaviorally infected adolescents with HIV—a qualitative study. *J Pediatr Psychol.* 2011;36(2):134–140. http://doi:10.1093/jpepsy/jsp051

Valera P, Chang Y, Lian Z. HIV risk inside U.S. prisons: a systematic review of risk reduction interventions conducted in U.S. prisons. *AIDS Care.* 2017;29(8):943–952. https://doi.org/10.1080/09540121.2016.1271102

Veracha V, Rukngan W, Chawanakrasaesin K, et al. Treatment of methamphetamine-induced psychosis: a double-blind randomized controlled trial comparing haloperidol and quetiapine. *Psychopharmacology.* 2014;231(16):3099–3108. http://doi: 10.1007/s00213-014-3485-6

Villanueva M, Miceli J, Speers S, et al. Advancing data to care strategies for persons with HIV using an innovative reconciliation process. *PLoS One.* 2022;17(5):e0267903. https://doi.org/10.1371/journal.pone.0267903

Vyavaharkar M, Glover S, Leonhirth D, et al. HIV in rural America: prevalence and service availability: a technical report by the South Carolina Rural Health Research Center. South Carolina Rural Health Research Center; 2013.

Wallace SA, McLellan-Lemal E, Harris MJ, et al. Why take an HIV test? Concerns, benefits, and strategies to promote HIV testing among low-income heterosexual African American young adults. *Health Educ Behav.* 2011;38(5):462–470. http://doi:10.1177/1090198110382501

Weiner LS, Battles HR, Wood LV. A longitudinal study of adolescents with perinatally or transfusion acquired HIV infection: sexual knowledge, risk reduction self-efficacy and sexual behavior. *AIDS Behav.* 2007;11:471–478.

Weyers S, Verstraelen H, Gerris J, et al. Microflora of the penile skin-lined neovagina of transsexual women. *BMC Microbiol.* 2009;9(1):102. http://doi.org/10.1186/1471-2180-9-102

White BL, Golin CE, Grodensky CA, et al. Effect of directly observed antiretroviral therapy compared to self-administered antiretroviral therapy on adherence and virological outcomes among HIV-infected prisoners: a randomized controlled pilot study. *AIDS Behav.* 2015;19(1):128–136. https://doi.org/10.1007/s10461-014-0850-8

White BL, Walsh J, Rayasam S, et al. What makes me screen for HIV? Perceived barriers and facilitators to conducting recommended routine HIV testing among primary care physicians in the Southeastern United States. *J Int Assoc Provid AIDS Care.* 2015;14(2):127–135. http://doi:10.1177/2325957414524025

Wiewel EW, Singh TP, Zhong Y, et al. Housing subsidies and housing stability are associated with better HIV medical outcomes among persons who experienced homelessness and live with HIV and mental illness or substance use disorder. *AIDS Behav.* 2020;24(11):3252–3263. http://doi:10.1007/s10461-020-02810-8

Williams RS, Stetten NE, Cook C, et al. The meaning and perceptions of HIV-related stigma in African American women living with HIV in rural Florida: a qualitative study. *J Assoc Nurses AIDS Care.* 2022;33(2):118–131. http://doi:10.1097/JNC.0000000000000252

Workowski K, Bachmann L, Chan P, et al. Sexually transmitted infections treatment guidelines, 2021. *MMWR Recomm Rep.* 2021;70(4):13–26.

World Health Organization (WHO). International classification of diseases, eleventh revision (ICD-11). 2019/2021. WHO. https://icd.who.int/browse11. Published 2022. Accessed September 1, 2022.

WHO. Social determinants of health. WHO. https://www.who.int/social_determinants/en/. Published 2022. Accessed September 20, 2022.

Woznica DM, Fernando NB, Bonomo EJ, et al. Interventions to improve HIV care continuum outcomes among individuals released from prison or jail: systematic literature review. *J Acquir Immune Defic Syndr.* 2021;86(3):271–285. https://doi.org/10.1097/QAI.0000000000002523

Xu Y, Chen X, Yu B, et al. The effects of self-efficacy in bifurcating the relationship of perceived benefit and cost with condom use among adolescents: a cusp catastrophe modeling analysis. *J Adolesc.* 2017;61:31–39. http://doi:10.1016/j.adolescence.2017.09.004

Yehia BR, Stewart L, Momplaisir F, et al. Barriers and facilitators to patient retention in HIV care. *BMC Infect Dis.* 2015;15:246. http://doi:10.1186/s12879-015-0990-0

Zanoni BC, Mayer KH. The adolescent and young adult HIV cascade of care in the United States: exaggerated health disparities. *AIDS Patient Care STDS.* March 2014;28(3):128–135. http://doi:10.1089/apc.2013.0345. PMID: 24601734; PMCID: PMC3948479.

Zash R, Caniglia EC, Diseko M, et al. Maternal weight and birth outcomes among women on antiretroviral treatment from conception in a birth surveillance study in Botswana. *J Int AIDS Soc.* 2021;24(6):e25763.

Zeidler Schreiter EA, Pandhi N, Fondow MDM, et al. Consulting psychiatry within an integrated primary care model. *Journal of Health Care for the Poor and Underserved.* 2013;24(4):1522–1530. https://doi.org/10.1353/hpu.2013.0178

Zhang X, Rhoads N, Rangel MG, et al. Understanding the impact of migration on HIV risk: an analysis of Mexican migrants' sexual practices, partners, and contexts by migration phase. *AIDS Behav.* 2017;21(3):935–948.

13.

COMPLEMENTARY AND ALTERNATIVE MEDICINE/ INTEGRATIVE MEDICINE APPROACHES

Yash Desai and Kalpana D. Shere-Wolfe

INTRODUCTION

LEARNING OBJECTIVES

- Discuss the fundamentals and practice of complementary and integrative medicine as it pertains to HIV medicine.

- Describe the established and evolving science of natural products, mind–body practices, and traditional medical systems.

WHAT'S NEW?

This edition contains updated information on the effects of micronutrient supplementation on CD4$^+$ T-cell counts and HIV disease progression as well fish oil supplementation. In addition, herb–drug interactions are reviewed, with new data presented on interactions with newer antiretroviral medications.

KEY POINTS

- CAM use is common in persons with HIV(PWH). Physicians caring for PWH should be aware of the high prevalence of CAM use and the failure of most PWH to disclose CAM use. Physicians need to routinely ask about CAM use, particularly herbal medicines, and supplements.

- Studies of nutritional supplementation with micronutrients—vitamins A, B, C, and E, and selenium—have shown mixed results with respect to markers of HIV progression and mortality.

- Natural health products (e.g., herbs, vitamins, and supplements) have the potential for significant drug interactions, which may lower the efficacy or increase the adverse effects of antiretroviral therapy.

- Fish oil supplementation remains controversial. The American Heart Association does not recommend fish oil for primary prevention, but there is evidence for its use in secondary prevention of cardiovascular disease and in hypertriglyceridemia.

- Evidence suggests gut microbiota changes in PWH, but, currently, the routine use of probiotics is not recommended in PWH.

- Some data suggest that stress, anxiety, and depression can affect HIV progression. Mind–body practices such as meditation, mindfulness, yoga, and tai chi can reduce stress, improve blood pressure, and improve quality of life. In addition, they may affect adverse health behaviors. The effects of these practices on CD4$^+$ T-cell count and disease progression are currently under investigation.

- Acupuncture may be of benefit in patients with musculoskeletal pain and sleep issues.

WHAT IS CAM AND INTEGRATIVE MEDICINE?

CAM is a group of diverse medical and health care systems, practices, and products that are not currently considered part of conventional medicine. Although the terms *complementary* and *alternative* are used simultaneously and interchangeably, they refer to different entities. Complementary practices are used together with conventional medicine, whereas alternative practices are nonmainstream practices that are used in place of conventional medicine. True alternative medicine is uncommon in developed countries but may be commonly found in resource-limited settings. Most people who use nonmainstream approaches use them along with conventional treatments (see the National Center for Complementary and Integrative Health (NCCIH) website at https://nccih.nih.gov). *Integrative medicine*, the increasingly more common term in use, refers to the use of CAM modalities with conventional medicine in an evidence-based integrated manner with emphasis on the importance of the relationship between practitioner and patient. Cornerstones of integrative medicine—nutrition, stress management, and exercise/movement—overlap those of conventional medicine but vary in their emphasis and approach.

Complementary and integrative health approaches can be classified upon their primary therapeutic input, such as, nutritional, psychological, physical, or combinations of psychological and physical approach (USDHHS/NIS, 2022). Nutritional approach, also known as natural products, include herbs or botanicals, vitamins and minerals, and probiotics. They are widely marketed, available, and typically sold as dietary supplements. Combinations of psychological and/or physical approach, also known as mind and body practices, include a large and diverse group of techniques typically administered by trained practitioners. They include yoga, chiropractic and osteopathic manipulation, meditation, massage therapy, acupuncture, relaxation techniques (e.g., breathing exercises, guided imagery, and progressive muscle relaxation), tai chi, gi qong, healing touch, movement therapies, and hypnotherapy. Traditional medical systems include various types of healers, Ayurvedic medicine, Chinese medicine, homeopathy, and naturopathy. The research on these various modalities varies widely. Although there are many studies on certain herbal products, acupuncture, yoga, spinal manipulation, and meditation, there have been fewer studies on other practices. Moreover, studies using these modalities in PWH are limited.

USE OF CAM BY PWH

In the HIV community, CAM gained tremendous popularity prior to the development of antiretroviral therapy (ART). Despite the effective treatments options available now, the popularity of CAM persists in the United States, Canada, Australia, many European countries, Asia, and Africa. Since life expectancy of PWH parallels that of people without HIV, CAM therapies are being sought for general wellness, mood disorders, stress reduction, and reduction of medication-associated side effects, as well as for boosting the immune system (Lorenc & Robinson, 2013; Thompson et al., 2012). For example, a survey of PWH demonstrated that 70% of participants who used any of the CAM therapies (exercise, lifestyle changes, dietary supplements, counseling, herbal medications, megavitamins, and prayer therapy) reported an improvement in their quality of life (Duggan et al., 2001). Importantly, one of the key reasons why CAM is being used by patients is because it enables them to have a more active role in their health care as well as a sense of control (Littlewood & Vanable, 2011).

There is variability in reports of CAM use owing to differences in study populations and definitions of CAM and CAM therapies. CAM is used by approximately 30%–60% of PWH; however, when restricted to practitioner-based CAM, the prevalence is approximately 15% or 16% (Bahall, 2017; Dhalla et al., 2006; Greene et al., 1999; Halpin et al., 2018; Josephs et al., 2007; Kelso- Chichetto et al., 2016; London et al., 2003; Lorenc & Robinson, 2013; Standish et al., 2001; Visser et al., 2002). CAM use is predicted by higher levels of education, men who have sex with men, female gender, longer disease duration, symptom severity and time on ART, and financial resources (Agnoletto et al., 2006; Halpin et al., 2018; Littlewood & Vanable, 2008; Lorenc & Robinson, 2013). Vitamins, herbs, and supplements are most common, followed by prayer, meditation, and spiritual approaches. In developing countries and areas with poor access to conventional HIV treatment, traditional culture-based systems are widely used. In general, patients have a high level of satisfaction with CAM modalities, with 50%–70% reporting

improvement in malaise, various symptoms, and quality of life (Agnoletto et al., 2003; Duggan et al., 2001).

There is insufficient data regarding adherence and CAM use. (Kelso-Chichetto, 2016; Owen-Smith et al., 2007). In general, most studies have found that CAM users do not have decreased adherence to conventional medication nor do they reject conventional ART. Rather, they use CAM in an integrated manner with their conventional HIV care (Littlewood & Vanable, 2008, 2014; Liu et al., 2009; Milan et al., 2008).

PHYSICIAN ATTITUDES TOWARD CAM

There are limited data on physician attitudes toward CAM. In one study of 89 HIV care providers, 63% believed that CAM and integrative medicine therapies may be helpful for PWH, and 36% had personally used one (Wynia et al., 1999). A national survey of ID physicians demonstrated that they are familiar with various CAM modalities, including vitamin and mineral supplementation, massage, acupuncture, chiropractic, yoga, and herbal medicine. They most recommended vitamin and mineral supplementation (80%) and massage (62%). Data regarding clinical efficacy, drug interactions, and safety appear to be important factors that influence ID physicians' use of these modalities for their patients (Shere-Wolfe et al., 2013). A study based in Italy, surveyed 438 physicians from different specialties, identified that oncologists were the physicians who were best informed on CAM, and physicians working at research institutes had a greater knowledge of CAM than those employed at general hospitals. The most well-known CAM intervention in this population of study was acupuncture, aloe vera, and high-dose vitamin C (Berretta et al., 2020).

PATIENT DISCLOSURE REGARDING CAM USE

Studies have shown that most physicians do not ask their patients about CAM use and that patients may not disclose CAM use for various reasons unless asked directly (Patel et al., 2017; Wahner-Roedler et al., 2014; Wynia et al., 1999). CAM use disclosure rates vary across studies from 38% to 90% (Littlewood & Vanable, 2008). CAM use disclosure rates vary across studies from 38% to 90% (Littlewood & Vanable, 2008). It is important that clinicians caring for PWH ask about CAM use to identify any potential drug interactions and safety issues.

Discussing CAM use is important, especially with respect to natural products. In the United States alone, there are over 20,000 different types of herbal products available to consumers (Xiong et al., 2021). Concerns regarding drug interaction are paramount; however, also important are issues related to contamination of natural products. One study found that 21% of Ayurvedic medicines purchased via the internet contained detectable levels of lead, mercury, and arsenic (Saper et al., 2008). Similarly, Chinese herbal medicines may have microbial and heavy metal contamination (Ting et al., 2013). Heavy metal toxicity and testing may be considered in patients with new symptoms after initiating Chinese or Ayurvedic medicines. Other safety issues include side effects from taking extremely large doses of vitamins. High doses of vitamin A can cause liver and bone damage as well as increase the risk of birth defects. High-dose vitamin C apparently increases the risk of kidney stones, and high doses of zinc (>75 mg/day) have been linked to copper deficiency.

Many patients may not be well informed about the products they are using. It may be helpful to direct patients to the National Institutes of Health's Medline Plus website for free, easy-to-understand, evidence-based information about many herbal products.

NATURAL HEALTH PRODUCTS TO CONSIDER FOR USE IN PWH

NUTRITIONAL SUPPLEMENTATION

Micronutrients (vitamin and minerals) are important for human development, disease prevention, and well-being. They are not produced in the body and must be derived from the diet. Vitamins A, D, E, C, and B, as well as zinc, iron, and selenium, play an important role in immunity. The PWH population has been found to have various micronutrient deficiencies that are prevalent before symptomatic disease and occur in patients who are ART naive as well as those taking ART (Baum et al., 1995; Beach et al., 1992; Hepburn et al., 2004; Remacha et al., 2003).

The data are unclear regarding the benefit of micronutrient supplementation in PWH. Several earlier randomized controlled studies demonstrated that micronutrient supplementation can improve markers of HIV progression (cluster of differentiation T-lymphocyte cell count (CD4 $^+$)) and/or viral load and mortality in both early (Baum et al., 2013) and late stages of HIV (Filteau et al., 2015; Jiamton et al., 2003; Kaiser et al., 2006; Range et al., 2006) as well as in pregnant women (Fawzi et al., 2004). A retrospective cohort study of 67,707 patients in Tanzania also demonstrated the effectiveness of routine vitamin B-complex, C, and E supplementation in PWH. Among the 48,207 ART-naive patients, MVI reduced the risk of mortality, incident tuberculosis, and meeting ART eligibility. Among 46,077 ART-experienced patients, MVI reduced risk of mortality, incident of tuberculosis, and immunological failure. The benefits of MVI were greatest in the first year of ART (Sudfeld et al., 2019).

However, more recent studies have shown mixed results. For example, micronutrients at higher doses compared to recommended daily allowance did not significantly improve CD4 $^+$ counts in a randomized, double-blinded study looking at a pediatric population in Nigeria (Esiowwa et al., 2021). A randomized, double-blinded study in India demonstrated no significant change in CD4 $^+$ counts in pediatric PWH receiving micronutrients but did show improvements in body mass index, hemoglobin, triglyceride levels, and intercurrent illnesses (Sucharita et al., 2022). Moreover, in a systemic review, micronutrient supplementations had little or no effect on mortality in adults PWH (Visser et al., 2017).

Zinc deficiency is common in PWH and is independently associated with disease progression (Baum et al., 1997, 2003;

Beach et al., 1992; Falutz et al., 1988; Graham et al., 1991; Jones et al., 2006). Again, the studies of zinc supplementation on CD4 $^+$ and viral load have had mixed results. A randomized, double-blinded, study of 146 HIV positive patients on ART receiving zinc supplement revealed a significant decrease in opportunistic infections (Hadadi et al., 2020). In a randomized, double-blind, placebo-controlled trial of 231 PWH with low plasma zinc levels, zinc supplementation at 12–15 mg of elemental zinc for 18 months resulted in a fourfold decrease in the likelihood of immunological failure, defined as a decrease in CD4 $^+$ T-cell count to 200 cells/mm^3, compared to placebo. Viral load was not affected by zinc supplementation. Zinc supplementation also significantly reduced diarrhea compared with placebo. Respiratory diseases and HIV-related mortality were not affected by supplementation.

A double-blinded placebo-controlled randomized clinical trial of 254 PWH who were ART naive with heavy alcohol consumption assessed if zinc gluconate supplementation (15 mg for men and 12 mg for women) taken daily for 18 months could change the Veterans Aging Cohort Study (VACS) Index score. A higher VACS Index score indicates higher mortality risk; however, the study concluded zinc supplementation did not decrease the Index score at 18 months or CD $^+$ 4 T-cell count, cardiovascular risk based on the Reynold Risk score, or inflammatory or microbial translocation biomarkers at 18 months (Freiberg et al., 2020).

A randomized, double-blinded, case control study evaluated the role of zinc in a trial of 40 PWH with immunovirological discordance compared to 40 PWH who achieved successful immune recovery. The study demonstrated that zinc supplementation in immunovirological discordance participants did not have statistically significant difference in CD4 $^+$ levels between cases and controls (Silva et al., 2021).

Zinc testing and supplementation should be considered in PWH with a high prevalence of zinc deficiency, such as drug users, children, men who have sex with men, and populations in developing countries (Baum et al., 2010).

Another single nutrient that has been studied in the PWH is selenium. A systematic review of randomized controlled trials comparing selenium with placebo and reporting outcomes of its effect on HIV viral load and CD4 $^+$ T-cell count concluded that daily supplementation with 200 mg of selenium can delay CD4 $^+$ T-cell count decline in HIV-infected patients but there was no quantifiable data that shows it suppresses or reduces viral load (Muzembo et al., 2019).

Pregnant PWH with selenium deficiency were noted to have eightfold higher risk for preterm delivery ($p = 0.03$) (Okunade et al., 2018). A randomized, placebo-controlled trial in Lagos analyzed the role of selenium in 90 participants who were living with HIV. The study demonstrated lower risk of preterm delivery (relative risk (RR) 0.32; 95% confidence interval (CI): 0.11–0.96) and a nonsignificant reduction in the risk of delivering term neonates with a low delivery weight (RR 0.24; 95% CI: 0.05–1.19). The study did not observe increase in the risk of perinatal death and adverse drug events (Okunade et al., 2021). However, selenium supplementation should be used with caution in primiparous women not receiving ART because at least one study has shown increased

HIV-1 RNA detection in the breast milk of these women with selenium supplementation (Sudfeld et al., 2014).

Vitamin D deficiency (VDD) is also common among PWH. The estimates range widely from 10% to 88% (Sherwood et al., 2012; Zhang et al., 2017). The wide range of estimates is likely due to differences in demographics, location, climate/season, and definitions. Etiology of VDD in PWH is likely multifactorial too. It includes both traditional risk factors such as dietary deficiency, darker skin, obesity, chronic kidney disease, lack of sun exposure, and malabsorption, as well as HIV-related factors such as ART regimens, especially those with efavirenz, which has been shown to interfere with vitamin D metabolism. Vitamin D plays an important role in osteoporosis, cardiovascular disease (CVD), and the immune system (Eckard et al., 2014). Some but not all data from randomized controlled trials in the general population demonstrate that vitamin D supplementation improves bone mineral density (BMD) and decreases fractures (Bischoff-Ferrari et al., 2005; Dawson-Hughes et al., 1997; Jackson et al., 2006). The degree to which contributes to osteopenia and osteoporosis, CVD, and disease progression in the PWH is unknown. The Endocrine Society recommends that at-risk persons be screened, including all persons receiving ART (Holick et al., 2011). The European AIDS Clinical Society also recommends screening for VDD in persons with the risk factors mentioned above, those with a history of low BMD and/or fracture, and those with a high risk for fracture (Holick, 2011).

Numerous studies have shown that vitamin D supplementation plays a beneficial role in bone health. For example, a trial demonstrated that for adolescents and young adults (n = 214) aged 16–24 years on TDF-containing regimen, monthly vitamin D supplementation (50,000 IU) improved vitamin D levels and lumbar spine BMD regardless of baseline vitamin D status (Havens et al., 2017). In adults aged 25–47 years, supplementation with high-dose vitamin D_3 (4,000 IU) and calcium carbonate (1,000 mg) with ART initiation (efavirenz, emtricitabine, and tenofovir) increased 25-(OH) D levels and attenuated increases in bone turnover markers and bone loss at the hip and lumbar spine by approximately 50% at 48 weeks (Overton et al., 2015). Lastly, a prospective, open-label, multicenter trial of 167 participants who were virologically suppressed, aged 60 years and older, and on a tenofovir disoproxil fumarate-containing regimen proved that BMD improved when the tenofovir disoproxil fumarate-containing regimen was switched to an elvitegravir, cobicistat, emtricitabine, and tenofovir alafenamide based regimen (Maggiolo et al., 2019).

The relationship between VDD in PWH and risk of tuberculosis (TB) is not clear. For example, in a diverse cohort of adults with advanced HIV infection in high-burden TB countries, VDD at ART initiation was found to be independently associated with increased risk of incident TB in next 96 weeks (Tenforde et al., 2017). Also, in Lima, Peru, a nested case control study, systemic review, and individual-participant data metanalysis showed vitamin D predicts TB disease in a dose-dependent manner and that the risk of TB disease is the highest among PWH with severe VDD (Aibana et al., 2019). However, a randomized, double-blind, placebo-controlled trial evaluated the role of vitamin D in 4,000 PWH who initiated ART and had serum 25-hydroxyvitamin D concentrations of less than 30 ng/mL. The trial revealed no overall effect of vitamin D3 supplementation on the risk of mortality (HR 1·04, p = 0·73). There was also no difference in the overall incidence of pulmonary tuberculosis between the vitamin D3 and placebo groups (p = 0·19) (Sudfeld et al., 2020).

Studies do not support the benefit of vitamin D supplementation on CD4 $^+$ T-cell count recovery. One trial of vitamin D supplementation in children with HIV on c-ART did not show an effect on CD4 $^+$ T-cell count (Ezeamama et al., 2016; Kakalia et al., 2011; Sudfield et al., 2012). In another double-blinded, randomized, and placebo-controlled trial in Ethiopia daily supplement with 5,000 IU of vitamin D3 and phenylbutyrate in treatment-naive PWH was shown to improve vitamin D3 status but did not reduce viral load, restore peripheral T-cell counts, improve body mass index, or middle-upper-arm circumference (Ashenafi et al., 2019). Given the data in the general population that support the use of vitamin D and calcium supplementation to decrease risk of fractures and improve BMD and the increasing number of studies in PWH, especially those on efavirenz (EFV)- and TDF-containing regimens that show improvement in BMD, it seems reasonable to screen high-risk PWH and provide supplementation to minimize HIV-related complications of osteoporosis and potentially affect immune function and disease progression. However, individuals on integrase strand transfer inhibitor (INSTI) containing regimens should be counseled on the drug interactions between INSTIs and MVI/minerals and the risk of potential treatment failure. They should be advised to take MVI/minerals either 2 hours before or 6 hours after INSTIs.

More recently, a systematic review of the effects of vitamin D, selenium, or zinc supplementation was conducted. Twenty-four single supplement trials involving 5,948 participants were included in the review. Seven vitamin D trials showed no harmful or beneficial effects of vitamin D supplementation on HIV progression. Six selenium trials found that selenium supplementation increased CD4 $^+$ T-cell counts and reduced the risk of diarrhea, and the hospital admission rate for HIV-related conditions. Eleven zinc trials showed a potential benefit of supplementation of diarrhea and immune function (Kayode & Anaba, 2020). Thus, it is recommended that each PWH be evaluated on an individual basis taking into account all the risks and benefits.

FISH OILS

According to the 2012 National Health Interview Survey, about 7.8 percent of adults and 1.1 percent of children have taken a fish oil supplement in the previous 30 days (Evans et al., 2012). Fish oils contain two different types of omega-3s, EPA (eicosapentaenoic acid) and DHA (docosahexaenoic acid), which are both found in seafood (fish and shellfish). There has been a significant interest in the role of fish oil omega 3 in terms of cardiovascular health over the last two decades. In a recent update from the American Heart Association (AHA), omega-3 supplements have not been shown reduce the risk of heart disease; however, they have been shown to reduce levels of triglycerides (Aung et al., 2018). A randomized placebo-controlled trial of 24,871 patients showed that supplementation with marine n-3 fatty acids did not result in lower incidence of major cardiovascular events or cancer than placebo (Manson et al., 2019). However, an updated meta-analysis of 13 trials concluded that marine omega-3 supplementation lowers risk for myocardial infarction, CHD death, total CHD, CVD death, and total CVD (Hu et al., 2019). Another randomized control study evaluated the role of marine omega 3 in 25,119 adults aged 50 years and older without the history of cardiovascular disease and its role in the incidence of atrial fibrillation. The study found no significant difference in the risk of incident atrial fibrillation over a median follow-up of more than 5 years (Albert et al., 2021). Therefore currently, data remain controversial on the benefit of omega 3s in cardiovascular health.

Omega-3s have been studied for many other conditions as well. For example, in a rheumatoid arthritis patient population, it has been shown to potentially decrease disease activity in rheumatoid arthritis (Kostoglou-Athanassiou et al., 2020). A meta-analysis evaluated the effectiveness of omega-3 fatty acids in bipolar personality disorder (BPD). This study analyzed five randomized controlled study ($n = 137$ patients with BPD) and demonstrated marine omega-3 fatty acids improve symptoms of BPD, particularly impulsive behavioral dyscontrol and affective dysregulation (Karaszewska et al., 2021). It is uncertain whether omega-3 fatty acid supplements are helpful for depression. For example, randomized controlled trial ($n = 18,353$) evaluated for effects of omega-3 supplementation on late-life depression risk and mood scores. The study found treatment with omega-3 supplements compared with placebo yielded small but statistically significant increase in risk of depression or clinically relevant depressive symptoms in the intervention group receiving omega-3 supplement compared to placebo group (HR 1.13; 95% CI: 1.01–1.26; P = .03).

A double-blinded, randomized control study evaluated the role of omega-3 in 128 critically ill, SARS-CoV-2-positive patients. It demonstrated higher 1-month survival rate in the intervention group receiving omega-3 compared to the placebo group (21% vs. 3%, P = 0.003). However, because of the small sample size, further studies are warranted (Doaei et al., 2021).

Data show that CVD mortality for the PWH has increased significantly from 1999 to 2013 (Feinstein et al., 2016). Currently, there are to date no studies looking at omega-3 fatty acids use for CVD in PWH.

There is evidence that inflammation and oxidative stress is important in the pathogenesis of CVD, which is particularly important in the HIV population. Nonetheless, a randomized parallel, placebo-controlled trial in Brazil of PWH on ART did not show any effect of 3 gm fish oils on high-sensitivity C-reactive protein (hs-CRP), fibrinogen, factor VIII, interleukin (IL)-6, IL 1-beta, or tumor necrosis factor (TNF)-alpha (Oliveira et al., 2014). In another randomized parallel controlled clinical trial of 70 PWH in Mexico were given 2.4 grams of omega-3 fatty acids, which was compared to a placebo. A reduction in markers for oxidative stress such as nitric oxide catabolites, lipoperoxides, or glutathione could not be proven in the treatment arm (Amador-Licona et al., 2015). Lastly, in a randomized, controlled, double-blinded clinical trial of 37 PWH aged between 40 and 70 years who were given fish oil 1.6 g/day for 12 weeks or a placebo, there was no significant differences between the treatment and control groups on any measures of inflammation or immunosenescence in both CD$^+$4 and CD$^+$8 T-cell counts (Swanson et al., 2018).

Omega-3 fatty acids supplementation has also been studied for depression in the general population with mixed results. Some studies have suggested that EPA may be more beneficial than DHA and that omega-3 fatty acids may best be used in addition to antidepressant medication rather than in place of it (Grosso et al., 2015). A randomized placebo-controlled trial of 100 PWH assigned to either omega-3 fatty acids (720 mg EPA and 480 mg DHA) daily treatment group versus placebo control group showed a reduction of depressive scores in the patients in the treatment group over time (Ravi et al., 2016).

Fish oils appear to be beneficial for the treatment of hypertriglyceridemia. A multicenter randomized trial involving patients with CVD or diabetes or other risk factors on a statin therapy with a fasting triglyceride (TG) level of 135 to 499 mg per deciliter and a low-density lipoprotein cholesterol level of 41–100 mg per deciliter were given 4 g of icosapent ethyl or placebo showed that the risk of ischemic events including cardiovascular death, was lower among those who received icosapent ethyl compared to placebo (Bhatt, 2019). Fish oils are relatively safe and do not have significant drug interactions with ART (De Truchis et al., 2005). In 100 PWH receiving ART with hypertriglyceridemia, fish oils at doses of approximately 6 g/day significantly reduced TG concentrations with no significant effect of fish oils on CD4$^+$ T-cell counts, immune function, or on lopinavir trough concentrations (Gerber et al., 2008). This result was confirmed in another RCT study of 48 PWH on ART as well as fenofibrate (Peters et al., 2012). In a study of PWH on combination ART with elevated fasting TG, the use of 3.0 g of fish oils combined with diet counseling and exercise resulted in a decrease in TG levels of 25% at 4 weeks versus a 2.8% increase in the control group (Wohl et al., 2005). Additionally, a meta-analysis of nine clinical studies compromising of 578 HIV-infected persons revealed that omega-3 fatty acids significantly reduced TG while increasing high-density lipoprotein cholesterol (Fogacci et al., 2020).

Doses greater than 3 g/day should be used with caution in patients with bleeding disorders or on anticoagulants. Unlike other supplements, fish oils are also available in prescription form (lovaza, omtryg, vascepa, and epanova) for use in hypertriglyceridemia. It is reasonable that fish oils—either as supplements or as fatty fish twice a week (salmon, mackerel, herring, lake trout, sardines, and albacore tuna)—be considered in PWH with hypertriglyceridemia and possibly those with CVD especially if they are not medically optimized.

PROBIOTICS

There has been a significant effort to elucidate the role of probiotics in terms of gastrointestinal health. A 2017 meta-analysis of 31 studies (n = 8,672 participants) concluded that probiotics could reduce the risk of *C. difficile* diarrhea in adults and children who are receiving antibiotics (number needed to treat for an additional beneficial outcome = 42 patients; 95% CI: 32–58) (Goldenberg et al., 2017). However, other studies demonstrate unclear role of probiotics in *C. difficile* infections as types of probiotics that would be most useful in reducing the risk of *C. difficile* diarrhea, the length of time for which they should be taken, and the most appropriate doses are uncertain. In 2020, American Gastroenterological Association (AGA) recommended against using probiotics for most digestive diseases. Currently, AGA recommends using probiotics for the following conditions: to reduce mortality and necrotizing enterocolitis in preterm and low-birthweight infants, certain probiotics for *C. difficile* infections (Su et al., 2020).

Intestinal microbiota serves to preserve the intestinal barrier, provide resistance to pathogenic colonization, and to stimulate the development of gut-associated lymphoid tissue. Gut microbiota is changed in PWH compared to the uninfected healthy population (Dillon et al., 2014; Dinh et al., 2015; Lozupone et al., 2013; Mutlu et al., 2014; Vujkovic-Cvijin et al., 2013); however, currently, probiotics cannot be recommended for PWH. They do deserve further investigation, particularly as immunomodulators.

INTERACTION OF NATURAL HEALTH PRODUCTS WITH ANTIRETROVIRAL AGENTS

Concurrent use of natural health products (NHPs) with ART is common among PWH. Of all the CAM modalities, herbal supplements have the greatest potential for adverse effects because of potential drug–drug interactions. With the development of newer ART agents, such as fostemsavir, ibalizumab, cabotegravir, bictegravir, and doravirine, it becomes essential to assess for drug–herb interactions. According to Natural Medicines, St. John's wart is strongly contraindicated with fostemsavir, bictegravir, and doravirine as St. John's wart induces CYP-3A, which is responsible for metabolism of these ARTs. However, there are currently no case studies published regarding drug–herb interactions of these new ART agents.

The following considerations add to the complexity and unpredictability of these interactions (MacDonald et al., 2009):

1. Many herbal remedies are complex products made of many different phytochemicals, some of which may not be fully characterized and standardized.

2. Some NHPs induce and inhibit gastrointestinal and hepatic enzymes simultaneously.

3. Many ART medications are substrates, inhibitors, or inducers of the drug-metabolizing enzymes (CYP family) and drug transporters (P-glycoprotein (P-gp)).

4. In vitro experiments may not predict in vivo effects because of various effects of intestinal enzymes, colonic microflora, and other factors.

5. Because of variations in extraction methods, constituents, and plant type/part, results from one study are not generalizable to other brands and formulation of NHPs.

For these reasons, it is difficult to state that any NHP is free from the possibility of potential drug–drug interactions. Most ART drug–drug interactions occur through the cytochrome P450 pathway and through drug transporters, which includes the P-gp efflux drug transporter (Brooks et al., 2017).

The major isoform responsible for protease inhibitor (PI) metabolism is CYP3A4 and are substrates of P-gp. Nonnucleoside reverse transcriptase inhibitors (NNRTIs) are metabolized by CYP3A4 and CYP2B6. PIs inhibit CYP3A4 whereas most NNRTIs induce CYP3A4. INSTIs (dolutegravir and raltegravir) neither induce nor inhibit CYP3A4. Conversely, nucleoside reverse transcriptase inhibitors and raltegravir are not inducers, inhibitors, or substrates of CYPs; therefore, they have less drug–drug interactions.

Thus, any medications, supplements, or herbs that interfere with CYP, P-gp, or uridine diphosphate glucuronosyltransferase (UGT) have the potential to result in changes in concentration of HIV and non-HIV drugs. ART–herbal interactions are bidirectional and ART may affect the concentrations, efficacy, and side/adverse effects of herbal medicines (Ladenheim, 2008; Lamorde, 2012).

GUIDE FOR NATURAL HEALTH PRODUCT–DRUG INTERACTION

Some commonly used CAM products, such as cod liver oil and flax/flaxseed oil have no known interactions with ART medications. Kava kava (*Piper methysticum*), black cohosh (*Cimicifuga racemose*), valerian (*Valeriana officinalis*), bitter orange (*Citrus aurantium*), saw palmetto (*Serenoa repens*), and Siberian ginseng (*Eleutheroccus senticosus*) have not been found to interact with CYP3A4. Therefore, it is unlikely that clinically significant pharmacokinetic interactions would occur with PIs or NNRTIs, but they may affect other ART (Lee et al., 2006).

Table 13.1 reviews potential CAM products that do interact with ART medications:

1. Red yeast rice extract (RYRE) is sometimes used by patients to lower cholesterol. It is made by fermenting a type of yeast called *Monascus purpureus* over red rice. RYRE contains several compounds known as monacolins, which block the production of cholesterol. One of these, monacolin K, has the same structure as the drugs lovastatin and mevinolin (Ma et al., 2000). Lovastatin is exclusively metabolized by CYP3A4 and is contraindicated in patients taking PIs. Red yeast rice was marketed in the United States as the dietary supplement Cholestin. The US Food and Drug Administration banned it in 1998. However, RYREs are still available, and some of them still contain lovastatin. Patients should be cautioned to avoid RYRE if on PIs or statins.

Table 13.1 POTENTIAL CAM PRODUCTS THAT INTERACT WITH ANTIRETROVIRAL MEDICATIONS

LIKELY SAFE	USE CAUTION BASED ON IN VITRO AND CASE REPORTS	AVOID	TO BE DETERMINED	ADJUST TIMING OF SUPPLEMENT
Cod liver oil	Ginseng	Red yeast rice extract	Evening primrose	Calcium carbonate
Flaxseed oil/flaxseed	Gingko	St. John's wort	Echinacea	Ferrous fumarate
Fish oils	Cat's claw		Cranberry	Multivitamins
Vitamin C	Goldenseal		Cancer bush	Other minerals: magnesium, zinc, copper, chromium, selenium
Aloe vera	Garlic		Goji	
	African potato		Green tea	
	Milk thistle		Harpagophyton	
	Echinacea		Horse chestnut	
	Piperine		Horsetail	
	Bitter orange		Moringa	
	Sweet orange		Saw palmetto	
	Borage		Milk thistle	
	Grapefruit		Red vine	
			Spirulina	
			Valerian	
			Wintergreen	

2. St. John's wort (*Hypericum perforatum*) is an herbal product used for depression. St. John's wort is known to be an inducer of CYP3A4 and P-gp. It also contains constituents that can affect other CYPs, including CYP2D6. It has been shown to alter levels of nevirapine, rilpivirine, and indinavir (de Maat et al., 2001; Hafner et al., 2010; Piscitelli et al., 2000). St. John's wort should be avoided by patients on ART.

3. Echinacea (*Echinacea angustifolia and Echinacea purpurea*) is commonly used for viral infections and immunologic boosting. Echinacea purpurea has been shown to induce CYP3A4 metabolism of darunavir but without effect on overall darunavir and ritonavir pharmacokinetics (Molto et al., 2011). Echinacea was also not found to affect etravirine concentrations (Molto et al., 2012b) or the pharmacokinetics of lopinavir/ritonavir (LPV/RTV) (Penzak et al., 2010).

4. Garlic is often taken to prevent heart disease, high cholesterol, and high blood pressure and to boost the immune system. However, garlic may induce intestinal CYP3A4 or P-gp (Berginc et al., 2010). In one study, garlic markedly reduced the concentration of saquinavir, although the results suggested that it affected the bioavailability of saquinavir rather than its systemic clearance (Piscitelli et al., 2002a). In single dose PK studies, garlic extract did not affect the area under the curve (AUC) or the maximum concentration recorded (C_{max}) of ritonavir or saquinavir (Gallicano et al., 2003; Jacek et al., 2004). Garlic should be avoided by patients on ART.

5. Milk thistle (*Silybum marianum*) inhibits CYP3A4 and P-gp activity in vitro but milk thistle has not been shown to significantly affect darunavir–ritonavir concentrations in one study (Molto, 2012a) or indinavir pharmacokinetics in three separate PK studies (DiCenzo et al., 2003; Mills et al., 2005; Piscitelli et al., 2002b).

6. Ginseng (*Panax ginseng*) may induce CYP3A4 activity in the liver and GI tract. Two multidose PK studies showed no effect of ginseng on LPV/RTV or indinavir levels (Andrade et al., 2008; Calderon et al., 2014). One case of an PWH on RAL + LPV/r therapy who developed liver failure after starting ginseng has been reported (Mateo-Carrasco et al., 2012).

7. *Ginkgo biloba* was not found to significantly alter raltegravir or LPV/RTV pharmacokinetics in healthy volunteers (Blonk et al., 2012; Robertson et al., 2008), but it was reported to potentially affect the efficacy of efavirenz (Naccarato et al., 2012; Wiegman et al., 2009).

8. Cat's claw (*Uncaria guianensis, U. tomentosa*), which is used for a wide variety of ailments including inflammatory and infectious diseases, may increase atazanavir, ritonavir, and saquinavir levels because of CYP3A4 inhibition (Galera et al., 2008).

9. Goldenseal (*Hydrastis candadensis*) has potent CYP3A4 inhibition properties but was not shown to affect indinavir levels (Sandhu et al., 2003). Patients taking goldenseal should be monitored for increased toxicity of CYP3A4 substrate drugs.

10. Fish oil in combination with LPV/RTV showed no significant decrease in ART level (Gerber et al., 2008).

11. Vitamin C decreased the AUC of indinavir by 15% and C_{max} by 23% in healthy volunteers. However, other studies in healthy individuals found no difference in CYP3A4 activity (Jalloh et al., 2017; Slain et al., 2005; van Heeswijk et al., 2005).

12. Two popular African herbs, African potato (*Hypoxis hermerocallidea*) and Cancer bush (*Lessertia frutescens*) have been shown to inhibit CY3A4 and P-gp in vitro (Awortwe et al., 2014). African potato (*Hypoxis hemerocallide, Hypoxoside obtuse*) was studied in two PK studies and was found to have no significant effect on AUC or C_{max} with efavirenz and lopinavir/ritonavir (Gwaza et al., 2013). Cancer bush can reduce the absorption and bioavailability of ARVs so patients should be monitored for plasma concentration and viral load (Bordes, 2020).

13. Evening primrose inhibits CYP3A4 and CYP2D6. There is one case report of evening primrose increasing LPV levels (Beukel van den Bout-van den, et al., 2008).

14. Calcium carbonate and ferrous fumarate significantly decrease serum levels of dolutegravir; chelation is suspected as the mechanism (Song et al., 2015). Patients on INSTI-based regimens taking calcium, magnesium, iron, zinc, copper, chromium, and selenium should be educated on this interaction and counseled on separating INSTI from supplement by 2 hours before or 6 hours after calcium or iron supplement (Brooks et al., 2017).

15. MVI decreased dolutegravir levels in healthy volunteers (Patel et al., 2011).

16. Black pepper contains active alkaloid piperine, which is often combined with turmeric to increase absorption. It has been shown to inhibit CYP3A4, P-gp, and UGT isoforms. Nevirapine levels increased significantly in individuals receiving 20 mg of piperine daily. Piperine may induce and/or inhibit other ART as well (Kasibhatta & Naidu, 2007). Piperine has been reported to inhibit CYP3A4 and P-gp, which in turn increases the bioavailability of nevirapine.

17. Grapefruit (*Citrus pardis, citrus maxima*) is also known to inhibit CYP3A4 and P-gp. There is a risk of increasing the absorption and bioavailability of certain ARVs, and a need to be cautious with PIs, NNRTIs, elvitegravir, bicgtegravir, dolutegravir, and maraviroc (Bordes et al., 2020).

18. Horse chestnut (*Aescuclus hippocastanum*) inhibits CYP3A4 and P-gp, and interacts with NNRTIs, elvitegravir, abacavir, tenofovir, indinavir, raltegravir, PIs, efavirenz, dolutegravir, bactegravir, and maraviroc (Bordes et al., 2020).

19. Horsetail (*Euisetum arvense)* inhibits CYP1A2 and CYP2D6 viral load, and interacts with lamivudine, zidovudine, efavirenz, emtricitabine, and tenofovir (Bordes et al., 2020).

20. Moringa (*Moringa oleifera*) inhibits CYP3A4, 1A2, 2D6, and interacts with nevirapine and efavirenz (Bordes et al., 2020).

21. Red vine (*Vitis vinifera*) inhibits CYP 2C9, 2D6, and 3A4, and interacts with PIs, NNRTIs, dolutegravir, elvitegravir, bictegravir, and maraviroc (Bordes et al., 2020).

22. Spirilina (*Anthrospira platensis*) inhibits CYP2C9, and interacts with etravirine (Bordes et al., 2020).

23. Sweet orange (Citrus sinensis) inhibits the OATP1A2 transporter, allowing intestinal absorption of substrate drugs for 4 hours. It interacts with saquinavir, lopinavir, and darunavir (Bordes et al., 2020).

24. Wintergreen causes renal toxicity and interacts with tenofovir (Bordes et al., 2020).

25. Licorice and its phytochemicals could affect the metabolism and clearance of certain drugs that are substrates of CYP3A4 and CYP1A2 such as rilpivirine and dolutegravir (Haron et al., 2022).

26. Jingyin granules significantly increases the plasma exposure of lopinavir by inhibiting human CES1A, CES2A, CYPs1A, 2A6, 2C8, 2C9, 2D6, and 2E1 (Zhang et al., 2022).

27. The lack of high-quality studies in humans and standardization of herbal formulations, among other factors, limits our knowledge on ART and herbal interactions. Other than a few herbal products such as St. John's wort, there is no simple guide to which NHP and ART combinations clearly have significant clinical interactions. In vitro testing may be helpful for identifying products to screen, but it is limited in its clinical extrapolation. Therefore, caution is advised and consultation with a pharmacist regarding any NHP and ART interaction is warranted. Resources for information on NHPs for both clinicians and patients are listed in Table 13.2. Particularly useful for clinicians is the Natural Medicines Database website (formerly known as Natural Standard and Natural Medicine Comprehensive Database), which has an extensive database on herbal medicines with in-depth information as well as a drug interaction checker. The database is available through subscription and is usually also available through most academic libraries or applications for smartphones. ART–herbal interactions can also be checked at http://www.hiv-druginteractions.org. The NCCIH also has concise evidence-based information on common herbs and links for information on herb–drug interactions.

HERBAL MEDICINES FOR HIV TREATMENT

In a meta-analysis of 12 RCTs involving 881 patients with advanced HIV disease, traditional Chinese medicine (TCM) interventions were associated with significantly reduced plasma viral load compared with placebo ($p = 0.04$). Patients receiving TCM interventions had significantly higher CD4[+] T-cell

Table 13.2 INTERNET RESOURCES FOR NATURAL HEALTH PRODUCTS INFORMATION AND NATURAL DRUG PRODUCT–DRUG INTERACTIONS

RESOURCE	WEBSITE
Natural Medicines	http://www.naturalmedicines.therapeuticresearch.com
National Center for Complementary and Integrative Health	https://nccih.nih.gov/health/herbsataglance.htm
HIV–Drug Interaction	http://www.hiv-druginteractions.org
National Institutes of Health, Office of Dietary Supplements Dietary Supplement Label Database	https:// //dsld.od.nih.gov
National Institutes of Health, Office of Dietary Supplements	https://ods.od.nih.gov
National Institutes of Health, MedlinePlus Herbs and Supplements Directory	https://nlm.nih.gov/medlineplus/druginfo/herb_All.html
Consumer Lab	http://www.consumerlab.com

counts compared with the placebo group ($p = 0.002$) as well as improved clinical symptoms ($p < 0.00001$). Additionally, TCM interventions were significantly more likely to result in improved clinical symptoms ($p < 0.00001$). TCM interventions conferred a similar risk of adverse events compared with control interventions ($p = 0.29$). Nonetheless, the reductions in plasma viral load significantly favored conventional Western medical therapy alone over integrated traditional Chinese and Western medical therapy ($p = 0.004$) (Deng et al., 2014).

MIND–BODY APPROACHES

Psychological and physical (mind and body) practices include a large and diverse group of procedures or techniques typically administered by trained practitioners or teachers rather than by physicians. They include yoga, chiropractic and osteopathic manipulation, meditation, massage therapy, acupuncture, relaxation techniques (e.g., breathing exercises, guided imagery, and progressive muscle relaxation), tai chi, gi qong, healing touch, and hypnotherapy. Central to these modalities is the elicitation of the relaxation response.

RELAXATION RESPONSE

The relaxation response can be described as a state of deep rest that changes the short- and long-term physical and emotional responses to stress (e.g., decreases in heart rate, blood pressure, rate of breathing, and muscle tension)—it is the opposite of the fight-or-flight response (Benson et al., 1974). Preliminary studies suggest that this response can affect gene expression related to energy metabolism, inflammatory response, and stress, as well affect telomere length, which is associated with premature

mortality and predicts a variety of health risks and diseases (Bhasin et al., 2013; Buric et al., 2017; Epel et al., 2004; Lavretsky et al., 2013). The clinical implications of these changes at the level of gene expression and telomeres is currently unknown.

A meta-analysis of 19 randomized control trials ($n = 1,300$) evaluated the efficacy of meditation and yoga on the immunological and psychological component of PWH. Eleven studies used mindfulness-based training, and eight studies adopted yoga. The study defined the intervention group as receiving mindfulness-based training and/or yoga, which it identified as mind–body therapy. Most of the mindfulness intervention included body scanning, mindfulness breathing, mindfulness to daily events, and gentle mindfulness stretching. Mind–body therapy significantly improved CD4$^+$ T-cell count (Cohen's d = 0.214, $p = .027$). mind–body therapy significantly reduced stress, depression, and anxiety symptoms (0.422, $p < .001$; 0.506, $p < .001$, and 0.709, $p < .001$, respectively) while improving quality of life (0.67, $p < .001$) (Jiang et al., 2021).

STRESS, DEPRESSION, AND HIV PROGRESSION

HIV infection presents many stresses and challenges—mental, emotional, and physical—that vary from time of diagnosis to coping with adherence and medication-related side effects, aging issues, and dealing with the loss of infected loved ones. Not surprisingly, PWH have higher incidences of depression and anxiety than the uninfected population (Pence et al., 2006; Whetten et al., 2008). Psychosocial variables and stress can affect measurable factors such as CD4$^+$ T-cell counts and viral loads in a variety of ways, including drug adherence, immune function, and health behaviors.

Stress has been shown in prospective human observational studies, animal studies, and laboratory experiments to be associated with depression, CVD, and progression of HIV/AIDS. This effect is generally thought to be mediated by negative affective states such as anxiety and depression, behavioral patterns (e.g., adherence, substance abuse), and stress-elicited endocrine responses mediated by the hypothalamic–pituitary–adrenocortical axis and the sympathetic–adrenal–medullary system (Cohen et al., 2007). In PWH, some studies have shown that stress may be associated with reductions in natural killer cell and cytotoxic T-lymphocyte phenotypes (Leserman et al., 1997).

Results from studies prior to 2000 were inconsistent with respect to the effect of stress and depression on HIV progression. However, several studies after 2000 have suggested a link between stress and HIV progression (Leserman et al., 2008). Among 96 asymptomatic, gay PWH not on antiretroviral medication at baseline who were followed every 6 months for up to 9 years, each additional moderately severe stress event increased risk of progression to AIDS by 50% and of developing an AIDS-related clinical condition by 2.5-fold after controlling for demographics, baseline CD4$^+$ T-cells and viral load, and antiretroviral medications (Leserman et al., 2002). In a study of 177 PWH men and women, baseline depression and hopelessness predicted slope of CD4$^+$ T-cells and viral load. High cumulative depression and avoidant coping were associated with approximately twice the rate of CD4$^+$

T-cell decline and greater increases in viral load (Ironson et al., 2005).

MEDITATIVE PRACTICES

Meditation is a practice of concentrating focus on a sound, object, visualization, the breath, movement, or attention itself in order to increase awareness of the present moment, reduce stress, promote relaxation, and enhance personal and spiritual growth. Examples include mantra meditation and mindfulness meditation. Yoga, tai chi, and chi gong are forms of breath coordinated movement meditations.

Research suggests that meditative practices may reduce blood pressure, symptoms of irritable bowel syndrome, anxiety and depression, and insomnia. (https://www.nccih.nih.gov/health/meditation-in-depth) In 2017, the AHA issued a scientific statement on meditation and cardiovascular disease risk reduction stating that overall, studies on meditation suggest a possible benefit on cardiovascular risk and may be considered as adjunctive therapy for cardiovascular risk reduction (Levine et al., 2017).

YOGA

Several yoga studies in the general population show possible benefits for stress management, mental/emotional health, sleep, and healthy lifestyle behaviors (NCCIH website https://www.nccih.nih.gov/health/yoga-what-you-need-to-know). In one large analysis of approximately 35,000 US adults, yoga practitioners reported high rates of health behavior outcomes such as motivation to exercise (~60%), eat healthier (~40%), cut back or stop drinking alcohol (12%), and cut back or stop smoking cigarettes (25%). More than 80% perceived reduced stress as a result of practicing yoga (Stussman et al., 2015).

Well-designed studies of yoga in the PWH are sparse. One prospective controlled study of yoga in PWH with CVD risk factors showed that 20 weeks of supervised yoga was effective in significantly reducing resting systolic and diastolic blood pressure by an average of 5/3 mm Hg—reductions similar to those achieved with the Dietary Approaches to Stop Hypertension diet. Studies suggest that a 10-mm reduction in systolic blood pressure and a 5-mm Hg reduction in diastolic blood pressure predict a 40%–50% lower risk of death from CAD. Extrapolating from these data in HIV-uninfected adults, yoga intervention would theoretically translate into a decreased risk of death from CAD by 20%–25% in PWH. Yoga did not affect body weight, fat mass, proatherogenic lipids, glucose tolerance, or immune or virologic status (Cade et al., 2010).

A 1-month yoga program was found to improve depression, anxiety, and CD4 $^+$ T-cell counts in 22 PWH on ART, as compared to 22 PWH controls (Naoroibam et al., 2016). Mantra meditation (i.e., repetition of a word or phrase) was found to be effective in reducing anger, improving quality of life (QOL), and improving spiritual well-being in a randomized controlled study of PWH (Bormann et al., 2006). Recent metanalyses of yoga studies in the HIV population demonstrated significant effects on stress, anxiety, positive affect (Dunne et al., 2019; Ramirez-Garcia et al., 2019).

MINDFULNESS-BASED STRESS REDUCTION

Mindfulness-based stress reduction (MBSR) is a technique that uses cultivation of nonjudgmental awareness in the present moment. It is usually taught as an 8-week structured program. MBSR has been shown to decrease the side effects of ART and alleviate symptoms. In one randomized wait-list controlled study of 76 PWH with ART-related side effects, MBSR was found to significantly reduced frequency of symptoms and distress related to symptoms (Duncan et al., 2012). In another RCT of 117 PWH, MBSR was found to result in a reduction in avoidance, higher positive affect, and improvement in depression at 6 months (Gayner et al., 2012). A recent trial in 72 PWH youth ages 14 to22 years showed significantly higher levels of mindfulness, problem-solving coping, and life satisfaction, as well as lower aggression, and were more likely to have or to maintain reductions in HIV viral load at 3 months (Webb et al., 2018).

Few studies have examined the effect of MBSR on CD4 $^+$ T-cell count. One small randomized, controlled short-term study of a diverse group of PWH suggested that MBSR could buffer CD4 $^+$ T-cell decline (Creswell et al., 2009). In a later RCT of 40 long-term diagnosed and treated PWH, mindfulness-based cognitive therapy (which combined elements of MBSR and CBT), patients were found to have decreased stress, anxiety, and depression and a significantly increased CD4 $^+$ T-cell count at week 20, compared to those receiving a placebo ($p < 0.001$), with no change in viral load (Gonzalez-Garcia et al., 2014). In contrast, a recent randomized, controlled rial of MBSR in PWH with CD4 $^+$ >350 cells/mm^3 not on ART, did not show benefit of MBSR with respect to CD4 $^+$ T-cell counts, CRP, IL-6, viral load, or d-dimer (Hecht et al., 2018).

TAI CHI

In the general population, studies suggest that tai chi may improve balance and stability in older people and those with Parkinson's, reduce pain from knee osteoarthritis, fibromyalgia and back pain, as well as promote QOL and mood in people with heart failure and cancer (NCCIH website, 2020). Data specific to PWH are limited. In a small study of 38 PWH randomly assigned to tai chi, exercise, and control groups, both tai chi and exercise were found to improve physiologic parameters, functional outcomes, and QOL. These patients were also noted to have improved social interactions (Galantino et al., 2005).

In a large group of 252 PWH, those randomly assigned to three 10-week stress-management approaches—cognitive–behavioral relaxation training, focused tai chi training, and spiritual growth—were compared to a wait-listed control group. Both the cognitive–behavioral relaxation and tai chi groups used less emotion-focused coping and had augmented lymphocyte proliferative function. Moreover, the tai chi group had an increase in QOL related mainly to an increase in emotional well-being (McCain et al., 2008).

Meditative practices can increase QOL; reduce stress, anxiety, and depression; and affect health-related behaviors. These practices have not been shown to have harmful side effects, and they should be considered for interested patients with stress, depression, anxiety, and adverse health behaviors. These practices may also be considered for patients who are unwilling to utilize psychological counseling, support, or cognitive–behavioral therapy. Many meditative practices are available. Which one is best depends on patient preference, which may be influenced by cultural factors, convenience, and finances. The practice most likely to be effective is the one that the patient is most likely to do.

ACUPUNCTURE

Pain is a frequently reported symptom in PWH (Vogl et al., 1999). Pain may be secondary to peripheral neuropathy or to musculoskeletal issues. Results from several studies suggest that acupuncture may help with chronic pain syndromes related to low-back pain, neck pain, and osteoarthritis/knee pain (Hinman et al., 2014; Linde et al., 2009; Manheimer et al., 2010; Vickers et al., 2012; Wit et al., 2006). Acupuncture may also help reduce the frequency of tension headaches and prevent migraine headaches. Clinical practice guidelines issued by the American Pain Society and the American College of Physicians in 2007 recommend acupuncture as one of several nonpharmacologic approaches that physicians should consider when patients with chronic low-back pain do not respond to practices such as remaining active, applying heat, and taking pain-relieving medications (Chou et al., 2007).

Few studies have examined the effect of acupuncture in PWH. A large multicenter, modified double-blind, randomized, placebo-controlled study comparing acupuncture and sham acupuncture for symptomatic treatment of HIV-related neuropathy revealed a modest decrease in average pain scores in both groups but no significant improvement with acupuncture (Shlay et al., 1998). In another small study of 23 PWH with sleep disturbances at least three times per week, patients received acupuncture two evenings a week for 5 weeks. Both sleep time and sleep quality were reported as improved (Phillips & Skelton, 2001). A recent meta-analysis of interventions for HIV-related neuropathic pain showed only a marginal benefit of acupuncture for this indication (Amaniti et al., 2019).

Although studies of acupuncture in PWH are limited, it seems reasonable to consider acupuncture in patients with musculoskeletal pain and perhaps those with sleep disturbances, especially in those who are either reluctant to take or intolerant of conventional medications.

EXERCISE

Substantial evidence indicates that regular physical activity contributes to the primary and secondary prevention of several chronic diseases, such as CVD, osteoporosis, and diabetes, and is associated with a reduced risk of premature death (Warburton et al., 2006). Moreover, studies have shown that in PWH, exercise can improve strength, endurance, time to fatigue, and body composition; increase QOL and sense of well-being; mitigate excessive bone loss; and

decrease depression and anxiety (Dudgeon et al., 2004; MacArthur et al., 1993; Rigsby et al., 1992; Stringer et al., 1998, Perazzo et al., 2018). It may also preserve or improve cognition in people living with HIV (Quigley et al., 2019). Given the increased risk of CVD, muscle wasting, and bone disease, it makes sense that some form of physical activity be encouraged for capable PWH. Physicians have an important role in educating and encouraging exercise as a measure for well-being and disease prevention.

MANUAL THERAPIES

Manual CAM therapies include massage, shiatsu, reiki, therapeutic touch, acupressure, and chiropractic manipulation. Manual modalities are often used by patients for their purported effects of increasing circulation, pain alleviation, relaxation, and stimulation of immune function (Power et al., 2002). One small RCT showed that massage therapy combined with stress management resulted in a decrease in medical care usage and an increase in health perceptions in PWH (Birk et al., 2000). A Cochrane review of massage in PWH showed that there appears to be a positive effect on the QOL of affected individuals, particularly when massage is combined with other interventions such as meditation and stress management (Hillier et al., 2010).

TRADITIONAL MEDICINE

It is beyond the scope of this chapter to review the major traditional medical systems of India, China, and Africa. These systems are broad and complex, and they often combine different therapeutic modalities discussed previously in this chapter, such as a combination of herbal remedies and mind–body practices. Reasons for the use of these traditional systems in the PWH stem from cultural beliefs, economic considerations, and limited accessibility to ART. Data from well-designed clinical trials regarding efficacy and safety of these systems are sparse.

Traditional Indian medicine consisting of Ayurveda, Unani medicine, Siddha medicine, homeopathy, and naturopathy is used by two-thirds of the Indian population—especially in rural areas—for both primary care needs and HIV (Fritts et al., 2008).

Similarly, in Africa, a large portion of the population uses herbs for primary health care, and HIV-related health problems (Calitz et al., 2014). Although there is increasing study of herbal medicines and their potential for drug interactions in vitro, clinical trials are lacking.

Traditional Chinese medicine has probably been the most studied of the traditional systems, with data showing potential efficacy of TCM herbs for HIV and HIV-associated conditions. To date, no data exist to support the use of these systems as primary treatment for HIV. Some data exist on efficacy, especially of TCM on end points such as CD4$^+$ T-cells and viral load; however, they have been inferior to ART. There may be a role for these systems in the management of symptoms, HIV-associated conditions, and delaying of HIV progression in those not on ART, but more data are needed with respect to their efficacy and herb–drug interactions.

Other aspects of traditional medical systems excluding herbal medicines, such as spiritual and healing practices and attitudes toward sickness and death (provided they do not harm), should be acknowledged and respected by physicians.

SUMMARY

Complementary, integrative, and alternative modalities are widely used by PWH. True alternative medicine for HIV is rare in developed countries but widespread in resource-limited areas. Physicians caring for PWH need to be aware of the prevalence of complementary therapies among their patients, the potential for herb–drug interactions, and the potential toxicities of herbal medicines.

Physicians can also play an important role in fostering partnerships with their patients who use CAM modalities by using nonjudgmental and open communication about their benefits and risks. Some NHPs, such as fish oils and MVI, should be considered for use in selected PWH. Strategies to delay HIV progression using micronutrients, probiotics, and traditional natural products in PWH with high CD4 + T-cell counts deserve further research, particularly in resource-limited settings in which access to ART is limited. Many mind–body techniques are useful for reducing stress, anxiety, and depression—all of which may affect HIV disease progression. These techniques may be especially useful in patients with adverse health behaviors who are unwilling to undergo formal therapy. They should also be considered in resource-limited settings as a self-empowering, low-cost means of coping with the emotional and physical challenges associated with HIV.

Treatment of HIV remains complex and multifactorial. Complementary and integrative modalities with low potential for adverse effects, such as mind–body techniques and certain natural products, should be considered in the balanced approach to dealing with the multidimensional aspects of HIV disease. The use of such practices will likely increase in the future. Therefore, it behooves physicians caring for these patients to understand the range of available options, their potential interactions with standard therapeutic regimens, and the ongoing data regarding their potential efficacy and safety.

RECOMMENDED READING

Baum MK, Campa A, Lai S, et al. Effect of micronutrient supplementation on disease progression in asymptomatic, antiretroviral-naive, PWH in Botswana: a randomized clinical trial. *JAMA*. 2013;310(20):2154–2163.

Bhasin MK, Dusek JA, Chang B, et al. Relaxation response induces temporal transcriptome changes in energy metabolism, insulin secretion and inflammatory pathways. *PLoS One*. 2013;, 8(5):e62817. http://doi:10.1371/journal.pone.0062817

Brooks KM, George JM, Kumar P. Drug interactions in HIV treatment: Complementary & alternative medicines and over-the-counter products. *Expert Review of Clinical Pharmacology*. 2017;10(1):59–79.

Buric I, Farias M, Jong J, Mee C, Brazil IA. What is the molecular signature of mind–body interventions? A systematic review of gene expression changes induced by meditation and related practices. *Frontiers in Immunology*. 2017;8:70670.

Cade W, Reeds DN, Mondy KE, et al. Yoga lifestyle intervention reduces blood pressure in HIV-infected adults with cardiovascular disease risk factors. *HIV Medicine*. 2010;11(6): 379–388.

Dinh DM, Volpe GE, Duffalo C, et al. Intestinal microbiota, microbial translocation, and systemic inflammation in chronic HIV infection. *Journal of Infectious Diseases*. 2015;211(1):19–27. http://doi:10.1093/infdis/jiu409

Halpin SN, Carruth EC, Rai RP, et al. Complementary and alternative medicine among persons living with HIV in the era of combined antiretroviral treatment. *AIDS and Behavior*. 2018;22(3):848–852.

Havens PL, Stephensen CB, Van Loan MD, et al. Vitamin D3 supplementation increases spine bone mineral density in adolescents and young adults with human immunodeficiency virus infection being treated with tenofovir disoproxil fumarate: a randomized, placebo-controlled trial. *Clinical Infectious Diseases*. 2017;66(2):220–228.

Jalloh MA, Gregory PJ, Hein D, Risoldi Cochrane Z, Rodriguez A. Dietary supplement interactions with antiretrovirals: A systematic review. *International Journal of STD & AIDS*. 2017;28(1):4–15. http://doi:10.1177/0956462416671087

Jiménez-Nácher I, Alvarez E, Morello J, et al. Approaches for understanding and predicting drug interactions in human immunodeficiency virus-infected patients. *Expert Opinion on Drug Metabolism & Toxicology*. 2011;7(4):457–477.

Klatt NR, Canary LA, Sun X, et al. Probiotic/prebiotic supplementation of antiretrovirals improves gastrointestinal immunity in SIV-infected macaques. *Journal of Clinical Investigation*. 2013;123(2):903–907. http://doi:10.1172/JCI66227

Lavretsky H, Epel E, Siddarth P, et al. A pilot study of yogic meditation for family dementia caregivers with depressive symptoms: effects on mental health, cognition, and telomerase activity. *International Journal of Geriatric Psychiatry*. 2013;28(1):57–65.

Saper RB, Phillips RS, Sehgal A, et al. Lead, mercury, and arsenic in US-and Indian-manufactured Ayurvedic medicines sold via the internet. *JAMA*. 2008;300(8):915–923.

REFERENCES

Agnoletto V, Chiaffarino F, Nasta P, et al. Reasons for complementary therapies and characteristics of users among HIV-infected people. *Int J STD AIDS*. 2003;14(7):482–486. http://doi:10.1258/095646203322025803

Agnoletto V, Chiaffarino F, Nasta P, et al. Use of complementary and alternative medicine in HIV-infected subjects. *Complement TherMed*. 2006;14(3):193–199.

Aibana O, Huang CC, Aboud S, et al. Vitamin D status and risk of incident tuberculosis disease: a nested case-control study, systematic review, and individual-participant data meta-analysis. *PLoS Med*. 2019;16(9):e1002907.

Albert CM, Cook NR, Pester J, et al. Effect of marine omega-3 fatty acid and vitamin D supplementation on incident atrial fibrillation: a randomized clinical trial. *JAMA*. 2021;325(11):1061–1073. http://doi:10.1001/jama.2021.1489

Amador-Licona N, Díaz-Murillo TA, Gabriel-Ortiz G, et al. Omega 3 fatty acids supplementation and oxidative stress in HIV-seropositive patients: a clinical trial. *PloS One*. 2016;11(3):e0151637.

Amaniti A, Sardeli C, Fyntanidou V, et al. Pharmacologic and non-pharmacologic interventions for HIV-neuropathy pain. a systematic review and a meta-analysis. *Medicina*. 2019;55:762.

Andrade AS, Hendrix C, Parsons T L, et al. Pharmacokinetic and metabolic effects of American ginseng (panax quinquefolius) in healthy volunteers receiving the HIV protease inhibitor indinavir. *BMC Complement Altern Med.* 2008;8:50. http://doi:10.1186/1472-6882-8-50

Ashenafi S, Amogne W, Kassa E, et al. Daily nutritional supplementation with vitamin D(3) and phenylbutyrate to treatment-naive HIV patients tested in a randomized placebo-controlled trial. *Nutrients.* 2019;11(1):133.

Aung T, Halsey J, Kromhout D, et al. Associations of omega-3 fatty acid supplement use with cardiovascular disease risks: meta-analysis of 10 trials involving 77 917 individuals. *JAMA Cardiology.* 2018; 3(3):225–234.

Awortwe C, Bouic PJ, Masimirembwa CM, et al. Inhibition of major drug metabolizing CYPs by common herbal medicines used by HIV/AIDS patients in Africa—implications for herb-drug interactions. *Drug Metabolism Letters.* 2014;7(2):83–95. http://doi:DML-EPUB-58874

Bahall M. Prevalence, patterns, and perceived value of complementary and alternative medicine among HIV patients: A descriptive study. *BMC Complementary and Alternative Medicine.* 2017;17(1):422.

Baum MK, Campa A, Lai S, et al. Zinc status in human immunodeficiency virus type 1 infection and illicit drug use. *Clin Infect Dis.* 2003;37(S2):S117–S123. http://doi:CID30489

Baum MK, Campa A, La, S, et al. Effect of micronutrient supplementation on disease progression in asymptomatic, antiretroviral-naive, HIV-infected adults in Botswana: a randomized clinical trial. *JAMA.* 2013;310(20):2154–2163.

Baum MK, Lai S, Sales S, et al. Randomized, controlled clinical trial of zinc supplementation to prevent immunological failure in HIV-infected adults. *Clin Infect Dis.* 2010;50(12):1653–1660. http://doi:10.1086/652864

Baum MK, Shor-Posner G, Lai S, et al. High risk of HIV-related mortality is associated with selenium deficiency. *J AIDS.* 1997;15(5):370–374.

Baum MK, Shor-Posner G, Lu Y, et al. Micronutrients and HIV-1 disease progression. *AIDS.* 1995;9(9):1051–1056.

Beach RS, Mantero-Atienza E, Shor-Posner G, et al. Specific nutrient abnormalities in asymptomatic HIV-1 infection. *AIDS.* 1992;6(7):701–708.

Benson H, Beary JF, Carol MP. The relaxation response. *Psychiatry.* 1974;37(1):37–46.

Berginc K, Trdan T, Trontelj J, et al. HIV protease inhibitors: garlic supplements and first-pass intestinal metabolism impact on the therapeutic efficacy. *Biopharm Drug Dispos.* 2010;31(8–9):495–505.

Berretta M, Rinaldi L, Taibi R, et al. Physician attitudes and perceptions of complementary and alternative medicine (CAM): a multi-centre Italian study. *Front Oncol.* 2020;10:594. http://doi:10.3389/fonc.2020.00594

Beukel van den Bout-van den CJ, Bosch ME, Burger DM, et al. Toxic lopinavir concentrations in an HIV-1 infected patient taking herbal medications. AIDS (London). 2008;22(10):1243–1244. http://doi:10.1097/QAD.0b013e32830261f4

Bhasin MK, Dusek JA, Chang B, et al. Relaxation response induces temporal transcriptome changes in energy metabolism, insulin secretion and inflammatory pathways. *PLoS One.* 2013;8(5):e62817. http://doi:10.1371/journal.pone.0062817

Bhatt DL, Steg PG, Miller M. Cardiovascular risk reduction with icosapent ethyl. *N Engl J Med.* 2019;380(17):1678.

Birk TJ, McGrady A, MacArthur RD, et al. The effects of massage therapy alone and in combination with other complementary therapies on immune system measures and quality of life in human immunodeficiency virus. *J Altern Complement Med.* 2000;6(5):405–414.

Bischoff-Ferrari HA, Willett W C, Wong JB, et al. Fracture prevention with vitamin D supplementation: a meta-analysis of randomized controlled trials. *JAMA.* 2009;293(18):2257–2264.

Blonk M, Colbers A, Poirters A, et al. Effect of ginkgo biloba on the pharmacokinetics of raltegravir in healthy volunteers. *Antimicrob Agents Chemother.* 2012;56(10):5070–5075. http://doi:10.1128/AAC.00672-12

Bordes C, Leguelinel-Blache G, Lavigne J-P, et al. Interactions between antiretroviral therapy and complementary and alternative medicine: a narrative review. *Clin Microbiol Infect.* 2020;26(9):1161–1170. http://doi:10.1016/j.cmi.2020.04.019

Bormann JE, Gifford AL, Shively M, et al. Effects of spiritual mantra repetition on HIV outcomes: a randomized controlled trial. *Journal of Behavioral Medicine.* 2006;29(4): 359–376.

Brooks KM, George JM, Kumar P. Drug interactions in HIV treatment: complementary & alternative medicines and over-the-counter products. *Exp Rev Clin Pharmacol.* 2017;10(1):59–79.

Buric I, Farias M, Jong J, et al. What is the molecular signature of mind–body interventions? A systematic review of gene expression changes induced by meditation and related practices. *Front Immunol.* 2017;8:670.

Cade W, Reeds DN, Mondy KE, et al. Yoga lifestyle intervention reduces blood pressure in HIV-infected adults with cardiovascular disease risk factors. *HIV Med.* 2010;11(6):379–388.

Calderón MM, Chairez CL, Gordon LA, et al. Influence of panax ginseng on the steady state pharmacokinetic profile of Lopinavir–Ritonavir in healthy volunteers. *Pharmacotherapy.* 2014;34(11):1151–1158.

Calitz C, Steenekamp JH, Steyn JD, et al. Impact of traditional African medicine on drug metabolism and transport. *Exp Opin Drug Metab Toxicol.* 2014;10(7):991–1003.

Chou R, Qaseem A, Snow V, et al. Diagnosis and treatment of low back pain: a joint clinical practice guideline from the American College of Physicians and the American Pain Society. *Ann Intern Med.* 2007;147(7):478–491.

Cohen S, Janicki-Deverts D, Miller GE. Psychological stress and disease. *JAMA.* 2007;298(14):1685–1687.

Creswell JD, Myers HF, Cole SW, et al. Mindfulness meditation training effects on CD4 + T cell T lymphocytes in HIV-1 infected adults: a small randomized controlled trial. *Brain Behav Immun.* 2009;23(2):184–188.

Dawson-Hughes B, Harris SS, Krall EA, Dallal GE. Effect of calcium and vitamin D supplementation on bone density in men and women 65 years of age or older. *N Engl J Med.* 1997;337(10):670–676.

de Maat MM, Hoetelmans RM, Mathôt RA, et al. Drug interaction between St. John's wort and nevirapine. *AIDS.* 2001;15(3):420–421.

De Truchis P, Kirstetter M, Perier A, et al. Treatment of hypertriglyceridemia in HIV-infected patients under HAART, by (n-3) polyunsaturated fatty acids: A double-blind randomized prospective trial in 122 patients [Abstract 39]. Paper presented at the 12th Conference on Retroviruses and Opportunistic Infections, Boston, February 22–25, 2005.

Deng X, Jiang M, Zhao X, et al. Efficacy and safety of traditional Chinese medicine for the treatment of acquired immunodeficiency syndrome: a systematic review. *J Tradit Chin Med.* 2014;34(1):1–9.

Dhalla S, Chan KJ, Montaner JS, et al. Complementary and alternative medicine use in British Columbia—a survey of HIV positive people on antiretroviral therapy. *Complement Ther Clin Pract.* 20016;12(4):242–248.

DiCenzo R, Shelton M, Jordan K, et al. Coadministration of milk thistle and indinavir in healthy subjects. *Pharmacotherapy.* 2003;23(7):866–870.

Dillon S, Lee E, Kotter C, et al. An altered intestinal mucosal microbiome in HIV-1 infection is associated with mucosal and systemic immune activation and endotoxemia. *Mucosal Immunol.* 2014;7(4):983–994.

Dinh DM, Volpe GE, Duffalo C, et al. Intestinal microbiota, microbial translocation, and systemic inflammation in chronic HIV infection. *J Inf Dis.* 2015;211(1):19–27. http://doi:10.1093/infdis/jiu409

Doaei S, Gholami S, Rastgoo S, et al. The effect of omega-3 fatty acid supplementation on clinical and biochemical parameters of critically ill patients with COVID-19: a randomized clinical trial. *J Transl Med.* 2021;19(1):128. http://doi:10.1186/s12967-021-02795-5

Dudgeon WD, Phillips KD, Bopp CM, et al. Physiological and psychological effects of exercise interventions in HIV disease. *AIDS Patient Care STDs.* 2004;18(2):81–98.

Duggan J, Peterson WS, Schutz M, et al. Use of complementary and alternative therapies in HIV-infected patients. *AIDS Patient Care STDs.* 2001;15(3):159–167.

Duncan LG, Moskowitz JT, Neilands TB, et al. Mindfulness-based stress reduction for HIV treatment side effects: a randomized, wait-list controlled trial. *J Pain Symptom Manage*. 2012;43(2):161–171.

Dunne EM, Balletto BL, Donahue ML, et al. The benefits of yoga for people living with HIV/AIDS: A systematic review and meta-analysis. *Complement Ther Clin Pract*. 2019;34:157–164. doi:10.1016/j.ctcp.2018.11.009. Epub 2018 Nov 8.

Eckard AR, McComsey, GA. Vitamin D deficiency and altered bone mineral metabolism in HIV-infected individuals. *Curr HIV/AIDS Rep*. 2014;11(3):263–270.

Epel ES, Blackburn EH, Lin J, et al. Accelerated telomere shortening in response to life stress. *Proc Natl Acad Sci US A*. 2004;101(49):17312–17315. http://doi:0407162101

Esiovwa R, Rankin J, David A, et al. The role of multimicronutrient supplementation in pediatric HIV management in Nigeria: a randomized controlled study. *J Pediatric Infect Dis Soc*. 2021;10(2):112–117. http://doi:10.1093/jpids/piaa025

Evans MW Jr, Ndetan H, Perko M, et al. Dietary supplement use by children and adolescents in the United States to enhance sport performance: results of the National Health Interview Survey. *J Prim Prev*. 2012;33(1):3–12. http://doi:10.1007/s10935-012-0261-4

Ezeamama AE, Guwatudde D, Wang M, et al. Vitamin-D deficiency impairs CD4 T-cell count recovery rate in HIV-positive adults on highly active antiretroviral therapy: a longitudinal study. *Clin Nutr*. 2016;35(5).1110–1117.

Falutz J, Tsoukas C, Gold P. Zinc as a cofactor in human immunodeficiency virus-induced immunosuppression. *JAMA*. 1988;259(19):2850–2851.

Fawzi WW, Msamanga GI, Spiegelman D, et al. A randomized trial of multivitamin supplements and HIV disease progression and mortality. *N Engl J Med*. 2004;351(1):23–32.

Feinstein MJ, Bahiru E, Achenbach C, et al. Patterns of cardiovascular mortality for PWH in the United States: 1999–2013. *Am J Card*. 2016;117(2):214–220.

Filteau S, PrayGod G, Kasonka L, et al.; NUSTART (Nutritional Support for Africans Starting Antiretroviral Therapy) Study Team. Effects on mortality of a nutritional intervention for malnourished HIV-infected adults referred for antiretroviral therapy: a randomised controlled trial. *BMC Medicine*. 2015;13:17-014-0253-8. http://doi:10.1186/s12916-014-0253-8

Fogacci F, Strocchi E, Veronesi M, et al. Effect of omega-3 polyunsaturated fatty acids treatment on lipid pattern of HIV patients: a meta-analysis of randomized clinical trials. *Mar Drugs*. 2020;18(6):292. Published 2020 Jun 1. http://doi:10.3390/md18060292

Freiberg MS, Cheng DM, Gnatienko N, et al. Effect of zinc supplementation vs placebo on mortality risk and HIV disease progression among HIV-positive adults with heavy alcohol use: a randomized clinical trial. *JAMA Netw Open*. 2020;3(5):e204330.

Fritts M, Crawford CC, Quibell D, et al. Traditional Indian medicine and homeopathy for HIV/AIDS: a review of the literature. *AIDS Res Ther*. 2008;5:25-6405-5-25. http://doi:10.1186/1742-6405-5-25

Galantino ML, Shepard K, Krafft L, et al. The effect of group aerobic exercise and t'ai chi on functional outcomes and quality of life for persons living with acquired immunodeficiency syndrome. *J Altern Complement Med*. 2005;11(6):1085–1092.

Galera RL, Pascuet ER, Mur JE, et al. Interaction between cat's claw and protease inhibitors atazanavir, ritonavir and saquinavir. *Eur J Clin Pharm*. 2008;64(12):1235–1236.

Gallicano K, Foster B, Choudhri S. Effect of short-term administration of garlic supplements on single-dose ritonavir pharmacokinetics in healthy volunteers. *Br J Clin Pharmacol*. 2003;55(2): 199–202.

Gayner B, Esplen MJ, DeRoche P, et al. A randomized controlled trial of mindfulness-based stress reduction to manage affective symptoms and improve quality of life in gay men living with HIV. *J Behav Med*. 2012;35(3):272–285.

Gerber JG, Kitch DW, Fichtenbaum CJ, et al. Fish oil and fenofibrate for the treatment of hypertriglyceridemia in HIV-infected subjects on antiretroviral therapy: results of ACTG A5186. *J AIDS*. 2008;47(4):459–466. http://doi:10.1097/QAI.0b013e31815bace2

Goldenberg JZ, Yap C, Lytvyn, L, et al. Probiotics for the prevention of Clostridium difficile-associated diarrhea in adults and children. *Cochrane Database Syst Rev*. 2017;12(12):Cd006095. http://doi:10.1002/14651858.CD006095.pub4

Gonzalez-Garcia M, Ferrer MJ, Borras X, et al. Effectiveness of mindfulness-based cognitive therapy on the quality of life, emotional status, and CD4 $^+$ T cell count of patients aging with HIV infection. *AIDS Behav*. 2014;18(4):676–685.

Graham NM, Sorensen D, Odaka N, et al. Relationship of serum copper and zinc levels to HIV-1 seropositivity and progression to AIDS. *JAIDS*. 1991;4(10):976–980.

Greene KB, Berger J, Reeves C, et al. Most frequently used alternative and complementary therapies and activities by participants in the AMCOA study. *J Assoc Nurses AIDS Care*. 1999;10(3):60–73.

Grosso G, Micek A, Marventano S, et al. Dietary n-3 PUFA, fish consumption and depression: a systematic review and meta-analysis of observational studies. *J Affect Disord*. 2016;205:269–281.

Gwaza L, Aweeka F, Greenblatt R, et al. Co-administration of a commonly used Zimbabwean herbal treatment (African potato) does not alter the pharmacokinetics of lopinavir/ritonavir. *Int J Infect Dis*. 2013;17(10):e857–e861.

Hadadi A, Ostovar A, Edalat Noor B, et al. The effect of selenium and zinc on CD4(+) count and opportunistic infections in HIV/AIDS patients: a randomized double blind trial. *Acta Clin Belg*. 2020;75(3):170–176. http://doi:10.1080/17843286.2019.1590023

Hafner V, Jager M, Matthee AK, et al. Effect of simultaneous induction and inhibition of CYP3A by St John's Wort and ritonavir on CYP3A activity. *Clin Pharmacol Ther*. 2010;8(2):191–196.

Halpin SN, Carruth EC, Rai RP, et al. Complementary and alternative medicine among persons living with HIV in the era of combined antiretroviral treatment. *AIDS Behav*. 2018;22(3):848–852.

Haron MH, Avula B, Ali Z, et al. Assessment of herb-drug interaction potential of five common species of licorice and their phytochemical constituents. *J Diet Suppl*. 2022;1–20. http://doi:10.1080/19390211.2022.2050875. Online ahead of print.

Havens PL, Stephensen CB, Van Loan MD, et al. Vitamin D3 supplementation increases spine bone mineral density in adolescents and young adults with human immunodeficiency virus infection being treated with tenofovir disoproxil fumarate: a randomized, placebo-controlled trial. *Clin Infect Dis*. 2017;66(2):220–228.

Hecht FM, Moskowitz JT, Moran P, et al. A randomized, controlled trial of mindfulness-based stress reduction in HIV infection. *Brain Behav Immun*. 2018;73:331–339. http://doi:S0889-1591(18)30190-9

Hepburn MJ, Dyal K, Runser LA, et al. Low serum vitamin B$_{12}$ levels in an outpatient HIV-infected population. *Int J STD AIDS*. 2004;15(2):127–133. http://doi:10.1258/095646204322764334

Hillier SL, Louw Q, Morris L, et al. Massage therapy for people with HIV/AIDS. *Cochrane Database Sys Rev*. 2010;1:CD007502.

Hinman RS, McCrory P, Pirotta M, et al. Acupuncture for chronic knee pain: a randomized clinical trial. *JAMA*. 2014;312(13):313–1322.

Holick MF, Binkley NC, Bischoff-Ferrari HA, et al. Evaluation, treatment, and prevention of vitamin D deficiency: an endocrine society clinical practice guideline. *J Clin Endocrin Metab*. 2011;96(7):1911–1930.

Hu Y, Hu FB, Manson JE. Marine omega-3 supplementation and cardiovascular disease: an updated meta-analysis of 13 randomized controlled trials involving 127 477 participants. *J Am Heart Assoc*. 2019;8(19):e013543. http://doi:10.1161/JAHA.119.013543

Ironson G, O'Cleirigh C, Fletcher MA, et al. Psychosocial factors predict CD4 $^+$ T cell and viral load change in men and women with human immunodeficiency virus in the era of highly active antiretroviral treatment. *Psychosom Med*. 2005;67(6):1013–1021. http://doi:67/6/1013

Jacek H, Rentsch KM, Steinert HC, et al. No effect of garlic extract on saquinavir kinetics and hepatic CYP3A4 function measured by the erythromycin breath test. *Clin Pharmacol Ther*. 2004;75(2):P80–P80. http://doi:10.1016/j.clpt.2003.11.304

Jackson RD, LaCroix AZ, Gass M, et al. Calcium plus vitamin D supplementation and the risk of fractures. *N Engl J Med.* 2006;354(7):669–683.

Jalloh MA, Gregory PJ, Hein D, et al. Dietary supplement interactions with antiretrovirals: a systematic review. *Int J STD AIDS.* 2017;28(1):4–15. http://doi:10.1177/0956462416671087

Jiamton S, Pepin J, Suttent R, et al. A randomized trial of the impact of multiple micronutrient supplementation on mortality among HIV-infected individuals. living in Bangkok. *AIDS.* 2003;17(17):2461–2469.

Jiang T, Hou J, Sun R, et al. Immunological and psychological efficacy of meditation/yoga intervention among people living with HIV (PLWH): a systematic review and meta-analyses of 19 randomized controlled trials. *Ann Behav Med.* 2011;55(6):505–519. http://doi:10.1093/abm/kaaa084

Jones CY, Tang AM, Forrester JE, et al. Micronutrient levels and HIV disease status in HIV-infected patients on highly active antiretroviral therapy in the nutrition for healthy living cohort. *J AIDS.* 2006;43(4):475–482. http://doi:10.1097/01.qai.0000243096.27029.fe

Josephs J, Fleishman J, Gaist P, et al. Use of complementary and alternative medicines among a multistate, multisite cohort of people living with HIV/AIDS. *HIV Med.* 2007;8(5):300–305.

Kaiser JD, Campa AM, Ondercin JP, et al. Micronutrient supplementation increases CD4$^+$ T cell count in PWH on highly active antiretroviral therapy: a prospective, double-blinded, placebo-controlled trial. *J AIDS.* 2006;42(5):523–528. http://doi:10.1097/01.qai.0000230529.25083.42

Kakalia S, Sochett EB, Stephens D, et al. Vitamin D supplementation and CD4 count in children infected with human immunodeficiency virus. *J Pediatr.* 2011;159(6):951–957.

Karaszewska DM, Ingenhoven T, Mocking RJT. Marine omega-3 fatty acid supplementation for borderline personality disorder: a meta-analysis. *J Clin Psychiatry.* 2021;82(3):20r13613. http://doi:10.4088/JCP.20r13613

Kasibhatta R, Naidu M. Influence of piperine on the pharmacokinetics of nevirapine under fasting conditions. *Drugs in R & D.* 2007;8(6):383–391.

Kayode I, Anaba U. Effect of vitamin D, selenium, or zinc supplementation in human immunodeficiency virus: a systematic review. *AIDS Reviews.* 2020;22:1–10.

Kelso-Chichetto NE, Okafor CN, Harman JS, et al. Complementary and alternative medicine use for HIV management in the state of Florida: medical monitoring project. *J Altern Complement Med.* 2016;22(11):880–886.

Kostoglou-Athanassiou I, Athanassiou L, Athanassiou P. The effect of omega-3 fatty acids on rheumatoid arthritis. *Mediterr J Rheumatol.* 2020;31(2):190–194.

Ladenheim D, Horn O, Werneke U, et al. Potential health risks of complementary alternative medicines in HIV patients. *HIV Medicine.* 2008;9(8):653–659.

Lamorde M, Byakika-Kibwika P, Merry C. Pharmacokinetic interactions between antiretroviral drugs and herbal medicines. *Br J Hosp Med.* 2012;73(3):132–136.

Lavretsky H, Epel E, Siddarth P, et al. A pilot study of yogic meditation for family dementia caregivers with depressive symptoms: effects on mental health, cognition, and telomerase activity. *Int J Geriatr Psychiatry.* 2013;28(1):57–65.

Lee LS, Andrade AS, Flexner C. Interactions between natural health products and antiretroviral drugs: pharmacokinetic and pharmacodynamic effects. *Clin Infect Dis.* 2006;43(8):1052–1059. http://doi:CID39658

Leserman, J. Role of depression, stress, and trauma in HIV disease progression. *Psychosom Med.* 2008;70(5):539–545. http://doi:10.1097/PSY.0b013e3181777a5f

Leserman J, Petitto J, Gu H, et al. Progression to AIDS, a clinical AIDS condition and mortality: psychosocial and physiological predictors. *Psychol Med.* 2002;32(06):1059–1073.

Leserman J, Petitto JM, Perkins DO, et al. Severe stress, depressive symptoms, and changes in lymphocyte subsets in human immunodeficiency virus-infected men: a 2-year follow-up study. *Arch Gen Psychiatry.* 1997;54(3):279–285.

Levine GN, Lange RA, Bairey-Merz CN, et al. Meditation and cardiovascular risk reduction: a scientific statement from the American Heart Association. *J Am Heart Assoc.* 2017;6(10):e002218.

Linde K, Allais G, Brinkhaus B, et al. Acupuncture for tension-type headache. *Cochrane Database Syst Rev.* 2009;1:CD007587.

Littlewood RA, Vanable PA. Complementary and alternative medicine use among HIV-positive people: research synthesis and implications for HIV care. *AIDS Care.* 2008;20(8):1002–1018.

Littlewood RA, Vanable PA. A global perspective on complementary and alternative medicine use among people living with HIV/AIDS in the era of antiretroviral treatment. *Curr HIV/AIDS Rep.* 2011;8(4):257–268.

Littlewood RA, Vanable PA. The relationship between CAM use and adherence to antiretroviral therapies among persons living with HIV. *Health Psychol.* 2014;33(7):660.

Liu C, Yang Y, Gange SJ., et al. Disclosure of complementary and alternative medicine use to health care providers among HIV-infected women. *AIDS Patient Care STDs.* 2009;23(11):965–971.

London AS, Foote-Ardah CE, Fleishman JA, et al. Use of alternative therapists among people in care for HIV in the United States. *Am J Public Health.* 2003;93(6):980–987.

Lorenc A, Robinson N. A review of the use of complementary and alternative medicine and HIV: issues for patient care. *AIDS Patient Care STDs.* 2013;27(9): 503–510.

Lozupone CA, Li M, Campbell TB, et al. Alterations in the gut microbiota associated with HIV-1 infection. *Cell Host Microbe.* 2013;14(3):329–339.

Ma J, Li Y, Ye Q, et al. Constituents of red yeast rice, a traditional Chinese food and medicine. *J Agric Food Chem.* 2000;48(11):5220–5225.

MacArthur RD, Levine SD, Birk TJ Supervised exercise training improves cardiopulmonary fitness in HIV-infected persons. *Med Sci Sports Exer.* 1993;25(6):684–688.

MacDonald L, Murty M, Foster BC. Antiviral drug disposition and natural health products: risk of therapeutic alteration and resistance. *Expert Opin Drug Metab Toxicol.* 2009;5(6):563–578. http://doi:10.1517/17425250902942302

Maggiolo F, Rizzardini G, Raffi F, et al. Bone mineral density in virologically suppressed people aged 60 years or older with HIV-1 switching from a regimen containing tenofovir disoproxil fumarate to an elvitegravir, cobicistat, emtricitabine, and tenofovir alafenamide single-tablet regimen: a multicentre, open-label, phase 3b, randomised trial. *Lancet HIV.* 2019;6(10):e655–e66.

Manheimer E, Cheng K, Linde K, et al. Acupuncture for peripheral joint osteoarthritis. *Cochrane Database Syst Rev.* 2010;1: CD001977.

Manson JE, Cook NR, Lee IM, et al. Marine n-3 fatty acids and prevention of cardiovascular disease and cancer. *N Engl J Med.* 2019;380(1):23–32.

Mateo-Carrasco H, Gálvez-Contreras MC, Fernández-Ginés FD, et al. A potential drug–herbal interaction between ginkgo biloba and efavirenz. *J Int Assoc Physicians AIDS Care.* 2012;11(2):98–100. http://doi:10.1177/1545109711435364

McCain NL, Gray DP, Elswick Jr R, et al. A randomized clinical trial of alternative stress management interventions in persons with HIV infection. *J Consult Clin Psychol.* 2008;76(3):431.

Milan FB, Arnsten JH., Klein RS, et al. Use of complementary and alternative medicine in inner-city persons with or at risk for HIV infection. *AIDS Patient Care STDs.* 2008:22(10):811–816.

Mills E, Wilson K, Clarke M, et al. Milk thistle and indinavir: A randomized controlled pharmacokinetics study and meta-analysis. *Eur J Clin Pharmacol.* 2005;61(1):1–7.

Molto J, Valle M, Miranda C, et al. Herb–drug interaction between echinacea purpurea and darunavir–ritonavir in HIV-infected patients. *Antimicrob Agents Chemother.* 2011;55(1):326–330. http://doi:10.1128/AAC.01082-10

Molto J, Valle M, Miranda C, et al. Effect of milk thistle on the pharmacokinetics of darunavir–ritonavir in HIV-infected patients.

Antimicrob Agents Chemother. 2012a;56(6):2837–2841. http://doi:10.1128/AAC.00025-12

Molto J, Valle M, Miranda C, et al. Herb–drug interaction between echinacea purpurea and etravirine in HIV-infected patients. *Antimicrob Agents Chemother.* 2012b;56(10):5328–5331. http://doi:10.1128/AAC.01205-12

Mutlu EA, Keshavarzian A, Losurdo J, et al. A compositional look at the human gastrointestinal microbiome and immune activation parameters in HIV infected subjects. *PLoS Pathog.* 2014;10(2):e1003829.

Muzembo BA, Ngatu NR, Januka K, et al. Selenium supplementation in HIV-infected individuals: a systematic review of randomized controlled trials. *Clin Nutr ESPEN.* 2019;34:1–7.

Naccarato M, Yoong D, Gough K. A potential drug–herbal interaction between ginkgo biloba and efavirenz. *J IAPAC (Chicago).* 2012;11(2):98–100. http://doi:10.1177/1545109711435364

Naoroibam R, Metri KG, Bhargav H, et al. Effect of integrated yoga (IY) on psychological states and CD4 counts of HIV-1 infected patients: a randomized controlled pilot study. *Int J Yoga.* 2016;9(1):57–61. http://doi:10.4103/0973-6131.171723

National Center for Complementary and Integrative Health (NCCIH). https://www.nccih.nih.gov/health/. Published 2022. Accessed August 15, 2022.

Okereke OI, Vyas CM, Mischoulon D. Effect of long-term supplementation with marine omega-3 fatty acids vs placebo on risk of depression or clinically relevant depressive symptoms and on change in mood scores: a randomized clinical trial. *JAMA.* 2021;326(23):2385–2394. http://doi:10.1001/jama.2021.21187

Okunade KS, Olowoselu OF, Osanyin GE, et al. Selenium deficiency and pregnancy outcome in pregnant women with HIV in Lagos, Nigeria. *Int J Gynaecol Obstet.* 2018;142(2):207–213.

Okunade KS, Olowoselu OF, John-Olabode S, et al. Effects of selenium supplementation on pregnancy outcomes and disease progression in HIV-infected pregnant women in Lagos: a randomized controlled trial. *Int J Gynaecol Obstet.* 2021;153(3):533–541. http://doi:10.1002/ijgo.13514

Oliveira JM, Rondó PH, Yudkin JS, et al. Effects of fish oil on lipid profile and other metabolic outcomes in HIV-infected patients on antiretroviral therapy: a randomized placebo-controlled trial. *Int J STD AIDS.* 2014;25(2):96–104.

Overton ET, Chan ES, Brown TT, et al. Vitamin D and calcium attenuate bone loss with antiretroviral therapy initiation: a randomized trial. *Ann Intern Med.* 2015;162(12):815–824.

Owen-Smith A, Diclemente R, Wingood G. Complementary and alternative medicine use decreases adherence to HAART in HIV-positive women. *AIDS Care.* 2007;19(5):589–593.

Patel P, Song I, Borland J, et al. Pharmacokinetics of the HIV integrase inhibitor S/GSK1349572 co-administered with acid-reducing agents and multivitamins in healthy volunteers. *J Antimicrob Chemother.* 2011;66(7):1567–1572. http://doi:10.1093/jac/dkr139

Patel SJ, Kemper KJ, Kitzmiller JP Physician perspectives on education, training, and implementation of complementary and alternative medicine. *Adv Med Educ Practice.* 2017;8:499.

Pence BW, Miller WC, Whetten K, et al. Prevalence of DSM-IV-defined mood, anxiety, and substance use disorders in an HIV clinic in the southeastern United States. *J AIDS.* 2006;42(3):298–306. http://doi:10.1097/01.qai.0000219773.82055.aa

Penzak SR, Robertson SM, Hunt JD, et al. Echinacea purpurea significantly induces cytochrome P450 3A activity but does not alter lopinavir–ritonavir exposure in healthy subjects. *Pharmacotherapy.* 2010;30(8):797–805. http://doi:10.1592/phco.30.8.797

Perazzo JD, Webel AR, Alam SK, et al. Relationships between physical activity and bone density in people living with HIV: results from the SATURN-HIV study. *J Assoc Nurses AIDS Care.* 2018;29(4):528–537.

Peters BS, Wierzbicki AS, Moyle G, et al. The effect of a 12-week course of omega-3 polyunsaturated fatty acids on lipid parameters in hypertriglyceridemic adult HIV-infected patients undergoing HAART: a randomized, placebo-controlled pilot trial. *Clin Ther.* 2012;34(1):67–76.

Phillips KD, Skelton WD. Effects of individualized acupuncture on sleep quality in HIV disease. *J Assoc Nurses AIDS Care.* 2001;12(1):27–39.

Piscitelli SC, Burstein AH, Chaitt D, et al. Indinavir concentrations and St. John's wort. *Lancet.* 2000;355(9203):547–548.

Piscitelli SC, Burstein AH, Welden N, et al. The effect of garlic supplements on the pharmacokinetics of saquinavir. *Clin Infect Dis.* 2002a;34(2):234–238. http://doi:CID010586

Piscitelli SC, Formentini E, Burstein AH, et al. Effect of milk thistle on the pharmacokinetics of indinavir in healthy volunteers. *Pharmacotherapy.* 2002b;22(5):551–556.

Power R, Gore-Felton C, Vosvick M, et al. HIV: effectiveness of complementary and alternative medicine. *Prim Care.* 2002;29(2):361–378.

Quigley A, O'Brien K, Parker K. Exercise and cognitive function in people living with HIV: a scoping review. *Disabil Rehabil.* 2019;41(12):1384–1395.

Ramirez-Garcia MP, Gagnon MP, Colson S, et al. Mind-body practices for people living with HIV: a systematic scoping review. *BMC Complement Altern Med.* 2019;19(1):125.

Range N, Changalucha J, Krarup H, et al. The effect of multi-vitamin/mineral supplementation on mortality during treatment of pulmonary tuberculosis: a randomised two-by-two factorial trial in Mwanza, Tanzania. *Br J Nutr.* 2006;95(4):762–770.

Ravi S, Khalili H, Abbasian L, et al. Effect of omega-3 fatty acids on depressive symptoms in HIV-positive individuals: a randomized, placebo-controlled clinical trial. *Ann Pharmacother.* 2016;50(10):797–807.

Remacha AF, Cadafalch J, Sarda P, et al. Vitamin B-12 metabolism in HIV-infected patients in the age of highly antiretroviral therapy: role of homocysteine in assessing vitamin B-12 status. *Am J Clin Nutr.* 2003;77(2):420–424.

Rigsby LW, Dishman R, Jackson AW, et al. Effects of exercise training on men seropositive for the human immunodeficiency virus-1. *Med Sci Sports Exercise.* 1992;24(1):6–12.

Robertson SM, Davey RT, Voell J, et al. Effect of ginkgo biloba extract on lopinavir, midazolam and fexofenadine pharmacokinetics in healthy subjects. *Curr Med Res Opin.* 2008;24(2):591–599. http://doi:10.1185/030079908X260871

Sandhu RS, Prescilla RP, Simonelli TM, et al. Influence of goldenseal root on the pharmacokinetics of indinavir. *J Clin Pharmacol.* 2003;43(11):1283–1288.

Saper RB, Phillips RS, Sehgal A, et al. Lead, mercury, and arsenic in US- and Indian-manufactured Ayurvedic medicines sold via the Internet. *JAMA.* 2008;300(8):915–923.

Shere-Wolfe KD, Tilburt JC, D'Adamo C, et al. Infectious diseases physicians' attitudes and practices related to complementary and integrative medicine: results of a national survey. *Evid Based Complement Altern Med.* 2013. Article ID 294381.

Sherwood JE, Mesner OC, Weintrob AC, et al. Vitamin D deficiency and its association with low bone mineral density, HIV-related factors, hospitalization, and death in a predominantly black HIV-infected cohort. *Clin Infect Dis.* 2012;55(12):1727–1736.

Shlay JC, Chaloner K, Max MB, et al. Acupuncture and amitriptyline for pain due to HIV-related peripheral neuropathy: a randomized controlled trial. *JAMA.* 1998;280(18):1590–1595.

Silva M, Montes CG, Canals A, et al. Role and effects of zinc supplementation in HIV-infected patients with immunovirological discordance: a randomized, double blind, case control study. *PLoS One.* 2021;16(1):e0244823. http://doi:10.1371/journal.pone.0244823

Slain D, Amsden JR, Khakoo RA, et al. Effect of high-dose vitamin C on the steady-state pharmacokinetics of the protease inhibitor indinavir in healthy volunteers. *Pharmacotherapy.* 2005;25(2):165–170.

Song I, Borland J, Arya N, et al. Pharmacokinetics of dolutegravir when administered with mineral supplements in healthy adult subjects. *J Clin Pharmacol.* 2015;55(5):490–496. http://doi:10.1002/jcph.439

Standish L, Greene K, Bain S, et al. Alternative medicine use in HIV-positive men and women: demographics, utilization patterns and health status. *AIDS Care.* 2001;13(2):197–208.

Stringer WW, Berezovskaya M, O'Brien WA, et al. The effect of exercise training on aerobic fitness, immune indices, and quality of life in HIV patients. *Med Sci Sports Exercise.* 1998;30(1):11–16.

Stussman BJ, Black LI, Barnes PM, et al. Wellness-related use of common complementary health approaches among adults: United States, 2012. *Natl Health Stat Rep.* 2015;85:1–12.

Su GL, Ko CW, Bercik P, et al. AGA clinical practice guidelines on the role of probiotics in the management of gastrointestinal disorders. *Gastroenterology.* 2020;159(2):697–705. http://doi:10.1053/j.gastro.2020.05.059

Sucharita PB, Reshmi YS, Basker MM, et al. Effect of nutritional supplementation on illness outcome in adolescents with HIV on HAART: a randomized, double-blind clinical trial. *Indian J Pediatr.* 2022;10:1007/s12098-022-04195-z. http://doi:10.1007/s12098-022-04195-z

Sudfeld CR, Buchanan A, Ulenga N, et al. Effectiveness of a multivitamin supplementation program among HIV-infected adults in Tanzania. *AIDS.* 2019;33(1):93–100.

Sudfeld CR, Aboud S, Kupka R, et al. Effect of selenium supplementation on HIV-1 RNA detection in breast milk of Tanzanian women. *Nutrition.* 2014;30(9):1081–1084. http://doi:10.1097/qad.0000000000002033

Sudfeld CR, Mugusi F, Muhihi A, et al. Efficacy of vitamin D(3) supplementation for the prevention of pulmonary tuberculosis and mortality in HIV: a randomised, double-blind, placebo-controlled trial. *Lancet HIV.* 2020;7(7):e463–e471. http://doi:10.1016/s2352-3018(20)30108-9

Sudfeld CR, Wang M, Aboud S, et al. Vitamin D and HIV progression among Tanzanian adults initiating antiretroviral therapy. *PloS One.* 2012;7(6):e40036.

Swanson B, Keithley J, Baum L, et al. Effects of fish oil on HIV-related inflammation and markers of immunosenescence: a randomized clinical trial. *J Altern Complement Med.* 2018;24(7):709–716. http://doi:10.1089/acm.2017.0222

Tenforde MW, Yadav A, Dowdy DW, et al. Vitamin A and D deficiencies associated with incident tuberculosis in HIV-infected patients initiating antiretroviral therapy in multinational case-cohort study. *J AIDS.* 2017;75(3):e71–e79.

Thompson MA, Aberg JA, Hoy JF, et al. Antiretroviral treatment of adult HIV infection: 2012 recommendations of the International Antiviral Society–USA panel. *JAMA.* 2012;308(4):387–402.

Ting A, Chow Y, Tan W. Microbial and heavy metal contamination in commonly consumed traditional Chinese herbal medicines. *J Tradit Chin Med.* 2013;33(1):119–124.

US Department of Health and Human Services, National Institutes of Health (USDHHS/NIS). Complementary, alternative, or integrative health: what's in a name? https://www.nccih.nih.gov/health/complementary-alternative-or-integrative-health-whats-in-a-name. Published 2022. Accessed August 15, 2022.

van Heeswijk RP, Cooper CL, Foster BC, et al. Effect of high-dose vitamin C on hepatic cytochrome P450 3A4 activity. *Pharmacotherapy.* 2005;25(12):1725–1728.

Vickers AJ, Cronin AM, Maschino AC, et al. Acupuncture for chronic pain: individual patient data meta-analysis. *Arch Intern Med.* 2012;172(19):1444–1453.

Visser ME, Durao S, Sinclair D, et al. Micronutrient supplementation in adults with HIV infection. *Cochrane Database Syst Rev.* 2017;5(5):Cd003650. http://doi:10.1002/14651858.CD003650.pub4

Visser RD, Grierson J. Use of alternative therapies by people living with HIV/AIDS in Australia. *AIDS Care.* 2002;14(5):599–606.

Vogl D, Rosenfeld B, Breitbart W, et al. Symptom prevalence, characteristics, and distress in AIDS outpatients. *J Pain Symptom Manage.* 1999;18(4):253–262.

Vujkovic-Cvijin I, Dunham RM, Iwai S, et al. Dysbiosis of the gut microbiota is associated with HIV disease progression and tryptophan catabolism. *Sci Transl Med.* 2013;5(193):193ra91. http://doi:10.1126/scitranslmed.3006438

Wahner-Roedler DL, Lee MC, Chon TY, et al. Physicians' attitudes toward complementary and alternative medicine and their knowledge of specific therapies: 8-year follow-up at an academic medical center. *Complement Ther Clin Practice.* 2014;20(1):54–60.

Warburton DE, Nicol CW, Bredin SS. Health benefits of physical activity: the evidence. *Can Med Assoc J.* 2006;174(6):801–809. http://doi:174/6/801

Webb L, Perry-Parrish C, Ellen J, Sibinga E. Mindfulness instruction for HIV-infected youth: a randomized controlled trial. *AIDS Care.* 2018;30(6):688–695.

Whetten K, Reif S, Whetten R, et al. Trauma, mental health, distrust, and stigma among HIV-positive persons: implications for effective care. *Psychosom Med.* 2008;70(5):531–538. http://doi:10.1097/PSY.0b013e31817749dc

Wiegman DJ, Brinkman K, Franssen EJ. Interaction of Ginkgo biloba with efavirenz. *AIDS.* 2009;23(9):1184–1185.

Witt CM, Jena S, Brinkhaus B, et al. Acupuncture for patients with chronic neck pain. *Pain.* 2006;125(1):98–106.

Wohl DA, Tien HC, Busby M, et al. Randomized study of the safety and efficacy of fish oil (omega-3 fatty acid) supplementation with dietary and exercise counseling for the treatment of antiretroviral therapy-associated hypertriglyceridemia. *Clin Infect Dis.* 2005;41(10):1498–1504. http://doi:CID37106

Wynia MK, Eisenberg DM, Wilson, IB. Physician–patient communication about complementary and alternative medical therapies: a survey of physicians caring for patients with human immunodeficiency virus infection. *J Altern Complement Med.* 1999;5(5):447–456.

Xiong Y, Gao M, van Duijn B, et al. International policies and challenges on the legalization of traditional medicine/herbal medicines in the fight against COVID-19. *Pharmacol Res.* 2021;166:105472. http://doi:10.1016/j.phrs.2021.105472

Zhang F, Liu W, Huang J, et al. Inhibition of drug-metabolizing enzymes by Jingyin granules: implications of herb–drug interactions in antiviral therapy. *Acta Pharmacologica Sinica.* 2022;43(4):1072–1081. http://doi:10.1038/s41401-021-00697-2

Zhang L, Tin A, Brown TT, et al. Vitamin D deficiency and metabolism in HIV-infected and HIV-uninfected men in the multicenter AIDS cohort study. *AIDS Res Hum Retroviruses.* 2017;33(3):261–270. http://doi:10.1089/AID.2016.0144

14.

HIV CARE COORDINATION

Margret O. Nelson

CHAPTER GOAL

Upon completion of this chapter, the reader should be able to:

- Demonstrate knowledge and the practice of interdisciplinary care coordination in the care of people living with HIV (PWH).

IMPORTANCE OF AN INTERDISCIPLINARY APPROACH TO HIV PATIENT CARE

LEARNING OBJECTIVE

Describe the importance of an interdisciplinary team approach to the optimal management of PWH.

KEY POINTS

- As PWH are surviving longer there is an increased prevalence of non–HIV-related comorbidities, which has resulted in an increasing need for chronic disease management.

- Coordination of care using a patient-centered interdisciplinary team model can be an effective strategy to increase engagement in care and reduce barriers, especially for complicated patients and/or those with few resources.

- When antiretroviral treatment is no longer effective, palliative care and hospice care teams focus on quality of life and comfort care, offering emotional and spiritual support.

Currently available antiretroviral therapies (ART) have higher efficacy and lower side-effect profiles and are associated with better adherence compared to ART available in previous decades. This has led to prolonged survival, approaching that of the general population (Samji et al., 2014; Wada et al., 2014). This prolonged survival, coupled with the fact that the US incidence of HIV has decreased only moderately over the past decade (Centers for Disease Control and Preventer (CDC), 2020), has resulted in an increased number of PWH needing complex medical care.

In 2018, over half of PWH were aged 50 years or older (CDC, 2020), and this segment of PWH is increasing. HIV accentuates the complications of aging, manifested by the earlier onset of cardiovascular disease, cognitive impairment, certain types of cancer, and diabetes in PWH relative to their HIV negative peers. As a result of both factors (i.e., increased age of PWH and increased risk of certain comorbidities), PWH often require chronic disease management in addition to the treatment of HIV infection (Chu & Selwyn, 2011; Guaraldi et al., 2018). Thus, optimal care for PWH is provided by clinicians with expertise in general medicine, behavioral health, and substance abuse treatment, in addition to HIV medicine and infectious diseases.

The HIV epidemic disproportionately affects people of color, as well as those with less education, lower income, lack of adequate insurance, lack of permanent housing, and those with a history of incarceration. Black men who have sex with men (MSM) have the highest rates of new infection (CDC, 2020). Ongoing stigma discourages HIV testing and may result in late presentations to care, and with more advanced disease. There may be real or perceived personal, cultural, or system-based barriers to care (Bauman et al., 2013; CDC, 2014; Irvine et al., 2014; Scanlon & Vreeman, 2013), which in some individuals can result in lower levels of continued engagement and result in suboptimal viral suppression (Gardner et al., 2011; White House Office of National AIDS Policy, 2014).

The social determinants of health play an important role in caring for PWH. Many PWH are facing the day-to-day struggles of poverty (e.g., unstable housing, lack of transportation and childcare, and inadequate medical insurance), which can impact their engagement in HIV care. These individuals are also likely to have more difficulty navigating the increasingly complicated US healthcare system, resulting in fragmented care or disengagement. If not addressed, these issues may result in lower levels of continued engagement and viral suppression.

THE HIV CONTINUUM OF CARE

The goals of HIV clinical care are to suppress viral replication, decrease HIV-related morbidities, improve immune status, prolong survival, improve quality of life, and decrease HIV transmission (US Department of Health and Human Services (USDHHS), 2021). The key steps needed to achieve

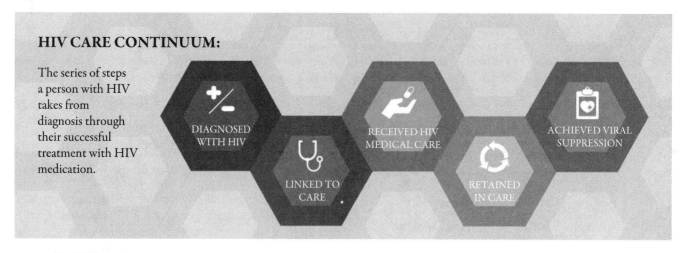

HIV CARE CONTINUUM:

The series of steps a person with HIV takes from diagnosis through their successful treatment with HIV medication.

DIAGNOSED WITH HIV

LINKED TO CARE

RECEIVED HIV MEDICAL CARE

RETAINED IN CARE

ACHIEVED VIRAL SUPPRESSION

Figure 14.1 The HIV care continuum   SOURCE: Centers for Disease Control and Prevention. HIV.Care.Continuum/HIV.gov. https://files.hiv.gov/s3fs-public/care-continuum-banner-v1.jpg. Published 2022. Accessed August 15, 2022.

these goals have been described as the HIV continuum of care, and include timely diagnosis, linkage to and subsequent retention in care, and finally, initiation and continuation of ART (CDC facts sheet, 2019). The steps in the HIV continuum are the basis of the recent US plan "Ending the HIV Epidemic: A Plan for America," which includes the goal to decrease HIV incidence by 90% by 2030 (USDHHS, 2021) (Figure 14.1).

The first step in the HIV continuum of care is the timely diagnosis of HIV infection. This requires a combination of targeted community outreach to increase testing in high-risk populations as well as routine HIV screening in the general population (USPSTF, 2019). The next step is prompt linkage to care, followed by engagement in care, and retention of the patient in care while ART is initiated. A growing body of literature supports the prolonged benefits of increased likelihood of viral suppression and retention in care with same-day or rapid (within 14 days of diagnosis) ART initiation (Ford et al., 2018). Once ART is initiated—and potentially for decades to follow—the patient needs to be effectively followed and supported in care to ensure durable virologic suppression. There are barriers to success at each step in the continuum, which need to be identified, anticipated, and addressed by clinicians and others providing care. The goals in the HIV continuum can be challenging and often require input and expertise from members of an interdisciplinary HIV care team working together to address potential barriers including depression, substance abuse, lack of housing, and lack of medical insurance (Dombrowski et al., 2015).

COMPLEXITY OF PWH CARE NEEDS

The following are illustrative case examples of the types of complex comorbidities and chronic conditions that currently characterize the care of PWH:

1. An obese 55-year-old woman has a history of major depression and prior inconsistent medication adherence, which led to virologic failure; she is currently taking ART and has an undetectable viral load.

This patient stopped seeing her therapist and psychiatrist one year ago because she felt she no longer required mental health treatment. However, she was recently divorced, lost her job (and thus her health insurance), and is not accepting of her new diagnosis of type 2 diabetes mellitus. Although this patient's HIV is currently controlled, the HIV provider is concerned about her recent major life events leading to a depressive episode, which may impact medication adherence, and thought this may have caused the decreased efficacy of her first HIV regimen (Crockett et al., 2020). This patient will need several issues addressed simultaneously including treatment of her depression, applying for Medicaid and the AIDS Drug Assistance Program (ADAP), and treatment of her obesity and diabetes. She would benefit from prompt referrals to behavioral health for treatment of her depression (both therapist and psychiatrist), to a case manager and financial counselor for assistance with ADAP and Medicaid, and to a nutritionist and endocrinologist for treatment of coexisting medical problems.

2. A 58-year-old man with multiple comorbidities including large granular lymphocytic leukemia, HIV on ART (CD4 >650 cells/mm^3, VL< 20 copies/log10), nonalcoholic fatty liver disease, type 2 diabetes mellitus, coronary artery disease, seizure disorder, anxiety, posttraumatic stress disorder, and chronic back pain. He presents to the Emergency Department with new pancytopenia and concern for myelodysplastic syndrome.

Despite having the benefit of stable housing and good insurance coverage, this patient has many needs that will challenge his team's ability to communicate between institutions. He was admitted to the hospital to work up his pancytopenia, manage his chronic back pain, and monitor and treat his escalating anxiety related to being hospitalized. His hospital-based oncology team can guide his new work up without introducing unfamiliar clinicians and aggravating his anxiety. His primary care team can provide rich historical and psychosocial information for the hospitalist team. Care coordination between sites will be very important for discharge planning and posthospitalization follow-up. The patient and his caregivers will need support through the stress of any new diagnosis. A palliative care consult would provide guidance and continuity across primary care and specialists, ensuring the treatment plan addresses the patient's complex needs.

PALLIATIVE CARE AND HOSPICE CARE

In the setting of advancements in ART and life expectancy for PWH, end-of-life care should be addressed as it would with any patient. Discussions about advanced care planning should be prioritized with all people diagnosed with serious illness to help lay the groundwork for choices later in care. These discussions should include intervention preferences, favored care settings, feelings about palliative/hospice care, and documented selection of a health care proxy. Studies have shown that patients who have participated in advance-care planning are more likely to be satisfied with their care.

The terms *palliative care* and *hospice care* are often used interchangeably. While both use an interdisciplinary approach and include a focus on comfort and symptom management and the inclusion of the person and their caregivers in decision-making, there are differences.

Palliative care is the broader term and *hospice care* is a component. Palliative care is designed to address suffering and improve quality of life at any stage of illness, from diagnosis to recovery or death. This whole person approach is most effective when engaged well before end-of-life care is needed. Symptom management interventions can be delivered while treatment for serious illness continues. Palliative care is meant to enhance a person's current care by focusing on quality of life (NIA, 2017). This level of care can be provided in hospitals, nursing homes, outpatient palliative care clinics, or at home.

Hospice care is a specialized form of palliative care that is delivered in the final months or weeks of life. Hospice care is focused on comfort and quality of life when curative treatment options are no longer effective and life expectancy is limited (typically 6 months or less). Like palliative care, hospice provides comprehensive comfort care and support for caregivers. When hospice care is delivered at home, a member of the hospice team visits regularly, and they are available by phone around the clock with individuals close to the patient often serving as primary caregivers. Dedicated hospice facilities, whether in hospitals or free-standing hospice homes, are staffed by licensed and unlicensed care givers. Unfortunately, many patients are enrolled in hospice care very late in their treatment course, missing the opportunity to benefit from hospice care. Beginning hospice care earlier can provide months of meaningful care and quality time with loved ones. Early enrollment in palliative and hospice care services can improve quality of life, reduce use of ineffective aggressive treatments, lower costs, and extend survival (Temel et al., 2010).

INTERDISCIPLINARY TEAM CARE

Because of the complexities of caring for the PWH, including the often concomitant diagnoses of substance use disorder and mental illness, coordinated, patient-centered care is optimally delivered in an ambulatory, chronic disease model by an interdisciplinary (multidisciplinary) team (Gallant et al., 2011; Mugavero et al., 2011; Ojikutu et al., 2014). In this integrated HIV care model, HIV primary care is combined with mental health and substance abuse services into a single coordinated program. The integrated HIV care model, which has been used effectively to meet the medical and social needs of PWH for decades (largely via Ryan White funding; see later discussion), is essentially a patient-centered medical home. In fact, it has been suggested that the HIV integrated care model can be used as a template for primary care clinic medical homes (Beane et al., 2014). In the integrated or coordinated care model, the goal is to treat the *patient* rather than the *disease*. Team members work together with the patient to clarify goals of care. This leads to improved outcomes by engaging various healthcare workers to work together to help the patient navigate through the complex healthcare system (Bauman et al., 2013; Boyd & Lucas, 2014; Chu & Selwyn, 2011).

Studies have demonstrated that shared and coordinated patient care among different disciplines can increase the efficiency of care without duplication of services among multiple healthcare service providers (Gallant et al., 2011; Horberg et al., 2012). A recent study of PWH on Medicaid and with chronic health problems (asthma, chronic obstructive pulmonary disease, diabetes, congestive heart failure) and psychiatric illness and/or substance use disorders found that patients in a medical home model of care had more efficient care, which resulted in substantial cost savings compared to patients not cared for in a medical home model (Crits-Christoph et al., 2018).

ROLES OF HIV PATIENT CARE TEAM

A comprehensive HIV care team will typically have a physician, nurse, case manager, advanced practitioner, mental health provider, social worker, nutritionist, health educator, clinical pharmacist, substance abuse treatment counselor, and financial counselor (Gallant et al., 2011; Horberget et al., 2012). The makeup of a particular HIV care team will be specific to the needs of the local patients served and the resources available. Some teams may not have all the listed positions, and some members of a care team may undertake tasks not traditionally part of their job description. In many cases the roles may overlap (see Table 14.1).

- Physicians and advanced practitioners diagnose, treat, refer to other specialists, and often lead interdisciplinary care teams.

Table 14.1 DIFFERENT ROLES OF HIV PATIENT CARE TEAM

	ROLES	RESPONSIBILITIES	POTENTIALLY INVOLVED PERSONNEL
Diagnosis (prevention)	Community outreach	Offer HIV screening Link patients to primary care "Test and Treat" (Offer PrEP if HIV negative)	Public health worker Researcher Nurse Health educator
Linkage to care	Patient navigation	Arrange appointments Function as a liaison between patient and the healthcare provider	Administrative staff Nurse Case manager
Linkage to care Prescribing ART	Insurance/social support	Link patients to available community resources Apply for medical insurance including ADAP Advocate for patient's needs	Social worker Financial adviser Case manager Advocacy group liaison
Engagement/retention	Retention/engagement	Outreach to out-of-care patients Outreach to public health and community-based organizations Gather patient data on retention	Administrative staff Nurse Case manager Public health worker
Engagement/retention	Mental health	Provide counseling Provide mental health treatment Provide psychosocial support	Social worker Psychologist Psychiatrist Substance abuse counselor
Prescribing ART Viral suppression	Medical care	Provide medical management Refer to appropriate specialist(s) Educate on medication adherence	HIV specialist or primary care clinician Advanced practice provider Pharmacist/local pharmacy worker Nurse
Viral suppression	Patient education	Provide education on nutrition, adherence, drug interaction, healthy lifestyle, etc.	Nurse Adherence counselor Nutritionist Health educator Pharmacist HIV specialist or primary care clinician
Linkage Engagement/retention Prescribing ART Viral suppression	Population health management	Gather data on each step of HIV continuum of care Conduct quality improvement Measure patient outcomes Evaluate projects/programs	Electronic medical record provider Administrative staff Data support staff Researcher HIV specialist or Primary care clinician Public health worker
All stages of care	Team lead	Provide system-based coordination Develop infrastructure	Any team member Commonly done by a clinician

- Public health workers, nurses, and health educators offer initial HIV screening, provide HIV prevention education including information on pre-exposure prophylaxis (PrEP) if HIV negative, and link PWH to an HIV provider.

- Administrative staff and case managers arrange appointments and serve as liaisons between the patient and healthcare providers.

- Social workers and financial advisers link patients to available community resources (e.g., housing, disability, and food assistance) and assist with applications for healthcare insurance, including ADAP.

- Clinical pharmacists and health educators provide assistance with medication information and adherence.

- Nursing staff and nutritionists provide education on nutrition, adherence, and healthy lifestyles.

- Psychiatrists, therapist/counselors, and substance abuse counselors respectfully provide mental health assessment and treatment, psychosocial support, and treatment of addiction (including substance use disorder).

The designated team leader, most often a physician or advanced practitioner should facilitate communication among the team members to support the goal of quality care for patients. Ongoing communication (via electronic health records (EHR), meetings, and phone consultation) between the interdisciplinary team and the patient is essential to ensure collaborative and patient-centered care (Gallant et al., 2011; Nancarrow et al., 2013). The patient's preference for mode of communication should be clearly visible in the EHR. Regular meetings to discuss the needs of patients and to reassess team member roles are important. The complexity of the patient's medical and psychosocial needs can often be overwhelming. Learning the patient's priorities and making partnered decisions with the patient can help interdisciplinary coordination of care among healthcare team and the patient (Gallant et al., 2011; Mugavero et al., 2011). There are limited data on standardized ways of measuring interdisciplinary team care (Boyd & Lucas, 2014). However, periodic internal review of the interdisciplinary member responsibilities and infrastructure can help improve and consolidate responsibilities, avoid duplication of tasks, and augment the efficiency and effectiveness of the team. One survey indicated that patients who received care in an interdisciplinary HIV care model had high levels of satisfaction (Vachirasudlekha et al., 2014).

Numerous factors, including the higher rates of homelessness, substance abuse, and mental illness, result in the need for more resources to manage PWH. Providing comprehensive care for these patients often requires referrals to other healthcare providers, financial counselors, social workers, and ancillary services. Depending on the model and scope of HIV care, the referrals may occur within the same interdisciplinary HIV team, to another provider in the same institution, or to someone outside the system. Effective referrals can be initiated and tracked through a structured referral process utilizing established referral sources. Making one team member responsible for tracking the status of referrals helps ensure their completion.

While there is no one approach that will work for all HIV providers or delivery models with regards to appropriate referrals, certain practices may be widely applicable. Initially, an assessment of the patient's referral needs should be performed, and objectives for those referrals should be clearly defined. Ideally, providers from different disciplines should work together to meet the identified patient healthcare needs. In the interdisciplinary team-based approach, decisions regarding referrals and patient care are shared. In collaborative arrangements, decision-making responsibilities are shared, and ownership of changes in care may shift depending on the level of expertise required at a given time. It is important to communicate changes to the interdisciplinary team and document clearly.

It is helpful for team members to become familiar with the various agencies in their community, especially those that maintain a core group of professionals committed to the care of PWH. This encourages further support and involvement in the patient's progress. Referral of patients to on-site providers is preferred but referrals off-site may be necessary. This can present its own set of challenges, especially regarding transportation, communication, and reimbursement. In some cases, if resources allow, the case manager may accompany the patient to ensure the patient attends the appointment and any recommendations are understood by the patient and are carried out. Clear two-way communication between the HIV provider and the specialist is important for the goals of care to be met. The referring provider should clearly identify the questions and objectives needed from the specialist. After the consult, the specialist should clearly communicate the plan of care to the referring provider and the patient. A shared EHR can help to alleviate the communication issue. However, direct communication between the referring provider and the specialist, as well as with other team members, is optimal.

Responsibility for the implementation and follow-up of recommended changes in the plan of care should be well outlined. Frequent and timely communication between the referring organization and the referral providers can decrease gaps in care and ensure continuity of quality care.

IMPORTANCE OF CLINICAL RESEARCH

Case management plays an important role in educating patients about the availability of clinical research trials. Having knowledge about local and regional clinical trials and how to access them should be the role of all members of the healthcare team. National resources for ongoing clinical trials such as https://clinicaltrials.gov/ should be made available to all patients.

INTERPRETING CLINICAL TRIAL RESULTS

PER-PROTOCOL (PP) VERSUS INTENT-TO-TREAT (ITT) ANALYSIS

In randomized trials, a per-protocol (PP) analysis (also known as as-treated analysis, observed analysis, or on treatment analysis) examines outcomes in only those study participants who remain on their assigned study regimen for the duration of the trial or, in the case of an interim analysis, up to a particular time point. In comparison, an ITT analysis evaluates each patient according to the treatment group to which they were originally randomly assigned, regardless of whether the participant received the treatment or completed the study. Both ITT and PP analyses are valuable in understanding the findings of a clinical trial.

By removing from the analysis those participants who were lost to follow-up, do not complete the study (for any reason), drop out because of side effects, or do not stay on their prescribed study regimen, a PP analysis selects for participants who tolerated study medication(s). This analysis method is, therefore, intrinsically biased toward a best-case scenario and may systematically bias results such that poor outcomes associated with a treatment that is not well tolerated may be hidden. The value of the ITT analysis is that it limits bias by evaluating the entire population of participants randomly assigned to a given study regimen. ITT analyses more completely encompass efficacy, tolerability, adverse events, and the myriad other reasons why participants do not remain on or deviate from the assigned drug regimen; therefore, it accounts for the influence of these factors on outcomes (Lang & Secic, 1997). The more rigorous ITT approach conveys a truer sense of a treatment's overall effectiveness and is less subject to bias.

Because of the inherent differences in these approaches, the PP analysis will frequently report better outcomes than will the ITT analysis (e.g., a higher proportion of participants achieving an undetectable HIV RNA level). PP analyses exclude participants who are noncompliant with study medications, procedures, and/or study visits and those who drop out because of intolerance of the assigned regimen. If more participants are excluded from one treatment arm than another, the PP analysis may report a clinical difference that is quite different from the actual treatment difference obtained when all subjects are analyzed. Conversely, a PP analysis may find no difference between two treatments, whereas an ITT analysis, which better accounts for tolerability, may find a superior outcome for a treatment because of less study drop out or discontinuation.

TIME TO LOSS OF VIROLOGIC RESPONSE VERSUS SNAPSHOT ANALYSIS

Achieving an undetectable HIV RNA level (viral load) is the most widely accepted endpoint for antiretroviral clinical trials, as it is the most clinically relevant surrogate marker for outcomes that may take years to occur (e.g., progression to AIDS and death). As such, investigational antiretroviral drug regimens are frequently evaluated by assessing the percentage of participants achieving low (suppressed) plasma levels of HIV RNA. Because assays that detect HIV RNA have different limits of detection, it is important to know which prespecified level of HIV RNA was considered "suppressed" or "undetectable." Often, trials will allow some "forgiveness" in statistical analysis to account for small elevations or "blips" in viral load that likely do not affect ultimate clinical outcome. In addition to measuring the failure to achieve or maintain HIV RNA suppression, the TLOVR analysis also considers the introduction of a new antiretroviral drug, death, or loss to follow-up as failures (US Food and Drug Administration (FDA), 2015). Depending on the patient population, the FDA suggests the Snapshot method of analyzing results with the goal of simplifying the evaluation of study results. Snapshot differs from TLOVR in that it primarily focuses on a virologic response at a predetermined endpoint (e.g., 24 or 48 weeks). Specifically, an outcome will be measured only if a participant is a responder with an HIV RNA< 50 copies/mL at week 48, (within a 1- to 2-week window) (Qaqish et al., 2010). Twenty-four weeks of follow-up data are often appropriate for drugs that have some benefit over existing options

(i.e., for patients with multiple ARV drug resistance where it may not be possible to construct a fully suppressive treatment regimen; or improved efficacy, tolerability, or ease of administration), while 48 weeks is recommended for investigational therapies with comparable characteristics to existing options (FDA, 2015). Both methods of analysis have value, and clinical trials often report results in both forms, although more recent analyses have favored the Snapshot algorithm.

NONINFERIORITY ANALYSIS

In contrast to statistical analyses used to demonstrate superiority, new drug regimens may be evaluated with the aim of demonstrating equivalence or noninferior efficacy relative to a standard drug regimen. The noninferiority trial is used mainly when the added value of a new drug/regimen is related to factors such as improved convenience, better tolerability, simpler dosing schedule, lower toxicity, or lower cost (Wittkop et al., 2010). FDA industry guidance regarding procedures for new drug approval has helped to standardize the statistical methods used in clinical trials. The proportion of treatment responders at 48 weeks is often used to assess noninferiority, as this provides sufficient time for emergence of loss of tolerability, ARV drug resistance, or other relevant measurable outcomes, using a specific margin of difference that is acceptable between study arms (FDA, 2015). In practical terms, a noninferiority analysis is a statistically rigorous way in which a clinical trial can demonstrate that a new therapy/regimen is at least as good as a currently available option. Often, efficacy results may appear numerically different, with one regimen achieving a slightly higher proportion of participants with undetectable viral loads at week 48, for example. In a noninferiority trial, numerical difference is less important than whether efficacy of both regimens falls within the prespecified "noninferiority margin," which then helps determine clinical equivalence. Trials are often powered differently, with larger numbers of participants if they aim to show superiority of one regimen over another rather than noninferiority. The FDA has tightened this noninferiority margin to ensure that new drugs are truly equivalent to existing therapies before coming to market.

CLINICAL VERSUS STATISTICAL SIGNIFICANCE

When evaluating research findings, clinicians should be aware of the difference between a statistically significant difference and a clinically significant difference. One of the most common errors in interpreting and reporting clinical trial results is not correctly distinguishing between clinical and statistical significance (Braitman, 1991). A *clinically significant finding* is one that has important implications for patient care. A *statistically significant finding* is a conclusion that there is evidence against the "null hypothesis"; that is, a low probability exists of getting a result as extreme or more extreme than the one observed in the study data by chance alone. *Statistical significance*, when applied to the terms *noninferiority* or *superiority*, indicates that the result of a clinical trial would be unlikely to occur by chance. It does not necessarily mean that the result will be important for treating patients (Braitman, 1991; Lang & Secic, 1997). Clinically significant findings typically must involve outcomes with particular relevance to clinical medicine and must have an effect size that is large enough to influence clinical decision-making.

QUALITY IMPROVEMENT

The goal of HIV care is to optimize patient health, decrease HIV transmission, and end the HIV epidemic. A clear vision with focused efforts to improve clinical outcomes and quality can help to develop, improve, and sustain effective patient care practices (Gallant et al., 2011; Mugavero et al., 2011). An up-to-date and available patient registry with relevant clinical and retention data can help monitor and measure patient care outcomes. Examples of relevant clinical and retention data include adherence, missed appointments, recent contact information and outreach, detectable viral load, status of ART, and evidence of failing or failed care (e.g., development of antiretroviral resistance, new opportunistic infections, onset or worsening of comorbid conditions, or clinical decline).

In a resource-limited setting, targeted data collection may be beneficial instead of attempting to obtain all data at once. For example, it may be beneficial to prioritize and focus resources to high-risk and vulnerable patients, such as those who have been out of care for more than 6 months or have a detectable viral load. A patient registry with clinical and laboratory data can also support the measurement of the quality of care delivered and improve patient outcomes by strategizing quality-improvement projects. Examples include annual influenza vaccination among patients with HIV and appropriate sexually transmitted disease screening.

FUNDING FOR HIV CARE

RYAN WHITE HIV/AIDS PROGRAM

The Ryan White HIV/AIDS Program (RWP) is an important component of HIV patient care (Health Resources and Service Administration (HRSA) HIV/AIDS, 2022; Sood et al., 2014). This federal program, which began in 1991, funds healthcare and services to PWH. Program funding is distributed among Parts A–F. Part A provides emergency assistance to eligible areas that are most severely affected by HIV/AIDS. Part B provides grants to all 50 states and US territories or associated jurisdictions. Part C provides outpatient-based comprehensive primary healthcare for PLWH. Part D provides family-centered care for women, infants, children, and youth with HIV/AIDS. Part F provides funds for a variety of programs, such as health information technology, social media, and outreach programs. The program also funds dental care, special projects, training programs, and minority AIDS initiatives.

The RWP funds cities, states, and local community-based organizations to provide HIV care and treatment services to more than half a million people each year and assists approximately 52% of all people diagnosed with HIV in the United States. In fiscal year 2021, the RWP provided $2.43 billion in funding (https://ryanwhite.hrsa.gov/about/budget). The program is known for its "wrap-around" services to patients with HIV. However, coverage and requirements of RWP-funded programs may vary state to state, and grantees of the program should review eligibility and criteria of renewal (including required data collection and conformance with standards of care) (HRSA, 2022). The RWP is always the "payer of last resort."

An important component of the RWP (under Part B) is ADAP, which provides medications approved by the FDA to low-income people living with HIV who have limited or no health coverage from private insurance, Medicaid, or Medicare. ADAP funds may also be used to purchase health insurance for eligible clients and for services that enhance access to, adherence to, and monitoring of drug treatments. Different states have varied eligibility criteria and renewal processes, including documentation of income status (15 states established income eligibility at 200% or less of the federal poverty level); diagnosis of HIV, opportunistic infections, and chronic medical conditions; and/or other service needs (HRSA, 2022).

Several studies have demonstrated better clinical outcomes for patients receiving care at RWP-funded clinics versus non-funded clinics. Wrap-around clinical and case management services provided by the RWP result in increased retention in care, and consequently in increased viral suppression (Kay et al., 2018). Assistance with necessities such as food and transportation (utilized by one in three patients served by the RWP) and housing (utilized by one in five patients) are key components to supporting people with HIV with incomes at or below the poverty level. In a study of 8,000 people with HIV, nearly 75% of patients receiving care at RWP-funded facilities achieved viral suppression despite a greater likelihood of poverty and unstable housing. Further, patients with incomes at or below the poverty level were more likely to achieve viral suppression if they received care at a RWP-funded facility (Weiser et al., 2015).

The RWP ensures access to ART among uninsured and underinsurance PWH and is thus associated with increase viral suppression among those groups. In an analysis of over 18,000 patients in which 41% of patients had RWP assistance, patients whose private or Medicaid coverage was supplemented by the RWP were both more likely to be prescribed ART and sustain viral suppression than those without RWP supplementation (Bradley et al., 2016). A recent study of over 3,000 MSM enrolled in the Miami-Dade County RWP demonstrated that nearly 85% of the men achieved sustained viral suppression (Sheehan et al., 2020). In this study, one of the factors associated with increased sustained viral suppression was having an HIV clinician who serves a larger volume of RWP clients. The central role of the medical case manager as part of the multidisciplinary RWP team was identified as one reason the rate of viral suppression was higher than expected.

ACKNOWLEDGMENTS

Special thanks to Amanda A. Westlake, Sally Spencer-Long, Daniel J Skiest, and Christian Ramers, who authored portions of this chapter in prior editions.

RECOMMENDED READING

Gardner LI, Giordano TP, Marks G, et al. Enhanced personal contact with HIV patients improves retention in primary care: a randomized trial in six US HIV clinics. *Clin Infect Dis.* 2014;59(5):725–734.

Newhouse RP, Spring B. Interdisciplinary evidence-based practice: moving from silos to synergy. *Nurs Outlook.* 2010;58(6):309–317.

Shah M, Risher K, Berry SA, et al. The epidemiologic and economic impact of improving HIV testing, linkage, and retention in care in the United States. *Clin Infect Dis.* 2016;62(2):220–229.

REFERENCES

Bauman LJ, Braunstein S, Calderon Y, et al. Barriers and facilitators of linkage to HIV primary care in New York City. *J AIDS.* 2013;64(1):S20–S26.

Beane SN, Culyba RJ, DeMayo M, Armstrong W. Exploring the medical home in Ryan White HIV care settings: a pilot study. *J Assoc Nurses AIDS Care.* May–June 2014;25(3):191–202.

Boyd CM, Lucas GM. Patient-centered care for people living with multimorbidity. *Curr Opin HIV AIDS.* 2014;9(4):419–427.

Bradley H, Viall AH, Wortley PM, et al. Ryan White HIV/AIDS program assistance and HIV treatment outcomes. *Clin Infect Dis.* January 1, 2016;62(1):90–98.

Braitman LE. Confidence intervals assess both clinical significance and statistical significance. *Ann Intern Med.* 1991;114:515–517.

Burchell AN, Raboud J, Donelle J, et al. Cause-specific mortality among HIV-infected people in Ontario, 1995–2014: a population-based retrospective cohort study. *CMAJ Open.* 2019;7(1):E1–E7. http://doi:10.9778/cmajo.20180159

Centers for Disease Control and Prevention (CDC). HIV surveillance report, 2018 (Updated); vol.31. cdc.gov. http://www.cdc.gov/hiv/library/reports/hiv-surveillance.html. Published May 2020. Accessed July 26, 2020.

Centers for Disease Control and Prevention (CDC). Understanding the HIV Care Continuum. https://www.cdc.gov/hiv/pdf/library/factsheets/cdc-hiv-care-continuum.pdf. 2019. Accessed March 9, 2023.

CDC, Division of HIV/AIDS Prevention. Understanding the HIV care continuum. cdc.gov. https://stacks.cdc.gov/view/cdc/26481. Published December 2014. Accessed November 3, 2015.

Chu C, Selwyn PA. An epidemic in evolution: the need for new models of HIV care in the chronic disease era. *J Urban Health.* 2011;88(3):556–566.

Crits-Christoph P, Gallop R, Noll E, et al. Impact of a medical home model on costs and utilization among comorbid HIV-positive Medicaid patients. *Am J Manag Care.* 2018;24:368–375.

Crockett KB, Entler KJ, Brodie E, et al. Brief report: linking depressive symptoms to viral nonsuppression among women with HIV through adherence self-efficacy and ART adherence. *J Acquir Immune Defic Syndr.* 2020;83(4):340–344.

Dombrowski JC, Simoni JM, Katz DA, et al. Barriers to HIV care and treatment among participants in a public health HIV care relinkage program. *AIDS Patient Care STDS.* 2015;29:279–287.

Ford N, Migone C, Calmy A, et al. Benefits and risks of rapid initiation of antiretroviral therapy. *AIDS.* 2018;32(1):17–23.

Gallant JE, Adimora AA, Carmichael JK, et al. Essential components of effective HIV care: a policy paper of the HIV Medicine Association of the Infectious Diseases Society of America and the Ryan White Medical Providers Coalition. *Clin Infect Dis.* 2011;53:1043–1050.

Gardner EM, McLees MP, Steiner JF, et al. The spectrum of engagement in HIV care and its relevance to test-and-treat strategies for prevention of HIV infection. *Clin Infect Dis.* 2011;52(6):793–800.

Guaraldi G, Malagoli A, Calcagno A, et al. The increasing burden and complexity of multi-morbidity and polypharmacy in geriatric HIV patients: a cross sectional study of people aged 65—74 years and more than 75 years. *BMC Geriatr.* 2018;18(1):99. http://doi:10.1186/s12877-018-0789-0

Health Resources and Services Administration (HRSA). The Ryan White HIV/AIDS Program. https://ryanwhite.hrsa.gov/. Published 2022. Accessed August 27, 2022.

HIV Care Continuum. What is the HIV Care Continuum? https:///HIV.gov. 2022. Accessed. August 15, 2022.

Horberg MA, Hurley LB, Towner WJ, et al. Determination of optimized multidisciplinary care team for maximal antiretroviral therapy adherence. *J AIDS.* 2012;60(2):183–190.

Irvine MK, Chamberlin SA, Robbins RS, et al. Improvements in HIV care engagement and viral load suppression following enrollment in a comprehensive HIV care coordination program. *Clin Infect Dis.* 2014;60:298–310.

Kay ES, Batey DS, Mugavero MJ. The Ryan White HIV/AIDS Program: supplementary service provision post-Affordable Care Act [published correction appears in AIDS Patient Care STDS. Aug 2019;33(8):379–380]. *AIDS Patient Care STDS.* 2018;32(7):265–271. http://doi:10.1089/apc.2018.0032

Lang TA, Secic M. *How to report statistics in medicine: annotated guidelines for authors, editors, and reviewers.* Philadelphia, PA: American College of Physicians; 1997.

Mugavero MJ, Norton WE, Saag MS. Health care system and policy factors influencing engagement in HIV medical care: piecing together the fragments of a fractured health care delivery system. *Clin Infect Dis.* 2011;52(Suppl 2):S238–S246.

Nancarrow SA, Booth A, Ariss S, et al. Ten principles of good interdisciplinary team work. *Hum Resour Health.* 2013;11:19.

National Institutes on Aging (NIA). What are palliative care and hospice care? National Institute on Aging. https://www.nia.nih.gov/health/what-are-palliative-care-and-hospice-care. Published May 17, 2017. Accessed January 25, 2023.

Ojikutu B, Holman J, Kunches L, et al. Interdisciplinary HIV care in a changing healthcare environment in the USA. *AIDS Care.* 2014;26(6):731–735.

Qaqish R, van Wyk J, King M. A comparison of the FDA TLOVR and FDA Snapshot algorithms based on studies evaluating once-daily vs. twice daily lopinavir /ritonavir (LPV/r) regimens. *J Intl AIDS Soc.* 2010;13.P58.

Samji H, Cescon A, Hogg RS, et al. Closing the gap: increases in life expectancy among treated HIV-positive individuals in the United States and Canada. *PLoS One.* 2014;8(12):e81355.

Scanlon ML, Vreeman RC. Current strategies for improving access and adherence to antiretroviral therapies in resource-limited settings. *HIV AIDS (Auckl).* 2013;5:1–17.

Sheehan DM, Dawit R, Gbadamosi SO, et al. Sustained HIV viral suppression among men who have sex with men in the Miami-Dade County Ryan White program: the effect of demographic, psychosocial, provider and neighborhood factors. *BMC Public Health.* 2020;20(1):326. http://doi:10.1186/s12889-020-8442-1

Sood N, Juday T, Vanderpuye-Orgle J, et al. HIV care providers emphasize the importance of the Ryan White program for access to quality of care. *Health Affairs.* 2014;33(3):394–400.

Temel JS, Greeg JA, Muzikansky A, et al. Early palliative care for patients with metastatic non-small-cell lung cancer. *N Engl J Med.* 2010;363(8):733–42.

US Food and Drug Administration (FDA). *Guidance for industry submitting select clinical trial data sets for drugs intended to treat human immunodeficiency virus-1 infection.* Washington, DC: US Department of Health and Human Services. https://www.fda.gov/media/112667/download. Published 2015. Accessed September 6, 2022.

US Department of Health and Human Services Administration (USDHHS). About ending the HIV Epidemic: Plan for America.

https://www.hiv.gov/federal-response/ending-the-hiv-epidemic/overview. Published 2020a. Accessed August 30, 2020.

US Preventive Services Task Force, Owens DK, Davidson KW, Krist AH, et al. Screening for HIV infection: US Preventive Services Task Force recommendation statement. *JAMA*. June 18, 2019;321(23):2326–2336.

Wada N, Jacobson LP, Cohen M, et al. Cause-specific mortality among HIV-infected individuals, by CD4+ cell count at HAART initiation, compared with HIV-uninfected individuals. *AIDS*. 2014;28:257–265.

Weiser J, Beer L, Frazier E, et al. Service delivery and patient outcomes in Ryan White HIV/AIDS program-funded and—nonfunded health care facilities in the United States. *JAMA Intern Med*. 2015;175(10):1650–1659.

White House Office of National AIDS Policy. *National HIV/AIDS strategy: update of 2014 federal actions to achieve national goals and improve outcomes along the HIV care continuum*. Washington, DC: The White House Office of National AIDS Policy; 2014.

Wittkop L, Smith C, Fox Z, et al. Methodological issues in the use of composite endpoints in clinical trials: examples from the HIV field. *Clin Trials*. February 2010;7(1):19–35.

Vachirasudlekha B, Cha A, Berkowitz L, et al. Interdisciplinary HIV care—patient perceptions. *Int J Health Care Qual Assur*. 2014;27(5):405–413.

15.

THE PHARMACIST'S ROLE IN HIV CARE

Jennifer Cocohoba

INTRODUCTION

Medications are essential tools used for prevention, treatment, and the management of co-occurring conditions in persons at risk for HIV and in persons living with HIV (PWH). A multidisciplinary approach to HIV care should consider the inclusion of a pharmacist because of pharmacists' broad expertise on medication therapy. Pharmacists play an important role across the spectrum of HIV care: they facilitate access to medications, ensure accurate dispensing, and provide patients with education on their medications. Pharmacist specialists have also become essential members of the HIV healthcare team because their expertise extends beyond dispensing to providing expert consultation, facilitating patient adherence, or co-managing HIV antiretroviral therapy (ART) and prevention services. When included on the healthcare team, HIV pharmacist expertise can be utilized to improve the selection, safety, efficacy, and overall quality of medication therapy.

LEARNING OBJECTIVES

- Describe common settings in which HIV pharmacists practice.

- List three potential ways in which pharmacists can contribute to HIV care.

WHAT'S NEW?

- Data and experience continue to accumulate on the innovative and meaningful ways that pharmacists contribute to improved HIV health outcomes along the care continuum and how pharmacists can help increase access to timely HIV-related services including testing and pre-exposure prophylaxis (PrEP).

KEY POINTS

- HIV pharmacists are a diverse group of healthcare providers who work to improve the health of PWH via medication therapy management, quality-assurance practices, research, and other avenues.

- HIV pharmacists may be particularly skilled at managing complex antiretroviral drug–drug interactions, recommending therapies for people with complex ART resistance patterns, and providing education and support with regard to adherence.

- If practicing with a physician under a collaborative drug therapy management agreement, an HIV pharmacist may be able to provide more direct disease state management (e.g., furnishing medications and ordering lab tests) including PrEP, HIV treatment, and medications for associated chronic conditions.

THE HIV CLINICAL PHARMACIST SPECIALIST

Medications for HIV have become more convenient but not less complex. Approximately half of people with HIV in the United States are over the age of 50 years, and a large proportion of them take five or more medications (Okoli et al., 2020). For this reason, having a clinical pharmacist as a part of the healthcare team can greatly enhance HIV care. HIV-specialized clinical pharmacists typically receive advanced training in HIV during postdoctorate residencies, infectious diseases fellowship programs, or HIV-specific fellowship programs, although some acquire their HIV knowledge through practice-based experience and intense self-study. Certification programs such as the American Academy of HIV Medicine's HIV Pharmacist (AAHIVP) certification program and the HIV Pharmacotherapy Continuing Education Program offered through the University of Buffalo can help distinguish pharmacists who are well-versed in many aspects of HIV pharmacotherapy (McLaughlin et al., 2018). Many HIV pharmacists also pursue Board of Pharmacy Specialties certification in infectious diseases (BCIDP) or ambulatory care (BCACP) owing to the wide knowledge base, roles, and responsibilities that can be associated with caring for PWH.

SETTINGS IN WHICH HIV PHARMACISTS PROVIDE PATIENT CARE

PWH encounter many different pharmacists who contribute to their care across the spectrum of their disease and medical visits. For patients who are acutely ill, the first setting in which they may interact with an HIV-specialized pharmacist is in the hospital. In many health systems, the infectious diseases (ID) team oversees consultative care for PWH, and HIV/ID pharmacists on these multidisciplinary teams contribute skills and knowledge to enhance HIV care. For example, the current paradigm of "test and treat" has increased the number of patients diagnosed with HIV and immediately initiated on ART during a hospital stay, but HIV pharmacotherapy is riddled with complex drug–drug interactions and requires close monitoring to dose adjust for renal insufficiency or hepatic dysfunction if present. HIV pharmacists on inpatient clinical services assist the team in selecting appropriate ART and opportunistic infection regimens, screen for interactions, may order and interpret resistance testing or therapeutic drug monitoring assays (if indicated), provide discharge counseling for patients initiating new ART, and may help coordinate transitions of care for persons with HIV who are entering or leaving the hospital (Durham et al., 2017).

Patients in a clinic may interact with HIV-specialized pharmacists who work as part of an interdisciplinary ambulatory care team. These HIV clinical pharmacists have a wide range of duties commensurate with their experience and level of expertise. Responsibilities can include dispensing medications in a clinic-associated pharmacy; performing medication-use evaluations to ensure optimal pharmacotherapy in a population; providing patient education; consulting with patients and medical providers regarding medication-related problems, adherence, or resistance testing results; initiating and managing ART or PrEP; administering vaccinations, ordering lab tests; and initiating, adjusting, or discontinuing medications for opportunistic infections and other concomitant disease states. HIV ambulatory care pharmacists have also taken on roles to facilitate patient access to clinic administered medications such as long-acting ART for treatment or prevention.

ART is typically dispensed by a community pharmacist. Nearly all people with HIV will interact with community pharmacists at some point; in fact, the community pharmacist may be the healthcare provider with whom a healthy PWH interacts most frequently. The act of picking up medication refills might seem simple, yet personal, intrapersonal, and system-related barriers may complicate the process for some patients (Johnson et al, 2020). In larger metropolitan areas, pharmacists and staff who are knowledgeable about HIV disease may frequently be found at pharmacies that specialize in HIV care. These HIV-focused pharmacies may belong to large retail chains, may be independently owned, may be integrated within a larger health system, or may assist patients through mail-order services. Pharmacies may elect to undergo an accreditation process to be officially recognized as a specialty pharmacy, although this designation typically indicates expertise in multiple disease states and not just HIV alone. Patient education and counseling, provision of reminder devices and adherence aids, managing the practical aspects of synchronizing and coordinating medication refills, facilitating procurement of antiretrovirals, and working with patients to address medication-related financial barriers (e.g., copay fees) are just a few of the activities conducted by HIV community pharmacists. As a testament to some of the less tangible but positive impact of community pharmacies, a large CDC demonstration project found a 12.9% improvement in retention in care when medical clinics partnered with community pharmacies in a patient-centered medical home model (Byrd et al., 2019).

PHARMACIST CONTRIBUTIONS TO HIV CARE: A SAMPLE OF SPECIFIC SKILLS

Pharmacists make ideal treatment facilitators because of their extensive training in comprehensive medication therapy management (MTM). The goal of MTM is for a pharmacist to optimize a patient's treatment through identification, resolution, and prevention of medication-related problems (American Pharmacists Association and the National Association of Chain Drug Stores Foundation, 2008). This definition of MTM is intentionally broad so that it may accommodate the wide variety of activities a pharmacist may perform to optimize a patient's therapy. For example, during a medication therapy review, a pharmacist may discover dangerous drug–drug interactions and poor patient adherence. The pharmacist may then work closely with the patient and their medical provider to create an action plan that addresses these issues. This section presents a sample of some of the evidence supporting the positive impact pharmacists have when caring for PWH.

AMELIORATING ANTIRETROVIRAL ERRORS

HIV-specialized pharmacists play an important role in preventing and ameliorating medication errors. Published literature suggests that PWH are at high risk of incurring medication errors when hospitalized and that these errors—including incorrect antiretroviral regimens, incorrect dosing strategies, incorrect scheduling, or drug–drug interactions—may occur at various points during their hospital stay.

Pharmacist-led antiretroviral stewardship programs have resulted in reduced ART medication errors in hospitalized persons with HIV. A joint statement endorsed by the American Academy of HIV Medicine, the HIV Medicine Association, and the Infectious Disease Society of America recommends inclusion of a clinical pharmacist on interdisciplinary antiretroviral stewardship teams and highlights the contributions of pharmacists in improving antiretroviral use in hospitalized patients (Koren et al., 2020). A Texas antiretroviral (ARV) stewardship program implemented pharmacist education, a pharmacist-led ART checklist, and modifications to the hospital order-entry and verification system to support prospective audit and feedback; this combination of interventions significantly reduced the number of ART-related errors from 208 to 24 (Shea et al., 2018). An ARV stewardship program in Philadelphia found that out of 567 hospital admissions involving persons with HIV, 43% required at least one stewardship intervention, and the cost savings associated with the program was estimated at $263,428 over a 1-year period (DePuy et al., 2019). Successful pharmacist-led stewardship programs may have wider impact beyond the immediate correction of medication errors. An ARV stewardship program in Chicago found statistically significant reductions in ARV error rates (17% to 6%) and 30-day hospital readmissions (27% to 12%) and increases in linkage to care for patients served (Brizzi et al., 2020). Similarly, a hospital system in North Carolina found significantly reduced ARV error rates and increased linkage to care with a pharmacist-led ARV stewardship program (Roshdy et al., 2021).

IDENTIFYING AND MANAGING DRUG–DRUG INTERACTIONS AND POLYPHARMACY

People with HIV take increasingly more medications as they age. The proportion of persons with HIV and polypharmacy (typically defined as taking five or more medications) has ranged from 36% to 94% when observed in various cohorts of elderly persons with HIV in the United States (Back & Catia, 2020). In a single center study, 248 persons with HIV were referred to a clinical pharmacist for medication review (McNicholl et al., 2017). Patients were taking an average of 11.6 +/- 5.7 medications in addition to their ART. The pharmacist identified medications that were potentially inappropriate (as defined by BEERS criteria) in 63% of the cohort, uncovered contraindicated drug interaction pairs in 20 patients, and was able to deprescribe at least one medication for 69% of patients in this study (Fick et al., 2019). Many antiretroviral agents strongly induce or inhibit the cytochrome P450 system, particularly the 3A4 isoform. Because approximately 60% of the most commonly prescribed drugs are also metabolized via cytochrome P450 3A4, pharmacists are trained to carefully review a patient's medication list to identify adverse drug interactions that may result in excess toxicity or subtherapeutic levels of the object drug or that may result in alterations in the HIV drug concentrations. Pharmacists provide management strategies for known interactions. For important theoretical interactions, pharmacists may suggest using therapeutic drug monitoring, and can help interpret the levels garnered from these tests.

SUPPORTING ADHERENCE AND PROVIDING PATIENT EDUCATION

In every setting, HIV pharmacists strive to support patient adherence to antiretroviral medications by addressing system-related and patient-related barriers to taking medications (Kibicho & Owczarzak, 2011). One very basic barrier PWH may face is difficulty adhering to medications because they cannot afford them. Pharmacists can provide patients with information and resources regarding pharmaceutical company–supported, patient assistance programs and state-run AIDS drug assistance programs to help them afford their regimens. In the modern era of broad utilization management practices, pharmacists and their technicians can play a critical role in selecting antiretroviral regimens that adhere to insurance formulary guidelines, providing clinical justification for prior authorizations, and managing those submissions so that patients do not have lapses in therapy.

Pharmacists have access to a wealth of reminder devices and tools that may improve medication adherence (Mahtani et al., 2011; Saberi & Johnson, 2011). Some pharmacies offer specialized unit-dose packaging in plastic "bubble packs" or on medication cards ("blister packs") to help patients remember to take their doses. Pharmacists can train patients on how to use weekly medication boxes. Some community and clinic pharmacists may offer text messaging or may work with patients to set up cell phone alarms to serve as automated medication reminders. Pharmacies may offer a variety of other adherence-enhancing services, such as online management of medications, automatic prescription refills, telephone refill reminders, and home mailing or courier medication delivery.

Pharmacist services also include patient counseling to enhance adherence. They offer personalized education regarding HIV as a chronic disease, HIV treatment and opportunistic infection prophylaxis, and management of adverse effects. Using evidence-based counseling techniques such as motivational interviewing, pharmacists may help assess a patient's readiness to initiate ART and can help motivate the patient toward that goal (D'Antonio, 2010; Krummenacher et al., 2011). Although these topics may be discussed during the treating clinician's visit rather than during a pharmacist visit, this type of assessment and information sharing often takes up more time than allowed in a brief clinic visit that is typically focused on acute medical problems. A visit with a pharmacist provides additional time for complementary education and serves as an extension of the provider's care.

Pharmacists may package all of these services into structured adherence programs that span the range of patient assessment, education, and counseling; offering reminder devices; dispensing medications; and providing continuity in the refill process. Although no two pharmacist-managed adherence programs are exactly alike, various studies have illustrated their benefits with regard to patient outcomes. A study of 10,801 PWH conducted at Kaiser Permanente in California compared different clinic team structures to determine the optimal combination of clinicians that would increase adherence (Horberg et al., 2012). For patients starting a new ART regimen, the largest adherence increases at 12 months were attributable to multidisciplinary teams composed of a clinical pharmacist, a social worker/benefits coordinator, and a non-HIV-specialized primary care provider (8.1% increase in mean adherence; 95% confidence interval (CI): 2.7%–13.5%). Kaiser Permanente also conducted an ecological study to assess the effects of its HIV clinical pharmacists on adherence, healthcare utilization, and HIV outcomes (Horberg et al., 2007). Refill adherence at 24 months was significantly higher for patients seen by an HIV clinical pharmacist (76.7% vs. 68.9%, $P = 0.02$). Odds of having a suppressed viral load or increase in CD4[+] T-cell count were modestly better for patients seen by HIV pharmacists, though the estimates did not achieve statistical significance. Evidence supporting the benefits of pharmacist-run HIV adherence programs continues to grow (Ahmed et al., 2022). These highly heterogeneous programs have been situated within community clinics, hospital clinics, and academic medical center clinics, and have found improvements in $CD4^+$ T-cell counts, increased rates of viral suppression, fewer acute medical visits, and increased adherence for patients who interact with an HIV clinical pharmacist. Future research should also focus on cost savings associated with pharmacist adherence support. One small study provided a cost-avoidance estimate of $49,702 for 16 PWH who completed a 6-month pharmacist-led adherence program (Dilworth et al., 2018). Adherence programs situated within community pharmacies may also have an important impact on antiretroviral adherence and patient outcomes. While ART adherence did not substantially change for a group of 765 persons with HIV who were cared for in a community pharmacy-medical clinic patient-centered medical home, rates of viral suppression improved from 75% preimplementation to 86% post-implementation ($P < 0.001$) (Byrd et al., 2020). The estimated incremental cost per virally suppressed patient was $5,039 (Shrestha et al., 2020). The estimated incremental cost per virally suppressed patient was $5,039 (Shrestha et al., 2020). These studies suggest potential for improvements in adherence and HIV viral suppression when patients use HIV-knowledgeable community pharmacies.

TESTING FOR HIV INFECTION

HIV testing is a service that is emerging predominantly in community pharmacies, although pharmacists in other settings are often included as members of multidisciplinary testing teams (Sherman et al., 2014). These models of care typically employ point-of-care "rapid" HIV tests, counseling, and linkage to confirmatory testing and/or care. In general, pharmacy-based testing appears to be acceptable to both patients and pharmacists (Amesty et al., 2015; Darin et al., 2015). In 2011 the CDC facilitated the development of an HIV testing model for adoption in community pharmacies (Weidle et al., 2014). A total of 1,540 point-of-care HIV tests were administered across 21 sites with pre- and posttest counseling requiring 3–4 minutes, and patients waited an average of 23 minutes for their test results. The average cost per person tested ranged from $32.17 to $47.21 (Lecher et al., 2015). This demonstration project resulted in the inclusion of testing in retail pharmacies as one of the CDC's effective interventions for enhancing diagnosis of HIV. A statewide HIV testing program implemented in pharmacies in Virginia also found that HIV testing in pharmacies was a successful way to connect with "hard-to-reach" populations (Collins et al., 2018). Of the 3,630 tests conducted over a two-year period, 46% of clients reported that they had either never been tested before or were unsure whether they had received an HIV test. Collectively, these studies, as well as others, demonstrate the importance of pharmacies serving as HIV testing sites and pharmacists as key personnel identifying new HIV infections.

EXPANDING PATIENT CARE VIA COLLABORATIVE PRACTICE AGREEMENTS

In the United States, most states have legislation that allows for pharmacists to engage in collaborative practice; however, the requirements and regulations vary from state to state. In some states, pharmacists may enhance the care of PWH via collaborative drug therapy management (CDTM) agreements. The specifics of any CDTM agreement depend on the collaborating physician and the qualifications and experience of the pharmacist.

The American College of Clinical Pharmacy defines a CDTM agreement as:

> . . . a collaborative practice agreement between one or more physicians and pharmacists wherein qualified pharmacists working within the context of a defined protocol are permitted to assume professional responsibility for performing patient assessments; ordering drug therapy-related laboratory tests; administering drugs; and selecting, initiating, monitoring, continuing, and adjusting drug regimens. (Hammond et al., 2003, p.1210)

The American Society of Health Systems Pharmacists published a statement on pharmacist involvement in HIV care that attempts to summarize the scope of practice for an HIV pharmacist (Schafer et al., 2016). Collaborative protocols with physicians may allow pharmacists to select and initiate ART or opportunistic infection prophylaxis, order and interpret pertinent labs that monitor efficacy or toxicity of a regimen, simplify regimens using fixed-dose combination tablets, and manage common antiretroviral-related side effects such as nausea and diarrhea. Knowledgeable pharmacists may order, interpret, and change a patient's ART based on resistance tests. In a cohort of 1255 persons with HIV, patients referred to the clinical pharmacist for treatment initiation were significantly more likely (HR 1.37) to achieve viral suppression during the first 2 years of therapy as compared to those who received standard of care initiation by a primary care provider (Nevo et al., 2015).

Effectively managing chronic conditions can become challenging as persons with HIV age. In addition to managing ART, some collaborative practice protocols can allow pharmacists to assess and adjust medication therapy for HIV-related and other comorbidities such as depression, diabetes, hypertension, hepatitis C, or dyslipidemia. One retrospective cohort study found that an interdisciplinary primary care team that included an HIV pharmacist produced significantly improved outcomes in lipid management and smoking cessation for patients with HIV and diabetes, hypertension, or hyperlipidemia ($n = 96$) compared to a control group ($n = 50$) that was managed by an individual healthcare provider (Cope et al., 2015). The interdisciplinary team achieved cost savings of approximately $3,000 per patient.

A collaborative, interdisciplinary practice coupled with good communication between providers can serves as an excellent model for enhancing HIV care and extends the provider's ability to reach the greatest number of patients. The roles, responsibilities, and impact of HIV pharmacists in clinical practice are likely to expand in the future as the profession advocates for all pharmacists to be recognized as healthcare providers under US federal law.

ENHANCING PREVENTION EFFORTS WITH PREP

Despite an increased focus on enhancing HIV prevention services to end the HIV epidemic, critical gaps in PrEP utilization remain (CDC, 2021). Some of these gaps may be related to clinician familiarity or time to discuss or manage PrEP, or lack of access to healthcare for certain populations who might benefit from PrEP. Pharmacists may offer unique access to some of these patient populations. CDTM agreements would allow pharmacists to screen for clinical appropriateness, prescribe PrEP under protocol, order and review monitoring labs, assess and support adherence, and refill as appropriate. The critical need to expand access to HIV prevention therapies has led to several states passing laws to widen pharmacist scope of practice to include furnishing of PrEP and postexposure prophylaxis under statewide protocols. These types of laws provide an alternative pathway for pharmacists to provide HIV prevention therapies when establishing individual pharmacist-physician CDTM agreements may be challenging. Widespread adoption and the ultimate success of these programs will depend upon many factors, including adequate pharmacy staffing, ease of performing HIV testing and drug therapy monitoring by pharmacists, and reimbursement for time and services rendered.

Various studies have confirmed patients' acceptability of pharmacists screening them for PrEP indications and for pharmacy-run PrEP programs (Crawford et al., 2020; Lutz et al., 2021; Zhu et al., 2020). The One-Step-PrEP program in Seattle, Washington, is an example of a pharmacy-run PrEP program operating under a CDTA (Tung et al., 2018). Over a three-year period from 2015 to 2018, 714 patients sought out this pharmacy-based PrEP service. Of those, 695 persons-initiated PrEP and most of these patients (98%) did not have to pay for their PrEP medication. An impressive retention rate of 75% was achieved over the first 3 years of operations. This study demonstrates that pharmacy-based PrEP services are feasible and desired and remain a promising avenue for pharmacists to contribute to the public health goal of preventing new infections. As additional biomedical options for PrEP are approved and become more widely available (i.e., long-acting injectable cabotegravir), the role of pharmacists in expanding PrEP access may develop even further.

A novel avenue for pharmacists to enhance HIV prevention efforts is to facilitate rapid ART and PrEP initiation. A pharmacist was the first point of contact for persons newly diagnosed with HIV for a pharmacist-driven rapid ART program at a Ryan White funded clinic in Rhode Island in 2019 (Brotherton et al., 2020). During the visit, the pharmacist assessed ART readiness, provided education, screened for drug interactions, facilitated ART access, recommended patient-specific ART to the triage physician for initiation, and called the client 2 weeks after initiation. A retrospective analysis of the program found significantly reduced time from intake to ART start (16 vs. 0 days, $P < 0.001$) and reduced time to viral suppression (81 vs. 34 days, $P = 0.001$). A pharmacist-led program at an HIV testing center in Mississippi facilitated PrEP initiation for 69 patients, 89% of whom received their prescriptions within the same day (Khosropour et al., 2020). Programs such as this one hold great potential to rapidly reduce viral loads and potentially impact HIV transmissions.

PHARMACISTS: UNLIMITED POTENTIAL

The benefit of having an HIV clinical pharmacist extends beyond direct patient services. Pharmacists are becoming increasingly essential members of HIV hospital or clinic quality-improvement teams. Performance measures often involve chart abstraction and generation of reports to benchmark rates of ART, viral suppression, opportunistic infection prophylaxis, and adherence. HIV pharmacists have the clinical background and skills to assess these and other key indicators quickly, accurately, and thoroughly. Pharmacists can also offer valuable insight for "plan–do–study–act" projects designed to improve any below-target performance measures.

Finally, an increasing number of trained HIV clinical pharmacist scientists are making a strong impact on HIV-related research. A solid understanding of study design, drug therapy monitoring, and pharmacotherapy makes HIV clinical pharmacists ideal study coordinators or project managers for research studies being conducted within clinical settings. Advanced training through master's degree programs and complementary PhD programs also places HIV clinical pharmacists in an optimal position to serve as principal investigators on research studies regarding pharmacokinetics, pharmacodynamics, investigational drugs, adherence, drug resistance, or provision of health services. As pharmacists become further trained in clinical research methods, they will continue to contribute valuable information to the body of HIV care knowledge.

CONCLUSION

HIV clinical pharmacists are a diverse group of healthcare practitioners with specialized skills and knowledge. Whether they are engaged in direct patient care, quality assurance, research, or a combination of these, they strive to benefit people with HIV through their efforts. Although not all clinics or hospitals have available resources or funding to house an HIV-specialized pharmacist, collaborations with HIV-focused community pharmacists can ensure that patients have access to this valuable healthcare team member and that they receive the highest-quality medication-management care possible.

RECOMMENDED READING

Durham SH, Badowski ME, Liedtke MD, Rathbun RC, Fulco PP. Acute care management of the HIV-infected patient: a report from the HIV Practice and Research Network of the American College of Clinical Pharmacy. *Pharmacotherapy.* 2017;37:611–629.

Hill LA, Ballard C, Cachay ER. The role of the clinical pharmacist in the management of people living with HIV in the modern antiretroviral era. *AIDS Rev.* 2019;21(4):195–210.

Koren DE, Scarsi KK, Farmer EK, et al. A call to action: the role of anti-retroviral stewardship in inpatient practice, a joint policy paper of the Infectious Diseases Society of America, HIV Medicine Association, and American Academy of HIV Medicine. *Clin Infect Dis.* May 23, 2020;70(11):2241–2246.

Schafer JJ, Cocohoba JM, Sherman EM, Tseng AL, (Eds.). *HIV pharmacotherapy: the pharmacist's role in care and treatment.* Bethesda, MD: American Society Of Health-System Pharmacists; 2018.

REFERENCES

Ahmed A, Dujaili JA, Rehman IU, et al. Effect of pharmacist care on clinical outcomes among people living with HIV/AIDS: a systematic review and meta-analysis. *Res Soc Admin Pharm.* 2022;18:2962–2980.

American Pharmacists Association and National Association of Chain Drug Stores Foundation. Medication therapy management in pharmacy practice: core elements of an MTM service model (version 2.0). *J Am Pharm Assoc (2003).* 2008;48(3):341–353.

Amesty S, Crawford ND, Nandi V, et al. Evaluation of pharmacy-based HIV testing in a high-risk New York City community. *AIDS Patient Care STDS.* August 2015;29(8):437–444. http://doi:10.1089/apc.2015.0017

Back D, Catia M. The challenge of HIV treatment in an era of polypharmacy. *J Int AIDS Soc.* 2020;23(2):e25449

Brizzi MB, Burgos RM, Chiampas TD, et al. Impact of pharmacist-driven antiretroviral stewardship and transitions of care interventions on persons with human immunodeficiency virus. *Open Forum Infect Dis.* 2020;24;7(8):ofaa073.

Brotherton AL, Shah RB, Garland J, et al. Pharmacist-driven rapid ART reduces time to virologic suppression in Rhode Island. [Abstract #498.] Conference on Retroviruses and Opportunistic Infections. Boston, MA; March 8–11, 2020.

Byrd KK, Hardnett F, Clay PG, et al. Retention in HIV care among participants in the patient-centered HIV care model: a collaboration between community-based pharmacists and primary medical providers. *AIDS Patient Care STDS.* February 2019;33(2):58–66.

Byrd KK, Hou JG, Bush T, et al. Adherence and viral suppression among participants of the patient-centered human immunodeficiency virus (HIV) care model project: a collaboration between community-based pharmacists and HIV clinical providers. *Clin Infect Dis.* February 14, 2020;70(5):789–797.

Centers for Disease Control and Prevention (CDC). Monitoring selected national HIV prevention and care objectives by using HIV surveillance data—United States and 6 dependent areas, 2019. *HIV Surveillance Supplemental Report.* 2021;26(2):34–35.

Collins B, Bronson H, Elamin F, Yerkes L, Martin E. The "no wrong door" approach to HIV testing: results from a statewide retail pharmacy-based HIV testing program in Virginia, 2014–2016. *Public Health Rep.* November/December 2018;133(Suppl 2):34S–42S.

Cope R, Berkowitz L, Arcebido R, et al. Evaluating the effects of an interdisciplinary practice model with pharmacist collaboration on HIV patient co-morbidities. *AIDS Patient Care STDS.* 2015;29(8):445–453.

Crawford ND, Albarran T, Chamberlain A, et al. Willingness to discuss and screen for pre-exposure prophylaxis in pharmacies among men who have sex with men. *J Pharm Pract.* 2021;34(5):734–740. doi:10.1177/0 2020:897190020904590. EPub: 18 February,2020.

D'Antonio N. Including motivational interviewing skills in the PharmD curriculum. *Am J Pharm Educ.* 2010;74(8):152d.

Darin KM, Scarsi KK, Klepser DG, et al. Consumer interest in community pharmacy HIV screening services. *J Am Pharm Assoc (2003).* January–February 2015;55(1):67–72.

DePuy AM, Samuel R, Mohrien KM, Clayton EB, Koren DE. Impact of an antiretroviral stewardship team on the care of patients with human immunodeficiency virus infection admitted to an academic medical center. *Open Forum Infect Dis.* July 2019;6(7): ofz290.

Dilworth TJ, Klein PW, Mercier RC, et al. Clinical and economic effects of a pharmacist-administered antiretroviral therapy adherence clinic for patients living with HIV. *JMCP.* 2018;24(2):165–172.

Fick DM, Semla TP, Steinman M, et al. American Geriatrics Society 2019 updated AGS Beers Criteria for potentially inappropriate medication use in older adults. *J Am Geriatr Soc.* April 2019;67(4):674–694.

Hammond RW, Schwartz AH, Campbell MJ, et al. Collaborative drug therapy management by pharmacists—2003. *Pharmacotherapy.* 2003;23(9):1210–1225.

Horberg MA, Bartemeier Hurley L, James Towner W, et al. Determination of optimized multidisciplinary care team for maximal antiretroviral therapy adherence. *J Acquir Immune Defic Syndr.* 2012;60(2):183–190.

Horberg MA, Hurley LB, Silverberg MJ, et al. Effect of clinical pharmacists on utilization of and clinical response to antiretroviral therapy. *J AIDS.* 2007;44(5):531–539.

Johnson SR, Giordano TP, Markham C, et al. Patients' experiences with refilling their HIV medicines: facilitators and barriers to on-time refills. *Perm J.* 2020;24:1–3.

Khosropour CM, Backus KV, Means AR, et al. A pharmacist-led, same-day, HIV pre-exposure prophylaxis initiation program to increase PrEP uptake and decrease time to PrEP initiation. *AIDS Patient Care STDS.* January 2020;34(1):1–6.

Kibicho J, Owczarzak J. Pharmacists' strategies for promoting medication adherence amongst patients with HIV. *J Am Pharm Assoc (2003).* 2011;51(6):746–755.

Koren DE, Scarsi KK, Farmer EK, et al. A call to action: the role of anti-retroviral stewardship in inpatient practice, a joint policy paper of the Infectious Diseases Society of America, HIV Medicine Association, and American Academy of HIV Medicine. *Clin Infect Dis.* May 23, 2020;70(11):2241–2246.

Krummenacher I, Cavassini M, Bugnon O, et al. An interdisciplinary HIV-adherence program combining motivational interviewing and electronic antiretroviral drug monitoring. *AIDS Care.* 2011;23(5):550–561.

Lecher SL, Shrestha RK, Botts LW, et al. Cost analysis of a novel HIV testing strategy in community pharmacies and retail clinics. *J Am Pharm Assoc (2003).* 2015;55(5):488–492.

Lutz S, Heberling, M, Goodlet KJ. Patient perspectives of pharmacists prescribing HIV pre-exposure prophylaxis: A survey of patients receiving antiretroviral therapy. *J Am Pharm Assoc (2003).* 2021;61(2):e75-e79

Mahtani KR, Heneghan CJ, Glasziou PP, et al. Reminder packaging for improving adherence to self-administered long-term medications. *Cochrane Database System Rev.* 2011;9:CD005025.

McLaughlin M, Gordon LA, Kleyn TJ, Lamsen M, Scott J. Assessment of the benefits of and barriers to HIV pharmacist credentialing. *J Am Pharm Assoc (2003).* March–April 2018;58(2):168–173.

McNicholl IR, Gandhi M, Hare CB, Greene M, Pierluissi E. A pharmacist-led program to evaluate and reduce polypharmacy and potentially inappropriate prescribing in older HIV-positive patients. *Pharmacotherapy.* December 2017;37(12):1498–1506.

Nevo ON, Lesko CR, Colwell B, et al. Outcomes of pharmacist-assisted management of antiretroviral therapy in patients with HIV infection: a risk-adjusted analysis. *Am J Health Syst Phasrm.* 2015;72:1463–1470.

Okoli C, de los Rios P, Eremin A, Brough G, Young B, Short D. Relationship between polypharmacy and quality of life among people in 24 countries living with HIV. *Prev Chronic Dis.* 2020;17:190359.

Rathbun RC, Farmer KC, Stephens JR, et al. Impact of an adherence clinic on behavioral outcomes and virologic response in the treatment of HIV infection: a prospective, randomized, controlled pilot study. *Clin Ther.* 2005;27(2):199–209.

Roshdy D, McCarter M, Meredith J, et al. Implementation of a comprehensive intervention focused on hospitalized patients with HIV by an existing stewardship program: successes and lessons learned. *Ther Adv Infect Dis.* 2021;19(8):20499361211010590.

Saberi P, Johnson MO. Technology-based self-care methods of improving antiretroviral adherence: a systematic review. *PLoS One.* 2011;6(11):e27533.

Schafer JJ, Gill TK, Sherman EM, McNicholl IR. ASHP guidelines on pharmacist involvement in HIV care. *Am J Health-Syst Pharm.* 2016;73:468–494. http://www.ajhp.org/content/73/7/468. Accessed July 7, 2018.

Shea KM, Hobbs AL, Shumake JD, Templet DJ, Padilla-Tolentino E, Mondy KE. Impact of an antiretroviral stewardship strategy on medication error rates. *Am J Health Syst Pharm.* June 15, 2018;75(12):876–885.

Sherman EM, Elrod S, Allen D, Eckardt P. Pharmacist testers in multidisciplinary health care team expand HIV point-of-care testing program. *J Pharm Pract.* December 2014;27(6):578–581.

Shrestha RK, Schommer JC, Taitel MS, et al. Costs and cost-effectiveness of the patient-centered HIV care model: a collaboration between community-based pharmacists and primary medical providers. *J Acquir Immune Defic Syndr.* 2020;85(3):e48–e54.

Tung EL, Thomas A, Eichner A, Shalit P. Implementation of a community pharmacy-based pre-exposure prophylaxis service: a novel model for pre-exposure prophylaxis care. *Sex Health.* November 2018;15(6):556–561.

Weidle PJ, Lecher S, Botts LW, et al. HIV testing in community pharmacies and retail clinics: a model to expand access to screening for HIV infection. *J Am Pharm Assoc (2003).* September–October 2014;54(5): 486–492.

Zhu V, Tran D, Banjo O, Onuegbu R, Seung H, Layson-Wolf C. Patient perception of community pharmacists prescribing pre-exposure prophylaxis for HIV prevention. *J Am Pharm Assoc (2003).* April 15, 2020:S1544–S3191(20):30128.

16.

VIROLOGY AND NATURAL HISTORY OF HIV

Poonam Mathur

CHAPTER GOALS

Upon completion of this chapter, the reader should be able to:

- Demonstrate and apply knowledge of the established and evolving science of human immunodeficiency virus (HIV) virology, both in the cell and in the host.

- Describe how HIV virology informs treatment aimed at various stages of the viral life cycle.

HIV STRUCTURE AND LIFE CYCLE

LEARNING OBJECTIVE

Discuss basic HIV virology and its relevance to current and potential drug targets.

WHAT'S NEW?

Expanded discussion of viral classification, entry, reverse transcription and integration is presented.

KEY POINTS

- HIV is a member of the lentivirus subfamily of retroviruses.

- The HIV life cycle can be divided into two phases: (1) virus entry, reverse transcription, entry into the nucleus, and integration of double-stranded DNA (the provirus), and (2) regulation of production of viral proteins and new infectious virions.

- HIV enters the human cell via the CD4 receptor and chemokine coreceptors, primarily CCR5 and CXCR4.

- The viral genome is transcribed from RNA to DNA by reverse transcriptase and integrated into the host genome by integrase.

- The HIV genome encodes 15 proteins comprising three categories: structural, regulatory, and accessory.

- After budding from the host cell, the virus matures into its infectious form through cleavage of viral precursor proteins by protease.

VIRAL CLASSIFICATION

HIV is a member of the lentivirus subfamily of retroviruses, differing from HTLV-1 and HTLV-2, which are oncoviruses. Two distinct groups of HIV lentiviruses are pathogenic in humans: HIV-1 and HIV-2, both of which cause immunodeficiency disease. HIV-2 is less pathogenic and epidemiologically distinct from HIV-1, and it was first isolated from people with HIV (PWH) in West Africa. HIV-2 differs from HIV-1 primarily in three ways: (1) a longer asymptomatic phase, (2) a slower rate of $CD4^+$ T-cell decline, and (3) lower plasma viral loads. Given these advantages, it has historically been associated with lower mortality compared to HIV-1 (Alabi et al., 2003; Berry et al., 1998). Subsequent discussion will focus on HIV-1 infection and pathogenesis.

HIV-1 is subclassified into three groups: M (major), O (outlier), and N (non-M, non-O) (Simon et al., 1998). The vast majority of HIV-1 infections belong to group M. Group M has at least nine known genetically distinct subtypes (or clades): A, B, C, D, F, G, H, J, and K. Subtype A remains the most prevalent strain in parts of East Africa, Russia, and the former Soviet Union; subtype B in Europe and the Americas; and subtype C in Southern Africa and India (Bbosa et al., 2019). Occasionally, genetic material from different clades of HIV-1 may recombine within the same host to form hybrid viruses, called *circulating recombinant forms* or *"CRFs"* (Salminen et al., 1997). Ninety intersubtype recombinants have been shown to be recurrent among circulating HIV-1, and recent studies based on nearly full-length genome sequencing have highlighted the growing importance of recombinant variants and subtype C viruses (Bbosa et al., 2019). Subtype C is the most prevalent form of HIV-1 globally, accounting for 46% of infections worldwide (Gartner et al., 2020). Currently of interest is whether subtype C leads to a faster progression to AIDS compared to other subtypes. In addition, the transmission and replication capacity of subtype C in genital and rectal lymphoid cells is under investigation to determine if those characteristics account for its high prevalence worldwide.

For a listing of current circulating recombinant forms (CRFs), see https://www.hiv.lanl.gov/content/sequence/HIV/CRFs/CRFs.html (Song et al., 2018).

VIRAL STRUCTURE

HIV-1 is an RNA virus, and its basic genomic structure is typical of other retroviruses. The integrated form of HIV is known as the *provirus*, which is flanked at both ends by a repeated sequence known as the *long terminal repeats* (LTRs). The genes of HIV are located in the central region of the proviral DNA and encode 15 distinct proteins divided into three classes: structural proteins (Gag, Pol, and Env), regulatory proteins (Tat and Rev), and accessory proteins (Vpu, Vpr, Vif, and Nef) (Klimkait et al., 1990; Willey et al., 1992). In the mature HIV-1 virion, the inner capsid contains two molecules of single-stranded RNA and key enzymes necessary for infection: reverse transcriptase, integrase, protease, and accessory proteins (Figure 16.1). Recent research has provided insight on the importance of the capsid protein in HIV-1 infection, as the capsid regulates several virus-host interactions in the HIV-1 life cycle (Rossi et al., 2021). The capsid is surrounded by structural matrix protein, itself contained within the viral envelope. Composed of a phospholipid bilayer derived from the host cell, the envelope contains trimers of the viral glycoproteins gp120 and gp41. The exposed surfaces of gp120 exhibit a high level of variability, limiting the humoral immune response to circulating virus (Tilton & Doms, 2010).

VIRAL ENTRY

The viral envelope contains the necessary proteins for cell fusion and viral entry, initiating infection of the host cell. HIV gains access to its target cells via multiple interactions of viral proteins with receptors on the cell membrane (Figure 16.2). The viral glycoprotein gp120 binds with high affinity to the CD4 receptor, which normally functions as a coreceptor in the activation of helper T-cells. CD4 binding induces a conformational change in gp120, exposing its binding sites for coreceptors (either CCR5 or CXCR4) on the host cell surface. Binding of gp120 to the coreceptor exposes the fusion domain of the viral glycoprotein gp41. Then, glycoprotein gp41 inserts its hydrophobic peptide into the target cell membrane, forming a pore through which the viral capsid enters (Tavasolli, 2011). This process is known as *fusion*. Gp41 is a target of drugs that bind to this glycoprotein and prevent formation of the fusion pore. In addition to infected T-cells, macrophages have become increasingly recognized as a target of HIV-1 infection, playing a role not just in pathogenesis, but also in persistence of infection (Han et al., 2022).

Viral strains vary in their coreceptor usage. Those that bind the chemokine receptors CCR5 or CXCR4 are classified as R5-tropic or X4-tropic, respectively. During HIV transmission and early infection, R5-tropic strains predominate. Individuals who do not express CCR5, by virtue of genetic mutation, are highly resistant to HIV infection by R5-tropic viruses (Reiche et al., 2007). Mutant alleles in the CCR5 gene have also been shown to prevent HIV infection by creating a partially nonfunctional coreceptor for HIV entry (Liu et al., 1996; Samson et al., 1996).

Drugs that target CCR5 and bind to the coreceptor alter its interaction with gp120. However, these drugs can only be used in PWH whose virus has been determined to be R5-tropic. Through evolution within the host, some HIV strains become X4-tropic, rendering them resistant to these agents. There have been five cases of PWH reported to achieve sustained HIV remission (cure) following stem cell transplantation with allogeneic, homozygous CCR5-Δ32 mutated donor cells, and efforts to modify CCR5 receptors to maintain HIV-1 remission in the absence of antiretroviral therapy are ongoing (Gupta et al., 2019). Downregulation of the CCR5 gene through genetic modification (gene therapy) of CD4[+] T-cells and hematopoietic stem/progenitor cells

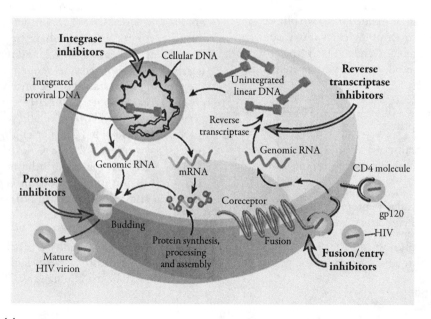

Figure 16.1 HIV life cycle and drug targets   SOURCE: Reproduced from Fauci 2003 with permission from Macmillan Publishers Ltd: Nat Med, copyright 2003.

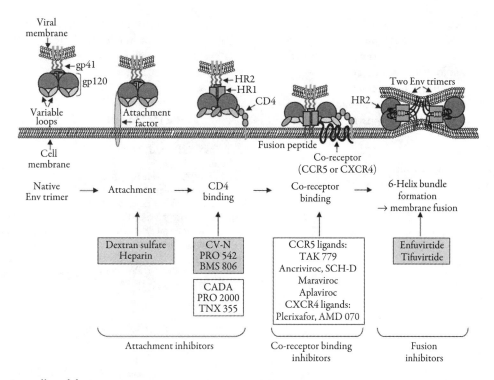

Figure 16.2 HIV entry into cells and drug targets   SOURCE: Reeves J, et al. Drugs. 2005;65(13):1747–1766, with permission from Springer Nature.

and autologous transplantation of these cells was proposed in 2012 as a mechanism for curing HIV without needing to find a donor with the homozygous CCR5-Δ32 mutated donor cells and developed as a phase 1 clinical trial in 2013 (Deeks et al., 2012, Mitsuyasu et al., 2020).

REVERSE TRANSCRIPTION AND INTEGRATION

After fusion, viral disassembly (which is distinct from and not merely the reverse of viral assembly) occurs before reverse transcription can take place. In order for HIV-1 to fully establish infection in a susceptible cell, the RNA must undergo reverse transcription into double-stranded DNA and integrate into the host genome (Tekeste et al., 2015). Reverse transcription starts when the viral RNA is released into the host cell cytoplasm, shedding associated proteins in a process known as *uncoating*. The viral enzyme reverse transcriptase (RT) then produces double-stranded DNA from the viral RNA template. RT is a heterodimer composed of a larger, functional subunit (p66) and a smaller, structural subunit (p51). At this stage, the host's natural antiviral immunity is activated, and the enzyme APOBEC3G, found in CD4 $^+$ T-cells and macrophages, terminates the elongating viral DNA by causing hypermutations. However, HIV has the protein Vif, which binds APOBEC3G and leads to its degradation, overriding the host's natural immunity and allowing propagation of viral DNA (Table 16.1) (Tavasolli, 2011).

The newly synthesized viral DNA then integrates into the host DNA. Integration is a vital step in the sustained propagation of the virus and its progeny; integrase-negative HIV mutants do not integrate and therefore do not produce infectious virions (Wiskerchen & Muesing, 1995). Integration is catalyzed by integrase (IN), in conjunction with the nuclear localization factor Vpr, to form the preintegration complex. Once in the nucleus, a critical interaction between integrase and the host protein LEDGF/p75 directs this complex to the host DNA (Tavasolli, 2011), and IN mediates strand transfer, linking viral and host DNA through covalent bonds. Co-opting host cell proteins, HIV relies on the cell's normal DNA repair mechanism to complete integration.

Table 16.1 VIRAL ACCESSORY AND REGULATORY PROTEIN FUNCTIONS

GENE	FUNCTION
Tat	Transcriptional transactivator
Rev	Allows unspliced viral genomes to leave the nucleus
Nef	Downregulates CD4 receptor and major histocompatibility complex class I, alters T-cell activation, aids viral infectivity
Vif	Counters the host restriction factor APOBEC3G
Vpr	Facilitates the nuclear localization of the viral genome
Vpr	Downregulates CD4 receptor, increases viral release

SOURCE: Adapted from Miller et al. *Trends Microbiol.* August 1994;2(8):294–298.

Integrase strand transfer inhibitors block the penultimate step of integration by preventing strand transfer to the host DNA. Also, since it has been demonstrated in vitro that the RT-IN interaction is biologically significant for reverse transcription (Tekeste et al., 2015), the interaction between these two enzymes has been a target for development of two-drug combination therapy, which has demonstrated viral suppression and a safety profile consistent with current ART regimens (Llibre et al., 2018).

Islatravir is a novel nucleoside analog in a new class of nucleoside reverse translocation inhibitors that was developed for the treatment and prevention of HIV-1 infection. In combination with doravirine in a phase IIb trial, the two-drug combination showed high efficacy and was well-tolerated regardless of dose (Molina et al., 2021). However, at the time of this publication, the FDA has placed a clinical hold on islatravir's clinical development because phase II and III trials have shown drops in CD4$^+$ T-cells and total lymphocyte counts.

VIRUS PRODUCTION

Once integrated into the host DNA, the viral genome can remain latent or undergo active expression. Active expression is dependent on cellular and viral factors that activate viral promotors, including coinfection with other agents, production of inflammatory cytokines, and cellular activation (Honda et al., 1998). In active infection, viral DNA is first transcribed into mRNA. Some of the early mRNA produced are 2-kb in size and serve as viral regulatory proteins. These mRNAs can be detected by Southern blot analysis (Kim et al., 1989) or even polymerase chain reaction within 6 hours of infection (Klotman et al., 1991). Many of the same transcription factors involved in CD4$^+$ T-cell activation also bind to the HIV LTR, promoting expression of the viral genome (Pereira et al., 2000). The resulting mRNA is spliced, processed, and ultimately translated into viral proteins by the host cell machinery. In a positive feedback loop, the viral protein Tat (transactivator) promotes further viral transcription by facilitating elongation of nascent viral transcripts (Kao et al., 1987).

The viral protein gag mediates assembly of progeny virions by packaging genomic RNA within virus particles. Finally, HIV protease catalyzes the cleavage of the gag-pol precursor polyprotein (p55), yielding the structural proteins that form the mature virion. Assembly of mature virus occurs at the cell membrane, and these virus particles exit the cell in a process known as *viral budding*. Budding occurs in areas called *lipid rafts*, located in the cell membrane, composed of high concentrations of cholesterol, sphingolipids, and glycolipids (Liao et al., 2001). HIV-1 generation time in vivo is 2 days, and the half-life of infected CD4$^+$ T-cells is 0.7 days (Markowitz et al., 2003). The ubiquitin proteasome system (UPS), which is a major protein degradation mechanism for eukaryotic cellular processes, may also play a critical role in in regulation of proteasomal degradation of viral and cellular counterparts during the HIV-1 life cycle, ultimately resulting in a contest for host or virus survival. However, the coordination and significance of viral protein degradation at different stages of the life cycle remains elusive and warrants further investigation (Rojas & Park, 2019).

RECOMMENDED READING

Fauci AS. HIV and AIDS: 20 years of science. *Nat Med*. 2003;9(7): 834–843.

Greene WC, Peterlin BM. *Molecular insights into HIV biology*. http://hivinsite.ucsf.edu/InSite?page=kb-02-01-01. University of California San Francisco. Published 2006. Accessed April 20, 2006.

Moore JP, Kitchen SG, Pugach P, et al. The CCR5 and CXCR4 coreceptors: central to understanding the transmission and pathogenesis of human immunodeficiency virus type 1 infection. *AIDS Res Hum Retroviruses*. 2004;20(1):111–126.

Reeves JD, Piefer AJ. Emerging drug targets for antiretroviral therapy. *Drugs*. 2005;65(13):1747–1766.

HIV NATURAL HISTORY

LEARNING OBJECTIVE

Discuss the course of HIV infection and its dynamics in the host over time.

WHAT'S NEW?

Establishment of the viral reservoir has been updated.

KEY POINTS

- In mucosal transmission, HIV crosses the epithelial barrier and establishes an expanding infection at the site of entry.

- During acute infection, HIV disseminates to lymphatic tissue throughout the body.

- The rate of fall in plasma viremia with ART reflects the kinetics of different types of infected host cells.

- HIV exhibits remarkable levels of diversity, both globally and within a single host.

- HIV establishes latent infection in a subset of host cells, allowing it to persist despite ART.

ESTABLISHMENT OF INFECTION

In sexual transmission, HIV must first breach the epithelial barrier of the genital or rectal mucosa. This may occur via physical breaks in the epithelium related to trauma or sexually transmitted infections, particularly herpes simplex virus. However, HIV can also cross intact mucosa via specialized dendritic cells in the genital tract or transcytosis in the gastrointestinal (GI) tract (Morrow et al., 2008). Upon crossing the epithelial barrier, the virus encounters multiple potential target cells. The major cellular receptor for fusion and entry of HIV is CD4 $^+$ T-cells, whose critical role in HIV infection was identified in 1984 (Dalgleish et al., 1984; Klatzmann et al., 1984). Initial infection is propagated by dendritic cells (especially the Langerhans cells), components of the innate immune system, which deliver HIV to CD4 $^+$ T-cells; or the virus may directly infect local CD4 $^+$ T-cells without the aid of dendritic cells. The initial proliferation of HIV represents a genetic bottleneck in which a large viral inoculum gives rise to a small founder population of infected cells. In heterosexual transmission, infection results from a single viral genotype in 80% of cases, with preference for the CCR5 coreceptor (Haase, 2010).

The *eclipse phase* refers to the period after mucosal exposure, when the virus remains undetectable in plasma, and lasts approximately 10 days. Once a founder viral population is established at the portal of entry, it must expand locally by rapid migration to regional lymph nodes and dissemination to distant draining lymph nodes via the bloodstream. In a chain reaction of cell-to-cell signaling, termed the *virologic synapse* (Piguet & Steinman, 2007), dendritic and Langerhans cell-type T-cells' exposure to HIV induces the recruitment of more plasmacytoid dendritic cells, and ultimately, more CD4 $^+$ T-cells (Haase, 2010). Therefore, in addition to the role that lymphoid tissue (in particular dendritic cells) plays in the initiation of HIV infection, it is also responsible for the dissemination of HIV infection. These early events may be altered to prevent infection, and they figure prominently in research on microbicides, pre-exposure and postexposure prophylaxis and preventive vaccines.

ACUTE INFECTION

Once infection is established in draining lymph nodes, activated CD4 $^+$ T lymphocytes become the predominant source of viral replication. Immune activation increases the pool of susceptible activated CD4 $^+$ T-cells, creating a positive feedback loop. An exponential increase in plasma viremia ensues, and PWH may develop symptoms of the acute retroviral syndrome. HIV disseminates and infects other lymphatic tissues throughout the body. The CD4 $^+$ T-cell count in peripheral blood declines markedly, thought to occur through several proposed mechanisms: increased destruction of cells by direct infection by HIV, activation of apoptosis, increased lymphocyte turnover, decreased production by reduced thymic output and redistribution of cells from peripheral blood to lymphoid tissue. A profound depletion of CD4 $^+$ T-cells also occurs in the gut-associated lymphatic tissue (GALT), causing permanent damage.

The events in acute infection have long-term consequences for the patient. Activation of CD4 $^+$ T-cells and HIV RNA replication causes fibrosis to occur in the lymphoid architecture, leading to incomplete immune reconstitution after initiation of ART (Brenchley et al., 2004). Damage to the GI epithelium and mucosal immune response allows an increase in microbial translocation (Haase, 2010), which may serve as a stimulus to systemic immune activation, magnifying the positive feedback loop for the virus. Over time, microbial translocation likely contributes to chronic immune activation and progression to AIDS. Finally, a reservoir of latently infected cells is established which later prevents viral eradication with ART. Important reservoir sites include the GALT and peripheral lymphoid tissues. In the rare cases in which HIV is diagnosed during primary infection, immediate ART may have potential to attenuate, although not reverse, these changes.

The establishment of the HIV reservoir and viral latency is widely discussed as the barrier to curing HIV (Castro-Gonzalez et al., 2018). Current therapies do not completely eliminate the reservoir after it has been established, since infected cells harbor replication-competent proviruses that are transcriptionally inactive, thus not utilizing the replication enzymes which are targets for ART. A more detailed discussion of this topic is included in Chapter 19.

VIRAL KINETICS AND LATENCY

Plasma HIV RNA levels reflect a dynamic interplay between the infection of susceptible cells and the destruction of infected cells. With initiation of ART, susceptible host cells are protected from infection. Consequently, the rate of decline in the viral load following initiation of ART reflects the kinetics of the death of HIV-infected cells (Figure 16.3) (Palmer et al., 2011).

Viral decay occurs in four distinct phases. The viral load declines dramatically in the first phase of 7–10 days, reflecting clearance of activated CD4 $^+$ T-cells ($t_{1/2}$ = 1 or 2 days), with roughly 90% of the decrease in plasma HIV occurring in these first weeks of therapy (Markowitz et al., 2003). The second phase, characterized by a more gradual decline in viral load and an average viral half-life of 14 days (Andrade et al., 2013), correlates with the intermediate half-lives of partially activated CD4 $^+$ T-cells, macrophages, and possibly dendritic cells. In the third phase, plasma HIV continues to decline, although at levels detectable only by ultrasensitive assays. This phase may represent decay of latently infected resting CD4 $^+$ T-cells that are producing HIV, but HIV RNA levels are unobserved since they have fallen below the limit of detection (Andrade et al., 2013). It is thought that during this phase, a first reservoir is maintained since there is suboptimal diffusion of ART into lymphoid tissues, allowing the virus to replicate at low levels. However, whether this phenomenon occurs in the majority of individuals on ART is controversial (Dufour et al., 2020). The fourth phase occurs 4–5 years after ART initiation and finally stabilizes at very low levels (< 1–5 copies/mL) (Siliciano et al., 2003). Research has focused on the resting memory CD4 $^+$ T-cell as the source of viral replication during these latter stages. In addition, monocytes and derivative macrophages or dendritic cells have been shown to play a role in the establishment latency (Tram, 2022). Despite fully suppressive ART, the proportion of resting CD4 $^+$ T-cells that are latently infected shows minimal decline over time, yielding an estimated half-life of 44 months (Siliciano et al., 2003).

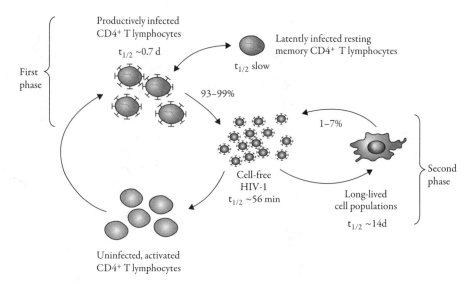

First phase

Productively infected
CD4+ T lymphocytes

$t_{1/2}$ ~0.7 d

Latently infected resting
memory CD4+ T lymphocytes

$t_{1/2}$ slow

93–99%

Cell-free
HIV-1

$t_{1/2}$ ~56 min

1–7%

Long-lived
cell populations

$t_{1/2}$ ~14d

Second
phase

Uninfected, activated
CD4+ T lymphocytes

Figure 16.3 Rates of clearance of different cell populations and viral turnover   SOURCE: Simon V, et al. Nat Rev Microbiol. 2003;1(3):181–90.

By this estimate, HIV eradication would require more than 70 years of uninterrupted ART.

Since HIV latency is the chief obstacle to eradicating HIV, increasing attention has turned to the mechanisms that maintain latent infection. In latent infection, proviral DNA is integrated into the host genome but remains in a transcriptionally silent, but inducible, state. Latently infected cells serve as a reservoir for virus that can reactivate and drive HIV viral loads to pretreatment levels if ART is interrupted (Rouzine et al., 2015). In rhesus macaque models, simian immunodeficiency virus (SIV) established latency in reservoir cells as early as 3 days after infection, before viremia was detected (Whitney et al., 2014). Different biological processes, such as host transcription factors, histone deacetylase-mediated epigenetic silencing, and cytokines, have been shown to play a role in HIV latency. The host transcription factors (NF-κB, NFAT, and P-TEFβ) and the viral protein Tat promote expression of proviral DNA, but they are present at low levels in resting CD4 + T-cells, thus maintaining latency. Histone deacetylation and DNA methylation at the HIV LTR alter the local chromatin environment, denying access to the machinery of transcription (Palmer et al., 2011). Establishment of the reservoir is also facilitated by cell-to-cell transmission of HIV, rather than cell-free transmission, which is more efficient and does not expose virus particles to the challenges of surviving in the extracellular environment (Pedro et al., 2019).

Therapies that promote expression of the proviral genome or activate resting CD4 + T-cells have the potential to speed decay of the latent reservoir. An observational study of two individuals on PrEP who started prophylactic ART an estimated 10 days after infection showed that after ART interruption, HIV viremia recurred despite initiation of ART at one of the earliest stages of acute HIV infection possible. Therefore, establishment of the reservoir occurs extremely early in infection (Henrich et al., 2017). Two animal studies demonstrated robust and persistent latency reversal in mice and SIV models in multiple tissues and peripheral blood

by activating the noncanonical NF-κB pathway (Nixon et al., 2020) and by interleukin-15 stimulation combined with CD8+ T-cells depletion (McBrien et al., 2020). Further investigations on latency reversal agents are reviewed in more detail in Chapter 19.

VIRAL DIVERSITY

During untreated infection, HIV replicates at an extraordinary rate, with roughly 10 billion new virions produced each day. RT, in contrast to DNA polymerases, lacks proofreading activity (Taylor et al., 2008). As a result, frequent mutations occur in the daughter viral genome, potentially altering the structure and function of viral proteins. HIV recombination is another means of viral diversity and occurs when one person is coinfected with two strains of the virus which replicate within the cell (Taylor et al., 2008). The rapid rate of production, combined with frequent mutations and recombination, leads to the production of diverse quasi-species. Strikingly, the genetic diversity observed in a single individual after six years of HIV infection is roughly equivalent to that observed worldwide in influenza A virus within a given year (Korber et al., 2001). However, the genetic diversity that occurs in acute infection occurs at a much higher rate than in chronic infection. The high number of replication cycles also allows for selection of resistant variants, either due to drug pressure or the immune system. Emergence of drug resistance mutations is governed by selection forces and drift (Maldarelli et al., 2013).

Viral diversity presents a unique challenge for producing an HIV vaccine. Historically, vaccines have prevented infection by stimulating antibody or cell-mediated immunity in susceptible PWH. Both HIV and SIV have been shown to escape from these host immune responses by virtue of their extreme diversity. An effective HIV vaccine may need to elicit broad immune responses that protect against multiple quasi-species and possibly other HIV subtypes. An international phase 3 study known as Mosaico (NCT03964415), was started in 2019 to investigate an experimental HIV vaccine that targets more strains of HIV than any other vaccine produced, and in vitro results indicate lasting immune response for at least two years after vaccine administration (Mega, 2019). The vaccine trial is ongoing, and results are pending.

The impact of viral diversity is well known to clinicians engaged in the treatment of HIV. The administration of multiple agents, initially called "drug cocktails," but now known as combination antiretroviral therapy, is required to suppress viral replication to levels at which drug-resistant strains are unlikely to emerge (i.e., viral diversity underpins the importance of strict adherence to HIV therapy). Similarly, the continuous evolution of HIV has required resistance testing in clinical practice and the continued development of antiretrovirals with novel therapeutic mechanisms.

RECOMMENDED READING

Finzi D, Blankson J, Siliciano JD, et al. Latent infection of CD4+ T cells provides a mechanism for lifelong persistence of HIV-1, even in patients on effective combination therapy. *Nat Med.* 1999;5(5):512–517.

Harris RS, Liddament MT. Retroviral restriction by APOBEC proteins. *Nat Rev Immunol.* 2004;4(11):868–877.

Mehandru S, Tenner-Racz K, Racz P, et al. The gastrointestinal tract is critical to the pathogenesis of acute HIV infection. *J Allergy Clin Immunol.* 2005;116(2):419–422.

Persaud D, Zhou Y, Siliciano JM, et al. Latency in human immunodeficiency virus type 1 infection: no easy answers. *J Virol.* 2003;77(3):1659–1665.

Simon V, Ho DD. HIV-1 dynamics in vivo: Implications for therapy. *Nat Rev Microbiol.* 2003;1(3):181–190.

ACKNOWLEDGMENT

This chapter was based on previous additions written by Schuyler Livingston, Martin Markowitz, William Wright, Benjamin Young, and Bruce L. Gilliam.

REFERENCES

Alabi AS, Jaffar S, Ariyoshi K, Blanchard T, et al. Plasma viral load, CD4 cell percentage, HLA and survival of HIV-1, HIV-2, and dually infected Gambian patients. *AIDS.* 2003;17(10):1513–1520.

Andrade A, Rosenkranz S, Cillo A, et al. Three distinct phases of HIV-1 RNA decay in treatment-naïve patients receiving raltegravir-based antiretroviral therapy: ACTG A5248. *J Inf Dis.* 2013;208(6):884–891.

Bbosa N, Kaleebu P, Sswemwanga D. HIV subtype diversity worldwide. *HIV and AIDS.* 2019;14(3):153–160.

Berry N, Ariyoshi K, Jaffar S et al. Low peripheral blood viral HIV-2 RNA in individuals with high CD4 percentage differentiates HIV-2 from HIV-1 infection. *J Hum Virol.* 1998;1(7):457–468.

Brenchley JM, Schacker TW, Ruff LE, et al. CD4\+ T cell depletion during all stages of HIV disease occurs predominantly in the gastrointestinal tract. *J Exp Med.* 2004;200(6):749–759.

Castro-Gonzalez S, Colomer-Lluch M, Serra-Moreno R. Barriers for HIV cure: the latent reservoir. *AIDS Res Hum Retroviruses.* 2018;34(9):739–759.

Dalgleish AG, Beverly PC, Clapham PR, et al. The CD4(T4) antigen is an essential component of the receptor for the AIDS retrovirus. *Nature.* 1984;312:763–767.

Deeks SG, Autran B, Berkhout B, et al.; International AIDS Society Scientific Working Group on HIV Cure. Towards an HIV cure: a global scientific strategy. *Nat Rev Immunol.* 2012;12:607–614.

Dufour C, Gantner P, Fromentin R. The multifaceted nature of HIV latency. *J Clin Invest.* 2020;130(7): e136227.

Gartner M, Roche M, Churchill M, et al. Understanding the mechanisms driving the spread of subtype C HIV-1. *Lancet.* 2020;53:102682.

Gupta RK, Abdul-Jawad S, McCoy LE, et al. HIV-1 remission following CCR5Δ32/Δ32 haematopoietic stem-cell transplantation. *Nature.* 2019;568(7751):244–248.

Haase A. Targeting early infection to prevent HIV-1 mucosal transmission. *Nature.* 2010;464:217–223.

Han M, Cantaloube-Ferrieu V, Xie M, et al. HIV-1 cell-to-cell spread overcomes the virus entry block of non-macrophage-tropic strains in macrophages. *Lancet HIV.* 2021;8(6):e324–e333.

Henrich T, Hatano H, Bacon O. HIV-1 persistence following extremely early initiation of antiretroviral therapy (ART) during acute HIV-1 infection: an observational study. *PLoS Med.* 2017;14(11):e1002417.

Honda Y, Rogers L, Nakata K, et al. Type I interferon induces inhibitory 16-kD CCAAT/enhancer binding protein (C/EBP) beta, repressing the HIV-1 long terminal repeat in macrophages: pulmonary tuberculosis alters C/EBP expression, enhancing HIV-1 replication. *J Exp Med.* 1998;188:1255–1265.

Kao SY, Calman AF, Luciw PA, et al. Anti-termination of transcription within the long terminal repeat of HIV-1 by tat gene product. *Nature.* 1987;330(6147):489–493.

Kim SY, Byrn R, Groopman J, et al. Temporal aspects of DNA and RNA synthesis during human immunodeficiency virus infection: evidence for differential gene expression. *J Virol.* 1989;63:3708–3713.

Klatzmann D, Champagne E, Chamaret S, et al. T-lymphocyte T4 molecule behaves as receptor for human retrovirus LAV. *Nature.* 1984;312:767–768.

Klimkait T, Strebel K, Hoggan MD, et al. The human immunodeficiency virus type 1-specific protein Vpu is required for efficient virus maturation and release. *J Virol.* 1990;64(2):621–629.

Klotman ME, Kim S, Buchbinder A, et al. Kinetics of expression of multiply spliced RNA in early human immunodeficiency virus type 1 infection of lymphocytes and monocytes. *Proc Natl Acad Sci U S A.* 1991;88:5011–5015.

Korber B, Gaschen B, Yusim K, et al. Evolutionary and immunological implications of contemporary HIV-1 variation. *Br Med Bull.* 2001;58:19–42.

Liao Z, Cimakasky LM, Hampton R, et al. Lipid rafts and HIV pathogenesis: host membrane cholesterol is required for infection by HIV type 1. *AIDS Res Hum Retroviruses.* 2001;17:1009–1019.

Liu R, Paxton W, Choe S, et al. Homozygous defect in HIV-1 coreceptor accounts for resistance of some multiply-exposed individuals to HIV-1 infection. *Cell.* 1996;86:367–377.

Llibre J, Chien-Ching H, Brinson C, et al. Efficacy, safety, and tolerability of dolutegravir-rilpivirine for the maintenance of virological suppression in adults with HIV-1: phase 3, randomised, non-inferiority SWORD-1 and SWORD-2 studies. *Lancet.* 2018;391(10123):839–849.

Maldarelli F, Kearney M, Palmer S, et al. HIV populations are large and accumulate high genetic diversity in a nonlinear fashion. *J Virol.* 2013;87(18):10313–10323.

Markowitz M, Louie M, Hurley A, et al. A novel antiviral intervention results in more accurate assessment of human immunodeficiency virus type 1 replication dynamics and T-cell decay in vivo. *J Virol.* 2003;77:5037–5038.

McBrien JB, Mavigner M, Franchitti L, et al. Robust and persistent reactivation of SIV and HIV by N-803 and depletion of CD8 + cells. *Nature.* 2020;578(7793):154–159.

Mega ER. Mosaic HIV vaccine to be tested in thousands of people across the world. *Nature*. 2019;572:165–166.

Mitsuyasu R, Lalezari J, Burke B, et al. Phase I Study of gene-modified CD4+ cells and CD34+ cells with or without busulfan in HIV+ adults. [CROI abstract 338]. In: Special issue: abstracts from the 2020 Conference on Retroviruses and Opportunistic Infections. *Top Antivir Med*. 2020;28(1):117.

Molina J-M, Yazdanpanah Y, Saud A, et al. Islatravir in combination with doravirine for treatment-naïve adults with HIV-1 infection receiving initial treatment with islatravir, doravirine, and lamivudine: a phase 2b, randomised, double-blind, dose-ranging trial. *Lancet HIV*. 2021;8(6):e324–e333.

Morrow G, Vachot L, Vagenas P, et al. Current concepts of HIV transmission. *Curr Infect Dis Rep*. May 2008;10(2):133–139.

Nixon CC, Mavigner M, Sampey GC, et al. Systemic HIV and SIV latency reversal via non-canonical NF-κB signaling in vivo. *Nature*. 2020;578(7793):160–165.

Palmer S, Josefsson L, Coffin JM. HIV reservoirs and the possibility of a cure for HIV infection [published online ahead of print October 27, 2011.] *J Intern Med*. 2011;270(6):550–560. http://doi:10.1111/j.1365-2796.2011.02457.x

Pedro K, Henderson A, Agosto L. Mechanisms of HIV-1 cell-to-cell transmission and the establishment of the latent reservoir. *Virus Res*. 2019: 265;115–121.

Pereira LA, Bentley K, Peeters A, et al. A compilation of cellular transcription factor interactions with the HIV-1 LTV promoter. *Nucleic Acids Res*. 2000;28(3):663–668.

Piguet V, Steinman RM. The interaction of HIV with dendritic cells: outcomes and pathways. *Trends Immunol*. 2007;28:503–510.

Reiche EM, Bonametti AM, Voltarelli JC, et al. Genetic polymorphisms in the chemokine and chemokine receptors: impact on clinical course and therapy of the human immunodeficiency virus type 1 infection (HIV-1). *Curr Med Chem*. 2007;14:1325–1334.

Rojas V, Park I-W. Role of the ubiquitin proteasome system (UPS) in the HIV-1 life cycle. *Int J Mol Sci*. 2019;20(12):2984.

Rossi E, Meuser E, Cunan C, et al. Structure, function and interactions of the HIV-1 capsid protein. *Life (Basel)*. 2021;11(2):100.

Rouzine I, Weinberger A, Weinberger L. An evolutionary role for HIV latency in enhancing viral transmission. *Cell*. 2015;160(5):1002–1012.

Salminen MO, Carr JK, Robertson DL, et al. Evolution and probably transmission of intersubtype recombinant human immunodeficiency virus type 1 in a Zambian couple. *J Virol*. 1997;71(4) 2647–2655.

Samson M, Libert F, Doranz B, et al. Resistance to HIV-1 infection in Caucasian individuals bearing mutant alleles of the CCR-5 chemokine receptor gene. *Nature*. 1996;382:722–725.

Schwartz O, Marechal V, Le Gall S, et al. Endocytosis of major histocompatibility complex class I molecules is induced by the HIV-1 Nef protein. *Nat Med*. 1996;2(3):338–342.

Siliciano JD, Kaidas J, Finzi D, et al. Long-term follow-up studies confirm the stability of the latent reservoir for HIV-1 in resting CD4\+ T cells [published online ahead of print May 18, 2003]. *Nat Med*. 2003;9(6):727–728. http://doi:10.1038/nm880

Simon F, Mauclere P, Roques P, et al. Identification of a new human immunodeficiency virus type 1 distinct from group M and group O. *Nat Med*. 1998;4(9):1032–1037.

Song H, Giorgi E, Ganusov V, et al. Tracking HIV-1 recombination to resolve its contribution to HIV-1 evolution in natural infection. *Nat Commun*. 2018;9:1928.

Tram MT, Malik S, Anderson E. Insights into persistent HIV-1 infection and functional cure: novel capabilities and strategies. *Front Microbiol*. 2022;13:862270. http://doi:10.3389/fmicb.2022.862270

Tavasolli A. Targeting the protein-protein interactions of the HIV lifecycle. *Chem Soc Rev*. 2011;40(3):1337–1346.

Taylor B, Sobieszczyk M, McCutchan F, et al. The challenge of HIV-1 subtype diversity. *N Engl J Med*. 2008;358(15):1590–1602.

Tekeste SS, Wilkonson TA, Weiner EM, et al. Interaction between reverse transcriptase and integrase is required for reverse transcription during HIV-1 replication. *J Virology*. 2015;89(23):12058–12069.

Tilton JC, Doms RW. Entry inhibitors in the treatment of HIV-1 infection [published online ahead of print August 14, 2009]. *Antiviral Res*. 2010;85(1):91–100. http://doi:10.1016/j.antiviral.2009.07.022

Whitney JB, Hill AL, Sanisetty S, et al. Rapid seeding of the viral reservoir prior to SIV viraemia in rhesus monkeys. *Nature*. 2014;512: 74–77.

Willey RL, Maldarelli F, Martin MA, et al. Human immunodeficiency virus type 1 Vpu protein regulates the formation of intracellular gp160-CD4 complexes. *J Virol*. January 1992;66(1):226–234.

Wiskerchen M, Muesing MA. Human immunodeficiency virus type 1 integrase: effects of mutations on viral ability to integrate, direct viral gene expression from unintegrated viral DNA templates, and sustain viral propagation in primary cells. *J Virol*. 1995;69:376–386.

17.

SCIENTIFIC BASIS OF ANTIRETROVIRAL THERAPY

David E. Koren, Neha Sheth Pandit, and Emily Heil

CHAPTER GOALS

Upon completion of this chapter, the reader should be able to:

- Describe the classes of antiretroviral (ARV) agents and their mechanisms of action.

- Discuss the clinical trials underpinning new trends in antiretroviral therapy (ART).

- Explain the basic principles of applied pharmacokinetics, pharmadynamics, and pharmagenomics of ARV agents.

- Recognize the benefits of coformulated ART regimens versus the need for tailored ARV dosing.

- Enumerate key principles of clinical trial design and expanded-access programs.

CLASSES AND MECHANISMS OF ANTIRETROVIRAL AGENTS

LEARNING OBJECTIVE

- Describe the mechanisms of action of the traditional and newer ARV classes.

WHAT'S NEW?

Long-acting intramuscular (LAI) cabotegravir and rilpivirine are a novel, two-drug regimen containing an integrase strand transfer inhibitor and nonnucleoside reverse transcriptase inhibitor (NNRTI), respectively, that can be administered to PWH virologically suppressed on an oral ARV regimen. The combination of these LAI ARVs is approved to be administered every month or every two months.

KEY POINTS

- There are five major categories of antiretroviral agents: inhibitors of viral entry, two types of HIV-1 reverse transcriptase inhibitors, inhibitors of HIV-1 protease, and inhibitors of HIV-1 integrase.

- Combination ART is recommended for all people living with HIV (PWH).

INTRODUCTION

Conventional terminology refers to individual antiretroviral agents as ARVs, whereas a combination of ARVs taken together to control HIV infection is known as antiretroviral therapy, or ART. As recommended by the United States Department of Health and Human Services (DHHS) since 2012 (DHHS, 2022) and as further validated by the START (INSIGHT START GROUP, 2015) and TEMPRANO (TEMPRANO ANRS 12136 STUDY GROUP, 2015) trials, ART is indicated for all persons living with HIV without regard to CD4 $^+$ T-cell count. There have been 30 unique US Food and Drug Administration (FDA)-approved agents to treat HIV, targeting the five major steps in the HIV replication cycle (Figure 17.1). Classes of ARVs can be divided into nucleoside/nucleotide reverse transcriptase inhibitors (NRTIs/NtRTIs), nonnucleoside reverse transcriptase inhibitors (NNRTIs), protease inhibitors (PIs), entry inhibitors (comprising an attachment inhibitor (AI), a fusion inhibitor (FI), a C-C chemokine receptor type 5 coreceptor antagonist (CCR5A), and a postattachment inhibitor (PAI)), and integrase strand transfer inhibitors (INSTIs). The primary goal of ART is to achieve and maintain viral suppression (DHHS, 2022).

NUCLEOSIDE/NUCLEOTIDE REVERSE TRANSCRIPTASE INHIBITORS

NRTIs inhibit the HIV-encoded reverse transcriptase enzyme in the host cell. This blocks the conversion of single-stranded viral RNA to double-stranded viral DNA, ultimately preventing incorporation of HIV genetic material into the host double-stranded DNA. NRTIs are nucleoside and nucleotide analogs; when reverse transcriptase incorporates them into the growing DNA, chain elongation is terminated. NRTIs must first be activated in the cell through three phosphorylation steps before they can become active chain terminators; NtRTIs require only two phosphorylation steps. NRTIs are poor substrates for human nuclear DNA polymerase alpha, but some NRTIs can be utilized by human mitochondrial DNA polymerase gamma and thus can cause mitochondrial toxicity. This class of antiretrovirals include the nucleosides abacavir (ABC), emtricitabine (FTC), lamivudine (3TC), and zidovudine (AZT) and the nucleotides tenofovir disoproxil

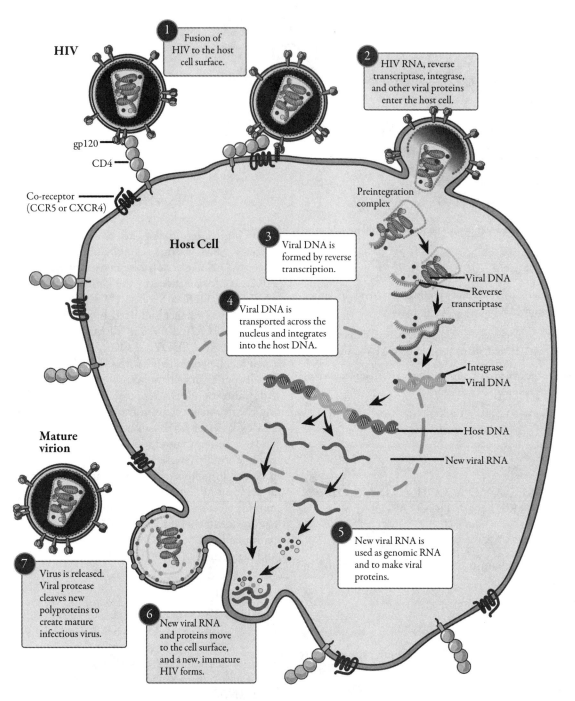

HIV

gp120

CD4

Co-receptor
(CCR5 or CXCR4)

Host Cell

**Mature
virion**

1. Fusion of HIV to the host cell surface.

2. HIV RNA, reverse transcriptase, integrase, and other viral proteins enter the host cell.

Preintegration complex

3. Viral DNA is formed by reverse transcription.

4. Viral DNA is transported across the nucleus and integrates into the host DNA.

Viral DNA
Reverse transcriptase

Integrase
Viral DNA

Host DNA

New viral RNA

5. New viral RNA is used as genomic RNA and to make viral proteins.

6. New viral RNA and proteins move to the cell surface, and a new, immature HIV forms.

7. Virus is released. Viral protease cleaves new polyproteins to create mature infectious virus.

Figure 17.1 HIV viral replication   SOURCE: NIH. https://www.niaid.nih.gov/diseases-conditions/hiv-replication-cycle. Published 2018. Accessed August 10, 2022.

fumarate (TDF) and tenofovir alafenamide (TAF), as well as three older NRTIs (didanosine (DDI), deoxycytidine (DDC), and stavudine (D4T)), which are no longer used clinically.

NONNUCLEOSIDE REVERSE TRANSCRIPTASE INHIBITORS

NNRTIs also inhibit viral reverse transcriptase in the host cell. They act at the same point in the HIV-1 replication cycle as do the NtRTIs, but NNRTIs bind the reverse transcriptase adjacent to the active site, causing structural alterations in the enzyme that sterically prevent it from adding any new nucleosides to the growing DNA chain. As the mechanism of action is different, the viral mutations that encode for resistance to NNRTIs are different from those that encode for resistance to N(t)RTIs. Doravirine (DOR), efavirenz (EFV), etravirine (ETR), nevirapine (NVP), and rilpivirine (RPV) make up the clinically relevant, FDA-approved NNRTIs.

PROTEASE INHIBITORS

PIs act when a nearly mature virion is budding from the surface of the infected host cell. These compounds bind HIV-1 protease, preventing it from cleaving the gag precursor polyproteins, an essential process for HIV core maturation. Thus, the viruses that bud from the cell have immature cores, rendering them defective and unable to infect further host cells. First-line PI regimens that include a pharmacologically boosted PI characteristically are associated with no to very low rates of treatment-emergent drug resistance at the time of virologic failure. While there are nine currently FDA-approved PIs, only two, atazanavir (ATV) and darunavir (DRV), are nine currently FDA-approved PIs, only two, atazanavir (ATV) and darunavir (DRV), are recommended in the DHHS guidelines (DHHS, 2022) in certain clinical situations. The remaining seven, saquinavir (SQV), ritonavir (RTV), indinavir (IDV), ritonavir-boosted lopinavir (LPV/r), nelfinavir (NFV), fosamprenavir (FPV), and tipranavir (TPV), are no longer recommended in the DHHS guidelines.

INTEGRASE STRAND TRANSFER INHIBITORS

INSTIs inhibit the viral enzyme integrase, which is responsible for inserting HIV proviral DNA into the host cell's DNA. There are five FDA-approved integrase inhibitors: bictegravir (BIC), cabotegravir (CAB), dolutegravir (DTG), elvitegravir (EVG), and raltegravir (RAL). Regimens that include an INSTI are associated with the most rapid viral load declines of all ARVs and greater $CD4^+$ T-cell increases compared to NNRTI- or PI-based regimens.

ENTRY INHIBITORS

HIV entry inhibitors are a diverse class with different mechanisms of action. Fostemsavir (FTR) is an attachment inhibitor that binds to the HIV envelope protein gp120 and prevents viral attachment to the CD4 cell surface receptor. Enfuvirtide (T-20), a fusion inhibitor, binds the HIV envelope protein gp41, preventing virus envelope–cell membrane fusion. Chemokine coreceptor antagonists act by binding to the CCR5 coreceptor, resulting in allosteric changes that prevent HIV gp120 binding and attachment. The only FDA-approved coreceptor antagonist is maraviroc (MVC), a CCR5 coreceptor antagonist, which requires testing for viral coreceptor tropism prior to utilization. Patients who harbor virus that partially or fully uses the alternative chemokine coreceptor, CXCR4, should not be prescribed maraviroc, because it will not antagonize this coreceptor. Ibalizumab (IBA), a monoclonal antibody characterized as a postattachment inhibitor, sterically inhibits post-CD4 receptor binding through attachment to domain 2 of the CD4 receptor of T cells.

KEY CHARACTERISTICS AND FINDINGS OF RECENT CLINICAL TRIALS OF US DHHS-RECOMMENDED REGIMENS

BICTEGRAVIR (BIC)- AND DOLUTEGRAVIR (DTG)-BASED REGIMENS

Bictegravir (BIC), an INSTI, is available only in a fixed-dose, single-tablet regimen with the NtRTI, tenofovir alafenamide, and NRTI emtricitabine. BIC/TAF/FTC is a regimen recommended by the DHHS for most PWH. BIC is generally well tolerated, and adverse drug reactions are uncommon. Characteristic adverse effects are diarrhea, nausea, and headache.

BIC is dosed once daily and has no dietary requirements. As with all INSTIs, oral absorption of BIC is affected by divalent cations, resulting in a recommended dose separation between BIC and divalent cation (aluminum, magnesium, iron, and calcium)–containing products. Alternatively, iron- and calcium-containing supplements can be taken at the same time as BIC or DTG if administered with food. BIC and DTG cause reversible inhibition of renal tubular transporters, resulting in predictable, minimal decreased tubular excretion of creatinine. This has the effect of increasing serum creatinine levels without impairment of glomerular filtration. Increases were seen in clinical trials after 4 weeks, averaging 0.1 mg/dL (0.03–0.17), and remained stable through week 48.

Two phase 3 clinical trials evaluated BIC- and DTG-containing treatments (with either TAF/FTC or ABC/3TC) for initial therapy in adults. GS-380-1489 was a multicenter, randomized, double-blind noninferiority study comparing once-daily BIC/TAF/FTC versus DTG/ABC/3TC in 631 patients. The primary endpoint at week 48 demonstrated noninferiority between the two regimens with regard to viral suppression (< 50 copies/mL) (Gallant et al., 2017).

GS-380-1490 was a similarly designed multicenter, randomized, double-blind noninferiority study comparing once-daily BIC/TAF/FTC versus DTG ± TAF/FTC in 657 treatment-naive adults. Overall, the two regimens performed very similarly at week 48, demonstrating noninferiority between the two regimens with regard to viral suppression (< 50 copies/mL) (Sax et al., 2017). These studies suggest that BIC, dosed as part of a single-tablet regimen, is a potent treatment option for persons initiating ART.

No treatment-emergent resistance mutations resulted at the time of virologic failure with any of the three regimens studied in the two trials. BIC retains in vitro activity against some viral strains resistant to other INSTIs (namely RAL and EVG), although cross-resistance is possible in isolates harboring certain resistance associated mutations. The clinical efficacy of BIC for treatment of PWH who have InSTI-resistant HIV has not been studied.

DTG-BASED REGIMENS

DTG is an INSTI commercially available as a stand-alone product (Tivicay), a fixed-dose, three-drug regimen with the two NRTIs, ABC and 3TC, (Triumeq), a fixed-dose, two-drug regimen with 3TC (Dovato), and as a fixed-dose, two-drug combination with the NNRTI, RPV (Juluca). DTG + TDF/FTC or TAF/FTC, DTG/ABC/3TC, and DTG/3TC are DHHS-recommended preferred initial treatment regimens (the latter depending on certain patient characteristics to meet eligibility for treatment). DTG is generally well tolerated, and adverse drug reactions, though uncommon, include diarrhea, nausea, and headache.

DTG has multiple dosing recommendations in adults: once daily in INSTI-naive patients or in those who are INSTI-experienced without associated resistance substitutions, and twice daily in patients who are INSTI-experienced with resistance associated mutations or who are receiving concurrent cytochrome P450-3A4 inducers (e.g., carbamazepine or rifampin). DTG has no dietary requirements, but oral absorption of INSTIs is affected by divalent cations as previously described in the BIC section. In order to reduce the risk of ABC hypersensitivity reaction, DTG/ABC/3TC should be administered only to individuals who test negative for the HLA-B*5701 allele. DTG causes reversible inhibition of the renal tubular transporter, resulting in decreased tubular excretion of creatinine. This has the effect of increasing serum creatinine levels without impairment of glomerular filtration as previously discussed for BIC.

Six phase 3 clinical trials evaluated DTG-containing treatments (with either TDF/FTC, ABC/3TC or in a 2-drug combination with 3TC) for initial therapy in adults. The SINGLE study was a randomized, double-blinded, 144-week study that compared DTG + TDF/FTC to single-tablet regimen, EFV/TDF/FTC, in approximately 800 treatment-naive adults (Pappa et al., 2014; Walmsley et al., 2013). The primary end point demonstrated statistical superiority of DTG + TDF/FTC, with the difference driven by discontinuations because of EFV-related side effects rather than differing rates of viral suppression between on-treatment groups. The superiority of the DTG study arm was maintained through 144 weeks of follow-up.

SPRING-2 was a randomized, double-blinded study comparing DTG to twice-daily RAL, paired with either an NRTI backbone, ABC/3TC, or TDF/FTC, in approximately 800 treatment-naive patients (Raffi et al., 2013). Overall, the two study arms performed similarly, with approximately 3% discontinuation because of treatment-related adverse effects and rare treatment-emergent drug resistance (none in the DTG arm), demonstrating noninferiority between the two INSTIs.

FLAMINGO was an open-label clinical trial comparing DTG to DRV/r (again with TDF/FTC or ABC/3TC) in treatment-naive adults (Clotet et al., 2014; Molina et al., 2014). The 48- and 96-week results demonstrated the superiority of DTG to DRV/r. The difference between the two study arms was driven by a combination of more frequent virologic and tolerability discontinuations in the DRV/r arm. Changes in fasting lipids were lower among subjects in the DTG arm.

ARIA was the first fully powered all-women's phase 3 clinical trial comparing DTG/ABC/3TC to ritonavir-boosted atazanavir (ATV/r) + TDF/FTC in 499 women (Orrell et al., 2017). After 48 weeks, DTG/ABC/3TC met

a predetermined statistical noninferiority endpoint of viral suppression of less than 50 copies/mL compared to the ritonavir-boosted protease inhibitor arm. Fewer patients receiving DTG reported drug-related adverse effects than with ATV/r (83 (33%) vs. 121 (41%)). Additionally, fewer patients receiving the INSTI-based regimen experienced adverse effects that led to discontinuation (10 (4%) vs. 17 (7%)).

Challenging the dogma of requiring three medications from two classes for initial ART, the GEMINI-1 and 2 trials determined the efficacy of a two-drug regimen among treatment-naive patients. These two identically designed, multicenter, double-blinded, randomized, noninferiority, phase 3 trials evaluated efficacy and safety of a once-daily, two-drug regimen comprising of DTG/3TC compared to DTG + TDF/FTC in ART-naive patients (Cahn et al., 2019). At week 48, 90% and 93% of patients receiving the two-drug or three-drug regimen across GEMINI-1 and 2, respectively, reached the primary end point of an HIV-1 RNA less than 50 copies/mL per intention-to-treat analysis; per protocol results were 92% and 94%, and noninferiority was met compared to a three-drug regimen. No emergence of INSTI or NRTI resistance-conferring mutations were detected in any patient meeting virological withdrawal criteria (< 1% of participants overall) through week 96 (Cahn et al., 2020). Of note, inclusion criteria for these studies consisted of initial viral loads greater than 1,000 but less than 500,000 copies/mL and excluded patients coinfected with hepatitis B or with known antiretroviral resistance mutations.

TANGO was an open-label, multicenter, phase 3 study that evaluated the efficacy and safety of a switch to DTG/3TC in adults living with suppressed HIV-1 on a three- or four-drug TAF-based regimen (van Wyk et al., 2020). At week 48, only one participant in the DTG/3TC group (0.3%) and two participants in the TAF-based regimen group (0.5%) had HIV RNA ≥50 copies/mL, demonstrating noninferiority. Zero participants in the DTG/3TC group and one in the TAF-based regimen group met confirmed virologic withdrawal criteria. Post hoc analysis described that all seven participants (4/322 in the DTG/3TC group and 3/321 in the TAF-based regimen group) who had preexisting archived M184V/I mutations (all mixtures with wild-type) maintained an HIV-1 RNA< 50 copies/mL at all on-treatment time points through week 48. Of note, a higher proportion of adverse events resulting in study withdrawal occurred in patients receiving DTG/3TC (3.5% vs. 0.5% in TAF-group). Weight gain was reported more frequently in patients receiving TAF; however, adjusted mean weight increase was only 0.8 kg in both groups (p = 0.863). A statistically significant difference was seen in the DTG/3TC group versus the TAF-containing regimen group with respect to improved lipid parameters.

Treatment-emergent resistance to DTG in treatment-naive clinical trials is exceptionally rare, with only one case reported with no corresponding decrease in DTG susceptibility (ViiV Healthcare, Tivicay package insert, 2022b). Moreover, resistance to NRTI components to initial therapy has not been reported in phase 3 clinical trials. DTG retains activity against some viral strains showing in vitro resistance to raltegravir and elvitegravir, although cross-resistance is possible in isolates harboring resistance mutations at integrase gene codon 148 (in combination with at least two other integrase inhibitor-resistance mutations).

In prior years, concern for adverse perinatal outcomes with dolutegravir use was prominent. In 2018, an interim analysis of the Tsepamo surveillance trial of birth outcomes in Botswana was released after four cases of neural tube defects were seen in infants from HIV-positive mothers who had received DTG prior to and through conception and pregnancy (Zash et al., 2017). Follow-up data published in 2019 analyzing 119,033 deliveries reported that among the 1,683 deliveries in which the mother was taking dolutegravir-based ART at conception, five neural tube defects were found (0.30% of deliveries), versus 15 defects among 14,792 (0.10%) infants born to mothers taking any nondolutegravir ART at conception (Zash et al., 2019). Study investigators stated that although the prevalence of neural tube defects was three times higher with dolutegravir than with non-dolutegravir antiretrovirals, this represented only approximately two excess defects per 1,000 exposures. An updated analysis of birth data from March 2019 to April 2020 found that 39,200 additional births had occurred. It was reported that newborns of mothers who were on DTG at the time of conception were not significantly more likely to have neural tube defects (0.19%) compared to newborns of mothers taking non-DTG antiretrovirals (0.12%) (Zash et al., 2020). More recently at IAS 2021 an additional 39,188 births were reported between April 2020 to March of 2021. It was again reported that the incidence of neural tube defects in newborns of mothers exposed to DTG during conception versus those not exposed to DTG did not differ at 0.15% and 0.1%, respectively (Zash et al., 2021).

As of December 2021, the DHHS guidelines list dolutegravir as the preferred treatment option in individuals trying to conceive and those already pregnant. Ultimately, given the changing nature of these recommendations, providers are recommended to check current DHHS or WHO guidance when starting DTG in women of child-bearing age (DHHS, 2022).

CAB-BASED REGIMENS

In March 2020, two studies were published in the New England Journal of Medicine evaluating the use of combination injectable long-active CAB, an INSTI and RPV, a NNRTI (Cabenuva) after oral induction for initial treatment HIV-1 treatment (FLAIR) and maintenance of suppression (ATLAS). The common focus of these studies was to evaluate the use of a long-acting, injectable, two-drug ART regimen to improve the overall antiretroviral adverse effects profile, decrease the burden of daily oral regimens, and improve engagement with care.

FLAIR was a phase 3, randomized, open-label trial that enrolled 629 ART-naive PWH (Orkin, et al., 2020). All participants were given 20 weeks of daily oral induction therapy with DTG/ABC/3TC, and at 16 weeks (once HIV-1 RNA levels were less than 50 copies/mL), randomly assigned to continue oral therapy or switch to oral cabotegravir plus rilpivirine for 1 month, followed by monthly injections of the same agents. Sixty-three participants withdrew from the trial before randomization, and the remaining 566 were randomly assigned to the two treatment groups. At week 48, an HIV-1 RNA level of 50 copies/mL or higher was found in six participants (2.1%) in the long-acting therapy arm and in seven participants (2.5%) in the oral therapy arm, meeting noninferiority criteria. At 96 weeks, an HIV-1 RNA of ≥50 copies/mL was found in nine participants (3%) in the long-acting therapy arm and in nine participants (3%) in the oral therapy arm, again demonstrating noninferiority (Orkin et al., 2021). The most common side effect was injection-site reaction (86% of participants). Virologic failure was seen in four participants in the long-acting therapy arm with possible correlations to body mass index >30, integrase polymorphisms, and low drug concentrations. Despite the reported adverse reactions, satisfaction scores were higher in the in the long-acting-therapy group.

ATLAS was a randomized, multicenter, parallel-group, open-label trial of long-acting CAB and RPV switch therapy compared to current oral therapy in virologically suppressed (HIV RNA < 50 copies/mL) participants with HIV-1 infection (Swindells et al., 2020). Participants were randomly assigned to continue their current oral therapy or switch to the long-acting regimen dosed every 4 weeks. At week 48, an HIV-1 RNA < 50 copies/mL was found in 92.5% of participants in the long-acting arm and 95.5% in the oral therapy arm, meeting criteria for noninferiority. At 52 weeks, participants had the opportunity to continue on long-acting CAB and RPV monthly (long-acting arm), switch from oral ART to long-acting CAB and RPV (switch arm), or transition to ATLAS-2M (to compare different administration schedules of CAB and RPV). At 96 weeks, 100% in the long-acting arm (23/23) and 97% in the switch arm (28/29) achieved an HIV RNA of < 50 copies/mL (Swindells et al., 2022). Injection-site reactions occurred in 83% of participants in the long-acting-therapy group, causing study withdrawal for four participants (1%). At week 44, participants in the long-acting-therapy group reported greater treatment satisfaction. Per the HIV Treatment Satisfaction Questionnaire assessment, 97% of participants in the long-acting-therapy group selected the injectable regimen over the daily oral therapy as their preferred HIV treatment.

ATLAS-2M was a randomized, multicenter, open-label study evaluating long-acting CAB and RPV administered every 8 weeks versus every 4 weeks. The study randomly assigned 1,0451045 participants, 522 in the every-8-weeks arm and 523 in the every-4-weeks arm. At 48 weeks, 94% of patients in the every-8-weeks group achieved HIV RNA< 50 copies/mL compared to 93% in the every-4-weeks group in the intention-to-treat analysis (Overton et al., 2020). At 96 weeks, 91% and 90% of patients maintained HIV RNA< 50 copies/mL in the every-8-weeks group and every-4-weeks group, respectively (Jaeger et al., 2021). No new safety signals were identified, and toxicities were similar to the ATLAS study.

CAB and RPV intramuscular injections were approved by the US FDA for monthly use in 2021 and for every-2-months dosing in 2022.

OTHER RECENTLY FDA-APPROVED ANTIRETROVIRAL AGENTS

Fostemsavir (FTR, Rukobia) is the prodrug of temsavir, an HIV-1 attachment inhibitor that binds directly to the viral envelope glycoprotein 120 (gp120), affecting the conformational change required for attachment and entry of the virus into the CD4 cell. FTR is an attractive treatment option for participants known to have multidrug-resistant HIV-1 infection as it has no in vitro cross-resistance with other classes of antiretroviral drugs, contains a favorable drug–drug interaction profile, and can be used regardless of HIV-1 CCR5 coreceptor tropism. The BRIGHTE trial is an ongoing phase 3 trial that enrolled 371 adult patients with a known history of multidrug-resistant HIV-1 infection who had failure of their current antiretroviral regimen and had exhausted at least 4–6 classes of antiretrovirals (Kozal et al., 2020). Patients were assigned to two study arms: the first arm consisted of patients with at least one to two fully active antiretroviral agents and were randomly assigned to receive FTR versus placebo + failing regimen the first 8 days, to be followed with open-label FTR combined with optimized background therapy ((OBT); most commonly used agents were dolutegravir, darunavir, and tenofovir) on day 9. The second arm had no fully active antiretroviral agents and received open-label FTR (600 mg twice daily) and OBT from day 1. The primary end point was defined as change in log10 level of HIV-1 RNA from day 1 through day 8 and was demonstrated to be statistically significant in the FTR groups (0.79 log10 decline). At week 48, the percentage of patients with an HIV-1 RNA level of < 40 and < 200 copies/mL was 62% and 84%, respectively. At week 96, an increase in virologic suppression of 53% at week 24 to 60% was seen in patients with one to two fully active agents. In the second arm, with no active agents, the viral suppression rate remained 37% at week 24 and week 96 (Lataillade et al., 2020). Adverse events and complications were associated with advanced AIDS (7% discontinuation rate associated with infections) and other drug-related events such as nausea and diarrhea. Virologic failure was seen in 18% of participants in the randomized group versus 46% in nonrandomized group and was associated with gp120 amino acid substitutions.

WHAT'S ON THE HORIZON?

Inhibition of the HIV-1 capsid is a novel mechanism of action that is currently being evaluated to help treat PWH with multidrug resistance. If approved, lenacapavir (LEN) would be the first in this class. This medication has the ability to be given every 6 months as subcutaneous injections after a 2-week oral lead-in. The CAPELLA study evaluated patients who were maintained on a failing ART regimen (defined as HIV RNA ≥400 copies/mL) for at least 8 weeks with resistance to two ARVs in 3 of 4 classes of HIV medications (NRTI, NNRTI, PI, or INSTI). Seventy-two patients were included in this study, and the group was divided into

two cohorts. The first cohort included those with persistent viremia and a HIV RNA >400 copies/mL. The first group in this cohort received oral LEN (600 mg on day 1 and 2, and then 300 mg on day 8) in addition to their failing regimen for 14 days (*n* = 24). The second group in this cohort received placebo in addition to their OBT for 14 days (*n* = 12). By day 15 it was noted that 88% of those in the LEN group achieved a HIV RNA 0.5 log decrease compared to 17% in the placebo group. After the 14 days on initial therapy, the LEN group was switched to subcutaneous LEN administered every 6 months and the placebo group was initiated on oral LEN and subsequently switched to subcutaneous injections as well. Both groups continued on OBT. The second cohort consisted of patients who achieved a HIV RNA< 400 copies/mL during the screening period. Patients in this cohort received oral LEN and OBT for 14 days and then transitioned to subcutaneous LEN every 6 months. By week 26 it was noted that 81% and 83% achieved a HIV RNA< 50 copies/mL in cohorts 1 and 2, respectively. Common adverse events noted in this study include injection-site reactions and GI related toxicities (Segal-Maurer et al., 2022).

At the 2022 Conference on Retroviruses and Opportunistic Infections, a study evaluating LEN in treatment-naive PWH was presented. One hundred and eighty-two patients were randomly assigned to one of four groups: (1) subcutaneous LEN plus TAF/FTC for 28 weeks then subcutaneous LEN plus TAF; (2) subcutaneous LEN plus TAF/FTC for 28 weeks then subcutaneous LEN plus BIC; (3) oral LEN plus TAF/FTC, then subcutaneous LEN plus oral TAF; or (4) oral BIC/TAF/FTC for 52 weeks. At week 28, 94%, 92%, 94%, and 100% achieved HIV RNA< 50 copies/mL in each group, respectively. At 54 weeks, 90%, 85%, 85%, and 92% achieved HIV RNA< 50 copies/mL in each group, respectively (Gupta et al., 2022).

A new drug application for LEN was submitted to the FDA in June 2022 by Gilead Sciences for PWH with multidrug resistance with an FDA prescription drug user free action date of December 2022.

RECOMMENDED READING

Cahn P, Madero J, Arribas J, et al. Dolutegravir plus lamivudine versus dolutegravir plus tenofovir disoproxil fumarate and emtricitabine in antiretroviral-naive adults with HIV-1 infection (GEMINI-1 and GEMINI-2): week 48 results from two multicentre, double-blind, randomised, non-inferiority, phase 3 trials. *Lancet.* 2019;393:143–55.

Kozal M, Aberg, J, Pialoux G, et al. Fostemsavir in adults with multidrug-resistant HIV-1 infection. N *Engl J Med.* March 2020;382:1232–1243.

Orkin C, Gorgolas M, et al. Long-acting cabotegravir and rilpivirine after oral induction for HIV-1 infection. *N Engl J Med.* 2020;382:1124–1135.

Segal-Maurer S, DeJesus E, Stellbrink HJ, et al. Capsid inhibition with lenacapavir in multidrug-resistant HIV-1 infection. *N Engl J Med.* 2022;386(19):1793–1803.

Swindells S, Andrade-Villanueva J et al. Long-acting cabotegravir and rilpivirine for maintenance of HIV-1 suppression, *N Engl J Med.* 2020;382:1112–1123

Van Wyk J, Ajana F, Bishop F, et al. Efficacy and safety of switching to dolutegravir/lamivudine fixed-dose 2-drug regimen vs continuing a tenofovir alafenamide–based 3- or 4-drug regimen for maintenance of virologic suppression in adults living with human immunodeficiency virus type 1: phase 3, randomized, noninferiority TANGO study. CID. http://doi:10.1093/cid/ciz1243. Published online January 6, 2020. Accessed September 15, 2022.

Zash R, Holmes LB, Diseko M, et al. Update on neural tube defects with antiretroviral exposure in the Tsepamo study, Botswana. [Abstract PEBLB14]. 11th International AIDS Society Conference. July 2021. Virtual.

PHARMACOKINETICS, PHARMACODYNAMICS, AND PHARMACOGENOMICS

LEARNING OBJECTIVE(S)

- Describe the basic pharmacokinetic properties of classes of ARV agents. Explain the benefits and shortcomings of using ritonavir or cobicistat (COBI) for pharmacokinetic enhancement of PIs and/or INSTIs.

- Review the potential role for therapeutic drug monitoring (TDM) for ARV agents.

- Demonstrate how pharmacogenomics are applied in the clinical management of PWH.

KEY POINTS

- Pharmacokinetics and local drug exposure can differ significantly within anatomical sanctuary sites compared with the systemic compartment.

- High variability in interpatient ARV concentrations is common, which makes population ARV pharmacokinetics difficult to interpret.

- Suboptimal ARV concentrations can result in drug resistance and virologic failure.

- TDM can be considered in certain cases.

- Pharmacogenomic testing for the HLA-B*5701 haplotype reduces the risk of abacavir hypersensitivity reaction and is recommended prior to the initiation of abacavir-containing therapy.

INTRODUCTION

The science of *pharmacokinetics* studies the amount of drug in various compartments of the body and attempts to explain the effect that the body has on the drug through the assessment of multiple factors known as **ADME**: (1) **a**bsorption or bioavailability of the drug, (2) **d**istribution of the drug throughout body compartments, (3) **m**etabolism of the drug, and (4) **e**limination or excretion of the drug from the body. Clinical pharmacokinetics is the application of these pharmacokinetic principles to the therapeutic management of a drug in a patient with the goal of enhancing efficacy while minimizing toxicity.

In contrast, *pharmacodynamics* examines the relationship between the drug concentration and response or the impact that the drug has on the body, which may have both intended and unintended pharmacologic effects. It also attempts to describe how drugs may interact with each other and display synergistic/multiplying or antagonistic effects. An example is the combination of AZT and ganciclovir causing additive bone marrow toxicity resulting in neutropenia. The combination of AZT and D4T is antagonistic as both drugs compete for the same site of action on the viral reverse transcriptase target. Similarly, FTC and 3TC should not be used together as they are unlikely to have additive antiviral activity due to similar chemical structures (DHHS, 2022).

Finally, *pharmacogenomics* is the practice of using host or viral genetic variation to individualize therapeutic decisions.

PHARMACOKINETICS

ABSORPTION

Medication absorption highly depends on the route of administration. Oral formulations of ARV medications have varying degrees of bioavailability that affect a patient's serum ARV concentration. Currently, AZT and ibalizumab are available in an intravenous formulation; enfuvirtide is available for subcutaneous injection; and cabotegravir and rilpivirine are administered as intramuscular injections. Ibalizumab, a humanized monoclonal antibody, is an intravenous infusion given every 14 days for heavily treatment-experienced patients (Emu et al., 2017). Long-acting injectable formulations of RPV and CAB are approved for administration every 4 weeks or every 8 weeks. For the solid dosage forms, absorption first requires the dissolution of the tablet or capsule, allowing the drug to be absorbed through the gastrointestinal (GI) tract and then into the systemic circulation from which it will be distributed to its site of action.

Drug absorption is a function of ionization and aqueous solubility, which can be impacted by factors such as gastric pH, gastric mobility (emptying), absorptive capacity, biliary function, GI enzymes, splanchnic blood flow, CYP enzyme expression in the gut, and transporters, such as P-glycoprotein. Absorption can be further affected under different patient conditions, such as use of nasogastric or percutaneous endoscopic gastrostomy tubes (g-tube) for medication administration, or when liquid formulations of medications are required, such as for pediatric patients or patients who have difficulty swallowing solid dosage forms. Many ARVs are available in oral solutions or suspensions to facilitate administration in these circumstances. The bioavailability of many ARV medications can be significantly compromised by manipulation of the dosage form, such as crushing tablets or opening up the contents of capsules (Bastiaans et al., 2014). For example, administration of crushed LPV/r tablets significantly decreased the exposure of both components, with a decrease in area under the plasma drug concentration–time curve (AUC) of 45% and 47%, respectively, compared to swallowing the tablets whole (Best et al., 2011). Additionally, certain medications like bictegravir and rilpivirine are insoluble in water so crushing these medications to mix in water for administration via g-tube could compromise drug concentrations (Gilead Sciences, 2021; Janssen Pharmaceuticals, Edurant Package Insert, 2022).

Food can impact the bioavailability and rates of absorption for certain medications because food increases the pH in the stomach and delays gastric emptying to the small intestine, which serves as the site of absorption for many medications. For example, the exposure of RPV is 40% lower when taken on an empty stomach compared to a food of at least 533 kcals (Janssen Pharmaceuticals, Edurant Package Insert, 2022). The solubility of a drug and surface area for absorption can be affected by gastric bypass procedures, which may impact the absorption of ART (Smith et al., 2011). In addition, the AUC and trough concentrations of INSTIs can be significantly reduced when coadministered with polyvalent cation products such as iron and calcium supplements or antacids containing aluminum, magnesium, or calcium. INSTIs should be given at least 2 hours before polyvalent cations under fasting conditions or at the same time if administered with food (DHHS, 2022).

Some antiretrovirals require an acidic environment for solubility to occur, and acid-reducing agents may impact the dissolution of these drugs. ATV is a PI whose absorption is dependent on a highly acidic environment. Up to 40 mg by mouth twice daily of famotidine with boosted and unboosted ATV was found to decrease ATV AUC by approximately 20% (Wang et al., 2011). A pharmacokinetic study of boosted ATV and omeprazole 20 mg reported a 42% reduction in ATV AUC and a 46% reduction in ATV trough concentration (C_{trough}) compared with boosted ATV alone (Zhu et al., 2011). Increased gastric pH by acid-reducing agents such as proton pump inhibitors (PPIs) do not cause changes in absorption with other PIs such as darunavir/ritonavir (DHHS, 2022). Increased gastric pH will also decrease RPV absorption, leading to suboptimal concentrations. RPV 150 mg was given with omeprazole 20 mg to 16 HIV-negative patients which resulted in an AUC and C_{max} decrease of 40%. Based on this study, PPIs are contraindicated with RPV, and H_2 antagonists should be taken 12 hours before or 4 hours after RPV ingestion (Crauwels et al., 2008).

DISTRIBUTION

After ARVs are absorbed into the bloodstream, they distribute into the interstitial and intracellular fluids depending on the individual physiochemical properties (pK, molecular weight/size, and lipophilicity) of each drug (Minuesa et al., 2011). Many of the ARVs circulate in the bloodstream reversibly bound to plasma proteins. Albumin primarily binds acidic drugs, and α_1 acid glycoprotein primarily binds basic drugs. Only free, or unbound, drug is pharmacologically active, and the greater the free fraction of the drug, the better it distributes into tissues or compartments. A decrease in plasma protein binding may be seen in patients with cirrhosis or cancer (Morse et al., 2006). Unbound drug can enter cells or tissues primarily through carrier-mediated transport mechanisms,

although some drugs can pass through via transcellular diffusion (Griffin et al., 2011).

The individual distribution characteristics of ARV compounds are under extensive investigation because each ARV drug may differ in the ability to penetrate into "sanctuary sites" throughout the body. These are areas where HIV can undergo compartmentalized viral replication with the potential to select resistant viral mutations due to suboptimal ARV drug concentrations within these sites, such as the male and female genital tract and/or the CNS (Pomerantz, 2002; Tseng et al., 2014). Drug distribution to the male and female genital tracts is influenced by many factors, including hormonal changes, inflammation, concomitant sexually transmitted infections, and drug factors such as protein binding and lipophilicity (Trezzan & Kashuba, 2014). Consequently, understanding drug distribution in the genital tract is essential for selecting agents for pre-exposure prophylaxis.

METABOLISM

Many ARV drugs, including CCR5 inhibitors, AIs, NNRTIs, and PIs are metabolized by CYP enzymes, which are located in the smooth endoplasmic reticulum in cells throughout the body, primarily the liver and intestines. Inhibition of gut CYP3A4 enzymes leads to increased bioavailability of these agents, whereas inhibition of liver CYP3A4 metabolism results in delayed elimination and a prolonged elimination half-life. RTV, an early protease inhibitor, is a highly potent CYP3A4 inhibitor, and coadministration of a subtherapeutic dose (~100 mg) of ritonavir is sufficient to enhance (or "boost") the pharmacokinetic profile of all but one (NFV) of the currently licensed PIs (Larson et al., 2014). COBI, a similarly potent inhibitor of CYP3A enzymes, is approved by the FDA to provide pharmacokinetic enhancement to PIs such as ATV and DRV and the INSTI, EVG. Because of its selective inhibition of CYP3A enzymes, COBI has less potential for off-target drug interactions compared to RTV. Unlike RTV, COBI has no anti-HIV activity; it is also more soluble than RTV, facilitating the development of coformulated products (Larson et al., 2014; Shah et al., 2013).

Pharmacokinetic enhancement of PI and INSTI concentrations with RTV or COBI, although increasing the risk of interactions with other agents, has several benefits, including:

- Higher C_{trough} levels, reducing the risk of selection for drug-resistant viral quasispecies;

- Higher plasma levels throughout the day, minimizing or eliminating:
  - the need for food requirements,
  - the significance of interactions with other agents that induce the metabolism of PIs and INSTIs, and
  - the effects of interpatient variations in drug levels due to factors such as sex, smoking, alcohol consumption, or liver disease;
- Increased plasma half-life, resulting in reduced dosing frequency and pill burden; and

- Increased levels of "forgiveness" with missed or late doses, potentially delaying/preventing the development of viral mutations.

P-glycoprotein (P-gp) is a cellular protein pump involved in transporting molecules in and out of the cell. P-gp is found extensively in the intestine, and its action is important in drug exposure and bioavailability. PIs are known to be substrates for P-gp. Overexpression of P-gp by certain individuals may result in lower intracellular concentrations of some PIs and thus decreased overall drug exposure (Sankatsing et al., 2004). RTV is a potent inhibitor of P-gp, whereas COBI is a weak P-gp substrate and inhibitor that does not lead to clinically relevant interactions (Larson et al., 2014; Shah et al., 2013).

EXCRETION

ARVs are eliminated from the body either unchanged by the process of excretion or converted to metabolites that may be more readily excreted. The kidney is the most important organ for the elimination of drugs and their metabolites, whereas the liver is the principal organ responsible for drug metabolism and biliary excretion (Verbeeck & Musuamba, 2009). Renal and hepatic diseases are progressive illnesses that may occur as comorbidities in PWH. Chronic kidney disease is a condition marked by deteriorating kidney function and subsequent decreases in medication elimination. NRTIs are primarily eliminated via the kidney, with the exception of ABC. If there is a decrease in the glomerular filtration rate (GFR) in chronic kidney disease, it may be necessary to decrease the NRTI dose or increase the dosing frequency interval to prevent high systemic drug concentrations that may lead to adverse drug reactions.

It is important for the clinician to routinely check kidney function at least every 6 months (DHHS, 2022). The National Kidney Foundation Kidney Disease Outcomes Quality Initiative recommends the use of kidney function estimating equations of either Cockroft–Gault or the Modification of Diet in Renal Disease for the routine estimation of GFR. Note that most FDA medication package-insert dosage guidelines for renal impairment are based on only the Cockroft–Gault estimating equation. Guidelines for renal dosage adjustments of ARV agents are provided in all prescribing information in addition to DHHS guidelines (DHHS, 2022).

PHARMACODYNAMICS AND THERAPEUTIC DRUG MONITORING

The need to maintain adequate drug concentrations that are effective in controlling HIV replication and preventing resistance has resulted in considerable interest in the relationship between ARV drug exposure, virologic response, and drug-related toxicity. The ideal ARV dosing strategy ensures the highest probability of success at maintaining viral suppression with the lowest possible dose. This relationship can be examined through TDM. A retrospective study of 1,807 samples found that the majority of concentrations for ARVs are above the upper therapeutic threshold and could likely benefit from dose optimization using TDM (Cattaneo et al., 2014). Currently, the only ARV approved at the lowest efficacious dose was RPV, but postapproval dose reduction has been seen ARVs such as AZT, DDI, D4T, and EFV. Other medications shown to be efficacious but not yet approved at lower doses include LPV, ATV, DRV, and RAL (Crawford et al., 2012).

DTG has predictable pharmacokinetics, with minimal intersubject variability and a defined exposure-response relationship (Cottrell et al., 2013). Early studies showed that dolutegravir toxicities occurred at dosing ranges used for evaluation (Boffito et al., 2020). A study of 43 people over the age of 60 years living with HIV showed a significantly higher C_{min} of DTG compared to control with many PWH presenting with toxicities of DTG (Elliot et al., 2019). Despite this, the use of TDM, for routine ART management has not been standard of care in most situations because of a lack of several key elements, including large prospective studies showing improved outcomes, established therapeutic concentration ranges for ARV agents, and laboratories that reliably perform ARV concentrations. These factors, plus intrapatient variability in drug concentrations, challenge the use of ARV TDM in clinical practice (DHHS, 2022; Pretorius et al., 2011).

Nevertheless, TDM of ARVs could be considered for patients who may have compromised ADME or in populations where pharmacokinetic studies are limited. For example, absorption may be disrupted in patients with drug interactions or impairment of GI, hepatic, and renal function. TDM of ARVs may be beneficial in pregnant, pediatric, obese, or elderly patients (Cattaneo et al., 2020; DHHS, 2022). Metabolism may be affected in patients on concurrent CYP P450-interacting ARVs, and excretion may be compromised, leading to toxicities for patients with hepatic or renal impairment (Cattaneo et al., 2020; DHHS, 2022). For patients who are experiencing virologic rebound, adherence to their treatment regimen should be thoroughly evaluated prior to TDM as noncompliance is the most common cause for treatment failure.

PISS

All PIs are CYP3A4 substrates, and most are CYP3A inhibitors; thus, there is a risk of drug interactions with commonly used medications that may be substrates of, induce or inhibit the same CYP enzymes. The most common example of this type of interaction is the boosting effect of RTV or COBI on other PIs or the INSTI, EVG, but many medications used for comorbidities common in PWH also have CYP3A4-based interactions. In addition, boosting can potentiate toxicity of the target drug. A retrospective analysis of 240 PWH on boosted and unboosted ATV found a direct correlation between ATV plasma concentrations and the incidence and severity of hyperbilirubinemia, percentage increase in triglycerides, and incidence of nephrolithiasis. These toxicities and increased plasma concentrations were seen mostly in the boosted ATV group, and the study suggested that concentrations greater than 800 ng/mL were likely the cause (Gervasoni et al., 2015).

NNRTISS

Like PiIs, NNRTIs are substrates of the CYP3A4 enzyme; unlike PiIs, however, most NNRTIs are CYP3A4 inducers, not inhibitors, and thus NNRTIs are also at high risk for drug interactions. Whereas PiIs have a high genetic barrier to resistance, single-point mutations such as K103N or Y181C can cause complete virologic resistance to first-generation NNRTIs. Second-generation NNRTIs, such as ETR, RPV, and DOR, have a higher genetic barrier to resistance (Usach et al., 2013) and maintain activity against K103N virus. As one might expect, the risk of virologic failure with EFV-based ART was associated with low EFV plasma levels in one small study (Marzolini et al., 2001). In a larger study, however, trough levels and AUC_{24} of NVP and EFV were not significantly predictive of virologic failure, although for EFV there was an association between these parameters and virologic failure (Van Leth et al., 2006). An analysis of ETR from the DUET trials failed to show any relationship between ETR pharmacokinetics and efficacy or toxicities (Kakuda et al., 2010). These studies suggest that when reliably taken at prescribed doses, NNRTIs retain full activity, with resistance occurring more because of improper adherence than pharmacokinetic issues.

Given intramuscularly, long-acting RPV avoids first pass metabolism and the gastric pH concerns for oral rilpivirine absorption are not a concern. LAI RPV has been approved to be administered every 4 or 8 weeks. The elimination half-life of LAI RPV is found to be 13 to 28 weeks (ViiV Healthcare, 2022a).

EFV-induced CNS toxicities have been correlated with elevated plasma concentrations (Marzolini et al., 2001). Through the use of TDM and dose adjustment, elevated plasma EFV concentrations were reduced to the recommended therapeutic range while maintaining undetectable viral loads (Mello et al., 2011). Although subjects in this trial were stable on long-term EFV, a significant improvement in anxiety scores and a trend toward lower stress scores were noted with the reduction in concentrations. EFV 400 mg was also compared to the standard 600 mg dose, and it was found that the lower 400 mg dose was noninferior to the standard 600 mg dose for virologic suppression and was associated with fewer EFV-related adverse events (ENCORE1 Study Group, 2015). A fixed-dose combination tablet including EFV 400 mg is FDA-approved to help minimize toxicities (Mylan Laboratories, 2019).

INSTISS

RAL, DTG, CAB, and BIC are metabolized by UGT1A1, whereas EVG acts similarly to a PI as a substrate of CYP3A4 requiring pharmacokinetic enhancing, with the attendant potential for drug interactions. BIC is a minor substrate of CYP3A4, so coadministration of potent inducers of CYP3A, P-gp, or UGT1A1 should be avoided (ViiV Healthcare, 2022b).

A study that evaluated RAL 800 mg once daily compared to 400 mg twice daily, both given with FTC/TDF, in treatment-naive individuals found that although PWH in both groups had similar AUCs, a sixfold decrease was seen in C_{trough} in the 800 mg group (Rizk et al., 2012). Even with the decrease in C_{trough}, similar response rates were seen in both groups with a baseline viral load of 100,000 copies/mL or less. However, the once-daily dosing arm was statistically inferior to the standard twice-daily dosing arm in those persons with a baseline viral load of more than 100,000 copies/mL and a CD4 [+] T-cell count 200 mm³ or less (Eron et al., 2011).

A different study comparing RAL 1200 mg once daily to 400 mg twice daily both in combination with TDF/FTC in ART-naive PWH found that the once-daily option was noninferior to twice-daily dosing. RAL HD 600 mg tablets are available and FDA approved for a total 1,200 mg dosage taken orally once daily (Deeks, 2017). A final feature seen with INSTIs has been a rapid decline in HIV viral load after initiation. DTG 50 mg daily was shown to achieve a 2.5 log decrease in HIV RNA after 10 days of therapy (Lalezari et al., 2009), and similar results were seen with the use of EVG, which resulted in a greater than 1 log decrease in HIV RNA after once- and twice-daily dosing (DeJesus et al., 2006).

The advent of long-acting ARVs has created alternatives for patients who are no longer able to maintain daily oral medication adherence. Intramuscular CAB allows for extended interval dosing due to its pharmacokinetic profile. Pharmacokinetic studies have shown that detectable concentration of LAI CAB can been seen up to 18 months after last dosing of intramuscular CAB administration. A study of 177 participants also found that that the terminal half-life of 1.33 times longer in females than in males. Higher body mass indexes also showed a statistically significant increase in terminal half-life (Landovitz et al., 2020). This extended half-life and elimination, also known as the pharmacokinetic tail, has the potential to lead to toxicities, resistance, and drug interactions if medications are not discontinued and monitored appropriately.

CNS EFFECTIVENESS OF ARVSS

The CNS is reached by considerable blood flow, but two anatomical barriers, the blood–brain barrier and the blood–cerebrospinal fluid (CSF) barrier, prevent the free passage of drugs into the brain (Calcagno et al., 2014). The CNS HIV Antiretroviral Therapy Effects Research (CHARTER) study group developed the CNS penetration-effectiveness (CPE) ranking scheme of CNS effectiveness of ARVs based partly on the physiochemical properties of the drug, such as lipophilicity, protein binding, and efflux substrate, that affect penetration into the CNS (Letendre et al., 2008). Regimens with higher CPE scores were proposed to have greater effectiveness in controlling HIV replication in the CSF. However, the use of CPE rankings to affect the course and severity of HIV-associated neurocognitive disorder (HAND) has not been demonstrated consistently (Caniglia et al., 2014; Ellis et al., 2014; Mukerji et al., 2018; Santos et al., 2019).

PHARMACOGENOMICS

Pharmacogenomics refers to the concept of using information about genetic variation to identify the most effective or well-tolerated ARV medications for an individual patient. Pharmacogenomic applications can be broadly categorized into the following areas: (1) ARV susceptibility, (2) explaining pharmacokinetic or pharmacodynamic variability, and (3) predicting adverse drug reactions. An example of the first category is genotypic resistance testing, which uses viral, not host genetic markers to predict susceptibility to ARV medications and is recommended prior to the initiation of treatment and in response to treatment failure. An example of the third category is seen with efavirenz, which is associated with characteristic neuropsychological side effects correlating with plasma levels. Its metabolism is variable, with higher levels associated with genetic polymorphisms of cytochrome CYP2B6 (Rotger et al., 2007). In one clinical trial from Japan, individuals harboring the CYP2B6*6 or -*26 allele successfully maintained plasma efavirenz levels despite dose reduction (Gatanaga et al., 2007).

Perhaps the best example, however, of using pharmacogenomic biomarkers to predict adverse drug reactions is the association between the HLA-B*5701 allele and ABC hypersensitivity. Without genetic screening, approximately 5%–8% of individuals exposed to abacavir develop a hypersensitivity reaction (HSR), which can be fatal upon drug rechallenge. Genetic screening identified the HLA-B*5701 allele as a predictor of HSR; subsequently, the PREDICT study (Mallal et al., 2008) randomized 1,956 predominantly white individuals who were treated with ABC-containing ART. The use of HLA genetic screening dramatically reduced clinically suspected HSR from 7.8% to 3.4%. Skin patch test immunologically confirmed HSR was reduced from 2.7% to 0%. In a large, racially diverse group of North American patients, HLA-B*5701 screening resulted in 0.8% of individuals having clinically suspected HSR and no immunologically confirmed cases (Young et al., 2008). HLA-B*5701 allele screening is now recommended prior to the use of abacavir by multiple national treatment guidelines (DHHS, 2022).

SUMMARY

Understanding the basic principles of applied clinical pharmacokinetics, pharmacodynamics, and pharmacogenomics can help the clinician gain insight into contemporary HIV pharmacotherapy and improve therapeutic responses. This information can be used to improve ART for the individual patient by gaining a fundamental working knowledge of concepts that contribute to the occurrence of drug–drug interactions, adverse drug reactions, poor adherence, decreased efficacy, and the selection of viral resistance. These factors, alone or in combination, can lead to treatment failure of ART and subsequent progression of HIV disease.

ARV DOSING AND COFORMULATIONS

LEARNING OBJECTIVE(S)

- Describe food requirements, typical dosing, and modified dosing according to weight, renal and hepatic clearance for FDA-approved ARV therapies.

- Identify coformulations used in HIV therapy.

WHAT'S NEW?

LAI CABO and RPV are now approved for administration every 4 or 8 weeks.

KEY POINTS

- The selection of an ARV dose should take into consideration the drug concentration that inhibits viral replication and the concentration that causes toxicity.

- Current oral ARV agents are dosed either once or twice daily without need for exact 24- or 12-hour dosing.

- Multiple factors affect drug exposures, including renal and/or hepatic insufficiency, ARV food requirements, and drug interactions.

- Coformulated medications reduce pill burden and improve adherence to ART.

The selection of an appropriate ARV dosage is based on the amount of drug needed to inhibit viral replication and the ability to physiologically obtain these concentrations without causing significant toxicities. Ideally, the maximum concentration should not cause adverse events, and the minimum drug concentrations at the end of a dosing interval should be in excess of the target concentration needed to inhibit viral replication.

Many ARV agents are metabolized by the liver and/or eliminated by the kidney; thus, changes in hepatic or renal function can cause drug accumulation. This increases the potential for adverse drug events and might necessitate dose changes. A single arm, open-label study by Eron and colleagues dosed EVG/COBI/TAF/FTC daily in patients with severe renal dysfunction (with estimated creatinine clearances < 15 mL/min) and in patients on intermittent hemodialysis; no significant adverse effects were seen (Eron et al., 2019). From these data, the FDA expanded dosing recommendations among several tablets that include these agents. However, in situations in which renal and/or hepatic impairment requires dosage modifications, the use of certain fixed-dose, single-tablet regimens (e.g., Atripla, Biktarvy, Complera, Delstrigo, Dovato, Genvoya, Odefsey, Stribild, and Triumeq) may not be possible; these situations may require the use of individual agents, when available, with the proper dosage adjustment for each agent. As of 2022, there are 23 coformulations licensed for use in HIV therapy in the United States (Table 17.1).

Counseling patients on optimal dosing and adherence is critical to the success of ART. Evidence-based guidelines for

Table 17.1 FDA-APPROVED COMBINATION ARV FORMULATIONS

TRADE NAME	COMPONENTS	CLASSES	DOSE
Combivir (1997)	AZT (300 mg) 3TC (150 mg)	2 NRTIs	1 tablet po daily
Trizivir (2000)	AZT (300 mg) 3TC (150 mg) ABC (300 mg)	3 NRTIs	1 tablet po BID
Kaletra (2000)	LPV (200 mg) RTV (50 mg)	2 PIs	2 tablets po BID For treatment-naive patients only: 4 tablets po daily
Truvada (2004)	FTC (200 mg) TDF (300 mg)	1 NRTI ± 1 NtRTI	1 tablet po daily
Epzicom (2004)	ABC (600 mg) 3TC (300 mg)	2 NRTI	1 tablet po daily
Atripla (2006)	FTC (200 mg) TDF (300 mg) EFV (600 mg)	1 NRTI ± 1 NtRTI ± 1 NNRTI	1 tablet po daily
Complera (2011)	FTC (200 mg) TDF (300 mg) RPV (25 mg)	1 NRTI ± 1 NtRTI ± 1 NNRTI	1 tablet po daily
Stribild (2012)	EVG (150 mg) COBI (150 mg) FTC (200 mg) TDF (300 mg)	1 NRTI ± 1 NtRTI ± 1 INSTI ± 1 PK booster	1 tablet po daily
Triumeq (2014)	ABC (600 mg) 3TC (300 mg) DTG (50 mg)	2 NRTI ± 1 INSTI	1 tablet po daily
Prezcobix (2015)	DRV (800 mg) COBI (150 mg)	1 PI ± 1 PK booster	1 tablet po daily
Evotaz (2015)	ATV (300 mg) COBI (150 mg)	1 PI ± 1 PK booster	1 tablet po daily
Genvoya (2015)	EVG (150 mg) COBI (150mg) FTC (200 mg) TAF (25 mg)	1 NRTI ± 1 NtRTI ± 1 INSTI ± 1 PK booster	1 tablet po daily
Dutrebis (2015)[a]	3TC (150 mg) RAL (300 mg)	1 NRTI ± 1 INSTI	1 tablet po BID
Odefsey (2016)	RPV (25 mg) TAF (25 mg) FTC (200 mg)	1 NRTI ± 1 NtRTI ± 1 NNRTI	1 tablet po daily
Descovy (2016)	TAF (25 mg) FTC (200 mg)	1 NRTI ± 1 NtRTI	1 tablet po daily
Juluca (2017)	RPV (25 mg) DTG (50 mg)	1 NNRTI ± 1 INSTI	1 tablet po daily
Biktarvy (2018)	TAF (25 mg) FTC (200 mg) BIC (50 mg)	1 NtRTI ± 1 NRTI ± 1 INSTI	1 tablet po daily
Cimduo (2018)	TDF (300 mg) 3TC (300 mg)	1 NtRTI ± 1 NRTI	1 tablet po daily
Symfi (2018)	TDF (300 mg) 3TC (300 mg) EFV (600 mg)	1 NtRTI ± 1 NRTI ± 1 NNRTI	1 tablet po daily

Table 17.1 CONTINUED

TRADE NAME	COMPONENTS	CLASSES	DOSE
Symfi Lo (2018)	TDF (300 mg) 3TC (300 mg) EFV (400 mg)	1 NtRTI ± 1 NRTI ± 1 NNRTI	1 tablet po daily
Symtuza (2018)	TAF (10 mg) FTC (200 mg) DRV (800 mg) COBI (150 mg)	1 NtRTI ± 1 NRTI ± 1 PI ± 1 PK booster	1 tablet po daily
Delstrigo (2018)	DOR (100 mg) TDF (300 mg) 3TC (300 mg)	1 NtRTI ± 1 NRTI ± 1 NNRTI	1 tablet po daily
Dovato (2019)	3TC (300 mg) DTG (50 mg)	1 NRTI ± 1 INSTI	1 tablet po daily
Cabenuva (2021)	<u>Every month:</u> Initial injection at month 1: CAB (600 mg) RPV (900 mg) Monthly maintenance injection starting at month 2: CAB (400 mg) RPV (600 mg) <u>Every 2 months:</u> Initial injection at month 1: CAB (600 mg) RPV (900 mg) Every 2 month maintenance injection starting at month 2: CAB (600 mg) RPV (900 mg)	1 NNRTI + 1 INSTI	CAB (600 mg) = 3 mL IM injection RPV (900 mg) = 3 mL IM injection CAB (400 mg) = 2 mL IM injection RPV (600 mg) = 2 mL IM injection

[a] Though FDA-approved, not commercially available in the United States.

ABC, abacavir; ARV, antiretroviral; ATV, atazanavir; AZT, zidovudine; BIC, bictegravir; BID, twice daily; CAB, cabotegravir; COBI, cobicistat; DOR, Doravirine; DRV, darunavir; DTG, dolutegravir; EFV, efavirenz; EVG, elvitegravir; FTC, emtricitabine; INSTI, integrase strand transfer inhibitor; LPV, lopinavir; NRTI, nucleoside reverse transcriptase inhibitor; NNRTI, nonnucleoside reverse transcriptase inhibitor; NtRTI, nucleotide reverse transcriptase inhibitor; PI, protease inhibitor; PK, pharmacokinetic; PO, oral; RAL, raltegravir; RPV, rilpivirine; RTV, ritonavir; 3TC, lamivudine; TAF, tenofovir alafenamide; TDF, tenofovir disoproxil fumarate.

improving adherence are available and include recommendations for the routine collection of self-reported adherence data and the use of pharmacy refill data adherence monitoring (International Advisory Panel on HIV Care Continuum Optimization, 2015). Nearly all ARV medications currently prescribed are dosed either once or twice daily. Note that this does not imply, nor require, that patients take their medications exactly every 24 or 12 hours; rather, they may aim to take their medications within a more generous time window.

Many ARV medications should be taken with food for optimal absorption. Some medications require an acidic stomach environment and may have negative drug interactions with acid-lowering agents such as PPIs (e.g., ATV and RPV). Others require dietary fat for optimal absorption (e.g., RPV). Counseling and patient adherence to dietary restrictions are important elements for optimal response to ART.

The adult and adolescent DHHS guidelines list the standard dose, food requirements, and dosage adjustments in renal and/or hepatic impairment for the FDA-approved ARVs (DHHS, 2022).

Coformulated ARV medications have been used for the treatment of HIV since 1997. The rationale for coformulation is to decrease pill burden, thereby facilitating treatment adherence while decreasing risk of selective nonadherence or supply chain gaps. A meta-analysis comparing STRs to multi-tablet ARV regimens (MTRs) concluded that STRs were associated with statistically significantly higher adherence compared to patients on MTRs of any frequency (odds ratio (OR) 2.37; 95% confidence interval (CI): 1.68–3.35; $p < 0.001$; four studies), twice-daily MTR (OR 2.53; 95% CI: 1.13–5.66; $p = 0.02$; two studies), and once-daily MTR (OR 1.81; 95% CI: 1.15–2.84; $p = 0.01$; two studies) (Clay, 2015). The relative risk (RR) for 48-week viral load suppression was improved with

STRs (RR 1.09; 95% CI: 1.04–1.15; p = 0.0003; three studies), whereas RR of grade 3 to 4 laboratory abnormalities was lower among patients on STRs (RR 0.68; 95% CI: 0.49–0.94; p = 0.02; two studies).

RECOMMENDED READING

Cattaneo D, Baldelli S, Cozzi V, Clementi E, Marriott DJE, Gervasoni C. Impact of therapeutic drug monitoring of antiretroviral drugs in routine clinical management of people living with HIV: a narrative review. *Ther Drug Monit.* 2020;42(1):64–74. http//:doi.10.1097/FTD.0000000000000684

Clay PG, Nag S, Graham CM, et al. Meta-analysis of studies comparing single and multi-tablet fixed dose combination HIV treatment regimens. *Medicine.* 2015;94(42):e1677.

CLINICAL TRIALS DESIGN AND ACCESS PROGRAMS

LEARNING OBJECTIVE

Describe the differences between phase 1, 2, 3, and 4 research clinical trials and expanded-access programs.

KEY POINTS

- Phase 1 studies are the earliest clinical trials, focusing mainly on safety and pharmacokinetics.

- Phase 2 studies further evaluate safety and begin to evaluate efficacy and dosing. Dose selection is done in early phase 2.

- Phase 3 studies focus on safety and efficacy in the target population.

- Phase 4 studies, sometimes referred to as *postmarketing trials*, occur after FDA approval and study the use of the drug in different patient populations and long-term safety.

- Expanded-access programs make a drug available to patients who are in particular need prior to the drug being available commercially. These programs are generally not established until after phase 3 studies have been fully enrolled.

PHASES OF CLINICAL TRIALS

In general, there are four phases to drug development, which are guided by procedures described in the US Code of Federal Regulations 21 CFR 314.126 (FDA, 2017):

- Phase 1 is the most preliminary clinical work in small numbers of human subjects and helps to determine safety/toxicity (FDA, 2017). Phase 1 studies usually start as single-dose studies and then progress to multiple-dose studies, mainly using healthy volunteers. They evaluate

a range of aspects, such as pharmacokinetics (including drug bioavailability), dosing interval, food effects, tolerability, and toxicity in order to define the maximum tolerated dose, sentinel adverse effects, and target organ toxicity.

- Phase 2 studies further evaluate toxicity and the effectiveness of the drug for a particular indication in a larger number of patients who have the disease or condition under study, and they potentially establish dosage (FDA, 2017). This is usually the initial assessment of activity or proof-of-concept study. It includes several doses and a short course of monotherapy or functional monotherapy. It may include randomized dosing and control or may be dose escalating. Phase 2 studies also collect data on pharmacokinetics, dose response, tolerability, and toxicity. In HIV, these studies are usually divided into phase 2a and phase 2b. Phase 2a trials are generally conducted in a small number of HIV-infected patients and usually are of short duration. Phase 2b trials usually involve longer term dosing, are almost always in combination with other agents, and have a control arm. Longer term tolerability, toxicity, and effectiveness are important outcomes.

- Phase 3 studies are primarily geared toward large cohort efficacy and, along with the accumulated weight of safety and toxicity studies, form the basis for submission to and approval by the FDA (FDA, 2017). Phase 3 studies are typically large, randomized studies that provide the core information for submission and regulatory approval. They frequently include blinded therapy. For ARVs, the end point for the most part has traditionally been some measurement of HIV-1 RNA response.

- Phase 4 studies are postmarketing or postapproval trials and may be mandated by the FDA to further determine long-term toxicities or may serve as vehicles for expanded indications or dosing changes (FDA, 2018a).

Expanded-access programs are often created for patients in particular need, to make a drug available before it is licensed. These programs are an outgrowth of the expedited review process for HIV drugs and are usually limited in the number of patients enrolled and the duration of availability. Typically, expanded-access programs are established after phase 3 studies have been fully enrolled and before drug approval. They are subject to FDA oversight (FDA, 2022), although considerably less so than are registrational trials. Because of the number of treatment options available today, expanded-access programs are much less common than in the past.

MECHANISMS FOR EXPANDED ACCESS

There are three general approaches to expanded access, whether it be for an individual patient, intermediate-size patient population, or widespread use (FDA 2018).

INDIVIDUAL PATIENT

For an emergency investigational new drug (E-IND) or protocol, a physician, on behalf of the patient, contacts the FDA and/or pharmaceutical manufacturer. In this type of emergency situation, a telephonic or electronic request/authorization may be used given the time-sensitive nature of the request and will either be submitted as a new IND or under the existing IND by the sponsor (manufacturer) as the situation allows. In such extreme emergency cases, institutional board (IRB) approval may not have been able to be acquired; however, this is expected to be reported to an IRB within 5 working days (FDA, 2018b).

INTERMEDIATE-SIZED PATIENT POPULATION

Access for use by more than one patient (but fewer patients than would otherwise be part of a normal IND, would be submitted as either a new IND or as a protocol addendum to the existing IND as the situation allows). Both FDA and IRB approval is required before treatment may begin. A request of this type may be submitted for an already approved medication or related product that would not otherwise normally be available because of extenuating circumstances (e.g., alternative manufacturers of products owing to drug shortages).

WIDESPREAD USE

Access for expanded/emergency widespread use must be submitted under either a new IND, or as a protocol addendum to the existing IND as the situation allows. The protocol must be approved by the FDA with a subsequent 30-day waiting period before treatment can begin, unless the FDA decides that treatment should begin at an earlier time.

RECOMMENDED READING

Food and Drug Administration, US (FDA). Expanded access. https://www.fda.gov/news-events/public-health-focus/expanded-access. Published 2022. Accessed August 15, 2022.

REFERENCES

Bastiaans DET, Cressey TR, Vromans H, Burger DM. The role of formulation on the pharmacokinetics of antiretroviral drugs. *Expert Opin Drug Metab Toxicol.* 2014;10(7):1019–1037. http://doi:10.1517/17425255.2014.925879

Best BM, Capparelli EV, Diep H, et al. Pharmacokinetics of lopinavir/ritonavir crushed versus whole tablets in children. *J AIDS.* 2011;58(4):385–391. doi:10.1097/ QAI.0b013e318232b057

Boffito M, Waters L, Cahn P, et al. Perspectives on the barrier to resistance for dolutegravir + lamivudine, a two-drug antiretroviral therapy for HIV-1infection. *AIDS Res Human Retroviruses.* 2020;36(1):13–18. http://doi:10.1089/AID.2019.0171

Cahn P, Madero J, Arribas J, et al. Dolutegravir plus lamivudine versus dolutegravir plus tenofovir disoproxil fumarate and emtricitabine in antiretroviral-naive adults with HIV-1 infection (GEMINI-1 and GEMINI-2): week 48 results from two multicentre, double-blind, randomised, non-inferiority, phase 3 trials. *Lancet.* 2019; 393: 143–155.

Cahn P, Madero JS, Arribas JR, et al. Durable efficacy of dolutegravir plus lamivudine in antiretroviral treatment-naive Adults with HIV-1 infection: 96-week results from the GEMINI-1 AND GEMINI-2 randomized clinical trials. *J Acquir Immune Defic Syndr.* 2020;83(3):310–318. http://doi:10.1097/QAI.0000000000002275

Calcagno A, Di Perri G, Bonora S. Pharmacokinetics and pharmacodynamics of antiretrovirals in the central nervous system. *Clin Pharmacokinet.* 2014;53(10):891–906. http://doi:10.1007/s40262-014-0171-0

Caniglia EC, Cain LE, Justice A, et al. Antiretroviral penetration into the CNS and incidence of AIDS-defining neurologic conditions. *Neurology.* 2014;83(2):134–141. http://doi:10.1212/WNL.0000000000000564

Cattaneo D, Baldelli S, Castoldi S, et al. Is it time to revise antiretrovirals dosing? A pharmacokinetic viewpoint. *AIDS.* 2014;28(16):2477–2479. http://doi:10.1097/qad.0000000000000440

Cattaneo D, Baldelli S, Cozzi V, Clementi E, Marriott DJE, Gervasoni C. Impact of therapeutic drug monitoring of antiretroviral drugs in routine clinical management of people living with HIV: a narrative review. *Ther Drug Monit.* 2020;42(1):64–74. http://doi:10.1097/FTD.0000000000000684

Clay PG, Nag S, Graham CM, Narayanan S. Meta-analysis of studies comparing single and multi-tablet fixed dose combination HIV treatment regimens. *Medicine (Baltimore).* 2015;94(42):e1677. http://doi:10.1097/MD.0000000000001677

Clotet B, Feinberg J, van Lunzen J, et al.; The ING114915 Study Team. Once-daily dolutegravir versus darunavir plus ritonavir in antiretroviral-naive adults with HIV-1 infection (FLAMINGO): 48-week results from the randomised open-label phase 3b study. *Lancet.* June 28, 2014;383(9936):2222–2231. [Erratum in: *Lancet.* June 27, 2015;385(9987):2576].

Cottrell ML, Hadzic T, Kashuba ADM. Clinical pharmacokinetic, pharmacodynamic, and drug interaction profile of the integrase inhibitor dolutegravir. *Clin Pharmacokinet.* 2013;52(11):981–994. http://doi:10.1007/s40262-013-0093-2

Crauwels HM, van Heeswijk RP, Kestens D, et al. The pharmacokinetic interaction between omeprazole and TMC 278, an investigational NNRTI. [Abstract P239]. Presented at the 9th International Congress on Drug Therapy in HIV Infection. Glasgow, Scotland; November 2008.

Crawford KW, Ripin DHB, Levin AD, et al. Optimising the manufacture, formulation, and dose of antiretroviral drugs for more cost-effective delivery in resource-limited settings: a consensus statement. *Lancet Infect Dis.* 2012;12(7):550–560. http://doi:10.1016/S1473-3099(12)70134-2

Deeks ED. Raltegravir once-daily tablet: a review in HIV-1 infection. *Drugs.* 2017;77(16):1789–1795. http://doi:10.1007/s40265-017-0827-9

DeJesus E, Berger D, Markowitz M, et al. Antiviral activity, pharmacokinetics, and dose response of the HIV-1 integrase inhibitor GS-9137 (JTK-303) in treatment-naive and treatment-experienced patients. *J Acquir Immune Defic Syndr.* 2006;43(1):1–5. http://doi doi:10.1097/01.qai.0000233308.82860.2f

Department of Health and Human Services (DHHS), Panel on Antiretroviral Guidelines for Adults and Adolescents. Guidelines for the use of antiretroviral agents in adults and adolescents. https://clinicalinfo.hiv.gov/en/guidelines/adult-and-adolescent-arv/whats-new-guidelines. Published 2022. Accessed August 12, 2022.

Elliot ER, Wang X, Singh S, et al. Increased dolutegravir peak concentrations in people living with human immunodeficiency virus aged 60 and over, and analysis of sleep quality and cognition. *Clin Infect Dis.* 2019;68(1):87–95. http://doi:10.1093/cid/ciy426

Ellis RJ, Letendre S, Vaida F, et al. Randomized trial of central nervous system-targeted antiretrovirals for HIV-associated neurocognitive disorder. *Clin Infect Dis.* 2014;58(7):1015–1022. http://doi:10.1093/cid/cit921

Emu B, Fessel WJ, Schrader S, et al. Forty-eight-week safety and efficacy on-treatment analysis of ibalizumab in patients with multi-drug resistant HIV-1. *Open Forum Infect Dis.* 2017;4(Suppl 1):S38–S39. http://doi:10.1093/ofid/ofx162.093

Eron JJ, Lelievre JD, Kalayjian R, et al. Safety of elvitegravir, cobicistat, emtricitabine, and tenofovir alafenamide in HIV-1-infected adults with end-stage renal disease on chronic haemodialysis: an open-label, single-arm, multicenter, phase 3b trial. *Lancet HIV.* 2019;6(1):e15–e24. http://doi:10.1016/S2352-3018(18)30296-0

Eron JJ, Rockstroh JK, Reynes J, et al. Raltegravir once daily or twice daily in previously untreated patients with HIV-1: a randomised, active-controlled, phase 3 non-inferiority trial. *Lancet Infect Dis.* 2011;11(12):907–915. http://doi:10.1016/S1473-3099(11)70196-7

Food and Drug Administration (FDA). FDA's drug review process. https://www.fda.gov/drugs/information-consumers-and-patients-drugs/fdas-drug-review-process-ensuring-drugs-are-safe-and-effective. Published 2017. Accessed September 15, 2022.

FDA. FDA post-market drug safety monitoring. https://www.fda.gov/patients/drug-development-process/step-5-fda-post-market-drug-safety-monitoring. Published 2018a. Accessed September 15, 2022.

FDA. Expanded access categories for drugs (including biologics). https://www.fda.gov/news-events/expanded-access/expanded-access-categories-drugs-including-biologics. Published 2018b. Accessed September 15, 2022.

FDA. Expanded access | information for physicians. https://www.fda.gov/news-events/expanded-access/expanded-access-information-physicians. Published 2022. Accessed September 15, 2022.

Gallant J, Lazzarin A, Mills A, et al. Bictegravir, emtricitabine, and tenofovir alafenamide versus dolutegravir, abacavir, and lamivudine for initial treatment of HIV-1 infection (GS-US-380–1489): A double-blind, multicenter, phase 3, randomized controlled noninferiority trial. *Lancet.* 2017;390(10107):2063–2072.

Gatanaga H, Hayashida T, Tsuchiya K, et al. Successful efavirenz dose reduction in HIV type 1-infected individuals with cytochrome P450 2B6*6 and *26. *Clin Infect Dis.* 2007;45(9):1230–1237. http://doi:10.1086/522175

Gervasoni C, Meraviglia P, Minisci D, et al. Metabolic and kidney disorders correlate with high atazanavir concentrations in HIV-infected patients: is it time to revise atazanavir dosage? *PLoS One.* 2015;10(4):1–12. http://doi:10.1371/journal.pone.0123670

Gilead Sciences. Biktarvy package insert. https://www.gilead.com/~/media/files/pdfs/medicines/hiv/biktarvy/biktarvy_pi.pdf, Published October 2021. Accessed September 15, 2022.

Griffin L, Annaert P, Brouwer KL. Influence of drug transport proteins on the pharmacokinetics and drug interactions of HIV protease inhibitors. *J Pharm Sci.* 2011;100(9):3636–3654. http://doi:10.1002/jps.22655

Gupta S, Sims J, Brinson C, et al. Leapai as part of a combination regimen in treatment naive PWH: week 54 results. [Abstract # 138]. Presented at the 29th Conference on Retroviruses and Opportunistic Infections. Virtual; February 2022.

INSIGHT START Study Group. Initiation of antiretroviral therapy in early asymptomatic HIV Infection. *N Engl J Med.* 2015;373(9):795–807. http://doi:10.1056/NEJMoa1506816.

International Advisory Panel on HIV Care Continuum Optimization. IAPAC guidelines for optimizing the HIV care continuum for adults and adolescents. *J Int Assoc Provide AIDS Care.* 2015;14(Suppl. 1):S3–S34. http://doi:10.1177/2325957415613442

Jaeger H, Overton ET, Richmond G, et al. Long-acting cabotegravir and rilpivirine dosed every 2 months in adults with HIV-1 infection (ATLAS-2M), 96-week results: a randomized, multicentre, open-label, phase 3b, non-inferiority study. *Lancet HIV.* 2021;8(11):e679–e689.

Janssen Therapeutics. Endurant package insert. https://janssenlabels.com/package-insert/product-monograph/prescribing-information/EDURANT-pi.pdf. Published March 2022.

Kakuda TN, Wade JR, Snoeck E, et al. Pharmacokinetics and pharmacodynamics of the non-nucleoside reverse-transcriptase inhibitor etravirine in treatment-experienced HIV-1-infected patients.

Clin Pharmacol Ther. 2010;88(5):695–703. http://doi:10.1038/clpt.2010.181

Kozal M, Aberg, J, Pialoux G, et al. Fostemsavir in adults with multidrug-resistant HIV-1 infection. *N Engl J Med.* March 2020;382:1232–1243.

Lalezari J, Sloan L, DeJesus E, et al. Potent antiviral activity of S/GSK1349572, a next generation integrase inhibitor (INI) in INI-naive HIV-1-infected patients: ING111521 protocol. [Abstract TUAB105]. Presented at the 5th Conference on HIV Pathogenesis, Treatment and Prevention. Cape Town, South Africa; July 19–22, 2009.

Landovitz RJ, Li S, Eron JJ, et al. Tail-phase safety, tolerability, and pharmacokinetics on long-acting injectable cabotegravir in HIV-uninfected adults: a secondary analysis of the HPTN 077 trial. *Lancet HIV.* 2020;7(7):e472–e481.

Larson KB, Wang K, Delille C, et al. Pharmacokinetic enhancers in HIV therapeutics. *Clin Pharmacokinet.* 2014;53(10):865–872. http://doi:10.1007/s40262-014-0167-9

Lataillade M, Lalezari JP, Kozal M, et al. Safety and efficacy of the HIV-1 attachment inhibitor prodrug fostemsavir in heavily treatment-experienced individuals: week 96 results of the phase 3 BRIGHTE study. *Lancet HIV.* 2020;7(11):e740–e751.

Letendre S, Marquie-Beck J, Capparelli E, et al. Validation of the CNS penetration-effectiveness rank for quantifying antiretroviral penetration into the central nervous system. *Arch Neurol.* 2008;65(1):65–70. http://doi:10.1001/archneurol.2007.31

Mallal S, Phillips E, Carosi G, et al. HLA-B*5701 screening for hypersensitivity to abacavir. *N Engl J Med.* 2008;358(6):568–579. http://doi:10.1056/NEJMoa0706135

Marzolini C, Telenti A, Decosterd LA, et al. Efavirenz plasma levels can predict treatment failure and central nervous system side effects in HIV-1-infected patients. *AIDS.* 2001;15(1):71–75. http://doi:10.1097/00002030-200101050-00011

Mello AF, Buclin T, Decosterd LA, et al. Successful efavirenz dose reduction guided by therapeutic drug monitoring. *Antivir Ther.* 2011;16(2):189–197. http://doi:10.3851/IMP1742

Minuesa G, Huber-Ruano I, Pastor-Anglada M, et al. Drug uptake transporters in antiretroviral therapy. *Pharmacol Ther.* 2011;132(3):268–279. http://doi:10.1016/j.pharmthera.2011.06.007

Molina JM, Clotet B, van Lunzen J, et al. Once-daily dolutegravir is superior to once-daily darunavir/ritonavir in treatment-naive HIV-1-positive individuals: 96-week results from FLAMINGO. *J Int AIDS Soc.* 2014;17(4 Suppl. 3):19490.

Morse GD, Catanzaro LM, Acosta EP. Clinical pharmacodynamics of HIV-1 protease inhibitors: use of inhibitory quotients to optimise pharmacotherapy. *Lancet Infect Dis.* 2006;6(4):215–225. http://doi:10.1016/S1473-3099(06)70436-4

Mukerji SS, Misra V, Lorenz DR, et al. Impact of antiretroviral regimens on cerebrospinal fluid viral escape in a prospective multicohort study of antiretroviral therapy-experienced human immunodeficiency virus-1-infected adults in the United States. *Clin Infect Dis.* 2018;67(8):1182–1190. http://doi:10.1093/cid/ciy267

Mylan Laboratories. Symfi Lo package insert. https://dailymed.nlm.nih.gov/dailymed/fda/fdaDrugXsl.cfm?setid=86aad85d-5460-4c38-9761-a225e6bce190&type=display. Published October 2019. Accessed September 19, 2022.

Orkin C, Keikawus A, Górgolas Hernández-Mora M, et al. Long-acting cabotegravir and rilpivirine after oral induction for HIV-1 infection. *N Engl J Med.* 2020;382:1124–1135.

Orkin C, Oka S, Philibert P, et al. Long-acting cabotegravir plus rilpivirine for treatment in adults with HIV-1 infection: 96-week results of the randomized, open-label, phase 3 FLAIR study. *Lancet HIV.* 2021;8(4):e185–e196.

Orrell C, Hagins DP, Belonosova E, et al. Fixed-dose combination dolutegravir, abacavir, and lamivudine versus ritonavir-boosted atazanavir plus tenofovir disoproxil fumarate and emtricitabine in previously untreated women with HIV-1 infection (ARIA): week 48 results from a randomized, open-label, noninferiority, phase 3b study. *Lancet HIV.* 2017;4(12):e536–e546.

Overton ET, Richmond G, Rizzardini G, et al. Long-acting cabotegravir and rilpivirine doses every 2 months in adults with HIV-1 infection (ATLAS-2M), 48-week results: a randomized, multicentre, open-label, phase 3b, non-inferiority study. *Lancet.* 2020;396(10267):1994–2005.

Pappa K, Baumgarten A, Felizarta F, et al. Dolutegravir (DTG) plus abacavir/lamivudine once daily superior to tenofovir/emtricitabine/efavirenz in treatment-naïve HIV subjects: 144-week results from SINGLE (ING114467). Paper presented at the Interscience Conference on Antimicrobial Agents and Chemotherapy (ICAAC), Washington, DC, 2014.

Pomerantz RJ. Reservoirs of human immunodeficiency virus type 1: the main obstacles to viral eradication. *Clin Infect Dis.* 2002;34(1):91–97. http://doi:10.1086/338256

Pretorius E, Klinker H, Rosenkranz B. The role of therapeutic drug monitoring in the management of patients with human immunodeficiency virus infection. *Ther Drug Monit.* 2011;33:265–274.

Raffi F, Jaeger H, Quiros-Roldan E, et al. Once-daily dolutegravir versus twice-daily raltegravir in antiretroviral-naive adults with HIV-1 infection (SPRING-2 study): 96-week results from a randomised, double-blind, noninferiority trial. *Lancet Infect Dis.* 2013;13(11):927–935.

Rizk ML, Hang Y, Luo WL, et al. Pharmacokinetics and pharmacodynamics of once-daily versus twice-daily raltegravir in treatment-naive HIV-infected patients. *Antimicrob Agents Chemother.* 2012;56(6):3101–3106. http://doi:10.1128/AAC.06417-11

Rotger M, Tegude H, Colombo S, et al. Predictive value of known and novel alleles of CYP2B6 for efavirenz plasma concentrations in HIV-infected individuals. *Clin Pharmacol Ther.* 2007;81(4):557–556. http://doi:10.1038/sj.clpt.6100072

Sankatsing SUC, Beijnen JH, Schinkel AH, et al. P glycoprotein in human immunodeficiency virus type 1 infection and therapy. *Antimicrob Agents Chemother.* 2004;48(4):1073–1081. http://doi:10.1128/aac.48.4.1073-1081.2004

Santos GMA, Locatelli I, Métral M, et al. Cross-sectional and cumulative longitudinal central nervous system penetration effectiveness scores are not associated with neurocognitive impairment in a well-treated aging human immunodeficiency virus-positive population in Switzerland. *Open Forum Infect Dis.* 2019;6(7):ofz277. https://doi.org/10.1093/ofid/ofz277

Sax PE, Pozniak A, Montes ML, et al. Coformulated bictegravir, emtricitabine, and tenofovir alafenamide versus dolutegravir with emtricitabine and tenofovir alafenamide, for initial treatment of HIV-1 infection (GS-US-380-1490): a randomized, double-blind, multicenter, phase 3, noninferiority trial. *Lancet.* 2017;390(10107):2073–2082

Segal-Maurer S, DeJesus E, Stellbrink HJ, et al. Capsid inhibition with lenacapavir in multidrug-resistant HIV-1 infection. *N Engl J Med.* 2022;386(19):1793–1803.

Shah BM, Schafer JJ, Priano J, Squires KE. Cobicistat: a new boost for the treatment of human immunodeficiency virus infection. *Pharmacotherapy.* 2013;33(10):1107–1116. http://doi:10.1002/phar.1237

Swindells S, Andrade-Villanueva J, Richmond GJ, et al. Long-acting cabotegravir and rilpivirine for maintenance of HIV-1 suppression. *N Engl J Med.* 2020;382(12):1112–1123. http://doi:10.1056/NEJMoa1904398

Swindells S, Lutz T, Van Zyl L, et al. Week 96 extension results of a Phase 3 study evaluating long-acting cabotegravir with rilpivirine for HIV-1 treatment. *AIDS.* 2022;36(2):185–194.

TEMPRANO ANRS 12136 Study Group. A trial of early antiretrovirals and isoniazid preventive therapy in Africa. *N Engl J Med.* 2015;373(9):808–822. http://doi:10.1056/NEJMoa1507198

Trezza CR, Kashuba AD. Pharmacokinetics of antiretrovirals in genital secretions and anatomic sites of HIV transmission: implications for HIV prevention. *Clin Pharmacokinet.* 2014;5(7)3:611–624. http://doi:10.1007/s40262-014-0148-z

Tseng A, Seet J, Phillips EJ. The evolution of three decades of antiretroviral therapy: challenges, triumphs and the promise of the future. *Br J Clin Pharmacol.* 2014;79(2):182–194. http://doi:10.1111/bcp.12403

Usach I, Melis V, Peris JE. Non-nucleoside reverse transcriptase inhibitors: a review on pharmacokinetics, pharmacodynamics, safety and tolerability. *J Int AIDS Soc.* 2013;16(1):1–14. http://doi:10.7448/IAS.16.1.18567

Van Leth F, Kappelhoff BS, Johnson D, et al. Pharmacokinetic parameters of nevirapine and efavirenz in relation to antiretroviral efficacy. *AIDS Res Hum Retroviruses.* 2006;22(3):232–239. http://doi:10.1089/aid.2006.22.232

van Wyk J, Ajana F, Bisshop F, et al. Efficacy and safety of switching to dolutegravir/lamivudine fixed-dose two-drug regimen versus continuing a tenofovir alafenamide-based three- or four-drug regimen for maintenance of virologic suppression in adults with HIV-1: phase 3, randomized, non-inferiority TANGO study. 2020;7(18):1920–1929. doi:10.1093/cid/ciz1243.

Verbeeck RK, Musuamba FT. Pharmacokinetics and dosage adjustment in patients with renal dysfunction. *Eur J Clin Pharmacol.* 2009;65(8):757–773. http://doi:10.1007/s00228-009-0678-8

ViiV Healthcare. Cabenuva package insert. https://viivhcmedinfo.com/search-medical-scientific-information/viiv-document-viewer?cmd=GSKMedicalInformation&token=23108-862a5aad-0610-40a2-95ac-0ef4073ff7be&dns=gsk-medcomms.veevavault.com&medcommid=REF--US-000964&product=Cabotegravir+and+Rilpivirine. Published March 2022a. Accessed September 15, 2022.

ViiV Healthcare. Tivicay package insert. https://viivhcmedinfo.com/search-medical-scientific-information/viiv-document-viewer?cmd=GSKMedicalInformation&token=23108-e1c4ef40-9430-4b30-b541-5fe2e93f53bd&dns=gsk-medcomms.veevavault.com&medcommid=REF--US-000284&product=Dolutegravir. Published June 2020b. Accessed September 15, 2022.

Walmsley SL, Antela A, Clumeck N, et al. Dolutegravir plus abacavir–lamivudine for the treatment of HIV-1 infection. *N Engl J Med.* 2013;369(19):1807–1818.

Young B, Squires K, Patel P, et al. First large, multicenter, open-label study utilizing HLA-B*5701 screening for abacavir hypersensitivity in North America. *AIDS.* 2008;22(13):1673–1681. http://doi:10.1097/QAD.0b013e32830719aa

Zash R, Holmes L, Diseko M, et al. Neural-tube defects and antiretroviral treatment regimens in Botswana. *N Engl J Med.* 2019;381:827–840.

Zash R, Holmes LB, Diseko M, et al. Updates on neural tube defects with antiretroviral exposure in the Tsepamo study, Botswana. [Abstract PEBLB14]. Presented at the 11th International AIDS Society Conference. July 2021. Virtual.

Zash R, Holmes L, Diseko M, et al. Update on neural tube defects with antiretroviral exposure in the Tsepamo study, Botswana. [Abstract OAXLB0102]. Presented at the 23rd International AIDS Conference. July 2020. Virtual.

Zash R, Jacobson D, Mayondi, GDM, et al. Dolutegravir/tenofovir/emtricitabine (DTG/TDF/FTC) started in pregnancy is as safe as efavirenz/tenofovir/emtricitabine (EFV/TDF/FTC) in nationwide birth outcomes surveillance in Botswana. 9th IAS. Paris, France; 2017.

Zhu L, Persson A, Mahnke L, et al. Effect of low-dose omeprazole (20 mg daily) on the pharmacokinetics of multiple dose atazanavir with ritonavir in health subjects. *J Clin Pharmacol.* 2011;51(3):368–377. http://doi:10.1177/0091270010367651

18.

PRESCRIBING ANTIRETROVIRAL THERAPY

Poonam Mathur, Steven Mudroch, Saira Ajmal, Zelalem Temesgen, and David E. Koren

---

CHAPTER GOALS

Upon completion of this chapter, the reader should be able to:

- Enumerate the goals of antiretroviral treatment (ART) and rationale for treatment as soon as possible of all persons with HIV (PWH).

- List the US Department of Health and Human Services (DHHS) panel's recommended initial HIV treatments.

- Describe important criteria in selecting an initial treatment regimen.

- Identify when ART should be switched and how to do so.

OVERVIEW OF ART

WHAT'S NEW?

- DHHS guidelines recommend starting ART immediately or as soon as possible after the diagnosis of HIV is made.

- HIV integrase inhibitors are the standard of care for initial therapy. Additional recommendations for certain clinical situations exist, including protease inhibitor (PI)- or NNRTI-based and NRTI-sparing regimens.

- Bictegravir (BIC), dolutegravir (DTG), or boosted darunavir (DRV/r) paired with tenofovir/emtricitabine (TDF/FTC) can be used for rapid ART initiation before initial lab results are available.

- The DHHS ART Guidelines recommend that the DTG + lamivudine (3TC) fixed-dose two-drug regimen be used for initial treatment except for individuals with HIV RNA >500,000 copies/mL, HBV coinfection, or in whom ART is to be started before the results of HIV genotypic resistance testing or HBV testing are available. The US Food and Drug Administration (FDA) does not make these recommendations.

KEY POINTS

- Uncontrolled HIV replication is associated with inflammation, accelerated aging, and a higher rate of comorbid illnesses, effects which have been shown to be reduced by earlier initiation of ART.

- Studies demonstrate improved clinical outcomes with treatment initiation at CD4$^+$ T-cell counts greater than 500/mm^3, and treatment is now recommended for all PWH regardless of CD4$^+$ T-cell count.

- Treatment of HIV with ART is highly effective at preventing HIV-1 transmission.

- ART regimen selection considers what is best suited for the patient to ensure adherence and long-term durability with regard to medication tolerability and toxicities, resistance, and patient comorbidities.

INTRODUCTION

Great strides have been made in ART since the introduction of zidovudine in 1987 and combination therapy in 1996. ART has reduced both HIV-associated and non-HIV-associated morbidity and mortality, making HIV a chronic disease that can be managed with potent and simple medication regimens, affording PWH a low risk of AIDS-related complications, few, if any, significant side effects from medications, and near-normal life expectancy (Samji et al., 2013; ATCC, 2017). In addition, treatment with ART has been shown to reduce HIV transmission. However, in 2018 only 65% of PWH in the United States had suppressed viral loads (HIV.gov, 2021) because of undiagnosed infections or difficulty linking PWH to and retaining them in care. Of note, in 2020, the number of PWH receiving regular ART had dropped to 56.8%. This drop in ART is thought to be attributable to the decreased availability of ARVs, and closed or reduced clinic hours owing to COVID-19.

Paramount to the success of ART is the patient's willingness and commitment to adhere to long-term therapy. In the past, acute and long-term adverse effects associated with ART limited adherence to therapy, often leading to treatment failure. However, current combinations are associated with less toxicity, reduced pill burden, and improved potency, allowing many PWH to achieve greater than 95% adherence required for stable, long-term viral suppression. Most patients can start with a single-pill or a two- or three-drug regimen, which includes an integrase strand transfer inhibitor. For the first time, guidelines now recommend a long-acting, two-drug, combination antiretroviral regimen injected (IM) once every 4 or every 8 weeks for patients with stable viral suppression. Nevertheless, PWH continue to face several factors which can have a significant impact on ART success, including access to and the cost of long-term ART, particularly in resource-limited areas; drug interactions; comorbid medical conditions such as hepatitis B and C, tuberculosis, cardiovascular and renal disease, diabetes, osteoporosis or osteopenia, psychological disorders and chemical dependency, weight gain, and other social, economic, geographic, racial, and gender-identity factors that disproportionately impact PWH. Recognizing and addressing the individual barriers to adherence for each patient prior to ART initiation, as well as long-term, can have a dramatic effect on treatment outcomes.

As reviewed in the last chapter, there are 23 FDA-approved individual antiretroviral (ARV) drugs classified based on their mechanism of action, plus one nonantiretroviral pharmacokinetic booster. A panel of leading HIV specialists, convened by the DHHS, has been developing and updating recommendations for use of ARV agents in PWH since the early days of the ART era. These guidelines and those published by the International Antiviral Society-USA (IAS-USA) (Gandhi et. al, 2023) are similar and are periodically updated to reflect the release of new medications and HIV treatment in special populations. The guidelines also address patient readiness for therapy, barriers to adherence and comorbid conditions, as well as providing information on dosing and drug interactions. At the time of this writing, the most recent DHHS guidelines update released on September 21, 2022, included key updates to several sections, including changes in recommendations for initial regimens for the ARV-naive patient and special considerations for women with HIV (DHHS, 2022).

CURRENT TREATMENT GUIDELINES: WHEN TO START

Both DHHS and IAS-USA guidelines recommend starting ART immediately or as soon as possible after the diagnosis of HIV is made, with an intent to improve the uptake of ART and linkage to care, decrease the time to virologic suppression, and reduce HIV transmission (DHHS, 2022; Gandhi et al., 2023). This guidance has not changed since the last publication, and it reflects data from the START and TEMPRANO (2015) trials supporting treatment in all PWH regardless of CD4$^+$ T-cell count to reduce the morbidity and mortality associated with HIV infection (ATCC, 2017; Lundgren et al., 2015). START and HPTN-052 (first in 2011, again in 2020) also demonstrated the power of ART-driven viral suppression to prevent HIV transmission (Cohen et al., 2011, 2020), a phenomenon known as "treatment as prevention," or TasP. Specifically, initiation of ART promptly may prevent sexual or perinatal transmission, especially when viral loads are suppressed to < 200 copies/mL (to prevent sexual transmission) and < 50 copies/mL (to prevent perinatal transmission) (Bavinton et al., 2018; Cohen et al., 2016; Rodger et al., 2016; Townsend et al., 2008; Tubiana et al., 2010). Lastly, the completeness of CD4$^+$ T-cell count recovery is related to the CD4$^+$ T-cell count at the time of treatment initiation, supporting the notion that ART should be started as soon as possible and not deferred. Many individuals who start treatment with CD4$^+$ T-cell counts < 350 cells/mm^3 do not achieve CD4$^+$ T-cell counts >500 cells/mm^3 even after 10 years of

ART, and they have a shorter life expectancy than those who initiate ART at higher CD4$^+$ T-cell counts (Moore & Keruly, 2007; Palella et al., 2016; Samji et al., 2013).

In some cases, ART initiation may be deferred because of psychosocial factors, but these cases should be the exception, and ART should be started as soon as psychosocial factors have stabilized and the patient is ready for treatment. The following conditions should be considered urgent and discourage deferral treatment initiation: pregnancy; CD4$^+$ T-cell count < 200 cells/mm^3; malignancies (both AIDS- and non-AIDS-defining), and opportunistic infections and conditions such as HIV-associated dementia, HIV-associated nephropathy, HBV or HCV coinfection, and acute or early HIV infection. Drug–drug interactions should be considered for patients with malignancies when selecting ART (DHHS, 2022; Gandhi et al., 2022).

An exception to starting ART immediately in the setting of opportunistic infections applies to individuals with tuberculosis or cryptococcal meningitis. For patients with tuberculosis without meningitis, ART should be started within 2 weeks of initiation of tuberculosis treatment if the CD4$^+$ count is < 50 cells/mm^3, and within 8 weeks if the CD4$^+$ count is ≥50 cells/mm^3. The timing of ART initiation in cases of tuberculous meningitis remains controversial, but DHHS recommends withholding ART until completion of 8 weeks of tuberculosis treatment, although it acknowledges that some experts advise ART initiation with very close monitoring after just 2 weeks of tuberculosis treatment for patients with CD4$^+$ < 50 cells/mm^3 (DHHS, 2022; Gandhi et al., 2023). In cases of cryptococcal meningitis, ART initiation should be deferred for 4–6 weeks after starting anticryptococcal therapy (DHHS, 2022). In cases of cryptococcal meningitis, ART initiation should be deferred for 4-6 weeks after starting anti-cryptococcal therapy (DHHS, 2022). Whether for acute or chronic HIV infection, DHHS guidelines also recommend not waiting for resistance test results in newly diagnosed PWH as long as an antiretroviral agent with a high genetic barrier to resistance such as BIC, DTG, or DRV/r is chosen (DHHS 2022).

"Rapid ART" refers to initiation of ART as soon as possible (i.e., within 7 days) after HIV diagnosis. "Immediate ART" and "Same-day ART" refer to starting HIV treatment on the day of diagnosis or during the first clinic visit (DHHS, 2022). Rapid ART is supported by randomized clinical trials conducted in South Africa (Rosen et al., 2016), Haiti (Koenig et al., 2017), and Lesotho (Labhardt et al., 2018). Additionally, clinic-based observational cohort studies in San Francisco (Rapid ART Program for Individuals with an HIV Diagnosis, or RAPID), Atlanta (Rapid Entry and ART in Clinic for HIV, or REACH), and San Diego demonstrated a significant decrease in time to viral suppression and time to initial provider appointment with immediate ART initiation (Coffey et al., 2019; Colasanti et al., 2018; Hoenigl et al., 2016; Pilcher et al., 2017).

These studies provide evidence that same-day HIV diagnosis and ART initiation is feasible and may be beneficial, whether in a resource-rich setting with a multidisciplinary support system or in more resource-limited settings.

Additionally, since persons recently infected with HIV often have very high viral loads during the first several weeks and are therefore at increased risk of infecting other persons, coupling early diagnosis with rapid ART initiation has great potential to reduce HIV transmission. However, data from the CASCADE study in Lesotho (Labhardt et al., 2018) suggested that favorable virologic outcomes with same-day ART are not sustainable after 12 months (Amstutz et al., 2019), a finding that needs further exploration in both resource-limited and resource-rich settings. Other data show that same-day ART in resource-limited settings is challenging, as it requires adequate resources, including staffing, readily available drugs, no payer concerns, and attention to housing and food challenges (Coffey et al., 2019). Although there are no randomized clinical trials demonstrating the success of same-day ART in resource-limited settings, observational studies have shown decreased time to viral suppression and high rates of viral suppression at 1 year compared with standard of care (Coffey et al., 2019; Seybolt et al., 2020). It is unclear, however, if same-day ART leads to improvement in retention in care or sustainable viral suppression after 1 year (Amstutz et al., 2019; Cuzin et al., 2019).

Overall, implementing rapid ART has been shown to reduce barriers to care (Cosalanti et al., 2018). The combination of data showing both personal and public health benefits of universal ART treatment for PWH creates a powerful impetus to improve all facets of the HIV care continuum discussed in the chapter on HIV Epidemiology (i.e., to diagnose all PWH and assist them in linkage, engagement and retention in health care that provides fully suppressive ART and comprehensive care for HIV comorbidities). High ART potency and low pill and side-effect/toxicity burdens make this more feasible than ever before, even to the point of starting treatment at the time of diagnosis for many patients.

CURRENT TREATMENT GUIDELINES: WHAT TO START

SELECTION OF AN INITIAL ANTIRETROVIRAL REGIMEN

Currently, there are over 30 different ARV agents comprising different mechanisms of action aimed at providing maximal viral suppression when used in combination (DHHS 2022; Gandhi et al., 2023). The available classes of agents and pharmacokinetic (PK) enhancers were reviewed extensively in the preceding chapter. Regimens that do not require boosting are favored in order to reduce the potential for drug interactions (Gandhi et al., 2023). Since 1996, effective combination ART regimens have been defined as a three-drug combination consisting of two NRTIs (NRTI backbone) with an NNRTI, PI, or integrase strand transfer inhibitors (INSTI) or with or without an added PK enhancer. Such regimens have resulted in favorable virologic and immunologic outcomes in most patients in clinical trials, as well as in clinical practice, particularly as pill burdens and toxicities decreased over the years. Additional data now support the use of the two-drug regimen DTG/3TC for initial treatment of some PWH (Cahn et al., 2018, 2020, 2022).

Per the latest DHHS HIV treatment guidelines from January 2022, four regimens, all INSTI-based, are recommended as initial therapy for most PWH. These recommendations are based on efficacy and toxicity, as evidenced from published reports of randomized, prospective clinical trials of an adequate sample size and duration. Raltegravir (RAL)-based regimens, which had previously been one of the preferred regimens for initial therapy, are now relegated to the category of "Recommended Initial Regimens in Certain Clinical Situations" based on evidence of lower barrier to resistance compared to other INSTIs (BIC, DTG), and a higher pill burden.

The previous guidelines recommended against the use of DTG during the first trimester of pregnancy and in those of childbearing potential who are trying to conceive or who are sexually active and not using effective contraception, because of preliminary data from Botswana suggesting an increased risk of neural tube defects (0.9%) (Zash et al., 2018). Updated results now show that the prevalence of neural tube defects in neonates with maternal exposure to DTG is substantially lower than suggested by preliminary data (Raesima et al., 2019; Zash et al., 2020), and not statistically significantly different compared to that noted with maternal exposure to non-DTG regimens. The DHHS now considers DTG a recommended option for people of childbearing potential, with the provision that the risks and benefits should be discussed with patients, allowing them to make an informed decision.

The most novel change in the latest version of the DHHS guidelines is arguably the addition of the long-acting, injectable, antiretroviral combination of cabotegravir (CAB) and rilpivirine (RPV) for treatment of PWH who have already achieved 3–6 months of virologic suppression on an oral ART regimen. It should be noted that while the 28-day, oral lead-in of oral cabotegravir and oral rilpivirine is now optional (straight to injections), a PWH must first be virally suppressed to begin Cabenuva, and, therefore, this combination is not approved as initial therapy at the time of this writing.

In general, when selecting an ART regimen, providers must consider comorbid conditions, past and present resistance test results, patient readiness, and barriers to adherence, such as cost and convenience (e.g., pill burden and dosing frequency); pregnancy state or potential among women of childbearing age; and the potential for drug interactions. A summary of patient and regimen-specific factors to consider when selecting an ARV regimen is provided in Table 18.1, and the four DHHS-recommended initial HIV regimens are shown in Box 18.1.

Weight gain can occur after initiation of any ART regimen because of ART-induced reversal of HIV-associated inflammation, catabolism, and anorexia (Gandhi et al., 2023). Weight gain can lead to obesity in individuals that are of normal weight or overweight prior to initiation of ART, increasing the risk of comorbidities. There are several risk factors for excess weight gain with ART initiation, including low pretreatment CD4$^+$ T-cell count, high pretreatment viral load, Black race, and female sex (Bares et al., 2018; Bhagwat et al., 2018; Sax et al., 2019). Differences in risk of weight gain are also seen among the ART classes (Sax, 2019). INSTI-containing regimens

Table 18.1 FACTORS FOR CONSIDERATION IN ART REGIMEN SELECTION

PATIENT CHARACTERISTICS	COMORBIDITIES	REGIMEN-SPECIFIC CONSIDERATIONS
Pretreatment HIV RNA level	Cardiovascular disease, hyperlipidemia, renal disease, osteoporosis, psychiatric illness, neurologic disease, need for opioid replacement therapy	Regimen's genetic barrier to resistance
Pretreatment CD4 $^+$ T-cells	Pregnancy or pregnancy potential	Potential adverse effects of medications
HIV genotypic drug resistance	Coinfections: hepatitis C, hepatitis B, tuberculosis	Drug interactions
HLA-B*5701 status	Concern for excess weight gain	Convenience—pill burden, dosing frequency, availability of fixed-dose combination products, food requirement
PWH anticipated compliance to regimen	–	Cost
PWH preference	–	Timing of initiation

Adapted from Adult Panel on Antiretroviral Guidelines for Adults and Adolescents. Guidelines for the use of antiretroviral agents in adults and adolescents with HIV. DHHS.

https:// clinicalinfo.hiv.gov/en/guidelines-search?guideline%5B0%5D=title_bookpart%3AHIV%20Clinical%20Guidelines%3A%20Adult%20and%20 Adolescent%20ARV.

Box 18.1 RECOMMENDED INITIAL ART REGIMENS

INSTI-BASED REGIMENS (IN ALPHABETICAL ORDER)

Bictegravir/emtricitabine/tenofovir alafenamide[b] (A1)

Dolutegravir/abacavir/lamivudine (DTG/ABC/3TC)[a,b]—if HLA-B*5701 negative (A1)

Dolutegravir plus tenofovir/emtricitabine (DTG + TDF/FTC or TAF/FTC)[a,c] (A1)

Dolutegravir/lamivudine -if HIV RNA< 500,000 copies/mL, no HBV coinfection, and able to wait for HIV genotypic resistance and HBV testing results (A1)

[a] Lamivudine (3TC) may be interchanged with emtricitabine (FTC) or vice versa.

INSTI, integrase strand transfer inhibitors.

[b] Single-pill, once-daily regimen.

[c] Fixed-dose coformulated product for nucleoside backbone.

[d] TAF and TDF are two forms of tenofovir approved by the FDA. TAF is associated with better bone demineralization and kidney toxicity biomarkers than TDF, while TDF is associated with lower lipid levels and lack of weight gain. Safety, cost, and access are among the factors to consider when choosing between these drugs.

SOURCE: Adapted from Adult Panel on Antiretroviral Guidelines for Adults and Adolescents. Guidelines for the use of antiretroviral agents in adults and adolescents with HIV. DHHS. https://clinicalinfo.hiv.gov/en/guidelines-search?guideline%5B0%5D=title_bookp art%3AHIV%20Clinical%20Guidelines%3A%20Adult%20and%20Adolescent%20ARV.

---

induce greater weight gain than comparator regimens, such as seen with regimens that include dolutegravir or bictegravir, which are associated with greater weight gain than regimens that include efavirenz or protease inhibitors (Bhagwat et al., 2018; Kouanfack et al., 2019; Venter et al., 2019). DRV-based regimens have also been implicated with more weight gain than EFV-based regimens when either was combined with FTC and tenofovir alafenamide fumarate (TAF) (Ruderman et al., 2021). Among NRTIs, TAF-containing regimens are associated with greater weight gain than tenofovir disoproxil fumarate (TDF)- or abacavir (ABC)-containing regimens.

The mechanisms underlying increased weight gain for certain ART classes versus others are unclear. For example, it is unknown if the greater weight gain seen with INSTIs is due to a direct effect on appetite or metabolism or because there are fewer adverse effects with INSTIs (Gandhi et al., 2023). In addition, further analysis of the ADVANCE study (Venter et al., 2019) showed that the weight gain observed with DTG-versus EFV-based regimens was primarily dependent on CYP2B6 polymorphisms associated with slow EFV metabolism (and presumably, higher EFV levels). Among those with rapid EFV metabolism genotype, there was no weight gain difference between the participants treated with DTG and EFV (Griesel et al., 2021). A placebo-controlled study of PrEP (Mayer et al., 2020) showed that TDF inhibited weight gain, which may explain why TAF is associated with greater weight gain when compared to TDF. The distribution of weight gain is also different for women with HIV compared to men with HIV on ART, with women gaining more fat than lean body mass compared to men, and more weight concentrated in the limbs and trunk (Kerchberger et al., 2020; Lake et al., 2020; Venter, 2020). Currently, the IAS does not recommend that the potential for weight gain drive the initial ART regimen selection; however, it may be addressed later in the course of therapy. The DHHS suggests considering weight gain in women (particularly Black women) with HIV even when choosing the initial ART regimen. Regardless, prior to initiation of ART, PWH should be educated on diet, exercise, and behavior modifications that can mitigate weight gain associated with initiation of ART.

CHOOSING BETWEEN RECOMMENDED NRTI BACKBONES

The NRTI combinations of TDF or tenofovir alafenamide (TAF/FTC, TDF/3TC, or TDF/FTC) or ABC/3TC comprise the nucleoside backbones in recommended and alternative regimens, with the exception of the two-drug regimens DTG/3TC/, DTG/RPV, or CAB/RPV. All of these NRTI combinations are available as coformulated, fixed-dose tablets and as components of coformulated single-tablet regimens. Choosing between the NRTI pairs or single NRTI is directed mainly by differences between TDF, TAF, and ABC. TDF and TAF are oral prodrugs of tenofovir (TFV) and are available in several coformulated single-tablet regimen (STR) preparations and as a single medication. ABC is available both as an STR with DTG and 3TC in Triumeq (DTG/ABC/3TC), dual NRTI tablet (ABC/3TC), or as a single medication.

Studies comparing the efficacy of ABC/3TC to that of TDF/FTC as components of three-drug regimens have yielded conflicting results. ACTG 5202 compared the efficacy and safety of ABC/3TC to that of TDF/FTC when each was used in combination with either efavirenz (EFV) or ritonavir-boosted atazanavir (ATV/r); significant differences in virologic efficacy favoring TDF/FTC were noted in those with baseline HIV RNA level greater than 100,000 copies/mL, leading to unblinding of this cohort (Sax et al., 2009). The ASSERT study compared ABC/3TC to TDF/FTC, with each also receiving EFV. The proportion of participants with HIV RNA less than 50 copies/mL was lower among ABC/3TC-treated participants compared to those who received TDF/FTC (Post et al., 2010). In contrast to these two trials, other studies have documented virologic equivalence between ABC/3TC and TDF/FTC. The HEAT study compared ABC/3TC to TDF/FTC, each in combination with ritonavir-boosted lopinavir (LPV/r); there was no difference in virologic efficacy, including in patients with baseline HIV RNA greater than 100,000 copies/mL (Smith et al., 2009). Similarly, ABC/3TC has shown comparable virologic efficacy to TDF/FTC when used in combination with DTG (Walmsley et al., 2013).

There are also differences in the safety profile of these NRTI drugs for certain PWH. The serious and potentially fatal ABC hypersensitivity reaction (HSR) was reviewed in the preceding chapter, but the importance of testing patients for the HLA-B*5701 allele before starting therapy to predict the risk of the ABC HSR bears repeating, as individuals who test positive should not take ABC (ViiV Healthcare, 2013). ABC has also been associated with myocardial infarction (MI) in some but not in all observational studies (Dorje et al., 2017; Monforte et al., 2013; Palella et al., 2015; Sabin et al., 2014; Worm et al., 2010; Young et al., 2015) and is therefore sometimes avoided in patients with increased cardiac risk profiles.

TDF has been associated with renal impairment and reduced bone mineral density, which may be exacerbated when TDF is used in regimens containing PIs boosted with ritonavir or cobicistat or elvitegravir boosted with cobicistat (McComsey et al., 2011; Mocroft et al., 2015). TAF is an oral prodrug of tenofovir (TFV) that was designed to enhance the pharmacokinetics (absorption from the gut) and pharmacodynamics (intracellular concentration) to achieve higher active metabolite (TFV-DP) concentrations inside peripheral blood $CD4^+$ mononuclear cells; it may therefore be administered at lower doses than TDF with comparable antiviral efficacy but less renal and bone mineral biomarker-based adverse effects. The approval of TAF and the two TAF-containing regimens—EVG 150 mg/COBI 150 mg/FTC 200 mg/TAF 10 mg (EVG/c/TAF/FTC) and RPV 2 5mg/TAF 25 mg/FTC 200 mg (RPV/TAF/FTC)—was supported by 48-week data from two pivotal phase 3 studies. In the first, EVG/c/TAF/FTC was found to be noninferior to elvitegravir 150 mg/cobicistat 150 mg/FTC 200 mg/TDF 300 mg (EVG/c/TDF/FTC) among treatment-naive adult patients. The safety and efficacy of TAF/FTC were also demonstrated in one switch study of virologically suppressed patients randomly assigned to continue TDF/FTC or switch to TAF/FTC (Gallant et al., 2016; Pozniak et al., 2016). Bioequivalence studies (which compare drug levels between approved and investigational drug products in humans without clinical safety or efficacy assessed) also demonstrated that stand-alone TAF/FTC achieved the same drug levels of TFV-DP in target cells as with EVG/c/TDF/FTC. Similar studies also demonstrated that RPV/TAF/FTC achieved similar drug levels of FTC and TFV in the blood as with EVG/c/TAF/FTC, and similar drug levels of RPV as stand-alone RPV. It is important to note, that for RPV/TAF/FTC and TAF/FTC, head-to-head comparison to a non-RTV or COBI-boosted regimen in treatment-naive patients has not been accomplished as with EVG/c/TAF/FTC compared to EVG/c/TDF/FTC, which included rigorous clinical follow-up.

TAF/FTC is now included as a component of the first-line recommended "for most patients" coformulated with bictegravir and emtricitabine (BIC/TAF/FTC). Of note, a very similar two-tablet regimen of DTG + TAF/FTC is also recommended by both the DHHS and IAS-USA ART Guidelines Panel "for most patients," based upon a large, phase 3 study comparing the two regimens which demonstrated noninferiority of the two treatments (GS-US-380-1490) (Sax, et al., 2017). Two doses of TAF have been FDA-approved: 25 and 10 mg, the latter intended for use in combination with ritonavir or cobicistat because of the "boosting" effect that cobicistat has on tenofovir to lessen the risk for renal and bone demineralization toxicity. A recent meta-analysis of 14 clinical trials involving almost 15,000 PWH on ART, showed TAF to have greater treatment efficacy compared to TDF, but only when used in ART regimens containing pharmacokinetic (PK) boosters (ritonavir or cobicistat). This difference in overall treatment efficacy was noted to be attributable to increased proximal renal tubular toxicity related to elevated levels of TFV associated with dose-unadjusted TDF further increased by the boosting agent. Of note, there was no difference overall in bone-related or proximal renal toxicity between TAF- and TDF-containing regimens. Of note, there was no efficacy or toxicity difference seen between TAF- and TDF-containing, unboosted ART regimens (Pilkington et al., 2020). The DISCOVER trial, a randomized, double-blind, phase 3 trial that compared the efficacy and safety of FTC/TAF to FTC/TDF for the prevention of HIV infection was the largest clinical trial to directly compare the adverse effects of these 2 NRTI pairs in HIV-negative persons at-risk for HIV. There was no difference in the incidence of new HIV infections between the two groups. However, FTC + TAF was associated with less bone demineralization and renal biomarkers (hip bone mineral density; spine bone mineral density; urine β2-microglobulin to creatinine ratio; retinol-binding protein to creatinine ratio, distribution of urine protein to creatine ratio above the clinically significant threshold of 22.6 mg/mmol, and change in serum creatinine from baseline). Weight gain was significantly greater in the TAF versus the TDF group. However, there were no statistically significant differences between the two groups in serious adverse events or discontinuation because of adverse events, including renal and bone demineralization toxicities (Mayer et al., 2020).

CHOOSING BETWEEN THIRD DRUG OPTIONS

The choice of the third drug in an initial ARV regimen lies between an INSTI, NNRTI, or PI, and is based on consideration of the regimens' efficacy, genetic barrier to resistance, safety profile, convenience, comorbidities, and potential for drug interactions. Based on these considerations, the following observations have been noted (complementing and reinforcing data presented in the preceding chapter):

- The efficacy and safety of DTG-based regimens with either ABC/3TC or TDF/FTC have been evaluated in three clinical trials (SPRING-2, SINGLE, and FLAMINGO), where they were found to be noninferior or superior to other INSTI-, NNRTI-, or PI-based regimens. Thus, DTG/ABC/3TC and DTG + TDF/FTC are among recommended first-line ART regimens (Clotet et al., 2014; Raffi et al., 2013; Walmsley et al., 2013).

- The two-drug regimen of DTG/3TC has been added as a recommended initial regimen, based on 96-week data from the GEMINI-1 and GEMINI-2 trials showing that the efficacy of the two-drug regimen was similar to the three-drug regimen of DTG plus TDF/FTC (Cahn et al., 2020). Extended 144-week analyses of GEMINI-1

and GEMINI-2 has provided evidence or the durable efficacy and long-term tolerability of DTG + 3TC (Cahn et al., 2022).

- The efficacy and safety of RAL (with either TDF/FTC or ABC/3TC) have been evaluated in a number of clinical trials, in which it was shown to be superior to EFV-, ATV/r-, and DRV/r-based regimens and noninferior to DTG-based regimens (Lennox et al., 2009, 2014; Raffi et al., 2013). However, this INSTI is no longer recommended for most people with HIV because of the pill burden and lower barrier to resistance.

- The fixed-dose combination EVG/c/TDF/FTC was evaluated in two randomized clinical trials and found to be noninferior to EFV/TDF/FTC or ATV/r plus TDF/FTC (Rockstroh et al., 2013; Zolopa et al., 2013). Similar to RAL, EVG-based regimens have a lower barrier to resistance than DTG- or BIC-containing regimens. In addition, EVG-requires pharmacokinetic boosting with cobicistat (a strong cytochrome P 3A4 inhibitor) for clinical use and, thus, has a greater potential for drug interactions.

- BIC is available only as part of a single-tablet, once-daily regimen that includes TAF and FTC (BIC/TAF/FTC). The efficacy of BIC in ART-naive adults was compared to DTG plus two NRTIs in two large phase 3 randomized, double-blind clinical trials (Gallant et al., 2017; Sax et al., 2017). The proportion of participants with plasma HIV RNA less than 50 copies/mL at week 48 in the BIC arms was noninferior to that noted in the DTG arms in both trials (89% vs. 93% and 92.4% vs. 93%, respectively). Longer term follow-up of these two studies have confirmed these results.

- Clinical studies of DRV/r + TDF/FTC have shown it to be noninferior to RAL and superior to LPV/r. Compared to DTG-based regimens in the FLAMINGO study, DRV/r was inferior to DTG, with adverse events being the primary driver for this difference (Clotet et al., 2014).

- Previously, ATV/r + TDF/FTC was among the preferred first-line ARV regimens based on its virologic efficacy, which is equivalent to that of a number of comparator regimens, including EFV/TDF/FTC, EFV + ABC/3TC, LPV/r + TDF/FTC, and EVG/c/TDF/FTC. However, a more recent study, ACTG 5257, compared ATV/r with DRV/r or RAL, each in combination with TDF/FTC. On-treatment virologic efficacy was comparable among the three groups; however, more adverse events and treatment discontinuations were noted among patients on ATV/r compared to the other two groups (Lennox et al., 2015). Thus, ATV/r has been relegated to the "Recommended Initial Regimens in Certain Clinical Situations" category.

- Historically, EFV, particularly the STR EFV/TDF/FTC (Atripla), played a central role in the preferred first-line ARV regimen category. This was based on its demonstrated superiority or noninferiority to all the regimens against which it was compared. However, more recent studies have shown superiority of DTG, RAL, and RPV (the latter in patients with baseline HIV RNA< 100,000 copies/mL and CD4 $^+$ cell count >200 cells/mm^3) to EFV; these results were primarily driven by differences in adverse events. Concern regarding EFV-related adverse events was further enhanced by a possible association with suicidality observed in one analysis of four clinical trials (Mollan et al., 2014). Thus, EFV/TDF/FTC was also moved to the alternative "Recommended Initial Regimens in Certain Clinical Situations" category.

- The DRIVE-AHEAD and DRIVE-FORWARD randomized controlled trials showed noninferiority of doravirine (DOR) to both EFV and DRV/r when either of these drugs was taken with two NRTIs (Molina et al., 2018; Orkin et al., 2019). Advantages of DOR include CNS tolerability (vs. EFV), lipid effects (vs. DRV/r, EFV), and drug interactions (vs. EFV, RPV). In addition, in a cross-trial analysis, DOR was not associated with weight gain compared with EFV (600 mg) or boosted DRV (Orkin et al., 2021).

RECOMMENDED INITIAL REGIMENS IN CERTAIN CLINICAL SITUATIONS

The US DHHS guidelines provide an evidence-based menu for selecting an initial ART regimen, and most patients will be eligible for one of the five recommended initial regimens. However, it remains the responsibility of clinicians to select the regimen most suited to the clinical scenario at hand. Other ART regimens listed as alternatives in Tables 6 and 7 of the DHHS guidelines are effective but may have some potential disadvantages (e.g., pill burden, dosing, schedule, toxicity profile, and baseline HIV RNA levels or CD4 $^+$ T-cell count restrictions) compared to the preferred regimens, or they may have fewer supporting data from randomized clinical trials. Nevertheless, there may be situations in which these agents might be preferred for an individual patient. These alternative regimens are categorized as INSTI-, NNRTI-, and PI-based regimens and regimens when ABC, TAF, and TDF cannot be used. These regimens and clinical scenarios that might prompt their use are shown here in Tables 18.2, 18.3 and 18.4.

Table 18.2 ALTERNATIVE ART REGIMENS

INSTI-BASED REGIMENS	NNRTI-BASED REGIMENS	PI-BASED REGIMENS	WHEN ABC, TAF AND TDF CANNOT BE USED
Elvitegravir/cobisistat/tenofovir/emtricitabine (EVG/c/TDF/FTC or TAF/FTC)[d] (B1)	Efavirenz/tenofovir/emtricitabine (EFV/TDF/FTC)[b,c] (EFV 400 mg or 600 mg with TDF/3TC) (B1)	Cobicistat-boosted atazanavir (ATV/c) plus tenofovir/emtricitabine (TDF/FTC)[a,c]—only if pretreatment estimated CrCl ≥70 mL/min (B1)	DTG/3TC—if HIV RNA< 500,000 copies/mL, no HBV coinfection, and able to wait for HIV genotypic resistance testing for reverse transcriptase/HBV testing (A1)
Raltegravir/tenofovir/emtricitabine or lamivudine (RAL/TDF/FTC or 3TC) (B1) or (RAL/TAF/FTC (BII)	Rilpivirine/tenofovir/emtricitabine (RPV/TDF/FTC)[a,b]—if pretreatment HIV RNA< 100,000 copies/mL and CD4 $^+$ T-cell count >200 cells/mm^3 [(B1)]	Ritonavir-boosted atazanavir (ATV/r) plus tenofovir/emtricitabine (TDF/FTC)[a,c] (B1)	DRV/r plus RAL twice daily—if pretreatment HIV RNA< 100,000 copies/mL and CD4 $^+$ T-cell count >200 cells/mm (C1)
–	–	Cobicistat-boosted darunavir (DRV/c) or ritonavir-boosted Darunavir (DRV/r) plus abacavir/lamivudine (ABC/3TC)[a,c]—if HLA-B*5701 negative (BII)	DRV/r plus 3TC (C1)
–	–	Cobicistat-boosted darunavir (DRV/c) plus tenofovir/emtricitabine (TDF/FTC)[a,c (A1)]	–

INSTI, integrase strand inhibitors; NNRTI, nonnucleoside analogue reverse transcriptase inhibitors; PI, protease inhibitor.

[a] Lamivudine (3TC) may be interchanged with emtricitabine (FTC) or vice versa.

[b] Single-pill, once-daily regimen.

[c] Fixed-dose coformulated product for nucleoside backbone.

[d] TAF and TDF are two forms of tenofovir approved by the FDA. TAF has fewer bone and kidney toxicities than TDF, while TDF is associated with lower lipid levels. Safety, cost, and access are among the factors to consider when choosing between these drugs.

SOURCE: Adapted from Adult Panel on Antiretroviral Guidelines for Adults and Adolescents. Guidelines for the use of antiretroviral agents in adults and adolescents with HIV. DHHS. https://clinicalinfo.hiv.gov/sites/default/files/guidelines/documents/adult-adolescent-arv/guidelines-adult-adolescent-arv.pdf.

Table 18.3 BASELINE CONDITIONS

SCENARIO	RECOMMENDED ACTION
Low CD4$^+$ T-cell count (< 200 cells/mm^3)	Do not use RPV or DRV/r plus RAL
Pretreatment HIV RNA >100,000 copies/mL	Do not use RPV, ABC/3TC with EFV or ATV/r, or DRV/r plus RAL
Pretreatment HIV RNA >500,000 copies/mL	Do not use RPV based regimens, ABC/3TC with ATV/r, DRV/r plus RAL, or DTG/3TC
ARV to be started before HIV-drug-resistance results are available	Recommended regimens: BIC/TAF/FTC, DTG plus (TAF or TDF) plus (3TC or FTC), (DRV/r or DRV/c) plus (TAF or TDF) plus (3TC or FTC) Avoid ABC, NNTRI-based regimen, and DTG/3TC

Adapted from Adult Panel on Antiretroviral Guidelines for Adults and Adolescents. Guidelines for the use of antiretrovirals in adults and adolescents with HIV. DHHS. https://clinicalinfo.hiv.gov/en/guidelines-search?guideline%5B0%5D=title_bookpart%3AHIV%20Clinical%20Guidelines%3A%20Adult%20and%20Adolescent%20ARV.

WHEN TO SWITCH OR SIMPLIFY ANTIRETROVIRAL THERAPY

The approach to changing ARV regimen for PWH can initially be considered in one of two broad categories: when PWH have attained viral suppression with their current regimen and when PWH are experiencing virologic failure.

In considering those PWH with viral suppression, the main goal of switching therapy is to maintain control of HIV infection avoid virologic failure and jeopardize the availability of future treatment options. Because PWH must take antiretroviral medications for life, side effects and toxicities must be addressed to avoid metabolic complications and adherence problems that can lead to virologic failure. A complete review of the patient's treatment history, resistance testing, treatment tolerance, and drug interactions should be conducted prior to designing a new regimen. According to the IAS-USA and DHHS, the following are some reasons to consider changing therapy (DHHS, 2022; Gandhi et al., 2023):

1. Reduce pill burden or dosing frequency.

2. Reduce short- or long-term toxicity and enhance tolerability.

3. Changes in food or fluid requirements.

4. Minimize drug–drug or drug-food interactions.

5. Optimize ART regimen for pregnancy or in case of pregnancy.

6. Reduce costs.

7. Change route of administration to meet patient's health or lifestyle needs.

Table 18.4 CONCOMITANT MEDICAL CONDITIONS

SCENARIO	RECOMMENDED ACTION
Cardiac disease	Consider avoiding ABC, LPV/r, and DRV/r.
Chronic kidney disease	Avoid TDF with a PK enhancer, in particular: EVG/cobi/TDF/FTC ATV/cobi with TDF DRV/cobi with TDF Avoid ATV. TAF may be used if CrCL >30 mL/min or if on chronic hemodialysis[b] ABC may be used if HLA-B*5701 negative. Options when ABC, TAF, or TDF cannot be used: DTC/3TC, DRV/r + 3TC, DRV/r + RAL.
HIV-associated dementia	Avoid EFV because its psychiatric effects may cloud the clinical picture. Favor use of DRV- or DTG-based regimens because of the possibility of increased central nervous system penetration.
Osteoporosis/osteopenia	Avoid TDF.
Hyperlipidemia	EFV, ABC, PI/r or PI/cobi, and EVG/cobi have been associated with increases in lipids. TDF lowers lipids, therefore switching from TDF to TAF is associated with increased lipids.
Psychiatric illness	Consider avoiding EFV, which can exacerbate psychiatric symptoms and may be associated with suicidality.
HBV coinfection	Use TDF or TAF/FTC or 3TC. If TDF use is contraindicated, recommend use of FTC or 3TC with entecavir.
Tuberculosis	If rifampin is used, EFV/TDF/FTC is the recommended regimen; however, DTG 50 mg BID has been shown to be effective. If a PI/r-based ART regimen is used, rifabutin is the rifamycin of choice in the tuberculosis regimen but requires dose adjustment.
Gastroesophageal reflux disease requiring proton pump inhibitors	Avoid ATV or RPV.
Situations when neither tenofovir nor abacavir can be used	DTG/3TC (no HBV coinfection, no history of resistance, and HIV RNA< 500,000 copies/mL). DRV/r plus RAL (treatment naive). LPV/r plus 3TC (treatment naive). DTG/RPV or CAB/RPV (virally suppressed with no previous virologic failure).

[a] Lamivudine (3TC) may be interchanged with emtricitabine (FTC) or vice versa.

[b] only studied with EVG/cobi/TAF/FTC.

Adapted from Adult Panel on Antiretroviral Guidelines for Adults and Adolescents. Guidelines for the use of antiretroviral agents in adults and adolescents with HIV. DHHS. https://clinicalinfo.hiv.gov/en/guidelines-search?guideline%5B0%5D=title_bookpart%3AHIV%20Clinical%20Guidelines%3A%20Adult%20and%20Adolescent%20ARV.

With the advent of newer agents with improved toxicity profiles, easier dosing schedules, and fewer pills, providers are often confronted with the question of whether to change individual agents or whole regimens. Because many medications are being manufactured in single tablets, simply changing one agent may not be possible. Switching to a simplified, less adverse effect-laden regimen in PWH with an extensive treatment history remains complex. Although the optimal time for changing therapy remains undetermined, most studies have investigated changes in therapy for PWH who have been controlled on an ART regimen for at least 6 months, but in most cases, the study participants are tolerating their current ART regimens well.

In general, the two approaches to changing therapy in virally suppressed PWH are changing one agent to another within the same class or to a different class (DHHS, 2022). Within-class simplification can decrease toxicity, dosing frequency, and pill burden, especially when coformulated agents are used. One example of a within-class change is switching from TDF to TAF for decreased long-term chances of bone and/or proximal renal tubular adverse effects (Gallant et al., 2016). Similar to NRTIs, within-class simplification of NNRTIs can reduce toxicities and adverse side effects. For example, switching efavirenz to rilpivirine (Hagins et al., 2018) or doravirine (Johnson et al., 2019) demonstrated noninferior efficacy for maintaining virologic suppression for 96 weeks and 48 weeks, respectively, and both rilpivirine and doravirine have fewer neuropsychiatric adverse effects when compared to efavirenz as shown in previous studies (Orkin et al., 2019; van Lunzen et al., 2016).

The majority of studies investigating class switches have evaluated the replacement of a boosted PI with an alternative class, such as an NNRTI or INSTI. This can be done to reduce toxicity or drug interactions or to change to a simpler, once-daily coformulated combination. Although this is generally successful in PWH without resistance, it can lead to virologic failure in PWH with previous underlying resistance. This was seen in the cases of the SWITCHMRK 1 and 2 studies, where PWH randomly assigned to change from LPV/r to RAL had improved serum lipid concentrations but also had a higher virologic failure rate than those who remained on LPV/r, leading to premature study termination at 24 weeks (Eron et al., 2010). Therefore, DHHS recommends a careful review of the drug-resistance profile and consultation with a clinician who has expertise in HIV drug resistance before ART changes in persons with a history of treatment failure and drug resistance (DHHS, 2022).

Over the past decade, there has been growing evidence for the use of two-drug ARV therapy for treatment-experienced patients. Each component's side effects and drug–drug interactions need to be reviewed prior to switching therapy. Also of note, patients should have no prior evidence of resistance to either drug in the combination prior to switching. Some of the most thoroughly investigated two-drug regimens have included DTG/3TC, DTG/RPV, and 3TC with a boosted PI. Noninferiority of switching to DTG/3TC through 144 weeks was observed when compared to continuing a three- or four-drug TAF-containing regimen in the TANGO study

(van Wyk et al., 2020) and through 48 weeks when compared to continuation of a three- or four-drug ART regimen containing two NRTIs plus an INSTI, NNRTI, or PI-based regimen in the SALSA study (Llibre et al., 2022). This is similar for DTG/RPV in the SWORD-1 and SWORD-2 studies. Noninferiority was demonstrated at week 100, when 89% of the early-switch arm (start of study) and 93% of the late switch arm (week 52) had maintained < 50 HIV RNA copies per mL (Aboud et al., 2019). Lastly, several smaller studies have found combinations of 3TC with a boosted protease inhibitor to be noninferior to the same boosted PI with two NRTIs. One example is the SALT study (Perez-Molina et al., 2017), which compared virologically controlled patients, randomized to either receive ATV/r + 3TC or ATV/r + 2NRTIs and found similar virologic response with observed rates of VL< 50 copies/mL of 74% for both groups at 96 weeks.

Another two-drug ARV combination was studied and is now FDA-approved, long-acting, injectable HIV therapy, which has the potential to transform the way that HIV is managed as an outpatient in the near future. Two phase 3 trials evaluated long-acting formulations of both the INSTI cabotegravir (CAB) plus a long-acting formulation of the NNRTI rilpivirine (RPV), delivered as gluteal intramuscular injections every 4 weeks and every 8 weeks. Both of these studies enrolled PWH who had achieved viral suppression. Participants in the FLAIR Trial (Orkin et al., 2020) were ART-naive at baseline, and initially achieved viral suppression with 20 weeks of DTG/ABC/3TC prior to initiation of LA CAB/RPV. PWH in the ATLAS Trial (Swindells et al., 2020) were stably virally suppressed for at least 6 months on an oral ART regimen prior to starting LA CAB/RPV. Ultimately, both studies found long-acting, injectable CAB/RPV therapy to be noninferior to oral ARV therapy with regards to HIV viral suppression at 48 weeks when administered at 4-week intervals. Further, the ATLAS-2M trial (Overton et al., 2020) found that an 8-week dosing schedule was noninferior to the 4-week dosing regimen in terms of viral suppression and risk of virologic failure. Injection site reactions (including pain in 70% and nodules in 10%–20%) were the most common adverse event, occurring in 75%–86% of patients (Swindells et al., 2020; Orkin et al., 2020). Of these episodes, 99% were reported as mild to moderate, and only about 1% of participants withdrew from the studies because of injection site reactions (Orkin et al., 2020).

Prior to committing patients to long-acting therapy, clinicians should consider hurdles they may encounter with more frequent patient visits, and they should explore some of potential changes to clinic infrastructure and operations to ensure successful delivery of long-acting medications on a monthly or every other month basis. The CUSTOMIZE trial (Czarnogorski et al., 2021) looked at effective strategies implemented within different types of clinics across the United States, noting useful changes included extending clinic hours, ensuring available rooms, dedicating refrigerator space for storage, and implementing a reminder system for patients.

Switching ART regimen in a patient who is experiencing virologic failure requires a somewhat different approach than ART changes for PWH who are virologically suppressed.

In such cases, one of the primary goals is to design an ART regimen with sufficient active agents to achieve virologic control, with particular attention to prior resistance testing. In an update to the previously held standard that PWH experiencing virologic failure should be switched to a regimen including three active drugs, the DHHS guidelines now say that a new regimen should strive to use two fully active ARV drugs if at least one with a high resistance barrier is included, such as DTG and boosted DRV (DHHS, 2022). BIC is also suspected of having this property but has not yet been fully studied as such. If a regimen cannot be crafted which satisfies these criteria, a provider should attempt to create a regimen including three fully active drugs.

If regimen switching is prompted by virologic failure or suboptimal viral load reduction, HIV drug-resistance testing must be performed to guide selection of active ARV drugs. For PWH with virologic failure while on an INSTI, genotype testing specifically for INSTI resistance should be performed, in addition to the standard genotyping performed on the protease and reverse transcription regions of the genome. Genotyping should be done while the patient is either on ART or within 4 weeks of discontinuation as the dominant viral strains may decrease in prevalence so that they become too low to detect. This is also commonly "reversion to wild-type virus" with fading of important mutations into the CD4$^+$ archive. The addition of phenotypic testing to genotypic testing traditionally was recommended for PWH with complex resistance patterns, although over time the sophistication and reliability of algorithmic genotype interpretations such as the Stanford Drug Resistance Database has largely obviated the need for phenotypic testing.

Several new medications may potentially be utilized for the treatment of multidrug-resistant HIV-1, though guidance from an HIV specialist is recommended. The attachment inhibitor fostemsavir is an option for patients expected to have incomplete activity from an optimized background regimen, helping 84% of such patients achieve HIV-1 RNA counts< 200 copies/ mL, at 48 weeks (Kozal et al., 2020). Ibalizumab is a humanized IgG4 monoclonal antibody that blocks entry of HIV-1 by targeting the CD4$^+$ extracellular domain 2. Fifty percent of the 40 patients with multidrug-resistant HIV-1 reached RNA count< 200 copies/mL at 25 weeks (Emu et al., 2018). Lastly, capsid inhibitors are a new class of ARV that are pending further investigation but have shown promise in virologic control for PWH with multidrug-resistant HIV-1 when combined with optimized background therapy (Segal-Maurer et al., 2022).

When switching regimens for someone with hepatitis B coinfection, a drug regimen effective for both HIV and HBV should be used; typically, this means using tenofovir, but if that is not possible, the patient should receive entecavir for HBV treatment in addition to their HIV ART regimen. Notably, none of the two-drug HIV ART regimens have adequate anti-HBV activity and are therefore not recommended by themselves for persons coinfected with HBV or whose HBV status is unknown (DHHS, 2022).

After switching regimens, PWH should be evaluated closely to ensure that no new side effects have emerged, and a repeat viral load 4–8 weeks after a regimen switch should be obtained to ensure the patient is virally suppressed. If pre-existing laboratory abnormalities were attributed to the prior ART regimen (e.g., hyperlipidemia assumed to be from PIs), these laboratory values should be rechecked 3 months after switching regimens (DHHS 2022).

SUMMARY

The DHHS, IAS-USA, World Health Organization, European AIDS Clinical Society, and British HIV Association guidelines now recommend treatment of all PWH regardless of the CD4$^+$ T-cell count. Currently, the critical issues in antiretroviral treatment are focused on optimizing regimens for the individual patient. Barriers to adherence and addressing those factors remain paramount, and resolution prior to treatment initiation is important to achieve treatment success. Once patients are ready for therapy, their ART regimen must be tailored to their to medical comorbidities, medication side effects, and lifestyle. Switching to newer agents must be done prudently, with careful consideration of the patient's resistance history and comorbidities. Finally, just as there has been enormous progress in the past, we will continue to witness significant change in the future as we seek to find the optimal treatments for PWH.

RECOMMENDED READING

Gandhi RT, Bedimo R, Hoy JF, et al. Antiretroviral drugs for treatment and prevention of HIV infection in adults: 2022 recommendations of the International Antiviral Society-USA Panel. *JAMA*. 2023 Jan 3;329(1):63–84.

US Department of Health and Human Services (USDHHS), Panel on Antiretroviral Guidelines for Adults and Adolescents. Guidelines for the use of antiretroviral agents in adults and adolescents with HIV. *DHHS*. https://clinicalinfo.hiv.gov/en/guidelines/adult-and-adolescent-arv. Published 2022. Accessed September 22, 2022.

REFERENCES

Aboud M, Orkin C, Podzamczer D, et al. Efficacy and safety of dolutegravir-rilpivirine for maintenance of virological suppression in adults with HIV-1: 100-week data from the randomised, open-label, phase 3 SWORD-1 and SWORD-2 studies. *Lancet HIV*. 2019;6(9):e576–e587.

Amstutz A, Brown J, Ringera I, et al. Engagement in care, viral suppression, drug resistance, and reasons for nonengagement after home-based, same-day antiretroviral therapy initiation in Lesotho: a two-year follow-up of the CASCADE trial. *Clinical Infectious Diseases*. 2019;71(10):2608–2614.

Antiretroviral Therapy Cohort C (ATC). Survival of HIV-positive patients starting antiretroviral therapy between 1996 and 2013: a collaborative analysis of cohort studies. *Lancet HIV*. 2017;4(8):e349–e356.

Bares SH, Smeaton LM, Xu A, et al. HIV-infected women gain more weight than HIV-infected men following the initiation of antiretroviral therapy. *J Womens Health (Larchmt)*. 2018;27(9):1162–1169.

Bavinton BR, Pinto AN, Phanuphak N, et al. Viral suppression and HIV transmission in serodiscordant male couples: an international, prospective, observational, cohort study. *Lancet HIV*. 2018;5(8):e438–e447.

Bhagwat P, Ofotokun I, McComsey GA, et al. Changes in waist circumference in HIV-infected individuals initiating a raltegravir or protease inhibitor regimen: effects of sex and race. *Open Forum Infect Dis.* 2018;5(11):ofy201.

Cahn P, Madero JS, Arribas JR, et al. Durable efficacy of dolutegravir plus lamivudine in antiretroviral treatment-naive adults with hiv-1 infection: 96-week results from the GEMINI-1 and GEMINI-2 randomized clinical trials. *J Acquir Immune Defic Syndr.* 2020;83(3):310–318.

Cahn P, Sierra Madero JS, Arribas JR, et al. Dolutegravir plus lamivudine versus dolutegravir plus tenofovir disoproxil fumarate and emtricitabine in antiretroviral-naïve adults with HIV-1 infection (GEMINI-1 and GEMINI-2): week 48 results from two multicenter, double-blind, randomized, non-inferiority, phase 3 trials. *Lancet.* 2018;393(10167):143–155. http://doi:10.1016/S0140-6736(18)32462-0

Cahn P, Sierra Madero J, Arribas JR, et al. Three-year durable efficacy of dolutegravir plus lamivudine in antiretroviral therapy—naive adults with HIV-1 infection. *AIDS.* 2022;36(1):39–48.

Clotet B, Feinberg J, van Lunzen J, et al. Once-daily dolutegravir versus darunavir plus ritonavir in antiretroviral-naive adults with HIV-1 infection (FLAMINGO): 48 week results from the randomised open-label phase 3b study. *Lancet.* 2014;383(9936):2222–2231.

Coffey S, Bacchetti P, Sachdev D, et al. RAPID antiretroviral therapy: high virologic suppression rates with immediateantiretroviral therapy initiation in a vulnerable urban clinic population. *AIDS.* 2019;33(5):825–832.

Cohen MS, Chen YQ, McCauley M, et al. Prevention of HIV-1 infection with early antiretroviral therapy. *N Engl J Med.* 2011;365:493–505.

Cohen MS, Gamble T, McCauley M. Prevention of HIV transmission and the HPTN 052 study. *Annu Rev Med.* 2020;71:347–360. http://doi:10.1146/annurev-med-110918-034551. Epub October 25, 2019. PMID: 31652410.

Cohen MS, Chen YQ, McCauley M, et al. Antiretroviral therapy for the prevention of HIV-1 transmission. *N Engl J Med.* 2016;375(9):830–839.

Colasanti J, Sumitani J, Mehta CC, et al. Implementation of a rapid entry program decreases time to viral suppression among vulnerable persons living with HIV in the Southern United States. *Open Forum Infect Dis.* January 27, 2018;5(6):ofy104. doi:10.1093/ofid/ofy104. eCollection 2018 Jun.

Cuzin L, Cotte L, Delpierre C, et al.; Dat'AIDS study group. Too fast to stay on track? Shorter time to first anti-retroviral regimen is not associated with better retention in care in the French Dat'AIDS cohort. *PLoS One.* 2019;14(9):e0222067.

Czarnogorski M, Garris C, D'Amico R, et al. Customize: overall results from a hybrid III implementation-effectiveness study examining implementation of cabotegravir and rilpivirine long-acting injectable for HIV treatment in US Healthcare settings; final patient and provider data. 11th IAS Conference on HIV Science. Virtual; July 18–21, 2021.

DHHS. US Department of Health and Human Services guidelines for the use of antiretroviral agents in adults and adolescents with HIV. https://clinicalinfo.hiv.gov/en/guidelines/adult-and-adolescent-arv/whats-new-guidelines. Published 2022. Accessed August 8, 2022.

DHHS. US Department of Health and Human Services guidelines for the prevention and treatment of opportunistic infections in adults and adolescents with HIV. https://clinicalinfo.hiv.gov/en/guidelines/hiv-clinical-guidelines-adult-and-adolescent-opportunistic-infections/whats-new. Published 2022. Accessed August 8, 2022.

Dorjee K, Baxi SM, Reingold AL, Hubbard A. Risk of cardiovascular events from current, recent, and cumulative exposure to ABC among persons living with HIV who were receiving antiretroviral therapy in the United States: a cohort study. *BMC Infect Dis.* 2017;17(1):708. h http://doi:10.1186/s12879-017-2808-8. PMID: 29078761; PMCID: PMC5660446.

Emu B, Fessel J, Schrader S, et al. Phase 3 study of Ibalizumab for multidrug-resistant HIV-1. *N Engl J Med.* 2018;379(7):645–654.

Eron JJ, Young B, Cooper DA, et al. The SWITCHMRK 1 and 2 investigators. Switch to a raltegravir-based regimen versus continuation of a lopinavir–ritonavir-based regimen in stable HIV-infected patients with suppressed viremia (SWITCHMRK 1 and 2): two multicentre, double-blind, randomized controlled trials. *Lancet.* 2010;375:396–407.

Gallant JE, Daar ES, Raffi F, et al. Efficacy and safety of tenofovir alafenamide versus tenofovir disoproxil fumarate given as fixed-dose combinations containing emtricitabine as backbones for treatment of HIV-1 infection in virologically suppressed adults: a randomised, double-blind, active-controlled phase 3 trial. *Lancet HIV.* 2016;3(4):e158–e165.

Gallant J, Lazzarin A, Mills A, et al. Bictegravir, emtricitabine, and tenofovir alafenamide versus dolutegravir, abacavir, and lamivudine for initial treatment of HIV-1 infection (GS-US-380-1489): a double-blind, multicentre, phase 3, randomised controlled non-inferiority trial. *Lancet.* 2017;390(10107):2063–2072.

Griesel R, Maartens G, Chirehwa M, et al. CYP2B6 genotype and weight gain differences between dolutegravir and efavirenz. *Clin Infect Dis.* 2021;73(11):e3902–e3909.

Hagins D, Orkin C, Daar ES, et al. Switching to coformulated rilpivirine (RPV), emtricitabine (FTC) and tenofovir alafenamide from either RPV, FTC and tenofovir disoproxil fumarate (TDF) or efavirenz, FTC and TDF: 96-week results from two randomized clinical trials. *HIV Med.* 2018;19(10):724–733.

HIV.gov. Overview: data and trends: US statistics. https://www.hiv.gov/hiv-basics/overview/data-and-trends/statistics. Published June 2, 2021. Accessed August 8, 2022.

Hoenigl M, Chaillon A, Moore DJ, et al. Rapid HIV viral load suppression in those initiating antiretroviral therapy at first visit after HIV diagnosis. *Sci Rep.* 2016;6:32947.

Johnson M, Kumar P, Molina JM, et al. Switching to doravirine/lamivudine/tenofovir disoproxil fumarate (DOR/3TC/TDF) maintains HIV-1 virologic suppression through 48 weeks: results of the DRIVE-SHIFT trial. *J Acquir Immune Defic Syndr.* 2019;81(4):463–472.

Kerchberger AM, Sheth AN, Angert CD, et al. Weight gain associated with integrase stand transfer inhibitor use in women. *Clin Infect Dis.* 2020;71(3):593–600.

Koenig SP, Dorvil N, Devieux JG, et al. Same-day HIV testing with initiation of antiretroviral therapy versus standard care for persons living with HIV: a randomized unblinded trial. *PLoS Med.* 2017;14(7)):e1002357.

Kouanfack C, Mpoudi-Etame M, Omgba Bassega P, et al; NAMSALANRS 12313 study group. Dolutegravir-based or low-dose efavirenz-based regimen for the treatment of HIV-1. *N Engl J Med.* 2019;381(9):816–826.

Kozal M, Aberg, J, Pialoux G, et al. Fostemsavir in adults with multidrug-resistant HIV-1 infection. *N Engl J Med.* March 2020; 382:1232–1243.

Labhardt ND, Ringera I, Lejone TI, et al. Effect of offering same-day ART vs usual health facility referral during home-based HIV testing on linkage to care and viral suppression among adults with HIV in Lesotho: the CASCADE randomized clinical trial. *JAMA.* 2018;319(11):1103–1112.

Lake JE, Wu K, Bares SH, et al. Risk Factors for weight gain following switch to integrase inhibitor-based antiretroviral therapy. *Clin Infect Dis.* 2020;71(9):e471–e477.

Lennox JL, DeJesus E, Lazzarin A, et al. Safety and efficacy of raltegravir-based versus efavirenz-based combination therapy in treatment-naïve patients with HIV-1 infection: a multicentre, double-blind randomised controlled trial. *Lancet.* September 5, 2009;374(9692):796–806.

Lennox JF, Landovitz RJ, Ribaudo HJ. Three nonnucleoside reverse transcriptase inhibitor-sparing antiretroviral regimens for treatment-naïve volunteers infected with HIV-1. *Ann Intern Med.* March 17, 2015;162(6):461–462.

Llibre JM, Brites C, Cheng CY, et al. Efficacy and safety of switching to the 2-drug regimen dolutegravir/lamivudine versus continuing a 3- or 4-drug regimen for maintaining virologic suppression in adults living with HIV-1: week 48 results from the phase 3, non-inferiority SALSA randomized trial. *Clin Infect Dis.* 2023;76(4):720–729. doi:10.1093/cid/ciac130. ePub online 2022 March 2.

Lundgren J, Babiker A et al. INSIGHT START Study Group. Initiation of antiretroviral therapy in early asymptomatic HIV infection. *N Engl J Med.* 2015;373(9):795–807.

Mayer KH, Molina JM, Thompson MA, et al. Emtricitabine and tenofovir alafenamide vs emtricitabine and tenofovir disoproxil fumarate for HIV pre-exposure prophylaxis (DISCOVER): primary results from a randomised, double-blind, multicentre, active-controlled, phase 3, non-inferiority trial. *Lancet.* 2020;396(10246):239254.

McComsey GA, Kitch D, Daar ES, et al. Bone mineral density and fractures in antiretroviral-naive persons randomized to receive abacavir-lamivudine or tenofovir disoproxil fumarate-emtricitabine along with efavirenz or atazanavir-ritonavir: AIDS Clinical Trials Group A5224s, a substudy of ACTG A5202. *J Infect Dis.* 2011;203(12):1791–1801.

Mocroft A, Lundgren JD, Ross M, et al. Exposure to antiretrovirals (ARVs) and development of chronic kidney disease (CKD). [Abstract 142]. Presented at the 2015 Conference on Retroviruses and Opportunistic Infections. Seattle, Washington; February 23–24, 2015.

Molina JM, Squires K, Sax PE, et al. Doravirine versus ritonavir-boosted darunavir in antiretroviral-naive adults with HIV-1 (DRIVE-FORWARD): 48-week results of a randomised, double-blind, phase 3, non-inferiority trial. *Lancet HIV.* 2018;5(5):e211–e220.

Mollan KR, Smurzynski M, Eron JJ, et al. Association between efavirenz as initial therapy for HIV-1 infection and increased risk for suicidal ideation or attempted or completed suicide: an analysis of trial data. *Ann Intern Med.* July 1, 2014;161(1):1–10.

Monforte Ad, Reiss P, Ryom L, et al. Atazanavir is not associated with an increased risk of cardio- or cerebrovascular disease events. *AIDS.* January 28, 2013;27(3):407–415.

Moore RD, Keruly JC. CD4 $^+$ cell count 6 years after commencement of highly active antiretroviral therapy in persons with sustained virologic suppression. *Clin Infect Dis.* 2007;44(3):441–446.

Orkin C, Arasteh K, Górgolas Hernández-Mora M, et al. Long-acting cabotegravir and rilpivirine after oral induction for HIV-1 infection. *N Engl J Med.* 2020;382(12):1124–1135.

Orkin C, Elion R, Thompson M, et al. Changes in weight and BMI with first-line doravirine based therapy. *AIDS.* 2021;35(1):91–99.

Orkin C, Squires KE, Molina JM, et al. Doravirine/lamivudine/tenofovir disoproxil fumarate is non-inferior to efavirenz/emtricitabine/tenofovir disoproxil fumarate in treatment-naive adults with human immunodeficiency virus-1 infection: week 48 results of the DRIVE-AHEAD trial. *Clin Infect Dis.* 2019;68(4):535–544.

Overton ET, Richmond G, Rizzardini G, et al. Long-acting cabotegravir and rilpivirine dosed every 2 months in adults with HIV-1 infection (ATLAS-2M), 48-week results: a randomised, multicentre, open-label, phase 3b, non-inferiority study. *Lancet.* 2021;396(10267):1994–2005.

Palella F, Althoff KN, Moore R, et al. NA-ACCORD: recent abacavir use and risk of MI. [Abstract 749 LB]. Presented at the 2015 Conference on Retroviruses and Opportunistic Infections. Seattle, Washington; February 23–26, 2015.

Palella FJJ, Armon C, Chmiel JS, et al. CD4 cell count at initiation of ART, long-term likelihood of achieving CD4 >750 cells/mm3 and mortality risk. *J Antimicrob Chemother.* 2016;71(9):2654–2662.

Perez-Molina JA, Rubio R, Rivero A, et al. Simplification to dual therapy (atazanavir/ritonavir + lamivudine) versus standard triple therapy [atazanavir/ritonavir + two nucleos(t)ides] in virologically stable patients on antiretroviral therapy: 96 week results from an open-label, non-inferiority, randomized clinical trial (SALT study). *J Antimicrob Chemother.* 2017;72(1):246–253.

Pilcher CD, Ospina-Norvell C, Dasgupta A, et al. The effect of same-day observed initiation of antiretroviral therapy on HIV viral load and treatment outcomes in a U.S. public health setting. *J Acquir Immune Defic Syndr.* 2017;74(1):44–51.

Pilkington V, Hughes SL, Pepperrell T, et al. Tenofovir alafenamide vs. tenofovir disoproxil fumarate: an updated meta-analysis of 14 894 patients across 14 trials. *AIDS.* 2020;34(15):2259–2268.

Post FA, Moyle GJ, Stellbrink HJ, et al. Randomized comparison of renal effects, efficacy, and safety with once-daily abacavir/lamivudine versus tenofovir/emtricitabine, administered with efavirenz, in antiretroviral-naive, HIV-1-infected adults: 48-week results from the ASSERT study. *J AIDS.* 2010;55(1):49–45.

Pozniak A, Arribas JR, Gathe J, et al. Switching to tenofovir alafenamide, coformulated with elvitegravir, cobicistat, and emtricitabine, in HIV-infected patients with renal impairment: 48-week results from a single-arm, multicenter, open-label phase 3 study. *J AIDS.* April 15, 2016;71(5):530–537.

Raesima MM, Ogbuabo CM, Thomas V, et al. Dolutegravir use at conception: additional surveillance data from Botswana. *N Engl J Med.* 2019;381(9):885–887.

Raffi F, Jaeger H, Quiros-Roldan E, et al. Once-daily dolutegravir versus twice-daily raltegravir in antiretroviral-naive adults with HIV-1 infection (SPRING-2 study): 96 week results from a randomised, double-blind, non-inferiority trial. *Lancet Infect Dis.* 2013;13(11):927–935.

Rockstroh J, DeJesus E, Henry K, et al. A randomized, double-blind comparison of coformulated elvitegravir/cobicistat/emtricitabine/tenofovir DF vs. ritonavir-boosted atazanavir plus coformulated emtricitabine and tenofovir DF for initial treatment of HIV-1 infection: analysis of week 96 results. *J AIDS.* 2013;62(5):483–486.

Rodger AJ, Cambiano V, Bruun T, et al. Sexual activity without condoms and risk of HIV transmission in serodifferent couples when the HIV-positive partner is using suppressive antiretroviral therapy. *JAMA.* 2016;316(2):171–181.

Rosen S, Maskew M, Fox MP, et al. Initiating antiretroviral therapy for HIV at a patient's first clinic visit: the RapIT randomized controlled trial. *PLoS Med.* 2016;13(5):e1002015. doi:10.1371/journal.pmed.1002015. eCollection 2016 May.

Ruderman S, Crane H, Nance, R, et al. Brief report: weight gain following ART initiation in ART-naïve people living with HIV in the current treatment era. *JAIDS.* 2021;86(3):339–343.

Saag MS, Gandhi RT, Hoy JF, et al. Antiretroviral drugs for treatment and prevention of HIV infection in adults: 2020 recommendations of the International Antiviral Society-USA panel. *JAMA.* 2020;324(16):1651–1669.

Sabin C, Reiss P, Ryom L, et al. Is there continued evidence for an association between abacavir and myocardial infarction risk? [Abstract 747]. Presented at the 21st Conference on Retroviruses and Opportunistic Infections. Boston, MA; 2014.

Samji H, Cescon A, Hogg RS, et al.; North American AIDS Cohort Collaboration on Research and Design (NA-ACCORD) of IeDEA. Closing the gap: increases in life expectancy among treated HIV-positive individuals in the United States and Canada. *PLoS One.* December 18, 2013;8(12):e81355. http://doi:10.1371/journal.pone.0081355. PMID: 24367482; PMCID: PMC3867319.

Sax PE, Erlandson KM, Lake JE, et al. Weight gain following initiation of antiretroviral therapy: risk factors in randomized comparative clinical trials. *Clin Infect Dis.* 2020;71(6):1379–1389. doi:10.1093/cid/ciz999.

Sax PE, Pozniak A, Montes ML, et al. Coformulated bictegravir, emtricitabine, and tenofovir alafenamide versus dolutegravir with emtricitabine and tenofovir alafenamide, for initial treatment of HIV-1 infection (GS-US-380-1490): a randomised, double-blind, multicentre, phase 3, non-inferiority trial. *Lancet.* 2017;390(10107):2073–2082.

Sax P, Tierney C, Collier A, et al. Abacavir–lamivudine versus tenofovir–emtricitabine for initial HIV-1 therapy. *N Engl J Med.* December 3, 2009;361(23):2230–2240.

Segal-Maurer S, DeJesus E, Stellbrink HJ, et al. Capsid inhibition with lenacapavir in multidrug-resistant HIV-1 infection. *N Engl J Med.* 2022;386(19):1793–1803.

Seybolt L, Conner K, Butler I et al. Rapid start lead to sustained viral suppression in young people in the South [Abstract 1073] in special issue: abstracts from the 2020 Conference on Retroviruses and Opportunistic Infections. *Top Antivir Med.* 2020;28(1):407.

Smith KY, Patel P, Fine D, et al. Randomized, double-blind, placebo-matched, multicenter trial of abacavir/lamivudine or tenofovir/emtricitabine with lopinavir/ritonavir for initial HIV treatment. *AIDS.* July 31, 2009;23(12):1547–1556.

Swindells S, Andrade-Villanueva JF, Richmond GJ, et al. Long-acting cabotegravir and rilpivirine for maintenance of HIV-1 suppression. *N Engl J Med.* 2020;382(12):1112–1123.

TEMPRANO ANRS 12136 Study Group. A trial of early antiretrovirals and isoniazid preventive therapy in Africa. *N Engl J Med.* 2015;373:808–822.

Townsend CL, Cortina-Borja M, Peckham CS, et al. Low rates of mother-to-child transmission of HIV following effective pregnancy interventions in the United Kingdom and Ireland, 2000–2006. *AIDS.* 2008;22(8):973–981.

Tubiana R, Le Chenadec J, Rouzioux C, et al. Factors associated with mother-to-child transmission of HIV-1 despite a maternal viral load < 500 copies/ml at delivery: a case-control study nested in the French perinatal cohort (EPF-ANRS CO1). *Clin Infect Dis.* 2010;50(4):585–596.

van Lunzen J, Antinori A, Cohen CJ, et al. Rilpivirine vs. efavirenz-based single-tablet regimens in treatment-naive adults: week 96 efficacy and safety from a randomized phase 3b study. *AIDS.* 2016;30(2):251–259.

van Wyk J, Ajana F, Bisshop F, et al. Efficacy and safety of switching to dolutegravir/lamivudine fixed-dose 2-drug regimen vs continuing a tenofovir alafenamide-based 3- or 4-drug regimen for maintenance of virologic suppression in adults living with human immunodeficiency virus type 1: phase 3, randomized, noninferiority TANGO study. *Clin Infect Dis.* 2020;71(8):1920–1929.

Venter WDF, Moorhouse M, Sokhela S, et al. Dolutegravir plus two different prodrugs of tenofovir to treat HIV. *N Engl J Med.* 2019;381(9):803–815.

ViiV Healthcare. Ziagen (abacavir) US prescribing information. http://www.accessdata.fda.gov/drugsatfda_docs/label/2012/020977s025,020978s029lbl.pdf. Published 2013. Accessed April 30, 2016.

Walmsley SL, Antela A, Clumeck N, et al. Dolutegravir plus abacavir–lamivudine for the treatment of HIV-1 infection. *N Engl J Med.* 2013;369(19):1807–1818.

Worm SW, Sabin C, Weber R, et al.; DAD Study Group. Risk of myocardial infarction in patients with HIV infection exposed to specific individual antiretroviral drugs from 3 major drug classes. *J Infect Dis.* 2010;201:318–330.

Young J, Xiao Y, Moodier EE, et al. Effect of cumulating exposure to abacavir on the risk of cardiovascular disease events in patients from the Swiss HIV cohort study. *J AIDS.* 2015;69(4):413–421.

Zash R, Holmes L, Diseko M, et al. Update on neural tube defects with antiretroviral exposure in the Tsepamo study, Botswana. Type presented at AIDS 2020, 23rd International AIDS Conference. Virtual; 2020.

Zash R, Makhema J, Shapiro RL. Neural-tube defects with dolutegravir treatment from the time of conception. *N Engl J Med.* 2018;379(10):979–981.

Zolopa A, Sax P, DeJesus E, et al. A randomized double-blind comparison of coformulated elvitegravir/cobicistat/emtricitabine/tenofovir disoproxil fumarate versus favirenz/emtricitabine/tenofovir disoproxil fumarate for initial treatment of HIV-1 infection: analysis of week 96 results. *J AIDS.* 2013;63:96–100.

19.

THE HIV RESERVOIR AND CURE AND REMISSION STRATEGIES

Boris Juelg, Rajesh T. Gandhi, and Nikolaus Jilg

CHAPTER GOALS

Upon completion of this chapter, the reader should be able to:

- Identify key hurdles for HIV eradication strategies and explain approaches that might overcome these challenges.

- Discuss new antiretroviral drugs in development.

- Discuss current research on preventive and therapeutic vaccines, immunomodulatory, and genetic agents.

THE HIV RESERVOIR AND CURE AND REMISSION STRATEGIES

WHAT'S NEW?

Novel strategies to promote HIV latency reversal and approaches to boost HIV-specific immunity are being evaluated in clinical trials aimed at eradicating HIV. A new generation of broadly neutralizing antibodies has demonstrated potency at suppressing HIV-1 viremia in clinical trials and may play a role in immunotherapy and prevention. Latency-reversing agents (e.g., histone deacetylase inhibitors) and gene therapy strategies using autologous CD4$^+$ T-cells and hematopoietic stem cells continue to be evaluated in trials.

KEY POINTS

- HIV-1 persists quiescently in cellular reservoirs not detected by the immune system because of the lack of active viral replication; these reservoirs represent the biggest obstacle to cure approaches.

- Reversal of HIV-1 latency and induction of virus expression by a variety of interventions may render infected cells susceptible to immune recognition and active clearance.

- Strategies to boost immune responses via active or passive immunization, immunomodulation, or gene therapy are being evaluated with the aim of achieving HIV-1 control or remission without antiretroviral therapy (ART), if not viral eradication.

INTRODUCTION

Currently available antiretroviral medications consistently achieve durable suppression of HIV but do not eliminate the latent reservoir of infection or significantly modulate host immune responses in a manner that improves clinical outcomes. In this chapter, we will discuss HIV reservoir reduction and cure/remission approaches, new antiretroviral drugs in development, and various strategies targeting immune dysregulation and T-cell homeostasis. We also update the status of clinical research evaluating immunomodulators and vaccines.

WHY SHOULD WE TRY TO CURE HIV?

Although current ART is highly effective at controlling HIV-1 replication, it does not eradicate or cure the infection. There are several compelling reasons for trying to cure HIV-1. First, despite efforts to expand access to treatment, many people with HIV (PWH) worldwide are not receiving ART, which leads to ongoing transmission of the virus. Second, because current ART does not eradicate HIV-1, PWH must take ART for many decades, which may eventuate in difficulties with adherence, substantial cost, and the potential for long-term side effects. Third, PWH have increased rates of cardiovascular disease, liver disease, neurocognitive disorders, and other noninfectious complications that may be driven by elevated levels of inflammation that persist despite suppressive ART. Fourth, many PWH treated with ART alone do not achieve immune restoration despite viral suppression; in a large trial of adults with HIV achieving virologic suppression for 3 years with CD4$^+$ T-cell counts of 200 cells/µL or less, these patients had significantly greater mortality compared to those with CD4$^+$ T-cell counts of more than 200 cells/µL (adjusted hazard ratio, 2.6) (Engsig et al., 2014). Given significant evidence that CD4$^+$ T-cell counts have been correlated with normal life expectancy (ART Collaboration Cohort, 2008; Lewden et al., 2007), attention has turned to strategies to control the chronic immune activation and loss of normal T-cell homeostasis seen in HIV. Finally, HIV-1 infection continues to be associated with stigma and social isolation, which adversely affects quality of life. Given these

211

limitations of current ART, there is a concerted effort to find a cure for HIV-1.

While complete viral eradication, or a "sterilizing cure," is the ultimate goal, the concept of a "functional cure" or "HIV-1 remission" has been introduced, which includes strategies aimed at achieving host control of the virus without the need for ART. Several clinical observations within the past few years have fueled the belief that one or the other of these types of "cure" might be possible. Certainly, the most compelling example is that of the "Berlin patient." This man with HIV-1 and virologic suppression on ART received, as treatment for acute myelogenous leukemia, allogeneic hematopoietic stem cell transplants from a donor who carried a homozygous deletion in CCR5 (CCR5Δ32/Δ32), the coreceptor for HIV-1, thereby making his new CD4 + T-cells resistant to infection (Hutter et al., 2009). Following discontinuation of ART, no HIV-1 RNA was subsequently detected in the Berlin patient's peripheral blood; moreover, multiple attempts to detect HIV-1 RNA or proviral DNA in cellular reservoirs and other tissue compartments were negative (Yukl et al., 2013).

These findings were replicated in the "London patient" who underwent a similar allogeneic stem cell transplantation with cells that did not express CCR5; following the transplant, no replication-competent virus in blood, CSF, intestinal tissue, or lymphoid tissue was detected at 30 months following ART discontinuation (Gupta et al., 2020). Since then, the "Duesseldorf patient," "the New York patient," and the "City of Hope patient" have been reported with similar outcomes. Because of the risk of stem cell transplantation, however, this intensive approach is not appropriate in PWH who do not have a hematologic malignancy.

Another notable "proof of concept" came from studies of early initiation of ART during acute HIV-1 infection. The VISCONTI study identified 14 PWH whose viremia remained controlled for years after the interruption of ART that had been initiated during primary infection (Saez-Cirion et al., 2013). Further, the CHAMP (Control of HIV after Antiretroviral Medication Pause) study, which combined more than 700 PWH who discontinued ART reported posttreatment controller (PTC) rates of up to 13% in early ART-treated individuals (Namazi et al., 2018); of note, < 5% of PTCs were identified in those who initiated ART during chronic stages of infection.

Along these lines, the "Mississippi baby," a child born to a woman with HIV, was started on ART 30 hours after delivery and quickly achieved virologic suppression (Persaud et al., 2013). The child was lost to follow-up, however, and ART was discontinued by the caregiver. Despite stopping ART, the virus remained undetectable for 27 months, but the child ultimately suffered virologic rebound (Luzuriaga et al., 2015).

These examples demonstrate that it is possible, under extraordinary circumstances, to eradicate HIV-1 (in the case of the "Berlin and London" patients) or control HIV-1 without ART (in the case of the VISCONTI and CHAMP cohorts and, temporarily, the "Mississippi child"). Now, the challenge is to extend the insights from these remarkable cases and cohorts to the development of practical interventions that will lead to ART-free remission in the large population of people living with HIV-1.

EARLY ESTABLISHMENT AND PERSISTENCE OF THE LATENT HIV-1 RESERVOIR

In 1995, Chun et al. identified integrated provirus as a persistent reservoir of infection in the resting CD4+ T-cells of PWH (Chun et al., 1995). While most activated memory CD4+ T-cells are destroyed during viral replication, a small fraction of infected cells survives to return to a resting and memory state. In the resting memory state, HIV-1 gene expression is shut down, resulting in latent infection of CD4+ T-cells (Nabel et al., 1987). As these cells do not express viral proteins, they remain hidden from the host immune response; moreover, without active replication, the currently approved antiretroviral drugs cannot act against the virus. While infected, resting cells leave the quiescent memory pool at a steady rate, the pool of infected cells persists, perhaps in part because of homeostatic proliferation. It has also been suggested that specific CD4+ T-cell memory subsets, including central memory (TCM), transitional memory (TTM), and memory stem cells (TSCM), harbor the majority of integrated HIV-1 DNA and that eradication therapies may require targeting of specific CD4+ T-cell populations (Buzon et al., 2014).

Reactivation of latently infected cells leads to viral gene expression and active viral replication. In patients on long-term ART, the percentage of latently infected cells is extremely low: less than 1 per million resting memory CD4+ T-cells harbor replication-competent HIV-1 (Finzi et al., 1997; Wong et al., 1997). Nevertheless, after a more rapid decline in the first year after infection, this latent pool decays very slowly: the mean half-life of this reservoir is approximately 44 months, and, as a result, suppressive ART would need to be maintained for more than 60 years to achieve viral eradication even if an infected person had only 100,000 latently infected cells (Besson et al., 2014; Finzi et al., 1999). Longitudinal studies of the reservoir are time-consuming, technically demanding, and challenged by in-person, between-person, and testing heterogeneity (e.g., expansion and contraction of infected T-cell clones was shown to occur even after years on ART), and difficulties in comparison of different testing methods (Einkauf et al., 2022; Guo et al., 2022; Inderbitzin et al., 2022). In addition, it is conceivable that latent infection may persist in cells other than CD4+ T-cells; however, this has yet to be proven.

It was initially believed that early suppression of viral replication during primary infection might prevent reservoir formation. However, Chun et al. demonstrated that ART initiated within 10 days of primary infection did not prevent the generation of latently infected CD4+ T-cells (Chun et al., 1998), pointing toward an early seeding of the reservoir. Newer data from the rhesus macaque model demonstrate that the latent reservoir is established within days of virus exposure, even before virus can be detected in peripheral blood (Whitney et al., 2014); the implication of this finding is that it may be practically impossible to treat or even diagnose HIV-1 infection early enough to avoid reservoir seeding. Several studies, however, have demonstrated that initiating ART during the acute/early phase of the infection results in a smaller HIV-1 reservoir (Ananworanich et al., 2012; Garcia-Broncano et al., 2019; Hocqueloux et al., 2013; Saez-Cirion et al., 2013), and may preserve functionality of CD8[+] T-cells (Takata et al., 2022), suggesting that early treatment could be beneficial by reducing the barrier to cure (Henrich & Gandhi, 2013; Strain et al., 2005).

Persistence of the HIV-1 latent reservoir represents the biggest obstacle for cure approaches. For this reason, a deeper understanding of how latency is maintained and how this state can be reversed is critical to inform HIV-1 eradication strategies (Richman et al., 2009).

"KICK AND KILL" AND "BLOCK AND LOCK"

In order to achieve viral eradication, or at least a state of HIV-1 suppression that does not require continuous ART, different strategies have been proposed, including modification of the host immune response to achieve enhanced control of viral replication, interventions to prevent reactivation of virus latency (Mousseau et al., 2015), and gene therapy to increase the resistance of target cells to HIV-1 infection (Tebas et al., 2014). Currently, the strategy that is receiving the most attention is the "shock and kill" or "kick and kill" approach (Deeks, 2012). In this strategy, the first step is to flush out HIV-1 from the latent reservoir by activating proviral DNA expression in resting cells, leading to de novo viral protein production (the "shock" or "kick"). If this "kick" is successful, the next step is to enhance immune recognition and elimination of infected cells (the "kill"). This two-step approach, however, requires a latency-reversing strategy and an antiviral immune response in order to clear infected cells; both tasks are encumbered by substantial challenges. A strategy that aims to achieve the opposite is named "Block -and -Lock." Here, HIV is locked into its latent form, eliminating or at least reducing the chance of viral reactivation and replication. This strategy does not require the help of the immune system as it does not seek viral eradication.

LATENCY REVERSAL APPROACHES

Latently infected CD4[+] T-cells evade immune surveillance as they do not express HIV-1 proteins (Hermankova et al., 2003). Reversal of HIV-1 latency and induction of virus expression may render infected cells susceptible to attack by cytolytic T lymphocytes or to destruction by viral cytopathic effects (Chun et al., 1997; Deeks, 2012). Several latency-reversing agents (LRAs) have been identified, perhaps the most promising being histone deacetylase inhibitors (HDACi) and toll-like receptor (TLR) agonists (Kim et al., 2018). HDACi are currently approved as anticancer drugs, and several have been evaluated in ART-suppressed PWH for their latency-reversing potential (Archin et al., 2014; Elliott et al., 2014;

Rasmussen et al., 2014). Vorinostat, the first HDACi to be studied in PWH on ART, was found to induce viral expression by an average of 4.8-fold in resting CD4[+] T-cells after a single dose (Archin et al., 2014). Two other HDACi agents—panobinostat and romidepsin—have also been found to induce virus expression in PWH on suppressive ART (Rasmussen et al., 2014; Sogaard et al., 2015). Following administration of romidepsin, plasma HIV-1 RNA levels became detectable in some individuals, suggesting the LRA was inducing virus production (Sogaard et al., 2015). However, the size of the HIV-1 reservoir, based on measurements of HIV-1 DNA and virus outgrowth assay, remained unchanged following three weekly infusions of romidepsin. In addition, in a recent trial, romidepsin alone failed to increase HIV-1 expression in persons on ART (McMahon et al., 2019), so clinical studies of romidepsin in combination with other agents or strategies are being explored (Mothe et al., 2020) and are discussed later in this chapter.

TLR agonists are another group of drugs being investigated. The TLR7 agonist vesatolimod was shown to induce transient increases in plasma viral load and decreases in cellular viral DNA levels in simian immunodeficiency virus (SIV)-infected rhesus macaques (Whitney et al., 2015). In a separate study in monkeys treated with ART during acute simian-human immunodeficiency virus (SHIV) infection, a combination of a TLR-7 agonist with a broadly neutralizing antibody (PGT121) led to virologic control in 5 of 11 animals even after the interventions and ART were stopped (Borducchi et al., 2018). Trials using vesatolimod in ART-treated HIV-1–infected humans are being conducted (Riddler et al., 2021; SenGupta et al., 2021); one study in ART-suppressed PWH with low pre-ART viral loads demonstrated a modest increase in time to viral rebound after ATI in the vesatolimod group (SenGupta et al., 2021). Further, the TLR9 agonist lefitolimod increased HIV-1 transcription and enhanced cytotoxic natural killer (NK) cell activation in a small group of ART-suppressed individuals, but subsequently failed to increase the time to viral rebound when ART was held during an analytical treatment interruption (Vibholm et al., 2017, 2019). Overall, it remains uncertain whether a single agent will be sufficient to effectively and completely purge the pool of replication-competent, integrated, latent HIV-1; rather a combination of LRAs targeting distinct pathways, and potentially different cell types, might be required (Laird et al., 2015).

LATENCY SILENCING

In contrast to activating latency, it has been proposed that reinforcing a deep state of latency by permanently silencing HIV transcription could be an alternative approach for a functional cure (Mori et al., 2020). This concept, also known as "block and lock" or "soothe and snooze" strategy, would apply latency-promoting agents to block the reactivation of latently infected HIV-1 proviruses. A potential agent that has been studied is the Tat inhibitor didehydro-cortistatin A, which, when added to ART, reduced viral mRNA in tissues of HIV-1–infected humanized mice and significantly delayed viral rebound following ART interruption (Kessing et al.,

2017). More in vivo studies are needed to further determine the role of these interventions in HIV cure.

IMMUNE ENHANCING AND/OR MODULATING STRATEGIES

While latency reversal will be crucial for eradication strategies, inducing viral replication alone will most likely not be sufficient to eliminate HIV infection. Indeed, in an in vitro model, reversal of latency alone did not result in clearance of infected cells (Shan et al., 2012). For this reason, it is anticipated that, following reactivation, cells harboring the reservoir will need to be actively cleared, perhaps through a second line of attack by the host immune system. Strategies to enhance immune responses via active or passive immunization or via immunomodulation have been proposed. For example, it has been hypothesized that boosting T-cell responses will lead to enhanced viral control—similar to what is seen in so-called HIV-1 elite controllers, individuals who maintain undetectable viral loads in the absence of ART, where antiviral T-cells have been associated with viral suppression (Deeks & Walker, 2007; McMichael et al., 2010). Vaccination strategies will be discussed later in this chapter; what follows next are other immunomodulatory approaches.

IMMUNE MODULATION: CHECKPOINT INHIBITORS

Given the challenge that the cellular dysfunction in PWH known as T-cell exhaustion poses for therapeutic vaccination strategies, novel immune-modulating concepts have been developed to reverse this state of exhaustion by inhibiting immune checkpoints. During progressive HIV-1 infection with persistent antigen exposure, increased expression of inhibitory receptors like PD-1 on HIV-1–specific T-cells is associated with greater immune dysfunction (Day et al., 2006; Khaitan et al., 2011), and it is thought that anti-–PD-1 antibodies may be able to restore the function of exhausted CD4+ and CD8+ T-cells by restoring host cell pathways needed for T- cell activation (Porichis & Kaufmann, 2012). Inhibiting the PD-1 pathway has shown efficacy in reversing T- cell exhaustion in the cancer field (Topalian et al., 2012), and recent data suggest that PD-1 blockade restores the ability of antiviral T-cells to inhibit HIV-1 replication in animal models, including nonhuman primates (Palmer et al., 2013; Velu et al., 2009, 2022). Moreover, PD-1 is believed to play an important role in the establishment and maintenance of latently infected cells (Evans et al., 2018) and PD1-blockade might therefore lead to increased HIV transcription, a key step in latency reversal, and this may be true for other immune checkpoint pathways as well (reviewed in Gubser et al., 2022). While, ex vivo, a PD-L1 antibody (BMS-936559) was not sufficient to increase latency reversal measured by HIV virion production from CD4+ T-cells (Bui et al., 2019). Dose-escalation of this antibody delayed viral load rebound after ARV cessation in rhesus macaques and significantly lowered the viral load setpoint (Mason et al., 2014). In a phase 1 randomized clinical trial in 8 HIV-1 patients on ART with CD4+ T-cell counts of greater than 350 cells/μL and detectable viral load who received a single infusion of BMS-936559, two patients demonstrated an increase in HIV-specific T-cell responses. However, the trial was stopped prior to full enrollment as there was concern about antibody-associated retinal toxicity in animal studies (Gay et al., 2017). Another checkpoint inhibitor trial (ACTG 5370) was stopped early because of concern for two possible immune-related adverse event complications (Hardy, 2020). However, while these drugs are no longer in clinical development, these studies did demonstrate, as a proof of concept, the potential utility of immune checkpoint inhibitors in targeting the HIV reservoir. Intriguingly, repeated doses of the anti-–PD-1 antibody pembrolizumab in a single individual with HIV and lung cancer were associated with an increase in functional HIV-specific CD8+ T-cells and a decline in cell-associated HIV-DNA (Guihot et al., 2018), and a recent trial in cancer patients on ART showed measurable latency reversal in the absence of clonal expansion after a single infusion of pembrolizumab (Uldrick et al., 2022).

Other immune checkpoint inhibitors have been approved as cancer therapies, including nivolumab, an anti-–PD-1 antibody, which, as described in a case report, appeared to decrease the HIV reservoir (as suggested by a decrease in cell-associated HIV-DNA, increase in HIV-RT and Nef-specific CD8+ cells, and increase in T-cell activation) in a 51-year-old man with non–small cell carcinoma and well-controlled HIV infection (Guihot et al., 2018). An observational study of 32 PWH who were treated for cancer with monoclonal antibodies against PD-1 failed to demonstrate increased immune responses to HIV, but found substantial induction of other immune checkpoint pathways, potentially indicating compensatory mechanism with inhibition of a single immune checkpoint pathway (Baron et al. 2022). In another study with either anti-PD-1 monotherapy or the combination of both anti-PD-1 and anti-CTLA-4, a modest increase in cell-associated HIV RNA was detected in the few participants receiving combination therapy (Rasmussen et al., 2021). Several studies evaluating PD-1 blockade in HIV-positive participants on suppressive ART regimens and their effect on the virus reservoir in PWH with concomitant malignant diseases are in progress (ClinicalTrials.gov identifiers: NCT02408861, NCT02595866, NCT03367754, and NCT04223804).

Remaining concerns with immune checkpoint inhibitors, mainly informed by experiences in treatment for malignant diseases, are variable response rates, development of resistance to therapy and, particularly, induction of autoimmune disease (Wykes & Lewin, 2018).

T-CELL TRAFFICKING

Early HIV infection of lymphocytes within gut-associated lymphoid tissue (GALT) and subsequent depletion of gut CD4+ T-cells appears to significantly contribute to the immune dysfunction observed in chronic HIV infection. Durable suppression of HIV replication with ART does not significantly reverse the damage caused to GALT during early infection. Accordingly, therapies aimed at attenuating HIV-mediated destruction of GALT may serve as an effective strategy to treat and/or prevent HIV-related immune dysfunction and has been suggested as a potential cure strategy. One such approach involves disruption of the interaction between $\alpha_4\beta_7$ gut-homing receptors on CD4$^+$ T-cells and the gut endothelial cell adhesion molecules to which these receptors bind via interaction with mucosal addressing cell adhesion molecules (MAdCAM). HIV interacts with $\alpha_4\beta_7$ via the V2 domain of the gp120 subunit, and CD4$^+$ T-cells with high expression of $\alpha_4\beta_7$ appear to be preferentially infected during acute HIV or SIV infection. Treatment of SIV-infected ART-suppressed macaques with an anti-$\alpha_4\beta_7$ integrin monoclonal antibody resulted in persistent viral control following ART cessation (Byrareddy et al., 2016). However, other studies in macaques were unable to show this effect (Abbink et al., 2019; Iwamoto et al., 2019).

A commercially available humanized anti-$\alpha_4\beta_7$ mAb, vedolizumab (Act-1), is currently FDA approved for use in inflammatory bowel disease. This antibody blocks binding to MAdCAM at the b7 chain of $\alpha_4\beta_7$, thereby inhibiting the migration of lymphocytes into the gastrointestinal tract and reducing local inflammatory responses. A phase 1 study evaluating vedolizumab in 20 participants with HIV infection undergoing analytical treatment interruption, the median duration of plasma viremia < 400 copies/mL was only 5.4 weeks, failing to show sustained viral suppression (Sneller et al., 2019); other studies are ongoing (ClinicalTrials.gov identifiers: NCT03147859 and NCT04120415).

In contrast to preventing trafficking of HIV target cells into anatomic sites of high viral replication, an alternative approach is promoting cytotoxic CD8$^+$ T-cell migration into lymph node follicles to clear infected cells. In the nonhuman primate model, administration of an interleukin-15 super-agonist resulted in an increase of CXCR5 expression on CD8$^+$ T-cells and increased frequency of such cells in the lymphoid tissues (Webb et al., 2018). A phase 1 trial that evaluated different doses of the IL-15 superagonist N-803 in ART-suppressed PWH demonstrated that while transcription in memory CD4$^+$ T-cells and intact proviral DNA initially increased after N-803 treatment, the frequency of PBMCs with an inducible HIV provirus shows a small but significant decrease that persisted for up to 6 months after therapy (Miller et al., 2022). This concept is now being further examined in humans, also combining IL15-agonists with monoclonal anti-HIV antibodies (ClinicalTrials.gov identifier: NCT04505501, NCT04340596, and NCT05245292).

CYTOKINES

IL-2, an autocrine T-cell growth factor, is produced by CD4$^+$ T-cells, and expression was found to be lower in PWH. Based on promising phase 2 trials showing increased CD4$^+$ T-cell counts in participants receiving recombinant IL-2 (rIL-2) (Pett et al., 2010), two phase 3 trials were performed. In the ESPRIT study, 4,111 HIV-positive patients with CD4$^+$ T-cell counts of 300 cells/µL or more were randomly assigned to receive SQ IL-2 (three 5-day cycles 8 weeks apart) with ART or ART alone (Abrams et al., 2009). Although the rIL-2 group had a significantly higher CD4$^+$ T-cell counts, this difference

declined with time, and clinical outcomes, including opportunistic infection/death and all-cause mortality, did not significantly differ between the two groups. In addition, there were more grade 4 adverse events in the group receiving IL-2, most notably deep venous thrombosis. Subsequent analysis also raised concern for an increased incidence of pneumonia in patients receiving rIL-2 less than 180 days previously (Pett et al., 2011). The second IL-2 phase 3 trial, SILCAAT, randomly assigned 1,695 patients with CD4$^+$ T-cell counts of 50–299 cells/mm^3 to similar treatment arms, except the IL-2 group received six cycles at a lower dose (Abrams, 2009). CD4$^+$ T-cell counts were again higher in the IL-2 group, but statistically significant differences in opportunistic infection/death, all-cause mortality, and grade 4 clinical events were not seen.

Additionally, IL-2 has been studied as a means to reduce the viral reservoir. One randomized trial did not show an impact of rIL-2 with ART on proviral DNA in blood, lymph nodes, and cerebrospinal fluid compared to ART alone (Stellbrink et al., 2002). Other potential uses of rIL-2, such as a means to delay ART initiation, facilitate ART treatment interruption or as a vaccine adjunct have also been studied. However, in the STALWART study, a phase 2 trial in patients not on ART with CD4$^+$ T-cell counts greater than 300 cells/µl, rIL-2 use was associated with more opportunistic disease and death and a statistically significant increase in grade 3 or grade 4 events (Tavel et al., 2010). In summary, IL-2 does currently not appear to confer clinical benefit to PWH, regardless of whether they are on ART, although this continues to be an area of investigation.

Other cytokines being studied for use in HIV include IL-7, IL-15, and IL-21. IL-7 plays a key role in T-cell homeostasis, leading to expansion and survival of naive and memory T-cells and preventing apoptosis of CD4$^+$ and CD8$^+$ T-cells in HIV-positive patients in vitro. In early clinical trials, human recombinant IL-7 therapy was well -tolerated and induced a significant and dose-dependent increase in functional naive and memory CD4$^+$ and CD8$^+$ T-cells in lymphopenic PWH on ART (Levy et al., 2009; Sereti et al., 2009). In a randomized, placebo-controlled trial of recombinant IL-7 in ARV-treated PWH, there were brisk T-cell increases of naive and central memory T-cells (averaging 323 cells/µL at 12 weeks) with a durable response seen up to 1 year (Levy et al., 2012). IL-7, however, appears to have a minimal impact on the HIV latent reservoir. A follow- up study of peripheral blood monocytes collected from ten participants who participated in an IL-7 treatment trial failed to demonstrate activation of latently infected resting memory CD4$^+$ T-cells (Vandergeeten et al., 2013).

In macaque models, IL-21 has demonstrated beneficial immune responses, such as improved NK and T-cell cytotoxicity and reduced levels of intestinal T- cell proliferation and microbial translocation. With this novel mechanism of action, it appears to be a promising treatment for augmenting immune response while ameliorating intestinal immune activation (Pallikkuth et al., 2011, 2013).

IL-15, like IL-2, has lymphocyte stimulatory activity and is significantly increased in HIV patients with a virologic and immunologic response to ART compared to ARV-naive patients (Forcina et al., 2004), which has prompted interest in its role in immune therapy (Harwood & O'Connor, 2021). A recent phase 1 study demonstrated safety of N-803, a long-acting IL-15 superagonist and a possible effect on the reservoir in PWH (Miller et al., 2022).

CHIMERIC ANTIGEN RECEPTOR T-CELLS

An alternative approach, which circumvents the problem of eliciting immune responses in PWH, is the adoptive transfer of T-cells with molecularly cloned high-affinity T- cell receptors and superior antiviral activity, targeting conserved and vulnerable regions of the virus (Varela-Rohena et al., 2008). Chimeric antigen receptor transduced T-cells, which combine the specificity of an antibody with the signaling of a T-cell receptor, have shown promise in cancer (Hombach et al., 2013) and are being studied in HIV (Choudhary et al., 2022; Lam & Bollard, 2013; Leibman et al., 2017). Clinical trials testing chimeric antigen receptor (CAR) T-cell therapy in ART-suppressed individuals include a bNAb (VRC01)-based CAR (ClinicalTrials.gov identifier: NCT03240328) and a CD4-CAR T-cell modified by zinc-finger nuclease CCR5 disruption to induce HIV resistance (ClinicalTrials.gov identifier: NCT03617198).

MONOCLONAL ANTIBODY THERAPY

During the past decade, multiple monoclonal antibodies (mAbs) have been developed against various viral targets, including viral membrane targets (e.g., gp120 and gp41), the CD4$^+$ receptor, and the CCR5 coreceptor (Chen & Dmitrov, 2012). Very few of these mAbs showed clinical benefit despite efficacy in nonhuman primate models, largely owing to the virus's ability to rapidly develop resistant variants. Nonetheless, several promising compounds and treatment approaches have evolved recently and are discussed here.

Leronlimab (PRO 140), a humanized CCR5 mAb, had potent activity in early clinical trials. Currently in phase 2 study, participants who are suppressed on a stable ART regimen are switched to weekly subcutaneous injections of leronlimab as a single agent maintenance therapy in patients with exclusively CCR5-tropic HIV-1. Preliminary results showed a failure rate of 65% in the 350 mg dose arm. (Dhody et al., 2018; Dhody & Kazempour, 2019). However, in phase 2b/3, PRO 140 subcutaneous injections were added to a failing ART regimen. Of 52 participants, 64% versus 23% ($P = 0.0032$) had at least 0.5 log viral load drop after 1 week (Mascolini et al., 2018) with no treatment-related resistance.

UB-421 is a humanized IgG1 monoclonal antibody that inhibits attachment of HIV-1 virus and entry into the cells by competitively binding to the CD4$^+$ receptor. In a phase 2 nonrandomized trial, 29 participants who had undetectable viral loads were enrolled and received either 10 mg/kg dosing every week or 25 mg/kg biweekly after stopping their ART for 8 weeks, with 94% of the patients maintaining virologic suppression (Wang et al., 2019). A phase 2 study that evaluated the efficacy of UB-421 in combination with standard ART in reducing the HIV reservoir in PWH was recently completed and results are pending (ClinicalTrials.gov identifier: NCT03743376).

BROADLY NEUTRALIZING ANTIBODIES

HIV-1 immunotherapy with first-generation mAbs in the preclinical and clinical settings was largely ineffective. However, the recent identification of novel broadly neutralizing anti-HIV-1 antibodies (bNAbs), which are able to neutralize the majority of viral strains at very low concentrations, may provide another approach to target the HIV-1 reservoir. In preclinical studies, administration of bNAbs was shown to reduce plasma viremia in chimeric SHIV-infected macaques (Barouch et al., 2013b; Shingai et al., 2013; Julg et al., 2017); in fact, one particular bNAb, PGT121, also resulted in substantial reductions of proviral DNA in peripheral blood, lymph nodes, and gastrointestinal mucosa (Barouch et al., 2013b). Multiple different bNAbs have been tested in PWH and have shown promising reductions in plasma viremia (Caskey, 2015, 2017; Lynch, 2015; Stephenson et al., 2021). As a potential mechanism, it has been suggested that clearance of infected cells expressing viral antigen on their surfaces (Lu et al., 2016) is mediated through interactions between the Fc component of the antibody and its receptor on innate immune effectors cells like NK cells and macrophages (Bruel et al., 2016).

VRC01 is a bNAb that targets the CD4-binding site of the HIV envelope glycoprotein. In phase 1 randomized placebo-controlled trial, VRC01 was safe and well tolerated, but did not have any significant effects on low-level plasma or cellular HIV-1 viremia in individuals on effective ART (Riddler et al., 2018); nevertheless, VCR01 is undergoing phase 2b studies. A phase 1 study evaluating a long-acting form of VRC01 (VRC01LS) demonstrated that VRC01LS was safe, well -tolerated, had a fourfold greater half-life, and elicited HIV-1 neutralizing activity (Gaudinski et al., 2018). Similarly, other bNAbs with half-life extending modifications, such as 3BNC117-LS, 10-1074-LS, PGT121.414.LS, and PGDM1400LS, are currently being evaluated (ClinicalTrials.gov Identifier: NCT04250636 and NCT05184452).

Administration of the antibodies 3BNC117 and VRC01 resulted in delayed viral rebound after ART cessation compared with historical controls, but the effects were modest and generally transient (Bar et al., 2016; Scheid et al., 2016). Not surprisingly, rapid selection of archived resistant viral strains reduced the therapeutic efficacy of single bNAbs; for this reason, bNAb combinations were proposed and a phase I clinical trial that combined the bNAbs 3BNC117 and 10–1074 demonstrated effective suppression of viral rebound for a median of 21 weeks (Mendoza et al., 2018). In addition, next-generation antibodies that incorporate the antigen specificity of different bNAbs by binding to multiple nonoverlapping sites on the virus or attaching to both virus and CD4$^+$ receptors have been engineered (Huang et al., 2016; Xu et al., 2017). The administration of three bNAbs targeting the CD4bs (VRC07-523LS), the V3-glycan (PGT121), and the V2 apex

(PGDM1400) resulted in robust reduction of plasma HIV RNA levels in viremic individuals not on ART. Viral rebound, however, occurred quickly and demonstrated partial to complete resistance to PGDM1400 and PGT121, suggesting rapid selection of viral escape variants (Julg et al., 2022). Triple combinations of bNAbs or a tri-specific antibody (Xu et al., 2017) are currently being evaluated in additional early phase clinical trials (ClinicalTrials.gov identifiers: NCT03721510 and NCT03705169).

These results will need to be studied further, especially with regard to impact on the latent reservoir and immune dysregulation, as chronic antigen stimulation should be reduced by these antibodies. Further, the lack of accessibility of antibodies to certain anatomic reservoir sites, such as the central nervous system, will need to be overcome.

DUAL-AFFINITY RETARGETING

A novel method to combine antibody and T-cell activity against HIV-1–infected cells is through bispecific protein constructs (dual-affinity retargeting (DARTs)), which are designed to latch onto HIV-1 envelope proteins on the surface of infected cells while also binding to CD3 on T-cells. This approach directs cytotoxic T-cells to eliminate infected cells while obviating the need for the T-cells to specifically bind to HIV-1 surface antigens (Sung et al., 2015; Pegu et al., 2015). Early in vitro studies of this approach are promising, and this concept has been explored in a phase 1 study and results are pending (ClinicalTrials.gov identifiers: NCT03570918).

COMBINATION STRATEGIES

The first randomized human trial using the "shock and kill" cure strategy was the RIVER study that combined a therapeutic vaccine ChAdV63.HIVconsv prime with MVA.HIVconsv boost, followed by administration of the LRA vorinostat. Disappointingly, no significant change in the viral reservoir was observed (Fidler et al., 2020). Another trial tested the combination of the HDACi romidepsin and the MVA.HIVconsv vaccine in early -treated PWH and a sustained suppression of viremia up to 32 weeks was reported (Mothe et al., 2020). In a randomized phase Ib/IIa trial, the impact of latency reservoir romidepsin followed by 3BNC117 on reservoir size, time to viral rebound was compared to romidepsin alone. Twenty patients were enrolled;, the combination did not reduce the reservoir size or delay viral rebound (Gruell et al., 2022). Another phase 2a trial is evaluating the efficacy of the TLR9-agonist lefitolimid with the bNAbs 3BNC117 and 10-1074 (ClinicalTrials.gov identifier: NCT03837756), while latter antibody in combination with the bNAb VRC07-523LS and the IL-15 superagonist N-803 is evaluated during an analytic treatment interruption (ClinicalTrials.gov identifier: NCT04340596). Another clinical trial is currently exploring the combination of (i) LRAs, (ii) therapeutic vaccines, and (iii) bNAbs (ClinicalTrials.gov Identifier: NCT04357821). There are also exciting results from a study combining a TLR-7 agonist with the broadly neutralizing antibody PGT121 in a nonhuman primate study, resulting in a subset of animals that did not have viral rebound upon ART interruption (Borducchi et al., 2018).

OTHER IMMUNOMODULATORY TREATMENTS

Because T- cell activation is controlled by several signaling pathways, inhibitors of these pathways may also play a role in reducing the size of the latent viral reservoir. Early preclinical research has shown that mTOR inhibitors (e.g., sirolimus, temsirolimus, and everolimus) may play a role in reducing T-cell activation and inflammation (Heredia et al., 2015; Martin et al., 2015; Palmer et al., 2015), although clinical trial data are lacking. A phase 4 study evaluated the impact of everolimus on HIV persistence post kidney or liver transplant in patients who are stable on ART. The study failed to demonstrate significant change in low-level viremia or CD4 $^+$ T-cell associated HIV-DNA or RNA levels 6 months after initiation of everolimus. However, the authors noted that participants who achieved a higher everolimus trough level of 5 during the first 2 months had significant sustained reduction in cellular RNA levels at 12 months. This study supported the hypothesis that there is a mechanistic interaction between mTOR inhibitor use and HIV persistence (Henrich et al., 2021).

GENE MODIFICATION

Gene therapy, also referred to as "intracellular immunization," involves the insertion of protective genes either mechanically or by viral vectors. Gene therapy research has focused on two areas: the disruption of cellular genes involved in HIV entry, such as the CCR5 coreceptor, and the introduction of genes to disrupt HIV replication. The goal of gene therapy in HIV is to have the target cells produce gene products that protect them and their progeny from HIV infection. The use of various technologies, including ribozymes, aptamers, RNA-based interference strategies, and zinc-finger nucleases, is currently being investigated.

RENDERING THE HOST'S CD4 $^+$ T-CELLS RESISTANT TO INFECTION

The Berlin patient, the London patient and others appear to be cured from HIV-1 after receiving stem cell transplants from CCR5Δ32 homozygous donor, which inspired attempts to generate HIV-1 resistant cells through gene therapy. Zinc-finger nucleases (ZFNs) are bioengineered restriction enzymes with two functional domains—one that recognizes DNA and another that cleaves it. ZFNs can bind specific DNA sequences, produce a double-stranded break, and then lead to permanent gene disruption when cellular repair pathways lead to the addition or deletion of nucleotides at the break site. ZFNs have been shown to disrupt CCR5 expression in human stem cells administered in a mouse model of HIV and to be associated with lower HIV viral loads after HIV challenge (Perez et al., 2008; Holt et al., 2010) and have entered evaluation in clinical trials.

SB-728T, an infusion of ZFN-modified autologous CD4$^+$ T-cells with the ability to knock out CCR5 expression, increased CD4$^+$ T-cell counts, decreased proviral DNA, and restored the CD4$^+$-depleted population of the gut mucosa in PWH with CD4$^+$ T-cell counts >200 cells/μL (June et al., 2012; Lalezar et al., 2012). One participant with the highest level of CCR5 modification had an undetectable viral load when ART treatment interruption occurred. Using the ZFN strategy, researchers modified the CCR5 gene ex vivo in autologous CD4$^+$ T-cells in 12 PWH and infused the cells back into the autologous donors (Tebas et al., 2014). The study found that genetically modified CD4$^+$ T-cells were significantly increased and persisted in vivo with a half-life of nearly a year. While no dramatic difference was seen in viral load set points following interruption of ART in six study participants, the modified cells appeared to be protected from HIV-1 infection as unmodified cells showed a faster depletion. Six of these patients underwent 12-week ART interruption, but in only one patient (heterozygous for the CCR5Δ32 mutation) did the viral load decline to an undetectable level prior to ART reinitiation.

Additional studies of SB-728T are under way, with one examining CCR5Δ32 heterozygotes and another examining the use of cytoxan prior to CD4$^+$ T-cell infusion to decrease the number of existing CD4$^+$ T-cells. Early data from the latter trial have demonstrated that cyclophosphamide treatment is well-tolerated with a dose-related increase in total CD4$^+$ T-cell count and engraftment of CCR5-modified cells (Blick et al., 2014). While this approach did not lead to durable suppression of HIV after cessation of ART, it did appear to delay viral load rebound in study participants (Tebas et al., 2021). Additional research investigating HIV-1 coreceptor modulation is ongoing.

Recent data in SHIV-infected and ART-suppressed pigtail macaques demonstrated that CCR5 gene-edited hematopoietic stem/progenitor cells (HSPCs) persisted following transplantation and expansion through virus-dependent positive selection, resulting in a significant reduction of tissue-associated SHIV DNA and RNA levels in the transplanted animals compared to controls (Peterson et al., 2018). Gene editing techniques carry a risk for off-target effects causing mutations at unintended sites in the genome, a currently relevant hurdle to their use in clinical trials (Cradick et al., 2013). The safety and feasibility of administration of clustered regularly interspaced short palindromic repeat (CRISPR)/Cas9 CCR5 gene-modified CD34$^+$ HSPC and ZFN CCR5 modified autologous CD4$^+$ T-cells in ART-suppressed HIV-positive individuals is currently being evaluated (ClinicalTrials.gov identifiers: NCT02500849 and NCT03164135, respectively). Of note, a 2019 report describes the case of an individual with HIV and acute lymphoblastic leukemia who was treated with an allogeneic bone marrow transplant in which the CCR5Δ32 mutation was introduced using CRISPR/Cas9. Cells with the deletion were only found in a small percentage of bone marrow engrafted cells. While the leukemia was subsequently in remission, the patient experienced viral rebound shortly after interrupting ART (Xu et al., 2019), perhaps because too few cells carried the protective mutation.

EXCISING THE HIV-1 PROVIRUS FROM THE HOST CELL GENOME

The CRISPR/Cas9 system permits targeted and precise genome editing in diverse cell types and organisms, including human cells (Cong et al., 2013; Maslennikova & Mazurov, 2022). Recently, several research groups have successfully applied gene editing technology to excise HIV-1 provirus from the host cell genome in vitro (Ebina et al., 2013; Hu et al., 2014; Liao et al., 2015). Importantly, the disruption of provirus expression not only restricted transcriptionally active provirus, but it also blocked the expression of latently integrated provirus (Ebina et al., 2013). Moreover, inserting the stably expressed CRISPR/Cas9 system into a T-cell line conferred long-term protection against HIV-1 infection (Liao et al., 2015). These results from in vitro cell culture models are promising, and this technology may open new avenues to developing antiviral therapies in the future.

RIBOZYMES, RNA-BASED INTERFERENCE, AND APTAMERS

Ribozymes are small, catalytically active RNA molecules that can be engineered to target specific RNA sequences. They target viral RNA during uncoating and after transcription of HIV, leading to RNA degradation. Although in vitro studies of ribozyme gene therapy have been promising, retroviral vectors delivering ribozymes targeting viral targets (e.g., Tat and Rev) have been plagued by problems with low transduction efficiency (Mitsuyasu et al., 2009).

RNA interference utilizes short RNAs that mediate the degradation of mRNAs in a sequence-specific manner: antisense oligonucleotides bind mRNA and trigger degradation through an RNase H-dependent pathway or block ribosome binding, thus preventing gene expression. Clinical research in this field has been limited by the ability to deliver the RNAs to the correct target cells, poor cellular uptake and stability, and viral escape (Zhou & Rossi, 2011). VRX496 (Lexgenleucel-T), antisense Env in a lentiviral vector, has been delivered via autologous CD4$^+$ T-cell infusion to both patients on failing regimens and patients on a fully suppressive ART regimen. In one trial, 17 patients received Lexgenleucel-T over 16 weeks, with ART interruption 1 month later in 13 of these patients (Tebas et al., 2013). Six of eight patients analyzed were noted to have a decrease in viral load set point. The use of a short-interfering RNA targeting a unique triple repeat of NF-κB was also shown to achieve long-term suppression of HIV-1 (Singh et al., 2014).

Aptamers are single-stranded RNA or DNA molecules that bind viral proteins, preventing them from carrying out their function in the viral life cycle (Figure 19.1). In clinical trials, when used alone, they have not been shown to be

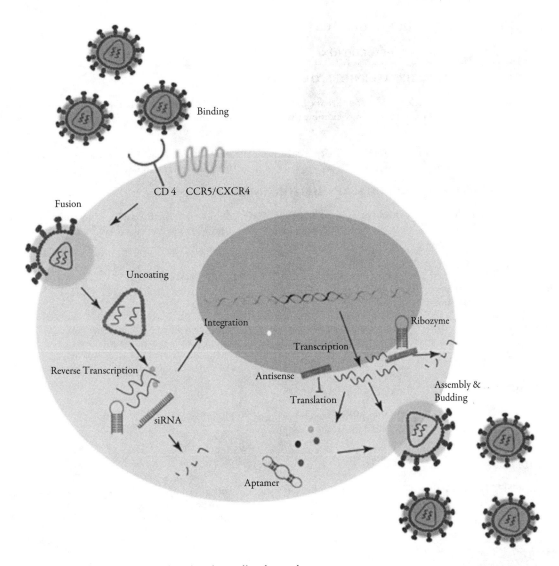

Figure 19.1 Schematic diagram of the HIV viral life cycle in host cell and gene therapy targets   SOURCE: Zeller S, Kumar P. RNA-based gene therapy for the treatment and prevention of HIV: from bench to bedside. *Yale J Biol Med*. 2011;84(3):301–309.

effective. However, strategies combining aptamers, ribozymes, and RNA interference, based on in vitro efficacy have shown potent inhibition of HIV-1 in vitro (Brake et al., 2008; Centlivre, 2013).

OTHER GENE STRATEGIES

A strategy to render T-cells resistant to HIV replication is the use of MazF-T (, i.e., autologous CD4 $^+$ T-cells modified with the MazF endoribonuclease gene) (Saito et al., 2014). Modified stem cells are being evaluated for PWH with hematologic malignancies. Although promising, it will be difficult to develop these and other gene strategies for widespread use because of high technical demands and costs. Gene therapy could also hypothetically be used to inhibit viral fusion. C46, a peptide with structural similarity to enfuvirtide, has been engineered for expression on autologous T-cells and was well tolerated in clinical trials, although clinical efficacy has not yet been demonstrated (van Lundzen et al., 2007).

A dual-cassette, lentiviral vector expressing CCR5 shRNA (knockdown) and C46 (CAL-1) has been shown in preclinical studies to be nontoxic and to protect gene-modified cells from both CXCR4- and CCR5-tropic HIV-1 strains (Wolstein, 2014). The results of a phase 1/2a clinical trial using autologous, CAL-1–modified CD4 $^+$ T-cells and hematopoietic progenitor/stem cells with and without bone marrow precondition (busulfan) in PLWH demonstrated safety, but only transient evidence of bone marrow engraftment (Mitsuyasu et al., 2020).

NOVEL NONCURATIVE ANTIRETROVIRAL DRUGS

Antiretroviral therapy (ART) remains the mainstay of treatment for PWH. Novel drugs, both within existing and new classes, are in various stages of development and testing (Table 19.1). Fostemsavir, an oral attachment inhibitor binding to HIV-1 gp120 and, thereby, blocking viral attachment

Table 19.1 ANTIRETROVIRAL DRUGS IN CLINICAL TRIALS

AGENT	DESCRIPTION	STAGE OF DEVELOPMENT
NUCLEOSIDE REVERSE TRANSCRIPTASE INHIBITORS (NRTIS)		
Elvucitabine (ELV)	Cytosine nucleoside analogue that can be used in cases of resistance to emtricitabine (ftc) or lamivudine (3tc)	Phase 2 trials completed. Drug out licensed for further development in China, Taiwan, and Hong Kong
Islatravir(MK-8591)	Nucleoside reverse transcriptase translocation inhibitor	Phase 3, placed on clinical hold in December 2021 (risk of lymphopenia); some studies continued with lower dosing
NONNUCLEOSIDE REVERSE TRANSCRIPTASE INHIBITORS (NNRTSS)		
Elsulfavirine (VM 1500)	Elsulfavirine is an oral prodrug of VM 1500; VM 1500 is available in a long-acting intramuscular formulation	Approved in Russia 2017 for combination art, ongoing clinical evaluation elsewhere
ENTRY AND FUSION INHIBITORS		
Fostemsavir (FTR)	Attaches to HIV GP120 to prevent HIV attachment to the host CD4 $^+$ T-cell	FDA approved in July 2020
Cenicriviroc (CVC)	Once-daily CCR5 antagonist that also HAS CCR2 activity (anti-inflammatory effect)	Phase 2 trial demonstrated improvement in neurocognition among participants with aids dementia complex; phase 3 trials in PWH planned, currently undergoing phase 3 clinical trials in participants with NASH
INHIBITORS OF REV-MEDIATED VIRAL RNA BIOGENESIS		
ABX464	Enhances viral MRNA splicing by interfering with these Rev-mediated functions (Campos, 2015)	Phase 2 trials
CAPSID INHIBITORS		
Lenacapavir (GS-6207)	Long-acting agent administered subcutaneously	Authorized by the European Commission (2022) for use in combination ART for resistant HIV and lack of alternatives, further approvals expected

CVC, Cenicriviroc; ELV, elvucitabine; FTC, emtricitabine; FTR, fostemsavir; INSTIs, integrase strand inhibitors; NNRTIs, nonnucleoside reverse transcriptase inhibitors; NRTIs, nucleoside reverse transcriptase inhibitors; 3TC, lamivudine.

to host CD4 $^+$ T-cells, was approved by the FDA in 2020 (Kozal et al., 2020).

Islatravir is a nucleoside reverse transcriptase translocation inhibitor in clinical development. MK-8591 triphosphate (MK-8591 TP) is the active phosphorylated form, which has a half-life of 78–128 hours in human peripheral blood mononuclear cells. In an open-label study, a single dose of MK-8591 in HIV-1 treatment-naiïve participants showed a greater than 1 $\log_{10}$ viral load decline after 7–10 days (Schurmann et al., 2020). A phase 2 randomized trial to evaluate the safety, tolerability, and ARV activity of MK-8591 in combination with doravirine and lamivudine was started. Primate studies have demonstrated clinically relevant drug exposures for more than 6 months after single a single dose of parenterally administered MK-8591, supporting evaluation of extended dosing formulations, which may have utility as PrEP or maintenance treatment (Barrett et al., 2018). Islatravir showed further promise in later stage clinical trials. As of October 2022, however, following multiple occurrences of mild-moderate lymphopenia, with decreased CD4 + T-cells, islatravir studies were first placed on clinical hold by the FDA and later reopened using reduced doses of islatravir in HIV treatment studies only. At the current time, islatravir will be developed for HIV treatment only and not HIV prophylaxis.

Cenicriviroc is a novel oral CCR5 and CCR2 antagonist that showed potent antiviral activity in treatment-experienced HIV-1 patients. In a phase 2 controlled trial, 143 treatment-naiïve patients were randomly assigned to cenicriviroc 100 mg or 200 mg or efavirenz. At 24 weeks, virologic suppression was achieved in 76%, 73%, and 71% of patients; and at 48 weeks, in 68%, 64%, and 50%, respectively (Thompson et al., 2016).

VM1500A (elsulfavirine) is a new oral prodrug NNRTI approved in Russia in 2017 for treatment of HIV-1 in combination with standard ART. A phase 1 study to assess the safety of a long-acting intramuscular formulation of VM1500A was recently presented at Conferences on Retroviruses and Opportunistic Infections (Yakubova et al., 2020).

Other novel ARV agents in early stage development include a Rev inhibitor (ABX 464) (Moron-Lopez et al., 2020); capsid inhibitor (GS-6207 or lenacapavir) (Link et al., 2020; Zheng et al., 2018); maturation inhibitor (GSK3640254) (Krystal et al., 2016); entry inhibitor (combinectin-GSK3732394); and a new NRTI active against resistant virus (GS-9131) (White et al., 2017). Phase 1 data of the capsid inhibitor lenacapavir demonstrated a significant reduction of 1.4 to 2.3 log viral load at day 10 after a single subcutaneous (SC) injection in patients who were experienced off ARV for 12 months. Owing to its unique mechanism of action blocking two stages of the viral life cycle, lenacapavir may have a higher threshold to development of resistance. Moreover, it is being used as a long-acting ARV (e.g., allowing for twice yearly dosing), and is available as an oral and subcutaneous formulation. Lenacapavir was more efficacious than placebo to reduce viral loads in heavily treated participants with multidrug-resistant HIV and led to high rates of virologic suppression in the phase 3 CAPELLA trial (Segal-Maurer et al., 2022). These results led to marketing authorization by the European Commission for lenacapavir in combination with other ARVs for multidrug-resistant HIV in the absence of alternative options. Another advantage of lenacapavir for certain situations is that it allows use as a long-acting antiretroviral (e.g., twice yearly dosing was used in the CAPELLA study).

CONCLUSION

Although antiretroviral medications effectively treat HIV-1 infection, there are many compelling reasons to attempt to cure HIV-1, not the least of which is the stigma and isolation experienced by many people with HIV. The major barrier to HIV-1 cure is the persistence of a long-lived population of latently infected cells in PWH on suppressive treatment. The latent reservoir is likely established very early during infection which has rendered attempts to prevent its formation futile to this point. Current efforts to cure HIV-1 infection are centered on flushing HIV-1 out of the latent reservoir along with enhancing immune mechanisms to clear infected cells. We are still in the early days of this massively difficult undertaking, and it is too soon to tell whether the approaches being pursued will be effective. That being said, just as the development of combination ART was based on a series of advances that culminated in our ability to successfully treat HIV-1, the stepwise progress being made today will hopefully lead us to an even greater breakthrough: the capability to eradicate or control HIV-1 without the need for lifelong therapy.

RECOMMENDED READING

Ahlensteil CL, Suzuki K, Marks K, et al. Controlling HIV-1: noncoding RNA gene therapy approaches a functional cure. *Front Immunol*. 2015;6:474.

Arthos JA, Cicala C, Nawaz F, et al. The role of integrin α4β7 in HIV pathogenesis and treatment. *Curr Opin HIV AIDS*. 2018;15:127–135.

Barouch DH, Deeks SG. Immunologic strategies for HIV-1 remission and eradication. *Science*. 2014; 45(6193):169–174.

Chomont N, El-Far M, Ancuta P, et al. HIV reservoir size and persistence are driven by T cell survival and homeostatic proliferation. *Nat Med*. 2009;15(8):893–900.

Choudhary MC, Cyktor JC, Riddler SA. Advances in HIV-1-specific chimeric antigen receptor cells to target the HIV-1 reservoir. *J Virus Erad*. 2022 Jun 18;8(2):100073.

Deeks SG, Archin N, Cannon P, et al. International AIDS Society (IAS) Global Scientific Strategy working group. Research priorities for an HIV cure: International AIDS Society Global Scientific Strategy 2021. *Nat Med*. December 2021;27(12):2085–2098.

Frater J. New approaches in HIV eradication research. *Curr Opin Infect Dis*. 2011;24(6):593–598.

Gubser C, Chiu C, Lewin SR, Rasmussen TA. Immune checkpoint blockade in HIV. *EBioMedicine*. February 2022;76:103840.

Kitchen SG, Shimizu S, A DS. Stem cell-based anti-HIV gene therapy. *Virology*. 2011;411:260–272.

Levy J. Not an HIV cure but encouraging new directions. *N Engl J Med*. 2009;360:724–725.

Lewin S, Rouzioux C. HIV cure and eradication: how will we get from the laboratory to effective clinical trials? *AIDS*. 2011;25:885–897.

Olender SA, Taylor BS, Wong M, et al. CROI 2015: advances in antiretroviral therapy. *Top Antivir Med*. 2015;23(1):28–45.

Pace P, Markowitz M. Monoclonal antibodies to host cellular receptors for the treatment and prevention of HIV-1 infection. *Curr Opin HIV AIDS*. 2015;10(3):144–150.

Richman DD, Margolis DM, Delaney M., et al. The challenge of finding a cure for HIV infection. *Science*. 2009;323(5919):1304–1307.

Wykes MN, Lewin SR. Immune checkpoint blockade in infectious diseases. *Nat Rev Immunol*. February 2018;18(2):91–104.

THERAPEUTIC AND PREVENTIVE VACCINES

LEARNING OBJECTIVE

Discuss the progression and status of research in HIV vaccines.

WHAT'S NEW?

HIV vaccine research has seen a resurgence in recent years with different classes of vaccines showing promise in clinical trials.

KEY POINTS

- Therapeutic immunization is a strategy for boosting anti-HIV-1 immunity in chronically infected PWH.

- Recent therapeutic vaccines under study have provided more durable and diverse immune responses and lowering of viral load set points.

- Many different types of vaccines have progressed to phase 2 trials, including DNA, subunit, and dendritic cell vaccines and novel vaccine concepts using mRNA are being explored in phase 1 studies.

OVERVIEW OF VACCINE TRIALS 1990–2015

Therapeutic immunization aims to induce a cellular immune response through vaccination with components of HIV-1 that will help contain viral replication through reconstitution of anti-HIV-1 immune responses. Data support the observation that the cellular immune response is critical in controlling HIV-1 replication, as reported in persons with primary HIV-1 infection and in HIV long-term nonprogressors (Borrow et al., 1994; Cao et al., 1995; Kroup et al., 1994; Rosenberg et al., 1997). Therapeutic vaccines can potentially be of benefit to ART-naive PWH by delaying progression to AIDS and time to initiation of ART. Among PWH on ART, development of a durable vaccine may intensify the effects of ART (accelerate response time to therapy, decrease risk of transmission, potentiate the immune effects of ART, and reduce proviral DNA), simplify ART regimens, and support regimens with treatment interruption (Ensoli et al., 2014).

Clinical therapeutic vaccine research for HIV started prior to the introduction of ART, first with a gp120-depleted inactivated HIV-1 preparation and then with vectors expressing viral proteins (e.g., Gag p17 and p24). Clinical trials of these agents largely failed to show efficacy and a sustained HIV-1-specific response (Hardy et al., 2007). Subsequent vaccines with recombinant HIV-1 glycoproteins (e.g., gp120 and gp160) also fared poorly, not altering the decline in CD4 $^+$ T-cell count or halting disease progression in HIV-1–infected individuals in phase 2 trials (Eron et al., 1996; Pontesilli et al., 1998; Sandstrom et al., 1999; Tsoukas et al., 1998). In one of the largest of these trials, 608 HIV-1–infected individuals with CD4$^+$ T-cell counts of greater than 400 cells/mm^3 were repeatedly immunized with a recombinant gp160 vaccine (VaxSyn HIV-1) or placebo and followed for 3–5 years. Although the vaccine had excellent immunogenicity (~70%), it failed to show a difference in reaching the primary clinical end points: a 50% decline in CD4 $^+$ T-cell count or disease progression to Walter Reed stages 4, 5, and 6 (Birx et al., 2000).

ANRS 093, a study of 70 PWH, compared ART to immunization with recombinant canarypox vector expressing several HIV genes (Env, Gag, Pol, and Nef) and lipo-6T (HIV-1 lipopepides) followed by SQ IL-2. The vaccine elicited a statistically significant INF-γ–producing CD8 $^+$ T-cell response that correlated with virologic control (Levy et al., 2005). The vaccine group had a lower viral set point and therefore a significantly greater number of days off ART (Levy et al., 2006), but the results of this study await validation in larger trials.

In ACTG 5197, administration of a replication-defective adenovirus type 5 HIV-1 Gag vaccine to PWH with CD4 $^+$ T-cell counts >500 cells/mm^3 failed to be sufficiently immunogenic and lacked statistically significant efficacy (Schooley et al., 2010). The finding that the plasma viral load was 0.5 log$_{10}$ lower in the vaccine arm at 16 weeks post-ART interruption prompted further analysis of the HLA class I alleles in all 110 participants because HLA classes have previously been shown to influence viral evolution and disease progression. Vaccinated PWH with neutral HLA alleles in this cohort had a lower plasma viral load than those of both PWH vaccinated with protective alleles and placebo participants with neutral alleles (Li et al., 2011).

A novel therapeutic vaccine strategy with promising results targeted Tat, a transactivator of HIV gene expression essential for viral replication which is relatively conserved among HIV-1 subtypes. This vaccine is aimed at PWH on ART with the hope of decreasing viral reservoirs and restoring immune homeostasis. In phase 2 trials, 168 PWH controlled on ART and anti-Tat antibody negative at baseline who were administered the vaccine three or five times monthly showed specific and durable immune responses when followed for up to 144 weeks (Ensoli et al., 2015). Most persons (79%) developed anti-Tat antibodies, which was associated with significant reduction of proviral DNA seen after week 72. The vaccine was also associated with a restoration of T, B, and NK cells and CD4 $^+$ and CD8 $^+$ T-cell central memory subsets.

A multinational phase 2 trial examined the safety and immunogenicity of Vacc-4x, a peptide-based HIV-1 therapeutic vaccine targeting the conserved domains of p24Gag (Pollard et al., 2014). In chronically infected PWH who were virologically suppressed on ART, the Vacc-4x vaccine did not alter time to ART resumption or lead to significant changes in CD4 $^+$ T-cell count at week 28 during treatment interruption. However, there was a statistically significant difference in HIV viral load at both week 48 (23,000 vs. 71,800 copies/mL) and week 52 (19,500 vs. 51,000 copies/mL).

T-CELL VACCINES

The ability to enhance the host's immune responses by therapeutic vaccination faces several key challenges. The majority of PWH have dysfunctional virus-specific effector cells (Sauce et al., 2013) as a result of continuous antigenic stimulation prior to treatment; indeed, ART only incompletely restores T-cell functionality on an epigentic level (Youngblood et al., 2013). Further, in PWH who initiate ART during chronic infection, almost all of the proviral sequences in the latent reservoir contain escape mutations that prevent killing of infected cells by cytotoxic T lymphocytes (Deng et al., 2015; Papuchon et al., 2013; Deng et al., 2015). The implication is that an effective vaccination strategy, instead of just expanding preexisting responses that already had failed to control the infection, would need to improve the quality and functionality of HIV-1-–specific immune response and elicit CD8 $^+$ T-cell responses against previously untargeted epitopes or unmutated regions of the virus to avoid escape (reviewed in Chen & Julg, 2020). To achieve this goal, multiple approaches are currently being tested in preclinical and clinical studies, including:

- Viral-vector–based vaccines, such as adenovirus, poxvirus modified vaccinia Ankara (MVA), vesicular stomatitis virus, and modified cytomegalovirus (CMV). Some of these approaches to deliver HIV-1 antigens have demonstrated robust immunogenicity, inducing broad and durable cellular immune responses, which were able to protect monkeys against SIV infection in preclinical challenge studies (Barouch et al., 2012, 2013a; Hansen, 2011, 2013), which were able to protect monkeys against SIV infection in preclinical challenge studies, but, more importantly, significantly reduced the viral load set points in SIV-infected macaques following ART cessation when combined with a TLR7 agonist (Borducchi et al., 2016). A phase I/IIa clinical trial of an Ad26 prime/MVA boost combination with mosaic HIV inserts in a cohort that initiated ART during the acute infection, however, did not lead to viremic control after treatment interruption (Colby et al., 2020). Studies in individuals who started ART during chronic infection are ongoing (ClinicalTrials.gov identifiers: NCT03307915). Another MVA-vectored vaccine trial expressing tHIVconsv3 and tHIVconsv4 immunogens evaluates its safety and efficacy in adults with HIV (ClinicalTrials.gov identifiers: NCT03844386). Furthermore, a prototype human CMV-based HIV vaccine is currently being tested (ClinicalTrials.gov Identifier: NCT04725877).

- Plasmid DNA expressing HIV-1 genes (Hallengard et al., 2011; Ramirez et al., 2013; Rodriguez et al., 2013; Sneller, 2017). A phase II trial is currently evaluating whether the PENNVAX-B vaccine, a synthetic plasmid expressing HIV Gag, Pol, and Env, leads to a significant reduction of HIV reservoir size (ClinicalTrials.gov identifier: NCT03606213). Another vaccine with HIV-derived conserved element (CE) p24 Gag DNA showed promising immunogenicity in macaques (Hu et al., 2016), and a human study just completed enrollment (ClinicalTrials.gov identifier: NCT03560258). The DNA plasmid vaccine GTU-multi-HIV-B, aimed at inducing immune responses to HIV-1 regulatory genes, has shown efficacy in HIV-1 subtype C PWH not on ART. In a population of 63 persons, the vaccine was deemed safe and was associated with a statistically significant decline in log pHIV-RNA with an increase in CD4$^+$ T-cell counts nearing significance compared to placebo, especially after intramuscular injections (Vardas et al., 2012). The GTU-multi-HIV-B DNA vaccine and LIPO-5 vaccine in a prime-boost strategy in PWH virologically suppressed on ART elicited strong and polyfunctional HIV-specific CD4 + and CD8 + T-cell responses, but these responses were not able to control viremia following antiretroviral treatment interruption (Levy et al., 2021).

- Dendritic cell–based vaccines to deliver HIV-1 antigens. Significant attention has also focused on dendritic cells as cellular adjuvants for therapeutic HIV-1 vaccines because they have been shown to elicit strong CD4$^+$ and CD8$^+$ T-cell responses in vivo. One uncontrolled study of immunization of 18 treatment-naive PWH with dendritic cells pulsed with inactivated autologous virus reported a 90% decrease in viral load during the course of a year (Lu et al., 2004). A subsequent randomized controlled trial of 24 treatment-naive participants with a similar vaccine, however, showed a weak HIV-1-specific response and a modest decrease in viral load compared to placebo (Garcia et al., 2011). In a trial of chronically infected PWH on ART with CD4$^+$ T-cell counts > 450 cells/mm^3, the use of a monocyte-derived dendritic cell pulse with heat-inactivated whole HIV helped lower plasma viral load set point after treatment interruption, with an associated increased in HIV-1–specific T-cell responses compared to placebo (Garcia et al., 2013). Recent trials have continued to demonstrate better vaccine responses and control of viral replication (Levy et al., 2014). Dendritic cells expressing the HIV proteins Gag, Tat, Rev, and Nef administered as a vaccine have been shown to elicit potent antiviral T-cell responses in PWH

on ART, including a Gag-specific IFN-γ response that correlated with HIV-1 inhibitory activity (van Gulck et al., 2012). An ongoing trial aims to test if autologous dendritic cells loaded with a conserved HIV Gag and Pol peptide pool or inactivated autologous HIV will yield broader T-cell responses (ClinicalTrials.gov identifier: NCT03758625).

Although no therapeutic vaccine is currently FDA approved, the future of therapeutic vaccine research for both naive and ART-treated PWH remains promising. Recent data have been encouraging, but the results of therapeutic vaccine trials have yet to yield a therapeutic vaccine strategy that can be implemented. In addition to further clinical trials of the vaccines discussed previously, additional studies investigating the heterogeneity of response to vaccines (e.g., genetic determinants) and the immunologic correlates of vaccine efficacy are needed for the field to advance. Some of the key vaccines in development are highlighted in Table 19.2.

PREVENTIVE VACCINES

Although a preventive HIV-1 vaccine would help control the worldwide AIDS pandemic, there have been many obstacles to its development. HIV-1 has significant genetic and antigenic diversity, making it difficult to target with a vaccine. The failure to induce broadly neutralizing antibodies against the virus and the lack of clear immune correlates of protection have also been challenges. Additionally, the SIV/SHIV nonhuman primate models on which preclinical testing of the vaccines is typically done have often showed promising results not reproduced in human clinical trials.

Multiple phase 1 and 2 vaccine trials were conducted dating back to 1987, but very few reached phase 2b/3. Initial trials used recombinant proteins to induce neutralizing antibodies. In two large randomized controlled trials, VAX003 and VAX004, involving vaccination with recombinant gp120 subunits, there were no statistically significant reductions in HIV infection in the vaccinated groups (Flynn et al., 2005; Pitisuttithum et al., 2006). In subsequent analysis, these vaccines seemed to fail due to a lack of a broad neutralizing antibody response.

Vaccine development subsequently shifted toward the use of live viral or bacterial vectors engineered to carry genes encoding the HIV antigens. These antigens are expressed in the cytoplasm of the target cell, broken down, and then presented on the surface of the cell, priming a CD8$^+$ response. In the STEP trial, HIV-negative participants received immunization with three injections of a replication-incompetent recombinant adenovirus vector expressing HIV-1 Gag, Pol, and Nef (Buchbinder et al., 2008). The vaccine did not show any benefit in preventing transmission or reducing early viral load after infection.

Surprisingly, however, vaccinated persons who were seropositive for AD-5 or uncircumcised had higher rates of HIV-1 infection than placebo, a finding prompting discontinuation of a contemporaneous clinical trial with the same vaccine. Subsequent genetic sequencing of the HIV-1 strains from the

Table 19.2 SELECT THERAPEUTIC VACCINE TRIALS

VACCINE*	DESCRIPTION	STAGE OF DEVELOPMENT	REGISTRATION NUMBER
MVA.HTI + ChAdOx1.HTI + vesatolimod	Viral vector vaccine + TLR7 agonist	Phase 2	NCT04364035
MVA HIV-B +/– vedolizumab	Viral vector vaccine +/– anti-$\alpha_4\beta_7$ integrin antibody	Phase 2	NCT04120415
ChAdV63.HIVconsv + MVA.HIVconsv + vorinostat	Viral vector vaccine + HDAC inhibitor	Phase 2	NCT02336074 UK CPMS18010
Ad26.Mos4.HIV, MVA-BN-HIV, PGT121, PGDM1400, VRC07-523LS	Viral vector vaccine +/– broadly neutralizing antibodies	Phase 1/2	NCT04983030
L-12 adjuvanted p24CE + MVA/HIV62B + lefitolimod + VRC07-523LS + 10-1074	Viral vector vaccine + TLR9 agonist + broadly neutralizing antibodies	Phase 1/2	NCT04357821
ChAdOx1.HTI, MVA.HTI, ConM SOSIP.v7 gp140	Viral vector vaccine + recombinant HIV-1 envelope protein	Phase 1	NCT05208125
HVRRICANE	DNA vaccine (HIVIS DNA) + viral vector vaccine (MVA-CMDR) +/– TLR4 agonist	Phase 1	NCT04301154
DC-HIV04	Dendritic cell vaccine (a1DC or pgDC) + inactivated whole autologous HIV or conserved HIV peptides	Phase 1	NCT03758625
NETI	Recombinant HIV envelope protein VRC-HIVRGP096-00-VP (Trimer 4571) therapeutic vaccination	Phase 1	NCT04985760

* https://www.treatmentactiongroup.org/cure/trials/.

vaccine and placebo groups revealed that the virus infecting the vaccine group had different epitopes from those in the placebo group (Rolland et al., 2011). The divergence was confined to the vaccine components of the virus, supporting the notion of selective pressure from vaccine-induced T-cell responses.

More recent vaccine strategies have used a heterologous prime-boost strategy to activate both cellular and humoral immune arms by priming with a certain vaccine (e.g., DNA vaccine) and then boosting the immune response with another type of vaccine (e.g., live vector vaccine) (Girard et al., 2011). The RV144 trial, a phase 3 randomized controlled trial, primed participants with two successive doses of a canarypox vector (ALVAC) encoding Gag/Pro and Env antigens followed by two additional immunizations with this vector and AIDSVAX B/E, a bivalent HIV gp120 envelope glycoprotein derived from a subtype B and subtype E envelope (Rerks-Ngarm et al., 2009). Seventy-four of 7,325 in the placebo group and 51 of 7,347 in the vaccine group developed HIV-1 infection at 96 weeks, offering a mildly statistically significant 31% efficacy. These results were encouraging, but there was not a significant broadly neutralizing antibody response, and the vaccine efficacy peaked in the first 6–12 months (50%–60%) only to decrease thereafter. Analysis of the RV144 trial, however, showed two immune correlates of infection risk after vaccination (Haynes et al., 2012). Binding of IgG antibodies to the variable regions of Env inversely correlated with infection rates, while plasma IgA binding to Env was directly correlated.

Building on the RV144 data, the HIV Vaccine Trials Network implemented HVTN 100, a phase 1/2, randomized controlled, double-blind trial in South Africa that compared a canarypox vector, ALVAC-HIV[vCP2438], in combination with an envelope glycoprotein (gp120), both adapted to circulating strains in South Africa and paired with a more potent adjuvant to placebo. This combination induced strong humoral and cellular responses (Bekker et al., 2018). These encouraging results led to the development of HVTN 702, a phase 2b/3 efficacy trial which randomly assigned 5,404 adults without HIV-1 infection to receive ALVAC-HIV/ bivalent subtype C gp120–MF59 adjuvant (2,704 participants) or placebo (2,700 participants). During an interim analysis, nonefficacy criteria were met and further vaccinations were subsequently halted (Gray et al., 2021).

Another strategy was evaluated in the APPROACH trial, a multicenter, randomized, double-blind, placebo-controlled phase 1/2a trial in Africa, South Africa, Thailand, and the United States (Barouch et al., 2018). The participants received Ad26.Mos.HIV expressing mosaic HIV-1 envelope (Env)/ Gag/Pol antigens and aluminum-adjuvanted clade C Env gp140 protein or placebo. Researchers evaluated the vaccine safety, tolerability, and antibody responses at weeks 28 and 52. A parallel study was also conducted in rhesus monkeys. It elicited Env-specific binding antibody responses (100%) and antibody-dependent cellular phagocytosis responses (80%) at week 52 and T- cell responses at week 50 (83%) in humans.

The most common adverse event was injection site reaction (69%–88%).

After these results, two2 large global trials were initiated to evaluate Ad 26 viral vaccines that express mosaic Env/Gag and Pol antigens. In Sub-Saharan Africa, the HVTN 705 (Imbokodo trial) investigated a trivalent Ad26 construct boosted with a clade C gp140 glycoprotein. Imbokodo recruited 2,600 young women in five southern African countries. There were 14% fewer infections in the women given the vaccine than in women given a placebo, but this did not reached statistical significance (press release: https://www.jnj.com/johnson-johnson-and-global-partners-announce-results-from-phase-2b-imbokodo-hiv-vaccine-clinical-trial-in-young-women-in-sub-saharan-africa). Correlates of protection analyses are ongoing at this point. In the Americas and Europe, HVTN 706 (Mosaico trial) is evaluating a tetravalent Ad26 vector boosted with a bivalent mosaic clade C gp140 glycoprotein with alum adjuvant (Mosaico study) (ClinicalTrials.gov Identifier: NCT03964415) Results are expected by 2024.

More recently, "germline-targeting" recombinant Env immunogen with the goal to specifically stimulate proliferation of B-cells expressing certain bNAb-like B-cell receptors are being explored (ClinicalTrials.gov Identifier: NCT05471076). Further, the HIV Vaccine Trial Network study HVTN302 is now evaluating three different HIV vaccines that are using the mRNA vaccine technology (ClinicalTrials.gov Identifier: NCT05217641).

In summary, recent progress has been made toward the development of a preventive HIV vaccine. Key issues in development remain the identification of the correlates of immunity, induction of broadly neutralizing antibody responses, and the durability of these responses. It is hoped that they will provide insight into the correlates of immunity and eventually lead to an effective preventive vaccine strategy.

RECOMMENDED READING

Ensoli B, Cafaro A, Monini P, et al. Challenges in HIV vaccine research for treatment and prevention. *Front Immunol*. 2014;5:417.

Gilliam BL, Redfield RR. Therapeutic HIV vaccines. *Curr Top Med Chem*. 2003;3(13):2536–1553.

Gotch FM, Imami N, Hardy G. Candidate vaccines for immunotherapy in HIV. *HIV Med*. 2001;2:260–265.

Haynes BF, Wiehe K, Borrow P, et al. Strategies for HIV-1 vaccines that induce broadly neutralizing antibodies. *Nat Rev Immunol*. 2023;23(3):142–158. doi:10.1038/s41577-022-00753-w. Epub 2022 Aug 12.

Levy Y. Therapeutic HIV vaccines: an update. *Curr HIV/AIDS Rep*. 2005;2(1):5–9.

Van Gulck E, Van Tendeloo VF, Berneman ZN, et al. Role of dendritic cells in HIV immunotherapy. *Curr HIV Res*. 2010;8(4):310–322.

ACKNOWLEDGMENTS

This chapter is based on previous versions with contributions from Drs. David Margolis, Adrian Majid, Bruce Gilliam, Niyati Jakharia, and Rohit Talwani.

REFERENCES

Abbink P, Mercado NB, Nkolola JP, et al. Lack of therapeutic efficacy of an antibody to α4β7 in SIVmac251-infected rhesus macaques. *Science*. 2019;365(6457):1029–1033. http://doi:10.1126/science.aaw8562

Abrams D, Levy Y, Losso MH, et al.; INSIGHT-ESPRIT Study Group; SILCAAT Scientific Committee. Interleukin 2 therapy in patients with HIV infection. *N Engl J Med*. 2009;361(16):1548–1559.

Ananworanich J, Schuetz A, Vandergeeten C, et al. Impact of multi-targeted antiretroviral treatment on gut T cell depletion and HIV reservoir seeding during acute HIV infection. *PLoS One*. 2012;7(3):e33948.

Archin NM, Bateson R, Tripathy MK, et al. HIV-1 expression within resting CD4\+\+ T cells after multiple doses of vorinostat. *J Infect Dis*. 2014;210(5):728–735.

ART Collaboration Cohort. Life expectancy of individuals on combination antiretroviral therapy in high-income countries: a collaborative analysis of 14 cohort studies. *Lancet*. 2008;372:293–299.

Bar KJ, Sneller MC, Harrison LJ, et al. Effect of HIV antibody VRC01 on viral rebound after treatment interruption. *N Engl J Med*. 2016;375:2037–2050.

Baron M, Soulie C, Lavole A, et al. Impact of anti-PD-1immunotherapy on HIV reservoir and anti-viral immune responses in people living with HIV and cancer. *Cells*. 2022;11(6):1015.

Barouch DH, Liu J, Li H, et al. Vaccine protection against acquisition of neutralization-resistant SIV challenges in rhesus monkeys. *Nature*. 2012;482(7383):89–93.

Barouch DH, Stephenson KE, Borducchi EN, et al. Protective efficacy of a global HIV-1 mosaic vaccine against heterologous SHIV challenges in rhesus monkeys. *Cell*. 2013a;155(3):531–539.

Barouch DH, Tomaka FL, Wegmann F, et al. Evaluation of a mosaic HIV-1 vaccine in a multicentre, randomised, double-blind, placebo-controlled, phase 1/2a clinical trial (APPROACH) and in rhesus monkeys (NHP 13–19). *Lancet*. 2018;392 (10143):232–243.

Barouch DH, Whitney JB, Moldt B, et al. Therapeutic efficacy of potent neutralizing HIV-1-specific monoclonal antibodies in SHIV-infected rhesus monkeys. *Nature*. 2013b;503(7475):224–228.

Barrett SE, Teller RS, Forster SP, et al. Extended-duration MK-8591-eluting implant as a candidate for HIV treatment and prevention. *Antimicrob Agents Chemother*. September 24, 2018;62(10):e01058–18. http://doi:10.1128/AAC.01058-18. PMID: 30012772; PMCID: PMC6153840.

Bekker L-G, Moodie Z, Grunenberg N, et al. Subtype C ALVAC-HIV and bivalent subtype C gp120/MF59 HIV-1 vaccine in low-risk, HIV-uninfected, South African adults: a phase 1/2 trial. *Lancet HIV*. 2018;5(7):PE366–E378.

Besson GJ, Lalama CM, Bosch RJ, et al. HIV-1 DNA decay dynamics in blood during more than a decade of suppressive antiretroviral therapy. *Clin Infect Dis*. 2014;59(9):1312–1321.

Birx D, Loomis-Price LD, Aronson N, et al. Efficacy of recombinant human immunodeficiency virus (HIV) gp160 as a therapeutic vaccine in early-stage HIV-1-infected volunteers. *J Infect Dis*. 2000;181:881–889.

Blick G, Lalezari J, Hsu R, et al. Cyclophosphamide enhances SB-728T engraftment to levels associated with HIV-RNA control. [Abstract 141]. Paper presented at the 21st Conference on Retroviruses and Opportunistic Infections. Boston, MA; March 2014.

Borducchi E, Abbink P, Nkolola J, et al. PGT121 combined with GS-9620 delays viral rebound in SHIV-infected rhesus monkeys. [Abstract 73LB]. The Conference on Retroviruses and Opportunistic Infections. Boston, MA; March 4–7, 2018.

Borducchi EN, Cabral C, Stephenson KE, et al. Ad26/MVA therapeutic vaccination with TLR7 stimulation in SIV-infected rhesus monkeys. *Nature*. December 8, 2016;540(7632):284–287.

Borrow P, Lewicki H, Hahn BH, et al. Virus specific CD8 cytotoxic T-lymphocyte activity associated with control of viremia in primary human immunodeficiency virus type 1 infection. *J Virol*. 1994;68:6103–6110.

Brake OT, Hooft K, Liu YP, et al. Lentiviral vector design for multiple shRNA expression and durable HIV-1 inhibition. *Mol Ther.* 2008;16:557–564

Bruel T, Guivel-Benhassine F, Amraoui S, et al. Elimination of HIV-1 infected cells by broadly neutralizing antibodies. *Nat Commun.* 2016;7:10844.

Buchbinder SP, Mehrotra DV, Duerr et al. Efficacy assessment of a cell-mediated immunity HIV-1 vaccine (the Step Study): a double-blind, randomised, placebo-controlled, test-of-concept trial. *Lancet.* November 29, 2008;372(9653):1881–1893.

Bui JK, Cyktor JC, Fyne E, et al. Blockade of the PD-1 axis alone is not sufficient to activate HIV-1 virion production from CD4+ T cells of individuals on suppressive ART. *PLoS One.* 2019;14(1):e0211112.

Buzon MJ, Sun H, Li C, et al. HIV-1 persistence in CD4\+\+ T cells with stem cell-like properties. *Nat Med.* 2014;20(2):139–142.

Byrareddy SN, Arthros J, Cicala C, et al. Sustained virologic control in SIV\+ macaques after antiretroviral and α4β7 antibody therapy. *Science.* 2016;354:197–202.

Cao Y, Qin L, Zhang L, et al. Virologic and immunologic characterization of long-term survivors of human immunodeficiency virus type 1 infection. *N Engl J Med.* 1995;332:201–208.

Caskey M, Klein F, Lorenzi JC, et al. Viraemia suppressed in HIV-1–infected humans by broadly neutralizing antibody 3BNC117. *Nature.* 2015;522(7557):487–491.

Caskey M, Schoofs T, Gruell H, et al. Antibody 10-1074 suppresses viremia in HIV-1-infected individuals. *Nat Med.* 2017;23(2):185–191.

Centlivre M, Legrand N, Klamer S, et al. Preclinical in vivo evaluation of the safety of a multi-shRNA-based gene therapy against HIV-1. *Mol Ther Nucleic Acids.* 2013; 2:e120.

Chen W, Dmitrov D. Monoclonal antibody-based candidate therapeutics against HIV type 1. *AIDS Res Hum Retroviruses.* May 2012;28(5):425–434.

Chen Z, Julg B. Therapeutic vaccines for the treatment of HIV. *Transl Res.* 2020;223:61–75.

Choudhary MC, Cyktor JC, Riddler SA. Advances in HIV-1-specific chimeric antigen receptor cells to target the HIV-1-reservoir. *J Virus Erad.* 2022;8(2):100073.

Chun TW, Engel D, Berrey MM, et al. Early establishment of a pool of latently infected, resting CD4\+(\+) T cells during primary HIV-1 infection. *Proc Natl Acad Sci U S A.* 1998;95(15):8869–8873.

Chun TW, Finzi D, Margolick J, et al. In vivo fate of HIV-1–infected T cells: quantitative analysis of the transition to stable latency. *Nat Med.* 1995;1(12):1284–1290.

Chun TW, Stuyver L, Mizell SB, et al. Presence of an inducible HIV-1 latent reservoir during highly active antiretroviral therapy. *Proc Natl Acad Sci U S A.* 1997;94(24):13193–13197.

ClinicalTrials.gov. NCT02500849.
ClinicalTrials.gov. NCT02595866.
ClinicalTrials.gov. NCT03147859.
ClinicalTrials.gov. NCT03164135.
ClinicalTrials.gov. NCT03240328.
ClinicalTrials.gov. NCT03307915.
ClinicalTrials.gov. NCT03367754.
ClinicalTrials.gov. NCT03560258.
ClinicalTrials.gov. NCT03570918.
ClinicalTrials.gov. NCT03617198.
ClinicalTrials.gov. NCT03705169.
ClinicalTrials.gov. NCT03721510.
ClinicalTrials.gov. NCT03743376.
ClinicalTrials.gov. NCT03758625.
ClinicalTrials.gov. NCT03837756.
ClinicalTrials.gov. NCT03844386.
ClinicalTrials.gov. NCT03964415
ClinicalTrials.gov. NCT04223804.
ClinicalTrials.gov. NCT04250636.
ClinicalTrials.gov. NCT04340596.
ClinicalTrials.gov. NCT04357821.
ClinicalTrials.gov. NCT04505501.
ClinicalTrials.gov. NCT04725877.

ClinicalTrials.gov. NCT05184452.
ClinicalTrials.gov. NCT05217641.
ClinicalTrials.gov. NCT05245292.
ClinicalTrials.gov. NCT05471076.
ClinicaltTrials.gov. NCT02408861.

Colby DJ, Sarnecki M, Barouch DH, et al. Safety and immunogenicity of Ad26 and MVA vaccines in acutely treated HIV and effect on viral rebound after antiretroviral therapy interruption. *Nat Med.* 2020;26(4):498–501.

Cong L, Ran FA, Cox D, et al. Multiplex genome engineering using CRISPR/Cas systems. *Science.* 2013;339(6121):819–823.

Cradick TJ, Fine EJ, Antico CJ, et al. CRISPR/Cas9 systems targeting β-globin and CCR5 genes have substantial off-target activity. *Nucleic Acids Res.* 2013;41(20):9584–9592.

Day CL, Kaufmann DE, Kiepiela P, et al. PD-1 expression on HIV-specific T cells is associated with T cell exhaustion and disease progression. *Nature.* 2006;443(7109):350–354.

Deeks SG, Walker BD. Human immunodeficiency virus controllers: mechanisms of durable virus control in the absence of antiretroviral therapy. *Immunity.* 2007;27(3):406–416.

Deeks SG. HIV: shock and kill. *Nature.* 2012;487(7408):439–440.

Deng K, Pertea M, Rongvaux A, et al. Broad CTL response is required to clear latent HIV-1 due to dominance of escape mutations. *Nature.* 2015;517(7534):381–385.

Dhody K, Kazempour K. PRO 140 SC: long-acting, single-agent, maintenance therapy for HIV-1 infection. [Abstract 486]. Paper presented at Conferences on Retroviruses and Opportunistic Infections (CROI). Seattle, WA; March 2019.

Dhody K, Pourhassan N, Kazempour K, et al. PRO 140, a monoclonal antibody targeting CCR5, as a long-acting, single-agent maintenance therapy for HIV-1 infection. *HIV Clin Trials.* 2018;19(3): 85–93.

Ebina H, Misawa N, Kanemura Y, et al. Harnessing the CRISPR/Cas9 system to disrupt latent HIV-1 provirus. *Sci Rep.* 2013;3:2510.

Einkauf KB, Osborn MR, Gao C, et al. Parallel analysis of transcription, integration, and sequence of single HIV-1 proviruses. *Cell.* 2022;185(2):266–282.e15.

Elliott JH, Wightman F, Solomon A, et al. Activation of HIV transcription with short-course vorinostat in HIV-positive patients on suppressive antiretroviral therapy. *PLoS Pathog.* 2014;10(10): e1004473.

Engsig FN, Zangerle R, Katsarou O, et al. Long-term mortality in HIV-positive individuals virally suppressed for >3 years with incomplete CD4 recovery. *Clin Infect Dis.* 2014;58(9):1312–1321.

Ensoli B, Cafaro A, Monini P, et al. Challenges in HIV vaccine research for treatment and prevention. *Front Immunol.* 2014;5:417.

Ensoli F, Cafaro A, Casabianco A, et al. HIV-1 Tat immunization restores immune homeostasis and attacks the HAART-resistant blood HIV DNA: results of a randomized phase II clinical exploratory clinical trial. *Retrovirology.* 2015;12:33.

Eron JJ Jr, Ashby MA, Giordano MF, et al. Randomized trial of MNrgp120 HIV-1 vaccine in symptomless HIV-1 infection. *Lancet.* 1996;348:1547–1551.

Evans VA, van der Sluis RM, Solomon A, et al. Programmed cell death-1 contributes to the establishment and maintenance of HIV-1 latency. *AIDS.* 2018;32(11):1491–1497.

Fidler S, Stöhr W, Pace M, et al; RIVER trial study group. Antiretroviral therapy alone versus antiretroviral therapy with a kick and kill approach, on measures of the HIV reservoir in participants with recent HIV infection (the RIVER trial): a phase 2, randomised trial. *Lancet.* 2020;395(10227):888–898. doi:10.1016/S0140-6736(19)32990-3. Epub 2020 Feb 19.

Finzi D, Blankson J, Siliciano JD, et al. Latent infection of CD4\+\+ T cells provides a mechanism for lifelong persistence of HIV-1, even in patients on effective combination therapy. *Nat Med.* 1999;5(5):512–517.

Finzi D, Hermankova M, Pierson T, et al. Identification of a reservoir for HIV-1 in patients on highly active antiretroviral therapy. *Science.* 1997;278(5341):1295–1300.

Flynn NM, Forthal DN, Harro CD, et al. Placebo-controlled phase 3 trial of a recombinant glycoprotein 120 vaccine to prevent HIV-1 infection. *J Infect Dis*. 2005;191:654–665

Forcina G, d'Ettorre G, Mastroianni C, et al. Interleukin-15 modulated interferon-γ and β-chemokine production in patients with HIV infection: implications for immune-based therapy. *Cytokine*. 2004;25:283–290.

Garcia F, Climent N, Assoumou L, et al. A therapeutic dendritic cell-based vaccine for HIV-1 infection. *J Infect Dis*. 2011;203:473–478.

Garcia F, Climent N, Guardo AC, et al. A dendritic cell-based vaccine elicits T cell responses associated with control of HIV-1 replication. *Sci Transl Med*. 2013;5:166ra62.

Garcia-Broncano P, Maddali S, Einkauf KB, et al. Early antiretroviral therapy in neonates with HIV-1 infection restricts viral reservoir size and induces a distinct innate immune profile. *Sci Transl Med*. 2019;11(520):eaax7350.

Gaudinski MR, Coates EE, Houser K, et al. Safety and pharmacokinetics of the Fc-modified HIV-1 human monoclonal antibody VRC01LS: a phase 1 open-label clinical trial in healthy adults. *PLoS Med*. January 24, 2018;15(1):e1002493. http://doi:10.1371/journal.pmed.1002493. eCollection January 2018.

Gay CL, Bosch RJ, Ritz J, et al. Clinical trial of the anti-PDL-L1 antibody BMS-936559 in HIV-1 infected participants on suppressive antiretroviral therapy. *J Infect Dis*. June 1, 2017;215(11):1725–1733.

Girard MP, Osmanov S, Assossou OM, Kieny MP. Human immunodeficiency virus (HIV) immunopathogenesis and vaccine development: a review. *Vaccine*. 2011;29:6191–6218

Gray GE, Bekker LG, Laher F, et al. Vaccine efficacy of ALVAC-HIV and bivalent subtype C gp120-MF59 in adults. *N Engl J Med*. 2021;384(12):1089–1100.

Gruell H, Gunst JD, Cohen YZ, et al. Effect of 3BNC117 and romidepsin on the HIV-1 reservoir in people taking suppressive antiretroviral therapy (ROADMAP): a randomised, open-label, phase 2A trial. *Lancet Microbe*. 2022;2(3):e203–e214.

Gubser C, Chiu C, Lewin SR, et al. Immune checkpoint blockade in HIV. *EBioMedicine*. 2022;76:103840.

Guihot A, Marcelin AG, Massiani MA, et al. Drastic decrease of the HIV reservoir in a patient treated with nivolumab for lung cancer. *Ann Oncol*. 2018;29:517–518.

Guo S, Luke BT, Henry AR, et al. HIV infected CD4+ T-cell clones are more stable than uninfected clones during long-term antiretroviral therapy. *PLoS Pathog*. 2022;18(8):e1010726.

Gupta RK, Peppa D, Hill AL, et al. Evidence for HIV-1 cure after CCR5Δ32/Δ32 allogeneic haemopoietic stem-cell transplantation 30 months post analytical treatment interruption: a case report. *Lancet HIV*. 2020;7(5):e340–e347.

Hallengard D, Haller BK, Maltais AK, et al. Comparison of plasmid vaccine immunization schedules using intradermal in vivo electroporation. *Clin Vaccine Immunol*. 2011;18(9):1577–1581.

Hansen SG, Ford JC, Lewis MS, et al. Profound early control of highly pathogenic SIV by an effector memory T cell vaccine. *Nature*. 2011;473(7348):523–527.

Hansen SG, Piatak M Jr, Ventura AB, et al. Immune clearance of highly pathogenic SIV infection. *Nature*. 2013;502(7469):100–104.

Hardy GA, Imami N, Nelson MR. A phase I, randomized study of combined IL-2 and therapeutic immunization with antiretroviral therapy. *J Immune Based Therapies Vaccines*. 2007;5:6.

Hardy WD. A5370. Safety and immunotherapeutic activity of an anti-PD-1antibody (cemiplimab) in HIV-1-diagnosed participants on suppressive cART: A phase I/II, double-blind, placebo-controlled, ascending multiple dose study. https://www.treatmentactiongroup.org/wp-content/uploads/2020/03/final_A5370_CROI_Presentations_030720.pdf. 2020. Published 2020. Accessed March 10, 2023.

Harwood O, O'Connor S. Therapeutic potential of IL-15 and N-803 in HIV/SIV infection. *Viruses*. 2021;13(9):1750.

Haynes BF, Gilbert PB, McElrath MJ, et al. Immune-correlates analysis of and HIV-1 vaccine efficacy trial. *N Engl J Med*. 2012;366:1275–1286.

Henrich TJ, Gandhi RT. Early treatment and HIV-1 reservoirs: a stitch in time? *J Infect Dis*. 2013;208(8):1189–1193.

Henrich TJ, Schreiner C, Cameron C, et al. Everolimus, an mTORC1/2 inhibitor, in ART-suppressed individuals who received solid organ transplantation: a prospective study. *Am J Transplant*. 2021;21(5):1765–1779.

Heredia A, Le N, Gartenhaus RB, et al. Targeting of mTOR catalytic site inhibits multiple steps of the HIV-1 lifecycle and suppresses HIV-1 viremia in humanized mice. *Proc Natl Acad Sci USA*. 2015;112(30):9412–9417.

Hermankova M, Siliciano JD, Zhou Y, et al. Analysis of human immunodeficiency virus type 1 gene expression in latently infected resting CD4\+ T lymphocytes in vivo. *J Virol*. 2003;77(13):7383–7392.

Hocqueloux L, Avettand-Fenoel V, Jacquot S, et al. Long-term antiretroviral therapy initiated during primary HIV-1 infection is key to achieving both low HIV reservoirs and normal T cell counts. *J Antimicrobial Chemother*. 2013;68(5):1169–1178.

Holt N, Wang J, Kim K, et al. Human hematopoietic stem/progenitor cells modified by zinc-finger nucleases targeted to CCR5 control HIV-1 in vivo. *Nat Biotechnol*. 2010;28(8):839–847.

Hombach AA, Holzinger A, Abken H. The weal and woe of costimulation in the adoptive therapy of cancer with chimeric antigen receptor (CAR)-redirected T cells. *Curr Mol Med*. 2013;13(7):1079–1088.

Hu W, Kaminski R, Yang F, et al. RNA-directed gene editing specifically eradicates latent and prevents new HIV-1 infection. *Proc Natl Acad Sci*. 2014;111(31):11461–11466.

Hu X, Valentin A, Dayton F, et al. DNA prime-boost vaccine regimen to increase breadth, magnitude, and cytotoxicity of the cellular immune responses to subdominant Gag epitopes of simian immunodeficiency virus and HIV. *J Immunol*. 2016;197(10):3999–4013

Huang Y, Yu J, Lanzi A, et al. Engineered bispecific antibodies with exquisite HIV-1-neutralizing activity. *Cell*. 2016;165:1621–1631.

Hutter G, Nowak D, Mossner M, et al. Long-term control of HIV by CCR5 Delta32/Delta32 stem-cell transplantation. *N Engl J Med*. 2009;360(7):692–698.

Inderbitzin A, Loosli T, Optiz L, et al. Transcriptome profiles of latently- and reactivated HIV-1 infected primary CD4+ T cells: a pooled data-analysis. *Front Immunol*. 2022;13:915805.

Iwamoto N, Mason RD, Song K, et al. Blocking α4β7 integrin binding to SIV does not improve virologic control. *Science*. 2019;365(6457):1033–1036.

Julg B, Pequ A, Abbink P, et al. Virologic control by the CD4-binding site antibody N6 in simian-human immunodeficiency virus-infected rhesus monkeys. *J Virol*. July 27, 2017;91(16):e00498–17.

Julg B, Stephenson KE, Wagh K, et al. Safety and antiviral activity of triple combination broadly neutralizing monocloncal antibody therapy against HIV-1: a phase 1 clinical trial. *Nat Med*. 2022;28(6):1288–1296.

June C, Tebas P, Stein D, et al. Induction of acquired CCR5 deficiency with zinc finger nuclease-modified autologous CD4 T cells (SB-728-T) correlates with increases in CD4 count and effects on viral load in HIV-infected subjects. [Abstract 155]. Paper presented at the 19th Conference on Retroviruses and Opportunistic Infection. Seattle, WA; February 2012.

Kessing CF, Nixon CC, Li C, et al. In vivo suppression of HIV rebound by didehydro-cortistatin A, a "block-and-lock" strategy for HIV-1 treatment. *Cell Rep*. October 17, 2017;21(3):600–611.

Khaitan A, Unutmaz D. Revisiting immune exhaustion during HIV infection. *Current HIV/AIDS Reports*. 2011;8(1):4–11.

Kim Y, Anderson JL, Lewin SR. Getting the "kill" into "shock and kill": strategies to eliminate latent HIV. *Cell Host Microbe*. 2018;23(1):14–26.

Kozal M, Aberg J, Pialoux G, et al. Fostemsavir in adults with multidrug-resistant HIV-1 infection. *N Engl J Med*. 2020;382(13):1232–1243.

Kroup RA, Safrit JT, Cao Y, et al. Temporal association of cellular immune responses with the initial control of viremia in primary human immunodeficiency virus type 1 syndrome. *J Virol*. 1994;68:4650–4655.

Krystal M, Wensel D, Sun Y, et al. HIV-1 Combinectin BMS-986197: a long-acting inhibitor with multiple modes of action. [Abstract 97].

Presented at the 23rd Conference on Retroviruses and Opportunistic Infection. Boston, MA: February 22–25, 2016.

Laird GM, Bullen CK, Rosenbloom DI, et al. Ex vivo analysis identifies effective HIV-1 latency-reversing drug combinations. *J Clin Invest*. 2015;125(5):1901–1912.

Lalezari J, Mitsuyasu R, Wang S, et al. A single infusion of zinc finger nuclease CCR5 modified autologous CD4 T cells (SB-728T) increased CD4 counts and leads to decrease in HIV proviral load in an aviremic HIV-infected subject. [Abstract 433]. Paper presented at the 19th Conference on Retroviruses and Opportunistic Infection. Seattle, WA; February 2012.

Lam S, Bollard C. T cell therapies for HIV. *Immunotherapy*. 2013;5(4):407–414.

Leibman RS, Richardson MW, Ellebrecht CT, et al. Supraphysiologic control over HIV-1 replication mediated by CD8 T cells expressing a re-engineered CD4-based chimeric antigen receptor. *PLoS Pathog*. October 12, 2017;13(10):e1006613.

Levy Y, Durier C, Lascaux AS, et al. Sustained control of viremia following therapeutic immunization in chronically HIV-1 infected individuals. *AIDS*. 2006;20:405–413.

Levy Y, Gahery-Segard H, Durier C, et al. Immunologic and virologic efficacy of therapeutic immunization combined with interleukin-2 in chronically HIV-1 infected patients. *AIDS*. 2005;19:279–286.

Levy Y, Lacabaratz C, Lhomme E, et al. A randomized placebo0controlled efficacy study of a prime boost therapeutic vaccination strategy in HIV-1-infected individuals: VRI01 ANRS 149 LIGHT phase II trial. *J Virol*. 2021;95(9):e02165–20.

Levy Y, Lacabaratz C, Weiss L, et al. Enhanced T cell recovery in HIV-1 infected adults through IL-7 treatment. *J Clin Invest*. 2009;119(4):997–1007.

Levy Y, Sereti I, Tambussi G, et al. Effects of recombinant human interleukin 7 on T-cell recovery and thymic output in HIV-infected patients receiving antiretroviral therapy: results of a phase I/ IIa randomized, placebo-controlled multicenter study. *Clin Infect Dis*. 2012;55(2):291–300.

Levy Y, Thiebaut R, Montes M, et al. Dendritic cell-based therapeutic vaccine elicits polyfunctional HIV-specific T-cell immunity associated with control of viral load. *Eur J Immunol*. 2014;44: 2802–2810.

Lewden C, Chene G, Morlat P, et al. HIV-infected adults with a CD4 cell count greater than 500 cells/µl on long-term combination antiretroviral therapy reach same mortality rates as the general population. *J AIDS*. 2007;46(1):72–77.

Li J, Brumme Z, Brumme C, et al. Factors associated with viral rebound in HIV-1 infected individuals enrolled in a therapeutic HIV-1 Gag vaccine trial. *J Infect Dis*. 2011;203:976–983.

Liao HK, Gu Y, Diaz A, et al. Use of the CRISPR/Cas9 system as an intracellular defense against HIV-1 infection in human cells. *Nat Commun*. 2015;6:6413.

Link JO, Rhee MS, Tse WC, et al. Clinical targeting of HIV capsid protein with a long-acting small molecule. *Nature*. 2020;584(7822):614–618.

Lu CL, Murakowski DK, Bournazos S, et al. Enhanced clearance of HIV-1–infected cells by broadly neutralizing antibodies against HIV-1 in vivo. *Science*. 2016;352:1001–1004.

Lu W, Arraes C, Ferreira WT, et al. Therapeutic dendritic cell vaccination for chronic HIV-1 infection. *Nat Med*. 2004;10:1359–1365.

Luzuriaga K, Gay H, Ziemniak C, et al. Viremic relapse after HIV-1 remission in a perinatally infected child. *N Engl J Med*. 2015;372(8):786–788.

Lynch RM, Boritz E, Coates EE, et al. Virologic effects of broadly neutralizing antibody VRC01 administration during chronic HIV-1 infection. *Sci Ttransl Med*. 2015;7(319):319ra206.

Martin AR, Siciliano RF. Immune modulation with rapamycin as a potential strategy for HIV-1 eradication. [Abstract 415]. Paper presented at the 22nd Conference on Retroviruses and Opportunistic Infections. Seattle, WA; February 2015.

Mascolini M. Primary efficacy results of PRO 140 SC in a pivotal phase 2b/3 study in heavily treatment-experienced HIV-1 patients. Paper presented at ASM Microbe. Atlanta, GA; June 2018.

Maslennikova A, Mazurov D. Application of CRISPR/Cas genomic editing tools for HIV therapy: toward precise modifications and multilevel protection. *Front Cell Infect Microbiol*. 2022;12:880030.

Mason SW, Sanisetty S, Osuna Gutierrez C, et al. Viral suppression was induced by anti-PD-L1 following ARV-interruption in SIV-infected monkeys. [Abstract 318LB]. Paper presented at the 21st Conference on Retroviruses and Opportunistic Infections. Boston, MA; March 2014.

McMahon DK, Zheng L, Cyktor JC, et al. Multidose IV romidepsin: no increased HIV-1 expression in persons on ART, ACTG A5315 [CROI Abstract 26]. In Special issue: abstracts from the 2019 Conference on Retroviruses and Opportunistic Infections. *Top Antivir Med*. 2019;27(Suppl 1):11s–12s.

McMichael AJ, Borrow P, Tomaras GD, The immune response during acute HIV-1 infection: clues for vaccine development. *Nat Rev Immunol*. 2010;10(1):11–23.

Mendoza P, Gruell H, Nogueira L, et al. Combination therapy with anti-HIV-1 antibodies maintains viral suppression. *Nature*. 2018;561(7724):479–484.

Miller JS, Davis BZ, Helgeson E, et al. Safety and virologic impact of the IL-15 superagonist N-803 in people with HIV-a phase 1 trial. *Nat Med*. 2022;28(2);3920402.

Mitsuyasu RT, Lalezari J, Burke B, et al. Phase I study of gene-modified CD4+ T cells and CD34+ cells with or without busulfan in HIV+ adults [CROI Abstract 338]. In Special issue: abstracts from the 2020 Conference on Retroviruses and Opportunistic Infections. *Top Antivir Med*. 2020;28(1):116.

Mitsuyasu RT, Merigan TC, Carr A, et al. Phase 2 gene therapy trial of anti-HIV ribozyme in autologous CD34\+ cells. *Nat Med*. 2009;15(3):285–292.

Mori L, Valente ST. Key players in HIV-1 transcriptional regulation: targets for a functional cure. *Viruses*. 2020;12(5):529.

Moron-Lopez S, Bernal S, Steens JM, et al. ABX464 decreases the total HIV reservoir and HIV transcription initiation in vivo. [Poster abstract 335]. CROI 2020. Boston, MA; 2020.

Mothe B, Rosás-Umbert M, Coll P, et al. HIVconsv vaccines and romidepsin in early-treated HIV-1-infected individuals: safety, immunogenicity and effect on the viral reservoir (study BCN02). *Front Immunol*. 2020;11:823.

Mousseau G, Kessing CF, Fromentin R, et al. The Tat inhibitor didehydro-cortistatin A prevents HIV-1 reactivation from latency. *MBio*. 2015;6(4):e00465.

Nabel G, Baltimore D. An inducible transcription factor activates expression of human immunodeficiency virus in T cells. *Nature*. 1987;326(6114):711–713.

Namazi G, Fajnzylber JM, Aga E, et al. The Control of HIV After Antiretroviral Medication Pause (CHAMP) Study: posttreatment controllers identified from 14 clinical studies. *J Infect Dis*. 2018;218(12):1954–1963.

Pallikkuth S, Micci L, Ende ZS, et al. Maintenance of intestinal Th17 cells and reduced microbial translocation in SIV-infected rhesus macaques treated with interleukin (IL)-21. *PLoS Pathog*. 2013;9:e1003471.

Pallikkuth, S, Rogers K, Villinger F, et al. Interleukin-21 administration to rhesus macaques chronically infected with simian immunodeficiency viruses increases cytotoxic effector molecules in T cells and NK cells and enhances B cell function without increasing immune activation or viral replication. *Vaccine*. 2011;29:9929–9938.

Palmer BE, Neff CP, Lecureux J, et al. In vivo blockade of the PD-1 receptor suppresses HIV-1 viral loads and improves CD4\+ T cell levels in humanized mice. *J Immunol*. 2013;190(1):211–219.

Palmer CS, Ostrowski M, Zhou J, et al. The mTORC1 inhibitors, temsirolimus and everolimus, suppress HIV-patient-derived CD4\+ T-cell death and activation in vitro. [Abstract 320]. Paper presented at the 22nd Conference on Retroviruses and Opportunistic Infections. Seattle, WA; February 2015.

Papuchon J, Pinson P, Lazaro E, et al. Resistance mutations and CTL epitopes in archived HIV-1 DNA of patients on antiviral treatment: toward a new concept of vaccine. *PLoS One*. 2013;8(7):e69029.

Pegu A, Asokan M, Wu L, et al. Activation and lysis of human CD4 cells latently infected with HIV-1. *Nature Commun.* 2015;6:8447.

Perez EE, Wang J, Miller JC, et al. Establishment of HIV-1 resistance in CD4\+ T cells by genome editing using zinc-finger nucleases. *Nat Biotechnol.* 2008;26(7):808–816.

Persaud D, Gay H, Ziemniak C, et al. Absence of detectable HIV-1 viremia after treatment cessation in an infant. *N Engl J Med.* 2013;369(19):1828–1835.

Peterson CW, Wang J, Deleage C, et al. Differential impact of transplantation on peripheral and tissue-associated viral reservoirs: implications for HIV gene therapy. *PLoS Pathog.* April 19, 2018;14(4):e1006956.

Pett SL, Carey C, Lin E, et al. Predictors of bacterial pneumonia in Evaluation of Subcutaneous Interleukin-2 in Randomized International TRIAL (ESPRIT). *HIV Med.* 2011;12(4):219–227.

Pett SL, Kelleher AD, Emery S. Role of interleukin-2 in patients with HIV infection. *Drugs.* 2010;70(9):1115–1130.

Pitisuttithum P, Gilbert P, Gurwith M, et al. Randomized, double-blind, placebo-controlled efficacy trial of a bivalent recombinant glycoprotein 120 HIV-1 vaccine among injection drug users in Bangkok, Thailand. *J Infect Dis.* 2006;194:1661–1671

Pollard RB, Rockstroh JK, Pantaleo G, et al. Safety and efficacy of the peptide-based therapeutic vaccine for HIV-1, Vacc-4x: a phase 2 randomised double-blind, placebo-controlled trial. *Lancet Infect Dis.* 2014;14(4):291–300.

Pontesilli I, Guerra ES, Ammassari A, et al. Phase II controlled trial of post-exposure immunization with recombinant gp160 versus antiretroviral therapy in asymptomatic HIV-1 infected adults. *AIDS.* 1998;12:473–480.

Porichis F, Kaufmann DE. Role of PD-1 in HIV pathogenesis and as a target for therapy. *Curr HIV/AID Rep.* 2012;9(1):81–90.

Ramirez LA, Arango T, Boyer J. Therapeutic and prophylactic DNA vaccines for HIV-1. *Expert Opin Biol Ther.* 2013;13(4):563–573.

Rasmussen TA, Brinkmann CR, Olesen R, et al. Panobinostat, a histone deacetylase inhibitor, for latent-virus reactivation in HIV-infected patients on suppressive antiretroviral therapy: a phase 1/2, single group, clinical trial. *Lancet HIV.* 2014;1(1):e14–e21.

Rasmussen TA, Rajdev L, Rhodes A, et al. Impact of anti-PD-1 and anti-CTLA-4 on the human immunodeficiency virus (HIV) reservoir in people living with HIV with cancer on antiretroviral therapy: the AIDS Malignancy Consortium 095 study. *Clin Infect Dis.* 2021;73(7):e1973–e1981.

Rerks-Ngarm S, Pitisuttithum P, Nitayaphan S, et al. Vaccination with ALVAC and AIDSVAX to prevent HIV-1 infection in Thailand. *N Engl J Med.* 2009;361(23):2209–2220.

Richman DD, Margolis DM, Delaney M, et al. The challenge of finding a cure for HIV infection. *Science.* 2009;323(5919):1304–1307.

Riddler SA, Para M, Benson CA, et al. Vesatolimod, a Toll-like receptor 7 agonist, induces immune activation in virally suppressed adults living with human immunodeficiency virus-1. *Clin Infect Dis.* 2021;72(11):e815–e824.

Riddler SA, Zheng L, Durand CM, et al. Randomized clinical trial to assess the impact of the broadly neutralizing HIV-1 monoclonal antibody VRC01 on HIV-1 persistence in individuals on effective ART. *Open Forum Infect Dis.* 2018;5(10):ofy242.

Rodriguez B, Asmuth DM, Matining RM, et al. Safety, tolerability, and immunogenicity of repeated doses of dermavir, a candidate therapeutic HIV vaccine, in HIV-infected patients receiving combination antiretroviral therapy: results of the ACTG 5176 trial. *J Acquir Immune Defic Syndr.* 2013;64(4):351–359.

Rolland M, Tovanabutra s, decamp AC et al. Genetic impact of vaccination on breakthrough HIV-1 sequences from the STEP trial. *Nat Med.* 2011;17(3):366–371

Rosenberg ES, Billingsley JM, Caliendo AM, et al. Vigorous HIV-1-specific CD4R T cell responses associated with control of viremia. *Science.* 1997;278:1447–1450.

SA, Boritz E, Busch M, et al. Challenges in detecting HIV persistence during potentially curative interventions: a study of the Berlin patient. *PLoS Pathog.* 2013;9(5):e1003347.

Saez-Cirion A, Bacchus C, Hocqueloux L, et al. Post-treatment HIV-1 controllers with a long-term virological remission after the interruption of early initiated antiretroviral therapy ANRS VISCONTI study. *PLoS Pathog.* 2013;9(3):e1003211.

Saito N, Chono H, Shibata H, et al. CD4\+ T cells modified by endoribonuclease MazF are safe and can persist in SHIV-infected rhesus macaques. *Mol Ther Nucleic Acids.* 2014;3(6):e168.

Sandstrom E, Wahren B; Nordic Vac-04 Study Group. Therapeutic immunization with recombinant gp160 in HIV-1 infection: a randomized double-blind placebo-controlled trial. *Lancet.* 1999;353:1735–1742.

Sauce D, Elbim C, Appay V. Monitoring cellular immune markers in HIV infection: from activation to exhaustion. *Curr Opin HIV AIDS.* 2013;8(2):125–131.

Scheid JF, Horwitz JA, Bar-On Y, et al. HIV-1 antibody 3BNC117 suppresses viral rebound in humans during treatment interruption. *Nature.* 2016;535(7613):556–560.

Schooley RT, Spritzler J, Wang H, et al.; AIDS Clinical Trials Group 5197. A placebo-controlled trial of immunization of HIV-1-infected persons with a replication-deficient adenovirus type 5 vaccine expressing the HIV-1 core protein. *J Infect Dis.* 2010;202(5):705–716.

Schürmann D, Rudd DJ, Zhang S, et al. Safety, pharmacokinetics, and antiretroviral activity of islatravir (ISL, MK-8591), a novel nucleoside reverse transcriptase translocation inhibitor, following single-dose administration to treatment-naive adults infected with HIV-1: an open-label, phase 1b, consecutive-panel trial. *Lancet HIV.* 2020;7(3):e164–e172.

Segal-Maurer S, DeJesus E, Stellbrink HJ, et al. Capsid inhibition with lenacapavir in multidrug-resistant HIV-1 infection. *N Engl J Med.* 2022;386(19):1793–1803.

SenGupta D, Brinson C, DeJesus E, et al. The TLR7 agonist vesatolimod induced a modest delay in viral rebound in HIV controllers after cessation of antiretroviral therapy. *Sci Transl Med.* 2021;13(599):eabg3071.

SenGupta D, Ramgopal M, Brinson C, et al. Safety and analytical treatment interruption outcomes of vesatolimod in HIV controllers [CROI Abstract 40]. In Special Issue: Abstracts from the 2020 Conference on Retroviruses and Opportunistic Infections. *Top Antivir Med.* 2020;28(1):13–14.

Sereti I, Dunham RM, Spritzler J, et al. IL-7 administration drives T cell entry and expansion in HIV-1 infection. *Blood.* 2009;113(25):6304–6314.

Shan L, Deng K, Shroff NS, et al. Stimulation of HIV-1-specific cytolytic T lymphocytes facilitates elimination of latent viral reservoir after virus reactivation. *Immunity.* 2012;36(3):491–501.

Shingai M, Nishimura Y, Klein F, et al. Antibody-mediated immunotherapy of macaques chronically infected with SHIV suppresses viraemia. *Nature.* 2013;503(7475):277–280.

Singh A, Palanichamy JK, Ramalingam P, et al. Long-term suppression of HIV-1 C virus production in human peripheral blood mononuclear cells by LTR heterochromatization with a short double-stranded RNA. *J Antimicrob Chemother.* 2014;69:405–415.

Sneller MC, Clarridge KE, Seamon C, et al. An open-label phase 1 clinical trial of the anti-α4β7 monoclonal antibody vedolizumab in HIV-infected individuals. *Science Translational Medicine.* 2019;11(509):eaax3447.

Sneller MC, Justement JS, Gittens KR, et al. A randomized controlled safety/efficacy trial of therapeutic vaccination in HIV-infected individuals who initiated antiretroviral therapy early in infection. *Sci Transl Med.* 2017;9(419):eaan8848.

Sogaard OS, Graversen ME, Leth S, et al. The depsipeptide romidepsin reverses HIV-1 latency in vivo. *PLoS Pathog.* 2015;11(9):e1005142.

Stellbrink HJ, van Lundzen J, Westby M, et al. Effects of interleukin-2 plus highly active antiretroviral therapy on HIV-1 replication and proviral DNA (COSMIC trial). *AIDS.* 2002;16:1479–1487.

Stephenson KE, Julg B, Tan CS, et al. Safety, pharmacokinetics and antiviral activity of PGT121, a broadly neutralizing monoclonal antibody against HIV-1: a randomized, placebo-controlled, phase 1 clinical trial. *Nat Med.* 2021;27(10):1718–1724.

Strain MC, Little SJ, Daar ES, et al. Effect of treatment, during primary infection, on establishment and clearance of cellular reservoirs of HIV-1. *J Infect Dis*. 2005;191(9):1410–1418.

Sung JA, Pickeral J, Liu L, et al. Dual-affinity re-targeting proteins direct T cell-mediated cytolysis of latently HIV-infected cells. *J Clin Invest*. 2015;125(11):4077–4090.

Takata H, Kakzau JC, Mitchell JL, et al. Long-term antiretroviral therapy initiated in acute HIV infection prevents residual dysfunction of HIV-specific CD8+ T cells. *EBioMedicine*. 2022;84:104253.

Tavel JA; INSIGHT STALWART Study Group. Effect of intermittent IL-2 alone or with peri-cycle antiretroviral therapy in early HIV-1 infection: the STALWART study. *PLoS One*. 2010;5(2):e9334.

Tebas P, Jadlowski J, Shaw P, et al. CCR5-edited CDr+ T cells augment HV-specific immunity to enable post-rebound control of HIV replication. *J Clin Invest*. 2021;131(7):e144486.

Tebas P, Stein D, Binder-Scholl G, et al. Antiviral effects of autologous CD4 T cells genetically modified with a conditionally replicating lentiviral vector expressing long antisense to HIV. *Blood*. 2013;121(9):1524–1533.

Tebas P, Stein D, Tang WW, et al. Gene editing of CCR5 in autologous CD4 T cells of persons infected with HIV. *N Engl J Med*. 2014;370(10):901–910.

Thompson M, Saag M, DeJesus E, et al. A 48-week randomized phase 2b study evaluating cenicriviroc versus efavirenz in treatment-naive HIV-infected adults with C-C chemokine receptor type 5-tropic virus. *AIDS*. 2016;30(6):869–878.

Topalian SL, Hodi FS, Brahmer JR, et al. Safety, activity, and immune correlates of anti-PD-1 antibody in cancer. *N Engl J Med*. 2012;366(26):2443–2454.

Tsoukas CM, Raboud J, Bernard NF, et al. Active immunization of patients with HIV infection: a study of VaxSyn, a recombinant HIV envelope subunit vaccine, on progression of immunodeficiency. *AIDS Res Hum Retroviruses*. 1998;14:483–490.

Uldrick TS, Adams SV, Fromentin R, et al. Pembrolizumab induces HIV latency reversal in people living with HIV and cancer on antiretroviral therapy. *Sci Transl Med*. 2022;14(629):eabl3836.

Van Gulck E, Vlieghe E, Vekemans M, et al. mRNA-based dendritic cell vaccination induced potent antiviral responses in HIV-1 infected patients. *AIDS*. 2012;26:F1–F12.

Van Lundzen J, Glausinger T, Stahmer I, et al. Transfer of autologous gene-modified T cells in HIV-infected patients with advanced immunodeficiency and drug-resistant virus. *Mol Ther*. 2007;15:1024–1033.

Vandergeeten C, Fromentin R, DaFronseca S, et. al. Interleukin-7 promotes HIV persistence during antiretroviral therapy. *Blood*. 2013;121(21):4321–4329.

Vardas E, Stanescu I, Leinonen M, et al. Indicators of a therapeutic effect in FIT-06, a phase II trial of a DNA vaccine, GTU-Multi-HIVB, in untreated HIV-1 infected subjects. *Vaccine*. 2012;30(27):4046–4054.

Varela-Rohena A, Molloy PE, Dunn SM, et al. Control of HIV-1 immune escape by CD8 T cells expressing enhanced T cell receptor. *Nat Med*. 2008;14(12):1390–1395.

Velu V, Titanji K, Ahmed H, et al. PD-1 blockade following ART interruption enhances control of pathogenic SIV in rhesus macaques. *Proc Natl Acad Sci U S A*. 2022;119(33):e2202148119.

Velu V, Titanji K, Zhu B, et al. Enhancing SIV-specific immunity in vivo by PD-1 blockade. *Nature*. 2009;458(7235):206–210.

Vibholm L, Konrad CV, Schleimann MH, et al. Effects of 24-week Toll-like receptor 9 agonist treatment in HIV type 1+ individuals. *AIDS*. 2019;33(8):1315–1325.

Vibholm L, Schleimann MH, Hojen JF, et al. Short-course toll-like receptor 9 agonist treatment impacts innate immunity and plasma viremia in individuals with human immunodeficiency virus infection. *Clin Infect Dis*. June 15, 2017;64(12):1686–1695.

Wang CY, Wong WW, Tsai HC, et al. Effect of anti-CD4 antibody UB-421 on HIV-1 rebound after treatment interruption. *N Engl J Med*. 2019;380(16):1535–1545.

Webb GM, Li S, Mwakalundwa G, et al. The human IL-15 superagonist ALT-803 directs SIV-specific CD8\+ T cells into B-cell follicles. *Blood Adv*. 2018;2:76–84.

White KL, Margot N, Stray K, et al. GS-9131 is a novel NRTI with activity against NRTI-resistant HIV-1. [Abstract 436]. Presented at the 24th Conference on Retroviruses and Opportunistic Infection. Seattle, WA; February 13–16, 2017.

Whitney JB, Hill AL, Sanisetty S, et al. Rapid seeding of the viral reservoir prior to SIV viraemia in rhesus monkeys. *Nature*. 2014;512(7512):74–77.

Whitney JB, Osuna CE, Sanisetty S, et al. Treatment with a TLR7 agonist induces transient viremia in SIV-infected ART-suppressed monkeys. Conference on Retroviruses and Opportunistic Infections. Seattle, WA; 2015.

Wolstein O, Boyd M, Millington M, et al. Preclinical safety and efficacy of an anti-HIV-1 lentiviral vector containing a short hairpin RNA to CCR5 and the C46 fusion inhibitor. *Mol Ther Methods Clin Dev*. 2014;1:11.

Wong JK, Hezareh M, Gunthard HF, et al. Recovery of replication-competent HIV despite prolonged suppression of plasma viremia. *Science*. 1997;278(5341):1291–1295.

Wykes MN, Lewin SR. Immune checkpoint blockade in infectious diseases. *Nat Rev Immunol*. 2018;18(2):91–104.

Xu L, Pequ A, Rao E, et al. Trispecific broadly neutralizing HIV antibodies mediate potent SHIV protection in macaques. *Science*. 2017;358:85–90.

Xu L, Wang J, Liu Y, et al. CRISPR-edited stem cells in a patient with HIV and acute lymphocytic leukemia. *N Engl J Med*. 2019;381(13):1240–1247.

Yakubova E et al. Safety and PK study of VM-1500A-LAI, a novel long-acting injectable therapy for HIV. [Late breaking poster abstract 473LB]. CROI 2020. Boston, MA; 2020.

Youngblood B, Noto A, Porichis F, et al. Cutting edge: prolonged exposure to HIV reinforces a poised epigenetic program for PD-1 expression in virus-specific CD8 T cells. *J Immunol*. 2013;191(2):540–544.

Yukl SA, Boritz E, Busch MB, et al. Challenges in detecting HIV persistence during potentially curative interventions: a study of the Berlin patient. *PLoS Pathog*. 2013;9(5):e1003347.

Zheng J, Yant SR, Ahmadyar S, et al. GS-CA2: a novel, potent and selective first-in-class inhibitor of HIV-1 capsid function displays nonclinical pharmacokinetics supporting long-acting potential in humans. [Abstract 539]. Presented at ID Week 2018. San Francisco, CA; October 3–7, 2018

Zhou J, Rossi JJ. Current progress in the development of RNAi based therapeutics for HIV-1. *Gene Ther*. 2011;18:1134–1138.

20.

HIV DRUG RESISTANCE
EVALUATION AND CLINICAL MANAGEMENT

Carolyn Chu, Lealah Pollock, and Robert W. Shafer

LEARNING OBJECTIVES

- Outline various types of HIV drug resistance (HIVDR) testing assays and clinical considerations for their use and interpretation.

- Define transmitted HIV drug resistance (TDR) and acquired HIV drug resistance (ADR), and general principles/approaches to their management.

- Describe unique considerations regarding HIVDR evaluation and management for select clinical scenarios including antiretroviral therapy (ART) switches/simplification, pregnancy, recent pre-exposure prophylaxis (PrEP) use, "rapid" ART initiation, and care of persons with HIV (PWH) in low- and middle-income countries.

WHAT'S NEW?

Approximately 35% of persons with diagnosed HIV infection in the United States do not have a suppressed viral load (Centers for Disease Control and Prevention, 2022), underscoring ongoing gaps in HIV care—many of which were exacerbated with the COVID-19 pandemic. Updated US guidelines continue to incorporate specific antiretroviral (ARV) recommendations after first- and second-line treatment failures, accounting for commonly observed resistance patterns that emerge across different treatment scenarios. Proviral DNA sequencing remains an area of high interest, given ongoing attention to regimen simplification and "switch" strategies, including the newly approved dual combination of long-acting injectable cabotegravir plus rilpivirine. For persons who acquire HIV in the setting of PrEP use (in particular long-acting injectable PrEP with cabotegravir), subsequent ART treatment selection should take into account potential transmitted and/or ADR.

KEY POINTS

- US treatment guidelines continue to recommend HIVDR testing at initial diagnosis and for persons who develop virologic failure on therapy.

- HIVDR testing is typically conducted with genotypic testing; simultaneous phenotypic testing may be considered if complex drug resistance mutation (DRM) patterns are of concern.

- ADR remains an important issue even with increasing use of second-generation INSTIs, thus clinicians should continue to emphasize treatment adherence and timely virologic monitoring.

- Proviral DNA resistance testing may be considered for regimen simplifications/switches particularly when a comprehensive history of prior plasma genotype testing results is not available. Results should be interpreted and applied carefully.

INTRODUCTION

Before highly active combination treatment, HIVDR was the main obstacle to successful therapy. As newer antiretroviral (ARV) drugs spanning different therapeutic classes have continued to be developed and approved, it has become possible to overcome HIVDR in many cases such that its management may be less of a clinical challenge in the current treatment era. However, because HIV is a chronic, lifelong infection, cumulative development of DRMs has the potential to limit treatment options over time for some people with HIV (PWH). HIVDR therefore remains an important concern, and providers should be aware of basic HIVDR prevention and management approaches. Ongoing trends in transmitted and acquired HIVDR, ARV drug development, advances in PrEP scale-up and medication options, and new dual regimen strategies all raise important clinical considerations. Table 20.1 includes a list of terms and definitions used in this chapter.

MECHANISMS OF HIV DRUG RESISTANCE

HIV mutates at a high rate during virus replication, resulting in nearly one nucleotide change during each replication cycle (Abram et al., 2010). Among PWH receiving incompletely suppressive ART, some mutations result in amino

Table 20.1 HIVDR-ASSOCIATED TERMS AND DEFINITIONS

Drug resistance mutations (DRMs)	Amino acid changes selected by ARV therapy, reducing ARV susceptibility in vitro, and/or reducing virological response to therapy.
Polymorphism	Amino acid changes in the targets of ARV therapy that are often present in ART-naive persons. Although most polymorphisms do not influence ARV susceptibility, some are selected by therapy and contribute to reduced ARV susceptibility nearly always in combination with nonpolymorphic DRMs.
Transmitted drug resistance	Presence of one or more nonpolymorphic DRMs in an ART-naive person.
Pretreatment drug resistance (PDR)	Presence of one or more nonpolymorphic DRMs in a PWH initiating or reinitiating ART in settings where pretherapy genotypic resistance testing is not routinely performed. Persons with PDR may include ART-naive persons, as well as pregnant persons who received ART for perinatal transmission prevention, persons receiving PrEP/PEP, and persons who discontinued first-line ART without a documented history of virological failure.
Acquired drug resistance	DRMs that are selected during ART, which can happen when viral replication is not fully suppressed in the presence of drug.
Genetic barrier to resistance	A function of the number of mutations required to reduce virus susceptibility to an ARV, the likelihood that these mutations will develop upon ARV drug exposure, and the impact of reduced ARV susceptibility on virological outcome. Some mutations rarely occur because they are associated with markedly reduced virus replication. The impact of reduced ARV susceptibility on virological outcome is highly heterogeneous.
Genotyping	Analysis for HIVDR through examination of viral genetic structure, specifically involving the sequencing of molecular targets of therapy to determine the presence of mutations known to confer decreased ARV drug susceptibility.
Phenotyping	Analysis for HIVDR which employs the measurement of drug susceptibility of virus by determining the concentration of drug which inhibits viral replication in tissue culture.
Sanger sequencing	Sequencing method of choice for commercially available genotypic resistance testing for over 20 years: DNA sequencing method used following reverse transcription of the viral ribonucleic acid genome (based on selective incorporation of chain-terminating dideoxynucleotides by DNA polymerase during in vitro DNA replication).
Next-generation HIVDR testing	High-throughput DNA sequencing technologies, where millions of DNA strands can be sequenced in parallel, yielding substantially more throughput and minimizing need for the fragment-cloning methods often used in Sanger sequencing.
Proviral DNA sequencing	Sequencing approach which samples the "archived" HIV viral reservoir found in PBMCs.
Wild-type virus	Naturally occurring, mutated strain of a virus.
Thymidine analogue mutations (TAM)	Polymorphic mutations selected by the thymidine analogs AZT and d4T: the accumulation of TAMs leads to progressive decrease in drug susceptibility for all approved NRTIs.

Adapted from Günthard et al. *Clin Infect Dis.* 2019;68(2):177–187.

acid changes that reduce susceptibility to one or more ARVs an individual is receiving (Coffin, 1995). In PWH on ART who do not maintain sufficiently high levels of medication adherence, viral variants possessing mutations that reduce ARV susceptibility will have a selective replication or "fitness" advantage. When strains harboring such mutations first emerge, they are part of a diverse swarm of viral variants (often referred to as a *quasispecies*). The complexity of the HIV-1 quasispecies is also increased by the high recombination rate occurring whenever more than one viral variant infects the same cell (Eberle & Gutler, 2012b; Levy et al., 2004). With sufficient selective ARV pressure, new variants will emerge and dominate the quasispecies (Figure 20.1). By contrast, if a person maintains virus suppression through consistent ART use, HIV is unable to replicate to a level high enough to support ongoing evolution

and development of HIVDR (Siliciano & Siliciano, 2013; van Zyl et al., 2018).

HIVDR is mediated almost entirely by mutations in the molecular targets of ART, including the reverse transcriptase (RT) gene in persons receiving nucleoside RT inhibitors (NRTIs) or nonnucleoside RT inhibitors (NNRTIs), the protease gene in persons receiving protease inhibitors (PIs), the integrase gene in persons receiving integrase strand transfer inhibitors (INSTIs); and the envelope genes (gp120 and gp41) in persons receiving entry inhibitors. The "genetic barrier to resistance" to an ARV is a useful concept which indicates that ARVs differ in their vulnerability to HIVDR by virtue of the number of mutations required for clinically significant reductions in drug susceptibility and the likelihood that these mutations will develop upon drug exposure (Figure 20.2). Further, some HIVDR-associated mutations

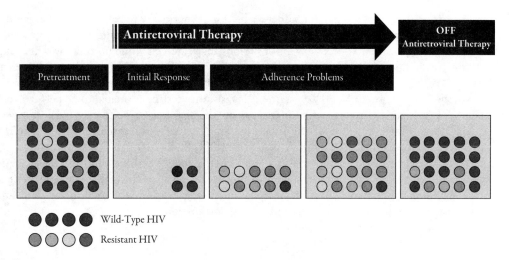

● ● ● ● Wild-Type HIV

○ ○ ○ ● Resistant HIV

Figure 20.1 Suboptimal ART and poor ART adherence lead to development of ARV-resistant strains　SOURCE: National HIV Curriculum. https://www.hiv.uw.edu/go/antiretroviral-therapy/evaluation-management-virologic-failure/core-concept/all. Published 2022. Accessed September 30, 2022.

occur rarely because they are associated with markedly reduced virus replication.

During its replication cycle, HIV-1 integrates into host chromosomal DNA and is then usually expressed leading to productive infection and cell killing. In resting memory CD4$^+$ T-cells, however, integrated proviral DNA may persist for many years forming a stable reservoir. As a result, proviral DNA levels in peripheral blood mononuclear cells (PBMCs) remain detectable even in PWH on ART who have undetectable plasma HIV-1 RNA levels. Therefore, in persons with stable virological suppression, the DRMs present in proviral DNA will often reflect resistance that emerged prior to the most recent regimen.

HIVDR is usually caused by "major" DRMs that reduce drug susceptibility by themselves, as well as accessory mutations that generally compensate for the reduced fitness associated with many of the major DRMs. With a few notable exceptions, major DRMs do not occur in previously untreated PWH, whereas accessory mutations are often polymorphic. HIVDR emerges in viruses from PWH exposed to suboptimal ARV inhibitory concentrations. As a result, most cases of virologic failure and drug resistance arise from incomplete adherence, which exposes viruses from PWH to incompletely suppressive ARV levels capable of exerting drug selective pressure. Accordingly, HIVDR appears to be less common in patients receiving fixed-dose combinations (FDCs) containing ARVs that have similar half-lives (and, ideally, a high genetic barrier to resistance) because incomplete adherence to these combinations is less likely to expose a virus to selective drug pressure (Llibre et al., 2011; Stella et al., 2022). Lower rates of HIVDR have also been associated with routine viral load monitoring programs/practices in which early detection

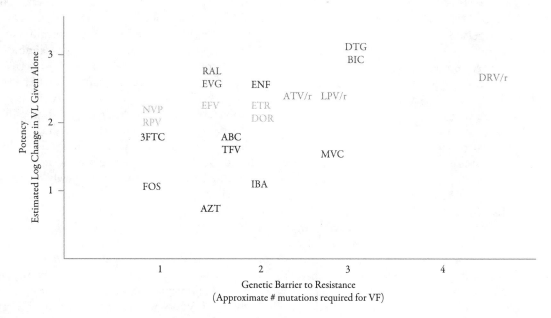

Figure 20.2 Schematic indicating genetic barrier to resistance (estimated) for select, approved ARV agents

of virological rebound provides the opportunity for adherence assessment and counseling, evaluation for drug–drug interactions, and/or regimen modification as necessary, prior to the evolution of multiple significant DRMs (Bachmann et al., 2019).

During its spread among humans, group M HIV-1 strains have evolved into many subtypes and circulating recombinant forms (Rambaut et al., 2004). However, none of the subtypes are intrinsically resistant to the main classes of ARVs (Günthard et al., 2019). Although viruses belonging to different subtypes occasionally differ in the frequency with which they develop different DRMs, the phenotypic effect of these mutations appear to be subtype independent, and it is, therefore, not necessary to know the subtype of a patient's virus to select therapy or to interpret the results of HIVDR testing (Günthard et al., 2019).

HIV DRUG RESISTANCE TESTING

INDICATIONS AND TIMING

Drug resistance testing is recommended at the time of initial diagnosis, regardless of whether someone starts ART soon thereafter—it is also recommended for people on therapy who are experiencing virologic failure and confirmed HIV-RNA levels >200 copies/mL (DHHS, 2022a; Günthard et al., 2019). For ART-naive PWH, the role of baseline resistance evaluation is to guide initial regimen selection. For ART-experienced persons with virologic failure, the role of resistance testing is to help ascertain the cause of virologic failure as well as to determine which ARVs may have been compromised and which agents still retain activity for potential incorporation into subsequent regimens.

With increasing use of first-line, INSTI-containing regimens for many newly diagnosed PWH in most settings, the cost-effectiveness of baseline resistance testing may be less than it once was (Hyle et al., 2019; Wood et al., 2022). Nonetheless, baseline testing remains the standard of care and is valuable not only for persons starting a standard, contemporary dual NRTI and INSTI-containing regimen, but also for many people who may require a subsequent regimen change, are considering a two-drug regimen, and who acquire HIV while on PrEP.

Timely resistance testing is recommended for all PWH because resistant variants are less fit in the absence of ARV selection pressure compared to wild-type susceptible virus variants. Retrospective studies involving stored samples have shown that transmitted drug-resistant variants are frequently outcompeted by wild-type revertants over time (Castro et al., 2013; Jain et al., 2011; Pingen et al., 2014; Yanik et al., 2012). The speed with which transmitted mutations are no longer detectable within plasma depends on the extent to which a mutation reduces virus fitness: some mutations are outcompeted by wild-type variants within several months, whereas others can persist as the dominant variant for years. In PWH experiencing virological failure, resistance testing should ideally be performed while the patient is still on ART because

in this scenario DRMs may no longer be detected within weeks of treatment discontinuation—specifically, the mutations that emerged while on therapy will rapidly be replaced by archived wild-type variants that were present before therapy was initiated (Deeks et al., 2001; Devereux et al., 1999). If resistance testing is unable to be performed while a person is on therapy, testing performed within 4 weeks after oral/non-long-acting ART discontinuation may still be informative (DHHS, 2022s). For PWH receiving long-acting ART, given the long half-lives of these drugs, resistance testing should be performed in all persons experiencing virologic failure—regardless of the amount of time since medication discontinuation.

GENOTYPIC AND PHENOTYPIC RESISTANCE TESTING

HIVDR testing can be performed genotypically (by sequencing the molecular targets of therapy) or phenotypically (by determining drug susceptibility in cell culture); both use PCR products directly amplified from cDNA that has been reverse-transcribed from plasma RNA. Genotypic resistance testing involves direct sequencing of the viral genome using conventional Sanger sequencing methodologies to identify mutations in the RT, protease (PR), and INSTI genes of circulating plasma RNA. Although genotypic tests are more complex than typical antimicrobial susceptibility tests, their ability to detect mutations present as mixtures (i.e., cocirculating with wild-type variants), even if the mutation is present at a level too low to affect drug susceptibility in a phenotypic assay, provides insight into the potential for resistance to emerge. Sequencing tests can also detect transitional mutations that do not cause drug resistance by themselves but indicate the presence of selective drug pressure. Compared to phenotypic testing, additional advantages of genotypic testing include lower cost and shorter turnaround time.

Phenotypic susceptibility testing involves the identification of ARV drug concentration that inhibits HIV replication by 50% (EC_{50}). The EC_{50} of a clinically sampled virus is then compared to that of a drug-susceptible laboratory reference strain and expressed as a ratio (referred to as *fold change*) of the EC_{50} of the sampled virus relative to the reference control (Figure 20.3). Most phenotypic tests use recombinant viruses created by inserting PCR-amplified clinical virus gene segments (protease/RT, integrase, envelope) into the backbone of a wild-type laboratory clone (Petropoulos et al., 2000). Phenotypic testing is not generally necessary as part of the baseline evaluation for newly diagnosed PWH. However, it may be a valuable complement to genotypic testing in persons who have experienced virologic failure on multiple treatment regimens and/or who have complicated DRM patterns (Günthard et al., 2019; DHHS, 2022a). It may also be useful in cases of acquired multiclass resistance. When phenotypic testing is indicated, it should be performed simultaneously with genotypic testing because of the ability of genotypic testing to detect emerging resistance as indicated above.

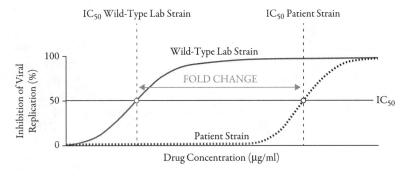

Figure 20.3 Calculating level of phenotypic resistance

This graph show the method for calculating the level of phenotypic resistance of a single ARV. The ARV is tested on a patient's HIV isolate and a laboratory reference (wild-type strain). The IC50 represents the concentration of the ARV required to cause 50% inhibition of HIV replication. The fold change is calculated by dividing the IC50 of the patient's isolate by the IC50 of the wild-type laboratory strain. As shown, as the curve shifts to the right, a higher concentration of ARV would be required to inhibit HIV replication and thus the strain of HIV would be more resistant. The further the curve shifts to the right (for the patient's HIV strain tested), the greater the level of resistance. **SOURCE:** National HIV Curriculum. https://www.hiv.uw.edu/go/antiretroviral-therapy/evaluation-management-virologic-failure/core-concept/all. Published 2022. Accessed September 30, 2022.

HIV THERAPEUTIC TARGETS FOR RESISTANCE TESTING

Sequencing of protease and the 5' part of RT usually constitutes one assay, whereas sequencing of integrase usually constitutes a second, distinct assay. Whereas RT/PR genotypic testing is routinely recommended for all newly diagnosed PWH and in patients with virologic failure, integrase genotypic testing is recommended primarily in persons with virologic failure on an INSTI-containing regimen or persons with an incomplete or delayed virologic response on an INSTI-based regimen. Baseline INSTI resistance testing should be considered in select persons with TDR such as those with reduced NRTI susceptibility or multiclass resistance and in persons who acquired HIV from a PWH failing an INSTI-containing regimen (Günthard et al., 2019). It is also recommended in persons who acquired HIV in the setting of prior cabotegravir-based PrEP use, as emergent INSTI-associated DRMs were detected in some clinical trial participants who were subsequently diagnosed with HIV (Marzinke et al., 2021; Eshleman et al., 2022; DHHS, 2022a).

Resistance testing for the four US FDA-approved entry inhibitors is less widely available. Genotypic testing for HIV-1 tropism (to evaluate activity of the CCR5 antagonist maraviroc) and for enfuvirtide susceptibility is available in several US-based reference laboratories including Quest, ARUP, and Monogram Biosciences/LabCorp; phenotypic testing for these two entry inhibitors is also available via Monogram Biosciences/LabCorp. Neither genotypic nor phenotypic resistance testing are yet commercially available for the attachment inhibitor fostemsavir or the postattachment inhibitor ibalizumab. To date, cross-resistance between attachment and entry inhibitors has not been described (Rose et al., 2022).

HIV-1 RNA THRESHOLDS FOR GENOTYPIC TESTING

Updated US treatment guidelines recommend HIVDR testing for PWH with virologic failure and confirmed HIV-1 RNA (i.e., viral load) levels greater than 200 copies/mL (DHHS, 2022a). Guidelines indicate resistance testing may be unsuccessful in people with confirmed viral load levels >200 copies/mL but < 500 copies/mL; however, it should still be considered. It is not uncommon for PWH to have repeated detectable viral load results between 50 to 500 copies/mL, and many studies have demonstrated that repeated viral loads between 200 to 500 copies/mL are associated with an increased risk of HIVDR and/or subsequent further viral load increases (Delaugerre et al., 2012b; Elvstam et al., 2017; Esber et al., 2019; Fleming et al., 2019; Hermans et al., 2018; Joya et al., 2019; Laprise et al., 2013; Li et al., 2012; Swenson, 2014; Vandenhende, 2015). For this reason, updated US guidelines have shifted the RNA threshold at which they recommend that resistance testing be pursued (i.e., from 500 to 200 copies/mL). Most nested PCR-based genotypic assays are able to yield interpretable results for many PWH with viral loads between 200 to 500 copies/mL (Gonzalez-Serra, 2014; Mackie et al., 2010; Swenson et al., 2014).

PROVIRAL DNA SEQUENCING

Proviral DNA sequencing is being increasingly employed in PWH who are planning to modify therapy while their virus levels are suppressed (Armenia et al., 2018; Ellis et al., 2019; Rodriguez et al., 2021; van Wyk et al., 2020). Current US guidelines support consideration of proviral DNA testing for PWH with viral suppression seeking regimen simplification, particularly if complex or semicomplex pre-existing HIVDR is suspected—for example, in persons who have experienced multiple prior treatment failures (DHHS, 2022a). Proviral DNA testing may be useful before switching to the dual therapy combination of long-acting cabotegravir plus rilpivirine, to exclude resistance-associated mutations, which have been associated with virologic failure (Cutrell et al., 2021). There is a strong but imperfect correlation between the DRMs in PBMC proviral DNA and plasma HIV-1 RNA from the same blood samples (Derache et al., 2015; Devereaux et al., 2000; Hoffman et al., 2022; Porter et al., 2016; Verhofstede et al.,

2004). Specifically, in patients with suppressed plasma viral load, proviral DNA genotyping will detect many but not all DRMs identified via historical plasma genotypic resistance testing (Allavena et al., 2018; Boukli et al., 2018; Delaugerre et al., 2012a; Margot, 2020; Wirden et al., 2011; Zaccarelli, 2016). This may occur particularly if previous episodes of virologic failure with emergent HIVDR were either not prolonged or associated with high-level viremia (Chu et al., 2022). Proviral DNA testing has also been studied in PWH with detectable viremia, including low-level viremia, but its clinical usefulness in this setting is less well characterized (Boukli et al., 2018; Curanovic et al., 2020; Lubke et al., 2015; Villalobos et al., 2020; Zaccarelli et al., 2016).

NEXT-GENERATION SEQUENCING

Newer sequencing technologies—collectively referred to as next-generation sequencing (NGS)—are replacing Sanger sequencing for many applications in diagnostic microbiology laboratories and continue to be used in research settings. The cost of NGS can be considerably lower than that of Sanger sequencing should a sufficient number of samples be tested in the same sequencing run (Lapointe et al., 2015; Noguera-Julian et al., 2017). Additionally, the ability of NGS to detect low-abundance DRMs (i.e., present at a prevalence below 15% to 20%) not detected by Sanger sequencing has potential advantages for improving patient outcomes particularly for the NNRTI class and for the detection of low levels of CXCR4 tropic viruses (Avila-Rios et al., 2016a; Boltz et al., 2011; Cozzi-Lepri et al., 2015; Li et al., 2011; Pou et al., 2014; Westby et al., 2006). Given the above, NGS may be useful for individual as well as population-level HIVDR evaluation in resource-limited settings (Baxter et al., 2021; Manyana et al., 2021). Nonetheless, Sanger sequencing has been used for over 2 decades to identify HIVDR and has been shown to be highly reproducible and interpretable in clinical

Table 20.2 SELECT RESOURCES ON HIVDR CLINICAL EVALUATION AND MANAGEMENT

US DHHS Guidelines	https://clinicalinfo. hiv.gov/en/guidelines/ adult-and-adolescent-arv/ whats-new-guidelines
IAS-USA: Drug resistance mutations in HIV-1	https://www.iasusa.org/resources/ hiv-drug-resistance-mutations/
Stanford HIV Database	https://hivdb.stanford.edu/
National HIV Curriculum (ART overview)	https://www.hiv.uw.edu/go/ antiretroviral-therapy
National Clinician Consultation Center	https://nccc.ucsf.edu/
HIV-ASSIST	https://hivassist.com
Clinical Care Options (HIV portfolio)	https://clinicaloptions.com/hiv

settings, whereas laboratory NGS procedures and approaches to sequence analysis continue to evolve (Avila-Rios et al., 2020; Mbunkah et al., 2020). Moreover, it has been difficult to translate the theoretical benefits of increased sensitivity for low-abundance variants into a practical clinical benefit, especially as ARV agents have become more potent and as most NGS assays have displayed reduced reproducibility at mutation detection thresholds below 5% (Avila-Rios et al., 2016a; Huber et al., 2017; Inzaule et al., 2018).

INTERPRETATION OF RESISTANCE TESTING RESULTS

Genotypic resistance testing produces a list of DRMs, which is accompanied by a prediction of which ARVs are likely to have reduced activity. As the many known HIV-associated DRMs occur in complex patterns and cause varying levels of reduced drug susceptibility, interpretation algorithms and systems are required to predict which ARVs are likely to retain activity. The four most commonly used publicly available interpretation systems include the Stanford HIVDB interpretation system (Paredes, 2017), ANRS system (Eberle & Gurtler, 2012a), Rega system (Eberle & Gutler, 2012a), and HIV-GRADE (Obermeier et al., 2012). The International AIDS Study-USA Antiviral Group also maintains a list of DRMs considered to be the most clinically relevant (Wensing et al., 2019).

Genotypic resistance interpretation system rules are usually developed by considering several types of published data including whether a DRM has been selected by a drug either in vitro or in PWH, whether a DRM reduces drug susceptibility in vitro, and whether there are data showing that a DRM interferes with virological response to an ART regimen containing the relevant drug. Although one might expect that DRMs present at low levels would have a lesser clinical impact than those present at higher levels, there are no interpretation systems that treat low-abundance DRMs differently from those present at higher levels. Further, interpretation systems often differ in the numbers of levels of resistance assigned. For example, most systems assign three levels: *susceptible, low-level/possible resistance*, and *resistance*. In contrast, the Stanford HIVDB system assigns five levels: *susceptible, potential low-level resistance, low-level resistance, intermediate resistance*, and *high-level resistance*. Overall, the systems are rarely completely discordant (i.e., a virus is rarely scored as being fully susceptible to a drug by one system but fully resistant by another system). Nonetheless, formal comparison of the various interpretation systems has found subtle differences (Rhee et al., 2009).

Phenotypic test results also require interpretation because the clinical significance of fold reductions in susceptibility differ among ARVs (de Meyer et al., 2008; Eron et al., 2013; Vingerhoets et al., 2010; Winters, 2009). Whenever possible, phenotypic tests provides three thresholds for fold reductions in drug susceptibility: (i) the reduction in susceptibility that exceeds the uppermost value for wild-type viruses often referred to as the *biological threshold* (Parkin et al., 2004); (ii) the lowest fold-reduction in susceptibility that indicates a PWH will have a reduced likelihood of responding to therapy (*lower clinical*

Table 20.3 COMMON HIVDR MUTATIONS AND IMPACT ON ARV SUSCEPTIBILITY, BY CLASS AND MEDICATION

ARV DRUGS	DRUG RESISTANCE MUTATIONS (DRMS)
NUCLEOSIDE/NUCLEOTIDE RT INHIBITORS	
Abacavir (ABC)	K65R, L74V/I, Y115F, M184V/I: one mutation confers low-level and two confer high-level resistance. T215Y/F + two additional TAMS: intermediate- to high-level resistance. MDR mutations: high-level resistance. K70E/Q/N/T: low-level phenotypic resistance.
Lamivudine (3TC); Emtricitabine (FTC)	M184V/I confer high-level resistance. K65R, MDR mutations, and 4-5 TAMS confer intermediate levels of resistance.
Tenofovir (TFV) disoproxil fumarate (TDF); Tenofovir alafenamide (TAF)	K65R: confers low-level phenotypic resistance but potentially high-level clinical resistance. T215Y/F + two additional TAMS: intermediate- to high-level resistance. MDR mutations: intermediate- to high-level resistance depending on the specific mutations. K70E/Q/N/T: low-level phenotypic resistance.
Zidovudine (AZT)	TAMs: confer intermediate- to high-level resistance. MDR mutations confer high-level resistance.
	TAMs (thymidine analog mutations) are defined as M41L, D67N, K70R, L210W, T215F/Y, K219Q/E. T215F/Y is the most important of these and the combination of M41L+L210W+T215Y has the greatest phenotypic and virological impact. MDR mutations are defined as (i) Q151M usually in combination with ≥2 of the following: A62V, V75I, F77L, and F116Y; (ii) An amino acid insertion at position 69, which nearly always occurs with ≥1 TAM. M184V/I increase susceptibility to AZT, TDF, and TAF; K65R increases susceptibility to AZT; TAF and TDF have similar resistance profiles. However, TAF achieves >fourfold higher intracellular levels of the active inhibitor TFV-diphosphate suggesting that it is likely to be more active than TDF at inhibiting both drug-susceptible and drug-resistant viruses. However, most genotypic resistance interpretation systems do not distinguish between the two TFV prodrugs. T215S/C/D/E/I/V are commonly transmitted mutations consistent with previous thymidine analog selection pressure. These mutations have much less clinical significance than T215Y/F.
NUCLEOSIDE RT INHIBITORS	
Efavirenz (EFV)	L100I, K101E/P, K103N/S, V106A/M, Y188L/C/H, G190A/S/E/Q, P225H, F227C, and M230L.
Etravirine (ETR)	L100I, K101E/P, Y181C/I/V, G190E/Q, F227C, and M230L.
Rilpivirine (RPV)	ETR + E138A/G/K/Q/R, H221Y, and Y188L.
Doravirine (DOR)	V106A/M, Y188L, G190E/Q, F227C/L, M230L, L234I, and F318Y.
General comments	Common accessory relatively nonpolymorphic DRMs: A98G, V106I, V108I, V179D/E/F, H221Y, and P225H. High-level DOR resistance in persons receiving DOR usually includes one of the following DRMs: V106A, Y188L, F227L/C, M230L, L234I, or Y318F. The common DRMs K103N, Y181C, and G190A are not associated with clinically significant reductions in DOR susceptibility. However, many combinations of ≥2 DRMs that emerge in persons receiving other NNRTIs can be associated with reductions in DOR susceptibility that are likely to be clinically significant. ETR usually requires ≥2 mutations for intermediate- or high-level resistance. Although E138K causes low-level RPV resistance, it is one of the most commonly emerging DRMs in persons developing virologic failure while receiving RPV. E138A, which is polymorphic in certain subtypes, minimally reduces RPV susceptibility but is of uncertain clinical significance.
PROTEASE INHIBITORS	
Atazanavir (ATV/r)	V32I, M46I/L, I47V, G48V/M, I50L, I54V/T/A/S/L/M, V82A/C/F/M/S/T, I84V/A/C, N88S, and L90M.
Darunavir (DRV/r)	V32I, I47V/A, I50V, I54L/M, L76V, V82F, and I84V/A/C.
Lopinavir (LPV/r)	L24I, V32I, M46I/L, I47V/A, G48V/M, I50V, I54V/T/A/S/L/M, L76V, V82A/C/F/M/S/T, I84A/C/V, and L90M.
General comments	Common accessory nonpolymorphic DRMs: L10F, V11I/L, K20T, L33F, G73/S/T/C/A, T74P, and L89V. DRV/r has the highest genetic barrier to resistance usually requiring two to three of the listed mutations and two to three of the accessory mutations to develop high-level resistance. LPV/r has a lower genetic barrier to resistance compared with DRV/r but likely a higher genetic barrier to resistance than ATV/r.

(continued)

Table 20.3 CONTINUED

INTEGRASE STRAND TRANSFER INHIBITORS

Raltegravir (RAL)	T66K, E92Q, G118R, F121Y, E138A/K/T, G140A/S/C, Y143CRH, Q148H/R/K, and N155H.
Elvitegravir (EVG)	T66A/I/K, E92Q, G118R, F121Y, E138A/K/T, G140A/S/C, S147G, Q148H/R/K, N155H, and R263K.
Dolutegravir (DTG)	G118R, E138A/K/T, G140A/S/C, Q148H/R/K, N155H, and R263K.
Bictegravir (BIC)	G118R, E138A/K/T, G140A/S/C, Q148H/R/K, N155H, and R263K.
Cabotegravir (CAB)	G118R, E138A/K/T, G140A/S/C/R, Q148H/R/K, N155H, and R263K.
Notes	Accessory uncommon nonpolymorphic DRMs: H51Y, G149A, S153Y/F, and S230R.
	Accessory polymorphic DRMs: L74M, T97A, E157Q, G163K/E, and D232N.
	Many of the EVG and RAL-associated DRMs appear to be DTG and BIC-accessory DRMs.
	There are three somewhat overlapping RAL-resistance mutational pathways: Y143C/R/H vs. Q148H/R/K vs. N155H often in combination with an additional mutation such as E92Q, E138K/A/T, G140S/A/C, and/or an accessory mutation.
	Persons receiving EVG are less likely to develop Y143 mutations and more likely to develop T66A/I/K, E92Q, and S147G. But there is a high-level of cross-resistance between RAL and EVG.
	There are somewhat overlapping DTG-resistance mutation pathways: Q148H/K/R + one to two additional mutations; N155H + ≥additional mutation; R263K; and G118R. Although R263K is the most commonly occurring DRM in persons developing DTG-associated virologic failure, it is associated with just a twofold reduction in susceptibility. BIC has a nearly identical resistance profile compared with DTG.
	High-level resistance to RAL and EVG usually requires just 1 to 2 DRMs while high-level resistance to DTG and BIC appears to require two to three DRMs. Additionally, DRMs emerge less frequently in persons receiving DTG or BIC compared with those receiving RAL or EVG. DRMs associated with reduced DTG or BID susceptibility generally have cause a greater reduction in CAB susceptibility.

ENTRY INHIBITORS

Enfuvirtide (fusion inhibitor)	Mutations in gp41 codons 36–45, the region to which enfuvirtide binds. The key mutations are G36D/E/V, V38E/A, Q40H, N42T, and N43D. A single mutation usually reduces susceptibility about tenfold, whereas two mutations usually reduce susceptibility about 100-fold.
Maraviroc (CCR5 inhibitor)	CXCR4-tropic gp120 variants: positively charged residues at positions 11 and 25 of the V3 loop of gp120, and several other combinations of mutations primarily but not exclusively within the V3 loop are associated with CXCR4 tropism. The most common mechanism of resistance is the expansion of pre-existing CXCR4-tropic variants that were not detected before therapy.
	Resistance can also emerge as a result of gp120 mutations that allow HIV-1 to bind to an altered CCR5 receptor. There is no consistent pattern of these mutations.
Ibalizumab (postattachment inhibitor)	Loss of potential N-linked glycosylation sites in the V5 loop of gp120 allows HIV-1 to bind CD4 and enter cells despite the presence of ibalizumab (Blair).
Fostemsavir	Several gp120 mutations including M426L and S375M are considered major fostemsavir-resistance mutations, while M434I and M475I are considered to have a lesser effect on susceptibility. The amino acids that explain why CRF01_AE viruses are usually resistant to fostemsavir map to 375H and 475I (Zhou, 2014).

threshold); and (iii) the lowest fold-reduction in susceptibility that indicates a drug will likely be completely inactive (*upper clinical threshold*). Upper and lower clinical thresholds have been developed for ARVs that have been used in salvage therapy situations for treatment of PWH with viruses containing DRMs affecting the same ARV class including abacavir (Lanier et al., 2004), tenofovir (Miller et al., 2004), etravirine (Vingerhoets et al., 2010), lopinavir (Kempf et al., 2002), darunavir (De Meyer et al., 2008), and dolutegravir (Eron et al., 2013).

Importantly, genotypic and phenotypic test interpretations alone do not contain sufficient information to construct a clinically appropriate ART regimen for an individual. In addition to the results of recent resistance testing, it is necessary to consider prior treatment history and previous resistance testing results. Genotypic and phenotypic resistance interpretation systems also vary in how they take into account differences in ARV potency, and thus do not incorporate fundamental principles of how treatment regimens should be constructed. Therefore, clinicians must place the results of drug resistance assays within the context of current treatment guidelines. Newly developed educational tools are available to inform clinical decision-making regarding ARV selection (Ramirez et al., 2020).

TRANSMITTED HIV DRUG RESISTANCE

EPIDEMIOLOGY

TDR is defined as the presence in an ART-naive person of one or more DRMs that are polymorphic in that they do not occur naturally in the absence of selective drug pressure. For practical purposes, polymorphic mutations have been defined as mutations that occur at a prevalence below 0.5% in all major HIV subtypes in ART-naive persons at times and in regions where TDR has been uncommon. The most common list of mutations used for surveillance of TDR was published in 2009 and is often referred to as the World Health Organization (WHO) list (Bennett et al., 2009). The US Centers for Disease Control and Prevention uses a more expansive list which includes mutations that may be polymorphic in non-B subtypes (Wheeler et al., 2010). A subset of major IAS-USA mutations has also been used in several surveillance studies (Wensing et al., 2019).

Over the past 10 years, TDR prevalence has been approximately 15% in the United States, 10%–15% in Europe and the Latin America and Caribbean regions, and 5%–10% in Sub-Saharan Africa and Asia (Avila-Rios et al., 2016b; Gupta et al., 2018; Kirichenko et al., 2022; McClung et al., 2022; Miranda et al., 2022; Rhee et al., 2015, 2020b). bTDR prevalence has been stable in most geographic regions except for Sub-Saharan Africa, where rates of transmitted NRTI and NNRTI resistance have been increasing, particularly among persons with pretreatment resistance (PDR), which includes ARV-naive persons, as well as PWH who have received prior ARVs to prevent perinatal HIV transmission or who are reinitiating therapy without a documented history of virologic failure; see "Resource-limited settings" below (Gupta et al., 2018; Rhee et al., 2020b).

Transmitted INSTI resistance has been below 1.0% in most regions, with one systematic review suggesting that prevalence of INSTI-associated surveillance DRMs has remained low even in regions where INSTIs have been widely used for several years (Bailey et al., 2021; McClung et al., 2022). In a study describing retrospective baseline genotype data obtained by NGS for clinical trials evaluating bictegravir/emtricitabine/tenofovir alafenamide, primary INSTI resistance substitutions were found in 1.3% of participants (Acosta et al., 2021). However, increases may be occurring in the United States: one study in Florida reported rates of 1.4% in 2015 and 2.2% in 2016 (McClung, 2019, 2020; Poschman & Spencer, 2020).

Samples obtained from PWH in upper-income countries with identified NRTI-, NNRTI-, and PI-associated TDR generally contain DRMs associated with ARVs that are now used infrequently such as thymidine analog mutations (TAMs), NNRTI-resistance mutations, and mutations associated with older PIs (Drescher, 2014; Machnowska et al., 2019; Margot, 2017; Pingen et al., 2014; Rhee et al., 2019a). Many of these circulating TDR strains are considered most likely to be established among ART-naive persons rather than reflecting direct transmission from persons experiencing virologic failure.

MANAGEMENT OF TDR

In the United States and other high-income countries, the risk posed by TDR to the success of first-line therapy is low because, as noted above, most of the currently transmitted DRMs do not compromise currently recommended first-line ART regimens. Moreover, the routine performance of genotypic resistance testing makes it possible to identify those transmitted DRMs that would compromise currently recommended first-line ART regimens and warrant consideration of an alternative initial combination.

Given the lack of clinical trials comparing treatment approaches for persons in whom baseline resistance testing reveals the presence of TDR, several retrospective studies provide useful insight. First, because there is no cross-resistance between drug classes, persons with transmitted NNRTI resistance are expected to have an undiminished response to treatment using an INSTI- or PI-containing first-line ART regimen. Second, the presence of the most commonly transmitted NRTI-associated DRMs—TAMs other than T215Y/F—do not appear to influence the virological response to first-line tenofovir disoproxil fumarate (TDF) or tenofovir alafenamide (TAF)-containing regimens (Margot et al., 2017; Sorstedt et al., 2018). Third, although the presence of baseline TDR-associated DRMs suggests the possible presence of additional undetected transmitted DRMs (i.e., those that have faded to low levels following competition with wild-type revertants) (Castro et al., 2013; Jain et al., 2011; Mbunkah et al., 2020; Pingen, 2014), such additional DRMs have not been detected frequently by sensitive NGS methods (Clutter, 2017; Dauwe et al., 2016; Toni et al., 2009; Varghese et al., 2009). Moreover, in retrospective studies, PWH with TDR detected by baseline genotypic resistance testing do not appear to have higher rates of virologic failure when the results of such testing is used to guide therapy (Borghetti et al., 2020; Geretti et al., 2019; Knyphausen et al., 2014; Margot et al., 2017; Metzner et al., 2010; Peuchant et al., 2008; Rhee et al., 2020a).

ACQUIRED HIV DRUG RESISTANCE

EPIDEMIOLOGY

The increased use of ARVs with a high genetic barrier to resistance, particularly the second-generation INSTIs, and the use of FDCs often administered in a single tablet regimen collectively make it less likely that medication adherence will result in a person's virus becoming exposed to an incompletely suppressive regimen. Many clinical trials and several longitudinal cohort studies in upper-income countries have reported that since 2000 fewer persons beginning ART have developed virologic failure or acquired HIVDR (ATCC, 2017; Carr et al., 2019; Davy-Mendez et al., 2018; Li et al., 2018; Lodi et al., 2018; Lombardi, 2021; Miranda, 2022; Nance et al., 2018; Rhee et al., 2020a; Scherrer, 2016). Additionally, several laboratory-based studies have observed a decline in the proportion of submitted viruses with HIVDR and multiclass resistance (Paquet et al., 2014; Kagan et al., 2019), although much of this decrease reflects the likelihood that an increasing proportion of resistance test samples are from persons with newly diagnosed HIV rather than those with virologic failure. This is also supported by the decreasing proportion of PWH with extensive treatment histories (Bajema et al., 2020).

Nonetheless, adherence to a daily treatment regimen is a continuing challenge, particularly in populations that face logistical, social, and financial barriers to obtaining HIV care and accessing lifelong ARVs (Rich et al., 2020; Siefried et al., 2017, 2018). Moreover, despite the increased use of FDCs and ARVs with a high genetic barrier to resistance, such regimens are not available to some PWH, particularly those who have experienced previous virologic failure or who have coexisting medical conditions such as advanced liver/kidney disease that might preclude use of certain agents. Additionally, the recent approval of long-acting ARV combinations may usher in a host of new questions regarding HIVDR management for which limited evidence is currently available to guide best practices. For example, new strategies will be required to determine how to minimize the risk of ADR in PWH receiving long-acting ARV combinations and how to best detect ADR in PWH who have recently received a long-acting ARV but are no longer virologically suppressed.

MANAGEMENT OF ADR

In PWH developing virologic failure on an initial ART regimen, those who develop HIVDR often have predictable patterns of DRMs. For example, persons receiving an NNRTI-containing regimen will usually have both NRTI and NNRTI-associated DRMs while those receiving a first-generation INSTI-containing regimen will often have both NRTI and INSTI-associated DRMs (DHHS, 2022a;

Gregson et al., 2016; Rhee et al., 2020a). In these two scenarios, the most common NRTI-associated DRMs are the 3TC/FTC mutations M184V/I; additionally, approximately 30% of PWH will also develop a tenofovir-associated DRM (usually K65R or K70E/Q). In low- and middle-income countries, the proportion of persons developing a tenofovir-associated DRM on a first-line NRTI/NNRTI-containing regimen is higher and approaches 60% (Gregson et al., 2016). In contrast, among PWH receiving an initial boosted PI or second-generation INSTI-containing regimen, those who develop HIVDR will usually just acquire M184V/I (DHHS, 2022; Dolling et al., 2013; El Bouzidi et al., 2014; Lathourwers et al., 2020; Rhee et al., 2019b, 2020b; Scarsi, 2020). As a result of these predictable patterns, the DHHS has developed recommendations for first-line treatment failure scenarios: specific recommendations most commonly involve modifying therapy to include at least one active NRTI and either a second-generation INSTI or boosted darunavir (Table 20.4).

In PWH who have experienced virologic failure on multiple ART regimens, the patterns of observed HIV-associated DRMs are often less predictable. In this scenario, the DHHS and IAS-USA guidelines recommend expert consultation and modification of therapy to include at least two fully active drugs from different ARV drug classes (DHHS, 2022a; Saag et al., 2020). The vast majority of clinical trials performed in heavily treated PWH have been registration trials designed to study the impact of "salvage therapy" with ART regimens containing either boosted darunavir, boosted tipranavir,

Table 20.4 TREATMENT OPTIONS FOR PWH WITH VIROLOGIC FAILURE ON A FIRST-LINE REGIMEN

CLINICAL SCENARIO	TYPE OF FAILING REGIMEN	HIVDR CONSIDERATIONS	NEW REGIMEN OPTIONS
First regimen failure	NNRTI plus two NRTIs	Likely resistance to NNRTI ± XTC (i.e., NNRTI mutations ± M184V/I). Additional NRTI mutations may be present.	Boosted PI plus two NRTIs (at least one active); *or* DTG (possibly BIC) plus two NRTIs (at least one active); *or* boosted PI plus INSTI
	Boosted PI plus two NRTIs	Most likely no resistance, or resistance limited to XTC (i.e., M184V/I without resistance to other NRTIs).	Continue same regimen; *or* Another boosted PI plus two NRTIs (at least one active); *or* INSTI plus two NRTIs (at least one active—if only one of the NRTIs is fully active or if adherence is a concern, DTG is preferred INSTI although BIC might be considered); *or* another boosted PI plus INSTI
	INSTI plus two NRTIs	No INSTI resistance (can have XTC resistance, i.e., only M184V/I, usually without resistance to other NRTIs).	Boosted PI plus two NRTIs (at least one active); *or* DTG (possibly BIC) plus two NRTIs (at least one active); *or* boosted PI plus INSTI
		RAL or EVG ± XTC resistance. Resistance to first-line BIC or DTG is rare.	Boosted PI plus 2 NRTIs (at least one active); *or* DTG twice daily or possibly BIC (if virus is sensitive) plus two active NRTIs; *or* DTG twice daily or possibly BIC (if virus is sensitive) plus boosted PI

XTC: 3TC/FTC; DTG = dolutegravir; RAL = raltegravir; EVG = elvitegravir; BIC = bictegravir; DRV = darunavir

SOURCE: Panel on Antiretroviral Guidelines for Adults and Adolescents. Guidelines for the use of antiretroviral agents in adults and adolescents with HIV. Department of Health and Human Services. Adapted from Table 11. https://clinicalinfo.hiv.gov/sites/default/files/inline-files/AdultandAdolescentGL.pdf. Accessed September 25, 2022.

etravirine, dolutegravir, enfuvirtide, maraviroc, ibalizumab, or fostemsavir (McCluskey et al., 2019).

With the demonstration that both dolutegravir and boosted darunavir plus a single active NRTI are fully suppressive ART regimens for many PWH, and with recent approval of several additional ARVs (e.g., doravirine, ibalizumab, and fostemsavir) and the likely imminent approval of the capsid inhibitor lenacapavir, the prospects for constructing a fully suppressive regimen in nearly all treatment experienced PWH with virologic failure are high (Bajema et al., 2020; Emu et al., 2018; Marcelin et al., 2022; Raymond et al., 2020; Paton et al., 2022; Puertas et al., 2020). Among INSTI-naive PWH or among INSTI-experienced persons with viruses retaining susceptibility to dolutegravir, the combination of dolutegravir plus one fully active NRTI and/or fully active NNRTI (e.g., rilpivirine or doravirine) may be sufficient. If etravirine will be used concurrently with dolutegravir, a boosted PI needs to be added because of drug interactions (DHHS, 2022a). For some PWH with INSTI-resistant viruses, susceptibility to dolutegravir may be retained if it is dosed twice a day (Akil et al., 2015; Castagna et al., 2014; Eron et al., 2013). Although guidelines indicate bictegravir may be considered rather than dolutegravir for treatment experienced PWH, it has not been studied for salvage therapy (in contrast to dolutegravir), and its dose cannot be doubled/adjusted to compensate for INSTI-related DRMs—therefore, careful consideration of its use in this scenario is warranted. Likewise, for PWH whose viruses retain complete or nearly complete susceptibility to boosted darunavir, the combination of boosted darunavir plus one fully active NRTI and/or fully active NNRTI (e.g., etravirine or doravirine) may be sufficient. Regimens including dolutegravir plus boosted darunavir have been increasingly used among treatment experienced PWH with viremia (Armenia et al., 2021; Capetti et al., 2018; Jablonowska et al., 2019)—this may reflect provider preferences for avoiding NNRTIs when their inclusion is considered to be of questionable benefit.

In the presence of pre-existing resistance to dolutegravir *and* boosted darunavir, current options for salvage therapy are more complicated. However, even in this scenario, there are several potentially useful treatment approaches including the use of two or more drugs from the four main ARV classes and possibly the use of one or more entry inhibitors (Puertas et al., 2020; Raymond et al., 2020). In most PWH, fostemsavir may have a similar degree of antiviral activity as ibalizumab; however, a small subset of persons will harbor intrinsically resistant viruses (Kozal et al., 2020).

ARV RESISTANCE CONSIDERATIONS FOR SPECIAL CIRCUMSTANCES

There are a number of circumstances in which HIV treatment guidelines offer limited information on specific recommendations for evaluation and management of HIVDR. A few of these are described briefly below.

ART SWITCH/SIMPLIFICATION (MODIFYING ART IN THE SETTING OF VIROLOGIC SUPPRESSION)

At times, providers and/or PWH may wish to consider changing to a fully suppressive ARV regimen. This may be due to concerns regarding safety profile, side effects, new drug–drug interactions, pill burden, pregnancy status/intentions, or cost/access (including formulary changes). In these situations, providers should consider the person's complete treatment history and comprehensive resistance testing history to construct a cumulative resistance profile (DHHS, 2022a; McCluskey et al., 2019; Saag et al., 2020). The fundamental clinical principle with regimen optimization/simplification is to maintain virologic suppression and not compromise future treatment options. If comprehensive resistance data are not available, clinicians may be able to extrapolate information from the treatment history—for example, a person with history of virologic failure while taking ARVs with relatively low barrier to resistance (most NNRTIs, first-generation INSTIs, lamivudine/emtricitabine) can be assumed to have accumulated resistance to these drugs (DHHS, 2022). Proviral DNA sequencing may be considered, but results should be interpreted in conjunction with the knowledge of HIVDR that may have emerged during past episodes of virological failure and previous genotypic resistance test results.

US guidelines list several specific optimization strategies that can be considered (Table 20.5), based on available data, taking into account the factors listed above as well as others (e.g., hepatitis B coinfection) (DHHS, 2022a; Saag et al., 2020). Individuals with no suspected or documented history of HIVDR generally have multiple options for switching ARV drugs in their regimen, either between classes or within classes. However, clinicians should still exercise caution and generally avoid switching to an agent with a lower genetic barrier to resistance, given the risk of virologic failure if the patient was primarily infected with a drug-resistant virus or previously ADR during a previous episode of virological failure (DHHS, 2022a; Eron, 2010). Of note, a number of two-drug regimens (including newly approved cabotegravir plus rilpivirine, both administered as long-acting injections) are currently identified as potential "switch" options—it would be especially prudent to have a high degree of confidence in a patient's full HIVDR profile when considering switching to a dual therapy regimen, to ensure that both ARV agents are active. For patients with a history of limited drug resistance, clinicians can consider a switch from one drug to another within the same class or in a different class, as long as the new drug has a high genetic barrier to resistance and there is no known or suspected resistance to the new agent. Based on data extrapolated from other studies, dolutegravir plus two NRTIs (one of which is fully active) should be effective as a switch strategy in virologically suppressed individuals without underlying dolutegravir resistance (DHHS, 2022a). Bictegravir/emtricitabine/tenofovir alafenamide has also been examined as a switch option in both clinical trials and real-world settings, including for treatment experienced PWH (Acosta et al., 2020; Armenia et al., 2022; Rolle et al.,

Table 20.5 TREATMENT OPTIONS FOR OPTIMIZING ART IN THE SETTING OF VIROLOGIC SUPPRESSION

CLINICAL SCENARIO	TYPE OF SWITCH	STRATEGIES THAT HAVE EVIDENCE FOR SUCCESS
No suspected or documented HIVDR	Within-class switch	• TDF or ABC to TAF • RAL to DTG • DTG, EVG/c, or RAL to BIC • EFV to RPV or DOR
	Between-class switch	• Replacing a boosted PI with an INSTI (other than RAL) • Replacing a boosted PI with RPV or DOR • Replacing an NNRTI with an INSTI
	Switch from three-drug to two-drug regimen (both drugs should be fully active)	• DTG + RPV • DTG + XTC • 3TC + boosted PI (e.g., DRV/r or DRV/cobi or ATV/r or LPV/r) • Boosted DRV + DTG • Long-acting CAB + RPV[a]
History of limited drug resistance	Within-class switch	• Switch from one drug with a high genetic barrier to resistance to another (i.e., from DTG to BIC) • Switch to a drug with a higher genetic barrier to resistance (i.e., from RAL to DTG or BIC)
	Between-class switch	• Switch from one drug with a high genetic barrier to resistance to another (i.e., from boosted PI to BIC or DTG) • Switch to a drug with a higher genetic barrier to resistance (i.e., from EFV to DTG or BIC or boosted PI)
History of complex underlying resistance	Proceed with caution; follow the same principles outlined under "Management of ADR" and consider expert consultation	

TDF = tenofovir disoproxil fumarate; ABC = abacavir; TAF = tenofovir alafenamide; RAL = raltegravir; DTG = dolutegravir; EVG/c = elvitegravir/cobicistat; BIC = bictegravir; EFV = efavirenz; RPV = rilpivirine; DOR = doravarine; ATV = atazanavir; 3TC = lamivudine; MVC = maraviroc; DRV = darunavir; ATV/r = ritonavir-boosted atazanavir; DRV/r = ritonavir-boosted darunavir; DRV/cobi = cobicistat-boosted darunavir; LPV/r = ritonavir-boosted lopinavir; CAB = cabotegravir. Footnote: [a]Given limited data and experience, US guidelines recommend that the dual regimen of long-acting CAB + RPV can be used to replace an existing, stable oral ARV regimen in PWH with sustained viral suppression for 3 to 6 months (optimal duration is not defined), who have good adherence and engagement in care, no known or suspected resistance to either medication and no prior treatment failures. If the person being considered for long-acting CAB + RVP has active or occult HBV infection, they should be receiving HBV therapy if indicated. Persons being considered for long-acting CAB + RPV should also not be receiving medications with significant drug interactions.

SOURCE: Panel on Antiretroviral Guidelines for Adults and Adolescents. Guidelines for the use of antiretroviral agents in adults and adolescents with HIV. Department of Health and Human Services. Adapted from text. http://www.aidsinfo.nih.gov/ContentFiles/AdultandAdolescentGL.pdf. Accessed September 25, 2022.

2021; Sax et al., 2022). Expert consultation may be especially helpful when considering regimen switching/simplification for PWH who are heavily ART experienced, as individuals who have undergone multiple regimen modifications have often done so because of virologic failure and ADR (and often multiclass HIVDR development) (DHHS, 2022a; Saag et al., 2020).

PREGNANCY

The fundamental principles of HIVDR testing/evaluation and management for pregnant people are the same as those in non-pregnant people (i.e., perform drug resistance testing at diagnosis, at initiation or reinitiation of ART, and in the event of virologic failure) (DHHS, 2022b). However, it is important to achieve virologic suppression as early as possible in pregnancy to reduce the likelihood of perinatal transmission. Because results of resistance testing may occasionally not be available for several weeks, US guidelines recommend immediate ART initiation if HIV is diagnosed in pregnancy

(DHHS, 2022b). In ART-experienced pregnant PWH, therapy reinitiation-initiation should be guided by what is known about the person's previous ART regimens and responses as well as previous resistance testing results. In both scenarios, ART should be modified if necessary once resistance testing results are available—taking into account ARV safety and dosing in pregnancy. Pregnant persons who have documented zidovudine (ZDV) resistance should still receive intravenous ZDV during labor when indicated (i.e., HIV RNA >1,000 copies/mL near delivery).

Unique pregnancy-associated factors may lead to incomplete viral suppression and HIVDR development, such as nausea and vomiting affecting adherence and pharmacokinetic changes such as increased plasma volume and renal clearance. Some ARVs require dose adjustment during pregnancy; US guidelines provide detailed information on use of specific ARVs in pregnancy (DHHS, 2022b). If perinatal/postnatal HIV transmission does occur in the setting of incomplete maternal viral suppression, maternal HIVDR can be transmitted to the infant, limiting treatment options for the infant (Boyce et al., 2022; Delaugerre et al., 2009; Weyland et al.,

2022). Decisions about ARV prophylaxis and/or treatment for infants exposed to a drug-resistant virus should therefore be made in consultation with a pediatric HIV specialist.

RAPID ART INITIATION AND RAPID ART REINITIATION

Rapid ART initiation immediately or very soon after HIV diagnosis is an approach that continues to hold widespread interest (Boyd et al., 2019). Individual clinical and public health benefits of rapid ART initiation include improved linkage to HIV medical care and ART uptake, decreased time to viral suppression, and decreased risk of HIV transmission to others (Ford et al., 2018; Mateo-Urdiales, 2019; Pilcher et al., 2017). Findings from several programs in the United States as well as resource-limited settings have demonstrated its feasibility and acceptability (Coffey et al., 2019; Colasanti et al., 2018; Martin et al., 2020; Rodriguez et al., 2019). One retrospective cohort analysis found no difference in probability of attaining virologic suppression by 48 weeks among people who initiated ART without baseline genotype vs. people who initiated ART guided by genotype results (Bavaro et al., 2022). US guidelines currently recommend initiating ART at the time of diagnosis (when possible) or soon afterwards "to increase the uptake of ART, decrease the time required to achieve linkage to care and virologic suppression, and improve the rate of virologic suppression among individuals who have recently received HIV diagnoses" (DHHS, 2022b).

Since regimen selection for rapid ART initiation occurs prior to the availability of baseline resistance testing results, options should have a suitably high likelihood of effectiveness and favorable safety and side effect profiles; local TDR patterns may also need to be considered. To date, the most commonly used rapid ART combination options in the United States include tenofovir (TDF or TAF) plus emtricitabine (or lamivudine), paired with either a second-generation integrase inhibitor (i.e., bictegravir or dolutegravir) or (less frequently) once-daily boosted darunavir (Bachelard et al., 2021; Huhn et al., 2022). If baseline resistance testing subsequently indicates potentially compromised ARV activity of any components of the selected regimen, providers are generally advised to consider treatment modification or, at minimum, frequent viral load monitoring until stable virologic suppression has been established. Most rapid ART studies have not provided detailed information on the frequency of, or reasons for, ART adjustments after initiation: one study indicated ART was modified in < 3% of participants after baseline genotype testing demonstrated transmitted resistance mutations (Coffey et al., 2019).

As of September 2022, the only specific medication recommendations provided in US guidelines on rapid ART selection were to avoid NNRTI-based regimens, abacavir, and the dual therapy combination of dolutegravir plus lamivudine. Given the potential impact of TDR on two-drug rapid ART initiation, additional evidence and real-world clinical experience are warranted (Kessler et al., 2020), although some interest exists in identifying rapid dual therapy approaches which might be feasible. For example, a single-arm study evaluating dolutegravir plus lamivudine as a "test and treat" strategy found that 78% of participants achieved HIV-1 RNA< 50 copies/mL by week 24, although initial treatment was modified in 4.6% because of subsequently identified HBV coinfection or baseline M184V (Rolle et al., 2021).

For patients with chronic HIV infection who have been out of care and/or off ART, "rapid ART re-initiation" decisions may not be straightforward, especially if limited history is available. Depending on the individual's prior HIV treatment, some providers would consider obtaining resistance testing at the first clinical re-engagement visit; however, as indicated above, testing performed in the absence of recent ART use may be of limited utility. Although it may provide useful information to guide therapy modification *after* rapid ART reinitiation-initiation (in the event that DRMs are identified), historically selected mutations may not be reflected accurately without the presence of selective drug pressure. In other words, the absence of detectable resistance must be viewed cautiously when interpreting results. In general, expert input is recommended for "rapid ART reinitiation" decisions (especially for heavily ART-experienced PWH) since multiple factors should be taken into account). After reinitiating therapy, and if the viral load does not decrease as anticipated, providers should have a low threshold to repeat resistance testing to guide further management.

HIV ACQUISITION IN THE SETTING OF PREP USE

There have been two main concerns regarding PrEP and HIVDR. The first is whether PrEP will remain effective in areas with high TDR prevalence and the second is whether PrEP will lead to an increased number of cases of HIVDR. Additionally, as more long-acting options become available, new considerations might arise as PrEP is further implemented globally (Parikh et al., 2022). Regarding the first issue, many studies have shown that the transmission of viruses resistant to tenofovir and/or 3TC/FTC is uncommon, with M184V/I occurring in 0.8% and K65R occurring in 0.1% of newly diagnosed PWH in the United States (McClung et al., 2020). However, one recent systematic review examining pretreatment HIVDR specifically among certain "key populations" found a high (>10%) prevalence of PDR among some groups (e.g., men who have sex with men, sex workers, and people in prisons), with differences across regions and by ARV class (Macdonald et al., 2020). Approximately 0.5% of newly diagnosed PWH in the United States are predicted to have cabotegravir resistance (McClung et al., 2020); low rates of cabotegravir resistance among ARV-naive PWH have also been reported from Europe (Charpentier et al., 2021). By contrast, among PWH experiencing virologic failure, approximately 15% have genotypic resistance to 3TC/FTC and/or tenofovir while approximately 5% have genotypic resistance to cabotegravir. Therefore, the risk of PrEP failure may be higher if a PrEP user acquires HIV from a PWH who is experiencing virologic failure. Regarding the second concern of whether widespread PrEP use will increase HIVDR, data from PrEP clinical trials have indicated that there are two scenarios in which HIVDR can emerge: persons who are undergoing acute infection at the time of PrEP initiation, and persons who acquire infection at a later time point (usually as a result of subtherapeutic PrEP drug exposure most commonly caused by low medication adherence) but continue to take PrEP. When HIVDR does occur with oral PrEP use, it is nearly always associated with M184V/I and 3TC/FTC resistance and rarely with K65R and tenofovir resistance (Gibas et al., 2019; Girometti et al., 2022; Johnson et al., 2021; Misra et al., 2019; Parikh et al., 2016). Of concern, cases of emergent INSTI-associated DRMs have been described among clinical trial participants who received long-acting cabotegravir and were subsequently diagnosed with HIV (Eshelman et al., 2022; Marzinke, 2021).

RESOURCE-LIMITED SETTINGS (LOW- AND MIDDLE-INCOME COUNTRIES)

The primary differences regarding evaluation and management of HIVDR between high-income countries and low-/middle-income countries include: (a) the absence of universal access to routine genotypic resistance testing; (b) less frequent viral load monitoring; (c) high prevalence of infants and children with perinatally- acquired HIV infection whose treatment options are limited because of transmitted or acquired DRMs; and (d) the large proportion of PWH who have failed previously recommended first-line therapy combinations (i.e., with resultant development of dual NRTI-NNRTI resistance) or who have failed first- *and* second-line therapy with subsequent three-class drug resistance.

Pretreatment drug resistance (PDR) refers to DRMs that are detected in PWH before they start ART. This may arise with either transmission of a drug-resistant strain (i.e., TDR) or DRMs, owing to previous ART exposure, such as with time-limited perinatal/postpartum ART use, PrEP or PEP, or interrupted first-line ART. For low- and middle-income countries (LMIC), global surveillance data have indicated a notable rise in pretreatment resistance to NNRTIs after initial ART scale-up, primarily because of use of first-generation NNRTIs with a low genetic barrier to resistance (Bertagnolio et al., 2022). Although the introduction of dolutegravir in many LMICs carries potential for improved individual and public health outcomes, further scale-up of viral load and resistance testing (as well as adherence monitoring and support) may also be necessary to avoid inadvertently placing ART-experienced PWH on functional dolutegravir monotherapy (McCluskey et al., 2021). The 2021 updated WHO HIV drug resistance strategy provides an overview of core WHO-recommended activities, including country-level monitoring of quality-of-care indicators associated with predicting HIVDR as well as implementation of HIV drug resistance surveys (World Health Organization, 2021).

HIV-2

HIV-2 infection (and HIV-1/-2 coinfection) remains rare in the United States; however, HIV-2 is endemic in many regions experiencing high overall HIV prevalence such as West Africa; HIV care providers should thus have some basic clinical knowledge of HIV-2. HIV-2 has demonstrated intrinsic, high-level resistance to NNRTIs and enfuvirtide. PIs exhibit variable activity against HIV-2: boosted lopinavir and darunavir are believed to have the most clinically useful potency. HIV-2 is susceptible to INSTIs, as well as all NRTIs currently in clinical use; however, data suggest differences in INSTI and NRTI mutation selection and HIVDR mechanisms/pathways between HIV-2 and HIV-1 (Boyer et al., 2012; Gottlieb et al., 2009; Requena et al., 2017; Tzou et al., 2020). Outcomes of trials involving first- and second-generation INSTIs and PI-based regimen algorithms will help provide more evidence to shape first-line HIV-2 treatment recommendations (Gottlieb et al., 2018; Raugi et al., 2021). HIV-2 drug resistance testing is not commercially available in the United States; some research laboratories (e.g., University of Washington) have limited capacity to perform genotype testing under research protocols.

CONCLUSION

ADR and, to a lesser extent, TDR continue to pose challenges to the successful treatment of PWH. In the absence of selective drug pressure, DRMs can quickly be replaced by wild-type variants, so resistance testing should be performed as close to HIV diagnosis as possible and, ideally, while patients are still on ART when virologic failure is identified. Any DRMs identified should be documented and taken into account when considering ART reinitiation or modification. PBMC DNA sequencing can be useful for ART switch/simplification in PWH who are virologically suppressed, but results should be interpreted with caution. Management of ADR and TDR should take into account HIV-specific factors and other key individual conditions and/or factors to construct a clinically appropriate regimen that includes at least two fully active drugs from different ARV drug classes. Rapid ART, HIV acquisition in the setting of recent PrEP use, virologic failure in highly treatment experienced patients, ART switch or simplification, and newly available long-acting ARV medications all pose unique challenges.

REFERENCES

Abram ME, Ferris AL, Shao W, et al. Nature, position, and frequency of mutations made in a single cycle of HIV-1 replication. *J Virology.* 2010;84(19):9864–9878.

Acosta RK, Chen GQ, Chang S, et al. Three-year study of pre-existing drug resistance substitutions and efficacy of bictegravir/emtricitabine/tenofovir alafenamide in HIV-1 treatment-naïve participants. *J Antimicrob Chemother*. 2021;76(8):2153–2157.

Acosta RK, Willkom M, Andreatta K, et al. Switching to bictegravir/emtricitabine/tenofovir alafenamide (B/F/TAF) from dolutegravir (DTG) + F/TAF or DTG + F/tenofovir disoproxil fumarate (TDF) in the presence of pre-existing NRTI resistance. *J Acquir Immune Defic Syndr*. 2020;85(3):363–371.

Akil B, Blick G, Hagins DP, et al. Dolutegravir versus placebo in subjects harbouring HIV-1 with integrase inhibitor resistance associated substitutions: 48-week results from VIKING-4, a randomized study. *Antivir Ther*. 2015;20:343–348.

Allavena C, Rodallec A, Leplat A, et al. Interest of proviral HIV-1 DNA genotypic resistance testing in virologically suppressed patients candidate for maintenance therapy. *J Virol Methods*. 2018;251:106–110.

Antiretroviral Therapy Cohort Collaboration. Survival of HIV-positive patients starting antiretroviral therapy between 1996 and 2013: a collaborative analysis of cohort studies. *Lancet HIV*. 2017;4:e349–e356.

Armenia D, Bouba Y, Gagliardini R, et al. Virological response and resistance profile in highly treatment-experienced HIV-1-infected patients switching to dolutegravir plus boosted darunavir in clinical practice. *HIV Med*. 2021;22(6):519–525.

Armenia D, Forbici F, Bertoli A, et al. Bictegravir/emtricitabine/tenofovir alafenamide ensures high rates of virological suppression maintenance despite previous resistance in PLWH who optimize treatment in clinical practice. *J Glob Antimicrob Resist*. 2022;30:326–334.

Armenia D, Zaccarelli M, Borghi V, et al. Resistance detected in PBMCs predicts virological rebound in HIV-1 suppressed patients switching treatment. *J Clin Virol*. July 2018;104:61–64.

Avila-Rios S, Garcia-Moralis C, Matias-Florentino M, et al; HIVDR MexNet Group. Pretreatment HIV-drug resistance in Mexico and its impact on the effectiveness of first-line antiretroviral therapy: a nationally representative 2015 WHO survey. *Lancet HIV*. 2016b;3:e579–591.

Avila-Rios S, Parkin N, Swanstrom R, et al. Next-generation sequencing for HIV drug resistance testing: laboratory, clinical, and implementation considerations. *Viruses*. 2020;12(6):617.

Avila-Rios S, Sued O, Rhee SY, et al. Surveillance of HIV transmitted drug resistance in Latin America and the Caribbean: a systematic review and meta-Analysis. *PLoS One*. 2016a;11:e0158560.

Bachelard A, Isernia V, Charpentier C, et al. Efficacy and safety of using bictegravir/emtricitabine/tenofovir alafenamide (BIC/F/TAF) in a test and treat model: the FAST Study. [Abstract PE2/7]. European AIDS Clinical Society. 2021. London, United Kingdom and Virtual. Abstr PE2/7.

Bachmann N, von Braun A, Labhardt ND, et al. Importance of routine viral load monitoring: higher levels of resistance at ART failure in Uganda and Lesotho compared with Switzerland. *J Antimicrob Chemother*. 2019;74(2):468–472.

Bailey AJ, Rhee SY, Shafer RW. Integrase strand transfer inhibitor resistance in integrase strand transfer inhibitor-naïve persons. *AIDS Res Hum Retroviruses*. 2021;37(10):736–743.

Bajema KL, Nance RM, Delaney JAC, et al. Substantial decline in heavily treated therapy-experienced persons with HIV with limited antiretroviral treatment options. *AIDS*. 2020;34(14):2051–2059.

Bavaro DF, De Vito A, Pasculli G, et al. Early versus delayed antiretroviral therapy based on genotypic resistance test: results from a large retrospective cohort study. *J Med Virol*. 2022;94(8):3890–3899.

Baxter JD, Dunn D, Tostevin A, et al. Transmitted HIV-1 drug resistance in a large international cohort using next-generation sequencing: results from the Strategic Timing of Antiretroviral Treatment (START) study. *HIV Med*. 2021;22(5):360–371.

Bennett DE, Camacho RJ, Otelea D, et al. Drug resistance mutations for surveillance of transmitted HIV-1 drug resistance: 2009 update. *PLoS One*. 2009;4(3):e4724.

Bertagnolio S, Jordan MR, Giron A, Inzaule S. Epidemiology of HIV drug resistance in low- and middle-income countries and WHO global strategy to monitor its emergence. *Curr Opin HIV AIDS*. 2022;17(4):229–239.

Boltz VF, Zheng Y, Lockman S, et al. Role of low-frequency HIV-1 variants in failure of nevirapine-containing antiviral therapy in women previously exposed to single-dose nevirapine. *Proc Natl Acad Sci USA*. 2011;108:9202–9207.

Borghetti A, Cicculo A, Lombardi F, et al. Transmitted drug resistance to NRTIs and risk of virological failure in naïve patients treated with integrase inhibitors. *HIV Med*. 2021;22(1):22–27. doi:10./1111/hiv.12956. Epub 2020 Sep 3. http://doi:10.1111/hv.12956

Boukli N, Boyd A, Collot M, Meynard JL, Girard PM, Morand-Joubert L. Utility of HIV-1 DNA genotype in determining antiretroviral resistance in patients with low or undetectable HIV RNA viral loads. *J Antimicrob Chemother*. 2018;73(11):3129–3136.

Boyce CL, Sils T, Ko D, et al. Maternal human immunodeficiency virus (HIV) drug resistance is associated with vertical transmission and is prevalent in infected infants. *Clin Infect Dis*. 2022;74(11):2001–2009.

Boyd MA, Boffito M, Castagna A, Estrada V. Rapid initiation of antiretroviral therapy at HIV diagnosis: definition, process, knowledge gaps. *HIV Medicine*. 2019;20(Suppl1):3–11.

Boyer PL, Clark PJ, Hughes SH. HIV-1 and HIV-2 reverse transcriptases: different mechanisms of resistance to nucleoside reverse transcriptase inhibitors. *J Virol*. 2012;86(10):5885–94.

Capetti AF, De Socio GV, Cossu MV, et al. Durability of dolutegravir plus boosted darunavir as salvage or simplification of salvage regimens in HIV-1 infected, highly treatment-experienced subjects. *HIV Clin Trials*. 2018;19(6):242–248.

Carr A, Richardson R, Liu Z. Success and failure of initial antiretroviral therapy in adult: an updated systematic review. *AIDS*. 2019;33(3):443–453.

Castagna A, Maggiolo F, Penco G, et al. Dolutegravir in antiretroviral-experienced patients with raltegravir-and/or elvitegravir-resistant HIV-1: 24-week results of the phase III VIKING-3 Study. *J Infect Dis*. 2014;210: 354–362.

Castro H, Pillay D, Cane P et al; UK Collaborative Group on HIV Drug Resistance. Persistence of HIV-1 transmitted drug resistance mutations. *J Infect Dis*. 2013;208:1459–1463.

Centers for Disease Control and Prevention (CDC). Monitoring selected national HIV prevention and care objectives by using HIV surveillance data—United States and 6 dependent areas, 2020. *HIV Surveillance Supplemental Report*. 2022;27(3). http://www.cdc.gov/hiv/library/reports/hiv-surveillance.html. Published May 2022. Accessed August 20, 2022.

Charpentier C, Storto A, Soulié C, et al. Prevalence of genotypic baseline risk factors for cabotegravir + rilpivirine failure among ARV-naïve patients. *J Antimicrob Chemother*. 2021;76(11):2983–2987.

Chu C, Armenia D, Walworth C, Santoro MM, Shafer RW. Genotypic resistance testing of HIV-1 DNA in peripheral blood mononuclear cells. *Clin Micro Rev*. 2022;35(4):e0005222. https://doi.org/10.1128/cmr.00052-22

Clutter DS, Zhou S, Varghese V, et al. Prevalence of drug resistant minority variants in untreated HIV-1-infected individuals with and those without transmitted drug resistance detected by Sanger sequencing. *J Infect Dis*. 2017;216(3):387–391.

Coffey S, Baccheti P, Sachdev D, et al. RAPID antiretroviral therapy: high virologic suppression rates with immediate antiretroviral therapy initiation in a vulnerable urban clinic population. *AIDS*. 2019;33(5):825–832.

Coffin JM. HIV population dynamics in vivo: implications for genetic variation, pathogenesis, and therapy. *Science*. 1995;267(5197):483–489.

Colasanti J, Sumitani J, Mehta CC, et al. Implementation of a rapid entry program decreases time to viral suppression among vulnerable persons living with HIV in the Southern United States. *Open Forum Infect Dis*. 2018;5(6):ofy104.

Cozzi-Lepri A, Noguera-Julian M, Di Giallonardo F; CHAIN Minority HIV-1 Variants Working Group. Low-frequency drug-resistant HIV-1 and risk of virological failure to first-line NNRTI-based ART: a multicohort European case-control study using centralized ultrasensitive 454 pyrosequencing. *J Antimicrob Chemother.* 2015;70:930–940.

Curanovic D, Martens S, Rodriguez M, et al. HIV-1 DNA testing in viremic patients demonstrates a greater ability to detect drug resistance compared to plasma virus testing. [PDB0402]. Presented at the 23rd International AIDS Conference 2020. Virtual; 2020. https://www.aids2020.org/

Cutrell AG, Schapiro JM, Perno CF, et al. Exploring predictors of HIV-1 virologic failure to long-acting cabotegravir and rilpivirine: a multivariable analysis. *AIDS.* 2021;35(9):1333–1342.

Dauwe K, Staelens D, Vancoillie L, et al. Deep sequencing of HIV-1 RNA and DNA in newly diagnosed patients with baseline drug resistance showed no indications for hidden resistance and is biased by strong interference of hypermutation. *J Clin Micro.* 2016;54:1605–1615.

Davy-Mendez T, Eron JJ, Brunet L, et al. New antiretroviral agent use affects prevalence of HIV drug resistance in clinical care populations. *AIDS.* 2018;32(17):2593–2603.

Deeks SF, Wrin T, Liegler T, et al. Virologic and immunologic consequences of discontinuing combination antiretroviral-drug therapy in HIV-infected patients with detectable viremia. *N Engl J Med.* 2001;344:472–480.

Delaugerre C, Bruan J, Charreau I, et al; ANRS 138-EASIER study group. Comparison of resistance mutation patterns in historical plasma HIV RNA genotypes with those in current proviral HIV DNA genotypes among extensively treated patients with suppressed replication. *HIV Medicine.* 2012a:13:517–525.

Delaugerre C, Chaix ML, Blanche S, et al; ANRS French Perinatal Cohort. Perinatal acquisition of drug-resistant HIV-1 infection mechanisms and long-term outcome. *Retrovirology.* 2009; 6:85.

Delaugerre C, Gallien S, Flandre P, et al. Impact of low-level viremia on HIV-1 drug resistance evolution among antiretroviral treated patients. *PLoS One.* 2012b;7(5):e36673.

De Meyer S, Vangeneugden T, Van Baelen B, et al. Resistance profile of darunavir: combined 24-week results from the POWER trials. *AIDS Res Human Retroviruses.* 2008;24(3):379–388.

Department of Health and Human Services (DHHS) Panel on Antiretroviral Guidelines for Adults and Adolescents. Guidelines for the use of antiretroviral agents in adults and adolescents with HIV. http://www.aidsinfo.nih.gov/ContentFiles/AdultandAdolescentGL.pdf. Published 2022a. Accessed September 25, 2022.

Department of Health and Human Services (DHHS) Panel on Treatment of Pregnant Women with HIV Infection and Prevention of Perinatal Transmission. Recommendations for the use of antiretroviral drugs in pregnant women with HIV infection and interventions to reduce perinatal HIV transmission in the United States. https://clinicalinfo.hiv.gov/sites/default/files/inline-files/PerinatalGL.pdf. Published 2022b. Accessed August 20, 2022.

Derache A, Shin HS, Balamane M et al. HIV drug resistance mutations in proviral DNA from a community treatment program. *PLoS One.* 2015;10(1):30117430.

Devereux HL, Loveday C, Youle M, et al. Substantial correlation between HIV type 1 drug-associated resistance mutations in plasma and peripheral blood mononuclear cells in treatment-experienced patients. *AIDS Res Human Retrovirus.* 2000;16(11):1025–1030.

Devereux HL, Youle M, Johnson MA, Loveday C. Rapid decline in detectability of HIV-1 drug resistance mutations after stopping therapy. *AIDS.* 1999;13:F123–127.

Dolling DI, Dunn DT, Sutherland KA, et al; UHDRD (UKHDRD) and the UCHCS (UK). Low frequency of genotypic resistance in HIV-1-infected patients failing an atazanavir-containing regimen: a clinical cohort study. *J Antimicrob Chemother.* 2013;68: 2339–2343.

Drescher SM, von Wyl V, Yang WL, et al. Treatment-naïve individuals are the major source of transmitted HIV-1 drug resistance in men who have sex with men in the Swiss HIV Cohort Study. *Clin Infect Dis.* 2014;58(2):285–94.

Eberle J, Gurtler L. HIV types, groups, subtypes and recombinant forms: errors in replication, selection pressure and quasispecies. *Intervirology.* 2012b;55:79–83.

Eberle J, Gurtler L. The evolution of drug resistance interpretation algorithms: ANRS, REGA and extension of resistance analysis to HIV-1 group O and HIV-2. *Intervirology.* 2012a;55(2):128–133.

El Bouzidi K, White E, Mbisa JL, et al. Protease mutations emerging on darunavir in protease inhibitor-naïve and experienced patients in the UK. *J Int AIDS Soc.* 2014;17:19739. http://doi:10.7448/IAS.17.4.19739

Ellis KE, Nawas GT, Chan C, et al. Clinical outcomes following the use of archived proviral HIV-1 DNA genotype to guide antiretroviral therapy adjustment. *Open Forum Inf Dis.* 2019;7(1):ofz533.

Elvstam O, Medstrand P, Yilmaz A, et al. Virological failure and all-cause mortality in HIV-positive adults with low-level viremia during antiretroviral treatment. *PLoS One.* 2017;12(7):e0180761.

Emu B, Fessel K, Schrader S, et al. Phase 3 study of ibalizumab for multidrug-resistant HIV-1. *N Engl J Med.* 2018;379:645–654.

Eron JJ, Clotet B, Durant J, et al; VIKING Study Group. Safety and efficacy of dolutegravir in treatment-experienced subjects with raltegravir-resistant HIV type 1 infection: 24-week results of the VIKING study. *J Infect Dis.* 2013;207:740–8.

Eron JJ, Young B, Cooper DA, et al. Switch to a raltegravir-based regimen versus continuation of a lopinavir-ritonavir-based regimen in stable HIV-infected patients with suppressed viraemic (SWITCHMRK 1 and 2): two multicenter-double-blind, randomized controlled trials. *Lancet.* 2010;375(9712):396–407.

Esber A, Polyak C, Kiweewa F, et al. Persistent low-level viremia predicts subsequent virologic failure: is it time to change the third 90? *Clin Infect Dis.* 2019;69(5):805–812.

Eshleman SH, Fogel JM, Piwowar-Manning E, et al. Characterization of human immunodeficiency virus (HIV) infections in women who received injectable cabotegravir or tenofovir disoproxil fumarate/emtricitabine for HIV prevention: HPTN084. *J Infect Dis.* 2022;225(10):1741–1749.

Fleming J, Mathews WC, Rutstein RM, et al; HIV Research Network. Low-level viremia and virologic failure in persons with HIV infection treated with antiretroviral therapy. *AIDS.* 2019;33:2005–2012.

Ford N, Migone C, Calmy A, et al. Benefits and risks of rapid initiation of antiretroviral therapy. *AIDS.* 2018;32(1):17–23.

Geretti AM, White E, Orkin C, et al. Virological outcomes of boosted protease inhibitor-based first-line ART in subjects harbouring thymidine analogue-association mutations as the sole form of transmitted drug resistance. *J Antimicrob Chemother.* 2019;74:746–753.

Gibas KM, van den Berg P, Powell VE, Krakower DS. Drug resistance during HIV pre-exposure prophylaxis. *Drugs.* 2019;79(6):609–619.

Girometti N, McCormack S, Tittle V, McOwan A, Whitlock G; 56 Dean Street Collaborative Group. Rising rates of recent preexposure prophylaxis exposure among men having sex with men newly diagnosed with HIV: antiviral resistance patterns and treatment outcomes. *AIDS.* 2022;36(4):561–566.

Gonzalez-Sefna A, Min JE, Woods C, et al. Performance of HIV-1 drug resistance testing at low-level viremia and its ability to predict future virologic outcomes and viral evolution in treatment-naïve individuals. *Clin Infect Dis.* 2014;58:1165–1173.

Gottlieb GS, Dia Badiane NM, Hawed SE, et al; University of Washington-Dakar HIV-2 Study Group. Emergence of multiclass drug resistance in HIV-2 in antiretroviral-treated individuals in Senegal: implications for HIV-2 treatment in resource-limited West Africa. *Clin Infect Dis.* 2009;48(4):476–483.

Gottlieb GS, Raugi DN, Smith RA. 90-90-90 for HIV-2? Ending the HIV-2 epidemic by enhancing care and clinical management of patients infected with HIV-2. *Lancet HIV.* 2018;5(7):e390–e399.

Gregson J, Tang M, Ndembi N, et al; TenoRes Study Group. Global epidemiology of drug resistance after failure of WHO recommended first-line regimens for adult HIV-1 infection: a multicentre retrospective cohort study. *Lancet Infect Dis.* 2016;16(5):565–575.

Günthard HF, Calvez V, Paredes R, et al. Human immunodeficiency virus drug resistance: 2018 recommendations of the International Antiviral Society–USA Panel. *Clin Infect Dis.* January 15, 2019; 68(2):177–187.

Gupta RK, Gregson J, Parkin N, et al. HIV-1 drug resistance before initiation or re-initiation of first-line antiretroviral therapy in low-income and middle-income countries: a systematic review and meta-regression analysis. *Lancet Inf Dis.* 2018;18:346–355.

Hermans LE, Moorhouse M, Carmona S, et al. Effect of HIV-1 low-level viraemia during antiretroviral therapy on treatment outcomes in WHO-guided South African treatment programmes: a muticentre cohort study. *Lancet Infect Dis.* 2018;18(2):130–131.

Hoffman C, Wolf E, Braun P, et al. Temporal variability of multi-class resistant HIV-1 in proviral DNA. [Abstract 513]. Presented at the Conference on Retroviruses and Opportunistic Infections. Virtual; 2022. https://www.croiconference.org/search-abstracts/

Huber M, Metzner KJ, Geissberger FD, et al. A rapid and versatile tool for HIV-1 drug resistance genotyping by deep sequencing. *J Virol Methods.* 2017;240:7–13.

Huhn GD, Crofoot G, Rampogal M, et al. Darunavir/cobicistat/emtricitabine/tenofovir alafenamide in a rapid-initiation model of care for human immunodeficiency virus type 1 infection: primary analysis of the DIAMOND study. *Clin Infect Dis.* 2020;71(12):3110–3117.

Hyle EP, Scott JA, Sax PE, et al. Clinical impact and cost-effectiveness of genotype testing at human immunodeficiency virus diagnosis in the US. *Clin Infect Dis.* March 17, 2020;70(7):1353–1363.

Inzaule SC, Hamers RL, Noguera-Julian M, et al. Clinically relevant thresholds for ultrasensitive HIV drug resistance testing: a multicountry nested case-control study. *Lancet HIV.* 2018;5:e638–e646.

Jablonowska E, Siwak E, Bociaga-Jasik M, et al. Real-life study of dual therapy based on dolutegravir and ritonavir-boosted darunavir in HIV-1-infected treatment-experienced patients. *PLoS One.* 2019;14(1):e0210476.

Jain V, Sucupira MC, Bacchetti P, et al. Differential persistence of transmitted HIV-1- drug resistance mutation classes. *J Infect Dis.* 2011;203:1174–1181.

Johnson KA, Chen MJ, Kohn R, et al. Acute HIV at the time of initiation of pre-exposure or post-exposure prophylaxis: impact on drug resistance and clinical outcomes. *J Acquir Immune Defic Syndr.* 2021;87(2):818–825.

Joya C, Won SH, Schofield C, et al. Persistent low-level viremia while on antiretroviral therapy is an independent risk factor for virologic failure. *Clin Infect Dis.* 2019;69(12):2145–2152.

Kagan RM, Dunn KJ, Snell GP, et al. Trends in HIV-1 drug resistance mutations from a US reference laboratory from 2006 to 2017. *AIDS Res Hum Retroviruses.* 2019;35(8):698–709.

Kempf DF, Isaacson JD. King MS, et al. Analysis of the virological response with respect to baseline viral phenotype and genotype in protease inhibitor-experienced HIV-1-infected patients receiving lopinavir/ritonavir therapy. *Antivir Ther.* 2002;7:165–174.

Kessler HH, Stelzl E, Blazic A, Mehta SR, et al. Antiretroviral treatment simplification with 2–drug regimens: impact of transmitted drug resistance mutations. *Open Forum Infect Dis.* January 2020;7(1):ofz535.

Kirichenko A, Kireev D, Lopatukhin A, et al. Prevalence of HIV-1 drug resistance in Eastern European and Central Asian countries. *PLoS One.* 2022;17(1):e0257731.

Knyphausen F, Scheufele R, Kücherer C, et al. First line treatment response in patients with transmitted HIV drug resistance and well-defined time point of HIV infection: updated results from the German HIV-1 Seroconverter Study. *PLoS One.* 2014;9:e95956.

Kozal M, Aberg J, Pialoux G, et al. Fostemsavir in adults with multidrug-resistant HIV-1 infection. *New Eng J Med.* 2020;382:1232–1243.

Lanier ER, Ait-Khaled M, Scott J, et al. Antiviral efficacy of abacavir in antiretroviral therapy-experienced adults harbouring HIV-1 with specific patterns of resistance to nucleoside reverse transcriptase inhibitors. *Antivir Ther.* 2004;9:37–45.

Lapointe HR, Dong W, Lee GQ, et al. High drug resistance testing by high-multiplex "wide" sequencing on the MiSeq instrument. *Antimicrobial Agents Chemo.* 2015;59:6824–6833.

Laprise C, de Pokomandy A, Baril JG, Dufresne S, Trottier H. Virologic failure following persistent low-level viremia in a cohort of HIV-positive patients: results from 12 years of observation. *Clin Infect Dis.* 2013;57(10):1489–1496.

Lathouwers E, Seyedkazemi S, Lou D, et al. Pooled resistance analyses of darunavir once-daily regimens and formulations across 10 clinical studies of treatment-naïve and treatment-experienced patients with human immunodeficiency virus-1 infection. *HIV Res Clin Prac.* 2020;21:83–89.

Levy DN, Aldrovandi GM, Kutsch O, Shaw GM. Dynamics of HIV-1 recombination in its natural target cells. *PNAS.* 2004;101:4204–4209.

Li JZ, Gallien S, Do TD, et al. Prevalence and significance of HIV-1 drug resistance mutations among patients on antiretroviral therapy with detectable low-level viremia. *Antimicrobial Agents Chemo.* 2012;56(11):5998–6000.

Li JZ, Paredes R, Ribaudo H, et al. Minority HIV-1 drug resistance mutations and the risk of NNRTI-based antiretroviral treatment failure: a systematic review and pooled analysis. *JAMA.* 2011;305(13):1327–1335.

Li X, Brown TT, Ho KS, et al. Recent trends and effectiveness of antiretroviral regimens among men who have sex with men living with HIV in the United States: the Multicenter AIDS Cohort Study (MACS) 2008–2017. *Open Forum Infect Dis.* 2019;6:ofz333. http://doi:10.1093/ofid/ofz333

Llibre JM, Arribas JR, Domingo P, et al. Clinical implications of fixed-dose coformulations of antiretrovirals on the outcome of HIV-1 therapy. *AIDS.* 2011;25(14):1683–1690.

Lodi S, Gunthard HF, Dunn D, et al. Effect of immediate initiation of antiretroviral treatment on the risk of acquired HIV drug resistance. *AIDS.* 2018;32(3):327–335.

Lombardi F, Giacomelli A, Armenia D, et al. Prevalence and factors associated with HIV-1 multi-drug resistance over the past two decades in the Italian ARCA database. *Int J Antimicrob Agents.* 2021;57(2):106252.

Lubke N, Di Cristanziano V, Sierra S, et al; Resina Study Group. Proviral DNA as a target for HIV-1 resistance analysis. *Intervirology.* 2015;58:184–189.

Macdonald V, Mbuagbaw L, Jordan MR, et al. Prevalence of pretreatment HIV drug resistance in key populations: a systematic review and meta-analysis. *J Int AIDS Soc.* 2020;23(12):e25656.

Machnowska P, Meixenberger K, Schmidt D, et al.; German HIV-1 Seroconverted Study Group. Prevalence and persistence of transmitted drug resistance mutations in the German HIV-1 Seroconverter Study Cohort. *PLoS One.* 2019;14(1):e0209605.

Mackie NE, Phillips AN, Kaye S, et. al; UK Resistance Database and the UK Collaborative HIV Cohort Study. Antiretroviral drug resistance in HIV-1-infected patients with low-level viremia. *J Infect Dis.* 2010;210(9):1303–1307.

Manyana S, Gounder L, Pillay M, et al. HIV-1 drug resistance genotyping in resource limited settings: current and future perspectives in sequencing technologies. *Viruses.* 2021;13(6):1125.

Marcelin AG, Charpentier C, Bellecave P, et al. Factors associated with the emergency of integrase resistance mutations in patients failing dual or triple integrase inhibitor-based regimens in a French national survey. *J Antimicrob Chemother.* 2021;76(9):2400–2406.

Margot N, Ram R, McNicholl I, et al. Differential detection of M184V/I between plasma historical HIV genotypes and HIV proviral DNA from PBMCs. *J Antimicrob Chemother.* 2020a;75:2249–2252.

Margot NA, Wong P, Kulkarni R, et al. Commonly transmitted HIV-1 drug resistance mutations in reverse-transcriptase and protease in antiretroviral treatment-naïve patients and response to regimens containing tenofovir disoproxil fumarate or tenofovir alafenamide. *J Infect Dis.* 2017;215(6):920–927.

Martin TCS, Abrams M, Anderson C, Little SJ. Rapid antiretroviral therapy among individuals with acute and early HIV. *Clin Inf Dis.* 2021;73(1):130–133. http://doi: 10.1093/cid/ciaa1174

Marzinke MA, Grinsztejn B, Fogel JM, et al. Characterization of human immunodeficiency virus (HIV) infection in cisgender men and transgender women who have sex with men receiving injectable cabotegravir for HIV prevention: HPTN083. *J Infect Dis.* 2021;224(9):1581–1592.

Mateo-Urdiales A, Johnson S, Smith R, Nachega JB, Eshun-Wilson I. Rapid initiation of antiretroviral therapy for people living with HIV. *Cochrane Database Syst Rev.* 2019;6(6):CD012962.

Mbunkah HA, Bertagnolio S, Hamers RL; WHO HIVResNet Working Group. Low-abundance drug-resistant HIV-1 variants in antiretroviral drug-native individuals: a systematic review of detection methods, prevalence, and clinical impact. *J Infect Dis.* 2020;221:1584–1597.

McClung RP, Ocfemia CB, Saduvala N, et al. Integrase and other transmitted HIV drug resistance: 23 US jurisdictions, 2013–2016. [Abstract 3337]. Presented at the Conference on Retroviruses and Opportunistic Infections. Seattle, WA; 2019. https://www.croiconference.org/search-abstracts/

McClung RP, Ocfemia CB, Saduvala N, et al. US HIV drug resistance: implications for current and future PrEP regimens. [Abstract 512]. Presented at the Conference on Retroviruses and Opportunistic Infections. Boston, MA; 2020. https://www.croiconference.org/search-abstracts/

McClung RP, Oster AM, Ocfemia MCB, et al. Transmitted drug resistance among human immunodeficiency virus (HIV)-1 diagnoses in the United States, 2014–2018. *Clin Infect Dis.* 2022;74(6):1055–1062.

McCluskey SM, Pepperrell T, Hill A, Venter WDF, Gupta RK, Siedner MJ. Adherence, resistance, and viral suppression on dolutegravir in sub-Saharan Africa: implications for the TLD era. *AIDS.* 2021;35(Suppl 2):S127–S135.

McCluskey SM, Siedner MJ, Marconi VC. Management of virologic failure and HIV drug resistance. *Infect Dis Clin North Am.* 2019;33(3):707–742.

Metzner KJ, Rauch P, von Wyl, et al. Efficient suppression of minority drug-resistant HIV type 1 (HIV-1) variants present at primary HIV-1 infection by ritonavir-boosted protease inhibitor-containing antiretroviral therapy. *J Infect Dis.* 2010;201:1063–1071.

Miller MD, Margot N, Lu B, et al. Genotypic and phenotypic predictors of the magnitude of response to tenofovir disoproxil fumarate treatment in antiretroviral-experienced patients. *J Infect Dis.* 2004;189:837–846.

Miranda MNS, Pingarilho M, Pimentel V, et al. Trends of transmitted and acquired drug resistance in Europe from 1981 to 2019; a comparison between the populations of late presenters and non-late presenters. *Front Microbiol.* 2022;13:846943.

Misra K, Huang J, Daskalakis DC, et al. Impact of PrEP on drug resistance and acute HIV infection, New York City, 2015–2017. [Abstract #107]. Presented at the Conference on Retroviruses and Opportunistic Infections. Seattle, WA; 2019. https://www.croiconference.org/search-abstracts/

Nance RM, Delaney JAC, Simoni JM, et al. HIV viral suppression trends over time among HIV-infected patients receiving care in the United States, 1997 to 2015. *Ann Int Med.* 2018;169:376–384.

Noguera-Julian M, Edgil D, Harrigan PR, et al. Next-generation human immunodeficiency virus sequencing for patient management and drug resistance surveillance. *J Infect Dis.* December 1, 2017;216(Suppl 9):S829–S833.

Obermeier M, Pironti A, Berg T, et al. HIV-GRADE: a publicly available, rules-based drug resistance interpretation algorithm integrating bioinformatics knowledge. *Intervirology.* 2012;55:102–107.

aquet A, Solberg OD, Napolitano LA, et al. A decade of HIV-1 drug resistance in the United States: trends and characteristics in a large protease/reverse transcriptase and co-receptor tropism database from 2003 to 2012. *Antivir Ther.* 2014;19(4):435–441.

Paredes R, Tzou PL, van Zyl G, et al. Collaborative update of a rule-based expert system for HIV-1genotypic resistance test interpretation. *PLoS One.* 2017;12(7):e0181357.

Parikh UM, Mellors JW. How could HIV-1 drug resistance impact pre-exposure prophylaxis for HIV prevention? *Curr Opin HIV AIDS.* 2022;17(4):213–221.

Parikh UM, Mellors JW. Should we fear resistance from tenofovir/emtricitabine preexposure prophylaxis? *Curr Opin HIV AIDS.* 2016;11:49–55.

Parkin NT, Hellmann NS, Whitcomb JM, et al. Natura variation of drug susceptibility in wild-type human immunodeficiency virus type 1. *Antimicrobial Agents Chemother.* 2004;48:437–443.

Paton NI, Musaazi J, Kityo C, et al. Efficacy and safety of dolutegravir or darunavir in combination with lamivudine plus either zidovudine or tenofovir for second-line treatment of HIV infection (NADIA): week 96 results from a prospective, multicentre, open-label, factorial, randomized, non-inferiority trial. *Lancet HIV.* 2022;9(6):e381–e393.

Petropoulos CJ, Parkin NT, Limoli KL, et al. A novel phenotypic drug susceptibility assay for human immunodeficiency virus type 1. *Antimicrob Agents Chemo.* 2000;44(4):920–928.

Peuchant O, Thiebaut R, Capdepont S, et al. Transmission of HIV-1 minority-resistance variants and response to first-line antiretroviral therapy: transmission of minority resistant HIV-1. *AIDS.* 2008;22(12):1417–1423.

Pilcher CD, Ospina-Norvell C, Dasgupta A, et al. The effect of same-day observed initiation of antiretroviral therapy on HIV viral load and treatment outcomes in a US public health setting. *J Acquir Immune Defic Syndr.* 2017;74(1):44–51.

Pingen M, Wensing A, Fransen K, et al. Persistence of frequently transmitted drug-resistant HIV-1 variants can be explained by high viral replication capacity. *Retrovirology.* 2014;11:105.

Porter DP, Toma J, Tan Y, et al. Clinical outcomes of virologically-suppressed patients with pre-existing HIV-1 drug resistance mutations switching to rilpivirine/emtricitabine/tenofovir disoproxil fumarate in the SPIRIT study. *HIV Clin Trials.* 2016;17(1):29–37.

Poschman K, Spencer EC. Prevalence of HIV-1 antiretroviral drug resistance in Florida, 2015–2016. [Abstract 526]. Presented at the Conference on Retroviruses and Opportunistic Infections. Boston, MA; 2020. https://www.croiconference.org/search-abstracts/

Pou C, Noguera-Julian M, Perez-Alvarez S, et al. Improved prediction of salvage antiretroviral therapy outcomes using ultrasensitive HIV-1 drug resistance testing. *Clin Infect Dis.* 2014;59(4):578–588.

Puertas MC, Ploumidis G, Ploumidis M, et al. Pan-resistant HIV-emergence in the era of integrase strand-transfer inhibitors: a case report. *Lancet Microbe.* 2020;1(3):e130–e135.

Rambaut A, Posada D, Crandall KA, Holmes EC. The causes and consequences of HIV evolution. *Nature Rev Gen.* 2004;5:52–61.

Ramirez JA, Maddali MV, Budak JZ, et al. Evaluating the concordance of clinician antiretroviral prescribing practices and HIV-ASSIST, an online clinical decision support tool. *J Gen Intern Med.* 2020;35(5):1498–1503.

Raugi DN, Diallo K, Baila Diallo M, et al. Resource and infrastructure challenges on the RESIST-2 Trial: an implementation study of drug resistance genotype-based algorithmic ART switches in HIV-2-infected adults in Senegal. *Trials.* 2021;22(1):931.

Raymond S, Piffaut M, Bigot J, et al. Sexual transmission of an extensively drug-resistance HIV-1 strain. *Lancet HIV.* 2020;7(8):e529–e530.

Requena S, Trevino A, Cabeza T; Spanish HIV-2 Study Group. Drug resistance mutations in HIV-2 patients failing raltegravir and influence on dolutegravir response. *J Antimicrob Chemother.* 2017;72(7):2083–2088.

Rhee S, Clutter D, Feddel WJ, et al. Trends in the molecular epidemiology and genetic mechanisms of transmitted Human Immunodeficiency Virus Type 1 drug resistance in a large US clinic population. *Clin Infect Dis.* 2019a;68(2):213–221.

Rhee SY, Blanco JL, Jordan MR, et al. Geographic and temporal trends in the molecular epidemiology and genetic mechanisms of transmitted HIV-1 drug resistance: an individual-patient-and sequence-level meta-analysis. *PLoS Med.* 2015;12(4):e1001810. http://doi:10.1371/journal.pmed.1001810

Rhee SY, Clutter D, Hare CB, et al. Virological failure and acquired genotypic resistance associated with contemporary antiretroviral treatment regimens. *Open Forum Infect Dis.* August 6, 2020a;7(9): ofaa316.

Rhee SY, Fessel WJ, Liu TF, et al. Predictive value of HIV-1 genotypic resistance test interpretation algorithms. *J Infect Dis.* 2009;200(3):453–463.

Rhee SY, Grant PM, Tzou PL, et al. A systematic review of the genetic mechanisms of dolutegravir resistance. *J Antimicrob Chemother.* 2019b;74:3135–3149.

Rhee SY, Kassaye SH, Barrow G et al. HIV-1 transmitted drug resistance surveillance: shifting trends in study design and prevalence estimates. *J Int AIDS Soc.* September 2020b;23(9):e25611.

Rich SN, Poschman K, Hu H, et al. Sociodemographic, ecological, and spatiotemporal factors associated with HIV drug resistance in Florida: a retrospective analysis. *J Infect Dis.* July 9, 2020;223(5):866–875.

Rodriguez AE, Wawrzyniak AJ, Tookes HE, et al. Implementation of an immediate HIV treatment initiation program in a public/academic medical center in the US South: the Miami Test and Treat Rapid Response Program. *AIDS Behav.* 2019;23(Suppl 3):287–295.

Rodriguez MA, Mills A, Stoker A, et al. HIV-1 DNA resistance testing informs the successful switch to a single tablet regimen. *J AIDS Clin Res.* 2020;12:828.

Rolle CP, Berhe M, Singh T, et al. Dolutegravir/lamivudine as a first-line regimen in a test-and-treat setting for newly diagnosed people living with HIV. *AIDS.* 2021;35(12):1957–1965.

Rolle CP, Nguyen V, Patel K, et al. Real-world efficacy and safety of switching to bictegravir/emtricitabine/tenofovir alafenamide in older people living with HIV. *Medicine (Baltimore).* 2021;100(38): e27330.

Rose R, Gartland M, Li Z, et al. Clinical evidence for a lack of cross-resistance between temsavir and ibalizumab or maraviroc. *AIDS.* 2022;36(1):11–18.

Saag MS, Gandhi RT, Hoy JF, et al. Antiretroviral drugs for treatment and prevention of HIV infection in adults: 2020 recommendations of the International Antiviral Society-USA Panel. *JAMA.* http://doi:10.1001/jama.2020.17025. Published October 14, 2020. Accessed January 29, 2023.

Sax PE, Andreatta K, Molina JM, et al. High efficacy of switching to bictegravir/emtricitabine/tenofovir alafenamide in people with suppressed HIV and pre-existing M184V/I. *AIDS.* 2022;36(11):1511–1520.

Scarsi KK, Havens JP, Podany AT, et al. HIV-1 integrase inhibitors: a comparative review of efficacy and safety. *Drugs.* 2020;80: 1649–1676.

Scherrer AU, von Wyl V, Yang WL, et al. Emergence of acquired HIV-1 drug resistance almost stopped in Switzerland: a 15-year prospective cohort analysis. *Clin Infect Dis.* 2016;62:1310–1317.

Siefried KJ, Mao L, Cysique LA, et al. Concomitant medication polypharmacy, interactions and imperfect adherence are common in Australian adults on suppressive antiretroviral therapy. *AIDS.* 2018;32:35–48.

Siefried KJ, Mao L, Kerr S, et al.; PAART study investigators. Socioeconomic factors explain suboptimal adherence to antiretroviral therapy among HIV-infected Australian adults with viral suppression. *PLoS One.* 2017;12:e0174613.

Siliciano JD, Siliciano RF. Recent trends in HIV-1 drug resistance. *Curr Opin Virology.* 2013;3:487–494.

Sörstedt E, Carlander C, Flamholc L, et al. Effect of dolutegravir in combination with nucleoside reverse transcriptase inhibitors (NRTIs) on people living with HIV who have pre-existing NRTI mutations. *Int J Antimicrob Agents.* 2018;51:733–738.

Stella G, Volpicelli L, Di Carlo D, et al. Impact of pre-existent drug resistance on virological efficacy of single-tablet regimens in people living with HIV. *Int J Antimicrob Agents.* 2022;60(3):106636.

Swenson LC, Min JE, Woods CK, et al. HIV drug resistance detected during low-level viremia is associated with subsequent virologic failure. *AIDS.* May 15, 2014;28(8):1125–1134.

Toni TA, Asahchop EL, Moisi D, et al. Detection of human immunodeficiency virus (HIV) type 1 M184V and K103N minority variants in patients with primary HIV infection. *Antimicrob Agents Chemother.* 2009;53:1670–1672.

Tzou PH, Rhee SY, Descamps, et al; WHO HIVResNet Working Groups. Integrase strand transfer inhibitor (INSTI)-resistance mutations for the surveillance of transmitted HIV-1 drug resistance. *J Antimicrob Chemother.* 2020;75:170–182.

Vandenhende MA, Perrier A, Bonnet F, et al. Risk of virological failure in HIV-1-infected patients experiencing low-level viraemia under active antiretroviral therapy (ANRS CO3 cohort study). *Antivir Ther.* 2015;20(6):655–660.

Van Wyk J, Orkin C, Rubio R, et al. Durable suppression and low rate of virologic failure 3 years after switch to dolutegravir + rilpivirine 2-drug regimen: 148-week results from the SWORD-1 and SWORD-2 randomized clinical trials. *J Acquir Immune Defic Syndr.* http://doi:10.1097/QAI. 0000000000002449. Published 2020. Accessed January 29, 2023.

Van Zyl G, Bale MJ, Kearney MF. HIV evolution and diversity in ART-treated patients. *Retrovirology.* 2018;15(1):14

Varghese V, Shahriar R, Rhee SY, et al. Minority variants associated with transmitted and acquired HIV-1 non-nucleoside RT (NNRTI) resistance: implications for the use of second generation NNRTIs. *J Acquir Immune Defic Syndr.* 2009;52(3):309–315.

Verhofstede C, Noe A, Demecheleer E, et al. Drug-resistance variants that evolve during nonsuppressive therapy persist in HIV-1-infected peripheral blood mononuclear cells after long-term highly active antiretroviral therapy. *J Acquir Immune Def Synd.* 2004;35:473–483.

Villalobos C, Ceballos ME, Ferres M, Palma C. Drug resistance mutations in proviral DNA of HIV-infected patients with low level of viremia. *J Clin Virol.* 2020;132:104657.

Vingerhoets J, Tambuyzer L, Azijn H, et al. Resistance profile of etravirine: combined analysis of baseline genotypic and phenotypic data from the randomized, controlled phase III clinical studies. *AIDS.* February 20, 2010;24(4):503–514.

Wensing AM, Calvez V, Ceccherini-Silberstein F, et al. 2019 update of the drug resistance mutations in HIV-1. *Top Antivir Med.* 2019;27(3):111–121.

Westby J, Lewis M, Whitcomb J, et al. Emergence of CXCR4-using human immunodeficiency virus type 1 (HIV-1) variants in a minority of HIV-1-infected patients following treatment with the CCR5 antagonist maraviroc is from a pretreatment CXCR4-using virus reservoir. *J Virol.* May 2006;80(10):4909–4920.

Weyland C, Mirani G, Gillespie SL, Paul ME. A case of in utero transmission of drug-resistant HIV in the United States. *Pediatr Infect Dis J.* 2022;41(1):57–59.

Wheeler WH, Ziebell RA, Zabina H, et al. Prevalence of transmitted drug resistance associated mutations and HIV-1 subtypes in new HIV-1 diagnoses, US—2006. *AIDS.* 2010;24:1203–1212.

Winters B, van Craenenbroeck E, van der Borght K, et al. Clinical cutoffs for HIV-1 phenotypic resistance estimates: update based on recent pivotal clinical trial data and a revised approach to viral mixtures. *J Virologic Methods.* 2009;162:101–108.

Wirden M, Soulie C, Valantin MA, et al. Historical HIV-RNA resistance test results are more informative than proviral DNA genotyping in cases of suppressed or residual viraemia. *Antimicrob Chemother.* 2011;66:709–712.

Wood BR, Stekler JD. Baseline HIV genotype drug resistance testing: is it time for more or less? *AIDS.* 2022;36(10):1449–1451.

World Health Organization (WHO). HIV drug resistance report 2021. https://www.who.int/publications/i/item/9789240038608. Published 2021. Accessed September 25, 2022.

Yanik EL, Napravnik S, Hurt CB, et al. Prevalence of transmitted antiretroviral drug resistance differs between acutely and chronically HIV-infected patients. *J Acquir Immun Defic Syndr.* 2012;61:258–262.

Zaccarelli M, Santoro MM, Armenia D, et al. Genotypic resistance test in proviral DNA can identify resistance mutations never detected in historical genotypic test in patients with low level or undetectable HIV-RNA. *J Clin Virol.* September 2016;82: 94–100.

Zhou N, Nowicka-Sans B, McAuliffe B, et al. Genotypic correlates of susceptibility to HIV1 attachment inhibitor BMS-626529, the active agent of the prodrug BMS-663068. *J Antimicrob Chemother.* 2014;69:573–581.

21.

ANTIRETROVIRAL TREATMENT AND STEWARDSHIP IN HOSPITAL SETTINGS

David E. Koren

CHAPTER GOALS

Upon completion of this chapter, the reader should be able to:

- Discuss issues in determining the relative priority of initiating and/or maintaining antiretroviral therapy (ART) in the context of hospitalized persons with HIV (PWH) with significant comorbid conditions, as well as issues of continuity of care after discharge from the inpatient setting.

- Define *antiretroviral stewardship* and understand its potential benefit in implementation.

- Describe important considerations in the perioperative care of a PWH.

GENERAL HOSPITALIZATION CONCERNS IN PWH INCLUDING ANTIRETROVIRAL STEWARDSHIP

LEARNING OBJECTIVE

Discuss issues in determining the relative priority of initiating and/or maintaining ART in the context of the hospitalized PWH with significant comorbid conditions, the new concept of antiretroviral stewardship, and issues of continuity of care after discharge from the inpatient setting.

WHAT'S NEW?

- An updated link to a reference table of available ART formulations is provided.

- New ART agents since last publication are incorporated.

- An additional resource regarding known absorption sites of ARVs, as well as pharmacokinetic effects of bariatric surgery on ARV, is provided.

The introduction of highly active antiretroviral therapy has changed many root causes for hospitalization among PWH. In the pre-ART era, progressive opportunistic infections (OIs) and end-stage AIDS were the main causes of recurrent hospitalizations; however, these causes (as well as hospitalization rates) have dramatically declined in the ART era. Recent drivers for hospitalization have diversified and are now associated with an increase incidence of chronic, noncommunicable

health conditions such as diabetes, cardiovascular disease, chronic kidney diseases, and malignancies (Paul et al., 2002). There are many considerations in the use of ART during hospitalization, and this issue can be divided into two main categories described here.

The first category consists of PWH not on ART at the time of admission, which may be due to nonadherence or not having been diagnosed with HIV until the hospitalization itself (possibly owing to presentation with an OI). The general question in this case is whether to start ART during hospitalization. Concerns regarding additional pill burden, increased potential for side effects and drug interactions, and possible immune reconstitution inflammatory syndrome must be weighed against faster OI improvement and ultimate morbidity/mortality benefits. A 2009 randomized controlled trial helped inform the issue, concluding that early ART initiation resulted in less AIDS progression/death with no increase in adverse events or loss of virologic response compared to deferred ART (Zolopa et al., 2009). Additionally, current US Department of Health and Human Service (DHHS) guidelines, supported by clinical literature including the START and TEMPRANO trials recommend "initiating ART immediately (or as soon as possible) after HIV diagnosis in order to increase the uptake of ART and linkage to care, decrease the time to viral suppression for individual patients, and improve the rate of virologic suppression among persons with HIV." This may occur in a rapid start scenario, in which antiretrovirals are initiated prior to return of all associated laboratory values (US DHHS, 2022). Additionally, in a multisite cohort of 801 persons living with both HIV and substance use disorder, initiation of ART while hospitalized was associated with a shorter time to first HIV care visit (29 days among those who initiated ART while hospitalized compared to 54 days among those who did not, $p = 0.0145$) (Jacobs et al., 2020). These data, however, did not reveal an association between inpatient ART initiation and either retention or viral suppression over 12 months, demonstrating that further interventions may be required in this population.

A critical additional factor in deciding whether to initiate ART during hospitalization is the importance of ensuring that the PWH will be able to access and continue ART upon discharge to prevent lapses in adherence and potential resistance. This issue involves both the immediate availability of ART on discharge (i.e., if the PWH has access to outpatient medications via insurance coverage or AIDS Drug Assistance

Program) and whether the PWH is in a position to continue with successful adherence (i.e., housing stability, substance abuse treatment needs, mental healthcare optimization, and willingness to take ART). In all cases, it is essential to ensure that PWH will have streamlined access to ongoing outpatient HIV specialty care and that people are linked before discharge to prevent adherence lapses.

The second category consists of PWH with a known HIV diagnosis who are on ART at the time of admission. PWH who are on stable ART and admitted to the hospital should continue taking their regimen with few exceptions. Issues that impact ART continuation include the reason for admission and if it impacts the ability to take oral medications—that is, severe gastrointestinal (GI) disturbances such as intractable vomiting, diarrhea, or GI obstruction. In such cases, ART use may need to be temporarily suspended until the PWH's GI symptoms resolve sufficiently to tolerate oral medications again to avoid intermittent absorption and subtherapeutic drug levels predisposing to resistance. In addition, temporary ART discontinuation may need to be considered in presentations of severe lactic acidosis, pancreatitis, severe hepatic enzyme elevations, obtundation, or emergent surgical issues. ART dosing should be resumed as soon as safely possible when the PWH clinically improves from these initial severe presentations.

If possible, PWH who are *nihil per OS* (NPO) should continue ART with water unless there is an acute GI problem that is rendering them NPO. PWH with nasogastric tubes should be given all ART in liquid form, when available, or crushed and reconstituted if no liquid form is available. An updated reference table based on a literature review for ARVs that can be crushed or sprinkled and also information on liquid formulation availability can be found at www.hiv-druginteracti ons.org/prescribing_resources/hiv-guidance-swallowing.

Drug interaction issues need to be considered routinely during hospitalization. Any new medications given need to be checked for interactions with the PWH's current ART regimen, and dose adjustments or medication changes should be made as needed, ideally in concert with an HIV specialty pharmacist. Particular attention should be paid to proton pump inhibitor (PPI) interactions because PPIs are often started for ulcer prophylaxis or other reasons during hospitalization. Atazanavir and rilpivirine are particularly susceptible to subtherapeutic drug levels because of PPI interaction; therefore, extra care should be taken to mitigate problematic interactions. Additionally, integrase strand inhibitor agents (bictegravir, dolutegravir, elvitegravir, and raltegravir) may have decreased activity in the context of simultaneous administration with medications containing di/poly-valent cations. These examples are only some of many potential pharmacokinetic/dynamic interactions. An updated reference for drug–drug interactions concerning ARV can be found at http://www.hiv-druginteractions.org.

Some other ART considerations during hospitalization include formulary availability, especially at smaller hospitals with less HIV experience, and adequate stock of all agents because the number and classes of ART medications have dramatically increased. It is important to work with the pharmacy to ensure that correct ART is available without delay in the correct dosing form and that, if there are any supply problems, appropriate class substitutions are given in consultation with an HIV expert. Recent approval of injectable cabotegravir-rilpivirine may cause unique issues during medication reconciliation, and clinicians not familiar with ART may require further education as to the long-acting nature of the formulations, particularly if a patient is hospitalized during an injection window. If a PWH is on an investigational medication via a research study, it is imperative that the treating physician and the research team administering the investigational drug are notified of the person's hospital admission because they must make arrangements to bring the drug to the hospital and arrange for its administration by the staff there.

Antiretroviral Stewardship

Given reported inpatient ARV error rates as high as 86% which may include, but are not limited to, incomplete ARV regimens and drug–drug interactions, the need has arisen for increased safety monitoring of PWH during transitions of care as well as in the hospital setting. To address issues of inpatient HIV management, a joint call to action was published in 2020 by the American Academy of HIV Medicine, HIV Medicine Association and Infectious Disease Society of America defining antiretroviral stewardship as, *"coordinated interventions designed to improve continuity of care of patients receiving ARVs through the utilization of evidence-based ARV practices including medication reconciliation, dosing, mitigation of drug interactions, and prevention of viral resistance."* These activities, tailored to the needs of the individual institution, are generally conducted by stakeholders with experience in ARV, and may consist of clinical checklists to ensure safe prescribing practices, standardized computerized physician order entry sets to prevent inadvertent errors, and/or prospective review strategies by physician-pharmacist collaborations to maintain safety throughout a hospitalization. In doing so, stewardship initiatives may prevent virologic failure, viral resistance, deleterious drug interactions, and adverse drug events. ARV stewardship activities should be routinely monitored for outcomes/efficacy and incorporated into reporting alongside other non-HIV related stewardship (Koren et al., 2020).

PERIOPERATIVE CARE, SURGICAL ISSUES, AND THE BARIATRIC PWH

KEY POINTS

- The balance of data shows no overall worse operation-associated morbidity and mortality in PWH undergoing surgical procedures.

- Perioperative complications may be more frequent or severe in very immunosuppressed PWH.

- There are some specific anesthesia considerations in PWH.

- Bariatric procedures may affect antiretroviral absorption. Considerations should be made regarding the person's specific ARV regimen and type of procedure during evaluative workup.

Overall, data suggest operation-associated morbidity and mortality in PWH are not different from those in uninfected people. Because of improvements in outcomes and overall, OI reduction in the early ART era, the number of operations for AIDS-related surgical illnesses has decreased considerably (Saltzman et al., 2005). Additionally, given available data from the ART era, general data supports that HIV infection does not increase the postoperative risk for complications or death (Cacala et al., 2006; Evron et al., 2004). Despite these positive attributes, given vastly improved survival and longevity of PWH alongside ongoing comorbidities that increase with an aging PWH population, the need for non-HIV related surgical operations and anesthesia has become far more commonplace.

POSTOPERATIVE COMPLICATIONS AND HIV INFECTION

Uncontrolled or advanced HIV infection may influence postoperative wound healing and complication rates (Rose et al., 1998). Additionally, advanced HIV infection accompanied by OIs or malignancies may complicate the perioperative course and management. This may be due to debility and wasting as much as immunosuppression. A CD4$^+$ T-cell count and viral load measurement are useful when calculating surgical risks and developing a prognosis in PWH (Evron et al., 2004; Saltzman et al., 2005). Postoperative CD4$^+$ T-cell counts of 200 cells/mm^3 or less are associated with higher mortality rates (Saltzman et al., 2005). Irrespective of surgical procedure, there is a 13.3% mortality rate with a CD4$^+$ T-cell count less than 50 cells/mm^3 and a 0.8% mortality rate with the CD4$^+$ T-cell count greater than 200 cells/mm^3 6 months postoperatively (Evron et al., 2004). Postoperative viral loads greater than 75,000 copies/mL are associated with higher complication and mortality rates (Saltzman et al., 2005). A 2006 Kaiser retrospective study showed that viral load suppression to less than 30,000 copies/mL reduced surgical complications (Horberg et al., 2006).

To mitigate operative complications, PWH with a history or signs of cardiac or pulmonary dysfunction should undergo a more thorough evaluation prior to surgery (e.g., blood gases, pulmonary function tests, echocardiography, further cardiac testing, or even cardiac catheterization as appropriate). Relevant history of past treatment with potentially cardiotoxic therapies, such as chemotherapy for Kaposi's sarcoma or lymphoma, should be considered in assessing operative risk. PWH may be in a relatively hypercoagulable state, with accelerated coronary atherosclerosis and possibly decreased left ventricular contractility (Evron et al., 2004).

ANESTHESIA CONSIDERATIONS AND DRUG INTERACTIONS

Information about the relative general hazards of anesthesia and surgery for PWH is scarce (Evron et al., 2004). Many ARVs may interact directly with anesthetic drugs and can cause side effects that influence which anesthetics are used and the way they are administered (Evron et al., 2004; Hughes, 2004). This issue is continually evolving given interaction profiles of each ARV or anesthetic agent.

Specific considerations when administering general anesthesia to PWH include the possible effects of anesthesia and opioids on the immune system, the cardiopulmonary and neurologic status of the person, and possible interactions with ART medications.

- *Opioids*: although there is laboratory evidence that opioids may detrimentally affect immune function, the clinical significance of short-term opioid administration during general anesthesia is unclear, and not enough clinical data are available to justify its avoidance.

- *Neurologic considerations*: neurologic manifestations, such as overt dementia, may impair the ability of PWH to provide preoperative consent and may increase brain sensitivity to sedative or psychoactive drugs such as opioids, benzodiazepines, and neuroleptics.

- *General central nervous system (CNS)*: increased intracranial pressure (ICP) and CNS infections (i.e., meningitis, encephalopathy, or myelopathy) are contraindications to neuraxial anesthesia.

- *Cerebrospinal fluid analysis and nerve or muscle biopsy* may be required, and radiological studies of the spinal cord should be performed as part of the neurological evaluation to exclude compressive lesions in symptomatic PWH. OIs may be associated with increased ICP, especially in the case of toxoplasmosis or cryptococcal meningitis. Because these infections respond to medical therapy, surgery should be postponed whenever possible if they are present.

- *Pulmonary considerations*: pulmonary complications can occur as a consequence of many OIs, leading to respiratory distress and hypoxemia.

Regional anesthesia has been shown to be associated with reduced morbidity and mortality in a wide range of patients, including PWH having cesarean delivery under spinal anesthesia. However, a high motor block with intercostal muscle paralysis may not be tolerated (Evron, 2004). Regional anesthesia is less likely to interfere with immune function or interact with ARV drugs. Sepsis and platelet abnormalities are contraindications to regional anesthesia, and neuropathy may also interfere. Post–dural puncture headache may occur after regional anesthesia and may necessitate epidural blood patch. No increase in neurologic abnormalities in six PWH receiving an epidural blood patch during a follow-up period of 2 years was observed, and there is no evidence to contraindicate the use of blood patch in PWH (Evron et al., 2004; Tom et al., 1992).

Some nonnucleoside reverse transcriptase inhibitors such as efavirenz or etravirine induce the cytochrome P450 enzyme system (CYP3A3/4) and may decrease serum levels of some anesthetic or sedative drugs that use this metabolic pathway, such as midazolam and fentanyl (Evron et al., 2004). Etomidate, atracurium, remifentanil, and desflurane are not dependent on CYP450 hepatic metabolism and may be preferable in persons receiving ART (Evron et al., 2004).

Protease inhibitors (PIs), primarily use the cytochrome P450 system as well (CYP3A4). Because PIs often inhibit, and may also induce this enzyme, they may increase or decrease the effects of other drugs using the same metabolic pathway; any anesthetics used concomitantly should be carefully titrated. Ritonavir is the most potent inhibitor of CYP3A4 and CYP2D6. Another CYP3A inhibitor, cobicistat, is commonly used as an ART boosting agent and has similar interactions to ritonavir with similar need for dosing considerations. Fentanyl is metabolized mainly by CYP3A4 (Evron et al., 2004); ritonavir can reduce fentanyl clearance by up to 67%. This strong interaction suggests that fentanyl (as well as other anesthetics) should be carefully titrated and monitored in a PWH on a concomitant boosting agent. These effects may be deleterious, respiratory monitoring should be maintained in the setting of this interaction as the risk of respiratory depression for an increased duration will likely be higher (Hughes, 2004). Integrase strand inhibitors themselves are neither inductive nor inhibitory to the cytochrome P450 system, though if used in combination with other products, such as elvitegravir with cobicistat, this will have the aforementioned inhibitory effects as above.

BARIATRIC SURGERY, PERSONS WITH HIV, AND ANTIRETROVIRAL THERAPY

Although bariatric surgeries have proven effective in both reducing obesity-related mortality and obesity-related comorbidities, they may bring about pharmacologic considerations/complications depending on the type of surgery performed on the PWH (e.g., Roux-en-Y gastric bypass or sleeve gastrectomy) (Cimino et al., 2018). Generally, these considerations consist of absorptive and dietary concerns. If the person's ART is known to be absorbed in the small intestine, and the small intestine is permanently bypassed because of a surgical procedure, the medication will not be absorbed. Additionally, if an antiretroviral requires a caloric and/or fat requirement, and the stomach volume is reduced significantly because of a procedure, this will inevitably result in subtherapeutic absorption. Minimal data exists on this issue, generally consisting of collections of case reports given the broad array of potential bariatric procedures and antiretroviral combinations. During evaluative workup prior to a procedure, considerations should be made as to available formulations of the PWH's antiretroviral regimen (including whether the medication can be crushed), potential for drug–drug interactions (including acid-suppression and di/polyvalent cations), and the type of bariatric procedure. While the exact site of absorption is only known among few ARVs, among those that are, many are absorbed in the small intestine, thus Roux-en-Y procedures may compromise absorption (Cimino et al., 2018). A summary of the known absorption sites of ARVs, as well as known pharmacokinetic effects of bariatric surgery on ARV concentrations, can be found at: www.hiv-druginteractions.org/prescribing_resources/hiv-guidance-gastric-surgery.

RECOMMENDED READING

Huesgen E, DeSear KE, Egelund EF, et al. A HAART-breaking review of alternative antiretroviral administration: practical considerations with crushing and enteral tube scenarios. Pharmacotherapy. 2016;36(11):1145–1165.

REFERENCES

Cacala SR, Mafana E, Thompson SR, et al. Prevalence of HIV status and CD4 counts in a surgical cohort: their relationship to clinical outcome. *Ann R Coll Surg Engl.* 2006;88(1):46–51.

Cimino C, Binkley A, Swisher R, et al. Antiretroviral considerations in HIV-infected patients undergoing bariatric surgery. *J Clin Pharm Ther.* 2018;43:757–767.

Evron S, Glezerman M, Harow E, et al. Human immunodeficiency virus: anesthetic and obstetric considerations. *Anesth Analg.* 2004;98(2):503–511.

Horberg MA, Hurley LB, Klein DB, et al. Surgical Outcomes in human immunodeficiency virus-infected patients in the era of highly active antiretroviral therapy. *Arch Surg.* 2006;141(12):1238–1245.

Hughes SC. HIV and anesthesia. *Anesthesiol Clin North Am.* 2004;22(3):379–404.

Jacobs P, Feaster DJ, Pan Y, et al. Initiation of antiretroviral therapy in the hospital is associated with linkage to human immunodeficiency virus (HIV) care for persons living with HIV and substance use disorder. *Clin Infect Dis.* 2020;73(7):e1982–e1990.

Koren DE, Scarsi KK, Farmer EK, et al. A call to action: the role of antiretroviral stewardship in inpatient practice, a joint policy paper of the Infectious Diseases Society of America, HIV Medicine Association, and American Academy of HIV Medicine. *Clin Infect Dis.* 2020;70(11):2241–2246.

Paul S, Gilbert HM, Lande L, et al. Impact of antiretroviral therapy on decreasing hospitalization rates of HIV-infected patients in 2001. *AIDS Res Hum Retroviruses.* 2002;18:501–506.

Rose D, Collins M, Kelban R. Complications of surgery in HIV-infected patients. *AIDS.* 1998;12:2243–2251.

Saltzman DJ, Williams RA, Gelfand DV, et al. The surgeon and AIDS: twenty years later. *Arch Surg.* 2005;140(10):961–967.

Tom DJ, Gulevich SJ, Shapiro HM, et al. Epidural blood patch in the HIV-positive patient. Review of clinical experience. San Diego HIV Neurobehavioral Research Center. *Anesthesiology.* 1992;76(6):943–947.

US Department of Health and Human Services (US DHHS). Panel on Antiretroviral Guidelines for Adults and Adolescents. Guidelines for the use of antiretroviral agents in adults and adolescents living with HIV. https://clinicalinfo.hiv.gov/sites/default/files/guidelines/documents/adult-adolescent-arv/guidelines-adult-adolescent-ar. Published 2022. Accessed March 9, 2023.

Zolopa AR, Anderson J, Powderly W, et al. Early Antiretroviral therapy reduces AIDS progression/death in individuals with acute opportunistic infections: a multicenter randomized strategy trial. *PLoS One.* 2009;4(5)e5575. http://doi.org/10.1371/journal.pone.0005575

22.

SOLID ORGAN TRANSPLANTATION IN PERSONS WITH HIV

Christine M. Durand

INTRODUCTION

The advent of effective combination antiretroviral therapy (ART) has resulted in increased life expectancy for people with HIV (PWH). With declining opportunistic infections, end-organ disease—both directly and indirectly associated with HIV—has become a major cause of morbidity and mortality in this population. Solid organ transplantation, once considered contraindicated for individuals with HIV, has demonstrated success and is now considered the standard of care for end-stage organ disease in this population.

This chapter focuses on kidney and liver transplantation in persons with HIV, which have the most evidence and experience to date. Relatively few studies have described cardiothoracic transplant and HIV-associated outcomes. One study of 75 heart transplant recipients with HIV demonstrated equivalent survival between matched recipients with and without HIV; similarly, a multicenter international study including 21 heart, 7 lung, and 1 heart/lung transplant recipients with HIV showed similar survival between recipients with and without HIV (Doberne et al., 2020; Koval et al., 2019).

Chronic kidney disease can develop as a direct consequence of the HIV virus itself (i.e., HIV-associated nephropathy (HIVAN)), long-term ART toxicities, and/or other comorbidities such as hypertension and diabetes, which are common in PWH (Abraham et al., 2015; Althoff et al., 2019; Mocroft, 2016). Liver disease can occur because of common coinfections such as hepatitis C virus and hepatitis B virus (Platt et al., 2016; Sun et al., 2014), alcoholic liver disease, or nonalcoholic fatty liver disease. Once end-stage kidney or liver disease has developed, the best treatment is organ transplantation and accordingly, there has been a growing need for kidney and liver transplantation among PWH (Locke et al., 2017b; Shaffer & Durand, 2018).

LEARNING OBJECTIVES

Discuss the evaluation and management of the kidney and liver transplant candidate with HIV and clinical outcomes for kidney and liver transplant recipients with HIV.

Explain key drug–drug interactions between immunosuppressive agents and ART in transplant recipients with HIV.

WHAT'S NEW?

- Studies have found that patient and graft survival rates in kidney transplant recipients with HIV are equivalent to kidney recipients without HIV.

- Studies have found that patient and graft survival rates in liver transplant recipients with HIV are lower than those without HIV, although outcomes are improving over time and with the advent of highly effective HCV treatment.

- With the increase in number and availability of integrase strand transfer inhibitors (InSTIs), clinicians and patients can often select an ART regimen, which minimizes risk of drug interactions while limiting side effects, maintaining ease of administration, and preserving a high barrier to ART resistance.

- The HIV Organ Policy Equity (HOPE) Act, which was signed into US law in 2013, allows the use of organs from donors with HIV to be used for transplant for recipients with HIV under research protocols. Early studies of HIV donor to HIV recipient (HIV D+/R+) kidney and liver transplantation are encouraging.

KEY POINTS

- End-organ disease has become a major cause of morbidity and mortality in people with HIV because of increased life expectancy, thus increasing the demand for organ transplantation in this population.

- The care of transplant recipients with HIV warrants a multidisciplinary team approach, including the specific organ transplant team, pharmacists, infectious disease/HIV specialists, nurses, patients, and their families.

- Transplant-related immunosuppression for recipients with HIV has not been associated with loss of virologic control or increased opportunistic infections.

- Protease inhibitors (PIs) and pharmacoenhancing ("boosting") agents are strong CYP3A4 inhibitors; their use results in clinically significant drug interactions with some transplant medications. Patients who receive these ART medications should be monitored carefully; for some, ART modification may be preferable to avoid problematic interactions. Use of older nonnucleoside reverse transcriptase inhibitors (NNRTIs) (; i.e., efavirenz, nevirapine, etravirine) also leads to significant drug interactions with some transplant medications.

- Kidney transplant recipients with HIV face an increased risk of allograft rejection after transplant.

- HCV treatment is essential to improve outcomes among liver and kidney transplant recipients with HIV and HCV coinfection.

PRETRANSPLANT EVALUATION

CRITERIA FOR TRANSPLANTATION

Many of the following recommendations are based on the National Institutes of Health (NIH)-funded Solid Organ Transplantation in HIV: Multi-site Study (HIVTR Study), which was a prospective observational study of kidney and liver transplantation in PWH conducted across 26 transplant centers in the United States between 2002 and 2013 (Roland et al., 2016; Stock et al., 2010; Terrault et al. 2012).

- Any opportunistic infections or malignancies should be completely treated prior to transplant. There are limited data on outcomes of transplant recipients who have a history of progressive multifocal leukoencephalopathy, visceral Kaposi's sarcoma, chronic cryptosporidiosis, or primary central nervous system lymphoma, as these individuals were excluded from clinical trials of kidney and liver transplantation for PWH.

- Transplant candidates with HIV should meet standard criteria for transplantation.

- Transplant candidates with HIV should be on a stable ART regimen.

Kidney Transplant Candidate Criteria

- CD4$^+$ T-cell count should generally be ≥200 cells/mm^3 prior to transplant.

- HIV RNA should be suppressed to below the assay's limit of detection (excluding viral "blips" of 20–200 copies/mL, which are common and unlikely to be clinically significant) (Nettles et al., 2005).

Liver Transplant Candidate Criteria

- CD4$^+$ T-cell count should generally be ≥100 cells/mm^3. A lower CD4$^+$ T-cell count criteria has been allowed for liver transplant candidates because of the impact of portal hypertension and splenomegaly on lowering overall lymphocyte counts.

- HIV RNA should be suppressed to below the limit of detection of the assay (excluding viral "blips" of 20–200 copies/mL, which are common and unlikely to be clinically significant) (Nettles et al., 2005).

PRETRANSPLANT INFECTION SCREENING AND VACCINATIONS

Latent Tuberculosis

- All candidates should be screened for latent tuberculosis (TB) prior to transplantation, with either a tuberculin skin test or interferon-gamma release assay (Blumberg & Roger, 2019; Centers for Disease Control and Prevention (CDC), 2020). Patients should be treated if they have evidence of latent TB. The preferred regimen is isoniazid (INH) ± vitamin B$_6$ for 9 months, completing at least 6 of the 9 months prior to transplantation. For liver transplantation, when prophylactic treatment cannot be completed prior to transplant, or if the risk of toxicity is too high, treatment should be completed as soon as possible after transplant.

Syphilis

- Test for and treat syphilis prior to transplant.

Other Infectious Conditions

- Test for cytomegalovirus (CMV), Epstein–Barr virus, herpes simplex virus, varicella zoster virus (VZV), and viral hepatitis serologies in all candidates. In addition, coccidioides and strongyloides serologies should be tested if the recipient has exposure to endemic areas.

Vaccinations

Whenever possible, vaccinations should be given pretransplant. Live vaccines such as varicella and mumps/measles/rubella (MMR) vaccines should not be given pretransplant if CD4$^+$ T-cell count is less than 300 cells/mm^3 (Miro et al., 2014). No live vaccines should be given post transplant.

- All candidates should be vaccinated against hepatitis A and B if not already immune.

- Inactivated influenza vaccine should be given yearly. The high-dose vaccine has demonstrated better immunogenicity and is safe in solid organ transplant recipients (Mombelli et al., 2018).

- Both the pneumococcal conjugate vaccine (PCV13) and polysaccharide vaccine (PPV23) should be given. PCV13 should be given for first vaccination and PPV23 can be given at least 8 weeks later. These vaccines should be administered every 3–5 years (Blumberg & Roger, 2019).

- Tdap vaccine should be given if not received in the past 10 years.

- HPV vaccine should be given for persons aged 9–45 years.

- Meningococcal conjugate vaccine (MenACWY) should be given to all candidates, and the serogroup B meningococcal vaccine should be given to candidates between 16 and 23 years of age.

- Varicella vaccine should be given to those who are VZV seronegative (and have CD4 ≥300 cells/mm^3) prior to transplant.

- Recombinant zoster vaccine (RSV, Shingrix) has shown safety and immunogenicity in immunocompromised populations (Berkowitz et al., 2015; Stadtmauer et al., 2014) and should be considered to prevent zoster reactivation, which is common among PWH and transplant recipients.

WHEN TO REFER

KIDNEY TRANSPLANT

- All individuals with HIV who have a glomerular filtration rate of 25 mL/min or less should be referred to a kidney transplant center.

LIVER TRANSPLANT

- All individuals with HIV who have decompensated or symptomatic cirrhosis or hepatocellular carcinoma should be referred for liver transplant evaluation. Patients with an albumin of less than 3 g/dL, prolonged prothrombin time, or a modified Child–Turcotte–Pugh score of 7 or higher should also be considered.

POSTTRANSPLANT MANAGEMENT AND CARE

All pre-, peri-, and posttransplant care should be coordinated among a multidisciplinary team consisting of the transplant surgeon, an ID or HIV specialist, a nephrologist or hepatologist, a primary care provider, a transplant coordinator, a transplant pharmacist, a social worker, and nursing staff.

IMMUNOSUPPRESSION THERAPY

Induction Immunosuppression for Kidney Transplantation

For kidney transplantation, induction immunosuppression at the time of transplant typically includes a lymphocyte depleting regimen with antithymocyte globulin (ATG) or a non-lymphocyte depleting regimen with an interleukin 2 receptor antagonist (anti-IL2R), a less potent monoclonal antibody that blocks early T-cell activation (Gabardi et al., 2011). There remains debate about which agent is optimal for transplant recipients with HIV. The multicenter HIVTR study suggested that the use of antithymocyte globulin was associated with a higher risk of graft loss and hospitalizations owing to infections (Stock et al., 2010). However, subsequent studies found a 2.6-fold lower risk of acute rejection and equivalent graft survival in transplant recipients with HIV who received ATG induction (Locke et al., 2014). A subsequent study of 830 renal transplant recipients with HIV found a 40% lower rate of rejection among those who received ATG for induction compared to either no induction or anti-IL-2R induction without evidence of increased infections (Kucirka et al., 2016). The choice of induction therapy should be made on a case-by-case basis, accounting for the individual's risk of rejection, although recent evidence suggests ATG is generally safe in PWH undergoing kidney transplantation.

Maintenance Immunosuppression

Maintenance immunosuppression generally consists of triple therapy including calcineurin inhibitors (CNIs) (e.g., cyclosporine and tacrolimus) with an antimetabolite (e.g., mycophenolate mofetil) and corticosteroids. A mammalian target of rapamycin (mTOR) inhibitor (e.g., sirolimus and everolimus) may be substituted if a patient is unable to tolerate CNIs or antimetabolites. The HIVTR study found an increased risk of rejection with the use of cyclosporine compared to tacrolimus (Stock et al., 2010), and sirolimus was found to be associated with a higher rate of rejection (Locke et al., 2014). Early steroid withdrawal has also been associated with a 60% higher risk of allograft rejection in kidney transplant recipients with HIV (Werbel et al., 2020).

ANTIRETROVIRAL THERAPY MANAGEMENT AMONG TRANSPLANT RECIPIENTS

Managing interactions between immunosuppressive agents and ART can be challenging. In ambulatory settings, clinicians will most frequently encounter maintenance immunosuppressive regimens consisting of a combination of a calcineurin inhibitor, antimetabolite, and corticosteroids as described above. In some individuals, an mTOR inhibitor will be used in place of one of these agents or as adjunctive therapy. Understanding the pharmacokinetics of each of these drug classes is crucial to safely manage transplant recipients with HIV. Calcineurin inhibitors are substrates, as well as weak inhibitors of cytochrome P450 3A4 (CYP3A4), and, therefore, have potential for significant interaction with antiretroviral agents that are CYP3A4 inhibitors or inducers. mTOR inhibitors are substrates of CYP3A4, and dosing must be adjusted in the presence of CYP3A4 inhibitors or inducers. The antimetabolites mycophenolate mofetil and azathioprine are not substrates for CYP3A4 and, therefore, have no expected or documented interactions with ART.

ART should not be interrupted in the posttransplant period. The optimal regimen for individual patients varies based on the person's ART resistance pattern and prior ART exposures as well as overall clinical profile. As indicated above, drug–drug interactions between CNIs, mTOR inhibitors, and some antiretroviral medications (i.e., protease inhibitors and some nonnucleoside reverse transcriptase inhibitors) may affect metabolism of immunosuppressant medications and potentially contribute to drug toxicity or rejection (Frasetto et al., 2007; Trullas et al., 2011; van Maarseveen et al., 2012). General guidelines by class are provided below. There are no absolute contraindications, as dosing modifications based on therapeutic drug monitoring of the immunosuppressants can compensate for the altered metabolism of these drugs.

Nucleoside Reverse Transcriptase Inhibitors (NRTIs)

When possible, older nucleoside reverse transcriptase inhibitors (NRTIs) with significant mitochondrial toxicity such as zidovudine and stavudine should be avoided because antagonism when used with mycophenolate and zidovudine may exacerbate bone marrow suppression. Tenofovir disoproxil fumarate should be avoided when possible because of nephrotoxicity, though its newer formulation (tenofovir alafenamide) may be a safer alternative.

NNRTIs

Older non-nucleoside reverse transcriptase inhibitors (NNRTIs) such as efavirenz, nevirapine, and etravirine are strong CYP3A4 inducers, thus increasing the metabolism of CNIs and decreasing their serum levels (mTOR levels may be similarly affected). The dose of these immunosuppressive agents frequently needs to be increased with close monitoring of drug levels. Newer NNRTIs such as rilpivirine and doravirine are not potent inducers and are not expected to impact CNI levels significantly (Spagnuolo et al., 2019). For transplant recipients taking proton pump inhibitors, rilpivirine should not be used.

PIs and Pharmacoenhancers

Protease inhibitors given in combination with low dose ritonavir or cobicistat, known as "boosted PIs," act both as strong CYP3A4 inhibitors (and sometimes also weak inducers) and decrease the metabolism of CNIs and mTOR inhibitors, resulting in higher levels of these agents. Thus, it is imperative that if boosted PIs or cobicistat must be used, the dosages of both CNIs and mTOR inhibitors commonly must be decreased and the dosing interval increased with close monitoring of drug levels, to avoid toxicity *and* maintain therapeutic immunosuppressive drug levels. Additionally, use of boosted PIs in kidney transplant recipients has been linked to an increased risk of graft loss and death in one recent study, while in another study it was found to actually be associated with reduced graft failure rates (Sawinski et al., 2017; Sparkes et al., 2018). This suggests that PIs should be used sparingly and with careful monitoring.

Boosted PIs also decrease the clearance of glucocorticoids, which may cause a Cushing-like syndrome. In addition, they may exacerbate hyperlipidemia post transplant and potentiate CNI-induced impaired glucose tolerance.

INSTIs

InSTIs have no or only minimal effects on CYP3A metabolism; thus, there are few potential drug interactions with immunosuppressants, making this class of ARVs well suited for use in PWH during solid organ transplantation. Although experience is greatest with raltegravir (Barau et al., 2014; Bickel et al., 2010; Miro et al., 2010; Di Biago et al., 2009), the absence of interaction and stability of immunosuppressant dosing are likely to be similar for other INSTIs, including dolutegravir and bictegravir. Because dolutegravir and bictegravir interfere with tubular secretion of creatinine, mild elevations of creatinine may be observed after dolutegravir (or bictegravir) initiation: these do not represent a decline in glomerular filtration rate (Lee et al., 2016). However, when INSTIs such as elvitegravir are given in combination with the pharmacoenhancer cobicistat, this will cause potent CYP3A4 inhibition (see "PIs and Pharmacoenhancers," above). Thus, cobicistat should be avoided, if possible, for the reasons discussed above.

CCR5 ANTAGONISTS

The CCR5 antagonist maraviroc does not have significant drug interactions with immunosuppressants and represent a good option for individuals with R5 tropic virus. Notably, blockade of CCR5 expression leads to a reduction in lymphocyte chemotaxis and has been hypothesized to reduce inflammation and potentially allograft rejection. It has been shown to reduce severe graft-versus-host-disease after bone marrow transplantation (Reshef et al., 2012) and is currently under study to reduce rejection among kidney transplant recipients with HIV (clinicaltrials.gov; NCT02741323).

Newer ART Agents

Ibalizumab is a monoclonal antibody for the CD4 T-cell receptor, which does not have drug–drug interactions with immunosuppressants. Fostemsavir is an HIV attachment inhibitor which blocks the interaction between the CD4 T-cell receptor and the HIV envelope protein gp120. Neither of these antiretroviral medications is expected to have problematic drug interactions with immunosuppressants, although there is limited experience with their use in transplant recipients at this time.

POSTTRANSPLANT INFECTION PROPHYLAXIS

In addition to standard posttransplant CMV prophylaxis, kidney and liver transplant recipients with HIV should receive the following prophylaxis:

- *Pneumocystis jiroveci*
  - Prophylaxis with trimethoprim/sulfamethoxazole (TMP/SMX) or dapsone (if sulfa allergic or bone marrow suppression is an issue, provided glucose-6-phosphate dehydrogenase (G-6PD) levels are normal).

Atovaquone can also be used as a secondary alternative to TMP/SMX.

- Prophylaxis is recommended for at least 1 year (Blumberg & Roger, 2019).

- *Mycobacterium avium* complex (MAC)

  - Some experts recommend primary prophylaxis against MAC with azithromycin for persons with CD4[+] T-cell count less than 50 cells/mm³ (Blumberg & Roger, 2019). However, recent opportunistic infection guidelines have eliminated CD4-directed prophylaxis for MAC generally for PWH, owing to low incidence (i.e., primary prophylaxis is no longer recommended for persons who immediately initiate ART, and may be discontinued in persons who are continuing on a fully suppressive ART regimen) (CDC, 2020; Saag et al., 2018). This may also extend to transplant recipient populations.
  - Toxoplasmosis
  - TMP/SMX should be used if CD4[+] T-cell count is less than 100 cells/mm³ and if either the recipient or the donor carries IgG antibodies against *Toxoplasma gondii*. Atovaquone can be used if a patient cannot tolerate TMP/SMX or dapsone (Blumberg & Roger, 2019).
  - Prior opportunistic infections (OIs)
  - Continue secondary prophylaxis for OIs such as cryptococcus or coccidioidomycosis until CD4[+] T-cell counts are above the discontinuation threshold (i.e., CD4[+] >200 cells/mm³) for approximately 3–6 months, although some providers may prefer lifelong secondary prophylaxis as data are limited (Blumberg & Roger, 2019).

OUTCOMES

PATIENT AND GRAFT SURVIVAL AND REJECTION

Kidney Transplantation

A review of over 1,400 individuals with HIV listed for kidney transplant showed a 79% reduction in the risk of death at 5 years for those who received a transplant, compared with those who remained on dialysis (Locke et al., 2017a). Several studies have shown patient and graft survival rates for kidney transplant recipients with HIV that are largely comparable to the transplant population as a whole. The HIVTR study, a prospective, nonrandomized investigation funded by the US National Institutes of Health, included 150 kidney transplant recipients with well-controlled HIV and demonstrated excellent 1- and 3-year patient and graft survival rates that were above the rates for recipients aged older than 65 years (Stock et al., 2010). The overall patient and graft survival rates of kidney transplant recipients with HIV in the HIVTR study were between the rates observed in HIV-uninfected, older recipients and all recipients, with rates of 94.6% ± 2% and 90.4% at

1 year, and 88.2% ± 3.8% and 73.7% at 3 years, respectively. Kidneys from living donors were associated with improved survival and the use of ATG, HCV coinfection, and older age were associated with decreased survival (Stock et al., 2010). Subsequently, the use of ATG induction was found to be associated with patient and graft survival rates equivalent to a cohort without HIV (Locke et al., 2014).

The HIVTR study also found the rate of acute rejection to be two- to threefold higher, and acute rejection was more aggressive, with a rate of 31% at 1 year and 41% at 3 years in kidney transplant recipients with HIV compared to rates in recipients without HIV (Stock et al., 2010). ATG induction was associated with a 2.6-fold decrease in the rate of acute rejection compared to that of patients who did not receive any induction (Locke et al., 2014), and a 40% lower rate of rejection compared to those who received either no induction or anti-IL-2R induction (Kucirka et al., 2016).

A study utilizing national data from the US Scientific Registry of Transplant Recipients (SRTR) that included 510 kidney transplant recipients with HIV showed that, in the absence of HCV coinfection, 5- and 10-year patient and graft survival for recipients with and without HIV was similar (Locke et al., 2015).

Liver Transplantation

Data also support liver transplantation in individuals with HIV. The HIVTR study included 125 liver transplant recipients with HIV and demonstrated a survival benefit of liver transplantation for individuals with ESLD and Model for End-Stage Liver Disease (MELD) score greater than 15 (Roland et al., 2016). In this study, overall survival was acceptable; however, it was lower for liver transplant recipients with HIV and HCV, with a 3-year survival of 60% versus 79% for those with HIV/HCV versus HCV, respectively (Terrault et al., 2012). The findings of lower survival in those with HCV coinfection was confirmed in a multicenter Spanish study (Miro et al., 2012) and a larger US national registry study (Locke et al., 2016). Studies have also shown that simultaneous liver and kidney transplantation, a lower pretransplant body mass index, older age, and HCV coinfection were associated with decreased patient survival, although there was a survival benefit for liver recipients with a pretransplant MELD score of 15 or higher (Roland et al., 2016). A recent study using combined data from the US and European registries between 2008 and 2015 shows that outcomes have significantly improved among liver transplant recipients with HIV and HCV in the recent era (Campos-Varela et al., 2019). This is likely due to the advent of highly effective direct-acting antivirals (DAAs) for HCV, which have demonstrated efficacy including in liver transplant recipients with HIV and HCV (Manzardo et al., 2018).

HIV/HCV COINFECTION

Kidney Transplantation

Kidney transplant recipients with HIV and HCV have lower 3-year patient survival and graft survival rates (73% and 60%, respectively) compared to recipients without infection (90% and 86%, respectively), with HIV infection only (89% and 81%, respectively), and with HCV infection only (84% and 78%, respectively) (Sawinski et al., 2015). Coinfected recipients are also at a higher risk of acute rejection at 1 year, and the use of induction in this population confers a survival benefit (Vivanco et al., 2013). These findings are consistent with those of other studies, suggesting that HCV coinfection has a negative impact on kidney transplantation outcomes. DAAs effectively cure HCV in kidney transplant recipients with HIV and HCV (Camargo et al., 2019) and with widespread use these disparities in outcomes are expected to improve.

Liver Transplantation

As discussed above, liver transplant recipients with both HIV and HCV have worse outcomes compared to recipients with either virus alone. Initial studies of liver transplantation in recipients with HIV showed that the 3-year patient and graft survival rates for HIV/HCV coinfected patients were lower (53% and 74%, respectively) than those for HCV mono-infected recipients (60% and 79%, respectively) (Terrault et al., 2012). One explanation is that many of these patients will have recurrent HCV infection that can be very aggressive, leading to graft loss and death. Previously reported 5-year survival of approximately 50%–55% may increase to 80% in coinfected liver recipients in whom HCV infection has been cleared (Miro et al., 2015). With the increasing use of DAAs, the negative patient and graft survival effects of HCV coinfection are predicted to decline, and more recent studies on temporal trends in liver transplant recipients with HIV have demonstrated this improvement (Campos-Varela et al., 2019).

HIV/HEPATITIS B VIRUS COINFECTION

Kidney Transplantation

Kidney recipients with hepatitis B virus (HBV) infection have overall lower survival rates compared to noninfected recipients. The 10-year patient survival rate was 51.4% in recipients with HBV compared to 82.8% in recipients without HBV, and graft survival rates were 44% for recipients with HBV compared to 74.2% for recipients without HBV (Lee et al., 2001).

LIVER TRANSPLANTATION

The overall outcomes for liver transplant recipients with HIV/HBV coinfection recipients appear to be equivalent to recipients with HBV only. One small study found that no patients developed clinical evidence of HBV recurrence despite low-grade viremia in 54% of coinfected recipients when treated with HBV immunoglobulin (HBIg) with or without anti-HBV antiviral therapy (Coffin et al., 2010). The recommended management for liver recipients with HBV includes a nucleos(t)ide analogue (e.g., lamivudine, tenofovir, and entecavir) posttransplant with or without hepatitis B immunoglobulin at the time of transplantation, with HBV

DNA monitoring every 6 months (Te & Doucette, 2019). This should be incorporated into or added to HIV/HBV coinfected recipients' ART regimen.

PROGRESSION OF HIV DISEASE

The HIVTR study reported five cases of new opportunistic infections, including two cases of cutaneous Kaposi's sarcoma, one case of cryptosporidiosis, one presumed case of *P. jiroveci*, and one case of candida esophagitis. Despite an initial decline in CD4$^+$ T-cell count posttransplant, which was more pronounced with ATG induction, there was no increase in complications associated with HIV disease or progression of HIV (Stock et al., 2010).

RISK OF INFECTION, IMMUNE RECOVERY, AND MALIGNANCY

Overall, 38% of kidney recipients had infections posttransplant in the HIVTR study. These infections consisted of predominantly genitourinary infections (26%), respiratory tract infections (20%), and bacteremia (19%). This study also found that HCV coinfected recipients had a higher rate of serious infections compared to recipients without HCV (Stock et al., 2010).

Another study found that individuals with pretransplant CD4$^+$ T-cell counts of less than 350 cells/mm^3 had a lower CD4$^+$ T-cell nadir 4-weeks posttransplant, which was associated with prolonged CD4$^+$ T-cell lymphopenia, and increased risk for serious infections (Suarez et al., 2016). Induction with ATG is associated with a more significant CD4$^+$ T-cell nadir posttransplant; however, larger observational studies have not identified an independent increased risk in infections with ATG use (Kucirka et al., 2016).

Based on available data, the incidence of new or recurrent cancer after transplantation in recipients with HIV is low and not significantly different from recipients without HIV. In the HIVTR study, 9% of patients (11.2% of liver recipients and 8.7% of kidney recipients) developed posttransplant malignancies (including skin cancer, cutaneous Kaposi's sarcoma, penile squamous cell cancer, head and neck cancer, renal cell cancer, lymphoma, recurrence of pretransplant hepatocellular carcinoma, and cholangiocarcinoma), and 3% of patients died from a cancer-related cause (Stock et al., 2010). The same study showed an increased risk of developing high-grade squamous intraepithelial lesions after transplantation in 89 patients followed for anal cytology; this requires further study (Nissen et al., 2012).

DONORS WITH HIV: THE HOPE ACT

With recognition of major advances in HIV and transplantation medicine, the HOPE Act of 2013 lifted the federal ban on the use of organs from donors with HIV. This legislation was also based on promising data from a cohort of transplant recipients in South Africa who had received organs from donors with HIV and who had good outcomes with overall survival of 84% at 1 year, 84% at 3 years, and 74% at 5 years, with graft survival rates of 93% at 1 year and 84% at both 3 and 5 years, and rejection rates of 8% at 1 year and 22% at 3 years (Muller et al., 2015). The HOPE Act allows transplantation from donors with HIV to recipients with HIV (D+/R+) within research protocols and was implemented in 2015. The HOPE in Action Multicenter Consortium is a multicenter transplant collaborative including more than 30 transplant centers performing HIV D+/R + within research studies to explore the safety and feasibility of this practice.

The HOPE Act has received widespread support among the community of people living with HIV, with high rates of willingness both to donate (Nguyen et al., 2018) and to receive organ from donors with HIV (Seaman et al., 2020). The first HIV D+/R + deceased donor kidney and liver transplants were performed in 2016 (Malani et al., 2016). Results of the HOPE in Action Multicenter Consortium kidney pilot study were published in 2021 (Durand et al., 2021). This study of 75 kidney recipients with HIV directly compared outcomes between recipients of kidneys from donors with and without HIV, finding excellent survival (100% in both arms) and no increased risk of graft failure, HIV viremia, opportunistic infections, or serious adverse events between groups. Results of the HOPE in Action Multicenter liver pilot study were published in 2022 (Durand et al., 2022). This study of 45 liver recipients with HIV also directly compared outcomes between recipients of livers from donors with and without HIV and found no differences in one-year graft survival (96% vs. 100%), rejection (10.8% vs. 18.2%), HIV breakthrough (8% vs. 10%), or serious adverse events (all p >0.05) (Durand et al., 2022). Overall patient survival was good (83% vs. 100%); however, there was a higher rate of viral infections (i.e., CMV, HHV8) and cancer in the recipients of livers from donors with HIV, which translated to a higher mortality. Larger NIH-funded studies of the HOPE in Action Multicenter Consortium to follow-up on these findings are ongoing (clinicaltrials.gov NCT03500315 and NCT0374393).

CONCLUSION

People living with HIV and end-stage organ disease can experience a survival benefit from transplantation, especially kidney transplantation, and in select cases, liver transplantation. Posttransplant immunosuppression does not appear to advance HIV disease or increase the risk of opportunistic infection. Recipients with HCV appear to have worse clinical outcomes, partially owing to a more aggressive posttransplant HCV recurrence, which emphasizes the importance of HCV cure with DAAs prior to or immediately posttransplant since newer, less toxic therapies are available. Anticipation and careful management of drug–drug interactions are crucial. Care of transplant recipients with HIV should include an integrated and coordinated group of providers, including the transplant team, pharmacists, infectious disease/HIV specialists, and nurses, in addition to patients and caregivers.

ACKNOWLEDGMENTS

This chapter is an extension of previous work and contributions made by authors involved with prior editions of this content: Jennifer Husson, Eurides Lopes, Carolyn Kramer, and Emily Blumberg.

REFERENCES

Abraham AG, Althoff KN, Jing Y, et al. End-stage renal disease among HIV-infected adults in North America. *Clin Infect Dis.* 2015;60(6):941–949.

Althoff KN, Gebo KA, Moore RD, et al. Contributions of traditional and HIV-related risk factors on non-AIDS-defining cancer, myocardial infarction, and end-stage liver and renal diseases in adults with HIV in the USA and Canada: a collaboration of cohort studies. *Lancet HIV.* 2019;6(2):e93–e104.

Barau C, Braun J, Vincent C, et al. Pharmacokinetic study of raltegravir in HIV-infected patients with end-stage liver disease: the LIVERAL-ANRS 148 study. *Clin Infect Dis.* 2014;59(8):1177–1184.

Berkowitz EM, Moyle G, Stellbrink H-J, et al. Safety and immunogenicity of an adjuvanted herpes zoster subunit candidate vaccine in HIV-positive adults: a phase 1/2a randomized, placebo-controlled study. *J Infect Dis.* 2015;211(8):1279–1287.

Bickel M, Anadol E, Vogel M, et al. Daily dosing of tacrolimus in patients treated with HIV-1 therapy containing a ritonavir-boosted protease inhibitor or raltegravir. *J Antimicrob Chemother.* 2010;65(5):999–1004.

Blumberg EA, Roger CC. Solid organ transplantation in the HIV-infected patient: guidelines from the American Society of Transplantation Infectious Diseases Community of Practice. *Clinical Transplantation.* 2019; 33:e13499.

Camargo JF, Anjan S, Chin-Beckford N, et al. Clinical outcomes in HIV+/HCV+ coinfected kidney transplant recipients in the pre- and post-direct-acting antiviral therapy eras: 10-Year single center experience. *Clin Transplant.* 2019;33(5)e13532.

Campos-Varela I, Dodge JL, Berenguer M et al. Temporal trends and outcomes in liver transplantation for recipients with human immunodeficiency virus infection in Europe and United States. *Transplantation.* 2020;104(10):2078–2086. http://doi:10.1097/TP.0000000000003107. Online ahead of print.

Coffin CS, Stock PG, Dove LM, et al. Virologic and clinical outcomes of hepatitis B virus infection in HIV–HBV co-infected transplant recipients. *Am J Transp.* 2010;10:1268–1275.

Di Biagio A, Rosso R, Siccardi M, et al. Lack of interaction between raltegravir and cyclosporine in an HIV-infected liver transplant recipient. *J Antimicrob Chemother.* 2009;64(4):874–875.

Doberne JW, Jawitz OK, Raman V, et al. Heart transplantation survival outcomes of HIV positive and negative recipients. *Ann Thorac Surg.* September 15, 2020;S0003-4975(20)31484–31483.

Durand CM, Zhang W, Brown DM, et al. A prospective multicenter pilot study of HIV-positive deceased donor to HIV-positive recipient kidney transplantation: HOPE in action. *Am J Transplant.* May 2021;21(5):1754–1764.

Durand CM, Florman S, Motter JD et al. HOPE in action: a prospective multicenter pilot study of liver transplantation from donors with HIV to recipients with HIV. *Am J Transplant.* March 2022;22(3):853–864.

Frasetto LA, Browne M, Cheng A, et al. Immunosuppressant pharmacokinetics and dosing modifications in HIV-1 infected liver and kidney transplant recipients. *Am J Transplant.* December 2007;7(12):2816–2820. https://www.ncbi.nlm.nih.gov/pubmed/17949460

Gabardi S, Martin ST, Roberts KL, Grafals M. Induction immunosuppressive therapies in renal transplantation. *Am J Health Syst Pharm.* 2011;68:211–218.

Koval CE, Farr J, Krisl J et al. Heart or lung transplant outcomes in HIV-infected recipients. *J Heart Lung Transplant*. December 2019;38(12):1296–1305.

Kucirka LM, Durand CM, Bae S, et al. Induction immunosuppression and clinical outcomes in kidney transplant recipients infected with human immunodeficiency virus. *Am J Transplant*. 2016;16(8):2368–2376.

Lee DH, Malat GE, Bias TE, et al. Serum creatinine elevation after switch to dolutegravir in a human immunodeficiency virus-positive kidney transplant recipient. *Trans Inf Disease*. 2016;18(4):625–627.

Lee WC, Shu KH, Cheng CH, et al. Long-term impact of hepatitis B, C virus infection on renal transplantation. *Am J Nephrol*. 2001;21:300–306.

Locke JE, Durand C, Reed RD, et al. Long-term outcomes after liver transplantation among human immunodeficiency virus-infected recipients. *Transplantation*. 2016;100(1):141–146.

Locke JE, Gustafson MD, Mehta S, et al. Survival benefit of kidney transplantation in HIV-infected patients. *Ann Surg*. 2017a;265(3):604–608.

Locke JE, James NT, Mannon RB, et al. Immunosuppression regimen and the risk of acute rejection in HIV-positive kidney transplant recipients. *Transplantation*. 2014;97(4):446–450.

Locke JE, Mehta S, Reed RD, et al. A national study of outcomes among HIV-infected kidney transplant recipients. *J Am Soc Nephrol*. 2015;265:2222–2229.

Locke JE, Mehta S, Sawinski D, et al. Access to kidney transplantation among HIV-infected waitlist candidates. *Clin J Am Soc Nephrol*. 2017b;12(3):467–475.

Malani P. HIV and transplantation: new reasons for HOPE. *JAMA*. 2016;316(2):136–138.

Manzardo C, Londoño MC, Castells L, et al. Direct-acting antivirals are effective and safe in HCV/HIV-coinfected liver transplant recipients who experience recurrence of hepatitis C: a prospective nationwide cohort study. *Am J Transplant*. 2018;18(10):2513–2522.

Miro JM, Agüero F, Duclos-Vallée JC, et al. Infections in solid organ transplant HIV-positive patients. *Clin Microbiol Infect*. 2014;20:119–130.

Miro JM, Montejo M, Castells L, et al. Outcomes of HCV/HIV-coinfected liver transplant recipients: a prospective and multicenter cohort study. *Am J of Transplant*. 2012;12:1866–1876

Miro JM, Ricart MJ, Trullas JC, et al. Simultaneous pancreas–kidney transplantation in HIV-infected patients: a case report and literature review. *Transplant Proc*. 2010;42(9):3887–3891.

Miro JM, Stock P, Teicher E, et al. Outcome and management of HCV/HIV coinfection pre- and post-liver transplantation: a 2015 update. *J Hepatol*. 2015;62:701–711.

Mocroft A, Lundgren JD, Ross M, et al. Cumulative and current exposure to potentially nephrotoxic antiretrovirals and development of chronic kidney disease in HIV-positive individuals with a normal baseline estimated glomerular filtration rate: a prospective international cohort study. *Lancet HIV*. 2016;3(1):e23–e32.

Mombelli M, Rettby N, Perreau M, et al. Immunogenicity and safety of double versus standard dose of the seasonal influenza vaccine in solid-organ transplant recipients: a randomized controlled trial. *Vaccine*. 2018;36(41):6163–6169.

Muller E, Barday Z, Kahn D. HIV-positive-to-HIV-positive kidney transplantation: results at 3 and 5 years. *N Engl J Med*. 2015;372:613–620.

Nettles RE, Kieffer TL, Kwon P, et al. Intermittent HIV-1 viremia (Blips) and drug resistance in patients receiving HAART. *JAMA*. 2005;293(7):817–829.

Nguyen AQ, Anjum SK, Halpern SE, et al. Willingness to donate organs among people living with HIV. *J Acquir Immune Defic Syndr*. 2018;79(1):e30–e36.

Nissen NN, Barin B, Stock PG. Malignancy in the HIV-positive patients undergoing liver and kidney transplantation. *Curr Opin Oncol*. 2012;24:517–521.

Platt L, Easterbrook P, Gower E, et al. Prevalence and burden of HCV co-infection in people living with HIV: a global systematic review and meta-analysis. *Lancet Infect Dis*. 2016;16:797–808.

Reshef R, Luger SM, Hexner E, et al. Blockade of lymphocyte chemotaxis in visceral graft-versus-host disease. *N Engl J Med*. 2012;367(2):135–145.

Roland ME, Barin B, Huprikar S, et al; HIVTR Study Team. Survival in HIV-positive transplant recipients compared with transplant candidates and with HIV-negative controls. *AIDS*. 2016;30(3):435–444.

Saag MS, Benson CA, Gandhi RT, et al. Antiretroviral drugs for treatment and prevention of HIV infection in adults. 2018 Recommendations of the International Antiviral Society–USA Panel. *JAMA*. 2018; 320(4):379–396.

Sawinski D, Forde KA, Eddinger K, et al. Superior outcomes in HIV-positive kidney transplant patients compared with HCV-infected or HIV/HCV co-infected recipients. *Kidney Int*. 2015;88:341–349.

Sawinski D, Goldberg DS, Blumberg E, et al. Beyond the NIH multicenter HIV transplant trial experience: outcomes of HIV\+ liver transplant recipients compared to HCV\+ or HIV\+/HCV\+ co-infected recipients in the United States. *Clin Infect Dis*. 2015;61(7):1054–1062.

Sawinski D, Shelton BA, Mehta S, et al. Impact of protease inhibitor-based anti-retroviral therapy on outcomes for HIV\+ kidney transplant recipients. *Am J Transplant*. 2017;17(12):3114–3122.

Seaman SM, Van Pilsum Rasmussen SE, Nguyen AQ, et al. Brief report: willingness to accept HIV-infected and increased infectious risk donor organs among transplant candidates living with HIV. *J Acquir Immune Defic Syndr*. 2020;85(1):88–92.

Shaffer AA, Durand CM. Solid organ transplantation for HIV-infected individuals. *Curr Treat Options Infect Dis*. 2018;10(1):107–120.

Spagnuolo V, Uberti-Foppa C, Castagna A. Pharmacotherapeutic management of HIV in transplant patients. *Expert Opin Pharmacother*. 2019;20(10):1235–1250.

Sparkes T, Manitpisitkul W, Masters B, et al. Impact of antiretroviral regimen on renal transplant outcomes in HIV-positive recipients. *Transpl Infect Dis*. 2018;20(6):e12992.

Stadtmauer EA, Sullivan KM, Marty FM, et al. A phase 1/2 study of an adjuvanted varicella-zoster virus subunit vaccine in autologous hematopoietic cell transplant recipients. *Blood*. 2014;124(19):2921–2929.

Stock P, Barin B, Murphy B, et al. Outcomes of kidney transplantation in HIV-positive recipients. *N Engl J Med*. 2010;363:2001–2014.

Suarez JF, Rosa R, Lorio MA, et al. Pretransplant CD4 count influences immune reconstitution and risk of infectious complications in human immunodeficiency virus-infected kidney allograft recipients. *Am J Transpl*. 2016;16(8):2463–2472.

Sun H-Y, Sheng W-H, Tsai M-S, et al. Hepatitis B virus coinfection in human immunodeficiency virus-infected patients: a review. *World J Gastroenterol*. 2014;20:14598–14614.

Te H, Doucette K. Viral hepatitis: guidelines by the American Society of Transplantation Infectious Disease Community of Practice. *Clinical Transplantation*. 2019;33:e13499.

Terrault N, Roland ME, Schiano T, et al. Outcomes of liver transplant recipients with hepatitis C and human immunodeficiency virus coinfection. *Liver Transpl*. 2012;18(6):716–726.

Trullas JC, Cofan F, Tuset M, et al. Renal transplantation in HIV-positive patients: 2010 update. *Kidney Int*. April 2011;79(8):825–842. https://www.ncbi.nlm.nih.gov/pubmed/21248716

van Maarseveen EM, Rogers CC, Trofe-Clark J, et al. Drug–drug interactions between antiretroviral and immunosuppressive agents in HIV-positive patients after solid organ transplantation: a review. *AIDS Patient Care STDs*. 2012;26(10):568–581.

Vivanco M, Friedmann P, Zia Y, et al. Campath induction in HCV and HCV/HIV-seropositive kidney transplant recipients. *Transpl Int*. 2013;26(10):1016–1026.

Werbel WA, Bae S, Yu S, et al. Early steroid withdrawal in HIV-infected kidney transplant recipients: utilization and outcomes. *Am J Transplant*. 2021;21(2):717–726. Online ahead of print.

23.

SELECT TOPICS IN THE CARE OF CIS-GENDER WOMEN WITH HIV

Jillian T. Baron, Christina E. Maguire, and William R. Short

CONTRACEPTION AND PREPREGANCY CARE

LEARNING OBJECTIVE

Discuss family planning and prepregancy care considerations in serodifferent couples living with HIV.

WHAT'S NEW?

- While this is a chapter focused on the care of cis-gender women, many of these topics including contraception and prepregnancy care relate to transgender and gender-diverse individuals. In recognition of that, gender inclusive language was used as much as possible. When reviewing data, results are discussed using gender-specific terminology as used by the publications. More research is needed on epidemiologic trends and prepregnancy care specific to transgender and gender-diverse individuals.

- The term *preconception* has been replaced with *prepregnancy*, consistent with terminology supported by the American College of Obstetricians and Gynecologists.

- Infant feeding guidance was added to reflect the importance of prepregnancy counseling. In the United States, breastfeeding is not recommended among individuals with HIV because of the nonzero risk of transmission among individuals with undetectable viral loads on antiretroviral therapy (ART). However, individuals should be offered evidence-based, patient-centered counseling, and individuals who desire to breastfeed should be supported with risk-reduction strategies.

KEY POINTS

- Healthcare providers need to be proactive in addressing issues related to prepregnancy care and contraception among individuals living with HIV who are of childbearing age and potential.

- Persons living with HIV should strive to achieve long-term, maximal suppression of viral load prior to attempts at conception. New recommendations have been made to address situations in which maximal suppression has been achieved, has not been achieved, or is unknown in serodifferent couples.

- HIV infection does not preclude the use of any methods of hormonal contraception; however, providers must make themselves aware of any potential drug–drug interactions between hormonal contraceptive methods and ART.

- Emergency contraception, including emergency contraceptive pills or the copper intrauterine devices (IUDs), may be offered to individuals with HIV when clinically appropriate. Drug–drug interactions must be considered when using hormonal emergency contraception in combination with ART.

Women account for approximately 23% of persons with HIV (PWH) in the United States, and 18% of new HIV diagnoses in the United States in 2020 were in women (CDC, 2020e). Because of this, there is continued emphasis placed on family planning and prepregancy care. The goals of family planning and prepregancy care are to promote conception planning, reduce unintended pregnancy, and support safer conception and pregnancy for the pregnant individual, fetus/infant, and partner without HIV. All individuals of childbearing age childbearing potential who are living with HIV should be offered comprehensive family planning and prepregancy care as part of routine primary medical care (ACOG, 2016).

THE IMPORTANCE OF FAMILY PLANNING AND PREPREGNANCY CARE

It is increasingly important for healthcare providers to be proactive in addressing issues related to prepregnancy care and contraception in PWH who are of childbearing age. In areas where ARVs are widely available and accessible, HIV has become a chronic disease with life expectancy comparable to that of persons without HIV (van Sighem et al., 2010), and perinatal transmission rates have been reduced to less than 1% (ACOG, 2016). Fertility desires in women with HIV in many studies show little difference from those in women without HIV (Craft et al., 2009; Finocchario-Kessler et al., 2012; Loutfy et al., 2009; Nattabi et al., 2009; Squires et al., 2011). In the Women's Interagency HIV Study cohort there was a 150% increase in live birth rates among women with HIV in the ART era when compared to the pre-ART era (Sharma et al., 2007). Current estimates are that there are 5000 women with HIV who give birth annually in the United States (Nesheim et al., 2018).

Studies among women with HIV suggest that unintended pregnancies are approximately 50% or higher (Craft et al., 2007; Loutfy et al., 2009; Massad et al., 2004). Many pregnancies among women with HIV occur despite use of contraception (Massad et al., 2004), implying that the pregnancies were unintended, and highlighting the importance of adequate and accurate counseling about use of effective birth control. Patients with unintended pregnancies are more likely than those without to not have received OB/GYN care or HIV monitoring in the past year (Sutton et al., 2018). Women living with HIV express the desire to talk about reproductive plans with their healthcare providers; however, data suggest that such counseling does not often occur until after conception (Finocchario-Kessler et al., 2010; Loufty et al., 2013; Panozzo et al., 2003; Squires, 2011).

COUNSELING AND ASSESSMENT ABOUT CHILDBEARING AND CONTRACEPTION

Because they may change over time, childbearing desires, and intentions, including timing of pregnancy, should be assessed during the initial evaluation and at intervals throughout the course of care. A comprehensive HIV, medical, and OB/GYN history and understanding of patient goals are important areas on which to focus counseling and assist in shared decision-making. Individuals who wish to prevent or delay pregnancy should receive information about contraceptive options and their efficacy, adverse effects, and other advantages or disadvantages, including noncontraceptive benefits. Individuals who wish to conceive should be given information about risk, rates, and prevention of perinatal transmission and the potential effects of HIV or its treatment on pregnancy course and outcomes. For couples in serodifferent relationships, the PWH should be counseled about the benefits of ART in reducing HIV transmission (Cohen et al., 2011). Disclosure and/or knowledge of HIV status for both partners is particularly important when conception is planned and should be encouraged and supported. It is also important to reinforce with patients that there may be legal ramifications for nondisclosure in certain jurisdictions. Knowledge of the disclosure laws in your area is suggested for review with patients during counseling sessions.

CARE FOR INDIVIDUALS WITH HIV WANTING TO BECOME PREGNANT

Interventions for individuals who want to become pregnant include the following:

- Overall health should be optimized with attention to standard primary care and management of chronic diseases, as well as treatment of drug and alcohol abuse.

- Benefits of smoking cessation and the elimination of other drugs and alcohol for the pregnant individuals and developing fetus should be reviewed, and referrals to cessation services should be offered.

- All current medications, including prescription, over-the-counter, and complementary/alternative medications should be reviewed, and potential adverse effects associated with use of these drugs in pregnancy should be assessed.

- The need to initiate or modify an ART regimen should be evaluated for all individuals living with HIV prior to conception. For individuals on ART, a stable, maximally suppressed viral load should be achieved prior to conception. The choice of ART regimen should take into account current treatment guidelines, what is known about the use of specific drugs in pregnancy, and the risk of teratogenicity or other adverse effects. The current guidelines for ART management during conception and the prenatal period can be found at: https://clinicalinfo.hiv.gov/guidelines/perinatal.

- Both partners should be screened for genital tract infections, and these should be treated if present. Genital tract inflammation is associated with genital tract shedding of HIV, even in the setting of fully suppressed HIV viral load and may additionally increase plasma viremia (Johnson & Lewis, 2008).

- Immunizations should be reviewed and updated as indicated, and folic acid supplementation should be started.

INFANT FEEDING COUNSELING

Part of pregnancy counseling should include counseling on infant feeding after birth. Current guidelines in the United States do not recommend breastfeeding in individuals with HIV because of the availability of sustainable and safe formula alternatives (National Institutes of Health (NIH)-CDC-HIVMA/IDSA, 2022). The recommendation against breastfeeding is due to studies showing that even in the setting of undetectable HIV viral load on ART in breastfeeding mothers, the risk of HIV transmission is very low (< 1%) but not zero (Flynn et al., 2021). However, despite this guidance many individuals continue to choose to breastfeed (Harbl et al., 2021; Tuthill et al., 2019; Yusuf et al., 2022). Individuals with questions regarding breastfeeding should be provided patient-centered, evidence-based counseling in a nonjudgmental manner. Those with HIV who opt to breastfeed should be supported and offered risk mitigation strategies that include but are not limited to supporting maternal ART adherence, close monitoring to ensure maternal viral suppression before delivery and throughout breastfeeding, and consideration of infant ARV prophylaxis (NIH-CDC-HIVMA/IDSA, 2022). The National Perinatal HIV Hotline (1-888-448-8765) is available for clinician consultation regarding infant feeding by individuals with HIV.

Dolutegravir

In 2018, preliminary data from an NIH observational study in Botswana identified an increased signal of neural tube defects (NTDs) in infants whose mothers initiated dolutegravir (DTG) prior to or when becoming pregnant and were receiving it at the time of conception (Zash et al., 2019). Of note, the analysis has been sequentially updated with additional pregnancies and the signal for increased incidence of NTDs associated with pregnancies in women receiving DTG at the time of conception has decreased to be statistically not different than women receiving non-DTG regimens (Zash et al., 2021). When counseling patients on the risk of birth defects, clinicians should highlight the overall rates of NTD among the general population, which in the United States is approximately 0.07%, and folic acid supplementation is recommended for women trying to conceive and in early pregnancy (Department of Health and Human Services (DHHS), 2022a).

The US DHHS now recommends DTG as a "preferred" ARV drug throughout pregnancy, regardless of trimester, and for individuals who are trying to conceive. A summary of the recommendations can be found here: https://clinicalinfo.hiv.gov/en/guidelines/perinatal/appendix-d-dolutegravir-counseling-guide-health-care-providers.

EFAVIRENZ

Animal models suggested an increased risk of NTDs with the use of efavirenz (EFV). Prospective follow-up trials have not detected an increased risk when EFV is used in the first trimester of pregnancy (ACOG, 2016). In prior updates to the US DHHS guidelines, the use of EFV prior to 8 weeks of pregnancy was not recommended because of the perceived risk of NTDs. Newer data from the Antiretroviral Pregnancy Registry (APR) identified defects in 35 of 1,173 first-trimester exposures to the drug (2.4%, 95% CI: 1.6–3.4) (January 2022). The same data revealed defects in 35 of 1,175 with late exposure (2.4%, 95% CI: 1.6–3.4) (APR, 2022). Current data on first-trimester exposures have been enough to rule out a twofold increase NTDs with use of the drug (NIH-CDC-HIVMA/IDSA, 2022). Data from a multicohort analysis showed 19 of 2,0002000 live births to women exposed to EFV at conception (1.6%, 95% CI: 0.96–2.5), with none of these birth defects being NTDs (Begoña, 2019). This has led to the US DHHS lifting its restriction on the use of EFV prior to 8-weeks' gestation. This decision is in line with both the World Health Organization (WHO) and British HIV Association recommendations. It is also recommended that women who are tolerating EFV well and have suppressed viral loads continue its use throughout their pregnancy. Of note, the caution remains in the package insert of the product.

HIV SERO-POSITIVE COUPLES

In couples where both partners are HIV-positive, a crucial aspect of the reproductive effort is ensuring that both partners have optimized their individual health. This should be accomplished from both the general and HIV perspective. This includes regular visits to their primary care provider, gynecologist, and HIV specialist for both partners as applicable. For both partners, sustained optimal viral suppression through ART is critical. Each partner should be evaluated and treated for sexually transmitted infections (STIs) because their presence can cause inflammation in the genital tract, which can lead to shedding of the virus even when the plasma viral load is undetectable (NIH-CDC-HIVMA/IDSA, 2022). Condomless intercourse should be timed to coincide with ovulation.

Along with discussions aimed at identifying potential fetal risks and benefits during pregnancy, it is also important to counsel patients on psychosocial issues. While there have been advances to allow couples to conceive with significantly lower risk of superinfection or viral mutation, other issues remain. Specifically, although ART has significantly extended life expectancy of PWH, it is unclear how well that correlates to life expectancy in uninfected control populations. Medication adherence, genetics, and other factors may still cause the loss of one or both parents with HIV prior to the child becoming an adult (American Society for Reproductive Medicine (ASRM), 2015). This in and of itself is not enough to counsel against conception but should be a part of conversations on the risk and benefits of conception in HIV-positive parents.

HIV SERODIFFERENT COUPLES

In couples where one partner is HIV-negative and natural conception is desired, the goal is to achieve pregnancy while minimizing the risk of HIV transmission to the HIV-negative partner and if this partner is pregnant, to the baby as well. Two large studies found no occurrences of genetically linked HIV transmissions between heterosexual couples while the PWH was virally suppressed (Cohen et al., 2016; Rodger et al., 2016). In light of this, the partner with HIV should receive ART to achieve sustained, maximal viral suppression prior to attempting conception (NIH-CDC-HIVMA/IDSA, 2020).

The PARTNERS 1 trial was conducted to investigate HIV transmission rates in serodifferent couples (both heterosexual and MSM) when maximal viral suppression (200 copies/mL) with ART was achieved in the partner living with HIV. A total of 1,166 couples in the trial practiced condomless sex. At the end of 1.3 years, no cases of HIV transmission to the HIV-negative partner were demonstrated (Rodger et al., 2016; NIH-CDC-HIVMA/IDSA, 2022). Similar results were found in a study of serodifferent couples attempting to conceive via natural means. The study included 161 couples attempting to conceive; 144 were successful; 107 babies were born; and no cases of vertical transmission or transmission of HIV to the uninfected partner were noted (NIH-CDC-HIVMA/IDSA, 2022; Del Romero et al., 2016).

Based on the results of these trials several new recommendations have been made regarding natural conception between serodifferent partners. They are summarized here:

1. Serodifferent couples who wish to conceive naturally, unprotected (condomless) intercourse in the peri-ovulatory period (2–3 days preceding ovulation) and the day of ovulation may be considered if the PWH is on ART and has maintained sustained viral suppression. This option for conception carries extremely low risk of transmission to the HIV-negative partner.

2. Serodifferent couples who wish to conceive naturally through unprotected (condomless) intercourse when the PWH has not maintained sustained viral suppression or their status is unknown, daily use of pre-exposure prophylaxis (PrEP) is recommended to reduce the risk of HIV transmission to the partner without HIV. Unprotected (condomless) sex should be limited to days of peak fertility.

3. For serodifferent couples who wish to conceive naturally through unprotected (condomless) intercourse during peak fertility, it is unclear whether the use of PrEP for the uninfected partner further reduces the risk of sexual transmission when the PWH has achieved viral suppression.

Providers may present the optional use of ovulation kits to couples to better predict peak fertility and assist in timing of unprotected intercourse.

In serodifferent couples who elect to use PrEP during the conception period, the CDC recommends that the partner without HIV begin treatment with daily combination tenofovir/emtricitabine 1 month prior to attempting conception and continue for 1 month beyond last vaginal intercourse (NIH-CDC-HIVMA/IDSA, 2022). As in patients who are using PrEP for routine HIV prophylaxis, baseline HIV and pregnancy testing should be drawn and repeated at 3-month intervals and renal function at baseline and 6-month intervals (NIH-CDC-HIVMA/IDSA, 2022).

CARE FOR INDIVIDUALS WISHING TO PREVENT OR DELAY PREGNANCY

An expert panel from the WHO (2014) reviewed the evidence on currently available methods of hormonal contraception and reaffirmed their 2009 statement that individuals living with HIV can potentially use all existing hormonal contraceptive methods without restriction. However, special care must still be taken to address any potential drug–drug interactions and alterations in pharmacokinetics that may occur when ART and contraceptives are used together.

The WHO and the CDC state that with use of methods involving spermicides containing nonoxynol-9, the risks generally outweigh advantages of the method because of potential disruption of cervical mucosa, which may increase viral shedding and HIV transmission to the HIV-negative partners. Both the copper IUD (Cu-IUD) and levonorgestrel-containing IUD can be initiated or continued in individuals living with HIV who are clinically doing well on ART therapy. Pharmacokinetic interactions between hormonal contraceptives (primarily studied with combined estrogen-progestin oral contraceptives) and

some PIs and NNRTIs may modify steroid levels and potentially decrease contraceptive effectiveness or increase risk of adverse effects, although the true clinical effect is not clear; an additional or alternative contraceptive method is generally advised if hormonal contraception is considered (Cohn et al., 2007; El-Ibiary & Cocohoba, 2008; NIH-CDC-HIVMA/IDSA, 2022; Vogler et al., 2010). Specifically, individuals on ritonavir-boosted protease inhibitors (PI) regimens should be placed on an additional or alternative method of contraception if using ART with combination hormonal contraceptives. These methods include patches, pills, rings, or progestin-only pills. Similarly, in patients taking EFV, an additional barrier contraceptive or alternative regimen can be considered in among those using etonogestrel or levonorgestrel contraceptive implants or combined oral contraceptives (Landolt et al., 2013; NIH-CDC-HIVMA/IDSA, 2022; Patel et al., 2015). For a detailed list of contraceptive drugs and their potential interactions with ARVs, please see the table labeled "Drug Interactions Between Antiretroviral Agents and Hormonal Contraceptives" in the most current US DHHS "Recommendations for Use of Antiretroviral Drug in Pregnant HIV-1 Infected Women for Maternal Health and Interventions to Reduce Perinatal HIV Transmission in the United States."

Emergency contraception, including emergency oral contraceptives or the copper IUD, may be offered to individuals with HIV if clinically appropriate. When oral contraceptives (either combination or levonorgestrel only) are used with ARVs, the potential for drug interactions seems to be similar to when they are used for routine contraception (NIH-CDC-HIVMA/IDSA, 2022).

Currently, there are no data on interactions between ART and ulipristal acetate, but interactions should be anticipated because of the metabolism of ulipristal acetate through the CYP3A4 pathways (NIH-CDC-HIVMA/IDSA, 2022).

Most studies have found no association between the use of hormonal contraception and HIV disease progression (Morrison et al., 2011; Polis et al., 2010: Stringer et al., 2009). Early observational studies indicated that certain types of hormonal contraception, particularly depot medroxyprogesterone acetate (DMPA), might increase risk of HIV infection among at risk seronegative individuals. However, the ECHO trial recently showed no significant difference in HIV acquisition among 7,800 women using intramuscular DMPA, copper IUDs, or levonorgestrel (LNG) implants (ECHO Trial Consortium, 2019). Based on this study, the WHO (2019) updated its recommendations to indicate that those at higher risk for HIV infection should have the option of using any reversible contraception method, including all hormonal options. Regardless of what hormonal contraception choice is made, family planning conversations should emphasize the importance of PrEP and condoms to prevent transmission of HIV and other STIs.

RECOMMENDED READING

Department of Health and Human Services, Panel on Treatment of Pregnant Women with HIV Infection and Prevention of Perinatal

Transmission. Recommendations for use of antiretroviral drugs in pregnant women with HIV infection and interventions to reduce perinatal HIV transmission in the United States. https://clinicalinfo.hiv.gov/en/guidelines/perinatal. Published 2022. Accessed August 14, 2022.

CERVICAL PAP SMEARS

LEARNING OBJECTIVE

Discuss the recommended frequency and specimen collection technique for cervical Pap smears in individuals with HIV, the role of human papillomavirus (HPV) testing, and indications for specialist referral for colposcopy.

WHAT'S NEW?

- The cervical cancer screening guidelines for individuals living with HIV have been updated to reflect that cervical cancer screening is no longer recommended prior to age 21 years.

KEY POINTS

- Cervical cancer screening should begin at time of diagnosis but no earlier but not earlier than 21 years of age.

- Between the ages of 21 to 29 years, a liquid-based Pap smear for cervical cancer screening is used without co-testing because of the high prevalence of HPV in this age group. If normal, the screening is repeated every 12 months. If the patient has three consecutive normal screenings, testing interval should be increased to every 3 years.

- At age 30 years and older, cervical cancer screening with either Pap alone or combined with HPV co-testing may be offered. The appropriate interval of follow-up screening is determined by the type of screening performed and the results returned.

- Unlike the general population, women living with HIV who are aged 65 years and older should continue cervical cancer screening.

CERVICAL HPV INFECTION IN WOMEN WITH HIV

In general, infection with HPV, the cause of cervical cancer, is quite common in the United States, with an estimated 24.9 million women between the ages of 14 to 59 having the infection (Dunne et al., 2007). Compared with HIV-negative women, women with HIV have a higher prevalence and incidence of HPV (Ahdieh et al., 2001; Branca et al., 2003), longer persistence of HPV (Ahdieh et al., 2001; Sun et al., 1997), higher HPV levels (Jamieson et al., 2002), higher prevalence of multiple HPV subtypes (Firnhaber et al., 2009; Jamieson et al., 2002; Sahasrabuddhe et al., 2007), and higher prevalence of oncogenic subtypes (Firnhaber et al., 2009; Minkoff

et al., 1998; Volkow et al., 2001). In addition, there is increased HPV prevalence and persistence of high-risk HPV with decreasing CD4$^+$ T-cell counts (Denny et al., 2008; Palefsky et al., 1999) and increasing HIV RNA levels (Palefsky et al., 1999). Also, compared to women without HIV, women with HIV are more likely to have abnormal cervical cytology (Denny et al., 2008; Ellerbrock et al., 2000), and both frequency and severity of cervical dysplasia increase with declining CD4$^+$ T-cell counts (Davis et al., 2001; Massad et al., 2001, 2008). Recurrent cervical dysplasia after treatment is more common among women with HIV (Boardman et al., 1999; Fruchter et al., 1996; Holcomb et al., 1999; Massad et al., 2001; Six et al., 1998). Rates of cervical cancer are also significantly higher among women with HIV compared to women in the general population (Chaturvedi et al., 2009; Clifford et al., 2005; Dal Maso et al., 2009; Grulich et al., 2007). Several HPV subtypes have been associated with the development of squamous intraepithelial lesions and cervical cancer, including most commonly HPV-16 (found in almost half of all cervical cancers) and HPV-18 (found in 10%–12% of cervical cancers) and less commonly HPV-31, -33, -35, -39, -45, -51, -52, -56, -58, -59, and -68 (each accounting for < 5% of cervical cancers) (Castle et al., 2009; Schiffman et al., 2009).

CERVICAL PAP SMEARS

Owing to the high level of HPV infection and higher prevalence of oncogenic subtypes, it is critical for women with HIV to be regularly screened for cervical dysplasia. Although a single Pap smear has historically been associated with high false-negative rates (10%–25%), regular screening can significantly improve accuracy (Anderson et al., 2012), and Pap smear screening programs have been associated with marked reductions in cervical cancer incidence (Eddy, 1990; Nygard et al., 2002).

In the setting of increased rates of cervical cancer among PWH, guidelines have typically recommended cervical cancer screening more frequently, at a younger age, and continued through older ages. More recently, data from the HIV/AIDS Cancer Match Study which including 164,084 women living with HIV, found the highest incidence rates of invasive cervical cancer among 35 to 39 year olds and 40 to 44 year olds. No cases of invasive cervical cancer occurred among < 25 year olds (Stier et al., 2021). Given the rarity of invasive cervical cancer among PWH aged younger than 25 years old, the NIH-CDC-HIVMA/IDSA now recommends starting cervical cancer screening at age 21 years, which permits sufficient time to identify early dysplastic changes prior to age 25. After age 25 years, risk of invasive cervical cancer among PWH consistently outpaces the general populations at all age groups. In the light of higher-than-normal risk of cervical cancer, screening should continue lifetime and not end at age 65 years among those with HIV. However, after age 65 clinicians should assess individual absolute risk of cervical and patient life expectancy to guide shared decision-making regarding ongoing screening.

The following table (Table 23.1) presents a summary of the cervical cancer screening recommendations from the

Table 23.1 CERVICAL CANCER SCREENING RECOMMENDATIONS FOR WOMEN WITH HIV

AGE, Y	SCHEDULE	FOLLOW-UP RECOMMENDATIONS FOR ABNORMAL RESULTS
< 21	• No Pap smear recommended	–

21–29	• Baseline liquid-based Pap at initial HIV diagnosis
	  • Co-testing not recommended because of high prevalence of HPV in this age group
	• Repeat screen 12 months after HIV diagnosis if screen is normal
	  • Note: some experts recommend screen after 6 months
	• Increase screening interval to 3 years after three consecutive normal tests
		• Reflex HPV test if atypical cells of undetermined significance (ASCUS) or greater
		  • Colposcopy if HPV positive
		  • If no reflex HPV, repeat cytology in 6–12 months; on repeat any result ASCUS or greater refer to colposcopy
		• Colposcopy if cytology shows low grade squamous intraepithelial lesion (LGSIL) or greater regardless of HPV status

≥30	• OPTION 1: Pap without HPV test at initial HIV diagnosis
	  • Repeat screen 12 months after HIV diagnosis if screen is normal
	  • Note: some experts recommend repeat screen after 6 months
	  • Increase screening interval to 3 years after three consecutive normal tests
	• OPTION 2: Pap with HPV co-test at HIV diagnosis
	  • Repeat in 3 years If both negative
	• Do not discontinue screening for either option at age 65 years—continue screening throughout lifetime in HIV-positive population
		• Repeat Pap in 6–12 months if Pap shows ASCUS and HPV is negative or unavailable. Colposcopy if ASCUS or greater on repeat cytology.
		• If normal Pap but positive HPV on co-test:
		  • Colposcopy if HPV subtype is HPV16 or HPV16/18 positive
		  • Otherwise, repeat co-test in 1 year. Colposcopy if repeat test abnormal (either Pap or HPV)
		• Colposcopy if cytology shows LGSIL or greater regardless of HPV status

SOURCE: DHHS. Panel on Guidelines for the Prevention and Treatment of Opportunistic Infections in Adults and Adolescents with HIV. Guidelines for the prevention and treatment of opportunistic infections in adults and adolescents with HIV. National Institutes of Health, Centers for Disease Control and Prevention, the HIV Medicine Association, and the Infectious Disease Society of America. https://clinicalinfo.hiv.gov/en/ guidelines/adult-and-adolescent-opportunistic-infection. Accessed September 30, 2022.

NIH-CDC-HIVMA/IDSA. The recommendations are categorized into three groups: women with HIV aged younger than 21 years, between 21 and 29 years, and 30 years and older.

CONSIDERATIONS FOR GENDER-DIVERSE PATIENTS

Transgender and gender-diverse individuals who have a cervix are at risk of HPV infection but are less likely than cisgender women to receive regular Pap tests (Hsiao, 2016). Transgender persons are also disproportionately affected by HIV (Clark et al., 2017). Transgender men and gender-diverse persons living with HIV should receive cervical cancer screenings on the same schedule as cis-gender women, as outlined above. Screening procedures should be performed in a supportive and culturally sensitive manner, and providers should be aware that exogenous testosterone use may increase the likelihood of unsatisfactory testing result (Hsiao, 2016). More specific recommendations for Pap smears in transgender patients can be found at: https://transcare.ucsf.edu/gui delines/cervical-cancer.

RECOMMENDED READING

American College of Obstetricians and Gynecologists. Gynecologic care for women and adolescents with human immunodeficiency virus. *ACOG Practice Bull*. No. 167. October 2016.

Bloomfield GS, Alenezi F, Barasa FA, et al. Human immunodeficiency virus and heart failure in low- and middle-income countries. *JACC Heart Fail*. 2015;3:579–590.

Carten ML, Kiser JJ, Kwara A, et al. Pharmacokinetic interactions between the hormonal emergency contraception, levonorgestrel (Plan B), and efavirenz. *Infect Dis Obstet Gynecol*. 2012;2012:137192.

Department of Health and Human Services, Panel on Opportunistic Infections in HIV-Infected Adults and Adolescents. Guidelines for the prevention and treatment of opportunistic infections in HIV-infected adults and adolescents: recommendations from the Centers for Disease Control and Prevention, the National Institutes of Health, and the HIV Medicine Association of the Infectious Diseases Society of America. https://clinicalinfo.hiv.gov/en/guideli nes/adult-and-adolescent-opportunistic-infection. Published 2022. Accessed September 30, 2022.

ART IN PREGNANCY

CHAPTER GOAL

Upon completion of this chapter, the reader should be able to describe the appropriate management of antiretroviral medications for pregnant individuals living with HIV.

INTRODUCTION

Over time, research has demonstrated that proper prevention strategies and interventions during pregnancy, labor, and delivery can significantly reduce the rate of mother-to-child transmission (MTCT) of HIV. In 1994, a pivotal study in the field of HIV medicine, the Pediatric AIDS

Clinical Trials Group 076, demonstrated that the use of zidovudine (ZDV) monotherapy during pregnancy substantially reduced the risk of HIV transmission to infants by 67% (Connor et al., 1994). The protocol is summarized in Table 23.2. It consisted of oral administration of ZDV initiated between 14 and 34 weeks of gestation and continued throughout pregnancy, followed by intrapartum administration of intravenous ZDV and oral administration of ZDV to the newborn for 6 weeks after delivery. Additional studies have demonstrated the effectiveness of the use of combination ART, further decreasing the risk of HIV transmission to 1%–2% (Cooper et al., 2002). Based on recent data, there have been modifications to the original protocol, including a more selective use of intravenous ZDV based on maternal viral load and changes to postpartum administration of ART to the newborn. With increased emphasis on early testing for HIV and modernized protocols for management antepartum, HIV MTCT has decreased significantly with only 32 infants born with perinatal HIV in the United States in 2019 (CDC, 2022). Prepregnancy ARVs, surgical delivery, and infant ARV prophylaxis/presumptive therapy are also key strategies to prevent perinatal HIV transmission.

LEARNING OBJECTIVE

Review the clinical management of pregnant individuals with HIV, including recommendations for use of ARVs and drug disposition.

WHAT'S NEW?

- The US Food and Drug Administration revised drug labeling for cobicistat products stating that cobicistat should not be used during pregnancy to boost other agents given rates of lower exposures of ART observed in pregnancy.

- Use of ritonavir-boosted PIs may be associated with increased risk of preterm birth. If PIs are needed, use of darunavir (DRV) or atazanavir (ATV) is recommended over use of lopinavir (LPV).

- Newer data suggests that DTG is not associated with an increased risk of NTDs in infants whose mother became pregnant while receiving a DTG-based regimen. DTG-based regimens are now recommended as preferred therapy in both pregnancy and individuals trying to conceive.

- Use of tenofovir alafenamide in pregnancy is now included as a preferred agent.

KEY POINTS

- ART should be initiated in all pregnant individuals with HIV regardless of CD4[+] T-cell count or HIV-1 RNA level. ARVs should be given as combination therapy, similar to that prescribed for nonpregnant individuals with HIV, with the goal of complete virologic suppression.

- ART changes during pregnancy have been associated with the loss of virologic control and are independently associated with MTCT of HIV.

- All cases of prenatal antiretroviral exposure should be reported to the APR (www.apregistry.com).

Table 23.2 THREE-PART ZDV CHEMOPROPHYLAXIS REGIMEN BASED ON PACTG 076

TIME OF ZDV ADMINISTRATION	REGIMEN
Antepartum	Oral administration of 100 mg ZDV five times daily,[a] initiated at 14–34-weeks' gestation and continued throughout pregnancy.
Intrapartum	During labor, intravenous administration of ZDV in a 1-hour initial dose of 2 mg/kg body weight, followed by a continuous infusion of 1 mg/kg body weight/hour until delivery.
Postpartum	Oral administration of ZDV to the newborn (ZDV syrup at 2 mg/kg body weight/dose every 6 hours) for the first 6 weeks of life, beginning at 8–12 hours after birth.[b]

[a] Oral ZDV administered as 200 mg three times daily or 300 mg twice daily is currently used in general clinical practice and is an acceptable alternative regimen to 100 mg five times daily.

[b] Intravenous dosage for full-term infants who cannot tolerate oral intake is 1.5 mg/kg body weight intravenously every 6 hours. ZDV dosing for infants of less than 35-weeks' gestation at birth is 1.5 mg/kg/dose intravenously, or 2.0 mg/kg/dose orally, every 12 hours, advancing to every 8 hours at 2 weeks of age if greater than 30-weeks' gestation at birth or at 4 weeks of age if less than 30-weeks' gestation at birth.

SOURCE: DHHS. Panel on Treatment of Pregnant Women with HIV Infection and Prevention of Perinatal Transmission. Recommendations for the use of antiretroviral drugs in pregnant women with HIV infection and interventions to reduce perinatal HIV transmission in the United States. https://clinicalinfo.hiv.gov/sites/default/files/guidelines/documents/perinatal-hiv/guidelines-perinatal.pdf. Published 2022a. Accessed September 30, 2022.

PHYSIOLOGIC CHANGES DURING PREGNANCY

There are physiologic changes that occur during pregnancy that may alter drug disposition and lead to decreased drug exposure. These changes may be associated with incomplete virologic suppression, virologic failure, and/or the development of drug resistance (Mirochnick et al., 2004). An understanding of the pharmacokinetic changes that can occur with ARVs during pregnancy is essential for making proper dose modifications to maintain efficacy and minimize toxicity. Summarized in Box 23.1 are some of the physiologic changes that occur during pregnancy that could affect drug disposition. Some pharmacokinetic changes during pregnancy can be overcome by maximizing dosing strategies of ARVs such as prescribing twice-daily DRV and RAL. An example of how physiologic changes can affect ARVs includes cobicistat boosted regimens and the increased activity of hepatic cytochrome P450 3A enzymes during pregnancy. A phase 4 pharmacokinetic study evaluating 14 women in their third trimester of pregnancy on regimens containing EVG/c found that 77% to 85% of women had troughs below the effective concentration needed to inhibit 90% of the virus. This is thought to be due to both increased clearance and shorter half-life of EVG as well as decreased cobicistat exposure (Bukkems et al., 2020). These results were echoed in the second trimester as well as with other cobicistat boosted regimens (Momper et al., 2018). DRV/c exposures were measured in six women, and an 89%–92% (total DRV) and 32%–41% (unbound DRV) decreased trough concentrations compared to postpartum exposures was noted. Cobicistat similarly had a trough that was 83% lower than postpartum exposures (Crauwells et al., 2019). The median ATV trough in 11 pregnant women was 0.21 mcg/mL in the second trimester, 0.21 mcg/mL in the third trimester, and 0.61 mcg/mL postpartum (Momper et al., 2022).

TRANSPLACENTAL TRANSFER OF ANTIRETROVIRAL DRUGS

Although the risk of perinatal transmission in mothers with undetectable viral load is low (approximately 0.04%), the use of agents that cross the placenta and act as PrEP to the fetus is an important facet of care to prevent perinatal transmission

(Warszawski et al., 2008; DHHS, 2022a, 2022b). In general, nucleoside reverse transcriptase inhibitors (NRTIs), NNRTIs, and integrase inhibitors (INSTIs) readily cross the placenta. PIs such as DRV/r, are highly protein bound, and, therefore, only a small percentage of drug that is unbound is free to transfer. Newer agents such as fostemsavir and ibalizumab do not have available human data on placental transfer (DHHS, 2022a).

BASIC PRINCIPLES OF USE OF ANTIRETROVIRALS IN PREGNANCY

- Antiretrovirals (ARVs) should be initiated in all pregnant women with HIV regardless of CD4 + T-cell count or HIV-1 viral load.

- The regimen should have optimal efficacy, safety and be well tolerated.

- The regimen should contain at least one drug with good placental passage.

- The provider should consider multiple factors when selecting a regimen, including baseline ARV resistance (determined by HIV genotype and treatment history), comorbidities, convenience, adverse effects, drug interactions, pharmacokinetics, and experience in pregnancy).

- Individuals entering pregnancy on ARVs should continue their regimen if it is effective, well tolerated, and does not contain agents that are teratogenic.

RECOMMENDATIONS
ARV-Naive Individuals

All individuals with HIV should receive a potent ARV regimen to reduce the risk of perinatal transmission. For an updated list please refer to the current US DHHS *preferred* and *alternate* regimens for women who have never received ART and are pregnant. Current preferred regimens include DTG, RAL, ATV/r, or DRV/r in combination with abacavir (ABC) plus lamivudine (3TC) or emtricitabine (FTC), tenofovir disoproxil fumarate (TDF) plus emtricitabine or 3TC, or tenofovir alafenamide (TAF) plus 3TC or FTC (Table 23.3). Note that DTG-based regimens are preferred in those with acute HIV during pregnancy. There is also a section on drug regimens that are no longer recommended and the rationale for the discontinuation of their use. See: http://clinicalinfo.hiv.gov/sites/default/files/guidelines/documents/perinatal-hiv/guidelines-perinatal.pdf/.

PREGNANCY WHILE ON ANTIRETROVIRAL THERAPY

HIV-positive pregnant individuals who present for care in the first trimester should be counseled about the risks and benefits of ART. If possible, they should be maintained on their

Table 23.3 ARV PRINCIPLES IN PREGNANCY, CONCEIVING, AND CONTRACEPTION

REGIMEN	USE IN ART-NAIVE PEOPLE	CONTINUING ART FOR PEOPLE WHO BECOME PREGNANT THAT ARE VIRALLY SUPPRESSED	ART FOR NONPREGNANT PEOPLE WHO ARE TRYING TO CONCEIVE	OTHER COMMENTS	EFFECTS ON CONTRACEPTION
NRTI BACKBONES					
ABC/3TC	Preferred	Continue	Preferred	Testing for the HLA-B*5701 allele should be performed and documented as negative before starting ABC, and women should be educated about symptoms of hypersensitivity reactions.	–
TAF/FTC	Preferred	Continue	Preferred	Associated with fewer adverse birth outcomes and higher gestational weight compared to TDF/FTC.	–
TAF + 3TC	Preferred	Continue	Preferred	–	–
TDF/FTC	Preferred	Continue	Preferred	–	–
TDF/3TC	Preferred	Continue	Preferred	–	–
INSTI					
BIC/TAF/FTC	Insufficient data	Insufficient data	Insufficient data	–	–
CAB/RPV	Not recommended	Insufficient data	Insufficient data	Not recommended owing to lack of data.	–
DTG	Preferred (early and late pregnancy)	Continue	Preferred	Only agent preferred in early pregnancy. Also preferred in late pregnancy.	–
EVG/c/TAF/FTC	Not recommended	Continue with frequent viral load monitoring or switch	Not recommended	Decreased levels of cobicistat in second and third trimester with increased risk for viral breakthroughs.	–
RAL	Preferred (late pregnancy); alternative (acute HIV)	Continue	Preferred	Must use 400 mg twice-daily strategy. No data available for 1,200 mg once daily extended-release tablets.	–
NNRTI					
DOR	Insufficient data	Insufficient data	Insufficient data	No data on use in pregnancy.	–
EFV	Alternative	Continue	Alternative	–	Consider alternative in addition to COC/P/R, POPs, etonogestrel implants.
ETV	Not recommended	Continue	Not recommended, except in special circumstances	Not recommended owing to limited data.	–

(continued)

Table 23.3 CONTINUED

REGIMEN	USE IN ART-NAIVE PEOPLE	CONTINUING ART FOR PEOPLE WHO BECOME PREGNANT THAT ARE VIRALLY SUPPRESSED	ART FOR NONPREGNANT PEOPLE WHO ARE TRYING TO CONCEIVE	OTHER COMMENTS	EFFECTS ON CONTRACEPTION
NVP	Not recommended	Continue	Not recommended, except in special circumstances	Not recommended because of high risk for adverse events, lead in dosing, and barrier to resistance.	–
RPV	Alternative	Continue	Alternative	Little experience in pregnancy and PK suggests lower levels in second and third trimesters with increased risk of viral rebound.	–
PROTEASE INHIBITORS					
ATV/r	Preferred	Continue	Preferred	Consider neonatal bilirubin monitoring when given throughout pregnancy.	–
DRV/r	Preferred	Continue	Preferred	Must use twice-daily dosing strategy.	Can consider alternative method of contraception in addition to COC/P/R, POPs, etonogestrel implants.
LPV/r	Not recommended except in special circumstances	Continue	Not recommended except in special circumstances	Must use twice-daily dosing strategy. Some experts recommend a higher dosing strategy during the second and third trimesters. Use of LPV/r is associated with increased risk of preterm delivery as well as more nausea.	–
ATV/c	Not recommended	Continue with frequent viral load monitoring or switch	Not recommended	Decreased levels of cobicistat in second and third trimester with increased risk for viral breakthroughs.	Contraindicated with drospirenone-containing hormonal contraceptives because of risk of hypokalemia. Consider alternative or additional method of contraception to COC/P/R, POPs, etonogestrel implants.
DRV/c	Not recommended	Continue with frequent viral load monitoring or switch	Not recommended	Decreased levels of cobicistat in second and third trimester with increased risk for viral breakthroughs.	Monitoring with drospirenone-containing hormonal contraceptives because of risk of hypokalemia. Consider alternative or additional method of contraception to COC/P/R, POPs, etonogestrel implants.

Table 23.3 CONTINUED

REGIMEN	USE IN ART-NAIVE PEOPLE	CONTINUING ART FOR PEOPLE WHO BECOME PREGNANT THAT ARE VIRALLY SUPPRESSED	ART FOR NONPREGNANT PEOPLE WHO ARE TRYING TO CONCEIVE	OTHER COMMENTS	EFFECTS ON CONTRACEPTION
ENTRY, ATTACHMENT, AND FUSION INHIBITORS					
FTR	Insufficient data	Insufficient data	Insufficient data	–	–
IBA	Insufficient data	Insufficient data	Insufficient data	No data on use in pregnancy.	–
MVC	Not recommended	Continue	Not recommended, except in special circumstances	Not recommended in nonpregnant patients given somewhat limited pharmacokinetic data in pregnancy.	–
T-20	Not recommended	Continue	Not recommended, except in special circumstances	–	–

COC/P/R: combined oral contraceptives/patch/ring.

SOURCE: DHHS. Panel on Treatment of Pregnant Women with HIV Infection and Prevention of Perinatal Transmission. Recommendations for the use of antiretroviral drugs in pregnant women with HIV infection and interventions to reduce perinatal HIV transmission in the United States. https://clinicalinfo.hiv.gov/en/guidelines/perinatal/overview-2?view=full. Published 2022a. Accessed August 11, 2022.

current ART regimen as discontinuations may lead to the loss of virologic control. This could adversely affect the health of the fetus, including HIV transmission. In a prospective cohort of 937 mother–infant pairs, interruption of ART during the first and third trimesters was independently associated with MTCT of HIV. The overall rate of MTCT of HIV was 1.3%, compared to the rate associated with first- and third-trimester interruptions of ART, which were 4.9% and 18.2%, respectively (Galli et al., 2009).

In the past, there has been concern over the teratogenic effects of EFV use in the first trimester of pregnancy. Preclinical primate data and retrospective reports raised concern about an increased risk of NTDs with EFV use in pregnancy. It is important to note that the neural tube closes at 36–39 days after the last menstrual period. Thus, the risk of NTDs is restricted to the first 5–6 weeks of pregnancy. A meta-analysis that included data on 1,437 first-trimester EFV exposures showed no overall increased risk of birth defects compared to women on other ARV drugs. There was one NTD, giving an incidence of 0.07% (Ford et al., 2011). The panel on treatment of pregnant women with HIV has updated its recommendation, noting that EFV is an alternative NNRTI regimen based on extensive experience in pregnancy. Coformulated EFV/TDF/FTC is a recommended regimen in women who require coadministration of drugs with significant interactions with preferred agents or those who need the convenience of a single tablet and are not eligible for RPV or DTG. It is important to screen for antenatal and postpartum depression (DHHS, 2022a, 2022b).

The Tsepamo birth outcome study is an ongoing observational study funded by the US NIH in Botswana comparing birth outcomes among pregnant women taking EFV- versus

DTG-based regimens. In 2018, an interim analysis was reported on women who were taking DTG-containing regimen before or during conception and revealed 4 out of 429 newborns (0.94%) had NTDs. In comparison, NTDs occurred in 14 out of 11,3000 (0.0012%) of infants born to women receiving non-DTG-based regimens at the time of conception, and 3 out of 5,787 (0.05%) of women on EFV-containing regimens (Zash et al., 2018). In an updated analysis, nine of out of 5,680 deliveries (0.15%) resulted in NTDs (Zash et al., 2019). This rate is not dissimilar from other studies suggesting a NTD rate of 0.10% in non-DTG-based regimens, 0.06% in EFV-based regimens, and 0.07% in mothers without HIV (Zash et al., 2021). The mechanism of DTG's association with NTD is unknown. As a result of the Tsepamo's recent findings, DTG is now recommended as a preferred agent in both pregnancy and women who are trying to conceive by the Panel on Antiretroviral Guidelines for Adults and Adolescents, the Panel on Antiretroviral Therapy and Medical Management of Children Living with HIV, and the Panel on Treatment of Pregnant Women Living with HIV and Prevention of Perinatal Transmission (DHHS, 2022a). Limited data are available regarding other INSTIs and their effect on NTDs. Surveillance data from the United Kingdom and Ireland indicate that RAL use in pregnancy was not associated with any NTDs and is listed as a preferred agent in pregnant women (Baxevanidi et al., 2021).

Current data raise the question of whether ritonavir-boosted PIs may increase the risk of preterm delivery (PTD), with the highest risk of PTD associated with lopinavir/ritonavir. Multiple studies have noted an association between PI regimens with the risk of PTD at an adjusted odds ratio of 1.32 (95% CI: 1.04–1.6) (Mesfin et al., 2016), but there are also multiple studies that suggest a lack of an effect. In a network meta-analysis of six randomized controlled trials, use of ZDV/3TC/LPV/r was associated with the highest risk of PTB, as compared to ZDV and other regimens (relative risk ranging from 1.43 to 1.81) (Tshivuila-Matala et al., 2020). That finding was mirrored when comparing lopinavir/ritonavir to atazanavir/ritonavir (unadjusted risk ratio 1.97; 95% CI: 1.2–3.4) (Rough et al., 2018). It remains uncertain the effect that boosted PIs have on PTD rates. However, given the data for this effect are strongest with the use of lopinavir/ritonavir, its use is not routinely recommended.

Historically TDF was the only tenofovir product recommended for use in pregnancy. However, newer data are available that suggest use of TAF is safe, and TAF is now listed as another agent that is preferred in pregnancy. When comparing initiation of DTG + TAF/FTC versus DTG + TDF/FTC starting between 14- and 28-weeks' gestation, use of TAF was associated with lower adverse pregnancy outcomes (24% vs. 44%, 95% CI: -17.3 to -0.3; $p = 0.043$) and no difference in infant adverse events, but was associated with higher maternal weight gain (0.378 kg/week vs. 0.319 kg/week, 95% CI: 0.013 –0.103; $p = 0.011$) (Lockman et al., 2021).There are multiple regimens that are listed as recommended regimens for nonpregnant people who are virally suppressed that are not recommended in pregnancy because of lack of sufficient data including oral and injectable two-drug regimens such as DTG/3TC, DTG/rilpivirine (RPV), and cabotegravir (CAB)/RPV. If patients have maintained viral suppression on a two-drug oral regimen, clinicians can consider continuing this regimen with increased frequency of viral load monitoring (every 1–2 months). Given limited data, patients on injectable CAB/RPV should switch to a three-drug regimen within 4 weeks of last injection.

PREGNANCY WITHOUT VIRAL SUPPRESSION

In late pregnancy, lack of virologic suppression could be due to either inadequate time on ART, poor adherence, or virologic failure. Providers must consider several things when evaluating a pregnant individual with lack of viral suppression including adherence, tolerability, correct dosing, drug interactions, and resistance. If there is a concern for resistance, ARV resistance studies should be sent and consultation with an expert is advised.

There have been case reports on the use of RAL-containing regimens in late pregnancy owing to the rapid viral decay that has been demonstrated with INSTIs. There are data demonstrating superior viral load suppression at the time of delivery in pregnant women with HIV receiving DTG-containing regimens versus those receiving EFV-based regimens (DHHS, 2022a).

INTRAPARTUM ZIDOVUDINE DURING LABOR

Those with HIV-1 RNA counts of greater than 1,000 copies/mL or an unknown viral load near delivery (within four weeks) should receive intravenous ZDV (Briand et al., 2013). In the past, all HIV-positive women were given intravenous ZDV during pregnancy regardless of viral load, as this was part of the PACTG 076 protocol noted earlier (Table 23.2).

The French Perinatal Cohort evaluated perinatal transmission in more than 11,000 pregnant women with HIV receiving ART. The overall rate of perinatal transmission was 0.9% in those who received intravenous ZDV and 1.8% without intravenous ZDV. Among women with HIV-1 RNA levels of more than 1,000 copies/mL, the risk of transmission without ZDV was 10.2% compared to 2.5% with intravenous ZDV if neonates received only ZDV for prophylaxis but was no different without or with intrapartum ZDV if the neonate received intensified prophylaxis with two or more ARV drugs. Among women with HIV-1 RNA levels of less than 1,000 copies/mL at delivery, zero transmissions occurred among 369 women who did not receive intravenous ZDV, compared to 0.6% of those receiving intravenous ZDV (Briand et al., 2013). A few additional studies were reported; based on these studies, intravenous ZDV should continue to be administered to women with HIV RNA counts of greater than 1,000 copies/mL near delivery regardless of intrapartum regimen. Intrapartum ZDV administration may be considered and assessed on a case-by-case basis in women with HIV-1 RNA levels in the range of 50 to 999 copies/mL as the risk of transmission is slightly higher (1%–2% vs. 1% or less). Additionally, patients with HIV-1 RNA levels greater than 1,000 copies/mL should be scheduled for cesarean delivery at 38-weeks' gestation to reduce the rate of perinatal transmission (ACOG, 2018).

ANTIRETROVIRAL PREGNANCY REGISTRY

Established in 1989, the APR collects data on pregnant individuals with HIV taking ARVs with the goal of detecting any major teratogenic effects. Registration is voluntary and confidential; however, providers are strongly encouraged to enroll pregnant patients in the registry at the time of the initial evaluation of the pregnant woman. This is an observational, exposure registration, and follow-up study. The APR is an international registry that has received reports from 67 countries, with the reports predominantly coming from the United States. More information can be obtained by visiting the registry website at: www.APRegistry.com.

REFERENCES

Aboulafia D M, Bundow D, Wilske K, Ochs UI. Etanercept for the treatment of human immunodeficiency virus-associated psoriatic arthritis. *Mayo Clin Proc.* 2000;75(10):1093–1098.

Altman K, Vanness E, Westergaard RP. Cutaneous manifestations of human immunodeficiency virus: a clinical update. *Curr Infect Dis Rep.* 2015;17(3):464.

Anton P, Soriano V, Jimenez-Nacher I, et al. Incidence of rash and discontinuation of nevirapine using two different escalating initial doses. *AIDS.* 1999;13(4):524–525.

Atkinson TM, Palefsky J, Li Y, et al.; ANCHOR HRQoL Implementation Group. Reliability and between-group stability of a health-related quality of life symptom index for persons with anal high-grade squamous intraepithelial lesions: an AIDS Malignancy Consortium study (AMC-A03). *Qual Life Res*. May 2019;28(5):1265–1269. http://doi:10.1007/s11136-018-2089-8. Epub January 7, 2019. PMID: 30617704; PMCID: PMC6472969.

Ball RA, Kinchelow T; ISR Substudy Group. Injection site reactions with the HIV-1 fusion inhibitor enfuvirtide. *J Am Acad Dermatol*. 2003;49(5):826–831.

Bartlett BL, Khambaty M, Mendoza N, et al. Dermatological management of human immunodeficiency virus (HIV). *Skin Therapy Lett*. 2007;12(8):1–3.

Baveewo S, Ssali F, Karamagi C, et al. Validation of World Health Organisation HIV/AIDS clinical staging in predicting initiation of antiretroviral therapy and clinical predictors of low CD4\++ T cell count in Uganda. *PLoS One*. 2011;6(5):e19089.

Bellavista S, D'Antuono A, Infusino SD, et al. Pruritic papular eruption in HIV: a case successfully treated with NB-UVB. *Dermatol Ther*. 2013;26(2):173–175.

Bennett JE, Dolin R, Blaser MJ, Peterson BW, Damon IK. In: Bennett J, Dolin R, Blaser MJ, (eds.), *Mandell, Douglas, and Bennett's principles and practice of infectious diseases*, Vol. 2. New York: Elsevier; 2020:1809–1817.

Bolognia JL, Jorizzo JL, Schaffer J. *Dermatology*. 3rd ed. New York: Elsevier; 2012.

Boonchai W, Laohasrisakul R, Manonukul J, Kulthanan K. Pruritic papular eruption in HIV seropositive patients: a cutaneous marker for immunosuppression. *Int J Dermatol*. 1999;38(5):348–350.

Boudhir H, Mael-Ainin M, Senouci K, et al. Kaposi's disease: an unusual side-effect of topical corticosteroids. *Ann Dermatol Venereol*. 2013;140(6–7):459–461.

Breuer-McHam J, Marshall G, Adu-Oppong A, et al. Alterations in HIV expression in AIDS patients with psoriasis or pruritus treated with phototherapy. *J Am Acad Dermatol*. 1999;40(1):48–60.

Calonje E, Brenn T, Lazar A, Mckee P. *McKee's pathology of the skin*, 4th ed. St. Louis, MO: Saunders; 2012.

Cambuim II, Macedo DP, Delgado M, et al. Clinical and mycological evaluation of onychomycosis among Brazilian HIV/AIDS patients [in Portuguese]. *Rev Soc Bras Med Trop*. 2011;44(1):40–42.

CDC. HIV surveillance report, 2020, vol. 33. cdc.gov. http://www.cdc.gov/hiv/library/reports/hiv-surveillance.html. Published May 2022e. Accessed August 14, 2022.

Centers for Disease Control and Prevention, US (CDC). Monkeypox: clinical recognition. https://www.cdc.gov/poxvirus/monkeypox/clinicians/clinical-recognition.html. Published 2022a. Accessed August 30, 2022.

CDC. Monkeypox: preparation and collection of specimens. https://www.cdc.gov/poxvirus/monkeypox/clinicians/prep-collection-specimens.html. Published 2022b. Accessed August 30, 2022.

CDC. Interim clinical considerations for use of JYNNEOS and ACAM2000 vaccines during the 2022 U.S. monkeypox outbreak. https://www.cdc.gov/poxvirus/monkeypox/health-departments/vaccine-considerations.html. Published 2022c. Accessed August 30, 2022.

CDC. Vaccination strategies. https://www.cdc.gov/poxvirus/monkeypox/interim-considerations/overview.html. Published 2022d. Accessed August 30, 2022.

Chandrasekar PH, Nandi PS, Fairfax MR, Crane LR. Cutaneous infections due to *Acanthamoeba* in patients with acquired immunodeficiency syndrome. *Arch Intern Med*. 1997;157(5):569–572.

Chaponda M, Pirmohamed M. Hypersensitivity reactions to HIV therapy. *Br J Clin Pharmacol*. 2011;71(5):659–671.

Cockerell C, Calame A. *Cutaneous manifestations of HIV disease*. London: Manson; 2013.

Crum-Cianflone NF, Burgi AA, Hale BR. Increasing rates of community-acquired methicillin-resistant *Staphylococcus aureus* infections among HIV-infected persons. *Int J STD AIDS*. 2007;18(8):521–526.

Cucinotta D, Vanelli M. WHO Declares COVID-19 a pandemic. *Acta bio-medica: Atenei Parmensis*. 2020;91(1):157–160. https://doi.org/10.23750/abm.v91i1.9397

Davis CM, Shearer WT. Diagnosis and management of HIV drug hypersensitivity. *J Allergy Clin Immunol*. 2008;121(4):826–832, e825.

de Berker D. Clinical practice: fungal nail disease. *N Engl J Med*. 2009;360(20):2108–2116.

de Moraes AP, de Arruda EA, Vitoriano MA, et al. An open-label efficacy pilot study with pimecrolimus cream 1% in adults with facial seborrhoeic dermatitis infected with HIV. *J Eur Acad Dermatol Venereol*. 2007;21(5):596–601.

Department of Health and Human Services (DHHS), Administration for Strategic Preparedness & Response. Determination that a public health emergency exists. 2022.

Department of Health and Human Services (DHHS). Panel on Guidelines for the Prevention and Treatment of Opportunistic Infections in Adults and Adolescents with HIV. Guidelines for the prevention and treatment of opportunistic infections in adults and adolescents with HIV. National Institutes of Health, Centers for Disease Control and Prevention, the HIV Medicine Association, and the Infectious Disease Society of America. https://clinicalinfo.hiv.gov/en/guidelines/adult-and-adolescent-opportunistic-infection. Published 2022b. Accessed September 30, 2022.

Department of Health and Human Services (DHHS). Panel on Treatment of HIV During Pregnancy and Prevention of Perinatal Transmission. Recommendations for the Use of Antiretroviral Drugs During Pregnancy and Interventions to Reduce Perinatal HIV Transmission in the United States. https://clinicalinfo.hiv.gov/sites/default/files/guidelines/documents/perinatal-hiv/guidelines-perinatal.pdf. Published 2022a. Accessed September 30, 2022.

Dogra S, Yadav S. Acitretin in psoriasis: an evolving scenario. *Int J Dermatol*. 2014;53(5):525–538.

Dover JS, Johnson RA. Cutaneous manifestations of human immunodeficiency virus infection: part II. *Arch Dermatol*. 1991;127(10):1549–1558.

Drain PK, Mosam A, Gounder L, et al. Recurrent giant molluscum contagiosum immune reconstitution inflammatory syndrome (IRIS) after initiation of antiretroviral therapy in an HIV-infected man. *Int J STD AIDS*. 2014;25(3):235–238.

Duvic M, Crane MM, Conant M, et al. Zidovudine improves psoriasis in human immunodeficiency virus-positive males. *Arch Dermatol*. 1994;130(4):447–451.

Duvic M. Immunology of AIDS related to psoriasis. *J Invest Dermatol*. 1990;95(5):38S–40S.

Eisman S. Pruritic papular eruption in HIV. *Dermatol Clin*. 2006;24(4):449–457, vi.

Farsani TT, Kore S, Nadol P, et al Etiology and risk factors associated with a pruritic papular eruption in people living with HIV in India. *J Int AIDS Soc*. September 3, 2013;16(1):17325. http://doi:10.7448/IAS.16.1.17325. PMID: 24004854; PMCID: PMC3763046.

Fearfield LA, Rowe A, Francis N, et al. Itchy folliculitis and human immunodeficiency virus infection: clinicopathological and immunological features, pathogenesis and treatment. *Br J Dermatol*. 1999;141(1):3–11.

Foissac M, Goehringer F, Ranaivo IM, et al. Efficacy and safety of intravenous cidofovir in the treatment of giant molluscum contagiosum in an immunosuppressed patient [in French]. *Ann Dermatol Venereol*. 2014;141(10):620–622.

Gasquet S, Maurin M, Brouqui P, et al. Bacillary angiomatosis in immunocompromised patients. *AIDS*. 1998;12(14):1793–1803.

Gelfand JM, Gladman DD, Mease PJ, et al. Epidemiology of psoriatic arthritis in the population of the United States. *J Am Acad Dermatol*. 2005;53(4):573.

Ghanem KG, Erbelding EJ, Wiener ZS, Rompalo AM. Serological response to syphilis treatment in HIV-positive and HIV-negative patients attending sexually transmitted diseases clinics. *Sex Transm Infect*. 2007;83(2):97–101.

Goldstein B, Berman B, Sukenik E, Frankel SJ. Correlation of skin disorders with CD4+ T cell lymphocyte counts in patients with HIV/AIDS. *J Am Acad Dermatol*. 1997;36(2 Pt 1):262–264.

Gompels MM, Simpson N, Snow M, et al. Desensitization to co-trimoxazole (trimethoprim-sulphamethoxazole) in HIV-infected patients: is patch testing a useful predictor of reaction? *J Infect.* 1999;38:111–115.

Hage CA, Azar MM, Bahr N, et al. Histoplasmosis: up-to-date evidence-based approach to diagnosis and management. *Semin Respir Crit Care Med.* 2015;36(5):729–745.

Hagensee ME, Cameron JE, Leigh JE, Clark RA. Human papillomavirus infection and disease in HIV-infected individuals. *Am J Med Sci.* 2004;328(1):57–63.

Hanifin JM, Reed ML, Eczema P, et al.; Impact Working Group. A population-based survey of eczema prevalence in the United States. *Dermatitis.* 2007;18(2):82–91.

Hemmige V, Arias CA, Pasalar S, Giordano TP. Skin and soft tissue infection in people living with human immunodeficiency virus in a large, urban, public healthcare system in Houston, Texas, 2009–2014. *Clin Infect Dis.* April 15, 2020;70(9):1985–1992. http://doi: 10.1093/cid/ciz509. PMID: 31209457; PMCID: PMC7156777.

Hevia O, Jimenez-Acosta F, Ceballos PI, et al. Pruritic papular eruption of the acquired immunodeficiency syndrome: a clinicopathologic study. *J Am Acad Dermatol.* 1991;24(2 Pt 1):231–235.

Hyle EP, Wood BR, Backman ES, et al. High frequency of hypothalamic–pituitary–adrenal axis dysfunction after local corticosteroid injection in HIV-infected patients on protease inhibitor therapy. *J AIDS.* 2013;63(5):602–608.

Iñigo Martínez J, Gil Montalbán E, Jiménez Bueno S, et al. Monkeypox outbreak predominantly affecting men who have sex with men, Madrid, Spain, 26 April to 16 June 2022. *Euro surveillance: bulletin Europeen sur les maladies transmissibles = European Communicable Disease Bulletin,* 2022;27(27):2200471. https://doi.org/10.2807/1560-7917.ES.2022.27.27.2200471

Introcaso CE, Hines JM, Kovarik CL. Cutaneous toxicities of antiretroviral therapy for HIV: part II. Nonnucleoside reverse transcriptase inhibitors, entry and fusion inhibitors, integrase inhibitors, and immune reconstitution syndrome. *J Am Acad Dermatol.* 2010;63(4):563–569; quiz 569–570.

Jagdeo J, Ho D, Lo A, Carruthers A. A systematic review of filler agents for aesthetic treatment of HIV facial lipoatrophy (FLA). *J Am Acad Dermatol.* 2015;73(6):1040–1054, e1014.

Kim CM, Vogel J, Jay G, Rhim JS. The HIV tat gene transforms human keratinocytes. *Oncogene.* 1992;7(8):1525–1529.

Knobel H, Miro JM, Domingo P, et al. Failure of a short-term prednisone regimen to prevent nevirapine-associated rash: a double-blind placebo-controlled trial: the GESIDA 09/99 study. *J AIDS.* 2001;28(1):14–18.

Krown SE, Lee JY, Dittmer DP; AIDS Malignancy Consortium. More on HIV-associated Kaposi's sarcoma. *N Engl J Med.* 2008;358(5):535–536; author reply 536.

Kuehnert MJ, Kruszon-Moran D, Hill HA, et al. Prevalence of *Staphylococcus aureus* nasal colonization in the United States, 2001–2002. *J Infect Dis.* 2006;193(2):172–179.

Leung AKC, Barankin B, Hon KLE. Molluscum contagiosum: an update. *Recent Pat Inflamm Allergy Drug Discov.* 2017;11(1):22–31. http://doi: 10.2174/1872213X11666170518114456. PMID: 28521677.

Lin RY, Lazarus TS. Asthma and related atopic disorders in outpatients attending an urban HIV clinic. *Ann Allergy Asthma Immunol.* 1995;74(6):510–515.

Liu Z, Xie Z, Zhang L, et al. Reliability and validity of dermatology life quality index: assessment of quality of life in human immunodeficiency virus/acquired immunodeficiency syndrome patients with pruritic papular eruption. *J Tradit Chin Med.* 2013;33(5):580–583.

Lolis MS, Gonzalez L, Cohen PJ, Schwartz RA. Drug-resistant herpes simplex virus in HIV infected patients. *Acta Dermatovenerol Croat.* 2008;16(4):204–208.

Lortholary O, Fontanet A, Memain N, et al.; Cryptococcosis Study Group. Incidence and risk factors of immune reconstitution inflammatory syndrome complicating HIV-associated cryptococcosis in France. *AIDS.* 2005;19(10):1043–1049.

Mallal S, Phillips E, Carosi G, et al. HLA-B*5701 screening for hypersensitivity to abacavir. *N Engl J Med.* 2008;358(6):568–579.

Mallon E, Bunker CB. HIV-associated psoriasis. *AIDS Patient Care STDS.* 2000; 14(5):239–246.

Maurer TA. Dermatologic manifestations of HIV infection. *Top HIV Med.* 2005;13(5):149–154.

Mayer PL, Larkin JA, Hennessy JM. Amebic encephalitis. *Surg Neurol Int.* 2011;2:50.

McCloskey JC, Metcalf C, French MA, et al. The frequency of high-grade intraepithelial neoplasia in anal/perianal warts is higher than previously recognized. *Int J STD AIDS.* 2007;18(8):538–542.

Menon K, Van Voorhees AS, Bebo BF, et al. Psoriasis in patients with HIV infection: from the medical board of the National Psoriasis Foundation. *J Am Acad Dermatol.* 2010;62(2):291–299.

Meola T, Soter NA, Ostreicher R, Sanchez M, Moy JA. The safety of UVB phototherapy in patients with HIV infection. *J Am Acad Dermatol.* 1993;29(2 Pt 1):216–220.

Mirmirani P, Maurer TA, Berger TG, et al. Skin-related quality of life in HIV-infected patients on highly active antiretroviral therapy. *J Cutan Med Surg.* 2002;6(1):10–15.

Mischo M, von Kobyletzki LB, Bründermann E, et al. Similar appearance, different mechanisms: xerosis in HIV, atopic dermatitis and ageing. *Exp Dermatol.* June 2014;23(6):446–448. http://doi:10.1111/exd.12425. PMID: 24758518.

Mohammed S, Vellaisamy SG, Gopalan K, et al. Prevalence of pruritic papular eruption among HIV patients: a cross-sectional study. *Indian J Sex Transm Dis AIDS.* July–December 2019;40(2):146–151. http://doi:10.4103/ijstd.IJSTD_69_18. PMID: 31922105; PMCID: PMC6896392.

Murphy M, Armstrong D, Sepkowitz KA, et al. Regression of AIDS-related Kaposi's sarcoma following treatment with an HIV-1 protease inhibitor. *AIDS.* 1997;11(2):261–262.

Murray H, Barber CJ, Foreman RM, et al.; GBD 2013 DALYs and HALE Collaborators. Global, regional, and national disability-adjusted life years (DALYs) for 306 diseases and injuries and healthy life expectancy (HALE) for 188 countries, 1990–2013: quantifying the epidemiological transition. *Lancet.* 2015;386:2145–2191.

Nakamura M, Abrouk M, Farahnik B, et al. Psoriasis treatment in HIV-positive patients: a systematic review of systemic immunosuppressive therapies. *Cutis.* January 2018;101(1):38;42;56. PMID: 29529104.

Nambudiri VE, Mutyambizi K, Walls AC, et al. Successful treatment of perianal giant condyloma acuminatum in an immunocompromised host with systemic interleukin 2 and topical cidofovir. *JAMA Dermatol.* 2013;149(9):1068–1070.

Nissen D, Nolte H, Permin H, et al. Evaluation of IgE-sensitization to fungi in HIV-positive patients with eczematous skin reactions. *Ann Allergy Asthma Immunol.* 1999;83(2):153–159.

Nomura T, Katoh M, Yamamoto Y, et al. Eosinophilic pustular folliculitis: a published work-based comprehensive analysis of therapeutic responsiveness. *J Dermatol.* August 2016;43(8):919–927. http://doi:10.1111/1346-8138.13287. Epub February 15, 2016. PMID: 26875627.

Oble DA, Collett E, Hsieh M, et al. A novel T cell receptor transgenic animal model of seborrheic dermatitis-like skin disease. *J Invest Dermatol.* 2005;124(1):151–159.

Obuch ML, Maurer TA, Becker B, Berger TG. Psoriasis and human immunodeficiency virus infection. *J Am Acad Dermatol.* 1992;27(5 Pt 1):667–673.

Okada S, Fujimura T, Furudate S, et al. Immunosuppression-associated eosinophilic pustular folliculitis (IS-EPF) developing after highly active anti-retroviral therapy (HAART): the possible mechanisms through CD163+ M2 macrophages. *Eur J Dermatol.* 2013;23(5):713–714.

Ortega-Loayza AG, McCall CO, Nunley JR. Crusted scabies and multiple dosages of ivermectin. *J Drugs Dermatol.* 2013;12(5):584–585.

Osborne GE, Taylor C, Fuller LC. The management of HIV-related skin disease. Part II: neoplasms and inflammatory disorders. *Int J STD AIDS* 2003;14:235.

Palefsky JM, Lee JY, Jay N, et al.; ANCHOR Investigators Group. Treatment of anal high-grade squamous intraepithelial lesions to prevent anal cancer. *N Engl J Med.* 2022;386(24):2273–2282. https://doi.org/10.1056/NEJMoa2201048

Panel on Guidelines for the Prevention and Treatment of Opportunistic Infections in Adults and Adolescents with HIV. Guidelines for the prevention and treatment of opportunistic infections in adults and adolescents with HIV. National Institutes of Health, Centers for Disease Control and Prevention, HIV Medicine Association, and Infectious Diseases Society of America. https://clinicalinfo.hiv.gov/en/guidelines/adult-and-adolescent-opportunistic-infection. Published 2022. Accessed August 29, 2022.

Pedrosa AF, Lisboa C, Goncalves Rodrigues A. Malassezia infections: a medical conundrum. *J Am Acad Dermatol*. 2014;71(1):170–176.

Philpott D, Hughes CM, Alroy KA, et al. Epidemiologic and clinical characteristics of monkeypox cases—United States, May 17–July 22, 2022. *MMWR Morb Mortal Wkly Rep*. 2022;71:1018–1022. http://dx.doi.org/10.15585/mmwr.mm7132e3

Ratnam I, Chiu C, Kandala NB, Easterbrook PJ. Incidence and risk factors for immune reconstitution inflammatory syndrome in an ethnically diverse HIV type 1-infected cohort. *Clin Infect Dis*. 2006;42(3):418–427.

Resneck JS Jr, Van Beek M, Furmanski L, et al. Etiology of pruritic papular eruption with HIV infection in Uganda. *JAMA*. 2004;292(21):2614–2621.

Rigopoulos D, Paparizos V, Katsambas A. Cutaneous markers of HIV infection. *Clin Dermatol*. 2004;22(6):487–498.

Rodrigues LK, Klencke BJ, Vin-Christian K, et al. Altered clinical course of malignant melanoma in HIV-positive patients. *Arch Dermatol*. 2002;138(6):765–770.

Rosen T, Friedlander SF, Kircik L. Onychomycosis: epidemiology, diagnosis, and treatment in a changing landscape. *J Drugs Dermatol*. 2015;14(3):223–233.

Rosenthal D, LeBoit PE, Klumpp L, Berger TG. Human immunodeficiency virus-associated eosinophilic folliculitis. A unique dermatosis associated with advanced human immunodeficiency virus infection. *Arch Dermatol*. 1991;127(2):206–209.

Sadick NS, McNutt NS, Kaplan MH. Papulosquamous dermatoses of AIDS. *J Am Acad Dermatol*. 1990;22(6 Pt 2):1270–1277.

Severson JL, Tyring SK. Relation between herpes simplex viruses and human immunodeficiency virus infections. *Arch Dermatol*. 1999;135(11):1393–1397.

Singh F, Rudikoff D. HIV-associated pruritus: etiology and management. *Am J Clin Dermatol*. 2003;4(3):177–188.

Sklenovská N, Van Ranst M. Emergence of monkeypox as the most important orthopoxvirus infection in humans. *Frontiers in Public Health*. 2018;6:241. https://doi.org/10.3389/fpubh.2018.00241

Smith G, Holman RP. The prozone phenomenon with syphilis and HIV-1 co-infection. *South Med J*. 2004;97(4):379–382.

Soeprono FF, Schinella RA, Cockerell CJ, Comite SL. Seborrheic-like dermatitis of acquired immunodeficiency syndrome: a clinicopathologic study. *J Am Acad Dermatol*. 1986;14(2 Pt 1):242–248.

Stanley SK, Folks TM, Fauci AS. Induction of expression of human immunodeficiency virus in a chronically infected promonocytic

cell line by ultraviolet irradiation. *AIDS Res Hum Retroviruses*. 1989;5(4):375–384.

Strick LB, Wald A, Celum C. Management of herpes simplex virus type 2 infection in HIV type 1-infected persons. *Clin Infect Dis*. 2006;43(3):347–356.

Suh KS, Han SH, Lee KH, et al. Mites and burrows are frequently found in nodular scabies by dermoscopy and histopathology. *J Am Acad Dermatol*. 2014;71(5):1022–1023.

Tarín-Vicente EJ, Alemany A, Agud-Dios M, et al. Clinical presentation and virological assessment of confirmed human monkeypox virus cases in Spain: a prospective observational cohort study. *Lancet (London, England)*. 2022;400(10353):661–669. https://doi.org/10.1016/S0140-6736(22)01436-2

Thornhill JP, Barkati S, Walmsley S, et al.; SHARE-net Clinical Group. Monkeypox virus infection in humans across 16 countries—April–June 2022. *N Engl J Med*. 2022;387(8):679–691. https://doi.org/10.1056/NEJMoa2207323

Toutous-Trellu L, Abraham S, Pechere M, et al. Topical tacrolimus for effective treatment of eosinophilic folliculitis associated with human immunodeficiency virus infection. *Arch Dermatol*. 2005;141(10):1203–1208.

van Sighem A, Gras L, Reiss P, et al. Life expectancy of recently diagnosed asymptomatic HIV-infected patients approaches that of uninfected individuals. *AIDS*. 2010;24(10):1527–1535.

Ward HA, Russo GG, Shrum J. Cutaneous manifestations of antiretroviral therapy. *J Am Acad Dermatol*. 2002;46(2):284–293.

Warren KJ, Boxwell DE, Kim NY, Drolet BA. Nevirapine-associated Stevens–Johnson syndrome. *Lancet*. 1998;351(9102):567.

Warshaw EM, Nelson D, Carver SM, et al. A pilot evaluation of pulse itraconazole vs. terbinafine for treatment of *Candida* toenail onychomycosis. *Int J Dermatol*. 2005;44(9):785–788.

Weinberg JL, Kovarik CL. The WHO clinical staging system for HIV/AIDS. *Virtual Mentor*. 2010;12(3):202–206.

Wheat LJ, Connolly-Stringfield PA, Baker RL, et al. Disseminated histoplasmosis in the acquired immune deficiency syndrome: clinical findings, diagnosis and treatment, and review of the literature. *Medicine (Baltimore)*. 1990;69(6):361–374.

Wilkins K, Turner R, Dolev JC, et al. Cutaneous malignancy and human immunodeficiency virus disease. *J Am Acad Dermatol*. 2006;54(2):189–206; quiz 207–110.

Workowski KA, Bolan GA. Sexually transmitted diseases treatment guidelines, 2015. *MMWR Recomm Rep*. 2015;64(RR-03):1–137.

Zancanaro PC, McGirt LY, Mamelak AJ, et al. Cutaneous manifestations of HIV in the era of highly active antiretroviral therapy: an institutional urban clinic experience. *J Am Acad Dermatol*. 2006;54(4):581–588.

Zeichner JA. New topical therapeutic options in the management of superficial fungal infections. *J Drugs Dermatol*. 2015;14(10):s35–s41.

Zheng Y, Niyonsaba F, Ushio H, et al. Cathelicidin LL-37 induces the generation of reactive oxygen species and release of human alpha-defensins from neutrophils. *Br J Dermatol*. 2007;157(6):1124–1131.

24.

ANTIRETROVIRAL THERAPY FOR CHILDREN AND NEWBORNS

Karin Nielsen-Saines

CHAPTER GOALS

Upon completion of this chapter, the reader should be able to:

- Understand the basics regarding pathogenesis of mother-to-child-transmission (MTCT) and be aware of landmark studies targeting prevention of HIV mother-to-child transmission.

- Understand the concept of HIV exposure versus HIV infection.

- Comprehend the specific challenges of early HIV diagnosis of infants and understand the importance of timing of transmission for diagnosis and pathogenesis.

- Be aware of the concept of HIV remission in early treated infants.

- Have a general idea of HIV disease course in children and surrogate markers of disease.

- Be aware of specific caveats guiding antiretroviral use in children, particularly in newborns receiving presumptive HIV therapy.

INTRODUCTION

In the absence of interventions to curtail mother-to-child HIV-1 transmission, HIV-1 infection in children parallels that of women of childbearing age. Perinatal transmission of HIV-1 accounts for nearly all worldwide cases of pediatric HIV-1 infection today, with the exception of adolescent acquisition of HIV-1 via adult risk behaviors. HIV-1 transmission from mother-to-child occurs in 25%–30% of cases when there is no maternal ARV treatment (Newell, 1991; Scott et al., 1989); if breastfeeding until 12 months of age is included, transmission risk can be as high as 40%. Infection may be transmitted during pregnancy, at the time of labor and delivery, and via breastfeeding. According to recent global estimates, 85% of pregnant women living with HIV in 2021 received antiretroviral therapy (ART) to prevent HIV vertical transmission through HIV Prevention of Mother to Child Transmission programs, preventing up to 220,000 new HIV infections (USAID). Global estimates indicate, however, that 11% of infants born to women living with HIV acquired HIV from perinatal or postpartum exposure through breastfeeding (USAID). The annual number of new HIV infections in children has continued to decline decreased by over 50% because of provision of combination ART to women living with HIV. In 2021, about 160,000 new HIV infections occurred in children aged younger than 5 years, in comparison to 320,000 cases reported in 2010 (UNICEF, 2021). Estimates of 150,000 new HIV infections in children in 2021 still match those reported from 2019 equating to 449 children infected per day per year. Further reduction in HIV MTCT was potentially adversely impacted by the COVID-19 pandemic which stalled preventive efforts across the globe. Although ART can reduce HIV MTCT transmission to less than 1% (Dorenbaum, 2002; Flynn et al., 2018; Fowler & Newell, 2016), failure to diagnose HIV-1 infection in women and/or unavailability of treatment still contributes to continuing mother-to-child HIV transmission worldwide. Management of HIV-1 infection in children has to take into consideration several factors. These include early diagnosis of infection, the natural history of HIV-1 infection in children and surrogate markers of disease, suitable pediatric drug formulations for children, drug metabolism and pharmacokinetics of antiretrovirals (ARVs) in children, and the general paucity of pediatric treatment data as compared to adult treatment data.

LEARNING OBJECTIVES

- Discuss advances in ART for the prevention of mother-to-child HIV transmission, particularly for postexposure infant prophylaxis.

- Review pediatric-specific issues of early HIV diagnosis, timing and pathogenesis of HIV disease, and use of surrogate markers of HIV infection in this population.

- Discuss current guidelines for management of antiretrovirals (ARVs) in children within the context of what drugs to use, when to start, and when to change ART.

WHAT'S NEW?

- US Department of Health and Human Services (DHHS) antiretroviral guidelines continue to recommend presumptive HIV therapy for infants who are at higher risk of perinatal HIV acquisition. This is intended to be preliminary HIV treatment for a newborn who may later be documented to have HIV infection; however, it may also serve as prophylaxis against HIV acquisition for infants who were exposed to HIV but did not acquire it perinatally. Presumptive HIV therapy differs from ARV prophylaxis, which is the administration of one or more ARV drugs to a newborn without documented HIV infection to reduce the risk of perinatal HIV acquisition. Presumptive HIV therapy on the other hand, is defined as administration of a three-drug ARV regimen at treatment doses for treatment of infants at higher risk of prenatal HIV acquisition. Presumptive HIV therapy is intended to be preliminary treatment of an infant who later is documented to have HIV infection, but also serves as prophylaxis against HIV acquisition in high-risk infants who later are not found to have HIV.

- Infants at risk for HIV acquisition include neonates whose mothers did not receive antepartum or intrapartum ARVs; or whose mothers only received intrapartum ARVs; infants whose mothers did not achieve virologic suppression within 4 weeks of delivery (HIV RNA< 50 copies/mL); and infants of mothers with acute HIV infection during pregnancy or acute HIV infection while breastfeeding.

- Presumptive HIV therapy should be provided to infants of mothers who acquire HIV while breastfeeding.

- Infants of mothers with previously unknown HIV status who are found to be HIV positive by point-of-care testing during labor or delivery should start presumptive HIV therapy. If supplemental testing excludes maternal HIV infection, the ARV regimen should be discontinued.

- ART should be initiated in all infants with confirmed HIV infection.

- A 4-week zidovudine (ZDV) ARV prophylaxis regimen continues to be recommended for HIV prophylaxis in newborns whose mothers received ART during pregnancy and had sustained viral suppression near delivery (defined as a confirmed HIV RNA level< 50 copies/mL) and for whom there are no concerns related to maternal adherence.

- Presumptive HIV therapy in the newborn period consists of three-drug HIV therapy including zidovudine, lamivudine, and nevirapine or raltegravir.

- Only ZDV, lamivudine, and nevirapine should be recommended in premature newborns of < 37 weeks of gestational age because of lack of dosing and safety data.

- Prepregnancy care should include testing of sexually active women for HIV. All pregnant women should be tested for HIV as early as possible during pregnancy. Partners of pregnant women should be encouraged to undergo HIV testing if their status is unknown.

- People who become pregnant while using tenofovir disoproxil fumarate (TDF)/FTC as PrEP can continue PrEP throughout their pregnancy. Risk for HIV acquisition should be reassessed, and people should be counseled regarding benefits and risks of PrEP use in pregnancy.

PrEP is not contraindicated for use in pregnancy and should be offered to patients with potential risk factors for HIV acquisition including multiple courses of post exposure prophylaxis and a history of partner violence. Repeat HIV testing in the third trimester of pregnancy is recommended for women with negative initial HIV antibody tests who are at increased risk of acquiring HIV. This includes women receiving care in facilities that have an HIV incidence of ≥1 case per 1,000 pregnant women per year, women who reside in jurisdictions with an elevated HIV incidence, or women who reside in states that require third-trimester testing.

- Women who were not tested for HIV before or during labor should undergo expedited HIV antibody testing during the immediate postpartum period (or their newborns should undergo expedited HIV antibody testing). If results for mother or infant are positive, an appropriate infant ARV drug regimen should be initiated immediately, and the mother should not breastfeed unless supplemental HIV testing is negative. Expedited HIV testing should be available 24 hours a day during labor and delivery for any pregnant woman with undocumented HIV status, and results should be available within 1 hour.

- HIV testing is recommended for infants and children in foster care and adoptees for whom maternal HIV infection status is unknown.

- HIV antibody tests should not be used in children aged < 18 months. For diagnosis of HIV in this younger population, virologic assays such as HIV RNA or HIV DNA nucleic acid tests are recommended. HIV RNA or HIV DNA nucleic acid tests are equally recommended.

- Assays that detect non-B subtype HIV or Group O HIV infections (HIV RNA NAT or a dual-target total DNA/ RNA test) are recommended for use in infants born to mothers with known or suspected non-B subtype virus or Group O infections. If a mother of an infant acquired HIV outside of the United States and has had repeated undetectable HIV RNA by standard testing, consultation with a clinical virologist on more sensitive HIV nucleic acid testing is suggested.

- Initial combination therapy for ARV treatment-naive children includes the use of integrase strand transfer inhibitor (INSTI)-based regimens as agents to be used in combination with two nucleoside analogue reverse transcriptase inhibitors (NRTIs). BIC/FTC/TAF is now recommended as a preferred InSTI-based regimen for children aged ≥2 years and weighing ≥14 kg. INSTI Doravirine plus a two NRTI backbone regimen is now recommended as an alternative NNRTI regimen for children and adolescents weighing ≥35 kg. FTC/TAF is recommended as a preferred dual NRTI combination in children and adolescents weighing >14 kg when used with an INSTI or NNRTI abacavir (ABC) plus lamivudine (3TC) or FTC are the preferred dual NRTI combinations in children aged >3 months and is also now approved for use in full-term children from the time of birth to 3 months of age as well. A negative test for the human leukocyte antigen (HLA) B5701 allele should be obtained before ABC initiation regardless of age. INSTI two-drug ART regimens and drugs such as cabotegravir (CAB), fostemsavir, and ibalizumab are not approved for treatment initiation in children and adolescents.

- The long-acting injectable regimen, Cabenuva (co-packaged CAB) and rilpivirine (RPV) suspensions) is recommended for treatment of HIV in children and adolescents aged ≥12 years and weighing ≥35 kg with HIV RNA levels < 50 copies/mL on a stable ARV regimen, no history of treatment failure, and no known or suspected resistance to CAB or RPV. The FDA has also approved the oral formulation of CAB for this group of children and adolescents. Oral lead-in dosing of CAB and RPV is now an option, rather than a requirement, when starting Cabenuva; patients may proceed to Cabenuva directly from their current ARV regimen.

- Vitamin D should be measured in children receiving efavirenz (EFV) and vitamin D supplementation should be prescribed for those with vitamin D deficiency. Studies in adults show that the use of EFV is associated with low vitamin D levels, while other studies found an association between EFV use and low bone mineral density.

- INSTI dolutegravir DTG is recommended as a preferred antiretroviral drug throughout pregnancy, and as an Alternative ARV drug in women who are trying to conceive. INSTI-based therapy continues to be the ART of choice during pregnancy.

- Oral cabotegravir (CAB) and the new long-acting injectable regimen of CAB and rilpivirine (RPV) have been classified as *Not Recommended* for use in pregnancy and as *Insufficient Data* for persons who are trying to conceive or who become pregnant while on this regimen.

KEY POINTS

- HIV-infected infants and children have a different, more progressive disease course as compared to adults, given that early infection leads to sustained, high-magnitude viremia with significant seeding of reservoirs in the first months of life, prior to full maturation of the immune system.

- Early diagnosis of HIV infection is pivotal in the management of infants and in the prevention of HIV-associated morbidity and mortality.

- The availability of potent pediatric ARV formulations encompassing different classes of drugs for infected infants and young children is still limited and needs further development.

- Infant postexposure HIV prophylaxis varies according to the risk scenario and in some situations, presumptive therapy may be implemented.

- Early ARV treatment (i.e., at the time of diagnosis) is the mainstay of pediatric HIV infection, particularly for infants younger than 12 months of age, but it is also highly recommended for older children.

- Early treatment of young infants diagnosed shortly after birth is the best approach to reduce the seeding of viral reservoirs and to potentially attain prolonged periods of HIV remission off ARVs, a strategy evaluated in prospective clinical trials recommended by current guidelines.

ANTIRETROVIRALS TO THE HIV-EXPOSED INFANT

Advances in perinatal primary ART and antepartum, peripartum, and postpartum delivery of zidovudine in non-breastfeeding, HIV-infected women without severe immunosuppression in the United States led to a decrease in perinatal transmission rates. The US Centers for Disease Control and Prevention (CDC) estimates that the number of infants born annually with HIV in the United States decreased from 1,650 in 1991 to 100–200 in 2004, with 91 cases of HIV in children younger than 13 years of age diagnosed in the United States in 2018 and 32 by 2019 (CDC, 2020). Although there has been a dramatic decline in pediatric HIV cases resulting from vertical transmission in the last two decades, HIV infection of adolescents and young adults is on the rise, with 57% of the new HIV diagnoses in the United States occurring in 13–34-year-old age group, and 20% occurring in the younger age bracket of 13–24 years of age. These individuals are the least likely of any age group to be aware of their infection status, be retained in care, or have a suppressed virus load (CDC, 2020). For pediatric cases, under 13 years of age, the provision of ARVs to infants born to HIV-infected mothers as prophylaxis has been standard of care in the Unites States since 1994, when results of Pediatric AIDS Clinical Trials Group study 076 were published (Connor et al., 1994). The study demonstrated that zidovudine monotherapy given to the mother starting at 16-weeks' gestation, accompanied by an intravenous zidovudine infusion during labor and delivery and followed by four times per day dosing of zidovudine to the infant from birth to 6 weeks of age was highly efficacious in preventing mother-to-child HIV transmission as compared to placebo (8% vs. 25% respectively, $p < 0.001$). In the developed country setting, 4–6 weeks of zidovudine to the infant initiated at birth, given at 2 mg/kg per dose four times a day or 4 mg/kg per dose twice a day became standard of care (Ruane et al., 2013). The major toxicities of zidovudine used as infant prophylaxis include anemia and neutropenia; however, these are dose-dependent and self-limiting, tend to occur toward the end of the course of treatment, and rarely require interruption of prophylaxis (Lahoz et al., 2010). In resource-limited settings, single-dose nevirapine to the infant (2 mg/kg) shortly after birth was used for many years as standard of care, following publication of HIVNET 012 (Guay et al., 1999), which documented the efficacy of this approach in reducing

MTCT when associated with single-dose nevirapine given to the mother at the time of labor. Nevertheless, this approach induced a large wave of ARV resistance in infants who ultimately became infected, rendering nevirapine use problematic for early infant treatment strategies in the developing world. Among HIV-infected infants whose mothers were not treated with ARVs throughout the course of pregnancy and are therefore at higher risk of HIV acquisition, double ARV prophylaxis initiated within 48 hours of birth with three doses of nevirapine in the first week of life concurrently with 6 weeks of zidovudine has been shown to be more efficacious for the prevention of HIV intrapartum infection than zidovudine alone (Nielsen-Saines, 2011). An alternative, equally efficacious regimen was the use of lamivudine and nelfinavir in the first 2 weeks of life concurrent with 6 weeks of zidovudine (Nielsen-Saines et al., 2011). Lopinavir/ritonavir suspension is currently not recommended by the FDA for use in infants younger than 2 weeks of age; however, raltegravir has been used in this setting and proven to be highly effective (Clarke et al., 2019). In resource-limited settings, the use of daily nevirapine prophylaxis to the HIV-exposed infant for prevention of MTCT has been evaluated up to 6 months of age and has been shown to be effective and safe in the prevention of postpartum HIV acquisition (Coovadia, 2012). Presently however, most settings in Sub-Saharan Africa have transitioned to WHO Options B+, which recommends treatment with ART to all HIV-infected women during pregnancy, lactation, and onward with no further treatment interruption (WHO, 2019).

The selection of ART to reduce perinatal HIV transmission must include consideration of optimal treatment for the infected pregnant women and balance potential for fetal harm. Maternal factors that should be considered include the mother's viral load, degree of immunosuppression, medications for use in treatment of comorbid conditions (e.g., tuberculosis, hepatitis C virus), and the potential for inducing viral resistance. Transmission of resistant HIV to infants has been described in the literature, but it is an infrequent event (de Lourdes Teixeira, 2015; Yeganeh, 2018). Other considerations to prevent perinatal transmission of HIV include scheduled delivery to minimize prolonged rupture of membranes, including a recommendation from the American College of Obstetrics for scheduled cesarean section for women with viral loads exceeding HIV RNA levels of 1,000 copies/mL (Committee on Obstetric Practice ACOG, 2001). In a meta-analysis of 15 North American and European cohorts of HIV-infected pregnant women ($n = 100$ women), vertical transmission rates differed by 5% for those with scheduled delivery by cesarean section (transmission rate, 2%) as compared with those with other delivery modes (transmission rate, 7.3%; International Perinatal HIV Group, 1999). Evaluation of the morbidity and mortality related to such scheduled cesarean sections suggests that HIV-infected pregnant women may have a higher incidence of postpartum hemorrhage with resultant transfusion, sepsis, pneumonia, and death than do their noninfected pregnant peers undergoing the same scheduled procedure (odds ratio 1.6) (Louis, 2007). HIV-infected pregnant women without detectable viral loads

should be informed preoperatively of their risk for having morbidity related to cesarean section performed to prevent perinatal HIV transmission. Although intravenous zidovudine was recommended in the past for use throughout labor and delivery, for women with an undetectable viral load during pregnancy, the current recommendation is to continue the current oral ARV regimen throughout labor delivery without the need for intravenous zidovudine.

InSTI-based ART regimens have become the treatment of choice during pregnancy, and treatment recommendations emphasize that the same ART regimen should be used in both pregnant and nonpregnant women, with DTG and RAL being the preferred INSTI drugs of choice. The only exception is in women trying to conceive, where RAL is the preferred regimen and DTG is an alternative recommended drug. Bictegravir is not recommended during pregnancy because of paucity of data, and EVG/c is not recommended because of the cobicistat component (DHHS Panel, 2022).

DIAGNOSIS

Early diagnosis of HIV-1 infection is crucial for identification of at-risk infants and consequent initiation of treatment. All HIV-1 exposed infants carry maternal HIV-1 antibodies until approximately 15–18 months of age. Thus, early pediatric diagnosis relies on identification of the virus, usually via HIV-1 DNA or RNA PCR techniques. The former measures integrated virus in the host genome, and the latter measures circulating plasma virus. HIV-1 co-culture is not routinely performed because of cost and time, although it is also a reliable diagnostic method. Infants infected in utero usually have positive PCR results within the first 48 hours of birth, while infants infected at the time of labor and delivery may have a negative HIV DNA or RNA PCR result at birth, followed by a positive result 1 week to 2 months following birth (Bryson et al., 1992). Breastfed infants have continuing HIV exposure and thus can develop a positive HIV DNA or RNA PCR result at any time. The risk of transmission by breastfeeding from an HIV-positive mother is approximately 16% (Fowler & Newell, 2002). Therefore, repeat PCR testing in the first few months of life is critical for determination of the timing of infection, with sensitivity of a PCR result reaching 96% by 4 weeks of life in the absence of breastfeeding (Dunn et al., 1992; Nielsen & Bryson, 2000). Infant HIV virologic diagnosis requires serial nucleic acid testing. Usually, infants are tested within the first 48 hours of life to detect in utero infection. Current guidelines recommend that infants be tested between 14 and 21 days, 1 and 2 months, and 4 and 6 months of life (DHHS Panel, 2022).

TIMING OF INFECTION

Acquisition of HIV infection may occur in utero, intrapartum, or through breastfeeding. Even before ARV treatment was recommended to pregnant women, two-thirds of HIV-exposed infants escaped HIV infection. Perinatal HIV infection rates have declined substantially in the developed world since 1994, following publication of the landmark PACTG 076 study which demonstrated reduction of perinatal HIV transmission in women who used zidovudine in pregnancy as compared to placebo (Connor et al., 1994). Approximately 30%–50% of infants who contract HIV infection will acquire it in utero, and 50%–70% will acquire the infection during the intrapartum period (Cao et al., 1997; Dickover et al., 1996; Mayaux et al., 1997). In order to characterize the timing of HIV infection, a working definition was created for acquisition of infection in utero and intrapartum (Bryson et al., 1992). An infant is considered to have in utero infection if virologic tests (HIV DNA or RNA PCR) are positive within 48 hours of life. Because of the risk of contamination with maternal blood, cord blood samples should not be used for diagnostic evaluations. Infants are considered to have intrapartum HIV infection if diagnostic tests within the first 48 hours of life are negative but further virologic testing after 1 week of life is positive. There is evidence that most cases of HIV transmission occur late in pregnancy or at delivery.

Postpartum transmission of HIV via breastfeeding has been a continuing problem for the prevention of MTCT of HIV efforts worldwide. HIV can be transmitted as cell-associated or cell-free virus in breastmilk (Lyimo et al., 2012). Mastitis, which triggers migration of inflammatory cells, is also a known risk factor for HIV breastmilk transmission (Semrau et al., 2013), as is nonexclusive breastfeeding (Coutsoudis et al., 1999) or the presence of oral thrush in the infant (Read et al., 2009). Longer duration of breastfeeding is also a well-known risk factor for transmission (Becquet et al., 2005), as is maternal primary infection during lactation (Morrison et al., 2015). In areas where safe alternatives to breastfeeding are not available; however, formula feeding is associated with higher morbidity and mortality. Provision of combination ART to lactating HIV-infected mothers has been demonstrated to significantly increase HIV-free survival in infants with improved infant outcomes in terms of growth and reduced infections (Marazzi et al., 2007, 2009, 2010). Successful screening of pregnant women with availability of ARV treatment for HIV-positive pregnant and lactating women through the WHO B\+ program (WHO, 2019) has decreased early and late postpartum HIV transmission via breastfeeding over time. In women with CD4$^+$ T-cell counts higher than 350/μL in Sub-Saharan Africa, the Promise Study observed a mother-to-child in utero transmission rate of HIV at 1 week of age of 0.5% when women received ART during pregnancy (Fowler et al., 2016). Further follow-up of the same infants revealed very low breastfeeding transmission rates when mothers received ART during lactation (HIV transmission 0.57%) or infants received prophylactic infant nevirapine (HIV transmission 0/58%) during the first 18 months of life or following cessation of breastfeeding, whichever occurred first (Flynn et al., 2018).

The timing of HIV-1 infection (in utero vs. intrapartum) is somewhat predictive of the patient's subsequent clinical course (Dickover et al., 1994). Early onset of AIDS-defining conditions is more frequently observed in in utero–infected

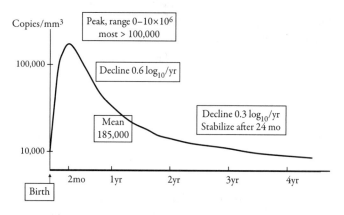

Figure 24.1 Natural course of HIV RNA viremia in children SOURCE: Figure courtesy of Palumbo PE, based on work from Palumbo PE, et al. Predictive value of quantitative plasma HIV RNA and CD4 + lymphocyte count in HIV-infected infants and children. *JAMA.* 1998;279(10):756–761.

infants who sustain early, prolonged elevated HIV RNA levels.

As in adults, prolonged periods of elevated HIV RNA levels are predictive of disease progression. HIV-infected infants undergo primary infection, either in utero or shortly after birth. Therefore, they tend to have very elevated virus loads in the first months of life (Figure 24.1).

MATERNAL RISK FACTORS FOR HIV TRANSMISSION

Maternal risk factors associated with enhanced perinatal HIV transmission identified include untreated HIV disease; seroconversion during pregnancy or breastfeeding; drug abuse; heterosexual infection by sexual partners with risk factors for acquiring HIV disease; presence of maternal syphilis (Yeganeh et al., 2015) and other STIs (Adachi et al., 2015, 2016, 2018a, 2018b); risk of cytomegalovirus (CMV) transmission (Adachi et al., 2017, 2018a, 2018b); and maternal transfusion before 1985. Prospective and retrospective evaluations of maternal predictors for perinatal HIV transmission have been the focus of multiple studies. Maternal transmission predictors identified to date include maternal viremia (measured as quantitative HIV RNA PCR or viral load) (Gabiano et al., 1992; Magder et al., 2005), maternal immunosuppression, or an inadequate immune response (measured by the CD4$^+$ T-cell count, neutralizing antibody production) (Magder et al., 2005), and viral characteristics (chemokine receptor tropism, resistance patterns of maternal virus at delivery or infant virus at birth) (Scarlatti, 2004). Pregnancy and placental variables (e.g., delivery mode, duration of rupture of membranes, and chorioamnionitis) may influence the risk for perinatal transmission of HIV (Mwanyumba et al., 2002; St Louis et al., 1993; International Perinatal HIV Group, 1999). Infant variables evaluated as predictors of transmission of HIV include specific HLA markers and the infant cellular immune response (cytokine production, activated T-cell function) (European Collaborative Study, 1991; Luzuriaga et al., 1991; Magder et al., 2005; Polycarpou et al.,

2002). In addition, immunogenetic factors (chemokine coreceptor expression) have been suggested to confer protection against progression of disease (Sei et al., 2001).

EARLY TREATMENT INITIATION AND HIV REMISSION IN HIV-EXPOSED INFANTS

ART to infants and children suppresses viremia, reduces the high infant mortality, and improves clinical outcome; however, children must continue lifelong ARV treatment. The major barrier to achieving HIV remission in children, as in adults, is the early establishment of long-lived latent cellular reservoirs in $CD4^+$ T-cells and other sites, with continued low-level replication and rebound viremia once taken off ARTs (Persaud et al., 2012). It is postulated that, through treatment of very early HIV infection, the establishment, quantity, or even elimination of latent reservoirs could be achieved by reducing viral spread into memory $CD4^+$ T-cell reservoirs, which would potentially allow patients to thrive off of ARTs without viral rebound, as evidenced by the "Mississippi baby" who remained in ARV-free viral remission for 27 months post early cART (Persaud et al., 2013; Siliciano & Silicano, 2014; Luzuriaga et al., 2015). Importantly, there are emerging data that very early therapy during acute HIV infection in both adults and children quantitatively modifies HIV persistence and may influence the rate of reservoir decay. This approach is presently being further evaluated in ongoing clinical trials such as IMPAACT P1115 (Persaud et al., 2022).

DISEASE COURSE

The natural history of pediatric HIV-1 infection is bimodal (Scott, 1991). Studies conducted in developed countries prior to the availability of ARVs demonstrate that approximately 20% of children exhibit very rapid disease progression, with rapid loss of $CD4^+$ T-cell counts and development of AIDS-defining conditions before 2 years of age (Nielsen et al., 1997). The majority of HIV-infected children, however (approximately 60%–65%) will have intermediate disease progression, with the presence of AIDS-defining events by 7–8 years of age. There is a small subset of children (as there is in adults), approximately 15%–20% of patients, who have very slow to no disease progression by age 8 years, and an even smaller set of elite controllers (< 5%). These children enter adolescence with minimal to no symptoms of HIV disease. Studies conducted in Africa have demonstrated an even faster pace of disease progression, with the majority of pediatric patients having AIDS-defining conditions by age 5 years (Newell et al., 2004). This might be due to the higher overall burden of disease and presence of multiple coinfections. ART makes it possible to alter the natural history of HIV disease and transform disease progressors into nonprogressors. This translates into improvements in the quality of life and reduction in HIV-associated disease morbidity and mortality.

Infants with in utero infection appear to have a more rapid disease course when compared to infants who acquire HIV infection intrapartum (Dickover et al., 1996). In utero–infected infants still have normal $CD4^+$ T-cell values at birth and are usually born with a low virus load (as measured by DNA or RNA PCR) (Mayaux et al., 1996). In addition, even in utero–HIV-infected infants are asymptomatic at birth. In utero HIV appears to result from transplacental passage of virus or ascending viral infection in patients with prolonged rupture of membranes (Minkoff et al., 1995). In the animal model, researchers have demonstrated that viral infection of the amniotic fluid with simian immunodeficiency virus resulted in infection of all the offspring (Van Rompay et al., 1995). Intrapartum transmission of HIV infection is responsible for the majority of perinatal cases. In a prospective study of 271 HIV-infected infants using HIV DNA PCR, 38% of children were found to be positive within 48 hours of life; 93% were positive by 14 days of age; and 96% of the total number of infected children were positive by 4 weeks of age (Dunn et al., 1992). There are infants who might not have detectable virus as late as 3 months following delivery in selected cases. Untreated infants tend to maintain a very high virus burden throughout their first year of life, and immunologic patterns of primary viremia in infants have long been described (Luzuriaga et al., 1997). High-level viremia might persist for a longer period of time in infants than in adults undergoing primary infection; untreated early infection is associated with a high mortality risk (Violari et al., 2008). Many years prior to the advent of cART, discordant twin infections were reported, with the firstborn twin having a higher risk of infection (Duliege et al., 1995).

SURROGATE MARKERS OF DISEASE

The goal of ART is to reduce the HIV-1 viral load as much as possible while restoring or preserving immune function. Viral load is generally measured via plasma HIV-1 RNA reverse transcriptase (RT) PCR (Roche Molecular Systems), HIV RNA quantitation by branched (b) DNA (Chiron Corporation), or nucleic acid sequence-based amplification (NASBA) HIV-1 RNA quantitative (QT) assay (Organon Teknika). All three methods are reliable parameters for the measurement of free virus in plasma, with new-generation assays being able to identify virus isolates of different subtypes. Immune function in HIV disease is measured primarily by evaluating T-cell subsets, particularly $CD4^+$ T-cell absolute numbers and percentages. Three-color flow cytometry is generally the methodology employed for this purpose. Declining counts parallel disease progression, with declines in $CD4^+$ T-cells usually following peak HIV RNA viremia. One important caveat in the management of HIV-infected children is that $CD4^+$ T-cell numbers, particularly in infants, differ significantly from adults and do not achieve similar levels until after 5 years. Therefore, an infant with a $CD4^+$ T-cell count of 750 cells/mm^3 or less is at significant risk for development of AIDS-defining conditions because normal values are generally greater than 2,000 cells/mm^3.

ANTIRETROVIRALS IN CHILDREN

One general principle in the use of ARV therapy is that continued viral replication in the presence of ARV drugs promotes development of drug resistance. Resistance to one specific ARV agent may in turn confer resistance to other drugs within the same class. Current standard of practice is that, once therapy is started, long-term or lifelong treatment is warranted. In children, the efficacy of ARV therapy often is extrapolated from data obtained from adult clinical trials because of lack of pediatric data. There are, however, significant age-related differences between children and adults. These encompass body composition, renal excretion, liver metabolism, and gastrointestinal function. This leads to differences in drug distribution and metabolism, drug clearance, drug dosing, and different toxicities between children and adults. In addition, protein binding and drug clearance of some specific ARVs may differ by race, owing to the presence of genetic polymorphisms. Nevertheless, often therapeutic doses for infants and children are not available. Liquid or palatable formulations for children do not exist for many ARVs, and adherence depends on adult caretakers. It is crucial when initiating ARV therapy to take into consideration the presence of comorbidities and concomitant medications in order to avoid overlapping drug toxicities. It is also important to consider cross-resistance and later therapeutic options.

GUIDELINES

Treatment guidelines have been developed over the years in order to address critical concerns about the use of ARV therapy in children. Major concerns have always included the optimal timing of initiation of ARV therapy, the preferred choice of ARVs, best ways to monitor efficacy and toxicities, and when to change therapy. There are decreased variations in guidelines between developed and developing countries. In the United States, traditionally, most children have been treated when identified as having HIV-1 infection, regardless of symptomatology. Given multiple therapeutic options and the general availability of viral load monitoring, guidelines in developed countries over the years have relied on virus load measures for predicting early switches in therapy (Panel on Antiretroviral Therapy and Medical Management of HIV-Infected Children, 2022). Randomized clinical trials, such as the Children with HIV Early Antiretroviral Therapy trial (CHER) in South Africa, demonstrated that early ARV treatment to infants diagnosed before 12 months of age is clearly beneficial in reducing morbidity and mortality (Violari et al., 2008).

The current US pediatric ARV treatment guidelines Panel has increased the strength of its recommendations for initiating ART in all children at the time of diagnosis and considers prompt initiation of treatment a medical emergency (Panel on Antiretroviral Therapy and Medical Management, 2022). Thus, the Panel recommends that all children receive ART, regardless of symptoms or CD4$^+$ T-cell count. WHO treatment guidelines for treatment of children with HIV infection also reflect the need for early treatment initiation (WHO, 2019).

TIMING OF INITIATION OF THERAPY

Early versus deferred initiation of ARV treatment in HIV-infected children was a controversial matter, but this is no longer a subject of debate. It is currently universally accepted in both the developed and developing world that ART should be started at the time of HIV diagnosis in all children, regardless of age. Starting therapy early in asymptomatic children controls viral replication before genetic mutations develop, leading to fewer number of circulating viral strains. It also prevents immune system destruction and avoids disease progression, including prevention of establishment of viral reservoirs in the brain. With this strategy, viral seeding of latent cells or CD4$^+$ T-cell reservoirs can often be circumvented. Given the significant repercussions to cognitive development when treatment is delayed, there is no justification at the present time to delay treatment to HIV-infected children.

CHANGE IN THERAPY

The decision to change ARVs varies slightly according to the pediatric guidelines employed. The variability is mostly due to the surrogate markers used. Nevertheless, most experts would agree that indicators of treatment failure include progression of HIV disease, growth failure, development of opportunistic infections while on established therapy, decline in CD4$^+$ percentiles, development or worsening HIV encephalopathy, and significant increases in virus load. Tolerability, palatability, and drug toxicities are also reasons why ARV regimens are switched in children, as in adults. Simplification of treatment regimens are recommended whenever possible, as the greatest predictor of achieving an undetectable plasma virus load is adherence.

SPECIFIC ANTIRETROVIRAL AGENTS

ARVs currently available for use in the United States are listed in Table 24.1. Optimal ARV combinations for children may differ slightly from that of adults. In infants, particularly those younger than 1 year of age, there is often a need to use very potent ARV regimens for reduction of persistently elevated viral loads (Luzuriaga et al., 2004; Palumbo et al., 2010). Therefore, in this scenario, four-drug combinations including a PI, two nucleoside analogs, and a nonnucleoside analog such as nevirapine may be indicated. The use of many ARVs is also limited in younger children (especially those younger than 4 years old) because of the lack of liquid formulations, as depicted in Table 24.1. Prevalent ART regimens in pediatrics include one PI such as ritonavir/lopinavir, or atazanavir or darunavir (in older children) in combination with a double NRTI backbone. The PIs may be substituted with NNRTIs such as nevirapine or efavirenz (the latter in older children). Specific ARV regimens to be avoided include any type of mono or dual therapy, and atazanavir without boosting. Treatment guidelines currently recommend use of integrase inhibitors in children as preferred regimens, contingent on availability

Table 24.1 ARVS AVAILABLE FOR TREATMENT IN THE UNITED STATES

NRTIs:	**PIs:**
Zidovudine (ZDV/AZT)[a]	Saquinavir mesylate (SQV)
Lamivudine (3TC)[a]	Ritonavir[a] (RTV)
Abacavir (ABC)[a]	Lopinavir/ritonavir[a] (LPV/r)
Tenofovir disoproxil fumarate (TDF)	Atazanavir ATV)
Tenofovir alafenamide (TAF)	Darunavir (DRV)
Emtricitabine (FTC)	Tipranavir (TPV)
NNRTIs:	**Fusion inhibitors:**
Nevirapine[a] (NVP)	Enfuvirtide (ENF)
Efavirenz (EFV)	**R-5 receptor inhibitors:**
Etravirine (ETR)	Maraviroc (MVC)
Rilpivirine (RPV)	**Attachment inhibitors:**
Doravirine (DOR)	Fostemsavir (FTR)
	Post-attachment Inhibitors:
	Ibalizumab-uiyk (IBA)
Combination ARVs[b]:	**Integrase inhibitors:**
ZDV/3TC	Raltegravir (RAL)
ZDV/3TC/ABC	Dolutegravir (DTG)
TDF/FTC or TAF/FTC	*Elvitegravir (EVG)*
3TC/TDF	*Bictegravir (BIC)*
ABC/3TC	*Cabotegravir (long-acting*
ABC/DTG/3TC	*injectable agent, CAB)*
EFV/TDF/FTC	
EFV/3TC/TDF	
FTC/RPV/TDF (or TAF)	
ATZ/cobi	
BIC/FTC/TAF	
DRV/cobi	
DRV/cobi/FTC/TAF	
DTG/3TC	
DTG/RPV	
DOR/3TC/TDF	
EVG/cobi/FTC/TDF (or TAF)	
LPV/r	
CAB/RPV	

[a]Pediatric formulations available.

[b]Additional formulations such as NVP/ZDV/3TC and NVP/D4T/3TC are available to children in pediatric formulations as generic drugs in resource-limited settings.

of pediatric formulations. In resource-limited settings, treatment studies have demonstrated greater durability of viral load suppression in children treated with ritonavir/lopinavir-based regimens as opposed to nevirapine-based regimens, although, interestingly, nevirapine has been shown to be associated with improved growth in this population (Chadwick et al., 2011). RAL and DTG have been increasingly recommended for use in the pediatric population in WHO guidelines. Pediatric US guidelines are extensively detailed in the following website: https://clinicalinfo.hiv.gov/en/guidelines/pediatric-arv.

TOXICITIES AND ADVERSE EFFECTS

The complications and side effects of specific ARV are multiple. The most frequent toxicities of zidovudine are hematologic, particularly, anemia and neutropenia. These may resolve with dose reduction. All NRTIs may cause some degree of mitochondrial toxicity. Zidovudine may cause myopathy, and peripheral neuropathy is seen with this drug and rarely with 3TC. Abacavir is uncommonly to rarely associated with a potentially fatal hypersensitivity reaction, which occurs in 1% of pediatric patients. It presents flu-like symptoms with or without a rash, abdominal pain, sore throat, and myalgias. If the drug has been interrupted in this scenario, shock will ensue when restarted. The NNRTIs most commonly cause skin rashes (about 40%) and have rarely been associated with Steven-Johnsons syndrome. There were concerns for the potential for efavirenz to be teratogenic inducing neural tube defects when used in the first trimester of pregnancy; however, they have not been demonstrated after large scale use of the drug worldwide (Ford et al., 2014). Efavirenz (EFV) can induce central nervous system findings such as dizziness, insomnia, and nightmares, which have been reported shortly after initiation of treatment with this drug. There was concern about the use of nevirapine during pregnancy in women with CD4 [+] T-cell counts greater than 250/mm^3 because of an increased risk of hepatic failure (Hitti, 2004), but additional studies failed to demonstrate an association (De Lazzari, 2008).

PIs have multiple drug–drug interactions because of their cytochrome P450 metabolism in the liver. Their most common side effects are gastrointestinal symptoms. Hepatitis and hyperbilirubinemia are not uncommon. In adults, they have been shown to induce lipodystrophy, diabetes, and increased atherosclerosis because of lipid abnormalities. These findings are now being recognized in children, although complications are to a lesser extent. There are also recent concerns about the potential for osteopenia and osteoporosis in children, either induced by ART (notably TDF) or HIV disease itself (Mora, 2004). With TAF increasingly replacing TDF use, it is likely that the concerns for osteopenia will decline over time.

Integrase inhibitors are generally well-tolerated medications with reduced toxicities. One major recent concern was the use of DTG during pregnancy and the potential for teratogenicity. Following the announcement of the launching of DTG to over 90 low- and middle-income countries at reduced pricing by UNAIDS and other partners in 2017, a report of neural tube defects following DTG treatment in pregnant women from the time of conception came forward in 2018 (Zash et al., 2018). This was data generated by the Tsepamo Study in Botswana with performed surveillance of birth outcomes at government maternity sites since 2014. The study was specifically designed to evaluate for potential neural tube defects following exposure to EFV at conception and for other adverse birth outcomes stratified by maternal HIV status and ART regimen. DTG was rolled out in Botswana in 2016. In May 2018, a prevalence of 0.94% of neural tube defects (4 cases in 426 participants) was noted in women who had been on DTG at conception. This contrasted with a prevalence of 0.12% for other women on non-DTG ART regimens at conception, 0.05% of women on EFV at conception, zero women who started DTG during pregnancy, and 0.09% of HIV negative women (Zash et al., 2018). An update of study results in March 2019 when 1683 participants who received DTG arm since the time of conception demonstrated an incidence of neural tube defects of 0.30% (5 in 1,683 cases) (Zash et al., 2019). More recent data reported until April 2020 has shown a decline in the incidence of neural tube defects in women receiving DTG at conception, with an incidence of 0.19% (7 cases in 3,591 exposures). Subsequent studies have failed to demonstrate neural tube defects associated with DTG use during conception, including the IMPAACT 2010 or the VESTED trial which compared regimens containing EFV and DTG during pregnancy (Chinula et al., 2020). Based on these findings, the WHO recommended DTG as the preferred HIV treatment option in all populations. DHHS guidelines also recommend the use of DTG during pregnancy, but list the drug as an alternative drug regimen for women planning to conceive, with RAL being the preferred INSTI in this scenario (DHHS, 2020).

IMMUNE RECONSTITUTION INFLAMMATORY SYNDROME

One recognized potential complication of potent ARV therapy is the immune reconstitution inflammatory syndrome. It is most frequently observed in patients who initiate ART with low CD4 $^+$ T-cell counts. It is associated with a wide range of reactivation of previously latent pathogens, with tuberculosis being a common underlying condition. The underlying pathogenesis appears to start with unrecognized, low-level colonization of opportunistic pathogens in patients who have moderate to severe immunosuppression. With the initiation of ART and subsequent recovery of immunity to the organism, there is a paradoxical clinical deterioration owing to a dysregulated, overly exuberant immune response. This syndrome usually presents in the first 6 weeks of ART and may resolve either with the use of steroids or temporary discontinuation of ART. It is infrequently seen in pediatric HIV practiced in developed countries, particularly because children are generally treated earlier. However, it is prevalent in the developing world and may carry high morbidity and mortality. As more children are treated early and soon after diagnosis, it should become an increasingly rare complication of ART use in pediatric populations.

BENEFITS OF THERAPY

Despite the complications and controversies, the benefits of ART in children with HIV are overwhelming. In the United States, the annual mortality in pediatric HIV patients decreased to less than 1% as of 1999 because of the availability of treatment (Gortmaker et al., 2001; Jeremy et al., 2005). ART decreases the virus load, preserves and restores the immune function, decreases the risk of comorbidities, decreases hospitalizations, improves survival, improves quality of life, and restores hope to children and their families. Many perinatally infected children who initiated treatment early in life are now adults who have families and children of their own. ART has also changed the AIDS paradigm. As one patient once said, HIV is no longer a disease you die from, but a disease you live with.

REFERENCES

Adachi K, Klausner JD, Bristow CC, et al.; NICHD HPTN 040 Study Team. Chlamydia and gonorrhea in HIV-infected pregnant women and infant HIV transmission. *Sex Transm Dis.* 2015;42(10):554–565.

Adachi K, Klausner JD, Xu J, et al.; NICHD HPTN 040 Study Team. Chlamydia trachomatis and Neisseria gonorrhoeae in HIV-infected pregnant women and adverse infant outcomes. *Pediatr Infect Dis J.* 2016;35(8):894–900.

Adachi K, Xu J, Ank B, et al.; NICHD HPTN 040 Study Team. Congenital cytomegalovirus and HIV perinatal transmission. *Pediatr Infect Dis J.* 2018b;37(10):1016–1021.

Adachi K, Xu J, Ank B, et al.; NICHD HPTN 040 Study Team. Cytomegalovirus urinary shedding in HIV-infected pregnant women and congenital cytomegalovirus infection. *Clin Infect Dis.* 2017;65(3):405–413.

Adachi K, Xu J, Yeganeh N, et al.; NICHD HPTN 040 Study Team. Combined evaluation of sexually transmitted infections in HIV-infected pregnant women and infant HIV transmission. *PLoS One.* 2018a;13(1):e0189851.

Becquet R, Ekouevi DK, Viho I, et al. Acceptability of exclusive breastfeeding with early cessation to prevent HIV transmission through breast milk, ANRS 1201/1202 ditrame plus, abidjan, Cote d'Ivoire. *J AIDS.* 2005;40(5):600–608.

Bryson YJ, Luzuriaga K, Sullivan JL, et al. Proposed definitions for in utero versus intrapartum transmission of HIV-1. *N Engl J Med.* 1992;327:1246–1247.

Cao Y, Krogstad P, Korber BT, et al. Maternal HIV-1 viral load and vertical transmission of infection: the Ariel Project for the prevention of HIV transmission from mother to infant. *Nat Med.* 1997;3(5):549–552.

CDC, HIV Surveillance Report. Diagnoses of HIV infection in the United States and dependent areas 2020. https://www.cdc.gov/hiv/library/reports/hiv-surveillance/vol-33/index.html. Published 2020. Accessed September 30, 2022.

Chadwick EG, Yogev R, Alvero CG, et al.; International Pediatric Adolescent Clinical Trials Group (IMPAACT) P1030 Team. Long-term outcomes for HIV-infected infants less than 6 months of age at initiation of lopinavir/ritonavir combination antiretroviral therapy. *AIDS.* 2011;25:643–649.

Chinula L, Brummel SS, Ziemba L, et al. Safety and efficacy of DTG vs EFV and TDF vs TAF in pregnancy: IMPAACT 2010 trial. [Abstract 130LB]. Presented at the *Conference on Retroviruses and Opportunistic Infections.* Boston, MA; March 8–11, 2020.

Clarke D, Acost EP, Cababasay M, et al.; International Pediatric Adolescent Clinical Trials Group (IMPAACT) P1110 Team. Raltegravir (RAL) in neonates: dosing, pharmacokinetics (PK), and safety in HIV-1–exposed neonates at risk of infection (IMPAACT P1110), *JAIDS.* 2020; 84:70–77.

Committee on Obstetric Practice. ACOG committee opinion scheduled cesarean delivery and the prevention of vertical transmission of HIV infection: number 234, May 2000 (replaces number 219, August 1999). *Int J Gynaecol Obstet.* 2001;73:279–281.

Connor EM, Sperling RS, Gelber R, et al. Reduction of maternal-infant transmission of human immunodeficiency virus type 1 with zidovudine treatment. Pediatric AIDS Clinical Trials Group Protocol 076 Study Group. *N Engl J Med.* 1994;331(18):1173–1180.

Coovadia HM, Brown ER, Fowler MG, et al.; HPTN 046 Protocol Team. Efficacy and safety of an extended nevirapine regimen in infant children of breastfeeding mothers with HIV-1 infection for prevention of postnatal HIV-1 transmission (HPTN 046): a randomised, double-blind, placebo-controlled trial. *Lancet.* 2012; 379(9812):221–228.

Coutsoudis A, Pillay K, Spooner E, et al. Influence of infant-feeding patterns on early mother-to-child transmission of HIV-1 in Durban, South Africa: a prospective cohort study. South African Vitamin A Study Group. *Lancet*. 1999;354(9177):471–476.

De Lazzari E, León A, Arnaiz JA, et al. Hepatotoxicity of nevirapine in virologically suppressed patients according to gender and CD4 cell counts. *HIV Med*. 2008;9:221–226.

de Lourdes Teixeira M, Nafea S, Yeganeh N, et al. High rates of baseline antiretroviral resistance among HIV-infected pregnant women in an HIV referral centre in Rio de Janeiro, Brazil. *Int J STD AIDS*. November 2015;26(13):922–928.

DHHS. Recommendations for the use of antiretroviral drugs in pregnant women with HIV infection and interventions to reduce perinatal HIV transmission in the United States. https://clinicalinfo.hiv.gov/en/guidelines/perinatal/whats-new-guidelines. Published 2020. Accessed October 1, 2020.

Dickover RE, Dillon M, Gillette SG, et al. Rapid increases in load of human immunodeficiency virus correlate with early disease progression and loss of CD4 cells in vertically infected infants. *J Infect Dis*. 1994;170:1279–1284.

Dickover RE, Garratty EM, Herman SA, et al. Identification of levels of maternal HIV-1 RNA associated with risk of perinatal transmission. Effect of maternal zidovudine treatment on viral load. *JAMA*. 1996;275(8):599–605.

Dorenbaum A, Cunningham CK, Gelber RD, et al. Two-dose intrapartum/newborn nevirapine and standard antiretroviral therapy to reduce perinatal HIV transmission: a randomized trial. *JAMA*. 2002;288:189–198.

Duliege AM, Amos CI, Felton S, et al. Birth order, delivery route, and concordance in the transmission of human immunodeficiency virus type 1 from mothers to twins. International Registry of HIV-Exposed Twins. *J Pediatr*. 1995;126:625–632.

Dunn DT, Newell ML, Ades AE, et al. Risk of human immunodeficiency virus type 1 transmission through breastfeeding. *Lancet*. 1992;340:585–588.

European Collaborative Study. Children born to women with HIV-1 infection: natural history and risk of transmission. *Lancet*. 1991;337:253–260.

Ford N, Mofenson L, Shubber Z, et al. Safety of efavirenz in the first trimester of pregnancy: an updated systematic review and meta-analysis, *AIDS*: 2014; 28:S123–S131.

Flynn PM, Taha TE, Cababasay M, et al. Prevention of HIV-1 transmission through breastfeeding: efficacy and safety of maternal antiretroviral therapy versus infant nevirapine prophylaxis for duration of breastfeeding in HIV-1-infected women with high CD4 cell count (IMPAACT PROMISE): a randomized, open-label, clinical trial. *J AIDS*. April 1, 2018;77(4):383–392.

Fowler MG, Newell ML. Breastfeeding and HIV-1 transmission in resource-limited settings. *J AIDS*. 2002;30:230–239.

Fowler MG, Qin M, Fiscus SA, et al. Benefits and risks of antiretroviral therapy for perinatal HIV prevention. *N Engl J Med*. 2016;375(18):1726–1737.

Gabiano C, Tovo PA, de Martino M, et al. Mother-to-child transmission of human immunodeficiency virus type 1: risk of infection and correlates of transmission. *Pediatrics*. 1992;90:369–374.

Gortmaker SL, Hughes M, Cervia J, et al.; Pediatric AIDS Clinical Trials Group Protocol 219 Team. Effect of combination therapy including protease inhibitors on mortality among children and adolescents infected with HIV-1. *N Engl J Med*. 2001;345(21):1522–1528.

Guay LA, Musoke P, Fleming T, et al. Intrapartum and neonatal single-dose nevirapine compared with zidovudine for prevention of mother-to-child transmission of HIV-1 in Kampala, Uganda: HIVNET 012 randomised trial. *Lancet*. 1999;354(9181):795–802.

Hitti J, Frenkel LM, Stek AM, et al.; PACTG 1022 Study Team. Maternal toxicity with continuous nevirapine in pregnancy: results from PACTG 1022. *J AIDS*. 2004;36:772–776.

International Perinatal HIV Group. The mode of delivery and the risk of vertical transmission of human immunodeficiency virus type 1—a meta-analysis of 15 prospective cohort studies. *N Engl J Med*. 1999;340(13):977–987.

Jeremy RJ, Kim S, Nozyce M, et al.; Pediatric AIDS Clinical Trials Group (PACTG) 338 & 377 Study Teams. Neuropsychological functioning and viral load in stable antiretroviral therapy-experienced HIV-infected children. *Pediatrics*. 2005;115:380–387.

Lahoz R, Noguera A, Rovira N, et al. Antiretroviral-related hematologic short-term toxicity in healthy infants: implications of the new neonatal 4-week zidovudine regimen. *Ped Inf Dis J*. 2010;29(4):376–379.

Louis J, Landon MB, Gersnoviez RJ, et al. Perioperative morbidity and mortality among human immunodeficiency virus infected women undergoing cesarean delivery. *Obstet Gynecol* 2007;110(2 Pt 1):385–390.

Luzuriaga K, Bryson Y, Krogstad P, et al. Combination treatment with zidovudine, didanosine, and nevirapine in infants with human immunodeficiency virus type 1 infection. *N Engl J Med*. 1997;336:1343–1349.

Luzuriaga K, Gay H, Ziemniak C, et al. Viremic relapse after HIV-1 remission in a perinatally infected child. *N Engl J Med*. 2015;372:786–788.

Luzuriaga K, Koup RA, Pikora CA, et al. Deficient human immunodeficiency virus type 1-specific cytotoxic T cell responses in vertically infected children. *J Pediatr*. 1991;119:230–236.

Luzuriaga K, McManus M, Mofenson L, et al.; PACTG 356 Investigators. A trial of three antiretroviral regimens in HIV-1-infected children. *N Engl J Med*. 2004; 350(24):2471–2480.

Lyimo MA, Mosi MN, Housman ML, et al. Breast milk from Tanzanian women has divergent effects on cell-free and cell-associated HIV-1 infection in vitro. *PLoS One*. 2012;7(8):e43815.

Magder LS, Mofenson L, Paul ME, et al. Risk factors for in utero and intrapartum transmission of HIV. *J AIDS*. 2005;38:87–95.

Marazzi CM, Germano P, Liotta G, et al. Implementing anti-retroviral triple therapy to prevent HIV mother-to-child transmission: a public health approach in resource-limited settings. *Eur J Pediatr*. 2007;166(12):1305–1307.

Marazzi MC, Liotta G, Nielsen-Saines K, et al. Extended antenatal antiretroviral use correlates with improved infant outcomes throughout the first year of life. *AIDS*. 2010;24(18):2819–2826.

Marazzi MC, Nielsen-Saines K, Buonomo E, et al. Increased infant human immunodeficiency virus-type one free survival at one year of age in sub-Saharan Africa with maternal use of highly active antiretroviral therapy during breast-feeding. *Ped Inf Dis J*. 2009;28(6):483–487.

Mayaux MJ, Burgard M, Teglas JP, et al. Neonatal characteristics in rapidly progressive perinatally acquired HIV-1 disease. The French Pediatric HIV Infection Study Group. *JAMA*. 1996;275:606–610.

Mayaux MJ, Dussaix E, Isopet J, et al. Maternal virus load during pregnancy and mother-to-child transmission of human immunodeficiency virus type 1: the French perinatal cohort studies. SEROGEST cohort group. *J Infect Dis*. 1997;175(1):172–175.

Minkoff H, Burns DN, Landesman S, et al. The relationship of the duration of ruptured membranes to vertical transmission of human immunodeficiency virus. *Am J Obstet Gynecol*. 1995;173:585–589.

Mora S, Zamproni I, Beccio S, et al. Longitudinal changes of bone mineral density and metabolism in antiretroviral-treated human immunodeficiency virus-infected children. *J Clin Endocrinol Metab*. 2004;89:24–28.

Morrison S, John-Stewart G, Egessa JJ, et al. Rapid antiretroviral therapy initiation for women in an HIV-1 prevention clinical trial experiencing primary HIV-1 infection during pregnancy or breastfeeding. *PLoS One*. 2015;10(10):e0140773.

Mwanyumba F, Gaillard P, Inion I, et al. Placental inflammation and perinatal transmission of HIV-1. *J AIDS*. 2002;29:262–269.

Newell ML. The natural history of vertically acquired HIV infection. The European Collaborative Study. *J Perinat Med*. 1991;19(Suppl 1):257–262.

Newell ML, Coovadia H, Cortina-Borja M, et al.; Ghent International AIDS Society (IAS) Working Group on HIV Infection in Women and Children. Mortality of infected and uninfected infants born to HIV-infected mothers in Africa: a pooled analysis. *Lancet*. 2004;364:1236–1243.

Nielsen K, Bryson YJ. Diagnosis of HIV infection in children. *Pediatr Clin N Am*. 2000;47:39–63.

Nielsen K, McSherry G, Petru A, et al. A descriptive survey of pediatric human immunodeficiency virus-infected long-term survivors. *Pediatrics*. 1997;99:pe4.

Nielsen-Saines K, Watts DH, Veloso VG, et al.; for the NICHD HPTN 040/ PACTG 1043 Protocol Team. Phase III randomized trial of the safety and efficacy of three neonatal antiretroviral regimens for prevention of intrapartum HIV-1 transmission (NICHD HPTN 040/ PACTG 1043). [Late Breaker Abstract 124LB]. Presented at the *18th Conference on Retroviruses and Opportunistic Infections*. Boston, MA; February 27–March 2, 2011.

Palumbo P, Lindsey JC, Hughes MD, et al. Antiretroviral treatment for children with peripartum nevirapine exposure. *N Engl J Med*. 2010;363:1510–1520.

Palumbo PE, Raskino C, Fiscus S, et al. Predictive value of quantitative plasma HIV RNA and CD4\+ lymphocyte count in HIV-infected infants and children. *JAMA*. 1998;279:756–761.

Panel on Antiretroviral Therapy and Medical Management of HIV-Infected Children. Guidelines for the use of antiretroviral agents in pediatric HIV infection. https:// clinicalinfo.hiv.gov/en/guidelines/pediatric-arv/whats-new-guidelines. Updated April 11, 2022. Accessed September 29, 2022.

Panel on Treatment of HIV During Pregnancy and Prevention of Perinatal Transmission. Recommendations for the use of antiretroviral drugs during pregnancy and interventions to reduce perinatal HIV transmission in the United States. https://clinicalinfo.hiv.gov/en/guidelines/perinatal/whats-new-guidelines. Updated March 17, 2022. Accessed September 29, 2022.

Persaud D, Gay G, Ziemniak C, et al. Absence of detectable HIV-1 viremia after treatment cessation in an infant. *N Engl J Med*. 2013;369:1828–1835.

Persaud D, Palumbo PE, Ziemniak C, et al. Dynamics of the resting CD4\+ T cell latent HIV reservoir in infants initiating highly active antiretroviral therapy less than six months of age. *AIDS*. July 31, 2012;26(12):1483–1490.

Persaud D, Chadwick E, Nelson B, et al. Two year virologic outcomes of very early ART for infants enrolled in P1115. *Conference on Retroviruses and Opportunistic Infections*. Abstract O-02. February 12–16, 2022. Virtual.

Polycarpou A, Ntais C, Korber BT, et al. Association between maternal and infant class I and II HLA alleles and of their concordance with the risk of perinatal HIV type 1 transmission. *AIDS. Res Hum Retroviruses*. 2002;18:741–746.

Read JS, Mwatha A, Richardson B, et al. Primary HIV-1 infection among infants in sub-Saharan Africa: HPTN 024. *J AIDS*. 2009;51(3):317–322.

Ruane PJ, DeJesus E, Berger D, et al. Antiviral activity, safety, and pharmacokinetics/pharmacodynamics of tenofovir alafenamide as 10-day monotherapy in HIV-1-positive adults. *J AIDS*. 2013;63(4):449–455.

Scarlatti G. Mother-to-child transmission of HIV-1: advances and controversies of the twentieth centuries. *AIDS Rev*. 2004;6:67–78.

Scott GB. HIV infection in children: clinical features and management. *J AIDS*. 1991;4:109–115.

Scott GB, Hutto C, Makuch RW, et al. Survival in children with perinatally acquired human immunodeficiency virus type 1 infection. *N Engl J Med*.1989;321:1791–1796.

Sei S, Boler AM, Nguyen GT, et al. Protective effect of CCR5 delta 32 heterozygosity is restricted by SDF-1 genotype in children with HIV-1 infection. *AIDS*. 2001;15:1343–1352.

Semrau K, Kuhn L, Brooks DR, et al. Dynamics of breast milk HIV-1 RNA with unilateral mastitis or abscess. *J AIDS*. 2013;62(3):348–355.

Siliciano JD, Siliciano RF. Recent developments in the search for a cure for HIV-1 infections: targeting the latent reservoir for HIV-1. *J Allergy Clin Immunol*. 2014;134:12–19.

St Louis ME, Kamenga M, Brown C, et al. Risk for perinatal HIV-1 transmission according to maternal immunologic, virologic, and placental factors. *JAMA*. 1993;269:2853–2859.

UNICEF. Elimination of mother to child HIV transmission. https://data.unicef.org/topic/hivaids/emtct/. Published 2022. Accessed September 29, 2022.

USAID. Prevention of mother to child transmission (PMTCT) | U.S. Agency for International Development. usaid.gov. https:// www.usaid.gov/global-health/health-areas/hiv-and-aids/technical-areas/pmtct. Published 2022. Assessed September 29, 2022.

Van Rompay KK, Otsyula MG, Marthas ML, et al. Immediate zidovudine treatment protects simian immunodeficiency virus-infected newborn macaques against rapid onset of AIDS. *Antimicrob Agents Chemother*. 1995;39:125–131.

Violari A, Cotton MF, Gibb DM, et al.; CHER Study Team. Early antiretroviral therapy and mortality among HIV-infected infants. *N Engl J Med*. 2008;359:2233–2244.

World Health Organization (WHO). Updated recommendations on first-line and second-line antiretroviral regimens July 2019. https://www.who.int/publications/i/item/WHO-CDS-HIV-19.15. Published July 2019. Accessed September 30, 2022.

Yeganeh N, Kerin T, Ank B, et al. HIV antiretroviral resistance and transmission in mother-infant pairs enrolled in a large perinatal study. *Clin Inf Dis*. 2018;66(11):1770–1777.

Yeganeh N, Watts HD, Camarca M, et al. Syphilis in HIV-infected mothers and infants: results from the NICHD/HPTN 040 study. *Pediatr Infect Dis J*. 2015;34(3):e52–e57.

Zash R, Holmes L, Diseko M, et al. Neural-tube defects and antiretroviral treatment regimens in Botswana. *N Engl J Med*. 2019;381(9):827–840.

Zash R, Makhema J, Shapiro RL. Neural-tube defects with dolutegravir treatment from the time of conception. *N Engl J Med*. 2018;379(10):979–981.

25.

UNDERSTANDING AND MANAGING ANTINEOPLASTIC AND ANTIRETROVIRAL THERAPY

Elizabeth M. Sherman and Taylor K. Gill

LEARNING OBJECTIVE

To review concepts regarding the safe and effective use of antineoplastic and antiretroviral therapy (ART) in people living with HIV and cancer.

WHAT'S NEW?

The disease states of HIV and cancer are constantly evolving. New therapies are introduced, and literature published advancing each area. Specifically, new oral agents and long-acting antiretrovirals for HIV and immunotherapy for cancer treatment bring exciting advancements.

KEY POINTS

- The use of combination ART in people with HIV and malignancies is associated with improved HIV- and cancer-related outcomes.

- Combining ART and antineoplastic therapy is often complicated by significant drug–drug interactions, drug–disease state monitoring interactions, and overlapping toxicities.

- Definitive studies including both antineoplastics and antiretrovirals are uncommon, and clinical judgment must often be used to determine the appropriate course of treatment.

- Adjusting ART in response to significant drug interactions or overlapping toxicities is often more feasible than modifying antineoplastic protocols.

- A multidisciplinary care team that includes primary care providers, infectious disease clinicians, hematologists/oncologists, and clinical pharmacists should be utilized to address the challenges of combining HIV and cancer treatment.

INTRODUCTION TO CANCER IN HIV

The incidence of cancer among persons with HIV (PWH) is nearly 50% greater than the general population (National Comprehensive Cancer Network (NCCN) Guidelines, 2022). The elevated risk of cancer in PWH is multifactorial and likely due to a combination of underlying immune deficiency, coinfection with oncogenic viruses, and a higher prevalence of other cancer-related risk factors such as the use of tobacco and alcohol products.

Before the widespread use of ART, AIDS-defining malignancies (ADMs) such as Kaposi's sarcoma, non-Hodgkin's lymphoma, and invasive cervical cancer accounted for the largest burden of cancer in PWH (Rubinstein et al., 2014). These malignancies occur most commonly in people with advanced HIV, and all are associated with oncogenic viruses. Following the widespread use of ART in the mid-1990s, there was a substantial decline in the number of new AIDS diagnoses and AIDS-related deaths (Rubinstein et al., 2014). The ability to reconstitute the immune system with ART also led to a decrease in ADMs. At the same time, the occurrence of non-AIDS-defining malignancies (NADMs) increased. These malignancies include Hodgkin's lymphoma, leukemia, and cancers of the head, neck, lung, kidney, liver, gastrointestinal tract, anus, and skin. Currently, NADMs cause more cancer-related morbidity and mortality than ADMs and will remain common among PWH, with lung and prostate cancer expected to emerge as the most prevalent cancer types in the next decade (Shiels et al., 2018).

Although ADMs most commonly occur in people with severe immune suppression, low CD4$^+$ T-cell counts (< 500 cells/mm^3) have been identified as a risk factor for both ADMs and NADMs (Torres and & Mulanovich, 2014). This suggests that initiating ART to suppress HIV replication and reconstituting CD4$^+$ T-cell counts may reduce the overall risk of malignancies in PWH. Recently, viral suppression, particularly long-term suppression with ART, has been linked with ADM and NADM prevention. Despite this, cancer risk can remain elevated even in virally suppressed

PWH in comparison to persons without HIV infection (Park et al., 2018).

In people with cancer, the use of ART alongside chemotherapy is routinely recommended to improve overall survival. The administration of chemotherapy and ART concurrently can be complicated by a number of factors (Rudek et al., 2011), including limited data regarding safe and effective therapy combinations; significant drug–drug interactions among ART, antineoplastics, and supportive care medications; drug–disease state monitoring interactions; and overlapping drug toxicities. The introduction of immunotherapy for cancer treatment advanced the treatment of many NADM including use of immune check point inhibitors and chimeric antigen receptor T-cell therapy. This chapter reviews contemporary information regarding the use of chemotherapy and ART in combination, including strategies for managing these complex situations.

GENERAL CONSIDERATIONS FOR COMBINING ANTINEOPLASTIC AND ANTIRETROVIRAL THERAPY

DRUG INTERACTIONS: CYP450

Drug interactions between ART and antineoplastic agents may occur via several different mechanisms. The most common are the interactions that occur during metabolism of medications from active to inactive substances via the cytochrome P450 enzyme system (CYP450). Medications may be substrates of CYP450, meaning that they use this system for metabolism, and their concentrations may be altered by concurrent administration with other agents. In addition, medications may be inducers or inhibitors of individual CYP450 isoenzymes, such as 3A4. CYP450 inducers will increase the metabolism of CYP450 substrates, thus decreasing the concentration of medication, which may lead to subtherapeutic medication levels. Conversely, CYP450 inhibitors will decrease the metabolism of CYP450 substrates, thus increasing the medication concentration, which may lead to toxicity. The timing of the CYP450 interactions may also vary as enzyme inhibition occurs rapidly, with maximum effect occurring when a medication is at steady state and enzyme induction occurring more slowly because of the need for enzyme synthesis (Di Francia et al., 2014). Many antiretroviral, antineoplastic, and supportive care medications utilize the CYP450 system for metabolism, and drug interactions are expected to be a challenge in this setting.

Several antineoplastic agents are substrates, inducers, or inhibitors of CYP3A4. The result is complex bidirectional interactions with ART (Rudek et al., 2011). Interacting chemotherapy agents include vinblastine, vincristine, paclitaxel, docetaxel, iphosphamide, cyclophosphamide, tyrosine kinase inhibitors, and corticosteroids that are metabolized by CYP3A4 (Rubinstein et al., 2014). HIV protease inhibitors, the integrase inhibitor elvitegravir, first generation nonnucleoside reverse transcriptase inhibitors, and the pharmacokinetic enhancers cobicistat and ritonavir have a higher likelihood

of drug interactions because of their CYP450 metabolism. However, nucleoside reverse transcriptase inhibitors, second generation non-nucleoside reverse transcriptase inhibitors (e.g., rilpivirine and doravirine) and integrase inhibitors have the least likelihood of causing significant interactions with chemotherapy (Navarro et al., 2021). ART regimens containing oral integrase inhibitors without pharmacologic boosters are favored in the setting of malignancy, owing to a lower potential for drug interactions (NCCN guidelines, 2022).

DRUG INTERACTIONS: P-GLYCOPROTEIN

To add to the complexity of interactions that occur with medication metabolism, there may also be absorption interactions with the p-glycoprotein efflux pump in the gastrointestinal tract. Like the CYP450 interactions, medications may be p-glycoprotein substrates, inducers, or inhibitors. P-glycoprotein inducers stimulate the efflux of medications back into the gastrointestinal lumen thus decreasing the absorption and plasma concentrations of these medications. Likewise, p-glycoprotein inhibitors will increase the absorption of medication and increase plasma concentrations of substrates, which could lead to toxicities. Antiretrovirals that effect, and are affected by, p-glycoprotein include maraviroc, nonnucleoside reverse transcriptase inhibitors, integrase inhibitors, and protease inhibitors. Long-acting injectable formulations of cabotegravir and rilpivirine do not rely on the gastrointestinal tract for absorption. Drug interactions with the injectable formulation of these agents may differ from oral formulations and these differences should be considered when combining these agents with chemotherapy (Nhean et al., 2021). Literature has shown that p-glycoprotein is highly expressed in HIV-associated malignancies such as non-Hodgkin's lymphoma and plays a significant role in the effectiveness of both ART and antineoplastic therapy (Klibanov & Clark-Vetril, 2007). Clinicians should be aware of ARV, antineoplastic, and supportive care agents that affect p-glycoprotein and should realize the potential for drug interactions with medications that influence, or are influenced by, this mechanism.

MEDICATION TOXICITIES

Clinicians will also need to consider overlapping toxicities of medication classes. Some ART and antineoplastic agents are known for causing severe adverse effects that may become additive when used in combination. For example, nucleoside reverse transcriptase inhibitors may cause neutropenia (e.g., zidovudine), peripheral neuropathy (e.g., didanosine), or nephrotoxicity (e.g., tenofovir). Utilizing newer nucleoside reverse transcriptase inhibitor formulations, such as tenofovir alafenamide, may minimize nephrotoxicity, especially in combination with nephrotoxic chemotherapy agents such as methotrexate and cisplatin (Navarro et al., 2021). Various nonnucleoside reverse transcriptase inhibitors are associated with rash and hepatic transaminase elevations and the entry inhibitor maraviroc may cause hepatotoxicity. Protease inhibitors may lead to greater gastrointestinal upset, including nausea, vomiting, and diarrhea, and may potentiate the myelosuppressive effects of certain chemotherapy (Torres & Mulanovich, 2014). Integrase inhibitors, however, are well-tolerated and overlapping toxicities with antineoplastic agents are not projected to be a major concern. It is vitally important when devising medication regimens that serious adverse effects of all agents be identified and overlapping toxicities minimized when possible.

DRUG–DISEASE INTERACTIONS

The presence of drug–disease interactions will need to be recognized when combining ARV and antineoplastic agents. Disease monitoring interactions are a concern because there are certain antiretroviral medications that increase oncologic disease markers such as bilirubin. Bilirubin is often used as a means for determining dosage adjustments for a number of chemotherapeutic agents, such as docetaxel, paclitaxel, doxorubicin, etoposide, irinotecan, imatinib, and vincristine (Beumer et al., 2014). Atazanavir may cause unconjugated hyperbilirubinemia secondary to UGT1A1 inhibition, leading to possible inaccuracies in chemotherapy dosage calculations.

Conversely, there are also concerns that antineoplastic agents may affect the level of CD4$^+$ T- cells, rendering the monitoring parameters of both disease states inaccurate (Klibanov & Clark-Vetril, 2007). This has especially been a concern with cancer immunotherapy, as this strategy utilizes a patient's immune system to detect and destroy cancer cells. While data are still evolving, cancer immunotherapy likely has similar effectiveness in PWH and has causes no significant impact on plasma HIV RNA or CD4 count (Abu Khalaf et al., 2022). Additionally, cancer immunotherapy may be more efficient in PWH compared to persons without HIV because of HIV infection upregulating immunotherapy targets (Bressan et al., 2021). When antineoplastic agents are combined with ARV agents, there may also be medication absorption concerns because of the presence of disease complications such as gastrointestinal tumors, mucositis, and graft-versus-host disease (Torres & Mulanovich, 2014). Clinicians may need to be creative in these situations, such as selecting medication regimens available in liquid formulations or alternative routes of administration.

The key concepts of drug interactions, overlapping toxicities, and drug–disease interactions are just a few examples of the complexity in utilizing combination ART and antineoplastic therapy. Specific literature and guideline recommendations to assist in the selection, dosing, and monitoring of these agents when used in combination are scarce. Thus, these concepts should be considered on a case-by-case basis and explored when crafting a medication regimen in the treatment of both HIV and oncologic diseases.

STRATEGIES FOR CLINICAL MANAGEMENT OF PEOPLE WITH CANCER AND HIV

Treatment of PWH and cancer is complex, and a variety of management strategies should be considered. Examples of management strategies include alterations to the ART or chemotherapy regimens, changes in monitoring frequency, and optimization of opportunistic infection prophylaxis. To address the challenges, PWH and cancer should be treated using a multidisciplinary approach including primary care providers, infectious disease clinicians, hematologists/oncologists, and clinical pharmacists. Communication among these professions is essential.

In combining ART and anticancer drug therapy, drug interactions and overlapping toxicities can be minimized or avoided by altering either the ART regimen or the chemotherapy regimen. In many instances, it is often simpler to substitute one or more components of a person's ART regimen in order to avoid risk of drug interactions or additive toxicity. When determining interaction potential, drug interaction resources such as the following should be consulted: the Toronto General Hospital Immunodeficiency Clinic's (https://hivclinic.ca/drug-information/antiretroviral-interactions-with-chemotherapy-regimens/) and the University of Liverpool HIV drug interaction website (http://www.hiv-druginteractions.org). ART regimen changes should always be carried out in conjunction with an HIV specialist utilizing the person's complete ARV treatment history, past adverse events, and resistance test results. Interruption of ART or a delay in ART initiation is not recommended because it has been associated with an increase in mortality. In addition, modifications to the medications in an antineoplastic regimen or their doses may also be considered based on a person's tolerance and response. Regardless, both ART and chemotherapy should be individualized according to a person's characteristics.

Increased monitoring for efficacy and toxicity is recommended when co-administering any ART regimen with chemotherapy. If an ARV regimen is modified, more intensive monitoring of tolerability, viral suppression, adherence, and laboratory changes is recommended during the first 3 months after a regimen switch. Identification and enhanced monitoring for toxicities is also recommended and should be assessed individually for each person.

Lastly, in PWH and cancer, opportunistic infection prophylaxis should be tailored and expanded with antimicrobials required for specific chemotherapy regimens or hematopoietic stem cell transplantation. The need for opportunistic infection prophylaxis should be re-evaluated on a regular basis and adjusted as needed via coordination among both the infectious disease and the oncology providers. Prophylaxis may need to be modified as the person's CD4$^+$ T-cell count decreases with some chemotherapy regimens or increases after completion of therapy.

REFERENCES

Abu Khalaf S, Dandachi D, Granwehr BP, et al. Cancer immunotherapy in adult patients with HIV. *J Investig Med*. April 2022;70(4):883–891.

Beumer JH, Venkataramanan R, Rudek MA. Pharmacotherapy in cancer patients with HIV/AIDS. *Clin Pharmcol Ther*. 2014;95(4):370–372.

Bressan S, Pierantoni A, Sharifi S, et al. Chemotherapy-induced hepatotoxicity in HIV patients. *Cells*. October 25, 2021;10(11):2871.

Di Francia R, Di Paolo M, Valente D, et al. Pharmacogenetic based drug–drug interactions between highly active antiretroviral therapy (HAART) and antiblastic chemotherapy. *WCRJ.* 2014;1(2): e386.

Klibanov OM, Clark-Vetril R. Oncologic complications of human immunodeficiency virus infection: changing epidemiology, treatments, and special considerations in the era of highly active antiretroviral therapy. *Pharmacotherapy.* 2007;27(1):122–136.

National Comprehensive Cancer Network (NCCN). Clinical practice guidelines in oncology. Cancer in people living with HIV. Version 1. https://www.nccn.org/guidelines/category_4. Published 2022. Accessed July 19, 2022.

Navarro JT, Moltó J, Tapia G, et al. Hodgkin lymphoma in people living with HIV. *Cancers.* August 29, 2021;13(17):4366.

Nhean S, Tseng A, Back D. The intersection of drug interactions and adverse reactions in contemporary antiretroviral therapy. *Curr Opin HIV AIDS.* November 1, 2021;16(6):292–302.

Park LS, Tate JP, Sigel K, et al. Association of viral suppression with lower AIDS-defining and non-AIDS-defining cancer incidence in HIV-infected veterans: a prospective cohort study. *Ann Intern Med.* 2018;169(2):87–96.

Rubinstein PG, Aboulafia DM, Zloza A. Malignancies in HIV/AIDS: from epidemiology to therapeutic challenges. *AIDS.* 2014;28(4):453–465.

Rudek MA, Flexner C, Ambinder RF. Use of antineoplastic agents in patients with cancer who have HIV/AIDS. *Lancet Oncol.* 2011;12(9):905–912.

Shiels MS, Islam JY, Rosenberg PS, et al. Projected cancer incidence rates and burden of incident cancer cases in HIV-infected adults in the United States through 2030. *Ann Intern Med.* 2018;168(12):866–873.

Torres HA, Mulanovich V. Management of HIV infection in patients with cancer receiving chemotherapy. *Clin Infect Dis.* 2014;59(1):106–114.

26.

SUBSTANCE USE IN HIV POPULATIONS

Thanh Thuy Truong and Elizabeth H. David

CHAPTER GOAL

Upon completion of this chapter, the reader should be able to:

- Discuss issues, implications, diagnosis, and treatment of substance use disorders in HIV-positive individuals.

INTRODUCTION

The relationship between substance use and HIV infection is complex and encompasses all stages, including transmission, diagnosis, progression, and treatment. Substance use can increase risk for exposure to HIV via needle-sharing or impairing judgment linked to risky sexual behaviors. Among men who have sex with men (MSM), substance use was associated with an increased risk of HIV infection, particularly with binge drinking, crack/cocaine, methamphetamine, and inhalant use. In the 2018 Centers for Disease Control and Prevention (CDC) report, MSM accounted for 66% of HIV diagnoses in the United States. HIV diagnoses attributed to injection drug use increased from 2014–2018, which was likely due to the increase in prescription opioid use and heroin (CDC, 2018). Among people with HIV (PWH), substance use can lead to a poor prognosis and progression to acquired immune deficiency syndrome (AIDS). Irregular follow-up with treatment, poor adherence to antiretroviral therapy (ART), and risk of acquiring other sexually transmitted infections (STIs) and hepatitis C through injection drug use increase morbidity and mortality (Cofrancesco et al., 2008; Stern et al., 2018).

Biological, psychological, and social factors influence the relationship between substance use disorders (SUD) and HIV infection. Risk of substance use involves interactions between genes and the environment. Approximately 40%–60% of vulnerability to addiction can be attributable to genetic variance. For example, in alcohol use disorder, while some genes have been associated with susceptibility to excess alcohol consumption, polymorphisms in alcohol metabolizing enzymes like alcohol dehydrogenases ADH1B and ALDH2 are protective against alcohol use disorder (AUD) (Chen et al., 1999). Moreover, periods of normal development have higher risk of drug use. During adolescence, normal behaviors of novelty-seeking, risk taking, and sensitivity to peer pressure may result in experimenting with legal and illegal substances. Adolescent brains have not completed development in areas involved in executive function, which is necessary for regulating impulses and emotions. Not surprisingly, rates of use for most substances occur between age 18 to 24 years, prior to full development of frontal lobes and functional networks at age 25 (Miller et al., 2019). Adolescent neurological development is also more vulnerable to long-term effects of chronic drug and alcohol exposure and can increase risk of developing SUDs later in life. This interaction between biological and psychological development leads to risky behaviors such as having multiple partners and inconsistent condom use that increase exposure to HIV (Hillfors, 2007). Socioeconomic disadvantage, low education, and unstable housing also contribute to unsafe sexual practices and limited access to preventive measures, thus increasing prevalence of HIV in these populations (Millett, 2007).

Psychiatric illnesses and substance use are separate and additive risk factors for HIV infection. Psychiatric illnesses are more prevalent in PWH. For example, personality disorders are highly represented among PWH, likely owing to traits such as impulsivity and maladaptive coping strategies to stress that perpetuate risky behaviors. Similarly, PWH are more likely to have a mental illness like anxiety or depression, whether resulting from HIV infection of neural tissue, or a distinct comorbidity (Stern et al., 2018). One study of PWH revealed that those who have a dual diagnosis of mental illness and substance use have an HIV prevalence of 4.7% as opposed to 2.4% for those with substance use disorder diagnosis alone—almost double the rate. Further, unhealthy substance use is associated with a host of medical sequelae (liver disease, infection, diabetes, cardiovascular disease, and neurocognitive changes) that add to the many potential medical complications associated with HIV and AIDS. Unfortunately, compounding these problems is inconsistent adherence to medical treatment in this population (Moore, 2008; Sullivan, 2011). This highlights the importance of a comprehensive approach in the treatment of individuals with multiple diagnoses. Despite advancement in diagnosis and treatment among PWH since the 1990s (Bhaskaran et al., 2008), stigma, shame, and complacency continue to be significant barriers to care in PWH and SUD.

Early detection and intervention can save lives and change the trajectory of the illness. Routine voluntary testing in all individuals aged 13–64 years is recommended by the CDC to facilitate early detection and treatment of HIV (Branson et al., 2006). Testing may be postponed in acute exacerbations of mental illness and substance use but should be offered once the person has capacity to consent to testing and treatment. A comprehensive and harm-reduction approach involving patient education and collaboration in therapeutic decisions are critical for this complex patient population. Persistent risky substance use should prompt referral to drug treatment services, and relapse prevention should be discussed at each patient encounter (CDC, 2003). Education about reducing risk of opportunistic infections should be provided. Resources may be limited in some areas for an interdisciplinary team approach, but, if possible, care is best managed concurrently with an HIV treatment expert.

LEARNING OBJECTIVES

- Describe the bidirectional interactions between HIV and unhealthy substance use.

- Recognize unhealthy substance use in PWH.

- Provide an initial outline of potential approaches to the treatment of SUD in this population.

WHAT'S NEW?

The chapter has been updated to reflect the terminology of the fifth edition of the *Diagnostic and statistical manual of mental disorders*, <u>text revision</u> (American Psychiatric Association, 2022). More thorough and specific treatment modalities and recommendations are included.

DIAGNOSIS AND TREATMENT OF SUBSTANCE USE DISORDERS

SCREENING AND DIAGNOSIS

Prior to conducting screening, assessment, or treatment planning, providers should evaluate their personal beliefs and attitudes toward PWH with SUD. Working with this complex population often elicits difficult feelings that can be emotionally and physically demanding for staff. Examining countertransference reactions and biases such as homophobia and fear of infection can help decrease burn out and facilitate a stronger therapeutic alliance with the PWH. Providers must be comfortable discussing taboo topics such as sex, drug use, shame, and trauma. Cultural competency is also important because people from different ethnic groups, socioeconomic class, genders, and cultures have varying levels of comfort in discussion of these topics. For example, asking personal questions about substance use and sexual risk factors may feel intrusive and disrespectful to some Asian and Pacific Islander individuals. Approaching screening with the least intrusive question may ease the person into more detailed questions later. While HIV/AIDS disproportionately affects African Americans, many may mistrust of the healthcare system because of a long history of exploitation of their community by medical institutions. Providers should be aware of social, economic, and political issues such as institutional racism that continue to affect the African American community. Working with the lesbian, gay, bisexual, and transgender (LGBTQ) populations requires understanding and sensitivity, as this population often faces stigma, trauma, low self-esteem, and lack of

family and social supports. Another group that needs special consideration is women. Women present differently and often at later stages in the HIV/AIDS disease process compared to men. Factors such as identity (e.g., as a caregiver), stigma (e.g., "unfit mother"), shame, and guilt over being HIV-positive may play a major role in a woman's care decisions. Lastly, while it is helpful to consider the common experiences of a group, providers should seek to understand the unique experience of each individual.

Although there are specific criteria for the diagnosis of SUD and physiologic dependence (American Psychiatric Association, 2022), assessing impact of a substance requires a comprehensive evaluation to understand the individual's unique experience. Historically, addiction was viewed as a voluntary moral failing by the individual, which led to stigmatization that has been a significant barrier to appropriate care. In recent decades research has advanced our understanding of the profound drug effects on neural networks involved in reward processing, motivation, and behavioral and emotional regulation that result in compulsive drug-seeking behaviors. Definitions of SUD in the literature now reflect biological, psychological, and social factors. After reviewing several definitions, one practical definition adopted by the European Monitoring Centre for Drugs and Drug Addiction (EMCDDA) is "a repeated powerful motivation to engage in a purposeful behavior that has no survival value, acquired as a result of engaging in that behavior, with significant potential for unintended harm" (West, 2013). The severity of substance use varies between individuals and encompasses low-risk, hazardous, and harmful addiction levels. Generally, an SUD is diagnosed when the use of a substance results in an impairment of functioning in multiple areas (occupational, social, and recreational), loss of control over intake, and the presence of a negative emotional state during abstinence.

Screening and brief intervention for tobacco and alcohol use disorders in a variety of clinical settings have demonstrated significant benefit in reducing use. Routine screening of all adults and pregnant women for alcohol and tobacco use is recommended by the US Preventative Services Task Force (USPSTF) (Campos-Outcalt, 2016). A variety of screening tools for unhealthy alcohol and illicit drug use are available through the National Institute on Alcohol Abuse and Alcoholism (NIAAA), the National Institute on Drug Abuse (NIDA), and other governmental agencies. The single question, *How many times in the past year have you used an illegal drug or used a prescription medication for nonmedical reasons?* has been shown to accurately identify drug use. A response of at least one time is positive for unhealthy drug use. To prescreen for any alcohol use, asking, *Do you sometimes drink beer, wine, or other alcoholic beverages?* can gently prepare the person for more detailed questions about unhealthy use. For heavy drinking, the question: *How many times in the past year have you had five or more (for men) or four or more (for women) drinks in a day?* is sensitive and specific for identifying unhealthy alcohol use in primary care settings (NIAAA, 2017). A positive screen prompts further assessment of severity and impact on the individual's functioning to determine risk level. Differentiating between at-risk use or a SUD is relevant to guide clinical recommendations for treatment. Brief intervention such as advice and motivational interviewing may be appropriate for at-risk use whereas more extensive follow-up and referral to an addiction specialist would be suitable for PWH meeting criteria for a SUD. Screening would be best accompanied by laboratory studies such as urine toxicology for drugs and serum carbohydrate and mean corpuscular volume for alcohol use.

TREATMENT

GENERAL PRINCIPLES

Successful treatment of PWH with SUD poses significant challenges and requires a multimodal approach. Chronic drug exposure leads to long-lasting neurological and behavioral changes that contribute to relapse, which can feel frustrating and demoralizing for PWH and their clinical team. Taking the approach of chronic disease management, such as diabetes or hypertension, with an expected long-term care model represents a shift in ideology toward harm-reduction. This involves recognizing that the illness will likely include periods of recovery and relapse depending on compliance and efficacy of treatment helps PWH and the treatment team approach care rationally. Rather than failure, a "relapse" can be reframed as a temporary setback as part of trial and error in achieving an effective care regimen. Some individuals may not be able to achieve abstinence despite appropriate treatment, thus setting attainable goals such as reducing frequency and severity of use and relapse can improve overall functioning. Clarifying and communicating these expectations to PWH and the treatment team can improve outcomes and retention in treatment (McLellan et al., 2000). The combination of psychosocial and pharmacological interventions is strongly recommended to target different facets of addiction. When possible, use of an interdisciplinary team with psychiatry, primary care, social work, substance use counselors, and case management is ideal for supporting the individual in their recovery and preventing relapse.

General principles of effective treatment of SUD include easy access to care, collaborating with the person to create a treatment plan to addresses their individual needs, monitoring for relapse, and treating psychiatric and medical comorbidities. Tests for HIV/AIDs, hepatitis B and C, tuberculosis, and other infectious diseases should be readily available. On-site availability of HIV testing can increase the likelihood of people being tested and receiving their results (NIDA, 1999). Even when individuals present for intoxication or withdrawal management, this can be viewed as an entry into treatment. The physician should establish rapport with the person and evoke their motivation for engaging in recommended addiction services. The appropriate treatment setting depends on the PWH's insight, physical and emotional ability to engage in care, and availability of necessary treatment (e.g., opioid-agonist therapy). Hospitalization is recommended for PWHs who are a danger to themselves or others because of intoxication or acute psychiatric disorder; need intensive withdrawal management; or have life-threatening medical conditions. Residential treatment programs are best for PWH who have fluctuating insight and need a highly structured and supportive environment. Partial hospitalization and intensive outpatient programs can be considered for persons who transition out of residential or hospital setting to a lower level of care, but still need close monitoring to manage risk of relapse. PWH who have a history of relapse after treatment completion or have plans to return to high-risk environments would be best continued in a highly structured setting. Finally, for PWH who demonstrate insight into their SUD and have high compliance with treatment and low severity of symptoms, outpatient programs are an appropriate, cost-effective option. Outpatient programs vary from low to high intensity, many of which have a multimodal approach that involves individual and group therapy and mental health and medical treatment (Miller et al., 2019).

THERAPY

Various psychotherapies have been shown to be effective for treatment of SUD through helping PWH modify behaviors, feelings, thoughts, and social contexts that drive compulsive substance use. Therapeutic intervention can increase motivation, improve mood, and build a strong social support network, all of which improve chances of recovery and prevent relapse. Motivational enhancement therapy is used to help PWH address ambivalence about drug use and engaging in treatment. Motivational interviewing techniques enhance motivation and commitment for change or maintaining progress. Cognitive behavioral therapy (CBT) has demonstrated efficacy in relapse prevention by helping individuals identify and correct behaviors and thoughts that precede cravings and increase risk of relapse. Studies have demonstrated retention of CBT skills at least a year after discharge from treatment (Carroll et al., 1994). Individual counseling focuses on reducing or stopping substance use, addresses various areas of impaired functioning, and connects PWH to community resources such as 12-step programs (Alcoholics Anonymous, Narcotics Anonymous), or Self-Management and Recovery Training recovery for patients who prefer a science-based and secular program. Supportive expressive psychotherapy has also been shown to improve outcomes among PWH with cocaine and opioid use disorders that are comorbid with psychiatric disorders (Woody, 1995). Another strategy that increases the duration of abstinence is voucher-based reinforcement therapy, where people are provided with a voucher that can be exchanged for retail goods and services consistent with a substance-free lifestyle each time they provide a drug-free urine sample. These voucher-based treatment approaches may be combined with individual, group, and family counseling; vocational counseling; and pharmacologic treatment.

PHARMACOLOGICAL MANAGEMENT

ALCOHOL

Excessive use of alcohol, especially binge drinking, is an important risk factor for HIV infection. Alcohol intoxication is linked to risky sexual behaviors (e.g., not using a condom, multiple partners) that increases risk of infection. AUD also leads to poorer treatment outcomes due to nonadherence to ART and medical morbidities like liver and cardiovascular disease.

INTOXICATION/WITHDRAWAL

Alcohol intoxication is characterized by reversible psychological and behavioral changes that occur after alcohol consumption. A blood alcohol concentration of 0.08 is the limit for legal intoxication. However, significant impairment may occur at much lower levels in some PWH (i.e., younger or medically/mentally ill), while others may be functional at much higher levels because of tolerance. Intoxication is associated with physical symptoms of nausea, vomiting, and neurological impairment (i.e., slurred speech, incoordination, and ataxia). Overdose can result in respiratory depression, hypotension, hypothermia, profound central nervous system (CNS) depression, coma, and death. Management of intoxication and overdose is supportive and may include IV fluids and airway protection to prevent aspiration. Presence of other forms of alcohol such as methanol and other substances like opioids and benzodiazepines should prompt adjustments to the clinical management. Clinicians should be on high alert for a possible thiamine deficiency in PWH with AUD, which can precipitate Wernicke's encephalopathy and Korsakoff psychosis. Thiamine 100–200 mg (IV or IM preferred) should thus be given before glucose to avoid central pontine myelinolysis. For behavioral dysregulation not responsive to verbal de-escalation, antipsychotics such as haloperidol (e.g., 2–5 mg IV/IM/PO) and olanzapine may be considered. Benzodiazepines are commonly used to treat agitation but should be used with caution as they can further disinhibit the person and worsen agitation and respiratory depression.

Alcohol withdrawal begins within 6–24 hours of abstinence or substantial reduction in amount of alcohol use. Early symptoms include anxiety, irritability/restlessness, insomnia, nausea, headache, diaphoresis, and fine tremor. PWH may experience visual, auditory, and tactile hallucinations that characterize alcoholic hallucinosis. Alcoholic hallucinosis may occur independently of other withdrawal symptoms. Alcohol withdrawal seizures may occur within 12–48 hours after the last drink, sometimes earlier. For most people, withdrawal does not progress beyond mild-to-moderate symptoms that remit after 48 hours. For a minority of individuals, withdrawal can progress to delirium tremens (DTs), which is characterized by autonomic dysfunction (tachycardia, fever, hypertension (HTN)) and delirium. Without proper management, DTs can be life-threatening. Pharmacologic treatment of alcohol withdrawal involves benzodiazepines. Selection of the benzodiazepine should consider pharmacokinetics, abuse potential, and presence of hepatic injury. For example, longer-acting agents (diazepam, chlordiazepoxide) have a smoother withdrawal course, but carry higher risks of excessive sedation in some individuals (e.g., elderly). For PWH with significant hepatic dysfunction, a benzodiazepine that does not undergo first-pass metabolism (lorazepam, oxazepam) is preferred.

Phenobarbital can be used in PWH who are not responding to benzodiazepines. Other agents that have shown efficacy and are well tolerated include anticonvulsants such as gabapentin, carbamazepine, and valproate (Minozzi et al., 2010). However, there are limited data on their ability to prevent DTs and withdrawal seizures. They may be added as augmenting agents, but benzodiazepines remain the first-line treatment.

PHARMACOTHERAPY FOR ALCOHOL USE DISORDER

Treatment for AUD involves medications that reduce the reinforcing effects of alcohol or deter use by causing adverse reactions when alcohol is consumed. Commonly used agents are summarized below:

- **Naltrexone** is a μ-opioid receptor antagonist that reduces the reinforcing effects of alcohol. This results in decreased craving as well as disruption of the euphoric feelings associated with alcohol intoxication. Naltrexone has been shown to reduce alcohol consumption and prevention of relapse to heavy drinking (Miller et al., 2019). Naltrexone use is contraindicated in PWH with significant liver disease (acute hepatitis and liver failure); therefore, all PWH with these risks should have liver function tested prior to initiation. Monitoring for liver toxicity is recommended in PWH, who may have concurrent liver disease from substance use, concurrent hepatitis infection, or liver impairment from ART. Naltrexone is often well tolerated and does not have documented interactions with ART. However, naltrexone should be avoided in individuals who require opioids for pain management or are in acute opioid withdrawal. PWH can be started on oral naltrexone at 50 mg to 100 mg/day. It is also available in the IM formulation (Vivitrol) at doses of 380 mg every 4 weeks. Common early side effects (nausea and other gastrointestinal symptoms, headache, dizziness) are usually mild and transient. For the IM formulation, swelling, pain, and other injection site reactions may occur.

- **Acamprosate** (Campral) reduces alcohol use via modulation of glutamate neurotransmission and increase in γ-aminobutyric acid (GABA) activity. It has been shown to reduce alcohol consumption and increase duration of abstinence (Stern et al., 2018). The medication is often well tolerated and safe in PWH with impaired liver function. However, because it is excreted renally, dose adjustments may be needed in persons with renal failure. Acamprosate is FDA-approved at a dosage of 1,998 mg/day in divided doses (333 mg capsule three times daily). The frequent dosing is a barrier to using this medication in many people. Common side effects are often mild and transient and may include gastrointestinal (e.g., nausea, diarrhea) and dermatological symptoms (e.g., itching). Acamprosate carries a warning for possible increase in suicidal behavior. However, many of these events occurred in the context of alcohol relapse, and no consistent pattern of relationship between the clinical course of recovery from alcoholism and the emergence of suicidality was identified (Forest Pharmaceuticals, 2004).

- **Disulfiram** (Antabuse) discourages drinking by causing an adverse physical reaction with alcohol consumption. It acts by inhibiting acetaldehyde dehydrogenase, which prevents metabolism of acetaldehyde, a byproduct of alcohol metabolism. Increased acetaldehyde concentration causes temporary flushing, sweating, palpitations, hypotension, nausea, and vomiting. Severe reactions have resulted in cardiovascular compromise and death. Because of these effects, it is often used in selected PWH who are highly motivated or are closely supervised for compliance and abstinence. The daily dose is limited to 250–500 mg/day, owing to the more adverse effects at higher doses. Disulfiram should not be administered to anyone who has not abstained from alcohol for at least 48 hours. It should also be avoided in PWH with a history of cardiovascular disease (e.g., myocardial infarction) or end-stage liver disease, or in pregnant women. Caution should be used in PWH with a history of psychosis because of disulfiram's inhibition of dopamine dehydroxylase, which may increase in dopamine concentrations and exacerbate psychotic symptoms. In PWH, disulfiram is often avoided because of a potential interaction with ART. However, a 2014 study indicated that there was no significant increase in adverse symptoms compared to baseline with coadministration of disulfiram and common antiretroviral (ARV) medications (i.e., ritonavir). With close monitoring, disulfiram should still be considered in some PWH to deter alcohol use (McCance-Katz et al., 2014).

- **Anticonvulsants** are commonly used off-label in treatment of AUD. Among these are gabapentin, topiramate, carbamazepine, and divalproex, all of which have demonstrated efficacy in reducing drinking and/or relapse in placebo-controlled trials. These medications have different mechanisms of action, though it is likely that they work for AUD by antagonism of glutamate receptors and potentiation of GABA receptors (Miller et al., 2019). Because of cognitive side effects, slow titration of topiramate is recommended (i.e., increase by 25 mg every week). Gabapentin has demonstrated efficacy in reducing cravings, amount consumed, and alcohol withdrawal symptoms at 900 mg to 1,800 mg/day in divided doses (Anton et al., 2020). Gabapentin may be additionally helpful for PWH with chronic pain. However, clinicians should regularly assess for potential misuse.

OPIOIDS

Use of opioid-based drugs (e.g., heroin, morphine, oxycodone, and fentanyl), particularly injection drug use, has long been associated with HIV infection and transmission. Opioids act on mu receptors and activate the reward system in the CNS, resulting in euphoria and dependence. The risk of developing an opioid use disorder (OUD) has been shown to be even higher in those who also have psychiatric illness and chronic pain. Depression in injection drug users has been linked to increased rates of sharing of needles and other paraphernalia, resulting in a greater risk for HIV infection. It is therefore crucial to treat both the psychiatric disorders and the behavioral risk factors in injection drug users (Ruiz, 2014).

THE US OPIOID EPIDEMIC AND HIV

In recent years, OUD has emerged as one of America's most pressing public health concerns, prompting greater consideration of how this growing epidemic could be impacting the transmission and treatment of HIV and other blood-borne infections, such as hepatitis C (HCV). In 2016, 2.1 million Americans were estimated to have an OUD, with nearly 12 million Americans estimated to have misused opioids during the preceding year (SAMHSA, 2016). Apart from the heightened morbidity and mortality associated with opioid overdose, this epidemic also places affected individuals at additional risk of contracting and transmitting infectious diseases during the course of their addiction. Research shows that people who misuse and abuse opioids commonly move from oral use to inhalation to injection use as they build tolerance to the drug's effects and require more potent concentrations to achieve their desired level of intoxication (Peters, 2016). Moreover, it is estimated that 10%–20% of people who misuse prescription opioids move on to inject either opioids or heroin (Van Handle, 2016). Given the long-standing association between injection drug use and transmission of HIV and HCV via needle-sharing, public health providers must necessarily remain vigilant in hopes of identifying co-occurring trends in these epidemics. One such instance was documented in 2015, in Scott County, Indiana, where opioid use was implicated in an HIV outbreak that resulted in 181 individuals being diagnosed with HIV, most of whom were co-infected with HCV (Van Handle, 2016). As individuals engaged in escalating drug use, they became more susceptible to transmission of HIV and HCV by way of high-risk sexual activity and injection drug use behaviors. This incident was integral in prompting the US Centers for Disease Control and Prevention (CDC) to identify 220 jurisdictions that might be equally vulnerable to similar co-occurring outbreaks owing to the preponderance of opioid addiction and high-risk needle-sharing, as well as limited access to care in those geographic areas (Van Handle, 2016). Targeted interventions such as these must be undertaken not only in hopes of preventing and rapidly identifying subsequent epidemics, but also as a means of ensuring that individuals with comorbid opioid dependence and HIV have adequate access to both medications for OUD (MOUD) and ART. In 2016, a systematic review and meta-analysis of 4,685 articles and 32 studies revealed that MOUD was associated with a 69% increase in recruitment into ART, a 54% increase in ART coverage, a twofold increase in ART adherence, a 23% decrease in the odds of attrition, and a 45% increase in odds of viral suppression (Low, 2016). Taken together, these striking statistics illustrate the importance of substance use recovery in both preventing the spread of HIV and improving the overall quality of life and treatment for persons living with HIV and OUD. It is imperative that individuals with opioid dependence are screened early for

HIV/HCV, then promptly referred for OUD treatment to reduce morbidity and mortality and mitigate the impact of these epidemics across the general population.

MANAGEMENT OF OPIOID USE DISORDER

INTOXICATION/WITHDRAWAL

Acute intoxication with opioids is characterized by euphoria, slurred speech, sedation, and analgesia. Physical signs include miosis, constipation, respiratory depression, and sedation. Overdoses result in respiratory arrest, cardiovascular compromise, coma, and death. Naloxone, a short-acting opioid antagonist, at doses of 0.5–2 mg IM/IV is used in all cases of suspected opioid overdose. Multiple doses may be required in the presence of fentanyl and other synthetic opioids. In severe cases, ICU care is required.

Opioid withdrawal is extremely uncomfortable and a reason for continued use in many individuals. Symptoms usually begin 8–12 hours after the last dose. Early symptoms include yawning, sweating, rhinorrhea, lacrimation, and irritability. More severe symptoms such as gastrointestinal disturbance (abdominal cramps, diarrhea, vomiting), insomnia, and tachycardia, and HTN may occur at 24–36 hours after the last dose. People on methadone (long half-life) may have a more protracted withdrawal lasting 2 to 4 weeks. This initial withdrawal phase is often followed by symptoms lasting for weeks or months. This "protracted abstinence syndrome" includes depressed mood, low energy, poor sleep, and anhedonia. Animal studies have implicated serotonin dysfunction in the development of this syndrome, which may respond to SSRIs (Goeldner et al., 2011).

Initial treatment of opioid dependence consists of a period of withdrawal management, which can be assisted by use of opioid agonists (e.g., methadone, buprenorphine) and/or supportive care for specific symptoms. Supportive care regimens may include acetaminophen for muscle aches, α2-adrenergic agonists (clonidine, guanfacine, lofexidine) for autonomic symptoms, ondansetron for nausea, dicyclomine for abdominal cramps, and lorazepam for anxiety/insomnia. Rapid and ultrarapid withdrawal protocols use an opioid antagonist to precipitate withdrawal, and then manage symptoms with supportive treatments (e.g., sedation procedures, anesthesia in ultrarapid protocol, and clonidine). Many PWH cannot tolerate withdrawal symptoms, and opioid-replacement therapy with methadone or buprenorphine is initiated and then tapered.

PHARMACOTHERAPY FOR MAINTENANCE OF OPIOID USE DISORDER

METHADONE

Developed in the 1960s, methadone is a μ-receptor agonist and a weak N-methyl-D-aspartate (NMDA) receptor antagonist that is very effective for OUD. The use of methadone has been shown to decrease the use of intravenous opioid drugs and the spread of communicable diseases such as HIV, hepatitis B virus, and hepatitis C virus by modifying behaviors such as intravenous drug use (Lollis, 2000). Methadone treatment for opioid dependence is provided in specialized opioid treatment programs (OTPs), which require federal licensing and certification. In addition to methadone treatment, OTP clinics also give counseling, drug testing, and vocational training/assistance. Studies have shown that methadone doses in the range of 20–40 mg/d are effective in suppressing symptoms of withdrawal, but they may not be effective in reducing or stopping symptoms of craving (Strain, 1993a, 1993b). Maintenance doses are carefully titrated to the needs of the individual (generally 60–100 mg/day).

Unfortunately, there are many issues with the use of methadone in HIV-positive individuals because of its side effects and drug–drug interactions. Methadone prolongs QT/QTc intervals and increases risk of torsade de pointes; therefore, close monitoring is required in persons who are taking other QT interval-prolonging drugs. Several ARV drugs induce CYP540 enzymes and may decrease serum methadone levels; they include lopinavir/ritonavir, efavirenz, nevirapine, doravirine, and abacavir. Other medications that have been shown to have drug–drug interaction with methadone include the anticonvulsants carbamazepine and phenytoin, as well as some antibiotics, such as rifampin. The combination of CNS depressants such as benzodiazepines with methadone may lead to severe CNS and respiratory depression. In general, caution should be used when combining these medications with methadone. If such medication combinations are required, then methadone doses may need to increase as needed for adequate management of withdrawal and cravings. Methadone has been shown to be safe during pregnancy (especially relative to opioid use or withdrawal) and safe with breastfeeding. Newborns exposed to methadone may experience neonatal abstinence syndrome, which consists of blotchy skin coloring (mottling), diarrhea, high-pitched crying, excessive sucking, fever, hyperactive reflexes, increased muscle tone, irritability, poor feeding, and, in rare cases, seizures.

BUPRENORPHINE (SUBUTEX) AND BUPRENORPHINE PLUS NALOXONE (SUBOXONE)

Buprenorphine is a partial agonist to the μ-opioid receptor and antagonist at the κ-opioid receptor. As a partial agonist, buprenorphine's effects plateaus at higher doses. It has a higher binding affinity to the μ-opioid receptor than most opioids, which allows it to displace or block other opioids from binding to the receptor. Therefore, PWH on buprenorphine will likely not feel greater euphoric effects from taking other opioids (i.e., heroin, oxycodone), which adds protection against overdose. In addition, buprenorphine may precipitate withdrawal in opioid users. Naloxone in the buprenorphine/naloxone formulation reduces the abuse potential of the drug by antagonizing buprenorphine's effects when it is injected. These medications require special certification for prescription, but they can be prescribed in an office setting. Initial doses are low (regardless of the person's wish to start at higher dose) to reduce risk of side effects and precipitation of withdrawal. Buprenorphine induction begins at 2 or 4 mg approximately 12–24 hours after the last dose of a short-acting opioid. Individuals should be in some form of opioid withdrawal assessed by a Clinical Opiate Withdrawal Scale (COWS) score of >10. Higher COWS scores (i.e., 14) may be needed for fentanyl users. If well tolerated and there are still signs of withdrawal, an additional 2–4 mg can be repeated 1 or 2 hours later. No more than 8 mg should be given on day 1. The procedure should be repeated for day 2, and buprenorphine can be titrated up to 16 mg/day. In the following weeks, titration should be based on cravings and withdrawal symptoms. Although up to 32 mg/d can be used, there is little evidence to support doses >24 mg/day having greater clinical advantage. Suboxone's effects plateau at 32 mg/d, and a higher dose has no therapeutic benefit. Overdose can still occur, and people with respiratory depression may require airway management. Other potential side effects include CNS depression and hepatitis. Those with a history of traumatic brain injury should be monitored for increased intracranial pressure because all potent opioids may elevate cerebrospinal fluid pressure. Buprenorphine is metabolized by CYP450 3A4 enzyme, and there are several clinically significant drug–drug interactions. Those taking CYP450 3A4 inhibitors such as nefazodone, fluvoxamine, fluoxetine, ketoconazole, itraconazole, erythromycin, clarithromycin, grapefruit juice, and most protease inhibitors (especially ritonavir) should take reduced doses of buprenorphine.

NALTREXONE

As a μ-opioid receptor antagonist, naltrexone blocks the reinforcing effects of opioids. Oral and intramuscular (IM) formulations of naltrexone are effective for highly motivated individuals who have completed withdrawal and can maintain abstinence from opioids. Oral naltrexone should be initiated after 5–7 days of abstinence from short-acting opioids, and 7–10 days for long-acting opioids to avoid precipitating withdrawal. It can be started at 25 mg, increased to 50 mg daily, or 350 mg weekly into three divided doses (100 mg, 100 mg, and 150 mg). In our experience, some patients benefit from doses of naltrexone up to 100 mg daily. While oral naltrexone is not effective for many people, the IM formulation can improve abstinence and retention in treatment. It can be given at 380 mg every 4 weeks. While the IM formulation is preferred, many patients will find it cost-prohibitive. See section on alcohol for more details on naltrexone. Baseline and periodic monitoring of liver function tests are recommended, especially in patients on higher doses of naltrexone. Because patients may increase the amount of opioid used to override the blockade from naltrexone, there is still a risk of opioid overdose. Discussing this possibility with patients may open a conversation about their motivations and ambivalence toward abstinence.

COCAINE/CRACK

In addition to the increased incidence of risk behaviors in cocaine abusers, studies have shown that cocaine use may have broad-ranging effects on human immunity. Regarding HIV infection, in vitro studies have shown that cocaine enhances infection of stimulated lymphocytes. Moreover, cohort studies in the pre- and post-highly active ART (HAART) era have linked stimulant abuse with increased HIV pathogenesis (Baum, 2009). It is therefore crucial to treat PWH with cocaine dependence.

Cocaine enhances activity of serotonin, norepinephrine, and dopamine (DA) by blocking reuptake of these neurotransmitters. Its addiction liability is thought to be secondary to increased dopamine levels in the nucleus accumbens. Cocaine effects depend on the mode of use, with smoked (crack) and intravenous administration having the quickest effects (seconds to 30 minutes; peak 15–30 minutes) and intranasal administration having slightly more delayed effects (5–90 minutes; peak 30 minutes). Mild-to-moderate intoxication produces sympathomimetic symptoms—generally increased heart rate and blood pressure, decreased appetite, insomnia, euphoria, hyper alertness, and irritability. With severe intoxication, dilation of the pupils, severe HTN, hyperthermia, cardiac arrhythmias/MIs, stroke, seizures, coma, and death may occur. At any level of intoxication, psychiatric symptoms may include auditory/visual/tactile hallucinations, delusions, paranoia, and aggression/violence. Individuals with severe cocaine intoxication (i.e., malignant HTN, hyperthermia, and seizure) will need medical stabilization. Phentolamine, cooling, and other supportive measures should be given for HTN crisis and hyperthermia; benzodiazepines should be given to terminate seizures and agitation. Antipsychotics may be considered for severe agitation/aggression/psychosis but should be used with caution because they increase the risk of neuroleptic malignant syndrome and seizures during stimulant intoxication.

Research into several medications for cocaine use disorder (CUD) has failed to show consistent evidence of effectiveness, but efforts are ongoing. Commonly used agents are summarized below:

- Anticonvulsants: Among anticonvulsants studied (carbamazepine, gabapentin, topiramate, lamotrigine, phenytoin, tiagabine, and vigabatrin), only topiramate showed significant treatment outcomes—it was better than placebo at maintaining 3 weeks of cocaine abstinence (Minozzi et al., 2015). Topiramate should be increased slowly (i.e., 25 mg/week) to reduce risk of cognitive impairment. Higher doses are more likely to cause impairment, which may be more pronounced in PWH who have HIV-associated neurocognitive decline.

- Stimulants: A metanalysis of stimulants as a class showed efficacy for promoting 3 weeks of abstinence compared to placebo, especially in people with comorbid ADHD (Castells et al., 2016). Methylphenidate may improve HIV-related cognitive impairment and depression in PWH (Hinkin et al., 2001). When using stimulants, extended-release formulations are preferred to reduce misuse potential.

- **Bupropion:** This is an antidepressant that inhibits the reuptake of dopamine and norepinephrine, bupropion has demonstrated therapeutic benefit in CUD. However, the response is less robust in patients with severe CUD (Chan et al., 2010). Bupropion is especially beneficial in PWH who also have tobacco use disorder.

- **Doxazosin:** This is an α1-adrenergic receptor antagonist that has shown some promise in decreasing cocaine use at doses of 8 mg per day in a small, clinically controlled trial (Shorter et al., 2013).

- **Disulfiram:** It has been studied as a potential treatment because of its inhibition of dopamine-β-hydroxylase, which prevents the conversion of dopamine to norepinephrine, thereby increasing dopamine levels. However, data have been inconsistent regarding its efficacy (Pani et al., 2010). Disulfiram is dosed at 250–500 mg/day.

- Other agents needing further study: these include ondansetron 4 mg twice daily (Blevins et al., 2021; Johnson et. al., 2006), and topiramate plus mixed amphetamine salts, which showed reduced cocaine use in small trials (Chan et al., 2019).

METHAMPHETAMINE

Methamphetamine use has grown exponentially in both rural and urban areas during the past few decades. It is an extremely potent stimulant that heightens sexual arousal with reduced inhibition and judgment, placing its users at risk of contracting STIs such as HIV. It can be smoked, eaten, snorted, injected, or rectally inserted. It has a rapid onset and long-lasting effects (half-life of 11–12 hours). Use induces the release of newly synthesized dopamine, norepinephrine, and serotonin. It is also an indirect catecholamine and serotonin (5-HT) agonist. Like cocaine, methamphetamine can deplete dopamine stores and lead to significant symptoms of depression and, in some cases, suicidal ideation and attempts. Other symptoms that may be experienced include psychosis (that may last weeks to months), aggression, thought disorders, and gum disease. Acute intoxication of methamphetamine is treated like cocaine intoxication with supportive care. Phentolamine, cooling, and other supportive treatments may be used for HTN crisis and hyperthermia; benzodiazepine is used for seizures and agitation. Antipsychotics may also be required to control severe aggression/agitation. The first-line treatments for methamphetamine use disorder are psychosocial and psychotherapeutic interventions such as contingency management, and the matrix model, which includes a variety of therapies that target use and relapse prevention. Pharmacological interventions are limited because there are currently no FDA-approved medications. Moreover, few medications have demonstrated consistent efficacy in controlled clinical trials. The following is a summary of medications that have demonstrated efficacy:

- **Antidepressants:** mirtazapine demonstrated efficacy in reduction of methamphetamine use and sexual risk behaviors in a small study with cis-gender men and transgender women who have sex with men (Coffin et al., 2020).

- **Antipsychotics:** Risperidone reduced MA use in small open-label trials (Meridith et al., 2007; Meridith et al., 2009). Paliperidone improved treatment retention, but did not reduce MA use in an RCT (Wang et al., 2019). Both antipsychotics were effective at improving psychotic symptoms. A case series of two patients taking cariprazine showed a reduction of cravings and frequency of use as well as longer time to relapse (Truong & Li, 2022). Taken together, for patients experiencing persistent methamphetamine-induced psychosis, use of long-acting injectable formulations of risperidone and paliperidone may be helpful to increase retention and engagement in treatment.

- **Anticonvulsants:** In a multicenter RCT, topiramate was more effective than placebo at reducing use and relapse rates, but not at promoting abstinence. Baclofen was effective at reducing use in highly adherent participants (Chan et al., 2019). Topiramate can be dosed 25–150 mg twice daily.

- **Atomoxetine 80 mg:** This is a nonstimulant medication for ADHD that inhibits the norepinephrine transporter to increase norepinephrine and dopamine (to a lower extent) in the prefrontal cortex. A small RCT in patients receiving buprenorphine/naloxone for OUD showed a reduction in methamphetamine cravings and use compared to placebo. A greater reduction in depressive symptoms was shown with atomoxetine than placebo (Schottenfeld et. al., 2018). It is important for clinicians and patients to know that atomoxetine may not have instantaneous effects as do stimulants, and may take a few weeks to show full benefit.

- **Stimulants:** Stimulants as a class has not shown greater efficacy than placebo. However, it is possible that the doses used in these studies were not sufficient. Among stimulants, methylphenidate has demonstrated efficacy in reducing use, cravings, and addiction severity among those with ADHD (Chan et. al., 2019). Methylphenidate may also improve cognitive symptoms in PWH. Extended-release formulations are preferred because of a lower risk of misuse.

- **Combination pharmacotherapy:** Bupropion 450 mg plus naltrexone 380 mg extended-release injectable every 3 weeks was more effective than placebo at reducing methamphetamine use in 13.6% of individuals (Trivedi et al., 2021).

ECSTASY OR MOLLY (MDMA)

Dubbed the "intimacy drug," ecstasy has been shown to produce profound feelings of closeness, which may lead to high-risk sexual behavior and HIV exposure. Some studies have shown that those using ecstasy may perceive less danger of contracting HIV and other STDs compared to nonusers of ecstasy (Theall, 2006). It is therefore critical that those with HIV and those at higher risk of contracting HIV be educated about the dangers of ecstasy use in addition to the other known health issues that may result from ecstasy use. Currently, there is no FDA-approved medication for treatment of MDMA use disorder, and acute management is geared toward treating life-threatening conditions such as serotonin syndrome and hyperthermia that are commonly seen in rave parties. The primary treatment of MDMA use disorder is cognitive behavioral interventions to help modify thought patterns and help PWH gain skills to cope with life stressors.

CANNABIS

The legalization and permissive attitudes toward cannabis has contributed to a rapid increase in availability and use of cannabis products. Cannabis is used by the public for recreational and medicinal purposes, the latter for a wide range of physical and mental conditions including anxiety, insomnia, and pain. In a study of 226 PWH from Canada, 97.7% reported recreational use, and 21.8% reported medicinal use for stress, anorexia, nausea, and pain. Although negative consequences were not as strongly reported as benefits, cannabis use was associated with other high-risk behaviors such as driving under the influence, ecstasy and tobacco use, paranoia, and greater financial expenditure (Harris et. al., 2014). Cognitive impairment has been well described among PWH who use cannabis. The impact of cannabis use on ARV adherence is inconsistent, with studies indicating negative, positive, or no effect. Data on safety and benefits of cannabis use for PWH is currently inconclusive. We recommend discouraging use and taking a harm-reduction approach in PWH who continue use (i.e., reduce to low-risk levels). Alternative interventions for appetite, anxiety, and sleep should be offered when indicated.

The most common cannabinoids found in the cannabis plant are Delta-9-tetrahydrocannabinol (THC) and cannabidiol (CBD). THC is a partial agonist at the cannabinoid receptors CB1 and CB2, activating the receptor up to 20%. THC use is associated with euphoria, laughter, increased appetite, altered perception of time, and relaxation. On the other hand, CBD is an antagonist at CB1 receptors, a partial agonist at CB2 receptors, and does carry similar euphoric effects to THC. These cannabinoids are smoked, vaped, or consumed as edibles. Cannabis withdrawal is associated with anxiety, irritability, insomnia, and depression. The mainstay of treatment is behavioral therapies such as CBT, motivational interviewing, and motivational enhancement therapy.

There is no well-established pharmacological intervention for cannabis use disorder. Some medications showing potential benefit include gabapentin, N-acetylcysteine (NAC), and cannabidiol. Gabapentin (1,200 mg or higher in divided doses) has shown benefit in reducing cannabis cravings, use, and withdrawal. Gabapentin may be beneficial for PWH who have HIV-associated polyneuropathy and pain. It is also often used off-label for anxiety and AUD. However, gabapentin has misuse potential and is now a controlled substance in several states. NAC 1,200 mg twice daily showed a use reduction in adolescents aged 15–21 years, but was not better than placebo in a group of adults aged 18–50 (Brezing & Levin, 2018). A 2020 study showed that participants receiving CBD 400 mg and 800 mg were more likely to use less cannabis and have more days abstinent (Freeman et al., 2020). However, more studies are needed to establish the safety and efficacy of CBD. A gradual transition from THC to CBD by slowly reducing THC concentration may be a harm-reduction approach for PWH who are still ambivalent about abstinence from cannabis.

MULTIPLE SUBSTANCE USE

Most people who use illicit substances use multiple substances, with tobacco/nicotine being the most common comorbid SUD. One study found that multisubstance use was present in 93.8% of heroin users (John et al., 2018). In our experience, multisubstance use is the rule rather than the exception in people with moderate-to-severe SUD. Overdose death rates have skyrocketed in recent years from the "speedball" combination of methamphetamine and opioids, particularly, fentanyl (NIH, 2021). Multisubstance use is associated with worse treatment outcomes and higher severity SUD. Therefore, it is important to address all SUD even when they may seem less impairing. For example, treatment of tobacco/nicotine use disorder may improve outcomes in patients with CUD (Winhusen et al., 2014). With such high rates of multisubstance use, we recommend providing all patients with illicit substance use, especially stimulant and opioids, with naloxone nasal spray for overdose prevention.

SPECIAL CONSIDERATIONS IN HIV POPULATIONS

Interactions between substances of abuse and ARV agents have been reported. The toxicity of amphetamines, MDMA, meperidine, and gamma hydroxybutyrate (GHB) is dangerously increased by ritonavir and other HIV medications that inhibit liver metabolism. Barbiturates induce the cytochrome systems responsible for metabolism of protease inhibitors (PI), nonnucleoside reverse transcriptase inhibitors (NNRTIs), maraviroc, elvitegravir, and dolutegravir, significantly decreasing their effectiveness. Oral midazolam and triazolam are contraindicated with PIs, NNRTIs, and efavirenz. The toxicity of ketamine and phencyclidine (PCP) is dangerously increased by PIs and etravirine.

All the agents listed for use in withdrawal management and maintenance of sobriety have utility in the HIV population, but special considerations include:

- Buprenorphine administration is office-based but requires special training and certification (an X-waiver). To increase treatment of OUD, recent reforms no longer require training to apply for an X-waiver to prescribe to 30 or fewer patients. Clinically, significant interactions occur with ARVs, including atazanavir, darunavir, and ritonavir (increased buprenorphine activity and sedation—especially with atazanavir) and etravirine, nevirapine, and tipranavir (decreased buprenorphine activity, with tipranavir levels also significantly decreased). Fluconazole can increase the activity of buprenorphine, whereas phenobarbital, phenytoin, rifabutin, and rifampin decrease the effective amounts, but sometimes cause withdrawal symptoms.

- Bupropion decreases the seizure threshold and increases risk of seizures in individuals with weight loss or electrolyte instability. Bupropion should be avoided in these patients until weight is restored and electrolyte abnormalities are corrected.

- Disulfiram (Antabuse) has a high risk of hepatotoxicity and may interact with tipranavir/ritonavir capsules (they contain alcohol).

- Methadone maintenance cannot be provided outside a registered clinic, and this agent has several clinically significant adverse interactions with ARVs (blood levels of abacavir are decreased; blood level of zidovudine is increased; abacavir increases blood levels of methadone, and dose adjustment may be required to avoid sedation; efavirenz, nevirapine, darunavir, lopinavir, ritonavir (even in boosting doses), and tipranavir all decrease methadone availability, and may precipitate withdrawal symptoms). Drug interactions with other medications frequently used in the HIV population are also reported (carbamazepine, phenobarbital, phenytoin, and rifampin sharply decrease methadone levels, and fluconazole significantly increases methadone blood levels).

- Naltrexone cannot be used in individuals requiring narcotic pain control but does not seem to interact with ARVs.

- Nirmatrelvir/ritonavir (Paxlovid) is used to treat COVID-19 infection. Ritonavir, as discussed in this chapter, may interact with medications for SUD.

- When selecting a medication for a SUD, consider comorbid conditions that may also benefit. For example, gabapentin may be considered for comorbid pain and cannabis use disorder. Methylphenidate may be preferred for HIV-associated cognitive impairment and stimulant use disorder.

SUBSTANCE USE AND HIV IN THE CORONAVIRUS (COVID-19) PANDEMIC

The COVID-19 pandemic has placed tremendous strain on the healthcare system, creating unique challenges for individuals with SUD. Currently there are limited data on the intersection between the COVID-19 pandemic, SUD, and HIV/AIDS. However, the pandemic involves social isolation, anxiety, stress, and boredom that can increase risk for substance use. Many individuals with SUD are homeless, incarcerated, or actively seeking drugs, putting them at greater risk for

contracting or transmitting COVID-19. As previously mentioned, substance use can increase exposure to HIV, which may be more likely with greater difficulty accessing community harm-reduction resources like syringe services programs that provide sterile injection equipment. In addition, people with SUD and comorbid medical conditions may be more likely to develop severe illness with COVID-19 infection. The virus's attack on the lungs could be a serious threat for PWH who smoke and vape tobacco and marijuana. Individuals with OUD may be vulnerable to hypoxemia with concurrent opioid use and respiratory infections. Methamphetamine can cause lung damage from constriction of blood vessels and pulmonary hypertension. Pre-existing respiratory conditions such as chronic obstructive pulmonary disease may increase mortality from viral illness. Data from the Chinese Center for Disease Control and Prevention showed that the fatality rate for COVID-19 was 6.3% for those with chronic respiratory disease compared to a rate of 2.3% overall (Wu & McGoogan, 2020). PWH may also be at risk of developing severe disease based on their age, comorbid medical conditions, and immune status. Thus, compliance with ART and medical follow-up should be discussed at each visit. PWH should be provided with education on these risks with practical recommendations to reduce or stop substance use. Those with ongoing substance use should be encouraged to practice harm-reduction behaviors such as using protective equipment (e.g., masks) when seeking drugs, practicing physical distancing when using, and using sterile needles when injecting. Although research is ongoing regarding impact of COVID-19 on various populations, PWH with respiratory diseases may experience discomfort with breathing while wearing a mask. Another consideration is history of trauma in this population, which mask-wearing—depending on the trauma—may elicit traumatic memories, feelings of suffocation and helplessness. Providers attuned to these issues may guide the individual in finding solutions to practice safe behaviors. Most importantly, all PWH should be offered the COVID vaccine and boosters.

Many residential/inpatient treatment centers have reduced the number of available beds to follow physical distancing guidelines. People who need residential treatment may have to be managed on an outpatient basis with close follow-up until space becomes available. Telehealth services have expanded in response to the pandemic, allowing continuation of care for those who need or want to maintain physical distancing. Collaboration between individuals and providers is key to determining if telehealth or in-person treatment is best. Careful balancing of risk of exposure to COVID-19 and benefits of in-person visits should be discussed with each person. PWH with ongoing substance use may require frequent in-person visits for comprehensive evaluation, physical exam, and urine toxicology screens, but stable PWH may be appropriate for a hybrid of telehealth and in-person management. Many clinics have adopted a hybrid telehealth/in-person model to provide care for different SUD populations. Whenever possible and appropriate, telehealth should be utilized if transportation and other barriers are impeding treatment. Providers are encouraged to check the CDC, SAMHSA, NIDA, and other trusted organizations for updates on recommendations and research.

SUMMARY

Substance use and SUDs are common in the HIV population, and require early and aggressive diagnosis and treatment, both to minimize further spread of the disease through ungoverned risk behaviors and to maximize the ability of the individual to fully participate in HIV treatment. Successful management will decrease morbidity and mortality from both conditions. Adequate treatment of substance use can improve adherence to HIV regimens (clinic visits and ART) to levels comparable to those seen in nonaddicted HIV populations. These principles apply even more stringently in those with "triple diagnosis"—substance abuse, mental illness, and HIV. As with any treatment process, success involves establishing a collaborative alliance—a therapeutic relationship between treatment staff and patients. This sets the stage for honest communication, mutual respect of boundaries, and continued participation in treatment (on both sides) despite temporary setbacks and failures. Integrated treatment of substance abuse and HIV (or substance abuse, HIV, and mental illness in the case of triple diagnosis) offers distinct advantages for these complex cases with multiple barriers to participation. Factors in a decision to start ART in individuals with active substance abuse are obviously complex, but substance use alone should not be an absolute contraindication to ART.

RECOMMENDED READING

Miller SC, Fiellin DA, Rosenthal RN, Saitz R. *The ASAM principles of addiction medicine*. Philadelphia: Wolters Kluwer; 2019.

Ruiz P, Strain EC. Alcohol abstinence pharmacotherapy treatment. In: Ruiz P, Strain EC (eds.), *The substance abuse handbook*. Philadelphia: Lippincott Williams & Wilkins; 2014.

Ruiz P, Strain EC. Amphetamines and other stimulants. In: Ruiz P, Strain EC (eds.), *The substance abuse handbook*. Philadelphia: Lippincott Williams & Wilkins; 2014.

Ruiz P, Strain EC. Buprenorphine treatment. In: Ruiz P, Strain EC (eds.), *The substance abuse handbook*. Philadelphia: Lippincott Williams & Wilkins; 2014.

Ruiz P, Strain EC. Cocaine and crack. In: Ruiz P, Strain EC (eds.), *The substance abuse handbook*. Philadelphia: Lippincott Williams & Wilkins; 2014.

Ruiz P, Strain EC. Methadone maintenance treatment. In: Ruiz P, Strain EC (eds.), *The substance abuse handbook*. Philadelphia: Lippincott Williams & Wilkins; 2014.

Ruiz P, Strain EC. Naltrexone and other pharmacotherapies for opioid dependence. In: Ruiz P, Strain EC (eds.), *The substance abuse handbook*. Philadelphia: Lippincott Williams & Wilkins; 2014.

REFERENCES

American Psychiatric Association. *Diagnostic and statistical manual of mental disorders, text revision*. 5th ed. Washington, DC: APA Press; 2022.

Anton RF, Latham P, Voronin K, et al. Efficacy of gabapentin for the treatment of alcohol use disorder in patients with alcohol withdrawal symptoms: a randomized clinical trial. *JAMA Intern Med*. 2020;180(5):728–736.

Bhaskaran K, Hamouda O, Sannes M, et al. Changes in the risk of death after HIV seroconversion compared with mortality in the general population. *JAMA*. 2008;300(1):51–59.

Baum MK, Rafie C, Lai S, et al. Crack-cocaine use accelerates HIV disease progression in a cohort of HIV-positive drug users. *J AIDS*. 2009;50(1):93–99.

Blevins D, Seneviratne C, Wang X.-Q, Johnson BA, Ait-Daoud N. A randomized, double-blind, placebo-controlled trial of ondansetron for the treatment of cocaine use disorder with post hoc pharmacogenetic analysis. *Drug and Alcohol Dependence*. 2021;228:109074.

Brezing CA, Levin FR. The current state of pharmacological treatments for cannabis use disorder and withdrawal. *Neuropsychopharmacology*. 2018;43(1):173–194.

Branson BM, Handsfield HH, Lampe MA, et al. Revised recommendations for HIV testing of adults, adolescents, and pregnant women in health-care settings. *MMWR Recomm Rep*. 2006;55(RR-14):1–17.

Carroll K, Rounsaville B, Nich C, et al. One-year follow-up of psycho-therapy and pharmacotherapy for cocaine dependence: delayed emergence of psychotherapy effects. *Arch Gen Psychiatry*. 1994;51:989–997.Campos-Outcalt D. 8 USPSTF recommendations FPs need to know about. *J Fam Pract*. 2016;65:338–342.

Castells X, Cunill R, Pérez-Mañá C, Vidal X, Capellà D. Psychostimulant drugs for cocaine dependence. *Cochrane Database of Systematic Reviews*. 2016;2016(9):CD007380.

Centers for Disease Control and Prevention (CDC). Incorporating HIV prevention into the medical care of persons living with HIV. Recommendations of CDC, the Health Resources and Services Administration, the National Institutes of Health, and the HIV Medicine Association of the Infectious Diseases Society of America. *MMWR Recomm Rep*. 2003;52(RR-12):1–24.

CDC. *HIV surveillance report, 2018 (Updated)*.Vol. 31. http://www.cdc.gov/hiv/library/reports/hiv-surveillance.html. Published May 2020.

Chan B, Freeman M, Kondo K, Ayers C, Montgomery J, Paynter R, Kansagara D. Pharmacotherapy for methamphetamine/amphetamine use disorder—a systematic review and meta-analysis. *Addiction*. 2019; 114(12):2122–2136.

Chen CC, Lu R-B, Chen Y-C, et al. Interaction between the functional polymorphisms of the alcohol metabolism genes in protection against alcoholism. *Am J Hum Genet*. 1999;65(3):795–807.

Coffin PO, Santos G-M, Hern J, et al. Effects of mirtazapine for methamphetamine use disorder among cisgender men and transgender women who have sex with men: a placebo-controlled randomized clinical trial. *JAMA Psychiatry*. 2020;77(3):246.

Cofrancesco J Jr, Scherzer R, Tien PC, et al. Illicit drug use and HIV treatment outcomes in a US cohort. *AIDS*. 2008;22:237–245.

Forest Pharmaceuticals. *Campral (Acamprosate calcium) delayed release tablets [product information]*. St. Louis, MO: Forest Pharmaceuticals; 2004.

Freeman TP, Hindocha C, Baio G, et al. Cannabidiol for the treatment of cannabis use disorder: a phase 2a, double-blind, placebo-controlled, randomised, adaptive Bayesian trial. *Lancet Psychiatry*. 2020; 7(10):865–874.

Goeldner C, Lutz PE, Darcq E, et al. Impaired emotional-like behavior and serotonergic function during protracted abstinence from chronic morphine. *Biol Psychiatry*. 2011;69(3):236–244.

Harris GE, Dupuis L, Mugford GJ, et al. Patterns and correlates of cannabis use among individuals with HIV/AIDS in maritime Canada. *Canadian Journal of Infectious Diseases & Medical Microbiology*. 2014;25(1):e1–e7.

Hillfors DD, Iritani BJ, Miller WC, et al. Sexual and drug behavior patterns and HIV and STD racial disparities: the need for new directions. *Am J Public Health*. 2007;97(1):125–132.

Hinkin CH, Castellon SA, Hardy DJ, Farinpour R, Newton T, Singer E. Methylphenidate improves HIV-1–associated cognitive slowing. *Journal of Neuropsychiatry and Clinical Neurosciences*. 2001;13(2):248–254.

John WS, Zhu H, Mannelli P, Schwartz RP, Subramaniam GA, Wu L-T. Prevalence, patterns, and correlates of multiple substance use disorders among adult primary care patients. *Drug and Alcohol Dependence*. 2018;187:79–87.

Johnson BA, Roache JD, Ait-Daoud N, et al. A preliminary randomized, double-blind, placebo-controlled study of the safety and efficacy of ondansetron in the treatment of cocaine dependence. *Drug and Alcohol Dependence*. 2006;84(3):256–263.

Lollis CM, Strothers HS, et al. Sex, drugs and HIV: does methadone maintenance reduce drug use and risky sexual behavior? *J Behav Med*. 2000;23(;6):545–557.

Low AJ, Mburu G, Welton NJ, et al. Impact of opioid substitution therapy on antiretroviral therapy outcomes: a systematic review and meta-analysis. *Clin Infect Dis*. 2016;63(8):1094–1104.

McCance-Katz EF, Gruber VA, Beatty G, et al. Interaction of disulfiram with antiretroviral medications: efavirenz increases while atazanavir decreases disulfiram effect on enzymes of alcohol metabolism. *American Journal on Addictions*. 2014;23(2):137–144.

McLellan AT, Lewis DC, O'Brien CP, Kleber HD. Drug dependence, a chronic medical illness: implications for treatment, insurance, and outcomes evaluation. *JAMA*. 2000;284:1689–1695.

Meredith CW, Jaffe C, Cherrier M, et al. Open trial of injectable risperidone for methamphetamine dependence. *Journal of Addiction Medicine*. 2009;3(2):55–65.

Meredith CW, Jaffe C, Yanasak E, Cherrier M, Saxon AJ. An open-label pilot study of risperidone in the treatment of methamphetamine dependence. *Journal of Psychoactive Drugs*. 2007;39(2):167–172.

Mille, SC, Fiellin DA, Rosenthal RN, Saitz R. *The ASAM principles of addiction medicine*. Philadelphia, PA: Wolters Kluwer; 2019.

Millett GA, Flores SA, Bakeman R. Explaining disparities in HIV infection among Black and White men who have sex with men: a meta-analysis of HIV risk behaviors. *AIDS*. 2007;21(15):2083–2091.

Minozzi S, Amato L, Vecchi S, et al. Anticonvulsants for alcohol withdrawal. *Cochrane Database Syst Rev*. 2010;3:CD005064.

Minozzi S, Cinquini M, Amato L, Davoli M, Farrell MF, Pani PP, Vecchi S. Anticonvulsants for cocaine dependence. *Cochrane Database of Systematic Reviews*. 2015;4:CD006754.

Moore RM, Gebo KA, Lucas GM, et al. Rate of co-morbidities not related to HIV infection or AIDS among HIV-positive patients by CD4 count and HAART use status. *Clin Infect Dis*. 2008;47(8):1102–1104.

National Institute on Alcohol Abuse and Alcoholism. *Helping patients who drink too much: a clinician's guide*. www.samhsa.gov/resource/ebp/helping-patients-who-drink-too-much-clinicians-guide. Published 2007. Accessed September 5, 2017.

NIDB. Overdose death rates. https://www.drugabuse.gov/drug-topics/trends-statistics/overdose-death-rates. January 29, 2021. Accessed September 30, 2022.

New York State Department of Health AIDS Institute. *Substance use in patients with HIV/AIDS*. Albany: New York State Department of Health; 2009.

Pani PP, Trogu E, Vacca, R, Amato L, Vecchi S, Davoli M. Disulfiram for the treatment of cocaine dependence. *Cochrane Database of Systematic Reviews*. 2010;1:CD007024.

Peters P, et al. HIV infection linked to injection use of oxymorphone in Indiana, 2014–2015. *N Engl J Med*. 2016;375:229–239.

Ruiz P, Strain EC. Psychiatric complications of HIV-1 infection and drug abuse. In: Ruiz P, Strain EC (eds.), *The substance abuse handbook*. Philadelphia: Lippincott Williams & Wilkins; 2014.

Schottenfeld RS, Chawarski MC, Sofuoglu M, et al. Atomoxetine for amphetamine-type stimulant dependence during buprenorphine treatment: a randomized controlled trial. *Drug and Alcohol Dependence*. 2018;186:130–137.

Shorter D, Lindsay JA, Kosten TR. The alpha-1 adrenergic antagonist doxazosin for treatment of cocaine dependence: a pilot study. *Drug Alcohol Depend*. 2013;131(1-2):66–70.

Stern TA, Freudenreich O, Smith FA, Fricchione G, Rosenbaum JF. *Massachusetts General Hospital handbook of general hospital psychiatry*. Philadelphia: Elsevier; 2018.

Strain EC, Stitzer ML, Lisbon IA, et al. Dose–response effects of methadone in the treatment of opioid dependence. *Ann Intern Med*. 1993a;119:23–27.

Strain EC, Stitzer ML, Lisbon IA, et al. Methadone dose and treatment outcome. *Drug Alcohol Depend* 1993b;33:105–117.

Substance Abuse and Mental Health Services Administration (SAMHSA). National survey of substance abuse treatment services: the N-SSATS report. February 25, 2010.

Substance Abuse and Mental Health Services Administration (SAMHSA). 2016 National survey on drug use and health. https://www.samhsa.gov/data/sites/default/files/NSDUH-FFR1-2016/NSDUH-FFR1-2016.pdf. Published 2017. Accessed September 30, 2023.

Sullivan LE, Goulet JL, Justice AC, et al. Alcohol consumption and depressive symptoms over time: a longitudinal study of patients with and without HIV infection. *Drug Alcohol Depend*. 2011;117:158–163.

Theall KP, Elifson KW, Sterk CE. Sex, touch, and HIV risk among ecstasy users. *AIDS Behav*. 2006;10(2):169–178.

Trivedi MH, Walker R, Ling W, et al. Bupropion and naltrexone in methamphetamine use disorder. *N Engl J Med*. 2021;384(2):140–153.

Truong TT, Li B. Case series: cariprazine for treatment of methamphetamine use disorder. *American Journal on Addictions*. 2022;31(1):85–88.

Van Handle M, et al. County-level vulnerability assessment for rapid dissemination of HIV or HCV infections among persons who inject drugs, United States. *J AIDS*. 2016;73(3):323–331.

Wang G, Ma L, Liu X, et al. Paliperidone extended-release tablets for the treatment of methamphetamine use disorder in Chinese patients after acute treatment: a randomized, double-blind, placebo-controlled exploratory study. *Frontiers in Psychiatry*. 2019;10:656. doi:10.3389/fpsyt.2019.00656.

West R. Models of addiction. European Moderating Centre for Drugs and Drug Addiction. 2013. Models of Addiction. | www.emcdda.europa.eu

Winhusen TM, Kropp F, Theobald J, Lewis DF. Achieving smoking abstinence is associated with decreased cocaine use in cocaine-dependent patients receiving smoking-cessation treatment. *Drug and Alcohol Dependence*. 2014;134:391–395.

Woody GE, McLellan AT, Luborsky L, et al. Psychotherapy in community methadone programs: a validation study. *Am J Psychiatry*. 1995;152(9):1302–1308.

Wu Z, McGoogan JM. Characteristics of and important lessons from the coronavirus disease 2019 (COVID-19) outbreak in China: summary of a report of 72 314 cases from the Chinese Center for Disease Control and Prevention. *JAMA*. 2020;323(13):1239–1242.

27.

CARING FOR OLDER PEOPLE WITH HIV

Aroonsiri Sangarlangkarn, John D. Zeuli, and Anchalee Avihingsanon

LEARNING OBJECTIVE

Describe how HIV care and management for persons with HIV (PWH) who are aged 50 years and older differs from the care and management for younger PWH.

WHAT'S NEW?

- Updated information regarding COVID-19 vaccine in PWH and updated Veterans Aging Cohort Study (VACS) index 2.0.

KEY POINTS

- Each older PWH is a unique and complex individual, and disease-centric guidelines should not be applied the same way in every patient.

- Management of diseases in older PWH should be individualized based on aging phenotypes, interactions with multimorbidity, and patient preferences.

- The VACS index may be used to identify aging phenotypes and can provide prognostic information to help prioritize interventions and guide shared decision-making with PWH and caregivers.

INTRODUCTION

There are increasing proportions of older PWH. It is estimated that at year-end 2018, persons aged 50–54 years made up the largest percentage of PWH (15%). From 2011–2015, the largest increase in rates of PWH was among persons aged 65 years and older (57%, from 94.2 in 2011 to 148.0 in 2015) (CDC, 2018). Part of this group consisted of individuals who have aged with chronic HIV infection, but a large proportion also resulted from new HIV diagnosis, with 16.6% of all new HIV transmissions in 2016 diagnosed in PWH aged 50 years and older (CDC, 2020).

Although many of the recommendations on the management of HIV infection are not age specific, PWH over the age of 50 years differ from their younger counterparts in many aspects, including diagnostic considerations, immune response to ART, and multimorbidity. In this chapter, we outline these differences, offer a strategy on how to care for this unique population, provide a practical guide on how to perform Comprehensive Geriatric Assessment (CGA), and describe special considerations for problem-based management of PWH over the age of 50.

DIFFERENCES IN OLDER PWH COMPARED TO YOUNGER PWH

The most common mode of HIV transmission among adults aged 50 years and older is through sexual contact. Among men, male-to-male sexual contact is the most common transmission risk, while heterosexual contact is the most common among women (CDC, 2013). This may be due to a false sense of security among older adults who view sexually transmitted illness (STI) as a condition of the young, and may forgo safe sex practices based on this perception (Pilowsky & Wu, 2015). They may also forgo barrier contraceptives when unwanted pregnancy is no longer a concern. Even though sexual exposure is the most common mode of HIV transmission among PWH aged 50 years and older, prior research has found that health care professionals often underestimate the level of sexual activity among older adults and their risk of STI exposure (Pilowsky & Wu, 2015; Lindau et al., 2007).

Moreover, many symptoms of early HIV transmissions mimic those of old age and may be difficult for clinicians to tease apart. Symptoms of acute HIV transmissions such as headache, loss of energy, loss of appetite, flu-like symptoms, or weight loss are common in older adults and can be caused by a myriad of conditions associated with old age, such as malignancy or frailty.

With inaccurate perception of HIV exposure risk and symptom mimicry, underdiagnoses and late diagnoses of HIV transmissions are common among older adults (Dai et al., 2015; Pilowsky & Wu, 2015). Late diagnosis is associated with delayed treatment, impaired response to ART, increased morbidity and mortality, lost opportunity to prevent onward transmission, and increased cost of health care (British HIV Assoc., 2016). As a result, it is essential that clinicians maintain a high suspicion and routinely screen older adults for HIV, regardless of risk perception. Although guidelines from the Centers for Disease Control and Prevention (CDC) recommends routine screening up to the age of 64 years old (CDC, 2006), the rationale or research evidence for this age cutoff was not included, and we recommend routine screening for all older adults as risk perception may be inaccurate in this population.

Despite successful viral suppression with ART, older adults have less robust immunologic recovery compared to their younger counterparts, with associated increase in mortality (Mpondo et al., 2016; Semeere et al., 2014; Vinikoor et al., 2014). Consequently, early HIV diagnosis and treatment is of great importance.

MULTIMORBIDITY

Older PWH are at increased risk of *multimorbidity* (Guaraldi et al., 2014), defined as the development of multiple chronic conditions that do not simply coexist, but together interact to worsen health outcomes. Compared to those without HIV, older PWH have higher burdens of cardiovascular, metabolic, pulmonary, renal, bone, and malignant diseases (Schouten et al., 2014). Multimorbidity is likely contributed by both lifestyle risk factors, as well as chronic HIV infection, with longer duration of severe immunodeficiency (CD4$^+$ counts< 200 cells/μL) correlating with higher comorbidity burden (Schouten et al., 2014).

Multimorbidity has important ramifications on health outcomes. It is associated with self-reported poor health, declines in self-rated health status, and increased mortality (adjusted odds ratio 11.87; 95% CI: 5.72–24.62). With increasing disease burden, PWH with multimorbidity are also at risk of fragmentation in care because of the involvement of multiple clinicians in multiple settings. Guidelines for one disease may clash with another, as most are disease-centric recommendations based on the ideal patient without multimorbidity (Tinetti et al., 2012). Treatments for one disease may inadvertently worsen other conditions, and increased treatment burden stemming from efforts to adhere to all relevant disease-centric guidelines without prioritization may not bring improvement in mortality or quality of life.

MANAGEMENT STRATEGY FOR THE CARE OF OLDER PWH

Each older PWH is a unique and complex individual. They cannot be described fully by one-dimensional classifications, such as chronological age or single disease entities. Aging occurs at different rates in different individuals, and within the same individual in different organs, resulting in different aging phenotypes that cannot be predicted by chronological age alone. Additionally, viewing PWH by a single disease entity ignores the importance of multimorbidity and the often-multifactorial nature of their diseases. Most importantly, different PWH have different goals and preferences. Consequently, applying disease-centric guidelines uniformly to every patient without considering aging phenotypes, multimorbidity, or individual preference ignores the unique care needs of each patient and likely will not lead to desirable patient-centered outcomes.

Understanding that not all PWH aged 50 years and older should be approached the same way, clinicians may utilize the VACS index (Justice et al., 2013b) to distinguish between those who are aging well and those who may appear phenotypically older than their chronological age. The VACS index has been shown to correlate with functional status (John et al., 2014), provide insight to clinician assessment of severity of illness (Justice et al., 2013b), and predict cause-specific (Justice et al., 2012) as well as all-cause mortality (Justice et al., 2013a). Based on prognosis predicted by the VACS index, clinicians can elicit patient preferences, identify diseases and risk factors that affect these goals, calculate the likely effects and lag time to benefit (Lee et al., 2013) of various disease-centric guidelines on these goals, and use this information to prioritize interventions and guide shared decision-making with patients and caregivers. The recently updated VACS index 2.0 is freely accessible on MDCalc (https://www.mdcalc.com/calc/10402/veterans-aging-cohort-study-vacs-2.0-index).

COMPREHENSIVE GERIATRIC ASSESSMENT

CGA is defined as a multidisciplinary diagnostic and treatment process that evaluates medical, psychosocial, and functional deficits in order to develop a coordinated intervention/plan to maximize overall health with aging (Stuck et al., 1993). CGA is based on the idea that a systematic evaluation of an older patient may lead to early detection of geriatric problems, help prevent complications, and aid the formation of comprehensive treatment plans (Bellera et al., 2012).

There is no peer-reviewed literature to demonstrate the efficacy of CGA in older PWH, although, owing to increased risks of geriatric syndromes in older PWH, many studies advocate for CGA in this population. In people without HIV, CGA in the home may improve functional status, prevent institutionalization, and reduce mortality (Huss et al., 2012). CGA in the hospital, especially in dedicated units, may improve survival (Ellis et al., 2017). However, CGA in the outpatient settings has not been found to consistently show benefits (Stuck et al., 1993), possibly because of the variability in adherence to recommendations in CGA. CGA as part of inpatient geriatric consultation (except for specific conditions such as hip fracture) have shown little benefit (Ellis et al., 2017; Stuck et al., 1993). Studies have shown that more complex CGA programs that address adherence or target patients at higher risk of admission may improve outcomes including physical functioning, social functioning, pain, mental/physical/emotional health, and overall well-being (Reuben et al., 1999).

PERFORMING CGA

Consider avoiding assessing all domains of CGA in a single visit—this could be overwhelming and tiring for an elderly patient and their family members. It may make sense to prioritize domains that are most likely to be abnormal or most urgent (likely to cause complications or catastrophic outcomes). Once the most urgent domains have been managed, patients can be brought back to complete the remaining non-urgent domains at subsequent visits. Various team members may be delegated to certain domains of the CGA based on their expertise or availability. For example, it may make sense for a pharmacist to assess patients for polypharmacy instead of a physician.

There is no consensus on selection criteria for patients who may benefit from CGA However, prior programs have used criteria such as age, medical comorbidities/complexity, specific geriatric syndromes such as falls/dementia, previous or predicted high utilization rates, or at times of transition, such as from hospital to home, or from home to nursing homes.

There is no consensus on what domains should be included in CGA and what tools are appropriate for each domain. However, most programs include some or all of the following domains. Except when noted, corresponding interventions are described in more details in the European AIDS Clinical Society guideline, accessible through website or mobile app (https://eacs.sanfordguide.com) (EACS, 2021).

FUNCTION

The Activity of Daily Living (ADL) and Instrumental Activity of Daily Living (IADL) have been utilized in PWH, are simple to perform and can readily identify essential deficits that may guide interventions. To assess function, providers may ask about ADL/IADL and determine who does them (patient or others). ADL consists of bathing, dressing, grooming, toileting, transferring, and eating. IADL consists of cooking, shopping, managing medications, using the phone, doing housework, doing laundry, driving or using public transportation, and managing finances (Katz et al., 1963).

MOBILITY/FALLS

For subjective measures. PWH may be asked if they had a *fall* in the past 12 months, defined as unexpectedly dropping to the floor or ground from a standing, walking, or bending position (Erlandson et al., 2012, 2016; Ruiz et al., 2013). For objective measures, providers may use the Timed Get-Up-and-Go (TUG) test (Podsiadlo & Richardson, 1991), in which the patient is timed while he/she/they rises from a chair, walks 3 meters, turns, walks back, and sits down again. The TUG has been used in prior HIV studies (Grinspoon et al., 1996; Grinspoon et al., 1998) and explores multiple components of mobility, including gait speed, balance, and proximal muscle strength. The TUG has also been shown to correlate with functional capacity and more formal tests on balance and gait speed (Podsiadlo & Richardson, 1991). Although various cutoffs have been used in prior studies, the CDC recommends that an older adult who takes ≥12 seconds to complete TUG should be considered at risk of falling (CDC, 2017).

FRAILTY

There is no consensus on the best tools to assess for frailty in older PWH (Conroy, 2009; Brothers & Rockwood, 2019).

The Fried frailty phenotype (Fried et al., 2001) is commonly used in HIV research and has been operationalize for clinical practice (Rockwood et al., 2007) to consist of five components (no items = robust; 1-2 = prefrail; 3–5 = frail):

1. *Weight loss*: defined as loss of either ≥10 pounds or ≥5% of body weight in the past year.

2. *Exhaustion* (poor endurance and energy): defined as self-reporting of feeling "tired all the time."

3. *Low physical activity levels and energy expenditure*: defined as needing assistance with walking to being unable to walk.

4. *Slowness*: defined as a time of ≥19 seconds on TUG test.

5. *Weakness*: defined as abnormal strength on physical examination.

The VACS index is another frailty tool specifically validated in PWH, with more details described previously. An online calculator is accessible on MDCalc at: (https://www.mdcalc.com/calc/10402/veterans-aging-cohort-study-vacs-2.0-index). Prior HIV studies have also used the frailty index. Because it follows the cumulative deficit approach and assesses for at least 30 and up to 75 health variables (Searle et al., 2008), this may prove cumbersome in clinical practice.

COGNITION/SAFETY CONCERNS

Age is a risk factor for cognitive impairment associated with HIV as well as other causes (Chan et al., 2014). It should be noted that many studies of cognitive impairment screening in PWH focus on the entity of HIV-associated neurocognitive disorder (HAND), although in clinical practice, providers would likely need to screen for cognitive impairment from all causes as older PWH are not immune from Alzheimer disease or vascular dementia. Providers may consider using the Montreal Cognitive Assessment, since it has been studied extensively in PWH (Rosca et al., 2019; Sangarlangkarn et al., 2019), and it is commonly used to screen for other causes of cognitive impairment. The HIV Dementia Scale (Power et al., 1995) and the International HIV Dementia Scale (Sacktor et al., 2005) were developed to screen for HAND, but their effectiveness in screening for other causes of dementia is unclear. Even though the Mini-Mental Status Exam is regularly used in HIV-negative individuals, it does not assess for executive function, which may be impaired in HAND (Valcour et al., 2011). Neuropsychological testing may be inaccessible or cumbersome for older PWH to complete.

MOOD

Depression and posttraumatic stress disorder (PTSD) are common in older PWH, especially women and men who have sex with men (Gallagher et al., 2008). Screening for depression and assessment of its severity are important since depression affects quality of life and medical compliance. Multiple tools have been used in PWH to screen for depression, including a screening Patient Health Questionnaire (PHQ-2) with subsequent diagnostic PHQ-9 (Chibanda et al., 2016; EACS, 2021), the Beck Depression Inventory II (BDI-II) (Rodkjaer et al., 2016), or the Center for Epidemiological Studies (CES-D) (Mueses-Marin et al., 2019). Although as many as 14 tools have been used to screen for PTSD in PWH (Gallagher et al., 2008), the posttraumatic stress disorder checklist (PCL-5) was validated for use in HIV primary care (Verhey et al., 2018). Because the understanding and perception of depression or other mental illnesses can be affected by culture, it is important to use tools that have been validated locally if available (Sangarlangkarn et al., 2019).

POLYPHARMACY

Older PWH face a unique challenge of managing the burden of HIV disease in the context of chronic multidrug antiretroviral therapy, increased risk of polypharmacy owing to multimorbidity, decreasing end organ function, and physiologic pharmacodynamic changes resulting in a narrower therapeutic index for many drug therapies. HIV providers need to be aware of polypharmacy in older PWH and take steps to optimize medication safety and effective medication use.

The term *polypharmacy* has been variably defined in the literature, usually meaning that a patient medication profile has reached a threshold number of medications (often six or more) with the degree of polypharmacy correlated to a larger number of absolute medications, though it has also been associated with duration of time on multiple medications, and characterized as to whether or not multiple medications were appropriate for a given condition (appropriate vs. inappropriate polypharmacy) (Masnoon et al., 2017). The nature of chronic combined antiretroviral therapy for PWH in an aging population already at risk of higher medication burden predisposes for potential drug therapy issues (e.g., drug interaction, additive adverse effects/toxicities, pharmacodynamic sensitivity, pill burden, and medication errors). Consequently, it has been shown that the burden of polypharmacy is greater in older PWH than older patients in the general population (Kong et al., 2019) and greater than in younger PWH (Holtzman et al., 2013; Marzolini, 2011).

ART-SPECIFIC CLINICAL CONSIDERATIONS

Multiple factors (e.g., ART history, viral resistance, history of adverse effects, drug interactions, and comorbid conditions) will dictate the selection of appropriate antiretroviral therapy and are covered in detail elsewhere, but considerations can be employed to mitigate age-related concerns in older PWH. Table 27.1 lists relevant class and drug-specific considerations for older PWH.

ADVERSE-EFFECT CONSIDERATIONS

We often have limited data on the prevalence of specific adverse-effect rates of antiretroviral therapy in older PWH, since these patients are often excluded from clinical trials on the basis of confounding illness/multimorbidity, decreased drug clearance, drug–drug interactions that may affect primary outcomes, discontinuation rates, or adverse effect assessment. Although more data evaluating antiretroviral therapy in older PWH are being published (Ramgopal et al., 2020), clinicians still need a heightened awareness of adverse effects of antiretroviral therapy, taking into account the extended duration of therapy, potential additive adverse effects from other drug therapy, historical toxicities from older antiretroviral therapy, and increased risk of complications owing to certain disease states (i.e., cardiovascular disease, diabetes, and osteopenia/osteoporosis).

MEDICATION CLEARANCE CONSIDERATIONS

Aging is associated with loss of function in both the kidney and liver, which can lead to reduced drug metabolism and excretion, increased drug exposure, and predisposition for potentially more drug toxicity (Knobel et al., 2001; Lindeman et al., 1985; Schmucker, 2001; Wellons et al., 2002). Declining drug clearance with age highlights the need to monitor glomerular filtration rate and dose adjust antiretroviral therapy as well as other drug therapy accordingly. The CKD-EPI equation has been postulated in a small subset of HIV patients on stable ART to best predict GFR (Vrouenraets et al., 2012), but the Cockcroft-Gault estimated creatinine clearance remains the standard in clinical trial evaluation and should be used for medication dosing where renal adjustments are required (Abrass et al., 2012). The Childs Pugh score should be calculated for those with chronic liver disease. The DHHS guidelines provides a summary table for dosing adjustments of ART based on estimated creatinine clearance and liver compromise (DHHS, 2022).

COMPREHENSIVE MEDICATION ASSESSMENT

A defined systematic approach to routine medication review will enable identification of medication concerns, guide intervention to address medication issues, optimize prescribing practices, and mitigate or prevent complications arising from polypharmacy in older PWH. Routine and regular medication review should be performed at every care visit, and detailed medication reconciliation should occur at least annually.

We recommend the following systematic approach to medication review in older PWH:

1. Obtain a comprehensive, accurate medication list to perform medication reconciliation.

2. Discontinue unnecessary medication therapy or supplements and optimize nonpharmacologic approaches to aid disease management.

3. Consider new medication therapy for needed indications.

4. Screen for drug interactions.

5. Confirm dosing appropriateness based on renal and liver function and relevant drug interactions.

6. Optimize and simplify the dosing regimen.

Table 27.1 CLASS AND DRUG-SPECIFIC CONSIDERATIONS FOR THE SELECTION OF ART IN OLDER PEOPLE WITH HIV

INSTIs	Often INSTIs are preferred agents given limited drug interactions (except for EVG/c) and favorable adverse effect profile. Potential association with weight gain. Possible neuropsychiatric adverse effects (e.g., dizziness, depression, and insomnia), though rare. Polyvalent mineral supplements (e.g., calcium, iron) should be spaced accordingly to avoid chelation. BIC and DTG inhibit tubular secretion of creatinine and may cause a stable 0.1–0.2 mg/dL increase in serum creatinine without effect on GFR. BIC and DTG have been associated with weight gain.
NNRTIs	EFZ may be a concern in older PWH because of the high incidence of neuropsychiatric adverse effects (e.g., dizziness, altered sensorium, worsening depression, and vivid dreams/nightmares), notable drug interactions (CYP2B6/3A4 inducer), and association with metabolic abnormalities (e.g., dysglycemia, lipid abnormalities). RPV has activity against the common EFZ-associated K103N mutation. However, acid suppression will decrease RPV absorption (PPIs are contraindicated with use), and the food requirement for RPV administration may be inconvenient for older patients. RPV has been associated with QT prolongation, which may be more relevant in older PWH. DOR has less clinical data but may be a favorable option given minimal AEs and activity in the setting of other NNRTI mutations (K103N/Y181C).
PIs	Notable drug interactions must be accounted for with the PI and boosting agent combinations. PIs as a class have both inhibition and induction effects on cytochrome P450 enzymes. The PI class is also associated with lipid abnormalities, metabolic abnormalities, and CV events. Both DRV and ATV require food for administration. ATV has been shown to have a lower association with CV events than DRV, but ATV absorption is reduced with acid suppression therapy. ATV inhibits UGT and leads to increased indirect serum bilirubin. Skin yellowing, scleral icterus, and bile salt deposition of the skin/consequent pruritis can occur in some patients. Risk is higher based on UGT1A1 genotype.
Boosting agents	Both agents pose noteworthy drug interactions as potent CYP3A4 and 2D6 inhibitors. Cobicistat lacks any relevant CYP induction (RTV induces several CYP enzymes) and may afford lower gastrointestinal adverse effects. Cobicistat may also have a lower risk of lipid effect given the independent association of ritonavir with hypertriglyceridemia. Cobicistat also inhibits tubular secretion of creatinine and may cause a stable 0.1–0.2 mg/dL increase in serum creatinine without effect on GFR.
NRTIs	Older NRTIs (DDI, D4T) should not be used given high risk of mitochondrial toxicity (lactic acidosis, hepatotoxicity, and lipodystrophy) and availability of alternatives. AZT can contribute to macrocytic anemia and peripheral neuropathy and should generally be avoided in older PWH. Tenofovir is associated with nephrotoxicity, Fanconi syndrome, and bone mineral density decreases. TAF affords a lower systemic exposure of tenofovir versus TDF, and TAF has demonstrated less effect on serum creatinine and lower bone mineral density changes during treatment, but it may increase lipids. TAF has been associated with weight gain. ABC has been associated with CV disease and CV associated mortality in some studies, though its role as a risk factor is unclear.

EVG/c, elvitegravir/cobicistat; BIC, bictegravir; DTG, dolutegravir; EFZ, efavirenz; RPV, rilpivirine; PI, protease inhibitor; CV, cardiovascular; DRV, darunavir; ATV, atazanavir; RTV, ritonavir; DDI, didanosine; D4T, stavudine; AZT, zidovudine; TAF, tenofovir alafenamide; TDF, tenofovir disoproxil fumarate; ABC, abacavir.

The "brown bag review" (Weiss et al., 2016) is a helpful approach to medication reconciliation, where patients are encouraged to bring all medications, herbal medications/supplements, creams/ointments, inhalers, and eye drops (essentially any item that they use regularly to optimize their health) in a brown bag to their appointment for discussion and review. An advantage to the brown bag approach is that patients can physically point out specific medications and describe how they physically take them, which is particularly helpful when actual administration differs from the instructions printed on the prescription label. Other helpful ways to garner the medication list can be: (1) To obtain a medication profile and dispensing history from their pharmacy for the last 3–6 months. (2) Screen health information networks (i.e., Surescripts) to garner medication dispensing histories, which can be viewed/pulled in by certain electronic health record systems.

After confirming an up-to-date medication list, providers need to align each medication with an indication for therapy, enabling assessment of appropriateness for the indication. Further, each indication for drug therapy can be assessed for

nonpharmacologic measures to reduce medication need. The BEERS criteria (AGS, 2019), medication appropriateness index (Hanlon & Schmader, 2013; Hanlon et al., 1992), and Screening Tool of Older Persons' Prescriptions (STOPP)/Screening Tool to Alert to Right Treatment (START) (Gallagher et al., 2008) can be utilized to effectively determine inappropriate medications in older PWH that can be discontinued or changed to safer alternatives. The BEERS criteria help provide guidance on inappropriate medication selection in older patients, while the medication appropriateness index utilizes a 10-item assessment to determine degree of medication appropriateness. The STOPP helps identify inappropriate medications in the setting of specific diseases and START advocates for utilizing appropriate, effective therapy for a given condition. While inappropriate or harmful medications should be removed, appropriate and indicated medications (e.g., aspirin for prophylaxis of CV stent thrombosis) should most certainly be added where appropriate.

Interaction screening will assess for additive toxicity of multiple therapies, determine if increased/decreased exposure of drugs is expected, or identify if efficacy concerns may arise from the medication profile. Electronic drug database platforms (Micromedex, Lexi-Comp, and Efacts) often have drug interaction screening tools to assist clinicians, though reviewing the metabolic pathways and the enzyme inhibitor/inducer status of profile medications will also help identify potential problems (see Table 23 of the DHHS (2022) guidelines). The DHHS guideline tables 24b-fa, 25a, and 25b, as well as the University of Liverpool website (www.hiv-druginteractions. org/), offer in-depth interaction details and recommendations for antiretroviral therapy.

Finally, medications need to be dosed appropriately for medication clearance (using estimated creatinine clearance and Child-Pugh scores where appropriate) with medication regimens simplified to reduce regimen complexity. Simplification may mean combining administration times to reduce the number of times in the day the patient takes medication and/or offering coformulated tablets to reduce pill burden.

The drug therapy evaluation will need to continually screen for adverse effects, toxicity, and barriers to adherence to maximize safe medication use, ensure efficacy of therapy, and reduce complications related to polypharmacy. This requires providers to:

1. Screen any new clinical sign/symptom as a potential adverse drug effect.

2. Monitor for changes in renal and liver function and dose adjust medication appropriately.

3. Monitor for socioeconomic barriers (i.e., loss of job, insurance, or income) to appropriate medication therapy, engaging social services as able.

4. Continue to discuss goals of care and perceived treatment burden, adjusting or stopping medication therapy that may no longer be congruent with the patient's wishes.

Clinically trained HIV pharmacists are key care team members that can aid in providing optimal care to older PWH (Schafer et al., 2016). Poised to assist in the provision of medication therapy management services, pharmacists are optimal providers to comprehensively reconcile patient medication profiles, screen for drug interaction, and assist with screening of antiretroviral and other drug related toxicities. When HIV clinical pharmacy services are available, we recommend integrating pharmacists into the care team to aid with the comprehensive and systemic medication review in older PWH.

SOCIAL/FINANCIAL ISSUES

A complete social history should be taken. Providers should also ask with whom the patient lives and what types of help/services (e.g., nursing, physical therapy, and home health aides) he/she/they has in the home at baseline to determine the types of support that are currently available and what additional services may be needed. Caregivers should be screened periodically for caregiver burnout (Adelman et al., 2014). Elder mistreatment or abuse should be evaluated when there are worrisome signs such as bruises, burn or bite marks, pressure ulcers, or malnutrition without clinical explanation (NCEA, 2022). A financial history should include determination of health insurance and identification of financial power of attorney in case patients become too ill to manage their finances.

NUTRITION/WEIGHT CHANGES

There is no consensus on an appropriate nutritional screening tool in older PWH since there are few studies in this area (Ruiz & Kammerman, 2010). The Rapid Nutrition Screening for HIV disease (RNS-H) is the only validated tool in PWH (Wright & Epps, 2020). It has seven questions, takes 10 minutes to administer, and includes important outcomes such as food security, anthropometric measures, and nutritional complications such as dysphagia or diarrhea.

SYMPTOM BURDEN/PAIN

The HIV Symptom Index (Justice et al., 2001) assesses bothersome HIV symptoms (Kilbourne et al., 2002; Ruiz & Kamerman, 2010; Whalen et al., 1994) and demonstrates strong associations with disease severity and physical and mental health (Justice et al., 2001). These scales can help providers determine the symptoms present, evaluate the overall symptom burden, and track the severity of the symptoms over time.

The first step in pain management involves assessing the characteristics of the pain and conducting biopsychosocial diagnostic evaluation of the pain, including assessing for associated conditions such as depression and anxiety or substance abuse. The Infectious Disease Society of America recommends using the Brief Pain Inventory-Short Form (BPI-SF) (Goodin et al., 2018) or the PEG (average Pain intensity, interference with Enjoyment of life, and interference with General activity) (Merlin et al., 2018) to understand the functional impact of pain. Using this information, providers can develop treatment plans that improve not only pain, but also physical as well as emotional functions.

ADVANCE CARE PLANNING

Advance care planning is defined as a process of communication between individuals and their healthcare agents to understand, reflect on, discuss, and plan for future healthcare decisions for a time when individuals are not able to make their own healthcare decisions in order to help maximize patient autonomy. With increased risk of neurocognitive impairment and debility from multimorbidity, advance care planning is essential among older PWH. Without clear documentation of surrogate decision-maker for health care and finances, decisions regarding emergent or end-of-life care may be legally deferred estranged family members who are unaware of the patient's preferences or HIV status (Sangarlangkarn et al., 2016). Although there are no specific guidelines for PWH, the National Institute of Aging recommends advance care planning in all patients with chronic life-limiting illness or anyone older than 55 years old regardless of health status (National Institute on Aging, 2018).

There is no formal guideline on the optimal time to initiate advance care planning in PWH. However, it is important to keep in mind that a conversation that is too early may result in changing patient preferences over time or the discussion becoming too abstract/far off in the future, while a conversation that is too late may result in patients being too sick or cognitively impaired to communicate preferences, leading to care that does not match patient preferences. With the lack of validated tools in PWH, providers may use the well-established "Respecting Choices" (Pecanac et al., 2014) paradigm detailing three stages of planning based on the patient's state of health. It should be noted that in cases of late diagnosis with advance disease at the time of ART initiation, short-term prognosis depends on the severity of the acute illness (such as opportunistic infections), while long-term prognosis depends on patient's adherence to ART and their retention in HIV primary care. As a result, advance care planning in this setting needs to balance the optimism surrounding the effectiveness of ART against the severity of acute illness and the long-term challenges of retention in HIV primary care.

If a patient appears to have cognitive impairment, either from baseline dementia or delirium related to other comorbid disease, capacity should be assessed. It should be noted that patients with cognitive impairment/delirium/dementia should not be dismissed as not having capacity. Any provider can determine capacity, not just psychiatrists or geriatricians. *Capacity* is treatment and scenario specific and is defined as the ability to use information regarding a proposed intervention to make a choice that is congruent with the patient's values and preferences. Despite cognitive impairment, if a patient can demonstrate understanding, expressing a choice, appreciation, and reasoning, then he/she/they is deemed to have capacity to make medical decisions.

SPECIAL CONSIDERATIONS FOR PROBLEM-BASED MANAGEMENT OF OLDER PWH

DIABETES

Although primary care guidelines for the management of PWH by the Infectious Disease Society of America (IDSA) did not include age-specific glycemic goals for PWH, AAVHIM recommends a target hemoglobin A1C of 8% for older PWH with frailty, less than 5-year life-expectancy, high risk for hypoglycemia, or high risk for polypharmacy (AAHIVM, 2014). This recommendation mirrors the guideline on standards of medical care in diabetes from the American Diabetes Association (ADA, 2022).

HYPERTENSION

Goal blood pressure for hypertensive patients in the general population remains controversial and presents a challenge for clinicians, with even less evidence to guide management among the HIV-positive population. The Systolic Blood Pressure Intervention Trial (SPRINT) was halted early in September 2015 because of benefits of lowering systolic blood pressure to below 120 mmHg (Ambrosius et al., 2014), and results of SPRINT have affected a change in guidelines in the United States and other countries. The American College of Cardiology and the American Heart Association guideline currently recommends a blood pressure cutoff of 130/80 mmHg (Whelton et al., 2017). The 2018 Canadian Hypertension Education Program Guidelines recommend a target systolic blood pressure ranging from < 120 to 140 mm Hg based on risk stratification with no specific guidelines on older adults or PWH (Hypertension Canada, 2022), while the 2016 Australian guideline (NHF, 2016) also recommends a target systolic blood pressure of ≤ 120 mm Hg (strong recommendation, Class II) for patients with high cardiovascular risk without diabetes, including patients with chronic kidney disease and those >75 years. However, the Eighth Joint National Committee (JNC8) recommendation has not been updated since SPRINT, and the goal remains < 150/90 mmHg in hypertensive adults aged 60 years and older, and a blood pressure goal of < 140/90 mmHg for all hypertensive adults with diabetes or nondiabetic chronic kidney disease (James, 2014). Current gaps include lack of specific recommendations for the HIV-positive population and lack of consensus among varying guidelines. A sensible approach may include a careful up titration of blood pressure medications to achieve the goal blood pressure of 125/90, as long as the patient does not experience medication side effects such as dizziness or falls.

BONE

Certain lifestyle and HIV-related factors put PWH at higher risk of osteoporosis, including smoking, alcohol abuse, glucocorticoid therapy, low consumption of calcium and vitamin D, low physical activity, immune dysfunction, persistent inflammation, and side effects of antiretroviral medications (Castronuovo et al., 2015). Modifiable risk factors should be addressed, and viral suppression should be achieved with ART. The IDSA recommends baseline bone densitometry (DXA) screening for osteoporosis in HIV-positive postmenopausal women and men aged ≥50 years (Thompson, 2021). If osteoporosis is detected, bisphosphonates may be considered, with a follow-up DXA 1 year afterwards to monitor response to therapy. Providers should also ensure patients ingest adequate amounts of calcium (1200 mg/day total diet plus supplement) and vitamin D (800 IU/day) (UpToDate, 2022).

PERIPHERAL NEUROPATHY

Age is a risk factor for peripheral neuropathy (Kaku & Simpaon, 2014). As a result, pain should be assessed at every visit. Currently, trials on symptomatic and disease-modifying treatments for HIV-associated distal symmetric polyneuropathy have had limited success, and there are no US Food and Drug Administration-approved treatments at this time.

AGE-RELATED SEXUAL CHANGES

Age-related sexual changes in PWH include menopause in women and hypogonadism in men.

The IDSA guideline advises that although hormone replacement therapy may be considered in patients with severe menopausal symptoms, it should be used only for a limited period of time at the lowest effective dose. This is because hormone replacement therapy has been associated with a small increased risk of breast cancer, cardiovascular disease, and thromboembolic morbidity (Thompson et al., 2021).

Morning serum testosterone level may be assessed in older HIV-positive men with decreased libido, erectile dysfunction, reduced bone mass or low trauma fractures, hot flashes, or sweats. Low levels should be confirmed with repeat testing. Full recommendations are included in the IDSA guidelines (Thompson, 2021).

MALIGNANCY

As with the uninfected population, age is a risk factor for multiple types of malignancies among PWH. According to the IDSA, mammography should be performed annually in HIV-positive women aged ≥50 years, and colorectal cancer screening should be performed beginning at age 45 years in asymptomatic PWH with average risk (Thompson et al., 2021). The United States Preventive Services Task Force recommends annual screening for lung cancer with low-dose computed tomography (CT) in adults aged 55–80 years who have a 30 pack-year smoking history and currently smoke or have quit within the past 15 years. The screening should be discontinued once the patient has not smoked for 15 years or develops a health problem that limits life-expectancy or the ability/willingness to have curative lung surgery (AHRQ, 2018). Although there was concern that PWH will have a higher false positive rate from chronic lung changes related to immunosuppression-related pulmonary infections, a prior study has shown that this may not be true (Sigel et al., 2014). There was a similar likelihood of pulmonary nodules meeting National Lung Screening Trial criteria for a positive CT scan among PWH and the uninfected population. There were also similar patterns of clinical evaluation triggered by the CT scan, suggesting the follow-up may not be more aggressive among PWH (Sigel et al., 2014).

IMMUNIZATIONS

Live-attenuated varicella vaccination can be given to adult PWH without evidence of immunity with CD4$^+$ T-cell counts ≥200 cells/µL (Grohskopf et al., 2019), as no transmission of vaccine strain varicella-zoster virus has been documented in PWH with CD4$^+$ T-cell counts above this threshold (Shafran, 2015).

Regarding zoster prevention, recombinant zoster vaccine (RZV) has higher and more long-lasting efficacy against herpes zoster and postherpetic neuralgia than herpes zoster live-attenuated vaccine, and the CDC preferentially recommends RZV in all persons aged ≥50 years. However, the efficacy studies did not include immunocompromised persons, and the CDC does not make recommendations regarding use of RZV in this population, although it may be reasonable to vaccinate PWH aged 50 years and older with CD4$^+$ T-cell counts ≥200 cells/µL (Thompson et al., 2021).

A recent study showed superior immunogenicity in adults aged 65 years and older who received high-dose inactivated influenza vaccine (Fluzone High-Dose HD-IIV3) compared to standard dosing (Fluzone SD-IIV3). Similar results were shown in a small clinical trial among PWH aged 18 years and older (McKittrick et al., 2013). Currently, the CDC recommends any IIV formulation (standard dose or high dose, trivalent or quadrivalent, unadjuvanted or adjuvanted) for patients aged 65 years and older regardless of HIV status (Grohskopf et al., 2019). We recommend high-dose IIV in older PWH because of its superior immunogenicity.

PWH aged 50 years and older should receive COVID-19 vaccine, including two booster shots based on age (CDC, 2022).

COVID-19

The severe acute respiratory syndrome coronavirus 2 (SARS-CoV-2) emerged in December 2019, causing the coronavirus disease 2019 (COVID-19). Preliminary studies found that although higher mortality from COVID-19 is reported among persons with immunosuppression, HIV infection was not identified as an important comorbid condition in hospitalized COVID-19 patients (del Amo et al., 2020). Moreover, despite risk factors for severe COVID-19 (e.g., older age, male sex, hypertension, diabetes mellitus, kidney disease, and chronic obstructive pulmonary disease) being common among older PWH, PWH do not seem to experience increased risk for serious COVID-19. It is speculated that PWH may not develop the intense immunologic response that leads to complications in COVID-19 (Borobia et al., 2020), despite preserved CD4$^+$ T-cells counts (Guo et al., 2020). ART may also provide a protective factor. Studies have shown that certain nucleos(t)ide reverse transcriptase inhibitors (NRTIs), such as TDF, TAF, abacavir (ABC), and lamivudine (3TC), may be effective against SARS-CoV-2 (del Amo et al., 2020). The relation between HIV and SARS-CoV-2 remains to be further investigated.

The psychosocial burden and limited healthcare access among older PWH are expected amidst social distancing and physical isolation recommended by the CDC to reduce the spread of COVID-19 among high-risk patients (Shiau et al., 2020). HIV infection and COVID-19 share many psychosocial drivers common among marginalized populations, including mental illness, illicit drug use, lower socioeconomic status, medical mistrust, food insecurity, and homelessness. These factors may worsen in older PWH with COVID-19, while limited access to care brought on by social distancing can also threaten ART adherence, successful viral suppression, and long-term health outcomes. The loneliness and social isolation experienced by older PWH will also likely be worsened by social distancing efforts.

CONCLUSION

There are increasing proportion of older PWH, and they differ from their younger counterparts in many ways, including the risk for late diagnoses or underdiagnoses, decreased immunologic recovery, and increased multimorbidity. However, each older PWH is a unique and complex individual, and disease-centric guidelines should not be applied the same way in every patient. Management of diseases in older PWH should be individualized based on aging phenotypes, interactions with multimorbidity, and patient preferences. The VACS index may be used to identify aging phenotypes and can provide useful prognostic information to help prioritize interventions and guide shared decision-making with patients and caregivers.

REFERENCES

Abrass C, Appelbaum J, Boyd C, et al. Summary report from the human immunodeficiency virus and aging consensus project: treatment strategies for clinicians managing older individuals with the human immunodeficiency virus. *J Am Geriatr Soc.* 2012;60(5):974–979.

Adelman RD, Tmanova LL, Delgado D, et al. Caregiver burden: a clinical review. *JAMA.* 2014;311(10):1052–1060. http://doi:10.1001/jama.2014.304

Agency for Health Research and Quality. Recommendations: screening for lung cancer. https://epss.ahrq.gov/ePSS/RecomDetail.do?method=search&sid=256&age=65&sex=Male&sexuallyActive=yes&tobacco=yes. Published 2018. Accessed October 7, 2022.

Ambrosius WT, Sink KM, Foy CG, et al. The design and rationale of a multicenter clinical trial comparing two strategies for control of systolic blood pressure: the Systolic Blood Pressure Intervention Trial (SPRINT). *Clin Trials.* 2014;11(5):532–546.

American Academy of HIV Medicine. Recommended treatment strategies for clinicians managing older patients with HIV. https://education.aahivm.org/product_bundles/2297. Published 2022. Accessed October 7, 2022.

American Diabetes Association. Standards of medical care in diabetes—older adults: *Standard of Medical Care in Diabetes—2022. Diabetes Care.* 2022;45(S1):S195–S207.

American Geriatrics Society. Updated AGS Beers criteria for potentially inappropriate medication use in older adults. *J Am Geriatr Soc.* 2019;67(4):674–694.

Bellera CA, Rainfray M, Mathoulin-Pelissier S, et al. Screening older cancer patients: first evaluation of the G-8 geriatric screening tool. *Ann Oncol.* 2012;23:2166–2172.

Borobia A, Carcas A, Arnalich F, et al. A cohort of patients with COVID-19 in a major teaching hospital in Europe. *J Clin Med.* 2020;9:1733. http://doi:10.3390/jcm9061733

British HIV Association. BHIVA guidelines for the treatment of HIV-1-positive adults with ART 2015 (2016 interim update). *Public Health.* https://www.bhiva.org/file/RVYKzFwyxpgiI/treatment-guidelines-2016-interim-update.pdf. Published 2016. Accessed October 7, 2022.

Brothers TD, Rockwood K. Frailty: a new vulnerability indicator in people aging with HIV. *Eur Geriatr Med.* 2019;10(2):219–226. http://doi:10.1007/s41999-018-0143-2

Castronuovo D, Pinzone MR, Moreno S, et al. HIV infection and bone disease: a review of the literature. *Infect Dis Trop Med.* 2015;1(2):e116.

Centers for Disease Control and Prevention (CDC). Assessment timed up & go (TUG). https://www.cdc.gov/steadi/pdf/TUG_Test-print.pdf. Published 2017. Accessed October 7, 2022.

CDC. COVID-19 vaccine boosters. cdc.gov. https://www.cdc.gov/coronavirus/2019-ncov/vaccines/booster-shot.html. Published 2022. Accessed on July 25, 2022.

CDC. Diagnoses of HIV infection among adults aged 50 years and older in the United States and dependent areas, 2011–2016. HIV surveillance supplemental report 2013;18(No. 3). cdc.gov. https://www.cdc.gov/hiv/pdf/library/reports/surveillance/cdc-hiv-surveillance-supplemental-report-vol-23-5.pdf. Published August 2018. Accessed on October 7, 2022.

CDC. HIV surveillance report, 2018 (updated). Vol. 31. http://www.cdc.gov/hiv/library/reports/hiv-surveillance.html. Published May 2020. Accessed October 7, 2022.

CDC. Revised recommendations for HIV testing of adults, adolescents, and pregnant women in health-care settings. www.cdc.gov/mmwr/preview/mmwrhtml/rr5514a1.htm. Published 2006. Accessed on October 7, 2022.

Chan P, Brew BJ. HIV associated neurocognitive disorders in the modern antiviral treatment era: prevalence, characteristics, biomarkers, and effects of treatment. *Curr HIV/AIDS Rep.* 2014;11(3):317–324. http://doi:10.1007/s11904-014-0221-0

Chibanda D, Verhey R, Gibson LJ, et al. Validation of screening tools for depression and anxiety disorders in a primary care population with high HIV prevalence in Zimbabwe. *J Affect Disord.* 2016;198:50–55. http://doi:10.1016/j.jad.2016.03.006

Conroy S. Defining frailty—the holy grail of geriatric medicine. *J Nutr Heal Aging.* 2009;13(4):389. http://doi:10.1007/s12603-009-0050-9

Dai SY, Liu JJ, Fan YG, et al. Prevalence and factors associated with late HIV diagnosis. *J Med Virol.* 2015;87(6):970–977. http://doi:10.1002/jmv.24066

del Amo J, Polo R, Moreno S, et al. Incidence and severity of COVID-19 in HIV-positive persons receiving antiretroviral therapy. *Ann Intern Med.* 2020;173(7):536–541.

Department of Health and Human Services (DHHS) Panel on Antiretroviral Guidelines for Adults and Adolescents. Guidelines for the use of antiretroviral agents in adults and adolescents with HIV. http://www.aidsinfo.nih.gov/ContentFiles/AdultandAdolescentGL.pdf. Published 2022. Accessed September 30, 2022.

Ellis G, Gardner M, Tsiachristas A, et al. Comprehensive geriatric assessment for older adults admitted to hospital. *Cochrane Database Syst Rev.* 2017; 9(9):CD006211. http://doi:10.1002/14651858.CD006211.pub3

Erlandson KM, Allshouse AA, Jankowski CM, et al. Risk factors for falls in HIV-infected persons. *J Acquir Immune Defic Syndr.* 2012;61:484–489.

Erlandson KM, Plankey MW, Springer G, et al. Fall frequency and associated factors among men and women with or at risk for HIV infection. *HIV Med.* 2016;17:740–748.

European AIDS Clinical Society. Guidelines version 11.0.https://eacs.sanfordguide.com. Published 2021. Accessed on October 7, 2022.

Fried LP, Tangen CM, Walston J, et al. Frailty in older adults: evidence for a phenotype. *J Gerontol A Biol Sci Med Sci.* 2001;56(3):M146–M157. http://doi:10.1093/gerona/56.3.M146

Gallagher P, Ryan C, Byrne S, et al. STOPP (Screening Tool of Older Person's Prescriptions) and START (Screening Tool to Alert doctors to Right Treatment). Consensus validation. *Int J Clin Pharmacol Ther.* 2008;46(2):72–83.

Goodin BR, Owens MA, White DM, et al. Intersectional health-related stigma in persons living with HIV and chronic pain: implications for depressive symptoms. *AIDS Care.* 2018;30(Suppl 2):66–73. http://doi:10.1080/09540121.2018.1468012

Grinspoon S, Corcoran C, Askari H, et al. Effects of androgen administration in men with the AIDS wasting syndrome. A randomized, double-blind, placebo-controlled trial. *Ann Intern Med.* 1998;129:18–26.

Grinspoon S, Corcoran C, Lee K, et al. Loss of lean body and muscle mass correlates with androgen levels in hypogonadal men with acquired immunodeficiency syndrome and wasting. *J Clin Endocrinol Metab.* 1996;81:4051–4058.

Grohskopf LA, Alyanak E, Broder KR, et al. Prevention and control of seasonal influenza with vaccines: recommendations of the Advisory

Committee on Immunization Practices—United States, 2019–20 influenza season. *MMWR Recomm Rep.* 2019;68(RR-3):1–21.

Guaraldi G, Silva AR, Stentarelli C. Multimorbidity and functional status assessment. *Curr Opin HIV AIDS.* 2014;9(4):386–397. http://doi:10.1097/COH.0000000000000079

Guo W, Ming F, Dong Y et al. A survey for COVID-19 among HIV/AIDS patients in two districts of Wuhan, China. *Lancet.* March 13, 2020. http://doi:10.2139/ ssrn.3550029

Hanlon JT, Schmader KE. The medication appropriateness index at 20: where it started, where it has been, and where it may be going. *Drugs Aging.* 2013;30(11):893–900.

Hanlon JT, Schmader KE, Samsa GP, et al. A method for assessing drug therapy appropriateness. *J Clin Epidemiol.* 1992;45(10):1045–1051.

Holtzman C, Armon C, Tedaldi E, et al. Polypharmacy and risk of antiretroviral drug interactions among the aging HIV-infected population. *J Gen Intern Med.* 2013;28(10):1302–1310.

Huss A, Stuck AE, Rubenstein LZ, et al. Multidimensional preventive home visit programs for community-dwelling older adults: a systematic review and meta-analysis of randomized controlled trials. *J Gerontol A Biol Sci Med Sci.* 2008;63(3):298.

Hypertension Canada. 2020–2022 hypertension highlights. https://hypertension.ca/wp-content/uploads/2020/10/2020-22-HT-Guidelines-E-WEB_v3b.pdf. Published 2022. Accessed July 25, 2022.

James PA, Oparil S, Carter BL, et al. 2014 Evidence-based guideline for the management of high blood pressure in adults: report from the panel members appointed to the eighth Joint National Committee (JNC 8). *JAMA.* 2014;311(5):507–520. http://doi:10.1001/jama.2013.284427

John M, Hessol N, Hare CB, et al. 1607: Veterans Aging Cohort Study (VACS) index, functional status, and other patient reported outcomes in older HIV-positive (HIV+) adults. *Open Forum Infect Dis.* 2014;1(Suppl 1):S428–S429. http://doi:10.1093/ofid/ofu052.1153

Justice A, Tate J, Brown S, et al. Can the Veterans Aging Cohort Study Index improve clinical judgment for both HIV infected and uninfected veterans? *J Gen Intern Med.* 2013b;28:S39–S39.

Justice AC, Holmes H, Gifford AL, et al., Development and validation of a self-completed HIV symptom index. *J Clin Epidemiol.* 2001;54(12):S77-S90.

Justice AC, Modur SP, Tate JP, et al. Predictive accuracy of the Veterans Aging Cohort Study index for mortality with HIV infection: a North American cross cohort analysis. *J Acquir Immune Defic Syndr.* 2013a;62(2):149–163. http://doi:10.1097/QAI.0b013e31827df36c

Justice AC, Tate J, Freiberg M, et al. Reply to Chow et al. *Clin Infect Dis.* 2012;55(5):751–752.

Kaku M, Simpson DM. HIV neuropathy. *Curr Opin HIV AIDS.* 2014;9(6):521–526. http://doi:10.1097/COH.0000000000000103

Katz S, Ford AB, Moskowitz RW, et al. Studies of illness in the aged. The index of ADL: a standardized measure of biological and psychosocial function. *JAMA.* 1963;185:914–919.

Kilbourne AM, Justice AC, Rollman BL, et al. Clinical importance of HIV and depressive symptoms among veterans with HIV infection. *JGIM.* 2002;17(7):512–520.

Knobel H, Guelar A, Valldecillo G et al. Response to highly active antiretroviral therapy in HIV-infected patients aged 60 years or older after 24 months follow-up. *AIDS.* 2001;15(12):1591–1593.

Kong AM, Pozen A, Anastos K, et al. Non-HIV comorbid conditions and polypharmacy among people living with HIV age 65 or older compared with HIV-negative individuals age 65 or older in the United States: a retrospective claims-based analysis. *AIDS Patient Care STDS.* 2019;33(3):93–103.

Koroukian SM, Warner DF, Owusu C, Given CW. Multimorbidity redefined: prospective health outcomes and the cumulative effect of co-occurring conditions. *Prev Chronic Dis.* 2015;12:E55. http://doi:10.5888/pcd12.140478

Lee SJ, Leipzig RM, Walter LC. Incorporating lag time to benefit into prevention decisions for older adults. *JAMA.* 2013;310(24):2609–2610.

Lindau ST, Schumm LP, Laumann EO, et al. A study of sexuality and health among older adults in the United States. *N Engl J Med.* 2007;357(8):762–774. http://doi:10.1056/NEJMoa067423

Lindeman RD, Tobin J, Shock NW. Longitudinal studies on the rate of decline in renal function with age. *J Am Geriatr Soc.* 1985;33(4):278–285.

Marzolini C, Back D, Weber R, et al. Ageing with HIV: medication use and risk for potential drug-drug interactions. *J Antimicrob Chemothe.r* 2011;66(9):2107–2111.

Masnoon N, Shakib S, Kalisch-Ellett L, et al. What is polypharmacy? A systematic review of definitions. *BMC Geriatr.* 2017;17(1):230.

McKittrick N, Frank I, Jacobson JM, et al. Improved immunogenicity with high-dose seasonal influenza vaccine in HIV-infected persons: a single-center, parallel, randomized trial. *Ann Intern Med.* 2013;158(1):19–26. http://doi:10.7326/0003-4819-158-1-201301010-00005

Merlin JS, Westfall AO, Long D, et al. A randomized pilot trial of a novel behavioral intervention for chronic pain tailored to individuals with HIV. *AIDS Behav.* 2018;22(8):2733–2742. http://doi:10.1007/s10461-018-2028-2

Mpondo BC, Gunda DW, Kilonzo SB, et al. Immunological and clinical responses following the use of antiretroviral therapy among elderly HIV-positive individuals attending care and treatment clinic in Northwestern Tanzania: a retrospective cohort study. *J Sex Transm Dis.* 2016;2016:5235269.

Mueses-Marín H, Montaño D, Galindo J, et al. Psychometric properties and validity of the Center for Epidemiological Studies Depression Scale (CES-D) in a population attending an HIV clinic in Cali, Colombia. *Biomedica.* 2019;39(1):33–45. http://doi:10.7705/biomedica.v39i1.3843

National Center on Elder Abuse (NCEA). NCEA website. https://ncea.acl.gov/. Published 2022. Accessed October 7, 2022.

National Heart Foundation. Guideline for the diagnosis and management of hypertension in adults—2016. Melbourne: National Heart Found. www.heartfoundation.org.au/getmedia/c83511ab-835a-4fcf-96f5-88d770582ddc/PRO-167_Hypertension-guideline-2016_WEB.pdf. Published 2016. Accessed October 7, 2022.

National Institute on Aging. Advance care planning. httpss://www.nia.nih.gov/health/advance-care-planning-health-care-directives. Published 2018. Accessed October 7, 2022.

Pecanac KE, Repenshek MF, Tennenbaum D, et al. Respecting Choices® and advance directives in a diverse community. *J Palliat Med.* 2014;17(3):282–287. http://doi:10.1089/jpm.2013.0047

Pilowsky D, Wu L-T. Sexual risk behaviors and HIV risk among Americans aged 50 years or older: a review. *Subst Abuse Rehabil.* 2015;6:51. http://doi:10.2147/sar.s78808

Podsiadlo D, Richardson S. The timed "Up & Go": a test of basic functional mobility for frail elderly persons. *J Am Geriatr Soc.* 1991;39:142–148.

Power C, Selnes OA, Grim JA, et al. HIV dementia scale: a rapid screening test. *J Acquir Immune Defic Syndr Hum Retrovirology.* 1995;8(3):273–278. http://doi:10.1097/00042560-199503010-00008

Ramgopal M, Maggiolo F, Ward D, et al. Pooled analysis of 4 international trials of bictegravir/emtricitabine/tenofovir alafenamide (B/F/Taf) in adults aged 65 or older demonstrating safety and efficacy: week 48 results. J *Int AIDS Soc.* 2020;23(Suppl 4):e25547.

Reuben DB, Frank JC, Hirsch SH, et al. A randomized clinical trial of outpatient comprehensive geriatric assessment coupled with an intervention to increase adherence to recommendations. *J Am Geriatr Soc.* 1999;47(3):269.

Rockwood K, Andrew M, Mitnitski A. A comparison of two approaches to measuring frailty in elderly people. *J Gerontol A Biol Sci Med Sci.* 2007;62(7):738–743. http://doi:10.1093/gerona/62.7.738

Rodkjaer L, Gabel C, Laursen T, et al. Simple and practical screening approach to identify HIV-infected individuals with depression or at risk of developing depression. *HIV Med.* 2016;17(10):749–757. http://doi:10.1111/hiv.12381

Rosca EC, Albarqouni L, Simu M. Montreal Cognitive Assessment (MoCA) for HIV-associated neurocognitive disorders. *Neuropsychol Rev.* 2019;29(3):313–327. http://doi:10.1007/s11065-019-09412-9

Ruiz M, Kamerman LA. Nutritional screening tools for HIV-infected patients: implications for elderly patients. *J Int Assoc Physicians AIDS Care*. 2010;9:362–367.

Ruiz MA, Reske T, Cefalu C, et al. Falls in HIV-infected patients: a geriatric syndrome in a susceptible population. *J Int Assoc Provid AIDS Care*. 2013;12:266–269.

Sacktor NC, Wong M, Nakasujja N, et al. The International HIV Dementia Scale: a new rapid screening test for HIV dementia. *AIDS*. 2005;19(13):1367–1374.

Sangarlangkarn A, Apornpong T, Justice AC, et al. Screening tools for targeted comprehensive geriatric assessment in HIV-infected patients 50 years and older. *Int J STD AIDS*. 2019;30(10):1009–1017. http://doi:10.1177/0956462419841478

Sangarlangkarn A, Merlin JS, Tucker RO, et al. Advance care planning and HIV infection in the era of antiretroviral therapy: a review. *Top Antivir Med*. 2016;23(5):174–180.

Schafer JJ, Gill TK, Sherman EM, et al. ASHP guidelines on pharmacist involvement in HIV care. *Am J Health Syst Pharm*. 2016;73(7):468–494.

Schmucker, D. L. Liver function and phase I drug metabolism in the elderly: a paradox. *Drugs Aging*. 2001;18(11):837–851.

Schouten J, Wit FW, Stolte IG, et al. Cross-sectional comparison of the prevalence of age-associated comorbidities and their risk factors between HIV-infected and uninfected individuals: the AGEHIV cohort study. *Clin Infect Dis*. 2014;59(12):1787–1797. http://doi:10.1093/cid/ciu701

Searle SD, Mitnitski A, Gahbauer EA, et al. A standard procedure for creating a frailty index. *BMC Geriatr*. 2008;8:24. http://doi:10.1186/1471-2318-8-24

Semeere AS, Lwanga I, Sempa J, et al. Mortality and immunological recovery among older adults on antiretroviral therapy at a large urban HIV clinic in Kampala, Uganda. *J Acquir Immune Defic Syndr*. 2014;67(4):382–389. http://doi:10.1097/QAI.0000000000000330

Shafran SD. Live attenuated herpes zoster vaccine for HIV-infected adults. *HIV Med*. 2016;17(4):305–310.

Shiau S, Krause KD, Valera P, et al. The burden of COVID-19 in people living with HIV: a syndemic perspective. *AIDS Behav*. 2020;24(8):2244–2249. http://doi:10.1007/s10461-020-02871-9

Sigel K, Wisnivesky J, Shahrir S, et al. Findings in asymptomatic HIV infected patients undergoing chest computed tomography testing: implications for lung cancer screening. *AIDS*. 2014;28(7):1007–1014.

Stuck AE, Siu AL, Wieland GD, et al. Comprehensive geriatric assessment: a meta-analysis of controlled trials. *Lancet*. 1993;342(8878):1032–1036. http://doi:10.1016/0140-6736(93)92884-V

Thompson MA, Horberg MA, Agwu AL et al. Primary care guidelines for the management of persons infected with human immunodeficiency virus: 2020 update by the HIV Medicine Association of the Infectious Diseases Society of America. *Clin Infect Dis*. 2021;73(11):e3572–e3605.

Tinetti ME, Fried TR, Boyd CM. Designing health care for the most common chronic condition--multimorbidity [published correction appears in *JAMA*. July 18, 2012;308(3):238]. *JAMA*. 2012;307(23):2493–2494. http://doi:10.1001/jama.2012.5265

UpToDate. Calcium and vitamin D supplementation in osteoporosis. https://www.uptodate.com/contents/calcium-and-vitamin-d-supplementation-in-osteoporosis?search=calcium%20vit%20d%20osteporosis&source=search_result&selectedTitle=3~150&usage_type=default&display_rank=3. Published 2022. Accessed October 7, 2022.

Valcour V, Paul R, Chiao S, et al. Screening for cognitive impairment in human immunodeficiency virus. *Clin Infect Dis*. 2011;53(8):836–842. http://doi:10.1093/cid/cir524

Verhey R, Chibanda D, Gibson L, et al. Validation of the posttraumatic stress disorder checklist—5 (PCL-5) in a primary care population with high HIV prevalence in Zimbabwe. *BMC Psychiatry*. 2018;18(1):109. http://doi:10.1186/s12888-018-1688-9

Vinikoor MJ, Joseph J, Mwale J, et al. Age at antiretroviral therapy initiation predicts immune recovery, death, and loss to follow-up among HIV-infected adults in urban Zambia. *AIDS Res Hum Retroviruses*. 2014;30(10):949–955. http://doi:10.1089/AID.2014.0046

Vrouenraets SM, Fux CA, Wit FW, et al. A comparison of measured and estimated glomerular filtration rate in successfully treated HIV-patients with preserved renal function. *Clin Nephrol*. 2012;77(4):311–320.

Weiss BD, Brega AG, LeBlanc WG, et al. Improving the effectiveness of medication review: guidance from the Health Literacy Universal Precautions Toolkit. *J Am Board Fam Med*. 2016;29(1):18–23.

Wellons, MF, Sanders L, Edwards LJ, et al. HIV infection: treatment outcomes in older and younger adults. *J Am Geriatr Soc*. 2002;50(4):603–607.

Whalen CC, Antani M, Carey J, et al. An index of symptoms for infection with human immunodeficiency virus: reliability and validity. *J Clin Epidemiol*. 1994;47(5):537–546.

Whelton PK, Carey RM, Aronow WS, et al. ACC/AHA/AAPA/ABC/ACPM/AGS/APhA/ASH/ASPC/NMA/PCNA guideline for the prevention, detection, evaluation, and management of high blood pressure in adults. *J Am Coll Cardiol*. 2018;71:e127–e248.

Wright L, Epps JB. Development and validation of a HIV disease–specific nutrition screening tool. *Top Clin Nutr*. 2020;35(3):264–269.

28.

OPPORTUNISTIC INFECTIONS

Lisa Y. Armitige, Karen J. Vigil, and Rita Wilson Dib

LEARNING OBJECTIVE

Upon completion of this chapter, the reader should be able to:

- Recognize and manage the most common opportunistic infections found in people living with HIV (PWH).

TIMING OF ANTIRETROVIRAL THERAPY INITIATION AND IMPACT ON OPPORTUNISTIC INFECTIONS

LEARNING OBJECTIVES

- Describe the issues concerning starting antiretroviral therapy (ART) in the setting of an opportunistic infection (OIs).

- Summarize the recommendations for starting ART in the setting of an OI.

KEY POINTS

- Early initiation of ART was associated with a decrease in AIDS progression and death in ACTG A5164.

- Early initiation of ART near the time of starting treatment for an OI should be considered for most patients, with the possible exception of patients with cryptococcal or tuberculous meningitis.

Timing of initiation of ART in the setting of an acute or ongoing OI has been debated. On the one hand, the immediate initiation of ART in the presence of an OI may provide better clinical outcomes as the immune system improves. On the other hand, rapidly decreasing HIV RNA levels have been associated with the immune reconstitution inflammatory syndrome (IRIS), which may lead to further complications in the setting of an OI. That is, in addition to concerns in regard to increasing pill burden, potential drug–drug interactions, additive toxicity and adverse events, and the more practical problem of continuity of care if ART is started in a hospital setting for a newly diagnosed patient with HIV, without established outpatient care already in place. This problem could be particularly troublesome for patients who do not

have health insurance or otherwise do not have affordable access to ART in the outpatient setting.

In the absence of pathogen specific therapies, some OIs, such as cryptosporidiosis, microsporidiosis, and progressive multifocal leukoencephalopathy (PML) can only be managed with ART. This mandates the early initiation of ART in the presence of concomitant OI. Further, patients with mild to moderate Kaposi's sarcoma (KS) may achieve remission through the receipt of ART without requiring chemotherapy. Opportunistic infections with available targeted therapies, however, may resolve with their corresponding therapies in the absence of ART. These include *Pneumocystis jirovecii* pneumonia (PJP), *Cryptococcus neoformans* meningitis, and *Mycobacterium tuberculosis* meningitis. It is for these patients that controversy has existed about the optimal time to start ART.

CLINICAL TRIAL RESULTS

The AIDS Clinical Trials Group (ACTG) A5164 study was designed to address the question of the optimal timing of ART initiation for individuals presenting with AIDS-defining OIs or serious bacterial infections (SBIs), other than tuberculosis, for which effective antimicrobial therapies were available. This was a randomized, open-label strategy trial to evaluate early (defined as within 14 days of starting acute OI treatment) versus deferred (given after OI treatment is completed) initiation of ART in patients starting treatment of acute OIs or SBIs, using clinical and virologic end points at 48 weeks (Zolopa et al., 2009). A total of 282 patients were evaluable, 141 in each arm. Most study participants were from racial/ethnic minority groups (73%), male (85%), with a median age of 38 years, a median CD4$^+$ T-cell count of 29 cells/mm^3, and a median HIV RNA level of 5.07 log$_{10}$ copies/mL. The most common recorded infections were PJP (63%), cryptococcal meningitis (12%), and SBIs (12%). ART was initiated at a mean of 12 days after starting OI treatment in the "early" arm and a mean of 45 days after OI treatment in the "deferred" arm.

The study found a statistically significant decrease in the proportion of participants experiencing a second AIDS-defining disease and/or death (composite endpoint) in the early treatment arm (14.2%) compared to the deferred arm (24.1%) (odds ratio (OR) 0.51; 95% CI: 0.27–0.94). The time to AIDS progression and death was also longer in the early treatment arm compared to the deferred group (hazard ratio 0.53; 95% CI: 0.30–0.92). The impact of these differences was seen most prominently in the first 6 months after the diagnosis of the OI. The rate of adverse events was not different in the two arms, and IRIS was reported in 8 participants in the early arm versus 12 participants in the deferred arm. These findings substantiated the fact that early initiation of ART during treatment for an acute OI or SBI is life-saving or, at least, serious morbidity–reducing if there are no major contraindications to starting ART. A cost-effectiveness analysis, supportive of this early treatment strategy, has also been published (Sax et al., 2010).

The overall rates of IRIS in the A5164 cohort were lower than those observed in previously published retrospective trials possibly because of the included types of the OIs, being largely secondary to PJP while excluding patients with *M. tuberculosis* infection. The presence of fungal infections (*Cryptococcus* or *Histoplasma*), lower baseline CD4 $^+$ T-cell counts, and higher baseline HIV RNA levels were found to be associated with IRIS in A5164. The occurrence of IRIS was also associated with higher CD4 $^+$ T-cell counts and lower HIV RNA levels while on ART. Early initiation of ART did not increase the incidence of IRIS in this study.

Recommendations regarding the timing of starting ART specifically in the setting of meningitis owing to *C. neoformans* or *M. tuberculosis* are more complex. In a study on *C. neoformans* meningitis related IRIS (Sungkanuparph et al., 2009), analysis of 101 participants employed a different methodology than ACTG 5164 and found no association between the timing of ART initiation and the diagnosis of IRIS. Rather, it found that an increased baseline serum cryptococcal antigen titer was a risk factor for IRIS. In contrast, a study of 54 participants in Zimbabwe showed that early initiation of ART (within 72 hours of diagnosis) versus delayed initiation (after 10 weeks of treatment with fluconazole alone) in persons with cryptococcal meningitis was associated with increased mortality. In this population, optimal management of increased intracranial pressure (i.e., decreasing cerebrospinal fluid (CSF) volume by lumbar puncture or other sterile procedure) was not always provided (Makadzange et al., 2010). Further, the 2014 Cryptococcal Optimal ART Timing Trial of 177 participants with HIV from Uganda and South Africa with cryptococcal meningitis reported increased mortality (hazard ratio, 1.73) at 26 weeks for participants who started ART within 1 or 2 weeks compared to those who had deferral of ART for 5 weeks (Boulware et al., 2014). Participants in the early group started ART at a median of 8 days after being on antifungal therapy while patients in the deferred group started ART at a median of 36 days. Most of the increase in mortality was observed within the first 8–30 days of the study. The differences in mortality were especially pronounced in patients who had white blood cell (WBC) counts of less than five cells/μL in their CSF, although, it was unclear if the increase in mortality in this study was due to progression of cryptococcal disease or IRIS. The current US Department of Health and Human Services (DHHS, 2022a) guidelines recommend a short delay in initiating ART in the presence of cryptococcal meningitis (discussed later).

Implementation of the findings of A5164 and similar studies may prove difficult in practice, particularly in settings in which patients may not have established linkage to primary care and limited access to ongoing treatment with ART after the resolution of the acute OI. However, effective implementation of early ART was accomplished and published by an academic medical center, and this may be a model for bringing early ART to a "real-world" population (Geng, 2011).

RECOMMENDATIONS OF GUIDELINES

The guidelines for prevention and treatment of OIs in adults and adolescents with HIV were last reviewed and updated in August 2022 and are available in the latest form online (https://clinicalinfo.hiv.gov/en/guidelines/hiv-clinical-guidelines-adult-and-adolescent-opportunistic-infections/whats-new, accessed August 10, 2022). These guidelines provide recommendations regarding the timing of initiation of ART in the setting of specific opportunistic conditions, and they should be referenced for guidance in the treatment of patients with those conditions. These guidelines generally reiterate the findings of A5164, suggesting that, unless contraindications are present, early initiation of ART near the time of treatment of an OI should be considered for most patients with an acute OI. Other elements that should be considered are degree of immunosuppression, availability of treatment for the OI, drug–drug interactions and overlapping toxicities, and the risk and potential consequences of IRIS.

In many instances, it is recommended that ART should be started as soon as possible. These conditions include PML, which is caused by the John Cunningham (JC) virus, cryptosporidiosis, microsporidiosis, and fungal infections other than meningitis caused by *C. neoformans*. For PJP and invasive SBIs, the guidelines recommend starting ART within 2 weeks of diagnosis, although the panel notes that no patients with respiratory failure requiring mechanical ventilation were enrolled in study A5164. For *Toxoplasma gondii* encephalitis, the panel cites expert opinion to start ART within 2 or 3 weeks after diagnosis and initiation of specific treatment for toxoplasmosis based on the data from A5164, which studied only 5% of participants diagnosed with toxoplasmosis. For disseminated *Mycobacterium avium* complex, the panel cites expert opinion to consider starting ART after the first 2 weeks of antimycobacterial therapy in order to decrease the overall initial pill burden and to decrease the possibility for IRIS. For cytomegalovirus (CMV) retinitis, the panel notes that many experts would not delay ART for more than 2 weeks after the start of CMV-specific treatment. The presence of disease caused by herpes simplex virus (HSV) or varicella zoster virus (VZV) does not preclude the initiation of ART.

Regarding cryptococcal meningitis, the panel notes that it would be prudent to defer ART at least until the initial 2-week antifungal induction is complete and possibly until the completion of the consolidation phase at 10 weeks, especially if the patient has increased intracranial pressure or a low CSF WBC count. The panel also notes that if ART is started prior to 10 weeks of antifungal treatment, the clinician should be prepared to promptly investigate and treat manifestations of IRIS, including increased intracranial pressure. Last, there is very limited randomized clinical trial evidence to guide the optimal time for initiation of ART in the setting of concomitant tuberculous meningitis. Expert opinion remains relevant in managing these patients.

SUMMARY

Although substantial barriers to early initiation of ART in the setting of an acute OI exist, the weight of the available evidence falls on the side of starting ART as soon as possible for most patients with acute OIs and invasive BIs, with the notable exception of meningitis due to *C. neoformans* or *M. tuberculosis*.

RECOMMENDED READING

Abdool Karim SS, Naidoo K, Grobler A, et al. Timing of initiation of antiretroviral drugs during tuberculosis therapy. *N Engl J Med.* February 25, 2010;362(8):697–706. http://www.ncbi.nlm.nih.gov/pubmed/20181971

Blanc FX, Sok T, Laureillard D, et al. Earlier versus later start of antiretroviral therapy in HIV-positive adults with tuberculosis. *N Engl J Med.* October 20, 2011;365(16):1471–1481. http://www.ncbi.nlm.nih.gov/pubmed/22010913

Boulware DR, Meya DB, Muzoora C, et al. Timing of antiretroviral therapy after diagnosis of cryptococcal meningitis. *N Engl J Med* June 26, 2014;370(26):2487–2498.

Mfinanga SG, Kirenga BJ, Chanda DM, et al. Early versus delayed initiation of highly active antiretroviral therapy for HIV-positive adults with newly diagnosed pulmonary tuberculosis (TB-HAART): a prospective, international, randomised, placebo-controlled trial. *Lancet Infect Dis.* July 2014;14(7):563–571. http://www.ncbi.nlm.nih.gov/pubmed/24810491

Temprano ANRS Study Group; Danel C, Moh R, Gabillard D, et al. A trial of early antiretrovirals and isoniazid preventive therapy in Africa. *N Engl J Med.* August 27, 2015;373(9):808–822. http://www.ncbi.nlm.nih.gov/pubmed/26193126

Zolopa A, Andersen J, Powderly W, et al. Early antiretroviral therapy reduces AIDS progression/death in individuals with acute opportunistic infections: a multicenter randomized strategy trial. *PLoS One.* 2009;4(5):e5575.

MYCOBACTERIAL INFECTIONS

LEARNING OBJECTIVE

Discuss the available tests and treatment modalities to appropriately manage people living with HIV (PWH) with *Mycobacterium tuberculosis, M. avium* complex, and *M. kansasii*, the most common mycobacterial diseases associated with HIV infection.

WHAT'S NEW?

- Shorter latent tuberculosis infection (LTBI) regimens such as 3 months of weekly INH-rifapentine or INH-rifampin are recommended over the longer INH regimen.

- One month of daily INH and rifapentine can be considered for treatment of LTBI.

- Primary prophylaxis to prevent disseminated Mycobacterium avium complex (MAC) disease is no longer recommended for PWH who immediately initiate antiretroviral therapy (ART).

KEY POINTS

- HIV infection markedly increases the likelihood of a person progressing from LTBI to active TB disease.

- Rifamycins are a critical component of effective TB therapy in PWH but have many drug–drug interactions.

- MAC should be treated with multidrug therapy, including clarithromycin and ethambutol optimally.

- Optimal treatment of MAC disease should include medications for both MAC and HIV (to reconstitute the immune system).

- *Mycobacterium kansasii* infection closely resembles TB with more frequent pulmonary presentation than MAC.

- Diagnosis and treatment of *M. kansasii* as outlined in the American Thoracic Society (2020) guidelines are the same for PWH and people without HIV.

MYCOBACTERIUM TUBERCULOSIS

Epidemiology

There were 10.0 million new cases of TB worldwide in 2020; PWH are 18-times more likely to develop active TB than the general population (WHO, 2021). Recognition of the vulnerability of the HIV population to TB and increased awareness of the need to rapidly diagnose and treat people with TB/HIV coinfection have led to a steady decrease in HIV-associated TB deaths since the numbers peaked globally in 2004. Deaths from TB in PWH declined from 540,000 in 2004 to 209,000 in 2019, which, despite these gains, remains substantial at 2.7 (2.4–3.1) per 100,000 PWH population. More concerning, deaths from TB-associated HIV increased for the first time since 2004, rising to 214,000 in 2020, reflecting the global impact of the COVID-19 pandemic on health care access worldwide (WHO, 2021).

The total number of TB cases in the United States peaked in 1992 and had been steadily declining with a slower progression noted in the year 2020 in the setting of the COVID-19 pandemic and a suspected state of underdiagnosis (CDC, 2020). The Centers for Disease Control and Prevention (CDC, 2012) recommends testing for HIV in all active persons with TB (CDC, 2012). HIV testing was completed for 89.8% of reported TB cases in the United States, with 4.8% of total cases reported with HIV coinfection in (CDC, 2020). This is down significantly from the peak in 1992, when nearly two-thirds of persons with TB aged 25–44 years had HIV. Attention to screening and treatment of tuberculosis as well as increasing focus on HIV treatment in the United States has resulted in a decrease in HIV-associated TB cases and a faster decline than in the general population (CDC, 2020).

Unlike other HIV-related opportunistic infections, CD4[+] T-cell count does not predict risk of TB infection. Rates of TB in PWH are higher than those in people without HIV at all CD4[+] T-cell counts.

Clinical Presentation

Infection with *M. tuberculosis* generally occurs after inhalation of infectious particles coughed into the air by a person with active pulmonary TB disease. A less common route of infection involves ingestion of unpasteurized dairy products produced from the milk from cows with *Mycobacterium bovis* (bovine TB). Once infected, individuals will either progress to active disease (progressive primary disease) or their immune system will contain growth of the organism but not kill it (LTBI). Host immune factors play a major role in which route initial infection will take. Host factors also play a role in whether individuals with LTBI will progress to active TB disease (postprimary or reactivation disease).

TB in people without HIV typically presents as pulmonary disease. Often, the upper lobes of the lung are involved, and cavitary lesions are characteristic. Pulmonary disease is frequently accompanied by constitutional symptoms such as fever, night sweats, and weight loss. These findings are more typical of reactivation disease rather than progressive primary infection found when there is poor containment of the infecting organism by the immune system.

CD4[+] T-cell count plays a pivotal role in the containment of *M. tuberculosis*. As HIV infection progresses and there is a decline in the number of these cells, there is less containment of infecting organisms. The clinical presentation of TB in PWH differs based on the CD4[+] T-cell count. PWH with CD4[+] T-cell counts >350 cells/mm³ often present with the classically described pulmonary presentation. As the CD4[+] T-cell count decreases, the clinical presentation can look more like progressive primary disease. In PWH with CD4[+] T-cell counts < 200 cells/mm³, pulmonary lesions may involve any lobe of the lungs and range from infiltrates to pneumonia. Cavitary lesions become less common with advanced HIV disease, and a number of persons with HIV and TB will have no abnormalities on chest radiograph at all.

Another feature of HIV-associated TB is extrapulmonary disease. Extrapulmonary disease is found in up to 50% of individuals in some series. Lymph node disease is the most common extrapulmonary site. Disseminated (miliary) disease and mycobacteremia are far more common in PWH with low CD4[+] T-cell counts.

Diagnosis

Diagnosis of TB infection in PWH requires a high index of suspicion. Recent advances in diagnostic testing modalities for TB, such as interferon-gamma release assays (IGRAs), have not translated into a major improvement in the diagnosis of TB infection in PWH. Diagnosis of TB disease requires the HIV physician to remain vigilant.

Traditionally, screening for TB infection has been performed with the tuberculin skin test (TST). The test involves injection of 0.1 ml (comprising five tuberculin units) of purified protein derivative subcutaneously into the volar surface of the forearm. Individuals who have been previously infected with *M. tuberculosis* develop a delayed-type hypersensitivity reaction to the injected proteins. Induration caused by this reaction is measured after 48–72 hours. A TST measurement of 5 mm of induration or greater is considered positive in PWH. Sensitivity of this test has always been poor in PWH, and it can be as low as 30% in patients with TB and CD4[+] T-cell counts < 200 cells/mm³. It is also important to note that the TST will not distinguish between persons with LTBI and those with active TB, and it may be falsely positive in persons vaccinated with Bacillus Calmette–Guérin (BCG) because of the cross-reaction with antigens found in the BCG vaccine.

IGRAs are diagnostic in vitro blood tests based on immune responses to antigens unique to *M. tuberculosis*. IGRAs have the benefits of negating the false positives seen with BCG vaccination and offering a blood draw that requires a single visit. There are two commercially available US Food and Drug Administration-approved IGRAs—the QuantiFERON-TB Plus (QFT-Plus) and the T.SPOT.*TB* (T-spot). The QFT-Plus assay replaced the QFT Gold In Tube (QFT-GIT) and tests the CD4[+] and CD8[+] cellular immune responses to *M. tuberculosis*-specific antigens. All indications are that the QFT-Plus and QFT-GIT assays perform similarly. Meta-analyses (Cattamanchi et al., 2011; Santin et al., 2012) showed the sensitivity to be approximately 60% for the QFT-GIT and 70% for the T-SPOT.TB assay in detecting *M. tuberculosis* infection. Although this appears to be an improvement over the TST, there was not a significant difference in head-to-head sensitivity with either test compared to the TST. The studies highlight the fact that there are still many cases of LTBI or active TB disease that may be missed by these tests and a high index of suspicion is still warranted. As highlighted in the recommendations on IGRAs outlined by the ATS/CDC/IDSA guidelines (Nahid et al., 2016), these tests are most useful in BCG-vaccinated populations (adding greater specificity) and in populations with poor rates of return (negating the need for a return visit for reading). These same guidelines state clearly that routine testing with both a TST and an IGRA is not generally recommended.

PWH should be screened for TB infection by a TST or IGRA at the time of HIV diagnosis and, if at high risk for exposure, regularly thereafter. Individuals who travel to countries with a high TB burden or who reside in areas with high rates of TB should be tested annually. All others should be tested when there is suspicion of exposure to an active case after their initial testing. Individuals with CD4[+] T-cell counts < 200 cells/mm³ at HIV diagnosis should be tested at baseline and, if they test negative, should have a repeat TB diagnostic test after CD4[+] T-cell count recovery to >200 cells/mm³ to confirm they are truly negative.

An individual with a positive TB diagnostic test (TST or IGRA) without evidence of active TB disease should be given a diagnosis of LTBI. PWH with LTBI are at very high risk for advancing to active TB. Individuals with LTBI without HIV have a 5%–10% lifetime risk of developing active TB, whereas PWH and LTBI are 18 (15–21)-times more likely to progress to active disease than persons without HIV (WHO, 2021b). LTBI treatment in this population is paramount and has formed the cornerstone of progress in reducing global HIV-associated TB cases and deaths.

Diagnosis of active TB disease requires the utilization of many pieces of data. A thorough history is useful in most cases. Important information to note includes exposure to an individual with active TB disease, residence in high-risk settings such as jail or homeless shelters, and a prior diagnosis of untreated LTBI. Signs and symptoms of active disease may include cough lasting longer than 3 weeks, unexplained weight loss, fevers, and/or night sweats. There are no physical exam findings specific for TB, but a thorough physical exam may reveal suspicious lymphadenopathy, draining fistulas, abnormal respiratory sounds, or signs of meningitis.

Diagnostic tests such as the TST and IGRA can add to available data but cannot be relied on entirely. One may also consider performing more than one of these tests to increase sensitivity, especially when the individual has a low CD4$^+$ T-cell count. In general, a positive TST or IGRA result should be taken as evidence of infection.

All PWH suspected of having active TB should receive a chest radiograph because the lungs are the most common entry point and a frequent site of infection. Though the chest radiograph can be normal in patients with culture-positive pulmonary TB, a high-resolution Computed tomography (CT) scan may show early miliary-type lesions. Any person with respiratory symptoms, regardless of chest radiograph findings, should have sputum collected (at least three specimens) 8–24 hours apart with at least one sputum being an early morning specimen and, preferably, at least one observed.

Individuals with low CD4$^+$ T-cell counts are more likely to have extrapulmonary TB with infected tissues that are more difficult to access and that have fewer organisms. It may be necessary to obtain biopsy specimens from lymph nodes, bone marrow, or pulmonary parenchyma to make the diagnosis. CSF, ascitic fluid, or abscess fluid may provide important diagnostic information. All tissue specimens from suspected sites of infection should be submitted for smear and culture analysis for acid-fast bacilli and, if indicated, histopathologic analysis searching for characteristic granulomas on pathology. When available, nucleic acid amplification tests significantly improve sensitivity in detecting *M. tuberculosis* organisms in patient specimens.

Treatment

Treatment of LTBI in PWH is essentially the same as that in people without HIV. The mainstay for treatment of LTBI in PWH has been 9 months of isoniazid (INH) dosed daily, self-administered, or intermittently (twice weekly) by directly observed therapy (DOT). Treatment with INH for 6–9 months has been shown to be effective in multiple studies. When used, INH doses should be supplemented with pyridoxine 25–50 mg to minimize the likelihood of peripheral neuropathy. While treatment with INH has the benefit of compatibility with nearly all HIV treatment regimens,

completion rates tend to be lower with longer courses of treatment for LTBI. Newer, shorter treatment regimens using rifamycins have been shown to be equally effective with increased rates of completion.

The most recently approved treatment regimens for LTBI include INH-rifapentine (3HP) dosed weekly and INH-rifampin (3HR) dosed daily. The 3HP regimen can be given by DOT or self-administered and is highly desirable as it can provide cure for LTBI with only 12 weekly doses. Initially, 3HP was contraindicated in any patients taking antiretroviral medication, but newer pharmacokinetic data showed rifapentine use to be compatible with raltegravir-, dolutegravir-, and efavirenz-based regimens in virally suppressed individuals (Borisov et al., 2018). The 3HR regimen can also cure LTBI in 12 weeks but requires daily dosing of both INH and rifampin. Both 3HP and 3HR showed similar effectiveness when compared with 9-month courses of INH. The 3HR regimen has more treatment limitations owing to the potential for drug–drug interactions between rifampin and most ARVs. Rifampin taken for 4 months is an acceptable and effective LTBI treatment, especially in patients who are intolerant of INH or who are exposed to an INH-resistant case. Rifampin interacts with almost all of the antiretrovirals. This interaction excludes all of the nucleoside analogues, EXCEPT tenofovir alafenamide (TAF). ***TAF use is contraindicated with all rifamycins.*** In many cases, rifabutin can be substituted for rifampin but there have been no studies utilizing rifabutin for the treatment of LTBI in PWH. The BRIEF-TB study evaluated 1 month of daily INH/rifapentine (1HR) for the treatment of LTBI in PWH. Endpoints of the study included progression to active TB disease, death from TB, or death from other causes. Though the outcomes of treatment with 1 month of daily INH/rifapentine were similar to treatment with 9 months of INH, only 21% of enrollees had a positive screening TST at baseline, indicating a low risk of progression in the study group as a whole (Swindells et al., 2019). While CDC does not endorse the use of 1HR, DHHS guidelines suggest its use as an alternate LTBI treatment regimen. When a rifamycin is used in the treatment of a patient on antiretroviral therapy, drug–drug interactions must be carefully considered. Guidance is available in a regularly updated document at https://hivinfo.nih.gov/.

Treatment of active TB disease in PWH is also essentially the same as that for people without HIV. All patients diagnosed in the United States with active TB should be started on a four-drug regimen consisting of isoniazid, rifampin, ethambutol, and pyrazinamide, unless there is known resistance or baseline severe impairment of hepatic or renal function. After 2 months of this four-drug therapy (initial phase) and if the patient's organism is not resistant, the regimen can be reduced to INH and rifampin for the duration of treatment (continuation phase). Length of treatment will depend on the site and extent of disease. Most cases can be treated with 6–9 months of total therapy, whereas infections involving the bones or meninges should be treated for a total of 9–12 months. Infections of the central nervous system should be treated with steroids in addition to anti-TB medications. Prior recommendations were to treat infectious of the pericardium with steroids; however, subsequent data suggested that the addition of steroids in these cases does not impact outcomes (Nahid et al., 2016).

The most significant differences between treatment of patients with and without HIV involve use of the rifamycins and frequency of dosing. As previously noted, there is significant interaction between rifampin and most antiretrovirals, so care must be taken in introducing this class of medications into the regimen. Treatment regimens for active TB that do not contain a rifamycin require extension to 18–24 months of therapy and have very high rates of relapse. Hence, every effort should be made to include a rifamycin in the treatment of PWH and TB. Regularly updated guidance on how to manage drug interactions can be found at https://hivinfo. nih.gov/.

DOT is highly recommended for all cases of active TB treated in the United States to support the individual's efforts at cure. Newer technologies involving directly observed therapy by synchronous or nonsynchronous video (VDOT) allow patients more freedoms while maintaining the support afforded by DOT. Patients can receive intermittent dosing but only if receiving DOT or VDOT. Highly intermittent dosing of TB therapy (once- or twice-weekly dosing) is associated with an increased risk of relapse with rifampin-resistant disease and should be avoided in PWH (Nahid et al., 2016). This is especially noted in patients with CD4$^+$ T-cell counts < 100 cells/mm^3. New cases of active TB disease in PWH should receive daily dosing for the first 2 months of therapy, and then daily or three-times weekly dosing to complete therapy (Nahid et al., 2016).

The question of when to initiate ART in a PWH and TB is not a trivial one. Treatment for both diseases simultaneously can result in a large pill burden, potential for multiple drug interactions, and potential for multiple drug toxicities. Although it is clear that patients who are diagnosed with TB should be started immediately on anti-TB medications, until recently the timing of adding ART was less clear. Several studies (Blanc et al., 2011; Havlir et al., 2011; Karim et al., 2011; Martinson et al., 2011) conducted at multiple sites have shown a survival benefit (reduced mortality) when starting ART within 2 weeks of starting TB medications in patients with CD4$^+$ T-cell counts < 50 cells/mm^3. Of note, a single study (Mfinanga et al., 2014) showed that ART could be delayed until completion of 6 months of TB therapy in patients with CD4$^+$ T-cell counts >220 cells/mm^3. At CD4$^+$ T-cell counts >50 cells/mm^3, the incidence of IRIS events increased. Although these same studies did not show a survival benefit to starting ART earlier in patients with CD4$^+$ T-cell counts ≥50 cells/mm^3, there was no demonstration of harm, and there were many other documented benefits to starting ART. Expert opinion is that ART should be started by 8 weeks of starting treatment for TB in patients with CD4$^+$ T-cell counts ≥50 cells/mm^3.

If IRIS does occur in the course of treatment, it is important that both antiretroviral and TB treatment be continued. Mild cases of IRIS can be observed or treated with nonsteroidal anti-inflammatory agents or, if more severe, a short course of steroids may be necessary. A randomized trial showed lower incidence of TB-associated IRIS in PWH, TB, and median CD4$^+$ T-cell counts 50 cells/mm^3 started empirically on steroids (Meintjes et al., 2018). In patients where TB-associated IRIS is likely, empiric steroids may be considered.

Special consideration should be given to PWH and TB meningitis. IRIS involving central nervous system disease leads to worse outcomes. PWH and TB meningitis must be monitored carefully and treated with steroid therapy and a slow wean to reduce the inflammatory effects associated with disease. Treatment with antiretroviral drugs should be added with careful monitoring of the patient with TB meningitis for any evidence of IRIS.

Drug-resistant disease in PWH requires individualized therapy and should be approached with an expert in drug-resistant TB. Patients with multidrug-resistant or extensively drug-resistant TB should have ART initiated within 2–4 weeks after initiation of second-line TB drug therapy. The treatment duration usually ranges from 18 to 24 months. It can be shortened to 6–12 months when bedaquiline is part of the regimen (Gill et al., 2022); however, bedaquiline has significant interactions with several antiretroviral agents or there are no data on its use with other medications for HIV.

Prevention

PWH should be screened for TB by a TST or IGRA at the time of diagnosis and as needed thereafter. PWH who are found to have a positive TST or IGRA without evidence of active disease should be treated for LTBI to prevent progression to active disease.

PWH who are contacts to a case with infectious pulmonary TB and have no evidence of active disease should be treated with a full course of therapy for LTBI, even with a negative diagnostic test. As outlined previously, available diagnostic tests are not sensitive enough to rule out TB infection, and patients exposed to an infectious case are highly susceptible. Active disease should be ruled out in all patients prior to initiation of treatment for LTBI.

Patients who have a history of untreated or inadequately treated TB who do not have evidence of currently active disease should receive treatment for LTBI. This may manifest as old fibrotic lesions on chest x-ray noted during routine screening.

MYCOBACTERIUM AVIUM COMPLEX

Epidemiology

MAC, also known as MAI, consists of *M. avium* and *M. intracellulare*, two organisms so similar that they can only be differentiated using DNA probes. MAC infections are the most common nontuberculous mycobacteria (NTM) infections in both PWH and people without HIV infection (Griffith, 2007).

These organisms are ubiquitous and are found environmentally in water, soil, and animal sources. Despite the many places from which the organisms can be isolated, the actual route of infection in PWH is unclear. There is no evidence for human-to-human or animal-to-human transmission.

Disseminated disease is the most common presentation of MAC infection associated with HIV and occurs almost exclusively in individuals with profound immunosuppression who are not yet receiving ART. Disseminated disease is most commonly found in PWH with CD4 $^+$ T-cell counts < 50 cells/mm^3. Having high HIV RNA levels (>100,000 copies/mm^3) has also been identified as a risk factor. The incidence of disseminated MAC has declined steadily since the introduction of combination ART, with most cases occurring in individuals who have not accessed care or poor adherence to ART.

Clinical Presentation

As stated previously, the most common presentation of MAC infection in PWH is disseminated disease. Symptoms tend to be nonspecific and typically include fever, night sweats, anorexia, weight loss, and gastrointestinal symptoms such as nausea, vomiting, diarrhea, and abdominal pain. It is important to remember that these same symptoms can be associated with other opportunistic infections, such as TB and fungal disease.

Disseminated MAC infection tends to involve the reticuloendothelial system, and, subsequently, physical exam findings may include hepatomegaly, splenomegaly, and lymphadenopathy. Pulmonary disease is rare, even with disseminated disease, but occasionally can manifest as nodules, infiltrates, cavities, or mediastinal/hilar adenopathy. Pulmonary findings are more likely to be associated with infection due to *M. tuberculosis* or *M. kansasii*.

Immune reconstitution in patients newly started on ART may "unmask" pre-existing, previously undetected disease. The presentation in this case may manifest as disseminated disease or perhaps localized disease.

Diagnosis

Isolation of MAC from a normally sterile site, such as the blood or tissue, should be considered diagnostic for disseminated disease. In the absence of a positive blood culture, other more invasive approaches, such as lymph node, liver, or bone marrow biopsy, may be necessary to obtain an adequate specimen for diagnosis.

Isolation of MAC from nonsterile sites such as the respiratory or gastrointestinal tracts may represent true pathology but can also represent colonization. In these cases, it is important to make an effort to determine if other pathogens may be at play.

Treatment

Optimally, the approach to treatment of disseminated MAC disease should include treatment of both MAC and HIV. Like treatment of TB and other NTM infections, treatment of MAC infection should include multidrug therapy, and ART should be started and optimized as soon as possible.

Drug susceptibility testing should be performed as macrolide susceptibility is associated with greater treatment success when using this class of drug. It should be noted that only macrolide and amikacin susceptibilities are associated with treatment outcomes.

Clarithromycin should be the first drug added to a MAC treatment regimen. Studies have shown treatment with clarithromycin to be associated with faster clearance of bacteremia than treatment with azithromycin. In the event of clarithromycin intolerance or a prohibiting drug interaction with other medications, azithromycin may constitute an alternative.

The second drug added should be ethambutol. Addition of ethambutol to a macrolide is associated with decreased relapse in the treatment of MAC. Rifabutin can also be added to the MAC treatment regimen, especially in situations where the risk of mortality is high and/or emergence of resistance is likely. Addition of rifabutin also adds the potential for significant interaction with many antiretrovirals and can lower the serum drug levels of clarithromycin when used in combination. Prior to the addition of rifabutin to the treatment of a mycobacterial infection, TB must be ruled out to prevent the emergence of rifampin-resistant TB disease.

Based on data from people without HIV, fluoroquinolones such as moxifloxacin or levofloxacin and injectable antibiotics such as amikacin and streptomycin can be utilized if there is a need for additional medication options owing to resistance, intolerance, or toxicity. While there are in vitro data showing susceptibility to these drugs, there are no randomized controlled trials evaluating their efficacy in the setting of macrolide susceptibility or effective ART.

The occurrence of IRIS has been documented with treatment of MAC disease, as it has with TB. The presentation generally manifests as a recurrence of fever and worsening lymphadenitis with negative blood cultures. Mild cases can be simply monitored or treated with a nonsteroidal anti-inflammatory agent or, in severe cases, a short course of steroids. Treatment for both MAC and HIV should be continued during management of IRIS reactions.

Treatment of disseminated disease should continue until there is a response to ART. Repeat blood cultures should be reserved for those without a clinical response after 4 to 8 weeks of treatment. PWH who complete a 12-month course of therapy, who remain free of signs or symptoms of disease, and who show a sustained increase in CD4$^+$ T-cell count to >100 cells/mm^3 for at least 6 months have a low risk of relapse. If a previously treated person experiences a decrease in CD4$^+$ T-cell count < 100 cells/mm^3 or is not on a fully suppressive ART regimen, the individual should reinitiate preventive (secondary) prophylactic treatment.

Prevention/Prophylaxis

No direct route for infection with MAC has been identified and, thus, there is no specific action known to prevent exposure to MAC. Primary prophylaxis to prevent disseminated MAC disease is no longer recommended for patients who immediately initiate ART. If primary prophylaxis is initiated, it should be discontinued once the patient is on a fully suppressive ART regimen. Primary prophylaxis for disseminated MAC is reserved for patients with a CD4 + T-cell count < 50 cells/mm³ who are not receiving ART, who remain viremic or for whom a fully suppressive ART regimen is not an option. Before starting primary prophylaxis, disseminated MAC should be ruled out.

Azithromycin dosed at 1,200 mg weekly is the preferred regimen for both primary and secondary prophylaxis. Clarithromycin dosed at 500 mg twice daily is effective but, because of the increased pill burden and higher number of drug interactions, is considered an alternative to azithromycin.

Rifabutin is an alternative when there is evidence of macrolide-resistant disease and secondary prophylaxis is needed or when there is macrolide intolerance, but rifabutin is less effective in this capacity and adds increased risk of drug interactions with many of the antiretrovirals. Before the use of rifabutin, every effort should be made to rule out active TB.

MYCOBACTERIUM KANSASII

Epidemiology

Mycobacterium kansasii infection is the second most common NTM infection in PWH (after MAC infection). Tap water appears to be the most likely environmental reservoir for strains causing human disease (Griffith, 2002). Lung disease caused by *M. kansasii* closely resembles disease caused by *M. tuberculosis* in both people with and without HIV. Despite its similarities to TB, there is no evidence of human-to-human transmission of *M. kansasii*. Similar to MAC, infection with *M. kansasii* is most commonly found in individuals with CD4 + T-cell counts < 50 cells/mm³.

Clinical Presentation

Unlike MAC disease, which is most commonly disseminated and rarely pulmonary, *M. kansasii* can be disseminated but is more commonly pulmonary. Radiographically, *M. kansasii* infection closely resembles infection with *M. tuberculosis*, with symptoms that include cough, fever, night sweats, weight loss, and hemoptysis.

Diagnosis

Diagnosis requires isolation of the organism from a sterile site or meeting the criterion outlined in the guidelines set forth by the American Thoracic Society (Griffith, 2007). Briefly, the ATS criteria for both people with and without HIV requires that the individual in question have pulmonary symptoms with suggestive radiography, exclusion of other diagnoses, positive culture results from two separate expectorated sputa, or at least one bronchoalveolar lavage specimen or bronchial biopsy with suggestive histopathology.

Mycobacterium kansasii, like other mycobacteria, will stain positive by acid-fast staining, which, when isolated from the sputum of a person with pulmonary lesions can trigger an unnecessary public health investigation for TB. Testing with a nucleic acid amplification test can rule out TB in these cases.

Treatment

Most studies guiding treatment of *Mycobacterium kansasii* infection are conducted in individuals without HIV. *Mycobacterium kansasii* responds well to anti-TB medications with the exception that the organism is widely resistant to pyrazinamide. Treatment with a rifamycin, ethambutol, and either isoniazid or a macrolide is recommended for at least 12 months. Prior studies suggested treatment for 12 months after culture conversion but there is no evidence that treatment for longer than 12 total months prevents relapse (Daley et al., 2020). Two studies demonstrated good outcomes with clarithromycin substituted for isoniazid (Daley et al., 2020). Rifamycins in the treatment regimen of *M. kansasii* patients (unlike those with MAC disease) provide clear benefit and prevent relapse. The choice and dose of rifamycin should be guided by the patient's antiretroviral treatment, with special attention to potential drug interactions.

As with infections caused by other mycobacteria, IRIS has been documented with treatment of *M. kansasii*. Mild cases can be simply monitored or treated with a nonsteroidal anti-inflammatory agent or, in severe cases, a short course of steroids. It is important that treatment for both *M. kansasii* and HIV be continued during management of IRIS reactions.

RECOMMENDED READING

Griffith DE, Aksamit T, Brown-Elliott BA, et al. An official ATS/IDSA statement: Diagnosis, treatment, and prevention of nontuberculous mycobacterial diseases. *Am J Respir Crit Care Med.* 2007;175:367–416.

US DHHS, Panel on Antiretroviral Guidelines for Adults and Adolescents. Guidelines for the use of antiretroviral agents in adults and adolescents with HIV. Department of Health and Human Services. https://clinicalinfo.hiv.gov/sites/default/files/guidelines/documents/adult-adolescent-arv/guidelines-adult-adolescent-arv.pdf. Published January 2022a. Accessed August 2022.

US Department of Health and Human Services. Guidelines for prevention and treatment of opportunistic infections in HIV-infected adults and adolescents. https://clinicalinfo.hiv.gov/sites/default/files/guidelines/documents/adult-adolescent-oi/guidelines-adult-adolescent-oi.pdf. Published 2022b. Accessed October 8, 2022.

OPPORTUNISTIC INFECTIONS: VIRAL INFECTIONS

LEARNING OBJECTIVE

Discuss the established and evolving science regarding diagnosis, treatment, and prophylaxis of opportunistic viral infections associated with HIV infection to improve quality of life and length of survival.

A new recombinant zoster vaccine (RZV) was approved in October 2017. In October 2021, the Advisory Committee on Immunization Practices (ACIP) recommended 2 RZV doses for prevention of herpes zoster and related complications in immunodeficient or immunosuppressed adults aged ≥19 years.

KEY POINTS

Herpes Simplex Virus

- HSV is a very common disease in PWH, typically presenting with orolabial, genital, and/or anorectal ulcers that may be very severe in the setting of advance immunosuppression. HSV could also manifest as proctitis (particularly in men who have sex with men), esophagitis, keratitis, meningitis, encephalitis, radiculitis, and retinitis (presenting as acute retinal necrosis).

- Treatment is generally with acyclovir or one of its derivatives. Acyclovir resistance is more common among PWH. HSV suppression should be considered for individuals with frequent or severe recurrent episodes.

Varicella Zoster Virus

- Varicella zoster reactivation disease in PWH is often more severe, multidermatomal, or disseminated. Severe complications such as progressive outer retinal necrosis must be treated quickly to prevent permanent sequelae. For mild disease, oral therapy with acyclovir or one of its derivatives is appropriate; in severe cases, however, intravenous therapy is required.

Cytomegalovirus

- Cytomegalovirus may cause a variety of clinical manifestations in PWH with CD4$^+$ T-cell counts of less than 50 cells/mm^3. Retinitis and colitis are the most common manifestations. Ganciclovir (or the oral prodrug valganciclovir), cidofovir, or foscarnet are the most common therapies, but they carry significant risk of toxicity. Primary prophylaxis is not recommended.

JC Virus

- Reactivation of the polyomavirus JC (JCV) causes PML, a progressive, demyelinating disease of the central nervous system that leads to relatively rapid accumulation of neurologic deficits with dementia, coma, and death. Diagnosis is generally made clinically with the support of typical magnetic resonance imaging (MRI) findings and JCV polymerase chain reaction (PCR) in the CSF. Definitive diagnosis is made by brain biopsy. No specific

antiviral therapy exists for JCV. ART often results in stabilization or regression of disease.

HERPESVIRUS

Herpes Simplex Virus

In the United States, the seroprevalence of HSV types 1 and 2 (HSV-1 and HSV-2) is 47.8 % and 11.9%, respectively, in the age-group 14 to 49 years (McQuillan et al., 2017). HSV-1 and HSV-2 are highly prevalent in PWH. Classically, HSV-1 is associated with oral ulcers, whereas HSV-2 causes genital ulcers; currently, however, both are recognized as a cause of genital infection, especially in young women and men who have sex with men (MSM). The incidence of primary HSV-1 genital infection has been increasing, with lesions identical to HSV-2 (Ryder et al., 2009).0.

HSV-2 is one of the most common sexually transmitted infections worldwide and remains as the primary cause of genital ulcer disease. The overall national HSV-2 prevalence was reported as 16.2% in 2010 (Xu et al., 2006); however, seroprevalence rates near 70% have been reported in PWH (Corey et al., 2004). The primary mode of transmission is through direct contact with oral or genital secretions. Clinical HSV disease is common in the absence of HIV infection, but manifestations are more common, more severe, or atypical in the setting of HIV infection.

Clinical Presentation

The classical presentation of herpes infection is large, painful, grouped vesicles with an erythematous base typically in the orolabial, genital, and anorectal regions; however, they may involve any area of the body. Inguinal lymphadenopathy is commonly seen in primary infection (Corey & Holmes, 1983). In patients with advanced HIV-associated immunosuppression, anogenital lesions may be severe, and they may be refractory to treatment or secondary to acyclovir-resistant virus (Safrin et al., 1994). Dissemination is possible, but it is rarely seen in PWH. Hypertrophic genital herpes, which is an atypical presentation, often resembles neoplasia and needs a biopsy to confirm the diagnosis (Yudin & Kaul, 2008). Proctitis, particularly in MSM, keratitis, meningitis, encephalitis, radiculitis, and retinitis (presenting as acute retinal necrosis) are possible complications. HSV esophagitis may occur in people with CD4$^+$ T-cell counts of less than 50 cells/mm^3 and typically presents with retrosternal chest pain and odynophagia.

Reactivation of HSV is more common in PWH. Recurrent lesions are often more frequent, more extensive, and of longer duration in this population. In addition, there is prolonged shedding of the virus even in the absence of lesions, especially in patients with lower CD4$^+$ T-cell counts and higher plasma HIV-1 RNA levels.

Diagnosis

HSV DNA PCR and viral culture are the recommended modalities for diagnosis for all suspected HSV mucosal infections with the PCR having the highest sensitivity (Workowski, 2021). Type-specific serological assays are available and recommended, but false positive HSV-2 serologic tests have been reported with enzyme immunoassay antibody tests with low index values (1.1 to 3.5), and repeat testing is recommended in such cases for confirmation (Workowski, 2021). Culture specimens can also be tested for antiviral drug susceptibility.

Prevention

Latex condoms, when consistently used, decrease acquisition of HSV-2 in HSV-2 discordant heterosexual couples (DHHS, 2022b). Suppressive therapy with oral acyclovir, valacyclovir, or famciclovir is recommended for severe or frequent recurrences in PWH. Annual assessment is recommended to determine the continuation of this therapy. There is no vaccine available for prevention of HSV infection.

Treatment

Table 28.1 shows the current treatment recommendations from the Guidelines for the Prevention and Treatment of in Adults and Adolescents with HIV (DHHS, 2022a). Oral acyclovir, valacyclovir, and famciclovir are comparable alternatives. In patients with extensive mucocutaneous lesions, it is recommended to use intravenous acyclovir. No sign of resolution of herpes lesions in 7 to 10 days after starting anti-HSV therapy raises suspicion for acyclovir resistance, and viral culture of the lesion with phenotypic testing and susceptibility testing should be performed (DHS, 2022b).

Resistance to acyclovir has been reported in up to 5% of PWH with HSV-2 infection and is more frequent in patients with prolonged acyclovir use. Acyclovir inhibits HSV-specific DNA polymerase after incorporation into the growing DNA, resulting in a chain termination owing to the absence of the 3′ hydroxyl group. It requires phosphorylation by a virally encoded thymidine kinase in order to be active. Altered, reduced, or absent thymidine kinase or altered viral DNA polymerase confers resistance to acyclovir and all the class, including ganciclovir. In these cases, foscarnet is the drug of choice. Cidofovir is a reasonable alternative for thymidine kinase negative HSV. Pritelivir, a helicase-primase inhibitor is a novel agent that is being studied in clinical trials for treatment of acyclovir-resistant herpes in the immunocompromised population. Prolonged application (21 to 28 days or longer) of topical agents like trifluridine, foscarnet, cidofovir, and imiquimod can effectively treat external lesions (OI guidelines CIII).

Prophylaxis

Condoms are recommended to prevent transmission of HSV-2. The use of 1% tenofovir vaginal gel has been shown to be associated with a 50% risk reduction of HSV-2 acquisition in women at high risk of HIV infection (Bender Ignacio et al., 2015). However, this has not been confirmed in other studies. In addition, in patients taking oral tenofovir, the rates of vaginal shedding of HSV-1 and HSV-2 are similar. Suppressive therapy with oral acyclovir, valacyclovir, or famciclovir is effective in preventing genital herpes recurrences, and it should be discussed with all patients with HSV-2 (Table 28.2). Immune

Table 28.1 HSV TREATMENT RECOMMENDATIONS

CONDITION	FIRST CHOICE TREATMENT	ALTERNATIVE TREATMENT
Orolabial lesions	Valacyclovir 1 g PO b.i.d. *or* Famciclovir 500 mg PO b.i.d. *or* Acyclovir 400 mg PO t.i.d. for 5–10 days	
Initial or recurrent genital lesions	Valacyclovir 1 g PO b.i.d. *or* Famciclovir 500 mg PO b.i.d. *or* Acyclovir 400 mg PO t.i.d. for 5–10 days	
Severe mucocutaneous lesions	Acyclovir 5 mg/kg IV every 8 hours until lesions regress, then switch to acyclovir 400 mg PO t.i.d. until lesions are healed	
Esophagitis	Valacyclovir 1 g PO t.i.d. *or* Famciclovir 500 mg PO t.i.d. *or* Acyclovir 400 mg PO five times daily for 14–21 days	
Encephalitis and hepatitis	Acyclovir 10–15 mg/kg IV every 8 hours for 21 days	
Acyclovir-resistant herpes	Foscarnet 90–120 mg/kg/day IV 2–3 times daily until clinical response Cidofovir 5 mg/kg/week IV for 3 weeks, then 5 mg/kg every other week with saline hydration and probenecid 2 g PO 3 hours before the dose followed by 1 g 2 hours and 8 hours after the dose (total of 4 g) until clinical response (off label)	Topical trifluridine, or Cidofovir 1% gel, or Topical imiquimod 5% three times weekly for 21–28 days or longer based on clinical response

Table 28.2 HSV SUPPRESSIVE THERAPY RECOMMENDATIONS

CONDITION	FIRST CHOICE TREATMENT
Genital lesions	Valacyclovir 500 mg PO b.i.d. *or* Famciclovir 500 mg PO b.i.d. *or* Acyclovir 400–800 mg PO b.i.d. or t.i.d.

reconstitution improves the frequency and severity of clinical episodes of genital herpes, but it does not decrease shedding.

In individuals with CD4$^+$ T-cell count of less than 250 cells/mm^3 who will start ART, there is an increased risk of HSV-2 shedding and genital ulcer diseases in the first 6 months. It is recommended to give suppressive antiviral therapy because it decreases the risk of genital ulcer diseases by 60%.

VARICELLA ZOSTER VIRUS

VZV causes initial infection in childhood (chickenpox) and later reactivates, causing herpes zoster. The prevalence of herpes zoster is 3%–5% in the general population, but it is 15–25-times higher in PWH (Buchbinder et al., 1992). Lower CD4$^+$ T-cell counts have been associated with atypical presentations of the disease, but not with increased incidence.

Clinical Presentation

The initial clinical presentation is similar to that of immunocompetent patients. It manifests as a prodrome of cutaneous burning or pain, followed by a cutaneous eruption of grouped vesicles on an erythematous base along a dermatome. However, PWH are at increased risk for multidermatomal or disseminated zoster, including neurologic and ophthalmologic complications. Approximately 20%–30% of PWH will experience subsequent episodes of herpes zoster, either in the same or in different dermatomes. The probability of a recurrence of herpes zoster within 1 year of the index episode is 10% (Gebo et al., 2005). Postherpetic neuralgia is reported in 10%–15% of PWH (Gebo et al., 2005; Harrison et al., 1999).

Atypical VZV presentations such as chronic hyperkeratotic lesions or chronic disseminated ecthyma have also been reported. Meningitis, multifocal leukoencephalitis, ventriculitis, myelitis, cranial nerve palsies, and focal brainstem lesions are possible neurological complications. Involvement of the ophthalmic division of the trigeminal nerve causes anterior uveitis, corneal scarring, and vision loss. Ocular involvement with acute retinal necrosis and progressive outer retinal necrosis are syndromes similar to CMV retinitis but of faster progression that typically occurs at CD4$^+$ T-cell counts of less than 100 cells/mm^3 and may result in retinal blindness (Engstrom et al., 1994).

Diagnosis

The diagnosis is made clinically. Laboratory confirmation could be done by viral culture, direct immunofluorescence testing, and the PCR assay, which is the most sensitive test.

Treatment

VZV treatment is summarized in Table 28.3.

Prevention

Long-term prophylaxis or suppressive treatment is not recommended. Postexposure prophylaxis is recommended for PWH susceptible to VZV and close contact with a person who has active varicella or herpes zoster. The preferred regimen is a single intramuscular dose of VariZIG dosed on body weight (maximum of 625 IU) administered as soon as possible and within 10 days after exposure. Alternatively, acyclovir or valacyclovir could be given starting 7–10 days after exposure.

Table 28.3 VZV TREATMENT RECOMMENDATIONS

CONDITION	FIRST CHOICE TREATMENT
VZV infection, immunocompromised patients	SEVERE: Acyclovir 10–15 mg/kg IV every 8 hours for 7–10 days. May switch to PO if no evidence of visceral involvement. UNCOMPLICATED: Valacyclovir (1 g PO 3 times daily), *or* famciclovir (500 mg PO 3 times daily) for 5 to 7 days.
Herpes zoster, acute localized dermatomal	Valacyclovir 1 g t.i.d. *or* Famciclovir 500 mg t.i.d. *or* Acyclovir 800 mg PO 5 times daily, each administered for 7–10 days. Consider longer duration if lesions slow to resolve.
Herpes zoster, extensive cutaneous lesion or visceral involvement	Acyclovir 10–15 mg/kg IV every 8 hours. After clinical improvement is evident, switch to oral therapy: Valacyclovir 1 g t.i.d. *or* Famciclovir 500 mg t.i.d. *or* Acyclovir 800 mg five times daily, each administered for 10–14 days.
Acute retinal necrosis	Acyclovir 10 mg/kg IV every 8 hours for 10–14 days; followed by oral valacyclovir 1 g t.i.d. for 6 weeks *plus* Ganciclovir 2 mg/0.05 mL intravitreal twice weekly × 1 or 2 doses.
Progressive outer retinal necrosis	Ganciclovir 5 mg/kg IV *and/or* Foscarnet 90 mg/kg IV every 12 hours *plus* Ganciclovir 2 mg/0.05 ml intravitreal twice weekly × 1 or 2 doses.
Acyclovir-resistant VZV infection	Foscarnet 90 mg/kg IV every 12 hours.

There are two vaccines available for the prevention of zoster: a live-attenuated virus zoster vaccine (ZVL) and a recombinant vaccine (RZV). ZVL was studied in a phase II, randomized, double-blind, placebo-controlled clinical trial designed to evaluate its safety, tolerability, and immunogenicity in PWH on ART with CD4$^+$ T-cell counts of 200 cells/mm^3 or higher and virologic suppression (Benson et al., 2018). A total of 295 participants received the vaccine. ZVL was safe and immunogenic. Those with CD4$^+$ T-cell counts of 350 cells/mm^3 or higher developed the highest zoster antibody levels post vaccination. A small phase 1/2a, randomized, observer-masked, placebo-controlled study evaluated the safety and immunogenicity of RZV in 123 PWH. The vaccine was found to have a clinically acceptable safety profile and elicited strong gE-specific cell-mediated and anti-gE humoral immune responses that persisted at least 1 year after the last vaccination (Berkowitz et al., 2015). In October 2021, the ACIP recommended 2 RZV doses for prevention of herpes zoster and related complications in immunodeficient or immunosuppressed adults aged ≥19 years. RZV is preferred over ZVL because of higher efficacy data in immunocompetent patients (OI guidelines AIII). ZVL can be given as an alternative to PWH with CD4$^+$ T-cell count >200 cells/mm^3 in case of unavailability of RZV or intolerance to it (OI guidelines BIII). It should be noted that ZVL is contraindicated in PWH with CD4$^+$ T-cell counts < 200 cells/mm^3 as it can lead to disseminated ZVL vaccine strain infection (OI guidelines AIII).

CYTOMEGALOVIRUS

CMV is a DNA herpesvirus and the largest among them with the longest genome. It is typically acquired from close contact during youth or adolescence. In the general population, the percentage of people with evidence of previous CMV infection ranges from 40% to 100% and varies with ethnicity and country. Active disease associated with HIV typically results from reactivation of latent infection in the setting of advanced immunosuppression with CD4$^+$ T-cell counts of less than 50 cells/mm^3 (Dieterich et al., 1991). Other risk factors for CMV disease include plasma HIV RNA levels of more than 100,000 copies/mL and the presence of other OIs.

Before the use of ART, CMV retinitis was the most common intraocular infection in patients with AIDS, occurring in up to 40% of patients (Whitcup, 2000). Currently, the incidence of new cases of CMV end-organ disease has declined to fewer than six cases/100 person-years (Jabs et al., 2007).

Clinical Presentation and Diagnosis

CMV can infect different organs of the body. Retinitis accounts for 85% of CMV manifestations and is the leading cause of vision loss among people with AIDS. Other CMV clinical syndromes include esophagitis, colitis, polyradiculopathy, ventriculoencephalitis, pneumonitis, adrenalitis, and pancreatitis.

Chorioretinitis

CMV chorioretinitis presents painless progressive loss of vision, floaters, and/or visual field cut defects. Symptoms are unilateral at first, but without treatment they can become bilateral. The diagnosis is exclusively made by recognition of typical retinal changes during a funduscopic examination: creamy or yellow-white granular areas with perivascular exudates and hemorrhage. These lesions initially are found in the periphery of the fundus but can later involve the macula and the optic disc, resulting in blindness.

Colitis

CMV colitis is the second most common manifestation of CMV infection in people with AIDS. Patients present with severe diarrhea, abdominal pain and cramping, anorexia, weight loss, and fever. The diagnosis is made by detection of mucosal ulcerations on endoscopic examination combined with colonoscopic or rectal biopsy. Pathology will reveal intracytoplasmic or intranuclear inclusions. A positive culture itself does not confirm the diagnosis. Mucosal hemorrhage and perforation rarely occur, but they are life-threatening.

Esophagitis

CMV esophagitis causes odynophagia, nausea, fever, and retrosternal pain. Diagnosis is made by endoscopic examination that reveals diffuse inflammation of the esophagus and/or esophageal ulcers. Biopsy specimens also reveal intranuclear inclusions. A positive culture itself does not make the diagnosis.

CMV Polyradiculopathy

CMV polyradiculopathy presents sacrolumbar radicular pain and lower limb paresthesia that may develop into progressive flaccid paralysis of the legs with decreasing and ultimately absent tendon reflexes. Urinary retention and stool incontinence may occur. If untreated, the condition rapidly advances up the spine, causing ascending sensory loss and growing flaccidity in the upper limbs, similar to Guillain–Barré paralysis. The CSF may reveal pleocytosis with a predominance of polymorphonuclear cells, elevated protein, and moderately low glucose. Lumbar MRI may show gadolinium enhancement of the cauda equina in 33% of patients. Diagnosis is made by viral culture, CMV antigen assays, and detection of CMV DNA by CSF PCR.

Ventriculoencephalitis

CMV ventriculoencephalitis is a late manifestation of CMV disease. It presents with fever, lethargy, confusion, and an acute course consisting of cranial nerve palsies, nystagmus, and other focal neurologic deficits that rapidly leads to death. CT and MRI scans show white matter enhancement. MRI with gadolinium may reveal a characteristic periventricular ring-like enhancement. Viral culture of the CSF is not always positive, although CMV DNA can often be detected in CSF using PCR.

Dementia

CMV dementia can present with fever, lethargy, and confusion, and it may be clinically similar to HIV-associated dementia. CSF analysis is significant for pleocytosis that may be polymorphonuclear with low to normal glucose, and normal to high protein. CT and MRI scans may show cerebral atrophy.

Pneumonia

CMV pneumonitis is uncommon in patients with AIDS. Symptoms include shortness of breath, dyspnea, dry nonproductive cough, and hypoxia. Imaging studies show diffuse interstitial infiltrates. A definitive diagnosis is made when multiple CMV inclusion bodies are seen in lung tissue. CMV may be isolated from bronchial washing or bronchoalveolar lavage fluid from approximately 50% of PWH undergoing bronchoscopy; however, the clinical significance of the CMV isolation from these fluids and respiratory secretions remains controversial due to the viral shedding.

CMV viremia is common in asymptomatic persons with low CD4 $^+$ T-cell counts (< 100 cells/mm^3). Viremia is typically present in active disease but may also be present in the absence of end-organ disease, so the tests are of limited value. The absence of CMV antibody may be helpful in excluding CMV disease; however, rarely, active disease can present during primary CMV infection with negative antibodies, and immunoglobin G antibody tests may revert to negative in individuals with advanced immunosuppression.

Treatment

Table 28.4 shows the current CMV treatment recommendations from the Guidelines for the Prevention and Treatment of Opportunistic Infections (DHHS, 2022b).

For CMV chorioretinitis, treatment consists of an induction phase of high-dose drug given for at least 2 weeks. Once retinitis is stable, patients are placed on chronic maintenance therapy until there is evidence of immune recovery (sustained CD4 $^+$ T-cell counts >100 cells/mm^3 for ≥6 months). In the absence of antiretroviral-mediated immune reconstitution, most patients will have a reactivation of CMV infection despite suppressive therapy and will require reinduction therapy. Intraocular treatment may be useful in salvage therapy for patients who cannot tolerate systemic antivirals. Otherwise, any local treatment should be accompanied by systemic anti-CMV therapy. Systemic therapy has been shown to decrease

Table 28.4 CMV TREATMENT RECOMMENDATIONS

CONDITION	FIRST CHOICE TREATMENT	ALTERNATIVE TREATMENT
CMV retinitis	*For sight-threatening lesions:* Intravitreal injections Ganciclovir or foscarnet *plus* Valganciclovir 900 mg PO b.i.d. for 14–21 days, then once daily *For small peripheral lesions:* Valganciclovir 900 mg PO bid for 14–21 days, then 900 mg once daily *or* any of the alternative treatments	Intravitreal injections Ganciclovir or foscarnet *plus* Ganciclovir 5 mg/kg IV every 12 hours for 14–21 days, then 5 mg/kg IV daily *or* Ganciclovir 5 mg/kg IV every 12 hours for 14–21 days, then valganciclovir 900 mg PO daily Foscarnet 60 mg/kg IV every 8 hours or Foscarnet 90 mg/kg IV every 12 hours for 14–21 days, then 90–120 mg/kg IV every 24 hours *or* Cidofovir 5 mg/kg/week IV for 2 weeks, then 5 mg/kg every other week with saline hydration and probenecid 2 g PO 3 hours before the dose followed by 1 g 2 hours and 8 hours after the dose (total of 4 g)
Secondary prophylaxis (previously called maintenance therapy) for CMV retinitis	Valganciclovir 900 mg PO daily *or* Ganciclovir implant (replaced every 6–8 months if CD4$^+$ count remains <100 cells/mm^3) *plus* Valganciclovir 900 mg PO daily until immune recovery	Ganciclovir 5 mg/kg IV 5–7 times weekly *or* Foscarnet 90–120 mg/kg body weight IV once daily *or* Cidofovir 5 mg/kg body weight IV every other week as above
CMV colitis or esophagitis	Ganciclovir IV *or* Foscarnet IV for 21–28 days	–
CMV neurological disease	Ganciclovir IV *plus* Foscarnet IV until symptomatic improvement	–

CMV, cytomegalovirus; IV, intravenous; PO, orally.

CMV involvement of the contralateral eye, to reduce the risk of CMV disease in other organs, and to increase survival rates. Intraocular therapy alone has been associated with progression of CMV to the contralateral eye, as well as with systemic disease (Martin et al., 1994).

Ganciclovir and valganciclovir, foscarnet, and cidofovir carry a significant toxicity risk. Ganciclovir and valganciclovir can cause neutropenia, thrombocytopenia, nausea, diarrhea, renal dysfunction, and central venous catheter infection. Foscarnet more commonly causes nephrotoxicity, electrolyte abnormalities seizures, genital ulcers, and central venous catheter infection. Cidofovir, when used, is associated with nephrotoxicity and intraocular hypotony.

Prevention/Prophylaxis

In patients with CD4 $^+$ T-cell count of less than 100 cells/mm^3, early recognition of the manifestations of end-organ CMV disease is the best modality for early diagnosis and prevention of further disease progression. Primary prophylaxis against CMV is not recommended. Patients with CD4 $^+$ T-cell counts of less than 100 cells/mm^3 should have an annual ophthalmology exam. Secondary prophylaxis is done with valganciclovir until CD4 $^+$ T-cell count has been greater than 100 cells/mm^3 for 3–6 months and the lesions are not life-threatening. If CD4 $^+$ T-cell count decreases to less than 100 cells/mm^3, secondary prophylaxis should be reinstituted.

HUMAN HERPESVIRUS-8

The prevalence of human herpesvirus-8 (HHV-8) ranges between 1% and 5% in the general population, but it is between 20% and 77% in MSM (Pauk et al., 2000). HHV-8 is associated with all forms of KS, primary effusion lymphoma, and lymphoproliferative disorders such as multicentric Castleman's disease (see Chapter 35).

JOHN CUNNINGHAM VIRUS (JCV)

Reactivation of the polyomavirus JC (JCV) causes PML, a disease characterized by focal demyelination. Approximately 85% of adults are seropositive for JC virus worldwide. Most individuals usually are exposed to JCV in childhood, which causes asymptomatic infection and a chronic asymptomatic carrier state (Antonsson et al., 2010; Knowles, 2006). The incidence of PML has decreased significantly since the widespread use of ART. However, PML has also been reported in PWH with CD4 $^+$ T-cell counts of greater than 300 cells/mm^3 and as a complication of IRIS (Berger et al., 1998; Cinque et al., 2003).

Clinical Presentation

The clinical presentation of PML depends on the location of brain lesions, and the specific deficits vary from patient to patient. Commonly involved areas include the occipital lobe, causing hemianopsia; the frontal and parietal lobes, leading

to aphasia, hemiparesis and hemisensory deficits; and the cerebellar peduncles and deep white matter, causing dysmetria and ataxia (Richardson & Webster, 1983). The spinal cord is rarely involved. Optic nerves are usually spared (Bernal-Cano et al., 2007). Patients can present with symptoms ranging from diffuse encephalopathy to focal deficits such as ataxia, hemiparesis, or speech difficulties. Symptoms tend to progress over several weeks to months. Seizures are seen in 20% of cases. Headache and fever are unusual in PML and if present, raises the possibility of another OI.

Diagnosis

MRI of the brain demonstrates distinct white matter lesions in areas of the brain corresponding to the clinical deficits. The lesions are usually white on T2 images, and they are also characteristically dark on T1 images. JCV DNAPCR in CSF is recommended to confirm the diagnosis and has a diagnostic sensitivity of 70%–80%, and specificity of 100% (Cinque, 1997). Brain biopsy, used to make a definitive diagnose, will reveal the typical findings of focal myelin loss with characteristic astrocytes and lipid-laden macrophages. Because of high JCV seroprevalence, serological testing is not recommended.

Prevention

Early initiation of ART, in order to prevent HIV-related immunosuppression, is the only effective modality for prevention of PML (OI guidelines AII).

Treatment

Initiation of effective ART is the treatment of choice. It prolongs survival and improves neurologic deficits when immune reconstitution is achieved. The early use of an optimized combination antiretroviral regimen with three or more drugs after PML diagnosis appeared to improve survival (Gasnault et al., 2011). Other treatments have been attempted with no improvement in survival. Recrudescence after remission of PML with ART is extremely rare, but a few cases have been reported (Cinque et al, 2001; Crossley et al., 2016).

PML-IMMUNE RECONSTITUTION INFLAMMATORY SYNDROME

PML-IRIS may occur after initiating ART in people with advanced HIV infection and low CD4 $^+$ T-cell counts. The patient may present with clinical and radiological findings different from the classical PML. Radiologic findings of lesions with contrast enhancement, edema and mass effect have been reported (Post et al., 2013). Both new onset and paradoxical worsening of PML can occur in ART-induced IRIS, and in many studies, empiric use of corticosteroids has been seen to be beneficial. The dose and duration of treatment with corticosteroids is yet to be established (Cinque et al., 2009; Fournier et al., 2017; Tan et al., 2009).

REFERENCES

American Thoracic Society. Targeted tuberculin testing and treatment of latent tuberculosis infection. http://www.cdc.gov/mmwr/preview/mmwrhtml/rr4906a1.htm. Published June 2000. Accessed August 15, 2022.

Antonsson A, Green AC, Mallitt KA, et al. Prevalence and stability of antibodies to the BK and JC polyomaviruses: a long-term longitudinal study of Australians. *J Gen Virol.* 2010;91(Pt 7):1849–1853.

Bender Ignacio RA, Perti T, Magaret AS, et al., Oral and vaginal tenofovir for genital herpes simplex virus type 2 shedding in immunocompetent women: a double-blind, randomized, cross-over trial. *J Infect Dis.* 2015 212(12): 1949–1956.

Benson CA, Andersen JW, Macatangay BJC, et al. Safety and immunogenicity of Zoster [JWOY1] vaccine live in HIV-positive adults with CD4$^+$ T-cell counts above 200 cells/mL virologically suppressed on antiretroviral therapy. *Clin Infect Dis.* 2018;67(11):1712–1719.

Berger JR, Levy RM, Flomenhoft D. Predictive factors for prolonged survival in acquired immunodeficiency syndrome-associated progressive multifocal leukoencephalopathy. *Ann Neurol.* 1998;44:341–349.

Berkowitz EM, Moyle G, Stellbrink HJ, et al. Safety and immunogenicity of an adjuvanted herpes zoster subunit candidate vaccine in HIV-positive adults: a phase 1/2a randomized, placebo-controlled study. *J Infect Dis.* 2015;211(8):1279–1287.

Bernal-Cano F, Joseph JT, Koralnik IJ. Spinal cord lesions of progressive multifocal leukoencephalopathy in an acquired immunodeficiency syndrome patient. *J Neurovirol.* 2007;13(5):474–476. https://www.ncbi.nlm.nih.gov/pubmed/17994433

Blanc FX, Sok T, Laureillard, D, et al. Earlier versus later start of antiretroviral therapy in HIV-positive adults with tuberculosis. *N Engl J Med.* 2011;365(16):1471–1481.

Borisov AS, Bamrah Morris S, et al. Update of recommendations for use of once-weekly isoniazid-rifapentine regimen to treat latent mycobacterium tuberculosis infection. *MMWR.* June 29, 2018:67(25):723–726.

Boulware DR, Meya DB, Muzoora C, et al. Timing of antiretroviral therapy after diagnosis of cryptococcal meningitis. *N Engl J Med.* 2014;370(26):2487–2498.

Buchbinder SP, Katz MH, Hessol NA, et al. Herpes zoster and human immunodeficiency virus infection. *J Infect Dis.* 1992;166(5):1153–116.

Cattamanchi A, Smith R, Steingart KR, et al. Interferon-gamma release assays for the diagnosis of latent tuberculosis infection in HIV-infected individuals: a systematic review and meta-analysis. *J Acquir Immune Defic Syndr.* 2011;56(3):230–238.

Centers for Disease Control and Prevention (CDC). *Recommendations for human immunodeficiency virus (HIV) Screening in tuberculosis (TB) clinics, factsheet.* Atlanta, GA: US Department of Health and Human Services, CDC; 2012. https://www.cdc.gov/tb/publications/factsheets/testing/HIVscreening.pdf

Centers for Disease Control and Prevention (CDC). *Reported tuberculosis in the United States, 2020.* Atlanta, GA: US Department of Health and Human Services, CDC; 2020.

Cinque P. Cytomegalovirus infections of the nervous system. *Intervirology.* 1997;40(2–3):85–97.

Cinque P, Bossolasco S, Brambilla AM, et al. The effect of highly active antiretroviral therapy-induced immune reconstitution on development and outcome of progressive multifocal leukoencephalopathy: study of 43 cases with review of the literature. *J Neurovirol.* 2003;9(Suppl 1):73–80.

Cinque P, Koralnik IJ, Gerevini S, et al. Progressive multifocal leukoencephalopathy in HIV-1 infection. *Lancet Infect Dis.* 2009;9(1):625–636.

Cinque P, Pierotti C, Vigano MG, et al. The good and evil of HAART in HIV-related progressive multifocal leukoencephalopathy. *J Neurovirol.* 2001;7(4):358–363.

Corey L, Holmes KK. Genital herpes simplex virus infections: current concepts in diagnosis, therapy and prevention. *Ann Intern Med.* 1983;98(6):973–983.

Corey L, Wald A, Patel R, et al. Once-daily valacyclovir to reduce the risk of transmission of genital herpes. *N Engl J Med.* 2004;350(1):11–20.

Crossley KM, Agnihotri S, Chaganti J, et al. Recurrence of progressive multifocal leukoencephalopathy despite immune recovery in two HIV seropositive individuals. *J Neurovirol.* 2016;22(4):541–545.

Daley CL, Iaccarino JM, Lang C et al. Treatment of nontuberculous mycobacterial pulmonary disease: an official ATS/ERS/ESCMID/IDSA clinical practice guideline. *Clin Infect Dis.* 2020;71(4):e1–e36.

Dieterich DT, Kim MH, McMeeding A, et al. Cytomegalovirus appendicitis in a patient with acquired immune deficiency syndrome. *Am J Gastroenterol.* 1991;86(7):904–906.

Engstrom RE, Holland GN, Margolis TP, et al. The progressive outer retinal necrosis syndrome. A variant of necrotizing herpetic retinopathy in patients with AIDS. *Ophthalmology.* 1994;101(9):1488–1502.

Fournier A, Martin-Blondel G, Lechapt-Zalcman E, et al. Immune reconstitution inflammatory syndrome unmasking or worsening AIDS-related progressive multifocal leukoencephalopathy: a literature review. *Front Immunol.* 2017;8:577.

Gasnault J, Costagliola D, Hendel-Chavez H, et al. Improved survival of HIV-1-infected patients with progressive multifocal leukoencephalopathy receiving early 5-drug combination antiretroviral therapy. *PLoS One.* 2011;6(6):e20967.

Gebo KA, Kalyani R, Moore RD, et al. The incidence of, risk factors for, and sequelae of herpes zoster among HIV patients in the highly active antiretroviral therapy era. *J Acquir Immune Defic Syndr.* 2005;40(2):169–174.

Geng EH, Kahn JS, Chang OC, et al. The Effect of AIDS Clinical Trials Group Protocol 5164 on the time from *Pneumocystis jirovecii* pneumonia diagnosis to antiretroviral initiation in routine clinical practice: a case study of diffusion, dissemination, and implementation, *Clin Infect Dis,* 2011;53(10):1008–1014.

Gill CM, Dolan L, Piggot LM, et al. New developments in tuberculosis diagnosis and treatment. *Breathe.* 2022;8(1):210149

Griffith DE. Management of disease due to *Mycobacterium kansasii. Clin Chest Med.* 2002;23:613–621.

Harrison RA, Soong S, Weiss HL, et al. A mixed model for factors predictive of pain in AIDS patients with herpes zoster. *J Pain Symptom Manage.* 1999;17(6):410–417.

Havlir DV, Kendall MA, Ive P, et al. Timing of antiretroviral therapy for HIV-1 infection and tuberculosis. *N Engl J Med.* October 20, 2011;365(16):1482–1491. http://www.ncbi.nlm.nih.gov/pubmed/22010914

Jabs DA, Van Natta ML, Holbrook JT, et al. Longitudinal study of the ocular complications of AIDS: ocular diagnoses at enrollment. *Ophthalmology.* 2007;114(4):780–786.

Karim SSA, Naidoo K, Grobler A, et al. Integration of antiretroviral therapy with tuberculosis treatment. *N Engl J Med.* 2011;365(16):1492–1501.

Makadzange AT, Ndhlovu CE, Takarina K, et al. Early versus delayed initiation of antiretroviral therapy for concurrent HIV infection and cryptococcal meningitis in Sub-Saharan Africa. *Clin Infect Dis.* 2010;50(11):1532–1538.

Martin DF, Parks DJ, Mellow SD, et al. Treatment of cytomegalovirus retinitis with an intraocular sustained-release ganciclovir implant. A randomized controlled clinical trial. *Arch Ophthalmol.* 1994;112(12):1531–1539.

Martinson NA, Hoffmann CJ, Chaisson RE. Epidemiology of tuberculosis and HIV. *Proc Am Thorac Soc.* 2011;8:288–293.

McQuillan G, Kruszon-Moran D, Markowitz LE, et al. The prevalence of HPV in adults aged 18–69: United States, 2011–2014. *NCHS Data Brief.* 2017;280:1–8.

Meintjes G, Stek C, Blumenthal L et al. Prednisone for the prevention of paradoxical tuberculosis-associated IRIS. *N Engl J Med* 2018;379:1915–1925.

Mfinanga SG, Kirenga BJ, Chanda DM, et al. Early versus delayed initiation of highly active antiretroviral therapy for HIV-positive adults with newly diagnosed pulmonary tuberculosis (TB-HAART): a prospective, international, randomised, placebo-controlled trial. *Lancet Infect Dis.* 2014; 14:563–571.

Nahid P, Dorman SE, Alipanah N, et al. Official American Thoracic Society/Centers for Disease Control and Prevention/Infectious Diseases Society of America clinical practice guidelines: treatment of drug-susceptible tuberculosis. *Clin Infect Dis*. 2016;63(7):e147–e195. http://doi:10.1093/cid/ciw376.

Pauk J, Huang ML, Brodie SJ, et al. Mucosal shedding of human herpesvirus 8 in men. *N Engl J Med*. 2000;343(19):1369–1377.

Post MJD, Thurnher MM, Clifford DB, et al. CNS-immune reconstitution inflammatory syndrome in the setting of HIV infection, part 2: discussion of neuro-immune reconstitution inflammatory syndrome with and without other pathogens. *AJNR Am J Neuroradiol*. 2013;34(7):1308–1318.

Richardson Jr, EP, Webster HD. Progressive multifocal leukoencephalopathy: its pathological features. *Prog Clin Biol Res*. 1983;105:191–203.

Ryder N, Jin F, McNulty AM et al. Increasing role of herpes simplex virus type 1 in first-episode anogenital herpes in heterosexual women and younger men who have sex with men, 1992–2006. *Sex Transm Infect*. 2009;85(6):416–419.

Safrin S, McKinley G, McKeough M, et al. Treatment of acyclovir-unresponsive cutaneous herpes simplex virus infection with topically applied SP-303. *Antiviral Res*. 1994;25(3–4):185–192.

Santin M, Munoz L, Rigau D. Interferon-γ release assays for the diagnosis of tuberculosis and tuberculosis infection in HIV-infected adults: a systematic review and meta-analysis. *PLoS One*. 2012;7(3):332482.

Sax PE, Sloan CE, Schackman BR, et al. Early antiretroviral therapy for patients with acute aids-related opportunistic infections: a cost-effectiveness analysis of ACTG A5164. *HIV Clin Trials*. 2010;11(5):248–259.

Sungkanuparph S, Filler SG, Chetchotisakd P, et al. Cryptococcal immune reconstitution inflammatory syndrome after antiretroviral therapy in AIDS patients with cryptococcal meningitis: a prospective multicenter study. *Clin Infect Dis*. 2009:49(6):931–934.

Swindells S, Ramchandani R, Gupta A et al. One month of rifapentine plus isoniazid to prevent HIV-related tuberculosis. *N Engl J Med*. 2019;380:1001–1011. http://doi10.1056/NEJMoa1806808

Tan K, Roda R, Ostrow L, et al. PML-IRIS in patients with HIV infection: clinical manifestations and treatment with steroids. *Neurology*. 2009;72(17):1458–1464.

Whitcup SM. Cytomegalovirus retinitis in the era of highly active antiretroviral therapy. *JAMA*. 2000;283(5):653–657.

Workowski KA, Bachmann LH, Chan PA, et al. Sexually transmitted infections treatment guidelines, 2021. *MMWR Recomm Rep*. 2021;20(4):1–187.

World Health Organization (WHO). Global tuberculosis report 2021. https://www.who.int/teams/global-tuberculosis-programme/data. Published 2021. Accessed September 15, 202.

Xu F, Sternberg MR, Kottiri BJ, et al. Trends in herpes simplex virus type 1 and type 2 seroprevalence in the United States. *JAMA*. 2006;296(8):964–973.

Yudin MH, Kaul R. Progressive hypertrophic genital herpes in an HIV-infected woman despite immune recovery on antiretroviral therapy. *Infect Dis Obstet Gynecol*. 2008;2008:592532.

Zolopa A, Andersen J, Powderly W, et al. Early antiretroviral therapy reduces AIDS progress/death in individuals with acute opportunistic infections: a multicenter randomized strategy trial. *PLoS One*. 2009;4(5):e5575.

29.

MALIGNANCIES IN HIV

Eva H. Clark and Elizabeth Y. Chiao

CHAPTER GOALS

- Review the epidemiology and role of antiretroviral therapy (ART) on the impact of AIDS-defining malignancies, which remain common among people with HIV (PWH).

- Discuss the role of human herpes virus-8 (HHV-8) in the development of Kaposi's sarcoma (KS), which remains the most common tumor associated with HIV infection.

- Discuss the role of Epstein–Barr virus (EBV) in primary central nervous system lymphoma (PCNSL) and other HIV-associated lymphomas.

- Review the role of human papillomavirus (HPV) vaccination in virally mediated anogenital squamous cell cancers in both men and women.

- Discuss non-AIDS-defining malignancies, including lung, prostate, oropharyngeal, liver, breast, and pancreatic cancer.

- Emphasize that ART initiation is of utmost importance for all AIDS-defining malignancies and non-AIDS-defining malignancies and summarize National Comprehensive Cancer Center Network (NCCN) guidelines for HIV malignancies.

INTRODUCTION

LEARNING OBJECTIVE

Discuss the role of virally mediated and non-virally mediated AIDS-associated and non-AIDS-associated malignancies.

WHAT'S NEW?

Immunotherapies, including immune check point inhibitors and chimeric antigen receptor (CAR) T-cell therapies are emerging as effective cancer treatments in PWH.

KEY POINTS

- Immunotherapies, including immune check point inhibitors and chimeric antigen receptor (CAR) T-cell therapies are emerging as effective cancer treatments in PWH.

- Malignancies in people with HIV (PWH) remain a major health concern and are among the leading causes of death among PWH.

- ART continues to contribute to decreasing malignancy rates overall.

Malignancies were one of the earliest recognized manifestations of the AIDS epidemic. KS became one of the first entities associated with AIDS (Ziegler et al., 1984). Subsequently, intermediate-grade and high-grade non-Hodgkin's lymphoma (NHL), invasive cervical cancer, and PCNSL were defined by the US Centers for Disease Control and Prevention (CDC) as "AIDS-defining conditions" (CDC, 2008). Since the advent of combination ART, several other cancers that are not AIDS-defining have been found to have an increased incidence in PWH. These include, but are not limited to, Hodgkin's disease and anal, liver, lung, oropharyngeal, colorectal, and renal cancers (Patel et al., 2008). They are generally referred to as "non-AIDS-defining cancers" (NADCs). The increasing longevity of PWH, as well as concurrent modifiable risk factors such as tobacco use, may also influence the epidemiology of these malignancies.

The introduction of combination ART in the mid-1990s significantly improved outcomes of PWH. In addition to changing the course of HIV disease in terms of survival and incidence of opportunistic infections, ART has dramatically decreased the incidence of viral-mediated HIV-associated malignancies, such as KS and PCNSL (Silverberg et al., 2015). Even so, cancer remains a significant concern for PWH. A large US registry linkage study during the post-ART era included 448,258 PWH from 1996 to 2012 and found an elevated risk for development of cancer overall (standardized incidence ratio (SIR) 1.69, 95% confidence interval (CI): 1.67–1.72)), AIDS-defining cancers (KS SIR 498.11, 95% CI: 477.82–519.03, NHL SIR 11.51, 95% CI: 11.14–11.89), and cervical cancer SIR 3.24, 95% CI: 2.94–3.56, most other virus-related cancers (e.g., anal SIR 19.06, 95% CI: 18.13–20.03), liver SIR 3.21, 95% CI: 3.02–3.41), and Hodgkin's lymphoma SIR 7.70, 95% CI: 7.20–8.23), as well as several virus–unrelated cancers (e.g., lung SIR 1.97, 95% CI: 1.89–2.05) (Hernández-Ramírez et al., 2017). However, their SIRs significantly decreased over the study period for KS, two subtypes of NHL, and cancers of the anus, liver, and lung, although they remained elevated above that of the general population. SIRs did not increase over time for any cancer. Additionally, older PWH seem to have a higher risk for most cancer types. When this same dataset was stratified by age, PWH aged older than 50 years were more likely to develop KS (SIR, 103.34), NHL (3.05), Hodgkin lymphoma (7.61), and cervical (2.02), anal (14.00), lung (1.71), liver (2.91), and oral cavity/pharyngeal (1.66) cancers, but were less likely to develop breast (0.61), prostate (0.47), and colon

(0.63) cancers (Mahale et al., 2018) compared to the general population. More recent studies indicate that PWH have an increased risk for not only these initial cancers, but also for developing a second primary cancer (Hessol et al., 2018; Mahale et al., 2020).

Although cancer mortality remains high in PWH, it has declined over time. One US population-based HIV and cancer registry study found cancer-attributed mortality for PWH was 386.9 per 100,000 person-years (including 9.2% of deaths from NADCs and 5.0% of deaths from AIDS-defining cancers) (Horner et al., 2021). In this study, most cancer deaths were due to NHL (3.5%), lung cancer (2.4%), KS (1.3%), liver cancer (1.1%), and anal cancer (0.6%), and cancer mortality was highest among PWH 60 years or older.

Management of malignancies in PWH presents the clinician with many challenges, including the risk of further compromise to the immune system of PWH receiving chemotherapy, toxicities of treatment, pharmacologic interaction between ART and chemotherapy drugs, and the risk of intercurrent opportunistic infections (Mandell et al., 2010; Reid et al., 2018). The safety profile and feasibility of ART administration with concurrent chemotherapy have improved with the introduction and increased use of integrase inhibitors during the past several years. Guidelines for managing cancer in PWH were released in 2018 by the National Comprehensive Cancer Network (NCCN, 2022a; Reid, 2018). They advise that PWH who develop cancer should be cared for by both an oncologist and an HIV specialist and should receive cancer therapy according to standard guidelines developed for the general population. The patient's ART may need to be modified if there are potential interactions with the proposed cancer therapy, but generally ART should be continued during cancer therapy.

This chapter reviews the malignancies most commonly associated with HIV, along with other non-HIV-associated cancers that PWH often develop.

RECOMMENDED READING

Horner MJ, Shiels MS, Pfeiffer RM, et al. Deaths attributable to cancer in the United States HIV population during 2001-2015. *Clin Infect Dis*. 2021;72(9):e224–e231. http://doi:10.1093/cid/ciaa1016

Reid E, Suneja G, Ambinder RF, et al. Cancer in people living with HIV, Version 1.2018, NCCN clinical practice guidelines in oncology. *J Natl Compr Canc Netw*. 2018;16(8):986–1017.

Shiels MS, Islam JY, Rosenberg PS, et al. Projected cancer incidence rates and burden of incident cancer cases in HIV-infected adults in the United States through 2030. *Ann Intern Med*. June 19, 2018;168(12):866–873. http://doi:10.7326/M17-2499. Epub May 8, 2018.

Silverberg MJ, Lau B, Achenbach CJ, et al. Cumulative incidence of cancer among persons with HIV in North America. *Ann Intern Med*. 2015;163(7):507–518.

Silverberg MJ, Leyden W, Hernandez-Ramirez RU, et al. Timing of antiretroviral therapy initiation and risk of cancer among persons living with HIV. *Clin Infect Dis*. 2021;72(11):1900–1909. http://doi:10.1093/cid/ciaa1046. Online ahead of print.

KAPOSI'S SARCOMA

LEARNING OBJECTIVES

- Discuss the epidemiology of KS.
- Discuss the pathogenesis and clinical manifestations.
- Review the treatments for KS, including local and systemic therapies.

WHAT'S NEW?

The incidence of KS continues to decline with the use of ART, but it remains significantly elevated in areas with endemic disease, such as Sub-Saharan Africa. Several novel therapies are emerging for HIV-related KS.

KEY POINTS

- The presence of human herpes virus-8 (HHV-8) and advanced immunosuppression are both associated with risk of KS development and other lymphoproliferative states, such as multicentric Castleman's disease (MCD) and primary effusion lymphoma (PEL).
- Treatment for KS includes ART, local therapy, and systemic therapy.
- The goals of treatment are suppressive and generally noncurative.

Chemotherapy and radiotherapy are palliative treatments for KS. In general, treatment decisions and referrals to oncology should be based on evidence of symptomatic or systemic disease. Radiotherapy should be avoided in the pelvis and lower extremities because of damage to the lymphatics and the potential for lymphedema and skin breakdown.

EPIDEMIOLOGY

KS was first described in 1872 by Moritz Kaposi, a Hungarian dermatologist. Four types of KS have been described: classic, endemic, transplant-associated, and AIDS-associated or epidemic KS. Classic KS is typically seen in elderly men of Mediterranean or Eastern European descent and is characterized by cutaneous lesions of the lower extremities (Iscovich et al., 2000). The endemic form, found primarily in Sub-Saharan Africa, often is more aggressive and morbid, with visceral involvement (Friedman-Kien & Saltzman, 1990). Transplant-associated KS was first described in the 1970s and is seen in immunosuppressed allograft recipients. Although cutaneous disease is the most common presentation, visceral disease has been described in multiple organs (Penn, 1979).

AIDS-associated KS was first described in men who have sex with men (MSM) in the early 1980s, at the advent of the HIV epidemic (Friedman-Kien, 1981). This malignancy disproportionately affected MSM with AIDS, who were estimated to have a 20-fold higher risk of developing KS compared to other HIV transmission risk groups (Beral et al., 1990; Hoover et al., 1993). KS is rarely reported in intravenous drug users or other HIV risk groups (Mitsuyasu et al., 1984; Safai, 1987).

The incidence of KS in high-income countries has declined markedly since the widespread use of ART began in the 1990s. Of 85,922 cases of KS in the United States evaluated by Shiels and colleagues between 1990 and 2007, the proportion of KS in persons with AIDS declined from 89% in 1990 to 1995 to 67% in 2001 to 2007 (*p* < 0.001) (Shiels et al., 2011b). Cumulative incidence of KS by age 75 years was among the highest compared to other cancers (lung, anal, colorectal, Hodgkin's lymphoma, liver, and oropharyngeal) from 1995 to 2009 at 4.1%. However, KS incidence decreased by 4% per year from 2005 to 2009 compared to 1996–1999 rates (*p* < 0.01) (Silverberg et al., 2015). Similarly, the Swiss HIV Cohort Study showed that the KS incidence was 33.3 per 1,000 patient-years (py) in 1984–1986 and did not change significantly in the subsequent periods until 1996–1998, when it declined to 5.1 per 1,000 py (95% CI: 3.9–6.5) and then further decreased to 1.4 per 1,000 py in 1999–2001 (Franceschi et al., 2008). A Brazilian retrospective cohort also described a decreased incidence of KS from 1998 to 2010, with an incidence rate ratio per year of 0.89 (95% CI: 0.83–0.97) (Castilho et al., 2015). In 2010, KS accounted for approximately 12% of cancers diagnosed in PWH (Robbins et al., 2015). Despite the overall decline in KS, there remain concerning differences in improvement in traditionally underserved racial and geographic groups. Between 2001 and 2013, Royse and colleagues evaluated 4,455 KS cases in US men and determined that the annual percent change (APC) for KS incidence significantly decreased for white men between 2001 and 2013 (APC −4.52, *p* = 0.02) (Royse et al., 2017). In contrast, the APC for Black men was not significant (APC −1.84, *p* = 0.09), and the APC among Southern Black men significantly increased (+3.0, *p* = 0.03). More recently, a study using the HIV/AIDS Cancer Registry Match found that the incidence of KS among young Black men with HIV was stable over time from 2008–2016 (Luo et al., 2021). Taken together, these epidemiologic studies suggest that rising KS in the young Black men is likely related to the increasing incidence of advanced HIV disease in this population.

In areas of southern Africa where KS is endemic, this cancer reached epidemic proportions during the initial AIDS epidemic owing to lack of ART. For instance, in Zimbabwe, KS was reported to represent 40% of all cancers in men (Chokunonga et al., 2000). A prospective cohort from 2004 to 2010 found that the incidence in Zimbabwe, Botswana, South Africa, and Zambia reached 413 per 100,000 py (95% CI: 342–497), with higher rates among groups aged older than 60 years (Rohner et al., 2014). Despite the increased availability of ART in these countries, estimates of KS have minimally decreased in the HIV population on ART, with the incidence of KS remaining high at 164 per 100,000 py (95% CI: 151–178) (Rohner et al., 2014). Of note, KS remains the leading cause of cancer incidence and death in men in several Sub-Saharan African countries (Sung et al., 2021).

PATHOGENESIS

In 1994, Chang and Moore (Chang et al., 1994) discovered a new herpesvirus, HHV-8 or KS herpes virus (KSHV), in more than 90% of AIDS-KS tissue samples. Although the KS types vary in epidemiology and clinical presentation, all are associated with HHV-8. In 2003, HHV-8 viremia was shown to be an early marker of KS, and the risk of developing disease was demonstrated to increase with HHV-8 antibody titers (Engels et al., 2003; Newton et al., 2003). HHV-8 also is associated with rare lymphoproliferative diseases most often seen in individuals with HIV, including MCD and a rare form of NHL called PEL. Although infection with KSHV is necessary for the development of KSHV-associated disease, it is not sufficient, and, in fact, HHV-8 viremia is prevalent only in a subset of cases. In an analysis of 335 patients with HIV-associated KS, only 130 (39%) were viremic, and the mean HHV-8 viral load was only 6,630 DNA copies/mL (Haq et al., 2016). Among PWH, immunosuppression confers the greatest risk and is most predictive of development of KS (Jacobson et al., 2000; Renwick et al., 1998).

The pathogenesis of KS is complex and involves viral processes and dysregulation of cytokine pathways. The HHV-8 genome encodes many homologues of human cellular gene products involved in inflammation, cell cycle regulation, and angiogenesis, such as viral cyclin-D1, vascular endothelial growth factor (VEGF), basic fibroblast growth factor, and interleukin-6 (IL-6) (Cannon, 2000). Much work has been done on the tumorigenesis of KS. KSHV infection leads to upregulation of Toll-like receptor 4 (TLR4), its adaptor MyD88, and coreceptors CD14 and MD2 (Gruffaz et al., 2018). The TLR4 pathway seems to be activated constitutively in KSHV-transformed cells, resulting in chronic induction of IL-6, IL-1β, and IL-18. IL-6 production in turn results in activation of the STAT3 pathway, an essential event for uncontrolled cellular proliferation and transformation. Gruffaz and colleagues have shown that TLR4 stimulation with lipopolysaccharides or live bacteria enhanced tumorigenesis while TLR4 antagonist CLI095 inhibited it. A regulatory transactivating (Tat) protein of HIV is released by infected cells and guards KS cells from apoptosis (Deregibus et al., 2002), stimulates growth and angiogenesis (Barillari & Ensoli, 2002; Ensoli et al., 1990), and increases the production and release of matrix metalloproteinases (MMPs) from endothelial and inflammatory cells. MMPs contribute to the angiogenesis found in KS lesions (Impola et al., 2003; Lafrenie et al., 1996), KSHV-mediated systemic inflammation that develops in patients with HHV-8 but without MCD is recognized as KSHV-inflammatory cytokine syndrome (KICS) (Polizzotto et al., 2016a).

The mechanism of HHV-8 transmission remains unclear. HHV-8 has been detected in semen, prostate tissue (Monini et al., 1996), and breast milk (Dedicoat et al., 2004). The virus is often shed from the oropharynx of both immunocompetent and immunocompromised men and women in areas where KSHV is endemic (Casper et al., 2004, 2007). Behaviors associated with exposure to saliva are correlated with a higher risk of KSHV infection, implicating both sexual and horizontal transmission (Casper et al., 2006; Plancoulaine et al., 2000). A relatively high KSHV seroprevalence has been described among injection drug users, and an increased incidence of KSHV infection has been noted among transfusion recipients in areas where KSHV is endemic, suggesting that parenteral transmission may be possible (Cannon et al., 2001; Hladik et al., 2006). Finally, transmission of KSHV from donors of solid organs has been described (Barozzi et al., 2003; Luppi et al., 2000).

CLINICAL MANIFESTATIONS

KS is an angioproliferative disease varying from an indolent to fulminant disease with potential for significant morbidity and mortality. The disease can occur in individuals with a wide range of CD4 $^+$ T- cell counts but becomes increasingly common as immune function declines. The progression of disease may be rapid or slow. PWH with limited disease and controlled HIV infection usually do reasonably well. However, in the setting of uncontrolled HIV viral replication and low CD4 $^+$ T-cell counts, KS progresses rapidly.

The skin is the most common site of presentation. Visceral involvement occurs less commonly, though as the disease progresses, KS frequently involves the gastrointestinal (GI) tract (see below). At autopsy, almost every organ system can show involvement. Visceral disease is rare in the absence of extensive cutaneous disease.

The cutaneous presentation of KS occurs in 95% of cases. Lesions may occur anywhere on the skin. Common sites include the face (particularly the periorbital area and tip of the nose), external ear, mouth, torso, and lower extremities. They can evolve from macules or nodular tumors to large plaque-like tumor masses that involve extensive cutaneous surfaces and eventually evolve into ulcerating tumors. Their color may vary from violaceous in light-skinned individuals to brownish-black in dark-skinned individuals. These lesions are generally nonblanching, and nonpruritic. Lesions of KS may be associated with some pain, particularly in the setting of immune reconstitution inflammatory syndrome (IRIS).

Lymphedema associated with KS usually appears in patients with visible cutaneous lesions, and edema may be out of proportion to the extent of visible lesions. Lymphedema also may occur in patients with no visible skin lesions. Common sites include the face, neck, external genitals, and lower extremities. A contiguous area of skin usually is involved as well.

Oral cavity involvement is seen in approximately one-third of people with KS and is the initial site of diagnosis 15% of the time (Dezube et al., 2004). These lesions may be flat or nodular and are red or purplish. They usually appear on the hard palate, but they may develop on the soft palate, gingival areas, and tongue. Oral lesions, if extensive, may cause tooth loss, pain, and ulceration. Involvement of the oral cavity correlates with KS in the GI tract.

Gastrointestinal (GI) KS has been reported in 40% of cases at initial diagnosis (Dezube et al., 2004) with any segment of the GI tract involved. Visceral spread of KS that involves the GI tract is rarely symptomatic. However, with disease progression, patients may have symptoms of abdominal pain, nausea, vomiting, or GI bleeding (Danzig et al., 1991). Rare cases of obstruction, perforation, or protein-losing enteropathy have been reported (Friedman, 1988). In those with advanced immunosuppression (CD4 $^+$ T-cell count < 100 cells/mm^3), GI KS may be more severe with complications. Some believe that screening endoscopy to detect occult disease may be warranted in these patients (Nagata et al., 2012).

Pulmonary KS also occurs; however, in contrast to KS at other visceral sites, lung involvement is generally symptomatic. Common symptoms include cough, bronchospasm, dyspnea, and hemoptysis. This complication tends to occur in the setting of advanced AIDS, with most individuals having CD4 $^+$ T-cell counts of less than 100 cells/mm^3 (Gill et al., 1989) and in patients with more extensive cutaneous disease (e.g., with >50 lesions). Of note, it can occur in patients with minimal and absent cutaneous KS. The disease is often rapidly progressive when it involves the lungs, with a median survival time of only 2–6 months in the pre-ART era (Kaplan et al., 1988). Respiratory failure is often the cause of death. The radiographic appearance is variable, with the characteristic reticulonodular pattern seen in approximately one-third of patients (Kaplan et al., 1988). Otherwise, diffuse interstitial infiltrates, pleural effusions, and hilar adenopathy may be seen (Levine & Tulpule, 2001).

Once KS is clinically suspected, diagnosis is made by biopsy and histologic examination or by presumptive diagnosis based on the endoscopic appearance of a visceral lesion (Aboulafia, 2001). A histologic confirmation is essential to exclude other conditions that can mimic KS. Endoscopically, the classic appearance of small submucosal vascular nodules establishes the diagnosis of GI KS. It may be difficult to establish a diagnosis of GI KS by biopsy because many of the lesions are submucosal (Hengge et al., 2002). In patients with suspected pulmonary KS, violaceous endobronchial lesions typically are observed on bronchoscopic examination. A presumptive diagnosis of pulmonary KS can be made based on characteristic radiographic and endobronchial findings in patients who have had KS at other sites (Kaplan et al., 1988). Endobronchial biopsy is discouraged because of the risk of hemorrhage. Gallium scanning may be helpful in differentiating KS from pulmonary infection because KS is not gallium-avid (Kaplan et al., 1988).

In the pre-ART era, the AIDS Clinical Trials Group (ACTG) developed a staging system based on tumor extent (T), severity of immunosuppression (I), and the presence of systemic illness (S) (Krown et al., 1997). Two different risk categories were noted based on this staging system: a good risk, defined as T0I0S0; and a poor risk, defined as T1I1S1 (Table 29.1).

Based on epidemiological, clinical, staging, and survival data of patients in two Italian prospective cohort studies (n = 211), Nasti and colleagues concluded that, in the ART era, a refinement of the ACTG staging system is needed (Nasti et al., 2003b). CD4 $^+$ T-cell counts in this study did not provide prognostic information, and only the combination of T1S1 identified patients with unfavorable prognosis. The 3-year survival rate for patients with T1S1 was 53%,

Table 29.1 AIDS CLINICAL TRIALS GROUP (ACTG) TUMOR STAGING SYSTEM

CHARACTERISTIC	GOOD RISK (0)	POOR RISK (1)
	All of the following:	Any of the following:
Tumor (T)	Tumor confined to skin and/or lymph nodes and/or minimal oral disease[a]	Tumor-associated edema or ulceration; extensive oral KS; GI KS; other visceral KS
Immune system (I)	CD4 count ≥150 cells/mm^3	CD4$^+$ T-cell count <150 cells/mm^3
Systemic illness (S)	No history of OI or thrush; no systemic symptoms; Karnofsky performance status ≥70	History of OI and/or thrush; systemic symptoms; Karnofsky performance status < 70; other HIV-related illnesses

[a]Nonnodular KS confined to the palate.

GI, gastrointestinal; KS, Kaposi's sarcoma; OI, opportunistic infection.

Adapted from Krown (1989) and incorporating revision by Krown (1997), with permission from the American Society of Clinical Oncology.

which was significantly lower compared to the 3-year survival rates of patients with T0S0, T1S0, and T0S1, which were 88%, 80%, and 81%, respectively. Several studies have found other prognostic markers for KS. Another study developed a prognostic index predicting poor survival, including not having KS as the AIDS-defining illness, decreasing CD4$^+$ T-cell count, being aged 50 years or older, and having another AIDS-associated illness at the same time (Stebbing et al., 2006). Other variables, including CD8$^+$ T-cell count (Stebbing et al., 2007) and detectable HHV-8 DNA in plasma at the time of diagnosis (El Amari et al., 2008) have also been associated with poor KS prognosis.

TREATMENT

Impact of Antiretroviral Therapy

ART is a key component in the treatment of KS and should be initiated or optimized to achieve complete HIV RNA suppression in all patients with AIDS-associated KS. The inhibition of HIV replication, decreased production of the Tat protein, restored immunity to HHV-8, and the direct antiangiogenic activity of some protease inhibitors (PIs) are among the many benefits of ART (Dubrow et al., 2017; Noy, 2003). Some older data suggested that PIs have an anti-KS effect (Sgadari et al., 2003); however, non-PI-containing ART regimens also lead to KS regression.

Combination ART has been associated with a lengthening of time to treatment failure with either local or systemic therapy for KS. A retrospective study found a median time of 20.4 months from the initiation of ART plus chemotherapy versus 6 months with just chemotherapy to detect treatment failure among PWH with KS (Bower et al., 1999). PWH who were receiving ART at KS diagnosis have a less aggressive presentation versus individuals who were ART-naive at the time of KS diagnosis (Nasti et al., 2003a). Another retrospective analysis from 1990 to 1999 found an 81% reduction in the risk of death among PWH with KS after the initiation of ART (Tam et al., 2002).

KS-associated IRIS has been well described. Some patients may experience painful enlarged lesions or progression of KS lesions during the first months of ART. In a prospective study of 69 patients with HIV and KSHV coinfection, approximately 12% of patients experienced IRIS-KS after initiation of ART (Letang et al., 2010).

Local Treatment

Local treatment should be reserved for patients with minimal or locally symptomatic disease. These patients should concurrently receive ART. Current options for local treatment include the following:

- Radiotherapy has been the mainstay of local therapy for KS. It is best suited for patients with a single or a few locally symptomatic areas or for symptomatic disease that requires rapid tumor reduction. Electron beam radiation applied to the entire face is highly effective in relief of facial edema. Radiotherapy also can be useful for treatment of dysphagia caused by pharyngeal lesions and tumor masses of the eye or the extremities (Hill, 1987). Radiotherapy, whether given as whole-body electron beam therapy, fractionated focal radiation therapy, or single treatments, has produced complete remissions in 50%–80% of patients (Cooper & Steinfeld, 1991; Pluda et al., 1992). Complications such as severe mucositis, radiotherapy fibrosis, loss of skin compliance, and chronic lymphedema may occur with these treatments. Radiotherapy is not recommended for the lower extremities because of potential skin changes and the high risk for cellulitis.

- With intralesional chemotherapy, vinblastine has been most commonly used, with a reported response rate of 70% in older studies (Boudreaux et al., 1993). Small cutaneous lesions can be treated with intralesional chemotherapy for cosmetic purposes. Repeated treatments may be necessary. Intralesional chemotherapy can cause significant pain and areas of hyperpigmentation after treatment.

- Alitretinoin gel (Panretin) is a topical treatment that may be used for relatively asymptomatic patients with KS lesions that do not respond to ART alone and for whom the KS is predominantly an issue of cosmesis. A response rate of 49% (*n* = 184) in a phase 3 study was reported

(Walmsley et al., 1999). Adverse effects include dry skin and light hypersensitivity.

- Cryotherapy with liquid nitrogen and laser therapy have been used successfully for the treatment of isolated small KS lesions. Given the significant mucosal toxicity associated with radiotherapy in the treatment of oral lesions, laser surgery may be substituted for radiation.

- There are several new therapies being explored for treatment of local KS, including a phase 1 trial of intralesional nivolumab, which is an immune checkpoint inhibitor (NCT03316274) (Bender-Ignacio et al., 2018).

Systemic Treatment

Treatment of KS is generally not considered curative and was not shown to have a significant impact on survival in the pre-ART era. An older retrospective review of 194 cases of KS (Volberding et al., 1989) showed no significant difference in survival time between patients treated with chemotherapy or interferon-α (IFN-α) and untreated patients. A South African randomized trial of ART alone versus ART plus chemotherapy demonstrated a significant difference in KS response but no difference in survival between the two arms (Mosam et al., 2012). Although starting ART is strongly recommended for all PWH with KS, adjunct therapies for patients with mild-to-moderate disease have not been well studied. One recent multicenter trial evaluated the use of oral etoposide (given "as needed" vs. immediately (as eight cycles of therapy)) and found that only about 30% of patients in both groups responded to therapy overall (Hosseinipour et al., 2018). Immediate treatment with oral etoposide resulted in early clinical benefits that were no longer observed 48 weeks post therapy. A post-hoc analysis of that study evaluated the effect of oral etoposide on the development of KS-IRIS and early progressive disease (KS-PD) after starting ART and found that etoposide decreased the development of KS-IRIS and KS-PD after ART initiation.

Systemic intravenous chemotherapy is used for disease that is more severe, including symptomatic visceral disease, extensive skin involvement, significant edema, or rapidly progressive KS. As described previously, the goal of systemic chemotherapy is mainly palliation of symptoms. Large, randomized studies have established liposomal anthracyclines (doxorubicin and daunorubicin) as first-line single-agent chemotherapy agents with promising results compared to combination chemotherapy treatment (Gill et al., 1996; Northfelt et al., 1998; Stewart et al., 1998). These studies found that liposomal anthracyclines alone can achieve response rates equal to or better than those of combination chemotherapy with a lower incidence of toxicity such as nausea, fatigue, alopecia, and neuropathy. Neutropenia, however, occurred as frequently with the liposomal agent as with the standard combination regimen. Prognosis is good; in one study of 140 patients with T1 disease who were treated with ART and liposomal anthracycline chemotherapy, the 5-year overall survival was 85% (Bower et al., 2014).

Paclitaxel is a highly active agent that is often used as second-line therapy. It has significant antitumor activity in patients with previously untreated (Gill et al., 1995) and refractory KS (Saville et al., 1995). Because liposomal doxorubicin is not available in many low-middle income countries (LMICs), other regimens including bleomycin and vincristine have been utilized for KS treatment. A three-arm randomized clinical trial conducted by the ACTG/AIDS Malignancy Consortium (AMC) in 11 sites in Brazil, Kenya, Malawi, South Africa, Uganda, and Zimbabwe compared oral etoposide plus ART and bleomycin plus vincristine plus ART to paclitaxel plus ART. The study was stopped early because the paclitaxel arm demonstrated superior progression-free survival at week 48 compared to the other two arms (Krown et al., 2020). The most significant side effects of paclitaxel are hypersensitivity, myelosuppression, peripheral neuropathy, alopecia, and drug interactions with ART. This agent is the treatment of choice for refractory KS or if there are contraindications to the use of anthracyclines. Regarding comparison of liposomal anthracyclines versus taxanes, a small, randomized trial of paclitaxel compared to liposomal doxorubicin and showed that both therapies improved symptoms such as pain and swelling in PWH with advanced KS (Cianfrocca et al., 2010). Additionally, they demonstrated comparable response rates, progression-free survival, and median survival between the two arms, though a slightly higher rate of grade 3 to 5 toxicity occurred in the paclitaxel arm (Cianfrocca et al., 2010). A 2014 Cochrane review indicated no observed difference between liposomal doxorubicin, liposomal daunorubicin, and paclitaxel for patients on ART (Gbabe et al., 2014).

In the United States, because a long-term cure of KS is difficult to measure given that hyperpigmented inactive lesions often persist, the primary goals of treatment for patients with KS are palliation of symptoms and improved cosmesis. Consultation with a KS-experienced oncologist or dermatologist should be considered for most patients diagnosed with this malignancy.

Several newer therapies are currently being studied for severe KS. Inhibition of the KS-activated mammalian target of rapamycin (mTOR) signaling pathway has been examined in an AMC study and has shown promising therapeutic results (Krown et al., 2012). Imatinib, a platelet-derived growth factor receptor/c-kit inhibitor, induced responses in 10 of 30 patients with KS when given up to 1 year in a multicenter phase 2 trial (Koon et al., 2014). The VEGF-A inhibitor, bevacizumab, was shown in another phase 2 trial to produce complete and partial responses in 3 and 2 of 16 patients, respectively (Uldrick et al., 2012). Two immunomodulatory agents with antiangiogenic effects, pomalidomide (oral) and lenalidomide (intravenous) have been evaluated in clinical trials. Pomalidomide was found to be well tolerated and active in KS regardless of HIV status (NCT02659930) (Polizzotto et al., 2016b; Ramaswami et al., 2022). Lenalidomide was well tolerated in ART-experienced patients with progressive KS previously treated with chemotherapy, but its phase 2 trial was halted due to lack of responses in this study population (Pourcher et al., 2017). Several other targeted therapies for KS are under evaluation in clinical trials (Bender-Ignacio et al., 2018).

RECOMMENDED READING

Cianfrocca M, Lee S, Von Roenn J, et al. Randomized trial of paclitaxel vs. pegylated liposomal doxorubicin for advanced human immunodeficiency virus-associated Kaposi sarcoma: evidence of symptom palliation from chemotherapy. *Cancer*. 2010;116(16):3969–3677.

Hosseinipour MC, Kang M, Krown SE, Bukuru A, et al. As-needed vs immediate etoposide chemotherapy in combination with antiretroviral therapy for mild-to-moderate AIDS-associated Kaposi sarcoma in resource-limited settings: A5264/AMC-067 randomized clinical trial. *Clin Infect Dis*. 2018;67(2):251–260.

Krown SE, Moser CB, MacPhail P, et al. Treatment of advanced AIDS-associated Kaposi sarcoma in resource-limited settings: a three-arm, open-label, randomised, non-inferiority trial. *Lancet*. 2020;395(10231):1195–1207. http://doi:10.1016/S0140-6736(19)33222-2

Luo Q, Johnson AS, Hall HI, et al. Kaposi sarcoma rates among persons living with human immunodeficiency virus in the United States: 2008–2016. *Clin Infect Dis*. 2021;73(7):e2226–e2233.

Ramaswami R, Polizzotto MN, Lurain K, et al. Safety, activity, and long-term outcomes of pomalidomide in the treatment of Kaposi sarcoma among individuals with or without HIV infection. *Clin Cancer Res*. 2022;28(5):840–850.

Reid E, Suneja G, Ambinder RF, et al. Cancer in people living with HIV, Version 1.2018, NCCN clinical practice guidelines in oncology. *J Natl Compr Canc Netw*. 2018;16(8):986–1017.

Shiels MS, Pfeiffer RM, Hall HI, et al. Proportions of Kaposi sarcoma, selected non-Hodgkin lymphomas, and cervical cancer in the United States occurring in persons with AIDS, 1980–2007. *JAMA*. 2011;305(14):1450–1459.

HIV-RELATED PRIMARY CENTRAL NERVOUS SYSTEM LYMPHOMA

LEARNING OBJECTIVES

- Review the epidemiology of PCNSL in PWH.

- Review the pathophysiology and clinical presentation of PCNSL in PWH.

- Review chemotherapeutic strategies for treatment PCNSL in PWH.

- Discuss survival among PWH with PCNSL.

WHAT'S NEW?

Fluorodeoxyglucose–positron emission tomography (FDG-PET) and magnetic resonance spectroscopy provide less-invasive strategies to characterize the invasiveness of disease and distinguish it from other pathologies.

KEY POINTS

- Epstein–Barr virus (EBV)-mediated oncogenesis in the setting of advanced immunosuppression is largely responsible for PCNSL.

- Treatment with ART should be initiated and maintained for all PWH with PCNSL.

- Despite improved survival in the ART era, overall survival remains poor.

Primary CNS lymphoma is a rare type of NHL, accounting for 1%–2% of all NHLs and less than 5% of all primary brain tumors (Lister et al., 2002). PCNSL has been diagnosed in 1.6%–9.0% of people with AIDS and represents the second most common intracranial mass lesion in this population (Rosenblum et al., 1988; Welch et al., 1984). The vast majority of PCNSL has been linked to EBV-infected B cells that reach the CNS during advanced immunodeficiency (Cingolani et al., 2005). MacMahon and colleagues (1991) noted that EBV genes important for oncogenesis are abundant in patients with PCNSL, suggesting a pathogenic role of EBV in this setting. This association suggests that the pathogenesis of PCNSL might differ from systemic NHL, which has a 40%–50% association with EBV (Ballerini et al., 1993; Hamilton-Dutoit et al., 1989).

EPIDEMIOLOGY

In the era before effective ART, the relative risk of PCNSL was approximately 1,000-fold and as high as 3,600-fold in people with AIDS compared to the general population (Cote et al., 1996).

The age-adjusted incidence of PCNSL in the United States had increased substantially since the 1970s, from 0.16 per 100,000 py in 1973–1984 to 0.48 per 100,000 py in 1985–1997 (Olson et al., 2002). However, with the introduction of ART in the mid to late 1990s, the incidence of PCNSL in PWH significantly decreased (Hoffman et al., 2001; Wolf et al., 2005). In the Multicenter AIDS Cohort Study (MACS), the incidence rate in 2,734 men with HIV declined from 4.3 to 0.4 per 100,000 py (Sacktor et al., 2001). In another study, PCNSL accounted for only 1% of lymphoma diagnoses in PWH in the period 2006–2015 (Gopal et al., 2013). Despite this dramatic decrease in incidence, survival rates have not significantly improved, especially compared to those of people without HIV (Bayraktar et al., 2011; Conti et al., 2000).

CLINICAL PRESENTATION

The clinical presentation of PCNL is similar irrespective of HIV status. Symptoms may include headaches, confusion, lethargy, memory loss, personality changes, and seizures. On examination, patients may present with hemiparesis, aphasia, and cranial nerve palsies. Lesions are most common in the cerebrum, basal ganglia, and brainstem. More diffuse and multifocal involvement is seen in HIV-related PCNSL (Gage et al., 2000). These lesions are contrast-enhancing on computed tomography (CT) and MRI. Before ART, the median $CD4^+$ T-cell count at presentation was less than 50 cells/mm^3 (Levine et al., 1991).

Polymerase chain reaction (PCR) to detect EBV DNA in the cerebrospinal fluid is useful for diagnosing

AIDS-associated PCNSL. Identification of EBV by PCR can detect most cases of AIDS-related PCNSL with a sensitivity of 80%––100% and specificity for lymphoma of 93%––100% (Bossolasco et al., 2002). Cerebrospinal fluid cytology alone has limited utility because of poor sensitivity and specificity (Ekstein et al., 2006).

Single-photon emission CT has been suggested as a less-invasive technique for diagnosis. However, because of conflicting results in terms of sensitivity and specificity, its role in the diagnosis of PCNSL remains limited (Licho et al., 2002; Ruiz et al., 1994). FDG-PET and magnetic resonance spectroscopy are two other imaging modalities that can aid in the diagnosis of cerebral PCNSL lesions apart from other infectious CNS pathologies such as toxoplasmosis. Magnetic resonance spectroscopy typically shows decreased N-acetylaspartate and increased choline, which reflects neoplastic cell proliferation (Westwood et al., 2013). FDG-PET can also help identify extracerebral systemic disease involvement (Lewitschnig et al., 2013). Currently, the gold standard for diagnosis of PCNSL is stereotactic brain biopsy. In patients in whom a brain biopsy is unobtainable, the combination of imaging, negative toxoplasma serology, previous toxoplasmosis prophylaxis, and positive EBV cerebrospinal fluid by PCR may be sufficient to make a presumptive diagnosis.

TREATMENT AND SURVIVAL

The relative rarity of PCNSL precludes large-scale randomized trials; therefore, the optimal treatment for PCNSL has not been determined. Norden et al. showed that HIV positivity significantly reduced median overall survival to 2 months versus 12 months in patients without HIV (Norden et al., 2011). Despite good initial response rates to treatment, median survival times with treatment remain only 2–5.5 months (Baumgartner et al., 1990). The previous standard treatment of patients with AIDS-related PCNSL was palliative corticosteroids and whole-brain radiation that achieved a complete response in 20%–50% of patients (Cote et al., 1996). Radiation alone can improve symptoms and extend median survival, but this is likely affected by a patient's baseline functional status and not the dose of radiation received (Goldstein et al., 1991).

Regarding chemotherapy for AIDS-related PCNSL, an uncontrolled pilot study published in 1997 used high-dose intravenous methotrexate in 15 patients, including 10 with histologically confirmed PCNSL. The median time since clinical onset was 27 days (range 7–69 days), and the mean CD4$^+$ T-cell count was 30 cells/mm^3. Complete responses, defined as clinical improvement and disappearance of contrast-enhancing brain abnormalities on CT or MRI, were obtained in 7 of 15 patients (3 of 10 patients with histological diagnosis and 4 of 5 patients without histological confirmation). One patient relapsed at 6 months. Six patients failed to respond, and two2 patients died of severe sepsis. The median survival time was 290 days for the 10 patients with histological diagnosis and 347 days for the 5 patients without histological confirmation. Corticosteroids were also administered, and individuals ultimately received ART including a PI (Jacomet et al., 1997). In a retrospective study, 20 PWH were treated with methotrexate-based regimens (Gupta et al., 2017). Some of these patients were treated with high-dose methotrexate alone, some with high-dose methotrexate and rituximab, and some with regimens that included a variety of other agents. The median survival in patients treated before ART and without high-dose methotrexate was 2 months, whereas with ART and high-dose methotrexate-based regimens the median survival had not yet been reached with a median follow-up of 27 months. In people without HIV and PCNSL, high-dose intravenous methotrexate remains the standard of care for those who can tolerate the therapy, and available evidence supports this strategy combined with ART in PWH. In 2016, the IELSG32 trial provided a high level of evidence supporting the use of matrix combination (methotrexate, cytarabine, and rituximab with or without thiotepa) as the new standard chemoimmunotherapy for patients aged up to 70 years old with newly diagnosed PCNSL (Ferreri et al., 2016). A phase 2 trial is under way evaluating induction with rituximab, high-dose methotrexate, and leucovorin every 2 weeks for 6 cycles, followed by consolidation with high-dose methotrexate alone (NCT00267865). Whole-brain radiation is traditionally reserved for those with poor performance status (NCCN PSCNL version 2.2022b); however, in the second randomization of the IELSG32 trial, both whole-brain radiotherapy and autologous stem cell transplantation were found to be feasible and effective as consolidation therapies after high-dose methotrexate-based chemoimmunotherapy (Ferreri et al., 2017). Finally, a small prospective series conducted by Lurain and colleagues at the National Cancer Institute demonstrated that 8 of the 12 PWH and PCNSL who received ART, rituximab, and high-dose methotrexate (R-HD-MTX) had sustained complete response (67%), including 3 participants who received second-line therapy without relapse at 2 years. The estimated 60-month overall survival was 67% (95% CI: 32–86), and, with median potential follow-up of 82 months, the median overall survival was not reached. They concluded that that treatment with ART and R-HD-MTX is associated with a high response rate, CD4$^+$ T-lymphocyte reconstitution, and long-term survival with preservation or improvement of neurocognitive function. In addition, the treatment regimen was tolerable, even for those with advanced HIV, significant comorbidities, and CNS infections (Lurain et al., 2020).

ROLE OF ANTIRETROVIRAL THERAPY

Combination ART should be initiated in all individuals with AIDS-related PCNSL who are undertaking treatment because it is associated with significant improvement in survival. In the pre-ART era, radiotherapy prolonged survival for 2–5.5 months compared to palliative care (Donahue et al., 1995). McGowan and Shaw (1998) were the first to describe a case of remission maintained for more than 2 years after treatment with ART alone in an individual who had PCNSL. Other case reports have also reported similar PCNSL response to ART (Aboulafia & Puswella, 2007; Corales et al., 2000; Travi et al., 2012). In a retrospective analysis, Hoffman and colleagues (2001) showed that survival times of patients receiving ART in addition to radiotherapy differed significantly from those of patients receiving radiotherapy or palliative care alone. Four of the six patients receiving ART survived for more than 1.5 years. In another retrospective analysis, Skiest and Crosby (2003) demonstrated a prolonged median survival of 667 days in individuals who received ART. These findings strongly suggest that immune recovery contributes to longer remission in PWH and PCNSL.

RECOMMENDED READING

Cingolani A, Fratino L, Scoppettuolo G, et al. Changing pattern of primary cerebral lymphoma in the highly active antiretroviral therapy era. *J Neurovirol*. 2005;11(Suppl 3):38–44.

Ferreri AJM, Cwynarski K, Pulczynski E, et al. Whole-brain radiotherapy or autologous stem-cell transplantation as consolidation strategies after high-dose methotrexate-based chemoimmunotherapy in patients with primary CNS lymphoma: results of the second randomisation of the International Extranodal Lymphoma Study Group-32 phase 2 trial. *Lancet Haematol*. November 2017;4(11):e510–e523.

Gupta NK, Nolan A, Omuro A, et al. Long-term survival in AIDS-related primary central nervous system lymphoma. *Neuro Oncol*. 2017;19:99–108

Westwood TD, Hogan C, Julyan PJ, et al. Utility of FDG-PETCT and magnetic resonance spectroscopy in differentiating between cerebral lymphoma and non-malignant CNS lesions in HIV-infected patients. *Eur J Radiol*. 2013;82(8):e374–e379.

SYSTEMIC NON-HODGKIN'S LYMPHOMA

LEARNING OBJECTIVES

- Review the epidemiology of NHL.

- Review the pathophysiology and clinical manifestations of NHL.

- Review the treatment of NHL and survival outcomes.

WHAT'S NEW?

- Survival for PWH and NHL continues to improve in the ART era; however, incidence remains significantly higher compared to that of people without HIV.

- Intensive chemotherapy and autologous hematopoietic cell transplantation (HCT) are safe in PWH and are associated with improved outcomes.

- CAR T-cell therapy is emerging as a safe and effective therapy for PWH and chemotherapy refractory NHL.

KEY POINTS

- NHL development is likely a multifactorial interplay among host immune factors as well as the presence of viral mediators including EBV and HHV-8. Disease can occur in a variety of nodal and extranodal sites, and some forms of NHL are more aggressive than others, such as PEL.

- Prognostic factors include host immunity, the presence of injection drug use, performance status, and the degree of tumor burden.

- Treatment with ART and intensive chemotherapy with consideration of HCT are cornerstones of NHL treatment.

The first cases of AIDS-related NHL were described in 1982 (Ziegler et al., 1982). In 1985, NHL was added to the list of AIDS-defining malignancies. Before the ART era, it was estimated to occur in approximately 8% of all HIV cases (Kaplan et al., 1989), and it is currently the second most common neoplasm occurring among PWH (Knowles, 2001).

The World Health Organization has divided AIDS-related lymphomas (ARLs) into three categories (Box 29.1):

1. Lymphomas also occurring in immunocompetent patients, such as Burkitt's lymphoma (BL) and diffuse large B-cell lymphoma (DLBCL).)

2. Lymphomas occurring specifically in PWH, such as PEL and plasmablastic lymphoma.

3. Lymphomas also occurring in other immunodeficiency states, such as polymorphic or posttransplant lymphoproliferative disorder-like B-cell lymphoma.

DLBCL and BL are the most common ARLs, representing approximately 90% of these malignancies (Besson et al., 2001). Only intermediate-grade or high-grade lymphomas are considered AIDS-defining.

EPIDEMIOLOGY

There are more than 30 types of NHLs, including DLBCL and BL. Individuals with impaired cell-mediated immunity

---

BOX 29.1 AIDS-RELATED LYMPHOMAS: WORLD HEALTH ORGANIZATION CLASSIFICATION

Lymphomas also occurring in immunocompetent people with HIV
Burkitt's lymphoma
Diffuse large B-cell lymphoma: centroblastic, immunoblastic, and anaplastic variants

Lymphomas occurring specifically in PWH
Primary effusion lymphoma
Plasmablastic lymphoma

Lymphomas also occurring in other immunodeficiency states
Polymorphic or posttransplant lymphoproliferative disorder-like B-cell lymphoma

SOURCE: Adapted from Raphael M, Said J, Dorisch B et al. Lymphomas associated with HIV infection. In: Swerdlow SH, Campo E, Harris NL et al., eds. *World Health Organization classification of tumours of haematopoietic and lymphoid tissue*. 4th ed. Lyon, France: IARC Press; 2008:

show a marked increase in the incidence of NHL. This has been best described in immunosuppressed allograft recipients. Similar trends were seen in PWH in the pre-ART era. The CDC examined data of 2,824 NHL cases occurring in 97,258 PLWH between 1981 and 1989 in the United States. The risk was 60 times greater in PWH (Beral et al., 1991). The risk also varies by histologic subtype, with up to 600-fold excess risk for immunoblastic lymphoma (IBL) (Cote et al., 1997). In a recent study evaluating the cumulative incidence of NHL in PWH living in the United States and Canada (n = 86,620), the incidence of NHL from 1996 to 2009 was 4.5% by age 75 years compared to only 0.7% in persons without HIV (n = 196,987) (Silverberg et al., 2015). Gopal and colleagues evaluated data from the US Centers for AIDS Research network including 23,050 PWH diagnosed between 1996 and 2011 and found that lymphomas developed in 2.1% of these patients (Gopal et al., 2013). Most of these were DLBCL (42.2%), followed by Hodgkin lymphoma (16.6%), Burkitt lymphoma (11.8%), PCNSL (11.3%), and other NHLs (18.1%).

PATHOGENESIS

The pathogenesis of HIV-related NHL is most likely multifactorial, involving HIV, immune dysfunction, cytokine dysregulation, and other viral antigens, including EBV and HHV-8 (Gates et al., 2003). EBV is present in approximately 40%–50% of cases of AIDS-related systemic NHL (Hamilton-Dutoit et al., 1989). This contrasts with a report by Ballerini and colleagues (1993), who reported 100% EBV coinfection in the immunoblastic lymphoma variant of DLBCL. The expression of the latent EBV transforming proteins EBNA-2 and LMP-1 is known to play a central role in the initiation and maintenance of EBV-induced B-cell growth and proliferation (Liebowitz & Kieff, 1989). Both EBNA-2 and LMP-1 can serve as targets for cytotoxic T- cells; thus, their expression induces T-cell immune surveillance and regulates lymphomagenesis in individuals who are immunocompetent. With immunodeficiency states such as late-stage HIV, EBNA-2 and LMP-1 expression may become unregulated and subsequently lead to uncontrolled proliferation of EBV-infected cells (Gaidano & Dalla-Favera, 1995). Genetic alterations involving oncogenes and tumor suppressor genes may also occur, and often *MYC* and *BCL6* translocations are implicated in neoplastic development (Chadburn et al., 2013).

Expression of HHV-8 also is associated with PEL, which presents as malignant pleural, peritoneal, or pericardial effusions with a paucity of nodal masses. It is aggressive and often refractory to chemotherapy. HHV-8 has been universally found in malignant cells, often in conjunction with EBV (Komanduri et al., 1996). Neoplastic cells have an immunoblastic to plasmablastic appearance. Most PELs have lymphocyte activation markers (CD30 and CD38) without normal B-cell markers (CD19 and CD20).

CLINICAL CHARACTERISTICS

Approximately two-thirds of ARLs are classified as DLBCL (Navarro & Kaplan, 2006). AIDS-related systemic NHL usually presented as widespread disease involving extranodal sites in the pre-ART era (Knowles et al., 1988). The most common sites of extranodal disease are the gastrointestinal tract, CNS, bone marrow, and liver. It has been reported that 95% of patients from several institutions had evidence of extranodal disease, including 42% with CNS involvement and 33% with bone marrow involvement (Ziegler et al., 1984). In a multicenter retrospective review of pooled data from 886 PWH with DLBCL, CNS involvement was found in 13% of patients and was not associated with reduced overall survival (Barta et al., 2016). However, CNS relapse was associated with a median overall survival of only 1.6 months. GI NHL occurs in approximately 30% of PWH with NHL. Most of these cases involve the stomach, but virtually any site in the GI tract or hepatobiliary tree can be involved (Burkes et al., 1986). Interestingly, most cases of plasmablastic lymphomas are associated with characteristic development of oral cavity lesions and predominate in mucosal sites (Chadburn et al., 2013). In the ART era, among patients with undetectable plasma HIV RNA levels, Gerard and colleagues found that NHL occurred at a median CD4$^+$ T-cell count of 297 cells/mm^3. In addition, they found that 65% of the cases occurred within 18 months of initiating HIV treatment with ART (Gerard et al., 2009). Other studies have shown that PEL and immunoblastic NHL are seen in patients with lower CD4$^+$ T-cell counts, of older age, and with a prior diagnosis of AIDS, whereas Burkitt NHL tends to occur in patients with more preserved immune function (Knowles, 1996). In a more recent study of 23,050 PWH diagnosed between 1996 and 2011, Gopal and colleagues found that patients with Hodgkin lymphoma and Burkitt NHL had the highest CD4$^+$ T-cell counts, while patients with PCNSL had the lowest (Gopal et al., 2013). In 2010, NHL accounted for approximately 21% of cancers diagnosed in PWH (Robbins et al., 2015).

PROGNOSTIC FEATURES

Historically, poor prognostic factors for patients with HIV-related NHL have included age older than 35 years, CD4$^+$ T-cell count of less than 100 cells/mm^3, history of injection drug use, history of AIDS-defining condition, poor performance status, elevated lactate dehydrogenase, tumor bulk or stage of disease, and International Prognostic Index (IPI) (Straus et al., 1998). The IPI includes clinical features that reflect the growth and invasive potential of the tumor (tumor stage, serum lactate dehydrogenase (LDH) level, and number of extranodal disease sites), the patient's response to the tumor (performance status), and the patient's ability to tolerate intensive therapy (age and performance status). The simplified model for younger patients (the age-adjusted IPI) uses a subgroup of these clinical features (tumor stage, LDH level, and performance status).

Lim and colleagues (2005) compared the prognostic factors for survival and the use of the IPI in pre- and post-ART PWH with DLBCL. In groups with low-, low-intermediate-, and high-intermediate-risk IPI disease, the 3-year overall survival rates were 20%, 22%, and 5% in the pre-ART era and improved to 64%, 64%, and 50% in the post-ART era, respectively.

Of note, PEL and extra-cavity PEL are known to be aggressive malignancies with a traditionally dismal prognosis. An early study found a median survival time of 6 months and few survivors beyond 12 months. Poor performance status and lack of ART portend worse prognosis (Boulanger et al., 2005). However, PEL prognosis may be improving. A 2015 single-center retrospective study of 15 patients found that complete remission was achieved in 14 (93.3%) (Cattaneo et al., 2015). Subsequently four patients relapsed, and two patients died. The overall survival rate at 3 years was 66.7%.

Barta and colleagues (2014) have developed an AIDS-related lymphoma IPI that combines the age-adjusted IPI with an HIV severity score including CD4$^+$ T-cell count, HIV RNA levels, and prior history of AIDS to risk-stratify HIV-related lymphomas. Using this scoring system, this group evaluated patients enrolled in HIV-associated lymphoma trials between 2005 and 2010 and found that individual HIV-related factors such as low CD4$^+$ T-cell counts (< 50 cells/mm^3) and prior history of AIDS were no longer associated with poorer outcomes (Barta et al., 2015).

TREATMENT

The treatment for AIDS-related lymphoma is similar to that of people without HIV, with some exceptions (Reid et al., 2018). Intrathecal chemotherapy prophylaxis is necessary because PWH are at an increased risk for CNS involvement. Those cases include lymphomas with aggressive pathologic features, including BL, plasmablastic lymphoma, and presentations consistent with possible CNS involvement (Chari et al., 2005). The use of hematopoietic stimulants such as granulocyte colony-stimulating factor (G-CSF) may aid in reducing chemotherapy-induced cytopenic complications. *Pneumocystis* jirovecii pneumonia prophylaxis is administered with standard-dose chemotherapy, irrespective of CD4$^+$ T-cell count.

Chemotherapy in the Pre-Art Era

In the pre-ART era, PWH with NHL had a poor prognosis, were managed on low-dose chemotherapy regimens because of concern for toxicity and had a median survival of 5–8 months (Kaplan et al., 1997; Sandler & Kaplan, 1996). In addition to persistent neoplasia contributing to death, many patients in this era died because of the infectious complications of opportunistic diseases (Lowenthal et al., 1988).

Chemotherapy in the Art Era

In the ART era, standard combination chemotherapy regimens are used successfully to treat NHL without excessive toxicity. The AMC reported on 65 patients given reduced doses of cyclophosphamide and doxorubicin combined with vincristine and prednisone (modified CHOP) or full doses of CHOP combined with G-CSF with concomitant ART. Complete response rates were 30% and 48% in the

reduced- and full-dose groups, respectively (Ratner et al., 2001). This study did not report long-term outcomes. Other studies of CHOP-based chemotherapy and concurrent ART describe median survival times of approximately 2 years. In patients with BL, a particularly aggressive form of NHL, intensive chemotherapy with cyclophosphamide, doxorubicin, high-dose methotrexate/ifosfamide, etoposide, and high-dose cytarabine (CODOX-M/IVAC) resulted in rates of event-free survival and remission similar to those of their counterparts without HIV (Wang et al., 2003).

Risk-adaptive chemotherapy has also been studied comparing the post- to pre-ART era. A total of 485 PWH were assigned randomly to chemotherapy after risk stratification based on an HIV score (comprised of performance status, prior AIDS, and CD4$^+$ T-cell counts < 100 cells/mm^3). Of these patients, 218 "good-risk" patients (HIV score 0) received doxorubicin, cyclophosphamide, vindesine, bleomycin, and prednisone (ACVBP) or CHOP; 177 "intermediate-risk" patients (HIV score 1) received CHOP or low-dose CHP; and 90 "poor-risk" patients (HIV score 2 or 3) received low-dose CHOP or vincristine and steroids. Five-year overall survival in the good-risk group was 51% for ACVBP versus 47% for CHOP ($p = 0.85$); that in the intermediate-risk group was 28% for CHOP versus 24% for low-dose CHOP ($p = 0.19$); that in the poor-risk group was 11% for low-dose CHOP versus 3% for vincristine and steroid ($p = 0.14$). The variables that significantly improved overall survival were ART (relative risk (RR) 1.6; $p = 0.0002$), HIV score (RR 1.7; $p = 0.0001$), and IPI score (RR 1.5; $p = 0.0012$) but not the intensity of chemotherapy (Mounier et al., 2006).

An infusional regimen of cyclophosphamide, doxorubicin, and etoposide with or without ART (only didanosine) resulted in a complete response rate of 45% and median overall survival of 12.8 months. At the time of the analysis, 30% in the pre-ART group were alive, compared with 47% in the ART group. Furthermore, patients in the ART group experienced less nonhematologic toxicity (22% vs. 42%), thrombocytopenia (31% vs. 52%), and anemia (9% vs. 27%) (Sparano et al., 2004). A similar regimen, etoposide, prednisone, vincristine, and doxorubicin (EPOCH) has been used more commonly and with perhaps even more success in the latter portion of the ART era. In two retrospective pooled analyses, Barta and colleagues (2012, 2013) concluded that EPOCH is superior to CHOP; however, these studies were limited by the potential confounder that experience with CHOP occurred in earlier time periods than that with EPOCH.

Regarding treatment of PEL, a 2012 multicenter retrospective study found no survival benefit from regimens that were more intensive than CHOP (Castillo et al., 2012). A 2015 retrospective single-institution study of 15 patients treated with CHOP or CHOP-like regimens found that complete remission was achieved in 14 patients (93.3%); four of these subsequently relapsed (Cattaneo et al., 2015).

Regimens That Include Rituximab

In the early 2000s, uncertainty existed around the use of rituximab in PWH with low CD4$^+$ T-cell counts because of concern for increased infection risk (Gates & Kaplan, 2003; Avivi et al., 2003). However, with subsequent experience there is now a general consensus that outcomes are improved when rituximab is added to the chemotherapy regimens discussed earlier; thus, rituximab should be regarded as the standard of care for both DLBCL and BL. Two multicenter retrospective analyses of DLBCL patients with and without HIV infection treated with rituximab plus CHOP (R-CHOP) completed in the early 2000s showed conflicting results. Coutinho and colleagues (2014) evaluated patients treated between 2003 and 2011 and found that HIV positivity was associated with an improved 5-year overall survival rate (78% compared with 64% in patients without HIV infection). In contrast, Baptista and colleagues (2015) evaluated patients treated between 2001 and 2011 and found that HIV positivity was associated with a worse 5-year survival rate (56% compared with 74% in patients without HIV). However, in the latter study PWH had a worse performance status and higher Ann Arbor stages than did patients without HIV, and, when complete response rates were compared among patients with high tumor burdens, there was no difference between the two groups. The safety and feasibility of R-CHOP in populations of LMICs is being established by studies such as a phase 2 trial of R-CHOP in patients with and without HIV and DLBCL in Malawi (Kimani et al., 2021) (NCT02660710).

Regarding other regimens for NHL in PWH, Sparano and colleagues examined rituximab plus infusional etoposide, vincristine, doxorubicin, cyclophosphamide, and prednisone (R-EPOCH) given either concurrently or sequentially. In the concurrent arm, 35 of 48 evaluable patients (73%; 95% CI: 58–85) had a complete response, whereas 29 of 53 evaluable patients in the sequential arm (55%; 95% CI: 41–68) had a complete response. Toxicity was comparable in the two arms, although patients with a baseline $CD4^+$ T-cell count of less than 50 cells/mm³ had a high infectious death rate in the concurrent arm (Sparano et al., 2010). A prospective, uncontrolled phase 2 trial of short-course R-EPOCH in PWH with untreated NHL indicated that low-intensity regimens can be effective (NCT00006436). A phase 2 trial of ibrutinib (a small molecule drug that binds permanently to Bruton's tyrosine kinase) in combination with R-EPOCH in stage II–IV DLBCL is ongoing (NCT03220022). Evidence remains unclear whether R-CHOP or R-EPOCH is best for patients with ARLs. A large multicenter trial addressed this question in the population without HIV and showed no difference between R-CHOP and dose-adjusted R-EPOCH in event-free survival or overall survival (Wilson et al., 2016). Despite a paucity of large studies in PWH, treatment with either R-CHOP or R-EPOCH is usually effective at achieving remission in PWH with DLBCL, and most patients who achieve remission remain lymphoma-free.

Regarding BL, a 2012 study examined CODOX-M, followed by IVAC with or without rituximab (Rodrigo et al., 2012). Most patients were on ART and had a median $CD4^+$ T-cell count of 375 cells/mm³. Of the 14 patients who received ART, intensive chemotherapy, and rituximab, 10 survived to the follow-up period of nearly 12 months. Complications included late neutropenia, which responded well to G-CSF.

Because of the predilection of herpesvirus reactivation with rituximab, study participants received prophylaxis for herpes simplex and varicella zoster and preemptive monitoring of cytomegalovirus. Similarly, a prospective multicenter trial showed that modified CODOX-M/IVAC with rituximab was safe and effective in PWH receiving ART, and the 2-year overall survival rate for 34 patients with HIV-related Burkitt lymphoma was 69.0% (Noy et al., 2015). A 2013 study of short-course low-intensity R-EPOCH in 13 patients with Burkitt lymphoma including 11 PWH found that the overall survival at a median follow-up of 73 months was even better, 90% (Dunleavy et al., 2013). No randomized data are available to determine which of the two regimens is best in PWH with BL; however, both appear to be effective, although the efficacy of R-EPOCH in patients with CNS involvement has not yet been established.

Intrathecal Chemotherapy for Aids-Related NHL

CNS involvement by systemic DLBCL has long been recognized as a problem, especially in PWH. To date there have not been any formal studies to evaluate the role of intrathecal prophylaxis in PWH and DLBCL. In the absence of definitive data, clinicians routinely administer intrathecal prophylaxis to patients with the following characteristics: extranodal involvement of two or more sites, elevated lactate dehydrogenase levels, or bone marrow or testicular involvement.

Alternative Therapies for Aids-Related NHL

Newer, targeted anticancer therapies are currently being explored for several types of uncommon but aggressive ARLs, but currently data are sparse. A 2017 systematic review evaluated the use of bortezomib (a 26S proteasome inhibitor that is used for multiple myeloma) in 21 patients with plasmablastic lymphoma, of whom 11 received bortezomib as initial treatment and 10 received bortezomib for relapsed disease. The study included 11 participants with and 10 without HIV. The overall response rate to bortezomib-containing regimens was 100% as initial therapy and 90% in the relapsed setting, and the 2-year survival of patients treated with bortezomib initially was 55% (Guerrero-Garcia et al., 2017). Daratumumab, a CD38-directed human IgG1κ monoclonal antibody also used for multiple myeloma, has been shown to be effective in controlling a case of refractory PEL (Shah et al., 2018). The biologic agent pembrolizumab has undergone phase 1 trials for patients with advanced NHL and seems to have an acceptable safety profile (Uldrick et al., 2019) (NCT02595866). Pembrolizumab has also been evaluated with and without pomalidomide in a retrospective review of stage IV relapsed and/or primary refractory HIV-associated NHL demonstrating a response rate of 50% in that setting (Lurain, et al., 2021).

Chimeric antigen receptor (CAR) T-cell therapy is increasingly used for treatment of refractory lymphomas in the general population and is emerging as an effective treatment for PWH as well. Abramson and colleagues (2019) reported two

PWH and high-grade B-cell lymphoma successfully treated with commercially available anti-CD19 CAR T-cells. Further, such therapies are being developed as potential cures for HIV (NCT03617198) (Rust et al., 2020).

Hematopoietic Cell Transplantation for Aids-Related NHL

Autologous HCT has long been the optimal therapy for high-risk and refractory NHL in patients without HIV, and now a sufficient number of PWH have undergone autologous HCT to determine that it is a safe and feasible approach for patients with ARLs who meet criteria for transplantation (Navarro & Kaplan, 2006). A multicenter study to evaluate the safety and efficacy of autologous HCT for PWH and lymphoma evaluated 40 patients with persistent or recurrent ARLs (DLBCL, plasmablastic lymphoma, Burkitt or Burkitt-like lymphoma, or classical Hodgkin lymphoma) (Alvarnas et al., 2016). Overall survival and time to progression were not different for PWH when compared with matched controls without HIV. Uninterrupted ART should be continued in these patients during the peri-transplant period, when feasible, to maintain virological suppression and avoid untoward effects of acute virological rebound, including acute retroviral syndrome and opportunistic infections (Woolfrey et al., 2008). Administration of ART is generally considered safe, with minimal effect on the transplantation course, including adverse drug–drug interactions or other significant adverse events (Johnston et al., 2016).

One study showed that low $CD4^+$ T-cell count, marrow involvement, and poor performance status independently affected survival with HCT (Re et al., 2009). Overall survival has been reported to be 50%–55% at 9 months (Gabarre et al., 2000; Re et al., 2003); 71% at 21 months (Diez-Martin et al., 2003); and 85% at 32 months (Krishnan et al., 2005). Most published studies (one exception is a French series, Diez-Martin et al., 2003) have required HIV disease to be under control for HCT, either by low to undetectable HIV RNA levels or by $CD4^+$ T-cell counts of more than 100 cells/mm³. In another study, they showed a similar incidence of relapse, overall survival, and progression-free survival in cohorts of patients with and without HIV and lymphoma who received HCT (Diez-Martin et al., 2009). Long-term survival of autologous HCT for relapsed/refractory lymphoma was examined in a 2015 retrospective review of survivors with HIV (Zanet et al., 2015). This study found a survival of 65% at 5 years for 37 patients. Among 26 patients who achieved complete remission, overall survival at 10 years was 91%,% and event-free survival was 36%. Nine patients developed opportunistic infections at a median of 0.4 years post HCT.

Regarding allogeneic bone marrow transplant (alloBMT), one famous case reported in 2009 demonstrated that allogeneic HCT with donor cells that are resistant to HIV infection (in this case, because of a homozygous deletion polymorphism in the donor's CCR5 gene) can cure HIV infection (Hutter et al., 2009). Although fascinating, this outcome is the exception rather than the rule with allogeneic HCT. Importantly,

caution must be observed because, in typical alloBMTs, the HIV reservoir disappears along with the patient's T-cells but can aggressively rebound if ART is discontinued (Henrich et al., 2014; Sugarman et al., 2016). More research is required to thoroughly explore the mechanism and frequency of this phenomenon. A prospective multicenter trial of matched related or unrelated allogeneic HCT in PWH included 17 patients with acute leukemias, myelodysplasia, Hodgkin lymphomas, and NHLs (Ambinder et al., 2017). No deaths occurred by 100 days posttransplant, and the overall survival rate at 1 year was 57%. Subsequent deaths were due to relapsed or progressive disease in five patients, acute graft-versus-host disease, adult respiratory distress syndrome, and liver failure. The overall conclusion from this trial was that allogeneic HCT should be considered the standard of care for PWH who meet usual transplant eligibility criteria. Other studies are currently being conducted to explore gene-modified autologous and allo-HSCT with HIV-resistant cells (Bender-Ignacio et al., 2018; DiGiusto et al., 2016; Lederman et al., 2016). Other recent studies have contributed important observations on the latent HIV reservoir dynamics post stem cell transplant. Eberhard and colleagues (2020) found strong $CD4^+$ and $CD8^+$ T-cell activation (as measured by coexpression of CD38 and HLA-DR) followed allo-HSCT that peaked between months 2 and 3 after HSCT, demonstrating that there is a period of high immune activation and a potential window of vulnerability for HIV reservoir re-seeding during that time. In another small study of allogeneic transplant patients where posttransplant cyclophosphamide was used for graft-versus-host disease prophylaxis to expand donor options, Durant and colleagues demonstrated that among six patients who had longitudinal measurements available, the HIV latent reservoir was not detected post-allo-HSCT in four patients with more than 95% donor chimerism, consistent with a 2.06–2.54 log_{10} reduction in the HIV latent reservoir. However, the HIV latent reservoir remained stable in the two patients with less than 95% donor chimerism. Although three of the six patients ultimately died after allo-HSCT, this study supports the use of allo-HSCT for PWH and reinforce the observation that allo-HSCT alone diminishes but does not completely eliminate the HIV latent reservoir (Durand et al., 2020).

Chemotherapy: Art Interactions

ART interruption during cancer treatment should generally be avoided because it increases the risk of severe consequences (including immunologic compromise, opportunistic infection, and death) (El-Sadr et al., 2006) and it improves tolerance and outcomes of cancer treatment. However, interactions between ART and proposed anticancer therapeutic options must always be checked as many medications used for chemotherapy (e.g., cyclophosphamide and vincristine) and immunotherapy are metabolized via the CYP3A4 isoenzyme. PIs (including ritonavir), nonnucleoside reverse transcriptase inhibitors (NNRTI), and pharmacokinetic boosters such as cobicistat inhibit and induce CYP3A4, with the potential for altered chemotherapeutic and cytotoxic effects. Thus, chemotherapy without antiretroviral drugs has been studied because of concerns of drug interactions with chemotherapy and nonadherence to ART resulting in increased resistance (Powles et al., 2000). Further, PIs (in ART regimens) have been associated with increased incidence of neutropenia with concomitant chemotherapy (Bower et al., 2004).

There are ART regimens that are unlikely to lead to problematic drug–drug interactions with chemotherapeutic agents. Among those with the fewest potential interactions are integrase strand transfer inhibitors (INSTIs) (e.g., raltegravir, elvitegravir, dolutegravir, bictegravir, and cabotegravir). Raltegravir, an INSTI metabolized via glucuronidation, has been given simultaneously with CHOP and with other antimetabolites such as gemcitabine and methotrexate, as well as with monoclonal antibodies rituximab and trastuzumab, with good tolerability and durable viral suppression (Bañon et al., 2014). ART regimens that include an INSTI improve virologic and immunologic responses in ART-naive patients and are considered in the US Department of Health and Human Services (USDHHS) ART guidelines for HIV disease as an acceptable first-line therapy (DHHS, 2022a); thus, ART regimens containing an INSTI should be leveraged for PWH undergoing cancer treatment (Fulco et al., 2010).

Impact of ART

Most studies have shown that the incidence of HIV-related NHL, like that for most other AIDS-defining cancers, has declined over time. In a meta-analysis by Appleby and colleagues (2000)) that included 47,936 PWH with NHL (including PCNSL), the incidence declined from 6.2 cases per 1,000 py in the pre-ART era to 3.6 cases per 1,000 py in the post-ART era ($p < 0.0001$).

In a population-based, record-linkage study of cancer in 472,378 people with AIDS from 1980 to 2006, the cumulative incidence of NHL declined from 3.8% during 1990–1995 to 2.2% during 1996–2006. Of note, NHL was the most common AIDS-defining cancer during the pre-ART era (53%) (Simard et al., 2011). In addition, the Swiss Cohort study examined 429 NHL cases of 12,959 PWH from 1993 to 2006. NHL incidence reached 13.6 per 1,000 py in 1993–1995 and declined to 1.8 in 2002–2006. Combination ART use was associated with a decline in NHL incidence (hazard ratio (HR) 0.26; 95% CI: 0.20–0.33) (Polesel et al., 2008).

A retrospective study using United States and Canadian data from 1996 to 2009 showed a significant decline in the annual hazard rate of NHL (–8%) in PWH compared to that of people without HIV, signifying a narrowing of the gap of NHL burden between people with and without HIV (Silverberg et al., 2015). This reduction also represents the benefit of immunological recovery and viral control.

RECOMMENDED READING

Abramson JS, Irwin KE, Frigault MJ, et al. Successful anti-CD19 CAR T-cell therapy in HIV-infected patients with refractory high-grade B-cell lymphoma. *Cancer.* 2019;125:3692–3698

Alvarnas JC, Le Rademacher J, Wang Y, et al. Autologous hematopoietic cell transplantation for HIV-related lymphoma: results of the BMT CTN 0803/AMC 071 trial. *Blood.* 2016;128:1050–1058.

Bañon S, Machuca I, Araujo S, et al. Efficacy, safety, and lack of interactions with the use of raltegravir in HIV-infected patients undergoing antineoplastic chemotherapy. *J Intern AIDS Soc.* 2014;17(4 Suppl 3):19590.

Kimani S, Painschab MS, Kaimila B, et al. Safety and efficacy of rituximab in patients with diffuse large B-cell lymphoma in Malawi: a prospective, single-arm, non-randomised phase 1/2 clinical trial. *Lancet Glob Health.* 2021;9(7):e1008–e1016. http://doi:10.1016/S2214-109X(21)00181-9

Lurain K, Ramaswami R, Mangusan R, et al. Use of pembrolizumab with or without pomalidomide in HIV-associated non-Hodgkin's lymphoma. *J Immunother Cancer.* 2021;9(2):e002097. http://doi:10.1136/jitc-2020-002097. PMID: 33608378; PMCID: PMC7898875.

Rust B, Kiem HP, Uldrick T. CAR T-cell therapy for cancer and HIV through novel approaches to HIV-associated haematological malignancies. *Lancet Haematol.* 2020;7(9):e690–e696. http://doi:10.1016/S2352-3026(20)30142-3

Uldrick TS, Gonçalves PH, Abdul-Hay M, et al. Assessment of the safety of pembrolizumab in patients with HIV and advanced cancer: a phase 1 study. *JAMA Oncol.* 2019;5(9):1332–1339. http://doi:10.1001/jamaoncol.2019.2244

Zanet E, Taborelli M, Rupolo M, et al. Postautologous stem cell transplantation long-term outcomes in 26 PLWH affected by relapsed/refractory lymphoma. *AIDS.* 2015;29(17):2303–2308.

NON-AIDS-DEFINING CANCERS

LEARNING OBJECTIVES

- Review the risk factors and epidemiology of NADCs.

- Review the impact of anogenital neoplasias and squamous cell cancer of the anus (SCCA) in men and women.

- Discuss treatment of anogenital neoplasias and SCCA, including the role of ART.

WHAT'S NEW?

- Women are recognized as a high-risk group for SCCA, and predisposing factors include positivity for high-risk human papilloma virus (HPV) serotypes. Some experts recommend screening all women with HIV ≥ 35 years old for HPV-related anal disease regardless of cervical cytology results.

- HPV vaccination in women with HIV (WWH) has demonstrated durable immunogenicity and safety.

- HPV vaccination for men with HIV beyond recommended ages may be beneficial and cost-effective in preventing invasive neoplasia.

KEY POINTS

- Owing to the aging HIV population, NADCs are responsible for an increasing number of deaths. Immunologic control with ART; however, has decreased the incidence of some cancers, including anogenital cancers.

- Screening with either cervical Papanicolaou (Pap) smear or high-risk HPV molecular testing in women is a key surveillance measure for detecting precancerous lesions. Screening with anal Pap smear in men and women with risk factors is also recommended, although uptake of this practice may be contingent on the availability of high-resolution anoscopy.

- HPV vaccination for PWH is safe and efficacious.

Since the advent of widely available ART in the United States, PWH have had significantly improved survival and decreased mortality from AIDS-related infections and AIDS-defining cancers (ADCs). However, with longer survival, it has become evident that PWH are now at increased risk for NADCs. Multiple risk factors for NADCs include degree and duration of viremia, low CD4$^+$ T-cell count nadir, coinfection with oncogenic viruses (e.g., HPV, EBV, HHV-8, HCV, and HBV), and personal carcinogenic exposure, which also should be considered when implementing risk mitigation strategies (Kowalkowski et al., 2014; Riedel et al., 2015b; Vallet-Prichard & Pol, 2004).

Simard and colleagues (2011) confirmed the benefits of immunological control in a population-based, record-linkage study examining cancers in 472,378 individuals with AIDS from 1980 to 2006. The cumulative incidence of ADCs declined sharply across three calendar periods (from 18% in 1980–1989 to 11% in 1990–1995 and 4.2% in 1996–2006). The cumulative incidence of NADC increased from 1.1% to 1.5%, with no change thereafter (1% in 1996–2006). However, the cumulative incidence increased steadily over time for specific NADCs (anal cancer, Hodgkin's lymphoma, and liver cancer) (Simard et al., 2011). Another study (Simard et al, 2010) showed an elevated incidence for the following NADCs in patients 3–10 years after the onset of AIDS: Hodgkin's lymphoma and cancers of the oral cavity and/or pharynx, tongue, anus, liver, larynx, lung and/or bronchus, and penis. These data demonstrate that having previously diagnosed advanced immunosuppression appears to increase the risk for NADCs as well as ADCs.

The increased risk of NADCs among PWH has been reported (Patel et al., 2008). The incidences of the following cancers were significantly higher: anal (standardized rate ratio (SRR) 42.9; 95% CI: 34.1–53.3), vaginal (SRR 21.0; CI: 11.2–35.9), Hodgkin's lymphoma (SRR 14.7; CI: 11.6–18.2), liver (SRR 7.7; CI: 5.7–10.1), lung (SRR 3.3; CI: 2.8–3.9), melanoma (SRR 2.6; CI: 1.9–3.6), oropharyngeal (SRR 2.6; CI: 1.9–3.4), leukemia (SRR 2.5; CI: 1.6–3.8), colorectal (SRR 2.3; CI: 1.8–2.9), and renal (SRR 1.8; CI: 1.1–2.7). The incidence of prostate cancer was significantly lower among PWH compared to the general population (SRR 0.6; CI: 0.4–0.8). Only the relative incidence of anal cancer increased over time (Patel et al., 2008). None of the AIDS–cancer match studies found an increased risk of breast, colon, or prostate cancer. It is unclear if a definite link exists between the level of immunodeficiency and certain NADCs. Some studies have failed to show such a relationship (Burgi et al., 2005). Conversely, another study utilized data from 4,453 patients in the prospective, multinational EuroSIDA cohort (Reekie et al., 2010). The incidence of NADCs in this cohort from 1994 to 2007 was 4.3 per 1,000 py of follow-up. After adjustment, a higher current CD4$^+$ T-cell count was independently associated with a decreased incidence of NADCs. In addition, an increased rate of virus-related cancers and non-virus-related epithelial cancers was found in immunodeficient patients. Hodgkin's lymphoma, anal cancer, and lung cancer were all found at higher rates in PWH with lower current CD4$^+$ T-cell counts after adjustment for other demographic and traditional risk factors (Reekie et al., 2010). More recently, a study of PWH in the US Veterans Aging Cohort Study (VACS) also showed that increased risk of lung cancer is associated with lower CD4$^+$ T-cell counts, lower CD4:CD8 ratios, and increased HIV RNA levels (Sigel et al., 2017).

PWH may be at higher risk for malignancies at younger ages. Shiels and colleagues (2010c) used the national US HIV/AIDS Cancer Match Study to demonstrate that PWH are not at increased risk for colon, prostate, or breast cancer at younger ages, but they were significantly (p < <0.001) younger at the time of diagnosis lung (median 50 vs. 54 years) and anal cancer (median 42 vs. 45 years). They also found that the age of diagnosis of Hodgkin's lymphoma was significantly older than that of the general population (median 42 vs. 40 years; P < 0.001). A study using data from the HIV/AIDS Cancer Match Study found that PWH with cancer tended to be younger than age 50 years compared to their counterparts without HIV, whose cancer occurred more often after age 60 years. This study also found that PWH presented with more advanced-stage cancers with distant disease (32.2%) compared to patients without HIV (17.7%), and they experienced higher cancer-specific mortality (Coghill et al., 2015). By comparing data from both the North American AIDS Cohort Collaboration on Research and Design (NAACCRD) and the US Cancer Statistics Surveillance, Epidemiology, and End Results (SEER) program, Shiels and colleagues (2017) found that PWH were diagnosed with lung cancer, anal cancer, head and neck cancer, kidney cancer, and myeloma at earlier ages than their counterparts without HIV. (Shiels et al., 2017). However, in a recent metanalysis from studies of women with breast cancer in North America and Sub-Saharan Africa, women with HIV (WWH) from both continents were more likely to be diagnosed with advanced-stage (3 and 4) disease and have poorer survival (Brandao et al., 2021).

NADCs are responsible for an increasingly large proportion of deaths in patients with HIV disease in the ART era, which is likely due to longer survival among PWH. A study conducted by the Data Collection on Adverse Events of Anti-HIV Drugs (D:A:D) evaluated factors associated with mortality owing to NADCs and ADCs (Monforte et al., 2008). The study included 23,437 patients followed from 1999 to 2001 and found that the overall mortality rate owing to NADCs was higher than that owing to ADCs. The death rate from NADCs was 1.8 per 1,000 py of follow-up (95% CI: 1.5–2.1) compared to 1.1 per 1,000 py of follow-up (95% CI: 0.9–1.2) for ADCs. In addition, the study found that low recent CD4$^+$ T-cell count and increasing age were associated with an increased risk of death from ADCs and NADCs.

Other factors, such as poor ART utilization, increased the risk of death for NADCs only. It is unlikely that HIV treatment itself increases the risk for NADCs. Rather, this finding underscores the complex relationship between prolonged survival with HIV, immunosuppression, and the diagnosis of and survival from NADCs.

The Mortalité study in France captured the changing patterns of AIDS-related deaths in that country (Bonnet et al., 2005; Lewden et al., 2005). Lewden reported on cancer deaths among PWH in the original study and found that, in 2000, NADCs were the third leading cause of death. They also found that as the patient population increased above age 45 years, deaths because of malignant disease eclipsed those attributed to infectious etiologies. The study was updated in 2005, demonstrating that the rate of death from non-AIDS/hepatitis-related cancers increased from 38% in 2000 to 50% in 2005. A subsequent follow-up study found that the combination of ADCs and NADCs has become the leading cause of death in French PWH (Morlat et al., 2014). Similarly, a more recent Tanzanian study showed that NADCs increased by 33.8% from 2002 to 2014, while the proportion of NADCs relative to all cancers significantly decreased from 6.8% in 2002 to 5.6% in 2014 (APC = –2.74%). (Campbell et al., 2016). Most of these increases were due to lung and liver cancers, although the number of head and neck cancers also increased. A large US population registry-based study found that most cancer deaths among PWH were due to NADCs, including lung cancer (2.4%), liver cancer (1.1%), and anal cancer (0.6%) (Horner et al., 2021).

Regardless of etiology, as the PWH population ages, the risk of NADCs will also undoubtedly increase. A US retrospective study found that cancer-related mortality among PWH compared to people without HIV (1996–2010) was significantly elevated for colorectal cancer (HR 1.49; 95% CI: 1.2–1.8), pancreatic cancer (HR 1.7; CI: 1.35–2.18), lung cancer (HR 1.28; CI: 1.17–1.3), melanoma (HR 1.72; CI: 1.09–2.7), breast cancer (HR 2.61; CI: 2.06–3.3), and prostate cancer (HR 1.57; CI: 1.02–2.41) (Coghill et al., 2015). Some evidence suggests that treatment of these individuals may be more difficult than that of the general population, that PWH may present with more advanced disease, and that PWH may not tolerate cancer therapies as well as patients without HIV (Bower et al., 2003). Screening for early signs of malignancy may be an important method for earlier diagnosis. However, no studies of screening approaches have been performed, and no specific recommendations for alternative screening practices different from what is recommended for the general population exist for PWH for most cancers.

Most studies of treatment outcomes for NADCs in the ART era demonstrate that PWH have outcomes similar to those without HIV. Simard and Engels (2010) evaluated cause of death in the pre-ART and ART eras and showed that death from NADCs (lung, Hodgkin's lymphoma, anal cancers, and other unspecified cancers) decreased steadily from 1980 to 2006. For all NADCs, the number of deaths per 1,000 py from 1980 to 1989 and then from 1996 to 2006 significantly declined from 2.21 to 0.84 (Simard & Engels, 2010). However, while more recent population-based studies, such as

that of Horner and colleagues, also show overall cancer mortality for PWH declining (from 484.0 per 100,000 person-year during 2001–2005 to 313.6 per 100,000 person-years during 2011–2015), their population attributable fractions for NADCs increased from 7.2% to 11.8% in 2011–2015. Because of the benefit of ART on cancer outcomes in PWH, it is recommended that most patients be treated similarly to those without HIV and that ART should be administered concurrently with chemotherapy or radiotherapy (Chiao et al., 2010; Reid et al., 2018).

ANOGENITAL NEOPLASIA

Anogenital neoplasia refers to anal and cervical carcinomas and their precursor lesions. One of the most important risk factors associated with anogenital neoplasia is HPV infection. HPV is a DNA virus that generally infects stratified squamous epithelium. More than 100 HPV serotypes have been identified to date, and at least 30 of these have a high predilection for the anogenital tract. HPV serotypes 6 and 11 have been associated with benign disease, whereas serotypes including 16, 18, 31, 33, 45, 52, and 58 are associated with high-grade cervical or anal squamous intraepithelial lesions (SILs) or cervical and anal carcinomas.

For PWH, HPV infection has a well-established relationship with the increased risk of developing anogenital neoplasia (Bjorge et al., 2002; Palefsky et al., 1991). Invasive and in situ forms of not only cervical and anal cancer but also vulvar/vaginal and penile cancers are reported among PWH (Frisch et al, et al., 2000a; Frish & Goodman, 2000b; Smith et al, et al., 2019).

PATHOGENESIS OF HPV IN HIV INFECTION

The increased prevalence of HPV disease associated with HIV infection may be mediated by impaired T-cell and antigen-presenting cell function. However, local effects of HIV infection may also upregulate HPV replication and oncogenesis. The HPV viral oncogenes E6 and E7 can immortalize primary keratinocytes and transform cells in culture (Barbosa et al., 1989; Munger et al., 1989). In an animal model of estrogen-stimulated HPV-induced cervical cancer, expression of E7 alone resulted in precancers and cancer, whereas the expression of E6 and E7 together resulted in larger cancers (Riley et al., 2003). Although the exact mechanisms of HIV-related immunosuppression and HPV coinfection have not been determined, several in vitro studies have shown that the HIV Tat protein can drive the replication of HPV-16 and HPV-18 through the overexpression of E7 and other genes in the early region (Tornesello et al., 1993; Vernone et al., 1993).

EPIDEMIOLOGY OF HIV-ASSOCIATED CERVICAL INTRAEPITHELIAL NEOPLASIA

The relationship between HIV infection and increased prevalence of cervical intraepithelial neoplasia (CIN) has been shown in many studies. Mandelblatt and colleagues (1999) performed a meta-analysis of 15 cross-sectional studies published between 1986 and 1998 that evaluated prevalence of cervical neoplasia, HPV infection, and HIV infection among women. They found that among women infected with HPV, WWH were significantly more likely to develop cervical neoplasia, and this effect was related to the degree of immunodeficiency. Several other studies have also shown that WWH are at higher risk for CIN, including that by Ahdieh and colleagues (2000), who found that 13% of WWH versus 2% of women without HIV had abnormal cytological findings. They also found that WWH had a much lower rate of HPV clearance on follow-up exams and that, in a multivariate model, the increased rate of CIN among WWH was fully accounted for by HPV persistence (Ahdieh et al., 2000). A 2016 study from the Kaiser group found that WWH had twofold higher odds of cervical intraepithelial neoplasia grade 2$^+$ (CIN2$^+$) and CIN3$^+$, but this was only in women with a recent CD4$^+$ T-cell count of less than 500 cells/mm^3 (Silverberg et al., 2016).

EPIDEMIOLOGY OF HIV-ASSOCIATED CERVICAL CARCINOMA

Since 1993, invasive cervical cancer has been listed by the CDC as an "AIDS-defining" condition. Globally, the risk of cervical cancer is higher in WWH (RR 6.07; 95% CI: 4.40–8.37) (Stelzle, 2021). In the United States, where the incidence of cervical cancer in general is relatively low, the incidence in WWH is 66% higher than in women without HIV (Brickman et al., 2015). However, in some areas of Africa, the cervical cancer incidence is much higher, nearly 168 per 100,000 women (Lince-Deroche, 2015). A recent systemic review and meta-analysis found that 63.8% (95% CI: 58.9–68.1) of women in southern Africa and 27.4% (95% CI: 23.7–31.7) of women in eastern Africa with cervical cancer were living with HIV (Stelzle et al., 2021). The same study demonstrated age-standardized incidence rates of HIV-attributable cervical cancer to be >20 per 100,000 in six countries, all in southern or eastern Africa. Cervical cancer incidence and mortality remains higher in WWH than in women without HIV, especially in resource-limited settings (Rohner, 2020). However, quantifying the contribution of HIV infection to the development of cervical cancer among WWH was challenging in the pre-ART era. A 1996 study that evaluated the relationship between HIV and cervical cancer found no conclusive evidence that HIV per se increased the risk of cervical cancer among WWH (International Agency for Research on Cancer, 1996). Subsequent studies continue to yield conflicting results. In LMICs with access to ART, several studies have shown an increased risk of cervical cancer. Using a national AIDS–cancer linked registry database of cases through 1998, researchers found a RR of 5.4 for invasive cervical cancer among WWH compared to the general population (Frisch et al., 2001). However, no increased risk in cervical cancer has been noted in case control studies from multiple Sub-Saharan African countries, where endemic rates of cervical cancer are higher and women have shorter survival (Gichangi et al., 2002; La Ruche et al., 1998; Patil et al., 1995).

As noted previously, with the use of ART since the mid-1990s, there have been definite declines in the incidence of AIDS-related cancers. This has been attributed to the improved immune function and control of oncogenic viruses seen with ART. This declining trend has not been consistently seen in AIDS-related cervical cancer. Researchers showed an increasing proportion of cervical cancers in persons with AIDS from 0.11% in 1980–1989 (95% CI: 0.08–0.13) to 0.69% in 2001–2007 (95% CI: 0.49–0.89) (Shiels et al., 2011b).

EFFECT OF ART ON HIV-ASSOCIATED CERVICAL DYSPLASIA

Although ART has significantly improved the survival of PWH through immune reconstitution and has decreased the incidence of opportunistic infections, the effects of ART on HPV infection and CIN among WWH remain unclear. Whereas three older studies did not find a significant reduction in risk of cervical dysplasia among women on ART (Lillo et al., 2001; Moore et al., 2002; Orlando et al., 1999), a more recent prospective study did find a reduction in cervical dysplasia risk related to ART (Minkoff et al., 2010).

The largest retrospective analysis performed by the Women's Interagency HIV Study (WIHS) group found that, among 741 WWH, those on ART were 40% (95% CI: 4–81) more likely to exhibit a regression of cervical lesions and were also significantly less likely to have progression of CIN (odds ratio (OR) 0.68) (Minkoff et al., 2001). The same group prospectively evaluated 286 WWH who initiated ART (Minkoff et al., 2010). They were assessed semiannually for HPV infection (by PCR) and SILs. Combination ART initiation among adherent women was associated with a significant reduction in HPV prevalence, incident detection of oncogenic HPV infection, and decreased prevalence and more rapid clearance of oncogenic HPV-positive SILs. Effects were smaller among nonadherent women (Minkoff et al., 2010). More recently, a large systematic review evaluated WWH with high-grade cervical lesions (high-grade squamous intraepithelial lesions (HSIL)-CIN2$^{\backslash+}$) (Kelly et al., 2018). WWH on ART had lower prevalence of high-risk HPV than did those not on ART. Their review included 17 studies that reported the association of ART with longitudinal cervical lesion outcomes and determined that ART was associated with a decreased risk of HSIL-CIN2$^+$ incidence, SIL progression, and increased likelihood of SIL or CIN regression. Further, three of their studies indicated that ART was associated with a reduction in invasive cervical cancer incidence. Collectively, the data suggest that treating HIV infection with ART has a beneficial effect on progression of HPV-related cervical disease.

SCREENING, TREATMENT, AND PREVENTION OF HIV-ASSOCIATED CERVICAL DYSPLASIA

Screening

Current US Public Health Service and Infectious Diseases Society of America guidelines recommend that WWH undergo a complete history and physical that includes a pelvic exam and Pap test at the time of initial evaluation. Screening for WWH should commence within 1 year of the onset of sexual activity regardless of mode of HIV transmission (e.g., sexual activity and perinatal exposure) but no later than age 21 years. Young women (i.e., those aged 21–29 years) should have only a Pap test at the time of initial diagnosis with HIV. Co-testing (Pap test and high-risk HPV molecular test) is not recommended for women with HIV younger than 30 years. If the initial Pap test for young (or newly diagnosed) WWH is normal, the next Pap test should be performed in 12 months (although some experts still recommend a repeat Pap test at 6 months after baseline testing). If the results of the three consecutive Pap tests are normal, follow-up Pap tests can be done every 3 years. For women aged 30 years or older, either Pap testing alone or co-testing with both Pap and HPV are acceptable screening strategies. For women who undergo Pap testing alone, the protocol is identical to that just described for women younger than 30. For women who undergo co-testing, Pap and HPV testing should be done at the time of HIV diagnosis (or starting at age 30 years). If the Pap is normal and the HPV screening test is negative, repeat cervical cancer screening can be done in 3 years. Women who have a normal Pap test but are positive for high-risk HPV should have repeat co-testing in one year (unless genotype testing for 16 or 16/18 is positive, in which case the patient should be referred for colposcopy). If either of the co-tests at 1 year is abnormal (i.e., abnormal cytology or positive HPV), referral to colposcopy is recommended. Any WWH with an abnormal Pap smear that shows atypical squamous cell of undetermined significance (ASCUS) or higher-grade lesions should undergo colposcopy (CDC, 2021). Cervical cancer screening in WWH should continue throughout their lifetime (and not end at age 65 years, as in the general population).

Treatment

Treatment options for CIN are similar for women with and without HIV and include cryotherapy, loop electrosurgical excision procedure (LEEP), and cold knife conization (Santesso et al., 2016). These options are generally safe and effective. Cryotherapy is an especially important option for women living in low-resource settings. A recent South African study evaluated 220 WWH who were randomly assigned to cryotherapy ($n = 112$) or no treatment ($n = 108$) (Firnhaber et al., 2017). Among participants, 94% were receiving ART, their median CD4[+] T-cell counts were 499 cells/mm^3, and 59% were high-risk HPV-positive. Cryotherapy reduced progression to HSIL (2 of 99 (2%) progressed in the cryotherapy group vs. 15 of 103 (15%)) in the no-treatment group; 86% reduction (95% CI: 41–97; $p = 0.002$). Participants in the cryotherapy arm experienced greater regression to normal histology and improved cytologic outcomes. Of note, endocervical extension is more frequent among WWH (Foulot et al., 2008). Therefore, LEEP is thought to be less effective and recurrence rates are higher in WWH than in women without HIV, although another recent South African study found that rates of cumulative CIN2[+] were lower after LEEP than cryotherapy treatment at 6 months (Smith et al., 2017). Importantly, in this study, both treatments appeared effective in reducing CIN2 + by more than 70% at 12 months.

Invasive cervical cancer diagnosed in WWH is treated using the same criteria and protocols as those for women without HIV if no other contraindications for treatment exist (Reid et al., 2018). Limited data exist on the treatment of cervical cancer in WWH (Ntekim et al., 2015). One prospective cohort study of 348 patients with cervical cancer in Botswana compared outcomes between women with (66%) and without HIV (Dryden-Peterson et al., 2016). The WWH group had a median CD4[+] T-cell count of 397 cells/mm^3 (interquartile range, 264–555). HIV infection was significantly associated with an increased risk of death among all women (HR 1.95; 95% CI: 1.20–3.17) and among the subset of those who received guideline-concordant curative therapy (HR 2.63; 95% CI: 1.05–6.55). These results suggest that HIV infection has an adverse effect on cervical cancer survival. That this effect was greater for women with a lower CD4[+] T-cell count ($p = 0.036$) suggests that immune suppression plays a significant role. Of note, the study was conducted in a resource-limited environment, and survival of both women with and without HIV and cervical cancer was lower than would be expected in most high-income countries. More recently, a prospective cohort study of 231 Botswanan WWH and cervical cancer indicated that larger improvement in CD4[+] T-cell count was significantly associated with lower mortality (Grover et al., 2020). Regarding newer therapies, a phase 3 trial that includes WWH in South Africa indicates that standard chemoradiotherapy with modulated electrohyperthermia (a noninvasive intervention using 13.56 MHz radiofrequency treatment) is effective for disease control of locally advanced cervical cancer and 6-month local disease-free survival (Minaar et al., 2019).

Prevention

There are currently three US Food and Drug Administration (FDA)-approved HPV vaccines: bivalent, quadrivalent, and nine-valent. All three prevent HPV-16 and HPV-18 infections and prevent precancers (and likely cancers) caused by HPV-16 and HPV-18. In addition, the quadrivalent and nine-valent HPV vaccines prevent HPV-6 and HPV-11 infections and genital warts attributed these types. The nine-valent vaccine also prevents infection and precancers attributed to five additional types (31, 33, 45, 52, and 58). The CDC currently recommends the HPV vaccine for PWH 9–26 years old. For individuals 9–14 years old, the vaccine can be given as two doses 6–12 months apart (CDC, 2021). Older individuals should receive the three-dose series (0, 2, and 6 months). Although the CDC has not yet released recommendations for older individuals, the FDA has approved the HPV vaccine for individuals aged up to 45 years old. Additionally, starting ART early likely reduces the risk of high-risk HPV infection and cervical cancer development.

EPIDEMIOLOGY OF HIV-ASSOCIATED ANAL INTRAEPITHELIAL NEOPLASIA

Unlike cervical HPV infection, which peaks in the third decade in women, anal HPV infection is highly prevalent throughout adult life among MSM well into the sixth decade (Chin-Hong et al., 2004; Schiffman & Kjaer, 2003). HPV-16 is the most common type of high-risk HPV among people with or without HIV (Lin & Chen, 2018). In a meta-analysis of 31 studies, Machalek showed that the pooled prevalence of anal HPV detected by PCR was 89% in men with HIV compared to 53.6% in men without HIV ($p = 0.047$) (Machalek et al., 2012). In addition, the prevalence of HPV-16 and HPV-18, associated with high-grade neoplasia and malignancy, was also significantly higher in men with compared to men without HIV.

Several studies report increasing prevalence of anal intraepithelial neoplasia (AIN) among men and women with HIV (Hessol et al., 2013; Islami et al., 2017; Palefsky, 2017). A recent multicenter trial reported a 27% prevalence of anal HSIL among women with HIV (Stier et al., 2020). Palefsky and colleagues (2001) found that the RR of developing HSIL was 3.7 for MSM with HIV compared MSM without HIV. Several studies indicate that between 41% and 97% of men with HIV have anal dysplasia on anal Pap smear screening (Kiviat et al., 2002; Palefsky et al., 2001; Piketty et al., 2008).

EPIDEMIOLOGY OF HIV-ASSOCIATED SQUAMOUS CELL CANCER OF THE ANUS

HIV seropositivity is associated with an increased incidence of anal cancer in both men (HR 20.73; 95% CI: 15.60–27.56) and women (HR 12.88; 95% CI: 8.69–19.07) (Michaud et al., 2020). Even before the HIV epidemic, anal cancer incidence among MSM was estimated to be as high as approximately 35 cases per 100,000 py. This rate is comparable to the incidence of cervical cancer in the United States before the advent of routine cervical cytology (Daling et al., 1987; Melbye et al., 1994). In the 1960s, the annual incidence of SCCA among men in the United States was relatively low and stable, with approximately 0.5 cases per 100,000 persons. Since then, studies have shown a steady increase. A US population-based analysis of the SEER program data found that the incidence of SCCA in the United States among men increased from 1.06 per 100,000 persons from 1973 to 1979 to 2.04 per 100,000 persons from 1996 to 2004 (Johnson et al., 2004).

Many studies have shown that the incidence of SCCA is higher in PWH. In a meta-analysis, researchers examined nine studies published before November 2011 reporting anal cancer incidence in MSM (Machalek et al., 2012). Six were linkage studies based on data obtained from HIV/AIDS and cancer registries, and three were observational cohort studies. The incidence of anal cancer was significantly higher in men with than without HIV ($p = 0.011$). This result has been mirrored in several studies in the United States and Europe, which show that the incidence of anal cancer among PWH ranges from 42 to 137 cases per 100,000 py, a rate 30–100-times higher than that of the general population (D'Souza et al., 2008; Patel et al., 2008; Piketty et al., 2008). Anal cancer incidence may be higher in Black MSM with HIV; one multicenter study found a weighted HR of 2.37 (95% CI: 1.17–4.82) compared to non-Black MSM (McNeil et al., 2022).

SCCA may be overlooked in the female population; however, the rate of HPV-related anal cancers among women appears to be higher than that in men (1.8 vs. 1.2 per 100,000 persons) (CDC, 2012). Other publications have found incidence rates as high as 18–30 per 100,000 persons (Piketty et al., 2012; Silverberg et al., 2012). Incidence of anal cancer in WWH in higher income countries is also high (3.9–30 per 100,000 persons) (Stier et al., 2015). Women with CD4$^+$ T-cell counts of less than 200 cells/mm^3 have a nearly 15-fold higher risk of developing invasive SCCA compared to the general population (SIR 14.5; 95% CI: 8.8–22.4) (Chaturvedi et al., 2009). Like the effects of HPV on cervical endothelium, the virus can lead to high-grade precancerous lesions and anal cancer. A systematic review of SCCA in women revealed higher prevalence of HPV in the anus versus cervix in most studies reviewed (16%–85% vs. 17%–70%, respectively) and that concordant HPV genotypes were found in 9%–16% of women. Risk factors for anal HPV included cervical HPV, low CD4$^+$ T-cell count, smoking, and perianal warts (Stier et al., 2015). Further, Machalek and colleagues found that the incidence of anal cancer was higher in the ART era. For example, from 1996 onward, the annual incidence of SCCA was 78 per 100,000 persons compared to 22 per 100,000 persons prior to this time. The reason for this increase is unclear. Improved survival associated with ART may allow for sufficient time for men with chronic HPV infection to develop anal cancer. Increases in screening are unlikely to explain this trend because routine screening is not yet currently recommended or routinely implemented in most clinical practice settings (Machalek et al., 2012). However, risk factors associated with SCCA have been shown to be associated with greater immunosuppression, including nadir CD4$^+$ T-cell count and median HIV RNA levels of greater than 500,000 copies/mL (Guiguet et al., 2009). A recent meta-analysis evaluating publications from 1996 to 2018 indicates that, though PWH have higher anal cancer-related mortality than people without HIV, the overall survival and anal cancer-specific survival HRs were not significantly different between the two groups (Sumner et al., 2021).

SCREENING, TREATMENT, AND PREVENTION OF HIV-ASSOCIATED ANAL DYSPLASIA

As discussed previously, PWH are at an increased risk for SCCA and AIN. While no national screening protocol for anal cancer is available yet, national recommendations are anticipated to be published soon, and the New York State Department of Health AIDS Institute published guidelines for screening for anal dysplasia and cancer in adults with HIV in 2022 (Hirsch et al., 2022). SCCA shares many biologic similarities with cervical cancer, including detectable dysplastic precursor lesions and high-risk HPV infection. In women, abnormal cervical cytology results are a risk factor for abnormal anal cytology results, though women may have anal dysplasia without concomitant cervical disease. Some studies show a higher prevalence of HPV-related anal disease than HPV-related cervical disease in women (Gaisa et al., 2017; Kojic et al., 2011; Liu et al., 2020). Consequently, many have recommended annual anal Pap screening for PWH (Bosch et al., 1995), and the New York State Department of Health AIDS Institute recommends annual screening for all PWH ≥35 years old for HPV-related anal disease (Hirsch et al., 2022). Anal Pap smears are acquired by randomly obtaining squamous cells from the anal canal using a Dacron swab. They are then fixed in liquid cytology media. Like cervical cytology protocols, abnormal anal cytologic findings are confirmed by high-resolution anoscopy-directed biopsy of visualized lesions (Figure 29.1). Screening via HPV molecular testing remains controversial because of the high prevalence of high-risk HPV infection in PWH (Benevolo et al., 2016; Berry et al., 2009). However, presence of high-risk HPV genotype 16 is associated with concurrent high-grade anal lesions in WWH (Heard et al., 2015, 2016). One study in which high-resolution anoscopy was performed on 156 PWH who tested negative for high-risk HPV by anal swab found that an approximately 8% risk of anal precancer remains for PWH who test high-risk HPV negative by anal swab (Wang et al., 2020). Anal cytology is categorized according to the Bethesda system for cervical cytology: ASCUS, low-grade squamous intraepithelial lesion, and HSIL. The New York State Health Department AIDS Institute recommends HPV testing only for PWH with anal cytology results of ASCUS (Hirsch et al., 2022); if HPV testing is negative then anal cytology should be repeated in lone year, and if HPV testing is positive for high-risk HPV, then the patient should be referred for high- resolution anoscopy. Anal Pap smears have a similar sensitivity and specificity as cervical Pap smears. Note that there are no definitive clinical studies showing that anal Pap smears decrease SCCA-related morbidity and mortality among PWH, though studies evaluating this and

related questions, such as the Anal Cancer/HSIL Outcomes Research (ANCHOR) study, are underway (Lee et al., 2022). Further, anal cytology should not be performed if evaluation with high-resolution anoscopy is not available for the patient. Women with a history of cervical or vulvar neoplasias are more likely to have anal HPV infection and abnormal anal cytology (Stier et al., 2015). The presence of anal warts or condyloma acuminata may also be an indicator for HPV infection of the anal canal and may warrant further screening. High-risk patients should be followed every 6 months for at least 5 years, ideally with periodic photographic documentation of the perianal region. There should be a low threshold to repeat biopsies of any changing lesion. Per the New York State Health Department AIDS Institute recommendations, anal cancer screening may be stopped for PWH with life expectancy less than 10 years and for non–sexually active PWH with two consecutive negative anal cytology specimens (Hirsch et al., 2022).

There is a lack of consensus and rigorous evidence regarding recommendations for performing annual digital rectal exam (DRE) in patients at risk for SCCA, such as MSM. The 2020 European AIDS Clinical Society (EACS) guidelines recommend DRE with or without an anal Pap smear every 1–3 years in MSM (EACS, 2021). The 2020 Guidelines for Prevention and Treatment of Opportunistic Infections in HIV-positive Adults and Adolescents suggest that annual DRE is only a class B, grade III recommendation (DHHS, 2022b). Most recently, the guidelines published by the New York State Department of Health AIDS Institute recommend annual DRE for all PWH aged ≥35 years old, to be used concomitantly with annual anal cytology. A phase 2 clinical trial assessed the feasibility of teaching MSM to recognize palpable masses in the anal canal using self or partner exams (Nyitray et al., 2018). Results indicated that tumors 3 mm or larger may be detectable by self or partner exams, which is significant as there is a high cure rate for tumors 10 mm or smaller.

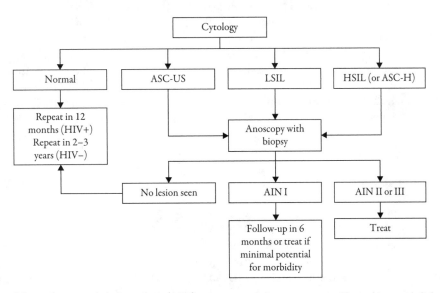

Figure 29.1 Screening protocol for anal intraepithelial neoplasia (AIN) Recommended screening protocol for anal intraepithelial neoplasia. ASC-H, atypical squamous cells, cannot rule out HSIL; ASC-US, atypical squamous cells of undetermined significance; HSIL, high-grade squamous intraepithelial lesion; LSIL, low-grade squamous intraepithelial lesion. SOURCE: Park IU, et al. *Curr Infect Dis Rep*. 2010 March;12(2):126–133.

Treatment

The surveillance of patients with AIN II and III is predominantly aimed at the identification of early invasive carcinoma that can be treated by local excision or localized chemo-/immune-therapy and/or radiation. Little data exist regarding the management of AIN, but it is thought that, like CIN, if AIN can be eradicated, then malignant transformation can be prevented. This is supported by results of the ANCHOR study (Palefsky et al., 2022) (NCT02135419). The ANCHOR study assigned more than 4,000 men aged 35 years and older with HIV and biopsy-proven anal HSIL to receive either HSIL treatment (which included office-based ablative procedures, ablation or excision under anesthesia, or the administration of topical fluorouracil or imiquimod) or active monitoring without treatment. This study found that, with a median follow-up of 25.8 months, 9 participants progressed to anal cancer in the treatment group (173 per 100,000 py; 95% CI: 90–332) and 21 in the active-monitoring group (402 per 100,000 py; 95% CI: 262–616). Targeted biopsies using high-resolution anoscopy and 3% acetic acid to the anal canal mucosa (like colposcopy) can help identify areas of AIN.

Treatment options for anal dysplasia are similar for people with and without HIV. These include topical trichloroacetic acid, liquid nitrogen, imiquimod, fluorouracil, infrared coagulation, electrocautery, carbon dioxide (CO_2) laser, and surgical excision. One randomized trial of 156 MSM with HIV showed that electrocautery is better than imiquimod and fluorouracil in the treatment of AIN but recognized that recurrence rates were substantial (Richel et al., 2013). Of note, there are several new therapies being evaluated for PWH with anal dysplasia. These include two Australian studies: a phase 2 trial evaluating the immunomodulator pomalidomide in anal HSIL (NCT03113942) and a phase 1 study evaluating a new topical drug with direct anti-HPV activity, ABI-1968 (NCT03202992).

The recommended treatment for PWH with anal cancer is the same as that recommended for the general population (Reid et al., 2018). In the general population, concurrent chemoradiotherapy with 5-fluorouracil (5-FU) infusion and mitomycin (or cisplatin) has been established as the standard-of-care regimen for nonmetastatic anal cancer (Leiker et al., 2020). In the ART era, reports on clinical outcomes of PWH with anal cancer have been conflicting. Some studies have shown that people with and without HIV had comparable disease control and survival (Blazy et al., 2005; Chiao et al., 2008; Fraunholz et al., 2011), whereas others have suggested that PWH (particularly those with increased time between anal cancer diagnosis and treatment and those with lower posttreatment CD4 [+] T-cell counts) may do worse in terms of treatment-related toxicity and/or an increased risk for local relapse (Grew et al., 2015; Oehler-Janne, 2008; Susko et al., 2020). Existing evidence is limited by mostly retrospective data as well as small numbers of patients studied, thus further investigation into this question is needed.

Prevention

Routine vaccination with quadrivalent HPV or the 9-valent HPV vaccine is now available for all individuals aged 9–45 years to prevent genital warts and the development of precancerous and cancerous HPV-mediated lesions. The CDC's Advisory Committee on Immunization Practices, however, still does not recommend routine vaccination of persons aged older than 26 years. Starting ART early likely reduces the risk of high-risk HPV infection and anal cancer development (Kelly et al., 2020).

EFFECT OF ART ON ANAL DYSPLASIA

Like studies evaluating the effect of ART on cervical dysplasia, studies evaluating the effect of ART on anal dysplasia have found conflicting results. This may be related to the significant design and methodological differences among these studies. There are two small case series ($n = 4$ and 26 patients, respectively) describing outcomes of HIV-associated SCCA, with 5-year survival rates of 47%–60% (Jephcott et al., 2004; Myerson et al., 2001). In studies that specifically compared survival among patients with SCCA in the pre-ART versus ART eras, there was a nonsignificant trend toward improved survival, better tolerability of chemoradiotherapy, and improved local tumor control in the ART era (Bower et al., 2004; Cleator et al., 2000; Stadler et al., 2004).

A study linking the New York State cancer registry with the New York City HIV/AIDS registry found that in the early ART era (1990–1996), the 24-month survival was 76% for patients with AIDS compared to 78% for patients without AIDS, suggesting that, at least during this time period, PWH with SCCA had equivalent survival with patients without HIV.

Palefsky and colleagues (2001) compared the rates of progression and regression of anal dysplasia after 6 months of ART. They found that the likelihood of lesion progression or regression was not affected by ART initiation, but they noted that, among the individuals starting ART at higher CD4 [+] T-cell counts, ART demonstrated a nonsignificant benefit on anal dysplasia lesions. In contrast, Wilkin and colleagues (2004) conducted a cross-sectional study evaluating anal HPV infection and anal dysplasia in 98 men with HIV. In a multivariate analysis, they found that ART and higher nadir CD4 [+] T-cell count were significantly protective for anal dysplasia by histology but were not protective of anal HPV infection. A Canadian study retrospectively evaluated 1,691 MSM with HIV and found that immunosuppression with nadir CD4 [+] T-cell count of less than 100 cells/mm^3 was a risk factor for anal cancer (OR 3.08; $p = 0.01$). They also found that men treated during the pre-ART era had a higher incidence (370 vs. 93 per 100,000 py) and shorter lead time to development of anal cancer compared to those in the post-ART era (Duncan et al., 2015). Therefore, it remains unclear if ART initiation influences the natural history of AIN in PWH. However, ART is beneficial for men undergoing treatment for HPV-related disease.

RECOMMENDED READING

Brandão M, Bruzzone M, Franzoi MA, et al. Impact of HIV infection on baseline characteristics and survival of women with breast cancer. *AIDS*. 2021;35(4):605–618. http://doi:10.1097/QAD.0000000000002810. PMID: 33394680.

Grover S, Mehta P, Wang Q, et al. Association between CD4 count and chemoradiation therapy outcomes among cervical cancer patients with HIV. *J Acquir Immune Defic Syndr*. 2020;85(2):201–208. http://doi:10.1097/QAI.0000000000002420

Hirsch BE, McGowan JP, Fine SM, et al. *Screening for anal dysplasia and cancer in adults with HIV*. Baltimore, MD: Johns Hopkins University; 2022.

Kojic EM, Kang M, Cespedes MS, et al. Immunogenicity and safety of the quadrivalent human papillomavirus vaccine in HIV-1-infected women. *Clin Infect Dis*. 2014;59(1):127–135.

Lee JY, Lensing SY, Berry-Lawhorn JM, et al. Design of the Anal Cancer/HSIL Outcomes Research study (ANCHOR study): a randomized study to prevent anal cancer among persons living with HIV. *Contemp Clin Trials*. February 2022;113:106679. http://doi:10.1016/j.cct.2022.106679

Leiker AJ, Wang CJ, Sanford NN, et al. Feasibility and outcome of routine use of concurrent chemoradiation in PLWH with squamous cell anal cancer. *Am J Clin Oncol*. 2020;43(10):701–708. http://doi:10.1097/COC.0000000000000736

McNeil CJ, Lee JS, Cole SR, et al. Anal cancer incidence in men with HIV who have sex with men: are Black men at higher risk? *AIDS*. 2022 Apr 1;36(5):657–664. http://doi:10.1097/QAD.0000000000003151

Palefsky JM, Lee JY, Jay N, et al. Treatment of anal high-grade squamous intraepithelial lesions to prevent anal cancer. *N Engl J Med*. June 16, 2022;386(24):2273–2282. http://doi:10.1056/NEJMoa2201048

Piketty C, Selinger-Leneman H, Grabar S, et al. Marked increase in the incidence of invasive anal cancer among HIV-infected patients despite treatment with combination antiretroviral therapy. *AIDS (London)*. 2008;22(10):1203–1211.

Rohner E, Bütikofer L, Schmidlin K, et al. Cervical cancer risk in women living with HIV across four continents: A multicohort study. *Int J Cancer*. 2020;146(3):601–609. http://doi:10.1002/ijc.32260

Smith AJB, Varma S, Rositch AF, et al. Gynecologic cancer in HIV-positive women: a systematic review and meta-analysis. *Am J Obstet Gynecol*. 2019;221(3):194–207. http://doi:10.1016/j.ajog.2019.02.022

Stelzle D, Tanaka LF, Lee KK, et al. Estimates of the global burden of cervical cancer associated with HIV. *Lancet Glob Health*. 2021;9(2):e161–e169. http://doi:10.1016/S2214-109X(20)30459-9

Stier EA, Sebring MC, Mendez AE, et al. Prevalence of anal human papillomavirus infection and anal HPV-related disorders in women: a systematic review. *Am J Ob Gyn*. 2015;213(3):278–309.

Sumner L, Kamitani E, Chase S, Wang Y. A systematic review and meta-analysis of mortality in anal cancer patients by HIV status. *Cancer Epidemiol*. 2022;76:102069. http://doi:10.1016/j.canep.2021.102069

LUNG CANCER

LEARNING OBJECTIVES

- Review the epidemiology and risks of lung cancer in PWH.

- Review the pathogenesis of lung cancer.

- Discuss the treatment of lung cancer.

- Discuss the treatment outcomes and mortality associated with lung cancer in PWH.

WHAT'S NEW?

- PWH have an increasing incidence of lung cancer during the ART era.

- Surgery, chemotherapy, and radiation are mainstays of standard treatment for PWH.

- Treatment disparities between people with and without HIV may contribute to poor survivability of those with lung cancer.

KEY POINTS

- Tobacco cessation is of utmost importance in preventing lung cancers in PWH.

- PWH have a higher incidence of lung cancer than the general population, although a predominant histology of non–small cell lung cancer (NSCLC) is common in both groups.

- PWH have worse survival, which may be due to frequent presentation with advanced disease.

- No specific guidelines for treating PWH and lung cancer exist, and more rigorous studies evaluating standards of care are needed.

Lung cancer is the leading cause of death attributed to cancer in the general US population, and it also represents the most common NADC (Frisch et al., 2001). Lung cancers in HIV are primarily non-small cell cancer (NSCLC) types, including adenocarcinoma and squamous cell carcinoma. This largely reflects the trend of histology types among the general population in Western settings (Cadranel et al., 2006). Mortality from lung cancer remains high in PWH compared to the general population, especially for patients presenting at advanced stages (Coghill et al., 2015; Shiels et al., 2010a).

The incidence of lung cancer, like that of other NADCs, has increased for several reasons, including increased life expectancy in the era of ART and longer cumulative exposure to carcinogens known to be associated with lung cancer development, namely tobacco smoke. Notably, tobacco exposure in the HIV population remains a significant health problem, with disproportionate use compared to the general population (Altekruse et al., 2018; Clifford et al., 2012; Rahmanian et al., 2011). Because of this increased risk, smoking cessation is of utmost importance (Shepherd et al., 2018). Immunosuppression may also be a contributing factor; however, this relationship is not clearly understood.

The US Preventive Services Task Force (USPSTF) recommends screening for lung cancer using chest CT in individuals aged 50–80 years with a ≥20-pack-year smoking history. Optimal screening criteria for PWH are unknown, but health care providers should follow the USPSTF recommendations for the general population while this question is studied further (Sellers et al., 2022).

EPIDEMIOLOGY OF LUNG CANCER IN HIV

Engels and colleagues examined data from large HIV and cancer registries in the United States to estimate the incidence of lung cancer. They found the incidence in the population with HIV to be 59 per 100,000 py during a period from 1991 to 2002 (Engels et al., 2008). This same study found that the incidence of lung cancer increased from 51 per 100,000 py to 126 per 100,000 py between people with HIV compared to people with AIDS diagnosis (Engels et al., 2008). In another study including Canadian data, researchers found that, from 1996 to 2009, the incidence of lung cancer in PWH was 129 per 100,000 py compared to 45.4 per 100,000 py in people without HIV. The incidence of lung cancer was higher for persons aged 75 years than for those aged 65 years (3.4% vs. 2.2%), which supports the increased risk of cancer development as the population ages (Silverberg et al., 2015). Researchers evaluated a Californian cohort of 24,768 PWH compared to 257,600 people without HIV between 1996 and 2011 and found that the lung cancer rate was 66 per 100,000 py for PWH and 33 per 100,000 py for people without HIV (rate ratio 2.0; 95% CI: 1.7–2.2) (Marcus et al., 2017).

A Ugandan study evaluating overall cancer incidence (ADC and NADCs) in PWH from 1988 to 2002 found the incidence over time to be increased, with a SIR of 5 (Mbulaiteye et al., 2006). Another study using the Swiss HIV Cohort Study and the Swiss Cancer Registries found that cancers of the trachea, lung, and bronchus were significantly elevated compared to those of the general population, with a SIR of 3.2 (Clifford et al., 2005).

The impact of ART on the incidence and risk of lung cancer remains unclear. Studies attempting to evaluate the incidence of lung cancer during the pre-ART and ART eras have found mixed results, with increased incidence in both eras. The previously cited study by Silverberg and colleagues (2015) showed that cumulative incidence of lung cancer in North America continues to increase in the ART era. They found a cumulative incidence of 3.7% from 2005 to 2009 compared to 1.8% from 1996 to 2009. Another study that examined data from 34 states showed similar results, with a steady increase in the number of lung cancers (35 to 283 cases) from 1991 to 2005, which largely occurred in persons older than 50 years (Shiels et al., 2011a). This phenomenon speaks to the increasing longevity of the population with HIV and accumulation of malignant comorbidities.

RISK FACTORS ASSOCIATED WITH LUNG CANCER IN HIV

Risk factors for lung cancer are multiple and include tobacco exposure, injection drug use, and possibly HIV infection itself. Other comorbid pulmonary diseases, such as chronic obstructive pulmonary disease and bacterial pneumonia, are more common in people with than without HIV and may place PWH at higher risk for cancer due to persistent states of inflammation (Crothers et al., 2011; Shebl et al., 2010). Inflammatory markers circulating in the blood have been associated with theoretical risk of lung cancer; these include C-reactive protein, serum amyloid, soluble tumor necrosis factor receptor-2 (sTNFR2), lymphoid differentiation cytokine interleukin-7 (IL-7), and various leukocyte-derived chemokines (Shiels, 2013). However, it remains to be determined exactly how these inflammatory states that are not confounded by smoking or other traditional risks factors like pneumonia impact the risk of lung cancer.

Cigarette smoking has repeatedly been implicated as a major risk factor for lung cancer in the general population as well as in the population with HIV (Altekruse et al., 2018; Shepherd et al., 2018). Prevalence of cigarette smoking among PWH is estimated to be between 42% and 59%, and it greatly exceeds that of the general population by two- to threefold (Altekruse et al., 2018; Mdodo et al., 2015; Tesoriero, 2010). In a Swiss study, Clifford and others reported that all persons with cancer of the respiratory tract were smokers, and there was a threefold higher excess risk of these cancers (Clifford et al., 2005). A similar finding was demonstrated in a US study that showed patients with HIV and lung cancer were 1.3 times more likely to be current or former smokers and to have greater pack-year tobacco consumption history compared to those with HIV but without cancer (D'Jaen et al., 2010). Shiels and colleagues also examined the role of cigarette smoking in the development of lung cancer in HIV. They found that those with HIV who smoked more than 1.43 packs per day had twice the risk of lung cancer compared to those with HIV who smoked less. Compared to patients without HIV who smoked less than 1.43 packs per day, those with HIV and who smoked more than 1.43 packs per day had a 7.2 times higher risk of developing lung cancer (Shiels et al., 2010a). A more recent study using the NAACCRD. A more recent study using the North (NA-ACCORD) consortium evaluated 52,441 PWH including 2,306 who were diagnosed with cancer between 2000 and 2015 (Altekruse et al., 2018). They found that PWH diagnosed with cancer were more likely to have been smokers (79%) compared to those without cancer (73%). Further, in PWH, smoking was associated with increased risk of cancer overall (HR 1.33; 95% CI: 1.18–1.49), smoking-related cancers (HR 2.31; CI: 1.80–2.98), and lung cancer (HR 17.80; CI: 5.60–56.63). Researcher recently used an HIV microsimulation model to evaluate cumulative lung cancer mortality by smoking exposure and found that PWH who continue to smoke have a 16.6–29.8% estimated mortality depending on sex and smoking intensity, while estimated mortality decreased to 3.7%–7.9% for those who quit smoking and to 1.2%–1.6% for never smokers (Reddy et al., 2017). Even PWH who were adherent to ART were 6–13 times more likely to die from lung cancer than from traditional AIDS-related causes. When the authors applied this model to the current US population with HIV, they found that 9.3% could die from lung cancer if their smoking habits do not change.

Other studies have not found the same association with smoking. In one, researchers studied 5,238 PWH and found that the overall smoking-adjusted SIR for lung cancer was 2.5 times higher than that of the general population (95% CI: 1.6–3.5) (Engels et al., 2006). However, in an analysis that assumed that all participants smoked, the smoking-adjusted SIR was only 1.7. This suggests that smoking did not account for all excess risk of lung cancer in HIV (Engels et al., 2006). In the mortality analysis by Shiels et al., it was found that, after adjusting for smoking and other patient characteristics, the risk of death was 3.8 times higher for people with versus without HIV (Shiels et al., 2010a). A large Veterans Administration study found that the incidence rate ratio (1.7) of lung cancer in patients with HIV remained significantly elevated after multivariable adjustment for confounders including smoking compared to persons without HIV (Sigel et al., 2012). These studies suggest that, independent of smoking, HIV positivity portends a higher incidence and mortality risk for lung cancer.

Injection drug use (IDU) among PWH has also been associated with an increased risk of lung cancer compared with that for nonusers in several studies. One study demonstrated that those with IDU, with or without HIV, had an increased risk of lung cancer, with SIRs of 14.3 and 6.2, respectively (Serraino et al., 2000). Other studies have found little evidence to support this risk factor, however. In another study that included 2,086 participants (the AIDS Link to the Intravenous Experience Study), IDU was not associated with increased risk of lung cancer (Kirk et al., 2007).

HIV itself may also be associated with the development of lung cancer because of directly acting oncogenic effects. HIV-1 replication depends on Tat protein expression, which can upregulate expression of proto-oncogenes *c-myc, c-fos,* and *c-jun* to enhance cellular proliferation, including human adenocarcinoma cell lines (El-Solh et al., 1997). Allelic loss and changes in microsatellites, which are short tandem repeat DNA sequences, have also been described in other malignancies, such as KS, NHL, and SCCA, and have been found in lung cancers of PWH (Wistuba et al., 1998). These genetic alterations may lead to activation of oncogenes and loss of tumor suppressor genes. However, the lack of HIV viral integration into cellular DNA of somatic neoplastic cells challenges this hypothesis of oncogenesis because cancer cells can have background genetic alterations and immunosuppression can also be associated with microsatellite changes (Bedi et al., 1995). Poor control of HIV also could contribute to the development of lung cancer. A study of PWH included in the US VACS found that increased risk of lung cancer was associated with low CD4$^+$ T-cell count, low CD4/CD8 ratio, high HIV RNA levels, and more cumulative episodes of bacterial pneumonia (Sigel et al., 2017). Another recent study similarly noted that a CD4$^+$ T-cell count of less than 200 cells/mm^3 was associated with a younger age at lung cancer diagnosis (Shiels et al., 2017). In contrast, a large Californian cohort study by Marcus et al. did not find an association between increased development of lung cancer and CD4$^+$ T- cell count of less than 200 cells/mm^3 (Marcus et al., 2017).

Although men historically have been considered at higher risk for lung cancer, women also share a significant proportion of lung cancer diagnoses. This may be due to the increase in women tobacco smokers in the population or the increase in the number of WWH. The WIHS compared data from the National Health and Nutritional Examination (NHANES) II and SEER. Researchers found that WWH have higher lifetime cigarette consumption as well as an elevated SIR of 3 (95% CI: 1.7–5.1) compared to the general population with a SIR of 2.11 (95% CI: 0.25–7.61). Further, these data did not vary by pre-ART versus ART era (Levine et al., 2010). A French study evaluating cancer in PWH in the pre-ART and ART eras found that the SIR of women was three-times higher than that of men in the ART era (6.28 vs. 2.12) (Herida et al., 2003). Several additional studies have shown greater incidence in women with SIR ranging from 1.6 to 16.7 (Calabresi et al., 2013; Clifford et al., 2005; Ramirez-Marrero et al., 2010).

DIAGNOSIS AND CLINICAL PRESENTATION OF LUNG CANCER IN HIV

Despite the increased risk of cancer with aging, PWH and lung cancer tend to be younger. In several studies, age at presentation ranged from 38 to 57 years. This is far below the age of presentation among the general population, which is closer to the seventh decade of life (Winstone et al., 2013). Stage at presentation also tends to be advanced in PWH, with a majority presenting with stages III or IV. This likely contributes to the poor survivability of these patients (Sigel et al., 2012; Winstone et al., 2013).

The majority of histological types mirror those of the general population, with greater than 50% consisting of non-small cell lung cancer (NSCLC.). Adenocarcinoma is the predominant NSCLC (36%), followed by squamous cell carcinoma (30%) (Sigel et al., 2012). Many patients present with advanced disease and have symptoms of persistent cough and chest pain (Karp et al., 1993). Early diagnosis of lung cancer improves prognosis; however, screening with plain chest radiography at any interval has not been shown to be effective and is not recommended. Use of low-dose chest CT (LDCT) may be beneficial in these patients. The recommendation of the US Preventive Services Task Force (USPTF) to screen high-risk patients for lung cancer with LDCT was based on the findings from the National Lung Screening Trial (National Lung Screening Trial Research Team, 2011). This was a large, randomized trial that found a 20% reduction in lung cancer mortality after implementing annual screening by LDCT in patients aged 55–74 years and at least a 30- pack-year smoking history. Because of improved mortality benefit, current USPTF guidelines recommend lung cancer screening with LDCT for people aged 55–80 in the general population with at least a 30 -pack-year smoking history and currently smoke or who have quit within 15 years, regardless of gender (Moyer, 2014). Of note, a handful of studies that have evaluated LDCT in PWH have suggested that these patients, especially those with low CD4$^+$ T-cell counts, are more likely to have false-positive LDCT findings owing prior lung infections (Sigel et al., 2014; Ronit et al., 2017). A recent modeling study evaluating patients with HIV with CD4$^+$ T-cell counts of at least 500 cells/mm^3 found that screening using the Centers for Medicare & Medicaid Services (CMS) criteria (i.e., age 55–77, 30-pack-years of smoking, and current smoker or quit within 15 years of screening) would reduce lung cancer mortality by 18.9% in this population, similar to the mortality reduction of people without HIV (Kong, 2018). Thus, the benefit and cost-effectiveness of LDCT in patients with HIV remain unknown, but following the USPTF and NCCN guidelines for the general population is reasonable after discussing risks (e.g., false positives and radiation exposure) and benefits (e.g., early detection and better prognosis) with patients (Reid et al., 2018). Currently, a French multicenter prospective pilot study (ANRS EP48 HIV-CHEST cohort) is evaluating the utility of LDCT in PWH (NCT01207986) (Makinson et al., 2015).

Understanding the mechanisms underlying the development of lung cancer in PWH could lead to improved lung cancer screening methodologies. Researchers recently studied the molecular mechanisms underlying the gene expression profiles of lung cancer in PWH and identified 758 differentially expressed genes in HIV-associated lung cancer (Zheng et al., 2018). Specifically, they found that the expression levels of SIX1 and TFAP2A mRNA are increased in HIV-associated lung cancer and that expression levels of ADH1B, INMT, and SYNPO2 mRNA are decreased.

TREATMENT OF LUNG CANCER

There are no alternative or specific treatment guidelines for lung cancer in the population with HIV. Most randomized trials for lung cancer have historically excluded PWH because of concerns regarding immune suppression, toxicity, and drug interactions with ART (Persad et al., 2008). Current treatment strategies are mainly with protocols for patients without HIV and depend on tumor histology, stage of disease, and underlying host factors such as comorbidities and pulmonary function. Patients with NSCLC are staged (I–IV) based on the tumor node metastasis system, with stage I disease confined to localized tumor without invasion into the chest wall, diaphragm, mediastinum, or surrounding structures and stage IV indicating metastatic disease (Shepherd et al., 2007). MRI of the brain should also be pursued for stage II or higher to identify intracranial metastasis. For localized, nonmetastatic disease, surgical resection is the preferred strategy with intent to cure those patients able to undergo surgery. Surgery (i.e., lobectomy, sublobular resection, and video-assisted thoracoscopy) may be followed by adjuvant chemotherapy or radiation for those with more advanced stages or invasion (NCCN, 2015b). For nonsurgical candidates, ablation with radiotherapy can be considered. Studies evaluating surgery in PWH have been described in mainly small case control series and case reports. Patients undergoing surgery for localized disease (stage I or stage II) tolerated surgery well with minimal complications (Cadranel et al., 2006).

For patients with advanced NSCLC or recurrence after initial definitive therapy, goals of therapy are largely palliative. For patients with solitary metastasis or recurrence, curative intention with additional surgery or radiotherapy may be indicated and beneficial to help prolong survival. However, risks and benefits must be weighed in advanced disease to avoid undue adverse events and toxicities. Systemic therapy with combination chemotherapy using a platinum-based regimen is the mainstay agent with or without additional agents, such as the VEGF inhibitor bevacizumab (NCCN, 2015b).

While HIV infection is often an exclusion criterion in lung cancer clinical trials, use of chemotherapy for lung cancer treatment in PWH is feasible, and it has been used in patients to treat metastatic disease and as an adjuvant therapy and in combination with radiation for locally advanced disease. One large retrospective study found similar rates of treatment modality between patient with and without HIV (Sigel et al., 2013). Limited data from case series have provided heterogeneous results regarding use of chemotherapeutic agents, efficacy, and drug toxicities in patients with HIV and lung cancer (Bower et al., 2003; Powles et al., 2003; Spano et al., 2004). Recently a French Phase II trial of PWH with advanced nonsquamous NSCLC showed that first-line four-cycle induction with carboplatin plus pemetrexed followed by pemetrexed maintenance was effective and reasonably well tolerated (Lavole et al., 2020). Additional studies to evaluate efficacy, tolerability, and safety of chemotherapy in patients with HIV are needed.

Additional molecular and genetic mutation analysis for potential genetic-directed therapy targets has been explored. These should be performed when possible in patients with advanced-stage NSCLC, namely for the presence of epidermal growth factor receptor (EGFR) and anaplasmic lymphoma kinase (NCCN, 2015b). Other targets include RAS family oncogenes, the mTOR signaling pathway, and the MEK signaling pathway. Treatment with EGFR tyrosine kinase inhibitors such as erlotinib may also be considered for patients with this specific EGFR mutation in the tumor. However, long-term survival has yet to be established with use of these agents (Okuma et al., 2014). Several novel treatment regimens are being studied in PWH with advanced lung cancer. Immunotherapies such as nivolumab, ipilimumab, and durvalumab are being evaluated in PWH and advanced solid tumors, including NSCLC (NCT03304093 and NCT02408861) (Rasmussen et al., 2021) and (Bender-Ignacio et al., 2018; Gonzalez-Cao, 2020) (NCT03094286). Nivolumab as second- or third-line treatment for PWH and NSCLC appears to be well tolerated (Lavole et al., 2021).

SURVIVAL OF LUNG CANCER IN HIV

Survival among PWH and lung cancer is worse compared to that of their counterparts without HIV. Researchers analyzed data from 1996 to 2010 and found that all-cause mortality and cancer-specific mortality risk were respectively 85% and 28% higher for PWH with lung cancer compared to patients without HIV (Coghill et al., 2015). For patients with local-stage NSCLC receiving standard cancer therapy, PWH continued to have greater cancer-related deaths compared to patients without HIV (HR 1.8; 95% CI: 1.21–2.7) (Coghill et al., 2015). Another large study utilizing SEER registry data compared 267 PWH to 1,428 patients without HIV with similar cancer stage and histology of NSCLC (Sigel et al., 2013). Both groups with stage I to IIIA disease received surgery, chemotherapy, and radiotherapy at similar rates. Among the PWH group, 82% died during follow-up compared to 66% of the group without HIV ($p < 0.001$). Median overall survival for PWH was only 6 months compared to 20 months for the cohort without HIV. Overall 5-year survival was also poor for PWH at 9% compared to 23% for the group without HIV. PWH and advanced disease (stage IIIB to IV) had the worst survival, with 9–20 times greater risk of death compared to PWH with only localized disease. Moreover, a major proportion of PWH also died from non-cancer-related causes (31% vs. 9%; $p < 0.001$).

Such disparity in outcomes in the previously discussed studies may be explained by several hypotheses, including the fact that PWH experience overall greater mortality than the general population. It may be that tumors behave more aggressively in PWH due to tumor effect or poor immunological surveillance due to lack of fully intact cellular immunity. Evaluation of the NA-ACCORD dataset found that PWH with a history of an AIDS-defining illness at lung cancer diagnosis had higher mortality and poorer survival after diagnosis compared to those without (Grover et al., 2018). Poor tolerability of surgery and chemotherapy may also contribute to worse outcomes. More studies are needed to clarify these issues.

Last, health disparities in treatment between PWH and populations without HIV may contribute to poor survivability. Data from the Texas Cancer Registry from 1995 to 2009 showed that PWH and NSCLC less frequently received any cancer treatments despite greater numbers presenting at younger ages and with distant-stage disease (Suneja et al., 2013). PWH and local-stage NSCLC were less likely to receive surgery (45.5% vs. 62.5%; $p = 0.04$) than patients without HIV. PWH with regional disease were less likely to receive systemic chemotherapy. For distant disease, PWH received less chemotherapy or radiation (31.1% vs. 45.5%; $p = 0.0009$) (Suneja et al., 2013).

RECOMMENDED READING

Coghill AE, Shiels MS, Suneja G, et al. Elevated cancer-specific mortality among HIV-infected patients in the United States. *J Clin Oncol.* 2015;33(21):2376–2383.

Gonzalez-Cao M, Morán T, Dalmau J, et al. Assessment of the feasibility and safety of durvalumab for treatment of solid tumors in patients with HIV-1 infection: the phase 2 DURVAST study. *JAMA Oncol.* 2020;7:1063–1067. http://doi:10.1001/jamaoncol.2020.0465

Grover S, Desir F, Jing Y, et al. Reduced cancer survival among adults with HIV and AIDS-defining illnesses despite no difference in cancer stage at diagnosis. *J AIDS.* 2018;79(4):421–429.

Lavole A, Greillier L, Mazieres J, et al. First-Line carboplatin plus pemetrexed with pemetrexed maintenance in HIV+ patients with advanced non-squamous non-small cell lung cancer: the phase II IFCT-1001 CHIVA trial. *Eur Respir J.* 2020;56(2):1902066. http://doi:10.1183/13993003.02066-2019

Lavole A, Mazieres J, Schneider S, et al. Assessment of nivolumab in HIV-Infected patients with advanced non-small cell lung cancer after prior chemotherapy. The IFCT-1602 CHIVA2 phase 2 clinical trial. *Lung Cancer.* 2021;158:146–150. http://doi:10.1016/j.lungcan.2021.05.031

Rasmussen TA, Rajdev L, Rhodes A, et al. Impact of anti-PD-1 and anti-CTLA-4 on the human immunodeficiency virus (HIV) reservoir in people living with HIV with cancer on antiretroviral therapy: the AIDS Malignancy Consortium 095 study. *Clin Infect Dis.* 2021;73(7):e1973–e1981. http://doi:10.1093/cid/ciaa1530

Sellers SA, Edmonds A, Ramirez C, et al. Optimal lung cancer screening criteria among persons living with HIV. *J Acquir Immune Defic Syndr.* 2022;90(2):184–192. http://doi:10.1097/QAI.0000000000002930

Sigel K, Crothers K, Dubrow R, et al. Prognosis in HIV-infected patients with non-small cell lung cancer. *Br J Cancer.* 2013;109:1974–1980.

Suneja G, Shiels MS, Melville SK. Disparities in the treatment and outcomes of lung cancer among HIV-infected Individuals. *AIDS.* 2013;27(3):459–468.

PROSTATE CANCER

LEARNING OBJECTIVES

- Review the epidemiology and risk factors for prostate cancer in men with HIV.

- Review the current screening recommendations for prostate cancer.

- Discuss the treatment options for prostate cancer in men with HIV.

WHAT'S NEW?

- Since the advent of prostate-specific antigen (PSA) testing, the incidence of prostate cancer has increased in men with HIV. However, the true incidence may be similar to that of men without HIV.

- Routine prostate cancer screening with PSA testing is not recommended.

KEY POINTS

- Prostate cancer represents a significant burden of neoplastic disease and mortality in men with and without HIV.

- Prostate cancer appears to be associated with states of immunological control.

- Screening with serum PSA testing should not routinely be implemented, having a "D" recommendation by the US Preventive Services Task Force.

- Decision to treat early-stage cancer versus watchful waiting should be carefully considered because evidence of long-term mortality benefits remains unclear.

- First-line therapies include radical prostatectomy and radiation.

Prostate cancer remains the leading cancer diagnosis among men in the United States and other high-income countries. It is the second leading cause of cancer deaths after lung cancer. Increased screening efforts in the United States led to increased incidence after the PSA test became widely available in 1992. However, screening and treatment are controversial because of the occult and often indolent nature of untreated prostate cancer, especially in older men with limited life expectancy. The mortality benefit of diagnosis and treatment of early-stage prostate cancer remains unproved; thus, emphasis on screening and early detection has waned in recent years. Compared to other NADCs, such as lung or anal cancer, some studies have demonstrated HIV infection to be associated with a reduced risk of prostate cancer (Sun, 2021). Regardless, diagnosis of prostate cancer carries a significant clinical impact on patients' sexual, genitourinary, and overall health.

EPIDEMIOLOGY OF PROSTATE CANCER IN HIV

Men with HIV in the United States experienced an increased incidence of prostate cancer after 1990 compared to the preceding decade, from 0.2% to 2.2% of all cancers in a retrospective study of population-based registry data (Engels et al., 2006). In the same study, the incidence increased during the pre-ART and post-ART eras, which may be explained by the introduction of the PSA screening test. Another study that was a large retrospective review also found that prostate cancer in men with HIV increased during the time from 1992 to 2003 (Patel et al., 2008). However, the group with HIV had significantly lower rates of cancer compared to the general population in the pre-ART era (15 vs. 47 per 100,000 py) and the ART era (38 vs. 61 per 100,000 py) (Patel et al., 2008). Another study that examined the PSA testing era (1992 to 2007) found an incidence of 28 per 100,000 py in men with HIV. However, the incidence in men with HIV compared to the expected rate in the general population during this same time period was significantly reduced, with a SIR of only 0.5 (95% CI: 0.44–0.57) (Shiels et al., 2010b). More recently, a study of the VACS between 2000 and -2015 found lower rates of PSA screening and prostate biopsies among PWH compared to the HIV-negative group (Leapman et al., 2022). Prostate cancer incidence was similar in both groups (IRR 0.93; 95% CI: 0.86–1.01). Of note, some disparity remains when prostate cancer diagnoses are compared among races. One study that evaluated men enrolled in the MACS from 1996 to 2010 found an incidence of 169 per 100,000 py among all men 40–70 years old compared to 276 per 100,000 py among African American men with HIV (Dutta et al., 2017). In this study prostate cancer risk was similar by HIV status (IRR 1.0; 95% CI: 0.55–1.82), but nearly threefold higher in African Americans compared to non-African Americans in adjusted models (IRRs 2.66 and 3.22; 95% CI: 1.36–5.18 and 1.27–8.16 for all or men with HIV, respectively).

RISK FACTORS FOR PROSTATE CANCER

Postulated risk factors that promote development of prostate cancer in men with HIV include exposure to carcinogens and use of androgen supplementation to treat hypogonadism. Coinfection with oncogenic viruses may also promote neoplasia (Montgomery et al., 2006). Chronic inflammatory states promoted by HIV systemically and localized to the prostate, as well as chronic prostatitis may contribute to cancer development (Leport et al., 1989; Smith et al., 2004).

Prostate cancer and risk of death have been associated with tobacco exposure in several studies. However, other studies have demonstrated conflicting data. Two large meta-analyses examined this issue and found similar results (Huncharek et al., 2010; Islami et al., 2014). Huncharek and colleagues found a dose-dependent relationship with incidence of prostate cancer in patients without HIV. The heaviest smokers had a 13% increased risk of cancer. These data were derived from seven7 prospective cohort studies. Based on 19 prospective studies, Islami and colleagues (2014) found smoking to be associated with an increased risk of death (RR 1.24) from prostate cancer, which was dose-dependent. The incidence of prostate cancer, however, was not statistically significant overall. In fact, baseline cigarette smoking was inversely associated with incidence of prostate cancer.

Unlike other malignancies in HIV, immunological control with increasing $CD4^+$ T-cell count has been associated with increased risk of prostate cancer, with a RR that is threefold greater in the ART era (Shiels et al., 2010b). In several studies, men with HIV and prostate cancer had robust $CD4^+$ T-cell counts of greater than 300 cells/mm^3 (Hsiao et al., 2009; Marcus et al., 2014; Pantanowitz et al., 2008). Overall, data from numerous studies suggest that variations in prostate cancer deficits in men with HIV are due to differential PSA screening in this population and not to immunologic status.

PROSTATE CANCER SCREENING

The primary tools for diagnosis of prostate cancer include serum PSA measurement, DRE, and, ultimately, prostate biopsy for definitive histologic diagnosis. Both European and US guidelines have recommended against routine screening with PSA in men regardless of HIV status (Heidenreich et al., 2014; Moyer et al., 2012). Rather, whether to perform individual screening with PSA for early detection should be a well-informed, mutual decision between physician and patient based on possible benefits and harms of a positive PSA test. Optimal interval of PSA screening has also not been established. DRE alone has limited sensitivity (6%–8%) of detecting prostate cancer (Gosselaar et al., 2009; Okotie et al., 2007). The combination of an abnormal DRE versus normal DRE with PSA level of higher than 3 ng/mL may enhance positive predictive value of cancer detection at 48% versus 22% (Gosselaar et al., 2008).

CLINICAL PRESENTATION

Prostate cancer diagnosis in HIV often occurs in the fifth and sixth decades of life, and patients often have a family history of prostate cancer (Hsiao et al., 2009; Ong et al., 2015; Shiels et al., 2010b). Men with HIV may present more often with late-stage disease compared to the general population, although this is supported by limited data (Shiels et al., 2015). A large California cohort found more localized cancer compared to regional or distant disease among men with HIV (88% vs. 7%), which was similar to the pattern found in men without HIV (Marcus et al., 2014). Other studies have found no difference in presentation with early or advanced disease (Hsiao et al., 2009; Riedel et al., 2015a). African Americans without HIV have a greater likelihood of presenting with advanced-stage prostate cancer in the general population (Siegel et al., 2012). Within the HIV population, African Americans may represent a higher risk group for prostate cancer because they comprise a large proportion of HIV prevalence and annual HIV diagnoses in the United States.

TREATMENT AND TREATMENT OUTCOMES OF PROSTATE CANCER

Treatment of prostate cancer in men with HIV is similar to that of men without HIV and is based on stage and grade of disease with use of the Gleason score (ranging from 2 to 10). For localized disease (stage I and stage II) not spread to lymph nodes or distant sites, strategies include active surveillance (PSA monitoring and/or repeat biopsy), radical prostatectomy, or radiation therapy (external beam radiation therapy (EBRT) and/or brachytherapy) with or without androgen deprivation. For locally advanced disease (stage III) that has spread outside the prostate gland, surgery or radiation with androgen deprivation therapy are alternatives. A Gleason score greater than 8 represents high-risk neoplasia, even if disease is localized. The optimal choice between surgical intervention and radiation is unclear for these patients, and careful consideration of individual risks and benefits should be discussed on a case-by-case basis (Grimm et al., 2012).

Treatment of disseminated disease, which often involves osteoblastic lesions, typically involves androgen deprivation therapy, castration (medical or surgical), and systemic chemotherapy. Two phase 3 trials examining the use of abiraterone and enzalutamide for treatment of metastatic, castration-resistant prostate cancer have shown clinical benefit with these agents, which target the androgen-synthesis pathway (Loriot et al., 2015; Ryan et al., 2015). Chemotherapy with taxane-based regimens has also shown success in prolonging survival in men with castration-resistant prostate cancer. Docetaxel plus prednisone is currently the standard, initial cytotoxic chemotherapy used in metastatic, castration-resistant disease (Berthold et al., 2008).

Few studies have evaluated the safety, tolerability, and efficacy of treatments for prostate cancer in men with HIV. Most studies have been small and limited to evaluation of EBRT with heterogeneity of dosing. One Veterans Administration study reported 15 patients who received an EBRT dose-escalation approach (75.6 Gy to 79.2 Gy) for localized disease. Of the 15 patients, 13 were treated with concomitant ART, and the 5-year event-free survival was 92.3% (Schreiber et al., 2014). Toxicities included urinary frequency and rectal bleeding. Eight patients on ART had a transient decline in CD4$^+$ T-cell count, which returned to near or above baseline in the follow-up period. Another study evaluating EBRT (72 Gy to 81 Gy) for localized prostate cancer in men with HIV compared to men without HIV found that 26% of men with HIV had biochemical failure compared to 12% of matched controls without HIV. At a mean of 36 months, there were no deaths in the HIV group. Genitourinary and anal adverse events were overall mild (Kahn et al., 2012).

The risk of death from prostate cancer is associated with advanced disease compared to local or regional prostate cancer (Shiels et al., 2010b). In a large retrospective study of HIV and cancer registries from 1996 to 2010, mortality of prostate cancer was significantly higher for men with HIV compared to that of men without HIV (HR 1.57; 95% CI: 1.02–2.41) even after adjusting for patient characteristics and cancer stage (Coghill et al., 2015). Cancer deaths were also greater in men with HIV after adjusting for treatment but not significantly so (HR 1.64; 95% CI: 0.93–2.89). One study that used data from 1996 to 2002 found a 2.1-fold increased risk of death from prostate cancer in men with HIV compared to men without HIV. Interestingly, in this study, men with HIV had more localized disease (Marcus et al., 2014).

RECOMMENDED READING

Coghill AE, Shiels MS, Suneja G, et al. Elevated cancer-specific mortality among HIV-infected patients in the United States. *J Clin Oncol*. 2015;33(21):2376–2383.

Leapman MS, Stone K, Wadia R, et al. Prostate cancer screening and incidence among aging persons living with HIV. *J Urol*. 2022;207(2):324–332.

Marcus JL, Chao CR, Leyden WA, et al. Prostate cancer incidence and prostate-specific antigen testing among HIV-positive and HIV-negative men. *J AIDS*. 2014;66:495–502.

Moyer VA. Screening for prostate cancer: US Preventive Services Task Force recommendation statement. *Ann Intern Med*. 2012;157(2):120–135.

Shiels MS, Goedert JJ, Moore RD, et al. Risk of prostate cancer in U.S. men with AIDS. *Cancer Epidemiol Biomarkers Prev*. 2010;19(11):2910–2915.

Sun D, Cao M, Li H, et al. Risk of prostate cancer in men with HIV/AIDS: a systematic review and meta-analysis. *Prostate Cancer Prostatic Dis*. 2021;24(1):24–34. http://doi:10.1038/s41391-020-00268-2

COLORECTAL ADENOCARCINOMA

LEARNING OBJECTIVES

- Review the epidemiology of colorectal cancer in the HIV population.

- Discuss the screening methods for colorectal cancer.

- Review treatment modalities and outcomes in patients with HIV and colorectal cancer.

WHAT'S NEW?

- The incidence of colon cancer has increased in the population with HIV compared to the general population in the ART era, and mortality remains high compared to that of the population without HIV.

- Patients with HIV disproportionately receive less colorectal cancer screening than the general population.

- Standard chemoradiation and surgical approaches for treating colorectal cancer appear to be well tolerated in PWH, although more research is needed in this area.

KEY POINTS

- Colorectal cancer presents a major health and mortality burden in the population with HIV.

- Colorectal cancer presentation occurs often in younger patients and with more advanced disease compared to the general population.

- Significant disparities exist in screening PWH for colorectal cancer compared to patients without HIV.

- Standard treatment includes surgery and neoadjuvant and/or adjuvant chemoradiation.

- Survival is significantly worse compared to that of patients without HIV and colorectal cancer.

In the United States, colorectal cancer (CRC) is the third leading cause of cancer death in the general population for both men and women. It has been the focus of large-scale primary prevention screening efforts to identify patients with early disease (Siegel et al., 2014). NADC such as colorectal adenocarcinoma in the population with HIV have become increasingly recognized as a significant health problem as patients are living longer and may accrue greater risk factors for cancer development. Vigilance for neoplastic processes such as colorectal cancer must be maintained in PWH because they are often diagnosed at advanced stages and can be overlooked because of presentation at a younger age and lack of traditional risk factors such as family history (Chapman et al., 2009; Yegüez et al., 2003). This phenomenon was characterized by early case reports of colorectal adenocarcinoma in PWH. Patients were often males, aged in their 20s to 40s, and with advanced immunosuppression (Cappell et al., 1988; Klugman et al., 1994; Ravalli et al., 1989).

PWH who are considered "average" risk are offered screening less frequently than the general population (Nayudu et al., 2012). Further, disparities in cancer treatment between individuals with and without HIV are also prevalent. PWH are less likely to receive treatment for colon cancer than their counterparts without HIV (Suneja et al., 2013). The lack of screening and treatment is likely to contribute to poorer outcomes and excess mortality in PWH.

EPIDEMIOLOGY OF COLON CANCER IN HIV

PWH have a higher incidence of CRC than the general population. A large US study that examined cancer incidence in PWH compared to the general population from 1992 to 2003 found an increased SIR during the early time period of 1992 to 1995 (39.9 per 100,000 py) compared to the later time period of 2000 to 2003 (66.2 per 100,000 py). During both time periods, the rates were greater than those of the general population (20.4 and 21.1 per 100,000 py, respectively) (Patel et al., 2008). In a more recent study using US and Canadian data from 2006 to 2009, the incidence rate of CRC in PWH was 36.4 per 100,000 py compared to 27.7 per 100,000 py in people without HIV. During this study period, the cumulative incidence declined by 6% per year for patients without

HIV but increased in those with HIV by 5% per year. This may reflect the declining death rate among PWH (Silverberg et al., 2015).

A large Taiwanese study that used the National Health Insurance Research Database from 1998 to 2009 found that, among 1,282 PWH and cancer, the incidence of CRC, excluding anal cancer, was 51 per 100,000 py with a SIR of 5.9 (95% CI: 4.15–8.37). Interestingly, colon cancer was the most common NADC in women, with an incidence of 156 per 100,000 py (Chen et al., 2014). In the US surveillance study using the HIV/AIDS Cancer Match Study registry data from 1991 to 2002, the incidence of CRC, excluding anal cancer, was 15 per 100,000 py (Engels et al., 2008).

Immunosuppression likely plays a role in the epidemiology of CRC, as demonstrated in the previously discussed case reports from the pre-ART era. A study by Silverberg et al. stratified groups by CD4[+] T-cell count and found that those with HIV and less than 200 cells/mm[3] had an 80% higher RR compared to a protective effect of higher CD4[+] T-cell counts (Silverberg et al., 2011). Another study that used flexible sigmoidoscopy for CRC screening in PWH found that patients with duration of HIV of greater than 10 years and CD4[+] T-cell counts of less than 200 cells/mm[3] had greater odds of having distal colon neoplastic lesions compared to those with higher CD4[+] T-cell counts (Bini et al., 2006). On the contrary, many other studies have not shown significant differences in rates among PWH or reduction of CRC in the ART era. Several studies support increases in CRC in the ART era. The lack of reporting of CRC in advanced immunosuppression coupled with the increase in CRC in the ART era may be explained by increased longevity of the population with HIV as well as an increase in screening measures allowing for more diagnoses.

An Australian study that used national HIV and cancer registry data in the pre-ART era evaluated the incidence of cancer among PWH. It did not find significantly increased incidence rates among PWH before and after developing advanced immunosuppression (Gulrich et al., 2002). A prospective study at the University of Alabama at Birmingham followed PWH from 1989 to 2002. It demonstrated an incidence during that period of 60 cases of NADC, with an increase in annual incidence of 0.65 cases per 1,000 py in the pre-ART era and 2.34 cases per 1,000 py in the ART era. Although the study found an increase in the incidence of the RR in the ART era of 3.6 (95% CI: 0.8–16.3), this difference was not statistically significant (Bedimo et al., 2004). These findings can likely be attributed to improved longevity and screening methods in the ART era. However, a lack of information on screening efforts reported in many of these studies is a major limitation in accurately measuring the true incidence of colorectal cancer in the population with HIV.

COLORECTAL CANCER SCREENING IN THE HIV POPULATION

Screening for CRC in PWH reflects that recommended for the general population with normal cancer risk. Normal cancer risk is defined as no personal history of CRC, adenomatous polyps, or inflammatory bowel disease and no first-degree relative with a history of CRC. The US Preventive Services Task Force recommends that for adults with an average risk of CRC, screening with fecal occult blood testing, flexible sigmoidoscopy, or colonoscopy should begin at age 45 years and continue until age 75 years. The current screening interval for colonoscopy is 10 years. These recommendations have been effective for reducing the incidence and mortality of CRC. For those with increased risk, such as an immediate family member with a history of CRC, screening should begin at age 40 years or 10 years prior to the relative's age at onset of CRC, whichever occurs first (Whitlock et al., 2008). Interestingly, even in the general population, screening is underutilized. The CDC found that only 64.5% of screening-eligible people aged 50–75 years surveyed in the Behavioral Risk Factor Surveillance System reported having one of the recommended tests (Joseph et al., 2012).

Screening PWH based on standard guidelines has been more challenging, with significant disparity compared to the general population. A retrospective study in New York identified 565 screening-eligible PWH with average risk and found that only 25% underwent screening colonoscopy within 10 years of the review. The median age was 58 years, and most of these patients had well-controlled HIV compared to those who did not have colonoscopy. Among those who had colonoscopy and biopsy, 32% of biopsies were of tubular adenomas, which exceeds the detection rate of tubular adenomas in the general population for men (34%) and women (27%) (Nayudu et al., 2012). A prospective study performed among New York veterans from 1998 to 2003 sought to describe the prevalence of adenomas or CRC in the distal colon with flexible sigmoidoscopy (Bini et al., 2006). The study included 2,217 controls without HIV and 165 PWH (85.5% on ART and 45.5% with undetectable HIV RNA levels). Among the PWH eligible for CRC screening, 91.9% underwent flexible sigmoidoscopy, which was similar to the percentage who underwent it in the cohort without HIV. More polyps were identified in the group with HIV compared to the control group (30.9% vs. 23%; $p = 0.2$), and polyps in the group with HIV were more likely to have neoplastic features compared to those of the controls (25.5% vs. 13.1%; $p < 0.001$; OR 2.27; 95% CI: 1.57–3.29). The study found that duration of HIV more than 10 years and lower $CD4^+$ T-cell count was significantly associated with having distal neoplasias. Those with positive sigmoidoscopy went on to have full colonoscopy, which showed a higher prevalence of proximal colon neoplastic lesions in the group with HIV compared to the controls without HIV (61.2% vs. 47.8%; $p = 0.07$) (Bini et al., 2006). Although not statistically significant, it appears that PWH are at high risk for malignant potential compared to their counterparts without HIV. Another study comparing CRC screening in PWH and controls demonstrated similar results as those obtained in the New York veterans' study. This study compared 302 PWH to 302 patients without HIV and found that PWH were significantly less likely to have any type of screening modality (55.6% vs. 77.8%; $p < 0.0001$). Undetectable HIV RNA levels, older age, and a family history were variables associated with having at least one CRC screening (Reinhold et al., 2005).

Appropriate use of screening for eligible persons is of utmost importance for PWH because polyps may have more high-risk features than those of the general population. Barriers to colonoscopy referral and screening should be identified and managed. Increased provider and patient education may also be beneficial. One pilot study randomizing screening-eligible PWH to receive educational material and in-person decision-making support showed increased screening colonoscopy uptake (Ferron et al., 2015). Based on this evidence, efforts to increase on-time screening in eligible PWH should be undertaken.

CLINICAL PRESENTATION

With regard to early presentations of CRC, one recent study compared the prevalence, type, and location of neoplastic lesions found on colonoscopy in 263 PWH matched with 657 patients without HIV and found that PWH were less likely to have any neoplastic lesions (21.3% vs. 27.7%, p < 0.05), adenoma (20.5% vs. 27.1%, $p = 0.04$), tubular adenomas greater than 10 mm (0.4% vs. 2.9%, $p = 0.02$), and serrated adenomas (0.0% vs. 2.6%, p < 0.01) (Fantry et al., 2016). They also found a nonsignificant increased prevalence of adenocarcinoma in PWH compared with people without HIV (1.5% vs. 0.8%, $p = 0.29$). However, at the time of diagnosis in PWH, CRC is often advanced and occurs in younger patients compared to the general population. Researchers from the Italian Cooperative Group AIDS and Tumors evaluated 27 PWH and 54 matched patients without HIV who were diagnosed with CRC between 1985 and 2003 (Berretta et al., 2009). The majority were diagnosed in the ART era, with a median age of 48 years in both groups. However, most patients in the HIV cohort were younger than 45 years old. Median $CD4^+$ T-cell count at the time of diagnosis was 325 cells/mm^3. In PWH, the stage was predominantly Dukes's stage D (distant metastasis) compared to those without HIV (74% vs. 35%; $p = 0.002$). Histopathology showed poorly differentiated adenocarcinoma in 66% of the cohort with HIV compared to 26% in the matched controls without HIV (Berretta et al., 2009).

A case control study from Southern California also found that CRC of PWH occurred mainly in those younger than age 50 years (72%) and with advanced disease (stages III and IV). PWH had a younger to older age ratio of 3:1 compared to the population controls, whose ratio was 1.33. In most patients, biopsy findings revealed poorly differentiated adenocarcinoma (64%). Of note, the mean $CD4^+$ T-cell count at time of diagnosis was robust at 467 cells/mm^3 (Wasserberg et al., 2007).

One multicenter retrospective study of 17 PWH and confirmed CRC from 1988 to 2003 reported a mean age of 43 years at diagnosis and most with $CD4^+$ T-cell counts of less than 500 cells/mm^3 (not specified further) (Chapman et al., 2009). Most tumors arose in the right side of the colon (57%) and with advanced-stage IV disease (47%) and histopathology with grade 2 or 3 adenocarcinomas (79%). Most metastatic sites were to the liver but also included lung, peritoneum, and subcutaneous sites (Chapman et al., 2009). Sigel and colleagues subsequently evaluated 184 patients with CRC (38 PWH and 146 patients without HIV) and found that PWH were more likely to have smoked ($p = 0.001$), have right-sided colorectal cancer (37% vs. 14%; $p = 0.003$), and tumor-infiltrating lymphocytes above 50/10 high-power fields (21% vs. 7%). They also evaluated mismatch repair protein (MMR) expression levels between the two groups (as MMR is a marker for microsatellite instability) but found no difference between the two groups ($p = 0.6$) (Sigel et al., 2016). Given the presence of right-sided colonic tumors, colonoscopy in PWH may have a greater diagnostic yield compared to flexible sigmoidoscopy. Further prospective studies should be performed to evaluate the various screening techniques in PWH.

TREATMENT FOR COLORECTAL CANCER IN HIV

Treatment for CRC in PWH is the same as that for those without HIV and primarily depends on clinical staging of the malignancy, which is determined by physical exam and radiographic imaging. CT scanning is mandatory for determining regional extension, nodal involvement, or distant metastasis in the tumor, nodal, and metastatic staging system. Stages range from stage I to stage IV as the disease advances from confined disease to the colonic mucosa, regional lymph node involvement, and involvement of one or more distant organs including peritoneal seeding. For patients with stage II to IV disease, imaging with CT scan of the chest, abdomen, and pelvis is recommended (NCCN, 2022a). Further imaging with MRI may be useful for better characterization of the liver for metastatic disease, especially in the setting of background steatosis (Shahani et al., 2014). Testing with the tumor marker carcinoembryonic antigen (CEA) should be performed prior to treatment to help serve as a guide in the posttreatment follow-up. This test has not been validated for use specifically in the population with HIV, nor has there been robust evidence supporting survival benefit in the general population, but CEA remains a standard pre- and posttreatment test for its prognostic utility (Locker, 2006).

Role of Surgery in Treatment of CRC

Treatment for localized disease can be curative with endoscopic resection of a carcinomatous polyp or surgical resection with simple colectomy and anastomosis. Surgery remains the cornerstone of therapy for localized disease, and margins should be free of cancer. Locally advanced disease or poorly differentiated polypoid lesions may warrant more invasive or radical surgery. If invasion involves surrounding structures, larger resection of contiguous, multivisceral structures is indicated to ensure negative margins in the affected noncolonic organs (NCCN, 2015c). This approach has yielded improved prognosis and outcomes in patients with locally advanced disease (Govindarajan et al., 2006; Lehnert et al., 2002). Tumor location is also an important aspect in consideration

of surgical approach because management of CRC involving the rectum (especially the lower rectum) may compromise anal sphincter tone and genitourinary function. If the anus is involved, sphincter-sparing surgery may be considered with adjuvant or neoadjuvant chemotherapy and radiation (NCCN, 2015a; Sauer et al., 2012).

Colorectal adenocarcinoma typically metastasizes to the liver, lung, lymph nodes, and peritoneum. With limited metastatic disease, curative surgery remains an option to improve survival; however, recurrence of disease is a reality for some patients (Neef et al., 2009; Shah et al., 2006).

Chemoradiotherapy in CRC

Neoadjuvant and adjuvant chemotherapies are generally considered for patients with advanced or metastatic disease when the expectation of noncurative surgery is present. Neoadjuvant chemoradiotherapy (CRT) is a standard approach to therapy in locally advanced rectal cancer (T3 or N1-2) prior to surgery or rectal cancer that is unresectable or medically inoperable. This consists of fractionated radiation therapy usually with a 5-fluorouracil (5-FU)-based regimen in combination with other agents, such as capecitabine or oxaliplatin and leucovorin (NCCN, 2015a; Sauer et al., 2012). Adjuvant CRT following resection to eliminate microscopic foci of tumors and promote recurrence-free survival has been most beneficial in patients with nodal involvement (stage III), which has been shown in randomized controlled trials (Smith et al., 2004). Typical regimens include 5-FU/leucovorin- or capecitabine-based regimens (NCCN 2015c). Other adjuvant therapies in metastatic disease include the vascular endothelial and epidermal growth factor inhibitor bevacizumab and cetuximab, respectively. Overall survival benefit of these agents remains controversial, and they may cause excess adverse events (da Gramont et al., 2012; Taieb et al., 2014).

TREATMENT OUTCOMES AND SURVIVAL OF PATIENTS WITH HIV AND CRC

There is a paucity of data on the efficacy, tolerability, and treatment outcomes of CRC for PWH. Case series have provided much of the data on this population. As previously discussed, PWH tend to present with more advanced disease, which may require both surgery and chemoradiation. In one case series, 10 PWH with stage III or IV disease underwent segmental colon or rectal resection. One of these patients underwent complete pelvic exenteration (Wasserberg et al., 2007). All patients also received first-line adjuvant chemotherapy with 5-FU/leucovorin. Four of the patients received additional CPT-11 or irinotecan for metastatic disease. Of the patients with rectal involvement, one patient received neoadjuvant 5-FU/leucovorin-based chemoradiation, and three patients received adjuvant radiation. Overall, chemotherapy was tolerated well, but some patients did experience grade 3 adverse events with neutropenia and anemia (Wasserberg et al., 2007).

Another case series from Italy reported on 27 PWH, the majority with metastatic CRC (Berretta et al., 2009). Of those with metastatic disease, three received neoadjuvant oxaliplatin-based chemotherapy for liver metastasis, seven underwent palliative chemotherapy, and two were treated with 5-FU chemoradiation. The remaining patients with metastatic disease underwent palliation. One patient who received radiation incurred hemorrhagic proctitis, which prompted treatment cessation (Berretta et al., 2009). Overall, chemotherapy was tolerated well in the group, with few grade 3 neutropenic events.

Surgical resection provides the best curative treatment for localized colon cancer, and this has been demonstrated with SEER data (2005–2011) showing 5-year survival rates of 90% for localized disease. However, survival declines steeply with regional or nodal involvement (70%) and with distant metastasis (13%) (Howlader et al., 2015). PWH may not receive surgery when indicated, giving them a survival disadvantage. This disparity was highlighted in a follow-up study by the previously mentioned Italian group. In 2010, the group released a brief report on its experience treating 14 PWH and CRC-related liver metastasis (Berretta et al., 2010). Only 3 PWH initially had unresectable liver metastasis as determined by a multidisciplinary team; however, the other 11 PWH underwent FOLFOX-4 treatment. Three people in the group that underwent surgery received neoadjuvant chemotherapy with FOLFOX-4 or FOLFIRI, followed by liver segmentectomy (two persons) or liver segmentectomy plus radiofrequency ablation (one person). These three PWH tolerated the treatments well, remained on ART without any grade 3 or 4 toxicities, and two of the three PWH remained disease-free at 21-month follow-up. Although the group was small, these researchers demonstrated that an aggressive surgical approach for metastatic CRC can be successfully performed in PWH. Narrowing the treatment gap between the population with HIV and the general population remains an important goal in the care of malignancies in HIV that may help improve survival outcomes for this group.

Mortality for PWH and CRC remains high compared to that for the general population. A large retrospective study estimated that PWH and CRC have a 50% higher risk of mortality compared to patients without HIV (Coghill et al., 2015). Smaller case control studies have shown markedly poorer survival for PWH compared to controls without HIV, with 4-year survival of 15% and 49%, respectively (Berretta et al., 2009). A more recent study found that PWH and CRC had reduced overall survival ($p = 0.02$) when compared to their counterparts without HIV, but no difference in progression-free survival (Sigel et al., 2016). It has been hypothesized that PWH are less likely to receive therapy and, therefore, on a population level, will have poorer survival. HIV positivity should not preclude delivery of the standard of care. Further studies are needed to rigorously evaluate the standard of care delivered to these patients. Disparities in screening and treatment of PWH and CRC are likely to perpetuate their less-than-optimal survival outcomes relative to those of patients without HIV.

RECOMMENDED READING

Berretta M, Cappellani A, Di Benedetto F, et al. Clinical presentation and outcome of colorectal cancer in PLWH: a clinical case–control study. *Onkologie*. 2009;32:319–324.

Bini EJ, Park J, Francois F. Use of flexible sigmoidoscopy to screen for colorectal cancer in HIV-infected patients 50 years of age or older. *JAMA Intern Med*. 2006;166(15):1626–1631.

IMMUNE CHECKPOINT INHIBITOR THERAPY FOR NADC

LEARNING OBJECTIVES

Review the mechanism and proposed use of immune check point inhibitor (ICPI) therapy for NADCs.

WHAT'S NEW?

ICPI therapy is currently being evaluated in PWH and, in patients with well-controlled HIV infection, is thought to be just as efficacious for the treatment of various NADCs as for the general population.

KEY POINTS

- ICPIs target key immune regulatory pathways and thus can untether T-cell-mediated antitumor responses, which could help target certain cancers in PWH.

- ICPIs like PD-1 inhibitors may also be able to help eliminate the cells that carry integrated HIV DNA, thus contributing to elimination of the patient's HIV reservoir.

- PD-1/PD-L1 inhibitors have been approved for melanoma, NSCLC and other lung cancers, renal cell carcinoma, Hodgkin's lymphoma, head and neck squamous cell cancers, several types of breast cancers, gastric cancer, urothelial cancer, and colorectal cancer in the general population; studies evaluating their use in PWH are ongoing.

ICPIs are a relatively new class of immunotherapy medications that inhibit suppression of effector T-cell responses. In other words, they help to turn on the cancer or infectious agent-suppressed cell-mediated immune again. Most of these are monoclonal antibodies directed against immune checkpoints that block the interaction between the immune checkpoint and their respective checkpoint ligands. One type of immune checkpoint is programmed cell death-1 (PD-1), which is predominantly expressed on T-cells. The interaction of PD-1 with its ligands (PD-L1 and -L2) expressed on antigen-presenting cells and tumors sends a negative signal to T-cells, which can lead to T-cell exhaustion or dysfunction. T-cell exhaustion is now recognized as a key mechanism contributing to impaired T-cell responses against tumors and some pathogens.

ICPI therapies are an appealing treatment option for many cancers that express PD-1 because they have broad activity with good response rates, they frequently induce long-term disease control, and they are relatively nontoxic. So far, six monoclonal antibodies that target PD-1 or PD-L1 have been approved by the FDA. The first, a PD-1 inhibitor, pembrolizumab, was approved in September 2014 for the treatment of advanced or unresectable melanoma in patients failing other treatments and was so successful it later became the first-line treatment (Robert et al., 2014). It is now approved for NSCLC (Garon et al., 2015), head and neck squamous cell cancers, refractory Hodgkin's lymphoma, primary mediastinal large B-cell lymphoma, advanced urothelial carcinoma, advanced gastric cancer, some types of colorectal cancers, and advanced cervical cancer. A second PD-1 inhibitor, nivolumab, was subsequently approved in 2015 for the treatment of melanoma and is now also approved for NSCLC, renal cell carcinoma, Hodgkin's lymphoma, head and neck squamous cell cancers, advanced urothelial carcinomas, certain colorectal cancers, and hepatocellular carcinoma. The third, fourth, and fifth approvals were for PD-L1 inhibitors (atezolizumab, durvalumab, and avelumab) for the treatment of various malignancies including bladder cancer, NSCLC, SCLC, breast cancer, melanoma, hepatocellular carcinoma, Merkel cell carcinoma, and renal cell carcinoma. The sixth approval (2018) was for cemiplimab, another PD-1 monoclonal antibody, for patients with metastatic or locally advanced cutaneous squamous cell carcinoma, and later for NSCLC and basal cell carcinoma (2021). Most recently, dostarlimab was approved in 2021 for the treatment of endometrial carcinoma and mismatch repair deficient (dMMR) solid cancers. Many more are in the pipeline.

Therapies with ICPIs are an exciting prospect for PWH because they have the potential to not only treat the patient's cancer but also to eliminate or reduce the HIV reservoirs that persist despite ART (Day et al., 2006; Trautmann et al., 2006). The concept behind this latter theoretical use is that HIV persistence is thought to stem primarily from the presence of integrated copies of the proviral genome within long-lived cells. Because active viral gene expression causes cell death due to viral cytopathic effects and the immune response, long-lived cells likely harbor transcriptionally silent, latent provirus, which is the remaining major barrier to finding a cure for HIV. Several studies offer evidence as to why PD-1 may be an important part of this process. PD-1 has been found to be upregulated on HIV-specific CD8[+] T-cells and has been correlated with disease progression (Day et al., 2006). Blockade of PD-L1 was shown to enhance IFN-γ secretion by HIV-specific CD8[+] T-cells, suggesting that PD-1 signaling might play a role in limiting T-cell responses against HIV (Petrovas et al., 2006; Zhang et al., 2007). Checkpoints that are considered markers of T-cell exhaustion, such as PD-1, TIM-3, and LAG-3, have been used to predict time of viremia rebound after treatment interruption (Hurst et al., 2015). Another study suggested a role for the immune checkpoint TIGIT in limiting antiviral T-cell responses in PWH (Chew et al., 2016). This study also showed that TIGIT expression was coexpressed with PD-1 and upregulated on T-cells from both PWH and simian immunodeficiency virus (SIV)-infected macaques. The AIDS Clinical Trials 5326 Study Team recently demonstrated that treatment with an anti-PD-L1 antibody enhanced HIV-specific CD8[+] T-cell

response in two of eight PWH on ART (Gay et al., 2017). Further, a recent subanalysis of the AMC 095: "Nivolumab and Ipilimumab in Treating Patients With HIV-Associated Relapsed or Refractory Classical Hodgkin Lymphoma or Solid Tumors That Are Metastatic or Cannot Be Removed by Surgery" evaluated the frequency of replication-competent HIV in participants before cycle 1 and after at least one dose of therapy (for all samples available) among participants who had suppressed HIV RNA levels. This study demonstrated that among 33 participants who received nivolumab alone, there was no effect on HIV latency or the latent HIV reservoir. However, in seven participants, a modest increase in cell associated unspliced RNA was induced (CA-US HIV RNA) and may potentially eliminate cells containing replication-competent HIV (Rasmussen et al., 2021). Although these studies suggest that immune checkpoints may limit T-cell responses during HIV infection and that immune checkpoint blockade might be beneficial in PWH, larger studies are required to determine the therapeutic benefit of immune checkpoint blockade in PWH on ART.

With regard to cancer therapy, treatment with PD-1/PD-L1 inhibitors may be even more useful in people with cancer with than without HIV because at least one study recently observed that, while PD-L1 expression is high in tumor cells from both people with and without HIV and NSCLC, it was associated with poor prognosis only in PWH (Okuma et al., 2018). However, to date, only a handful of case reports and small case series offer data about PWH treated with these new medications (Guihot et al., 2018; Heppt et al., 2017; Le Garff et al., 2018; Wightman et al., 2015). Many of the PD-1/PDL-1 inhibitor therapies currently in use or being tested in PWH have been mentioned throughout the text of this chapter. In addition, there are several larger clinical trials under way that will be emphasized here (Bender-Ignacio et al., 2018). The Cancer Immunotherapy Trials Network conducted a trial of pembrolizumab in PWH with solid tumors and Hodgkin lymphoma (NCT02595866). They accrued 30 PWH and multiple different types of both AIDS-defining and NADCs and found that pembrolizumab had acceptable safety in patients with cancer, treated with ART and a CD4[+] T-cell count of greater than 100 cells/μL. Despite the report of a treatment-emergent episode of B-cell clonal proliferation in a patient with KS, there was a clinical benefit to participants with lung cancer, NHL, and KS. (Uldrick et al., 2019). Other trials are still pending, including one that will evaluate pembrolizumab in PWH and advanced cancers, although it requires patients to have a CD4[+] T-cell count of greater than 200 cells/mm³ (NCT02595866). A French trial will evaluate therapy with nivolumab in PWH with NSCLC; they are accepting patients with any CD4[+] T-cell count but require a HIV RNA levels less than 200 copies/mL (NCT03304093). Another French study is following PWH who receive ICPIs as part of routine cancer care to evaluate their safety and effects on the HIV reservoir (NCT03354936). Pending the results of these trials, HIV positivity is not thought to be a contraindication to treatment with PD-1 inhibitors, although PWH with low CD4[+] T-cell counts should be monitored closely both for treatment response and for IRIS.

REFERENCES

Abramson JS, Irwin KE, Frigault MJ, et al. Successful anti-CD19 CAR T-cell therapy in HIV-infected patients with refractory high-grade B-cell lymphoma. *Cancer*. 2019;125: 3692–3698.

Aboulafia DM. Kaposi's sarcoma. *Clinics Derm*. 2001;19(3):269–283.

Aboulafia DM, Puswella AL. Highly active antiretroviral therapy as the sole treatment for AIDS-related primary central nervous system lymphoma: a case report with implications for treatment. *AIDS Patient Care STDS*. 2007;21(12):900–907.

Ahdieh L, Munoz A, Vlahov D, et al. Cervical neoplasia and repeated positivity of human papillomavirus infection in human immunodeficiency virus-seropositive and -seronegative women. *Am J Epidemiol*. 2000;151(12):1148–1157.

Altekruse SF, Shiels MS, Modur SP, et al. Cancer burden attributable to cigarette smoking among HIV-infected people in North America. *AIDS*. 2018;32(4):513–521.

Alvarnas JC, Le Rademacher J, Wang Y, et al. Autologous hematopoietic cell transplantation for HIV-related lymphoma: results of the BMT CTN 0803/AMC 071 trial. *Blood*. 2016;128:1050–1058.

Ambinder RF, Wu J, Logan B, et al. Allogeneic hematopoietic cell transplant (alloHCT) for hematologic malignancies in human immunodeficiency virus infected (HIV) patients (pts): Blood and Marrow Transplant Clinical Trials Network (BMT CTN 0903)/AIDS Malignancy Consortium (AMC-080) trial. *J Clin Oncol*. 2017;35(Suppl 15):7006.

Appleby P, Beral V, Newton R, et al. Highly active antiretroviral therapy and incidence of cancer in human immunodeficiency virus-infected adults. *Cancer Inst*. 2000;92:1823–1830.

Avivi I, Robinson S, Goldstone A. Clinical use of rituximab in hematological malignancies. *Br J Cancer*. 2003;89(8):1389–1394.

Ballerini P, Gaidano G, Gong JZ, et al. Multiple genetic lesions in acquired immunodeficiency syndrome-related non-Hodgkin's lymphoma. *Blood*. 1993;81(1):166–176.

Barillari G, Ensoli B. Angiogenic effects of extracellular human immunodeficiency virus type 1 Tat protein and its role in the pathogenesis of AIDS-associated Kaposi's sarcoma. *Clin Microbiol Rev*. 2002;15(2):310–326.

Bañon S, Machuca I, Araujo S, et al. Efficacy, safety, and lack of interactions with the use of raltegravir in HIV-infected patients undergoing antineoplastic chemotherapy. *J Intern AIDS Soc*. 2014;17(4 Suppl 3):19590.

Baptista MJ, Garcia O, Morgades M, et al. HIV-infection impact on clinical-biological features and outcome of diffuse large B-cell lymphoma treated with R-CHOP in the combination antiretroviral therapy era. *AIDS*. 2015;29:811–818.

Barbosa MS, Schlegel R. The E6 and E7 genes of HPV-18 are sufficient for inducing two-stage in vitro transformation of human keratinocytes. *Oncogene*. 1989;4(12):1529–1532.

Barozzi P, Luppi M, Facchetti F, et al. Post-transplant Kaposi sarcoma originates from the seeding of donor-derived progenitors. *Nature Med*. 2003;9(5):554–561.

Barta SK, Joshi J, Mounier N, et al. Central nervous system involvement in AIDS-related lymphomas. *Br J Haematol*. 2016;173:857–866.

Barta SK, Lee JY, Kaplan LD, et al. Pooled analysis of AIDS malignancy consortium trials evaluating rituximab plus CHOP or infusional EPOCH chemotherapy in HIV-associated non-Hodgkin lymphoma. *Cancer*. 2012;118:3977–3983.

Barta SK, Samuel MS, Xue X, et al. Changes in the influence of lymphoma- and HIV-specific factors on outcomes in AIDS-related non-Hodgkin lymphoma. *Ann Oncol*. 2015;26:958–966.

Barta SK, Xue X, Wang D, et al. Treatment factors affecting outcomes in HIV-associated non-Hodgkin lymphomas: a pooled analysis of 1546 patients. *Blood*. 2013;122:3251–3262.

Barta SK, Xue X, Wang D, et al. A new prognostic score for AIDS-related lymphomas in the rituximab-era. *Haematologica*. 2014;99:1731–1737.

Baumgartner JE, Rachlin JR, Beckstead JH, et al. Primary central nervous system lymphomas: natural history and response to radiation therapy in 55 patients with acquired immunodeficiency syndrome. *J Neurosurg*. 1990;73(2):206–211.

Bayraktar S, Bayraktar UD, Ramos JC, et al. Primary CNS lymphoma in HIV positive and negative patients: comparison of clinical characteristics, outcome and prognostic factors. *J Neurooncol*. 2011;101:257–265.

Bedi GC, Westra WH, Farzedegan H, et al. Microsatellite instability in primary neoplasms from HIV\+ patients. *Nature Med*. 1995;1(1):65–68.

Bedimo R, Chen RY, Accortt NA, et al. Trends in AIDS-defining and non-AIDS defining malignancies among HIV-infected patients: 1989–2002. *Clin Infect Dis*. 2004;39(9):1380–1384.

Bender-Ignacio R, Lin LL, Rajdev L, et al. Evolving paradigms in HIV malignancies: review of ongoing clinical trials. *J Natl Compr Canc Netw*. 2018;16(8):1018–1026.

Benevolo M, Donà MG, Ravenda PS, et al. Anal human papillomavirus infection: prevalence, diagnosis and treatment of related lesions. *Expert Rev Anti Infect Ther*. 2016;14(5):465–477.

Beral V, Peterman TA, Berkelman RL, et al. Kaposi's sarcoma among persons with AIDS: a sexually transmitted infection? *Lancet*. 1990;335(8682):123–128.

Beral V, Peterman T, Berkelman R, et al. AIDS-associated non-Hodgkin lymphoma. *Lancet*. 1991;337(8745):805–809.

Berretta M, Cappellani A, Di Benedetto F, et al. Clinical presentation and outcome of colorectal cancer in PLWH: a clinical case–control study. *Onkologie*. 2009;32:319–324.

Berretta M, Zanet E, Basile F, et al. HIV positive patients with liver metastasis from colorectal cancer deserve the same therapeutic approach as the general population. *Onkkologie*. 2010;33:203–204.

Berry JM, Palefsky JM, Jay N, et al. Performance characteristics of anal cytology and human papillomavirus testing in patients with high-resolution anoscopy-guided biopsy of high-grade anal intraepithelial neoplasia. *Dis Colon Rectum*. 2009;52(2):239–247.

Berthold DR, Pond GR, Soban F, et al. Docetaxel plus prednisone or mitoxantrone plus prednisone for advanced prostate cancer: updated survival in the TAX 327 study. *J Clin Oncol*. 2008;26(2):242–245.

Besson C, Goubar A, Gabarre J, et al. Changes in AIDS-related lymphoma since the era of highly active antiretroviral therapy. *Blood*. 2001;98(8):2339–2344.

Bini EJ, Park J, Francois F. Use of flexible sigmoidoscopy to screen for colorectal cancer in HIV-infected patients 50 years of age or older. *JAMA Intern Med*. 2006;166(15):1626–1631.

Bjorge T, Engeland A, Luostarinen T, et al. Human papillomavirus infection as a risk factor for anal and perianal skin cancer in a prospective study. *Br J Cancer*. 2002;87(1):61–64.

Blazy A, Hennequin C, Gornet JM, et al. Anal carcinomas in PLWH: high-dose chemoradiotherapy is feasible in the era of highly active antiretroviral therapy. *Dis Colon Rectum*. 2005;48(6):1176–1181.

Bonnet F, Burty C, Lewden C, et al. Changes in cancer mortality among HIV-infected patients: the Mortalite 2005 Survey. *Clin Infect Dis*. 2009;48(5):633–639.

Bosch FX, Manos MM, Munoz N, et al. Prevalence of human papillomavirus in cervical cancer: a worldwide perspective. *J Natl Cancer Inst*. 1995;87(11):796–802.

Bossolasco S, Cinque P, Ponzoni M, et al. Epstein–Barr virus DNA load in cerebrospinal fluid and plasma of patients with AIDS-related lymphoma. *J Neurovirol*. 2002;8(5):432–438.

Boudreaux AA, Smith LL, Cosby CD, et al. Intralesional vinblastine for cutaneous Kaposi's sarcoma associated with acquired immunodeficiency syndrome: a clinical trial to evaluate efficacy and discomfort associated with infection. *J Am Acad Derm*. 1993;28(1):61–65.

Boulanger E, Gerard L, Gabarre J, et al. Prognostic factors and outcome of human herpesvirus 8-associated primary effusion lymphoma in patients with AIDS. *J Clin Oncol*. 2005;23(19):4372–4380.

Bower M, Dalla Pria A, Coyle C, et al. Prospective stage-stratified approach to AIDS-related Kaposi's sarcoma. *J Clin Oncol*. 2014;32:409–414.

Bower M, Fox P, Fife K, et al. Highly active anti-retroviral therapy (HAART) prolongs time to treatment failure in Kaposi's sarcoma. *AIDS*. 1999;13(15):2105–2111.

Bower M, McCall-Peat N, Ryan N, et al. Protease inhibitors potentiate chemotherapy-induced neutropenia. *Blood*. 2004;104(9):2943–2946.

Bower M, Powles T, Nelson M, et al. HIV-related lung cancer in the era of highly active antiretroviral therapy. *AIDS (London)*. 2003;17(3):371–375.

Bower M, Powles T, Newsom-Davis T, et al. HIV-associated anal cancer: has highly active antiretroviral therapy reduced the incidence or improved the outcome? *J AIDS*. 2004;37(5):1563–1565.

Brandão M, Bruzzone M, Franzoi MA, et al. Impact of HIV infection on baseline characteristics and survival of women with breast cancer. *AIDS*. 2021;35(4):605–618. http://doi:10.1097/QAD.0000000000002810. PMID: 33394680.

Brickman C, Palefsky JM. Review: human papillomavirus in the HIV-infected host: epidemiology and pathogenesis in the antiretroviral era. *Curr HIV/AIDS Rep*. 2015;12(1):6–15.

Burgi A, Brodine S, Wegner S, et al. Incidence and risk factors for the occurrence of non-AIDS-defining cancers among human immunodeficiency virus-infected individuals. *Cancer*. 2005;104(7):1505–1511.

Burkes RL, Meyer PR, Gill PS, et al. Rectal lymphoma in homosexual men. *Arch Intern Med*. 1986;146(5):913–915.

Cadranel J, Garfield D, Lavole A, et al. Lung cancer in HIV infected patients: facts, questions, and challenges. *Thorax*. 2006;61:1000–1008.

Calabresi A, Ferraresi A, Festa A, et al. Incidence of AIDS-defining cancers and virus-related and non-virus-related non-AIDS-defining cancers among HIV-infected patients compared with the general population in a large health district of northern Italy, 1999–2000. *HIV Med*. 2013;14(8):481–490.

Campbell JA, Soliman AS, Kahesa C, et al. Changing patterns of lung, liver, and head and neck non-AIDS-defining cancers relative to HIV status in Tanzania between 2002–2014. *Infect Agent Cancer*. 2016;11:58.

Cannon MJ. Kaposi's sarcoma-associated herpesvirus and acquired immunodeficiency syndrome-related malignancy. *Semin Oncol*. 2000;27:408–419.

Cannon MJ, Dollard SC, Smith DK, et al. Blood-borne and sexual transmission of human herpesvirus 8 in women with or at risk for human immunodeficiency virus infection. *N Engl J Med*. 2001;344(9):637–643.

Cappell MS, Yao F, Cho KC. Colonic adenocarcinoma associated with the acquired immune deficiency syndrome. *Cancer*. 1988;62:616–619.

Casper C, Carrell D, Miller KG, et al. HIV serodiscordant sex partners and the prevalence of human herpesvirus 8 infection among HIV negative men who have sex with men: baseline data from the EXPLORE study. *Sex Transm Infect*. 2006;82(3):229–235.

Casper C, Krantz E, Selke S, et al. Frequent and asymptomatic oropharyngeal shedding of human herpesvirus 8 among immunocompetent men. *J Infect Dis*. 2007;195(1):30–36.

Casper C, Redman M, Huang ML, et al. HIV infection and human herpesvirus-8 oral shedding among men who have sex with men. *J AIDS*. 2004;35(3):233–238.

Castillo JJ, Furman M, Beltrán BE, et al. Human immunodeficiency virus–associated plasmablastic lymphoma. *Cancer*. 2012;118:5270–5277.

Castilho JL, Luz PM, Shepherd BE, et al. HIV and cancer: a comparative retrospective study of Brazilian and US clinical cohorts. *Infect Agent Cancer*. 2015;10(4):1–10.

Cattaneo C, Re A, Ungari M, et al. Plasmablastic lymphoma among human immunodeficiency virus-positive patients: results of a single center's experience. *Leuk Lymphoma*. 2015;56:267–269.

Centers for Disease Control and Prevention (CDC). AIDS-defining conditions. https://www.cdc.gov/mmwr/preview/mmwrhtml/rr5710a2.htm. Published 2008. Accessed October 8, 2022.

CDC. Human papillomavirus-associated cancers—United States, 2004–2008. *Morbid Mortal Wkly Rep*. 2012;61(15):258–261.

CDC. Human papilloma virus (HPV) fact sheet. Available at www.cdc.gov/std/hpv. Published July 22, 2021. Accessed September 30, 2022.

Chadburn A, Abdul-Nabi AM, Teruya BS, et al. Lymphoid proliferations associated with human immunodeficiency virus infection. *Arch Path Lab Med*. 2013;137(3):360–370.

Chang Y, Cesarman E, Pessin MS, et al. Identification of herpesvirus-like DNA sequences in AIDS-associated Kaposi's sarcoma. *Science*. 1994;266(5192):1865–1869.

Chapman C, Aboulafia DM, Dezube BJ, et al. Human immunodeficiency virus-associated adenocarcinoma of the colon: clinicopathologic findings and outcome. *Clin Colorectal Cancer*. 2009;8(4):215–219.

Chari A, Kaplan L, Volberding PA, et al. Diagnosis and management of non-Hodgkin's lymphoma and Hodgkin's lymphoma. 2005.

Chaturvedi AK, Madeleine MM, Biggar RJ, et al. Risk of human papillomavirus-associated cancers among persons with AIDS. *J Natl Cancer Inst*. 2009;101(16):1120–1130.

Chen YH, Lin MW, Bhatia K, et al. Cancer incidence in a nationwide HIV/AIDS patient cohort in Taiwan in 1998–2000. *J AIDS*. 2014;65(4):463–472.

Chew GM, Fujita T, Webb GM, et al. TIGIT marks exhausted T cells, correlates with disease progression, and serves as a target for immune restoration in HIV and SIV infection. *PLoS Pathog*. 2016;12:e1005349.

Chiao EY, Dezube BJ, Krown SE, et al. Time for oncologists to opt in for routine opt-out HIV testing? *JAMA*. 2010;304(3):334–339.

Chiao EY, Giordano TP, Richardson P, et al. Human immunodeficiency virus-associated squamous cell cancer of the anus: epidemiology and outcomes in the highly active antiretroviral therapy era. *J Clin Oncol*. 2008;26(3):474–479.

Chin-Hong PV, Vittinghoff E, Cranston RD, et al. Age-specific prevalence of anal human papillomavirus infection in HIV-negative sexually active men who have sex with men: the EXPLORE study. *J Infect Dis*. 2004;190(12):2070–2076.

Chokunonga E, Levy LM, Bassett MT, et al. Cancer incidence in the African population of Harare, Zimbabwe: second results from the cancer registry 1993–1995. *Int J Cancer*. 2000;85(1):54–59.

Cianfrocca M, Lee S, Von Roenn J, et al. Randomized trial of paclitaxel vs. pegylated liposomal doxorubicin for advanced human immunodeficiency virus-associated Kaposi sarcoma: evidence of symptom palliation from chemotherapy. *Cancer*. 2010;116(16):3969–3977.

Cingolani A, Fratino L, Scoppettuolo G, et al. Changing pattern of primary cerebral lymphoma in the highly active antiretroviral therapy era. *J Neurovirol*. 2005; 11(Suppl 3):38–44.

Cleator S, Fife K, Nelson M, et al. Treatment of HIV-associated invasive anal cancer with combined chemoradiation. *Eur J Cancer (Oxford: 1990)*. 2000;36(6):754–758.

Clifford GM, Lise M, Franceschi S, et al. Lung cancer in the Swiss HIV Cohort Study: role of smoking, immunodeficiency, and pulmonary infection. *Br J Cancer*. 2012;106:448–452.

Clifford GM, Polesel J, Richenbach M, et al. Cancer risk in the Swiss HIV Cohort Study: associations with immunodeficiency, smoking, and highly active antiretroviral therapy. *J Natl Cancer Inst*. 2005;97(6):425–432.

Coghill AE, Shiels MS, Suneja G, et al. Elevated cancer-specific mortality among HIV-infected patients in the United States. *J Clin Oncol*. 2015;33(21):2376–2383.

Conti S, Masocco M, Pezzotti P, et al. Differential impact of combined antiretroviral therapy on the survival of Italian patients with specific AIDS-defining illnesses. *J AIDS*. 2000;25(5):451–458.

Cooper JS, Steinfeld AD, Lerch I. Intentions and outcomes in the radiotherapeutic management of epidemic Kaposi's sarcoma. *Int J Radiat Oncol Biol Phys*. 1991;20(3):419–422.

Corales R, Taege A, Rehm S, et al. Regression of AIDS-related CNS lymphoma with HAART. [Abstract MoPpB1086]. Proceedings of the XIII International AIDS Conference. Durban, South Africa; 2000.

Cote TR, Biggar RJ, Rosenberg PS, et al. Non-Hodgkin's lymphoma among people with AIDS: incidence, presentation and public health burden. *Int J Cancer*. 1997;73(5):645–650.

Cote TR, Manns A, Hardy CR, et al.; AIDS/Cancer Study Group. Epidemiology of brain lymphoma among people with or without acquired immunodeficiency syndrome. *J Natl Cancer Inst.* 1996;88(10):675–679.

Coutinho R, Pria AD, Gandhi S, et al. HIV status does not impair the outcome of patients diagnosed with diffuse large B-cell lymphoma treated with R-CHOP in the cART era. *AIDS.* 2014;28:689–697.

Crothers K, Huang, L, Goulet JL, et al. HIV infection and risk for incident pulmonary diseases in the combination antiretroviral therapy era. *Am J Respir Crit Care Med.* 2011;183(3):388–395.

Da Gramont A, Van Cutsem E, Schmoll HJ, et al. Bevacizumab plus oxaliplatin-based chemotherapy as adjuvant treatment for colon cancer (AVANT): a phase 3 randomised controlled trial. *Lancet Oncol.* 2012;13(12):1225–1233.

Daling JR, Weiss NS, Hislop TG, et al. Sexual practices, sexually transmitted diseases, and the incidence of anal cancer. *N Engl J Med.* 1987;317(16):973–977.

Danzig JB, Brandt LJ, Reinus JF, et al. Gastrointestinal malignancy in patients with AIDS. *Am J Gastroenterol.* 1991;86(6):715–718.

Day CL, Kaufmann DE, Kiepiela P, et al. PD-1 expression on HIV-specific T cells is associated with T-cell exhaustion and disease progression. *Nature.* 2006;443:350–354.

Dedicoat M, Newton R, Alkharsah KR, et al. Mother-to-child transmission of human herpesvirus-8 in South Africa. *J Infect Dis.* 2004;190(6):1068–1075.

Deregibus M, Cantalupp IV, Doublier S, et al. HIV-1-Tat protein activates phosphatidylinositol 3-kinase/AKT-dependent survival pathways in Kaposi's sarcoma cells. *J Biol Chem.* 2002;277(28):25195–25202.

Dezube BJ, Pantanowitz L, Aboulafia DM. Management of AIDS-related Kaposi sarcoma: advances in target discovery and treatment. *AIDS Reader.* 2004;14(5):236–238, 243.

Diez-Martin J, Balsalobre P, Carrion R. et al. Long-term survival after autologous stem cell transplant (ASCT) in AIDS related lymphoma patients (Abstract 868). *Blood.* 2003;247a:102.

Diez-Martin JL, Balsalobre P, Re A, et al. Comparable survival between HIV\+ and HIV–non-Hodgkin and Hodgkin lymphoma patients undergoing autologous peripheral blood stem cell transplantation. *Blood.* 2009;113(23):6011–6014.

DiGiusto DL, Cannon PM, Holmes MC, et al. Preclinical development and qualification of ZFN-mediated CCR5 disruption in human hematopoietic stem/progenitor cells. *Mol Ther Methods Clin Dev.* 2016;3:16067.

D'Jaen GA, Pantanowitz L, Bower M, et al. Human immunodeficiency virus-associated primary lung cancer in the era of highly active antiretroviral therapy: a multi-institutional collaboration. *Clin Lung Cancer.* 2010;11(6):396–404.

Donahue BR, Sullivan JW, Cooper JS. Additional experience with empiric radiotherapy for presumed human immunodeficiency virus-associated primary central nervous system lymphoma. *Cancer.* 1995;76(2):328–332.

Dryden-Peterson S, Bvochora-Nsingo M, Suneja G, et al. HIV infection and survival among women with cervical cancer. *J Clin Oncol.* 2016;34:3749–3757.

D'Souza G, Wiley D, Li X, et al. Incidence and epidemiology of anal cancer in the multicenter AIDS cohort study. *J AIDS.* 2008;48:491–499.

Dubrow R, Qin L, Lin H, et al. Association of CD4\+ T-cell count, HIV-1 RNA viral load, and antiretroviral therapy with Kaposi sarcoma risk among HIV-infected persons in the United States and Canada. *J AIDS.* 2017;75(4):382–390.

Duncan KC, Chan KJ, Chiu CG, et al. HAART slows progression to anal cancer in HIV-infected MSM. *AIDS.* 2015;29:305–311.

Dunleavy K, Pittaluga S, Shovlin M, et al. Low-intensity therapy in adults with Burkitt's lymphoma. *N Engl J Med.* 2013;369:1915–1925.

Durand CM, Capoferri AA, Redd AD, et al. Allogeneic bone marrow transplantation with post-transplant cyclophosphamide for patients with HIV and haematological malignancies: a feasibility study. *Lancet HIV.* 2020;7(9):e602–e610. http://doi:10.1016/S2352-3018(20)30073-4

Dutta A, Uno H, Holman A, et al. Racial differences in prostate cancer risk in young HIV-positive and HIV-negative men: a prospective cohort study. *Cancer Causes Control.* 2017;28(7):767–777.

Eberhard JM, Angin M, Passaes C, et al. Vulnerability to reservoir reseeding due to high immune activation after allogeneic hematopoietic stem cell transplantation in individuals with HIV-1. *Sci Transl Med.* 2020;12(542):eaay9355. http://doi:10.1126/scitranslmed.aay9355

Ekstein D, Ben-Yehuda D, Slyusarevsky E, et al. CSF analysis of IgH gene rearrangement in CNS lymphoma: relationship to the disease course. *J Neurol Sci.* 2006;247:39–46.

El Amari EB, Toutous-Trellu L, Gayet-Ageron A, et al. Predicting the evolution of Kaposi sarcoma in the highly active antiretroviral therapy era. *AIDS.* 2008;22(9):1019–1028.

El-Sadr WM, Lundgren J, Neaton JD, et al. CD4\+ count-guided interruption of antiretroviral treatment. *N Engl J Med.* 2006;355:2283–2296.

El-Solh A, Kumar NM, Nair MP, et al. An RDG-containing peptide from HIV-1 TAT-(65–80) modulates protooncogene expression in human bronchoalveolar carcinoma cell line, A549. *Immunol Invest.* 1997;26(3):351–370.

Engels EA, Biggar RJ, Hall I, et al. Cancer risk in people infected with human immunodeficiency virus in the United States. *Intern J Cancer.* 2008;123:187–194.

Engels EA, Biggar RJ, Marshall VA, et al. Detection and quantification of Kaposi's sarcoma-associated herpesvirus to predict AIDS-associated Kaposi's sarcoma. *AIDS (London).* 2003;17(12):1847–1851.

Engels EA, Brock MV, Chen J, et al. Elevated incidence of lung cancer among HIV-infected individuals. *J Clin Oncol.* 2006;24(9):1383–1388.

Ensoli B, Barillari G, Salahuddin S, et al. Tat protein of HIV-1 stimulates growth of cells derived from Kaposi's sarcoma lesions of AIDS patients. *Nature.* 1990;345(6270):84–86.

European AIDS Clinical Society (EACS). Guidelines version 11.0 https://eacs.sanfordguide.com. Published October 2021. Accessed October 8, 2022.

Fantry LE, Nowak RG, Fisher LH, et al. Colonoscopy findings in HIV-infected men and women from an urban US cohort compared with non-HIV-infected men and women. *AIDS Res Hum Retroviruses.* 2016;32(9):860–867

Ferreri AJM, Cwynarski K, Pulczynski E, et al. Chemoimmunotherapy with methotrexate, cytarabine, thiotepa, and rituximab (MATRix regimen) in patients with primary CNS lymphoma: results of the first randomisation of the International Extranodal Lymphoma Study Group-32 (IELSG32) phase 2 trial. *Lancet Haematol.* 2016;3(5):e217–e227.

Ferreri AJM, Cwynarski K, Pulczynski E, et al. Whole-brain radiotherapy or autologous stem-cell transplantation as consolidation strategies after high-dose methotrexate-based chemoimmunotherapy in patients with primary CNS lymphoma: results of the second randomisation of the International Extranodal Lymphoma Study Group-32 phase 2 trial. *Lancet Haematol.* 2017;4(11):e510–e523.

Ferron P, Asfour SS, Metsch LR, et al. Impact of a multifaceted intervention on promoting adherence to screening colonoscopy among persons in HIV primary care: a pilot study. *Clin Transl Sci.* 2015;8(4):290–297.

Firnhaber C, Swarts A, Goeieman B, et al. Cryotherapy reduces progression of cervical intraepithelial neoplasia grade 1 in South African HIV-infected women: a randomized, controlled trial. *J AIDS.* 2017;76(5):532–538.

Foulot H, Heard I, Potard V, et al. Surgical management of cervical intraepithelial neoplasia in HIV-infected women. *Eur J Obstet Gynecol Reprod Biol.* 2008;141:153–157.

Franceschi S, Dal Maso L, Rickenbach M, et al. Kaposi sarcoma incidence in the Swiss HIV Cohort Study before and after highly active antiretroviral therapy. *Br J Cancer.* 2008;99(5):800–804.

Fraunholz I, Rabeneck D, Gerstein J, et al. Concurrent chemoradiotherapy with 5-fluorouracil and mitomycin C for anal carcinoma: are
there differences between HIV-positive and HIV-negative patients
in the era of highly active antiretroviral therapy? *Radiother Oncol.*
2011;98(1):99–104.

Friedman SL. Gastrointestinal and hepatobiliary neoplasms in AIDS.
Gastroenterol Clin North Am. 1988;17(3):465–486.

Friedman-Kien AE. Disseminated Kaposi's sarcoma syndrome in young
homosexual men. *J Am Acad Dermatol.* 1981;5(4):468–471.

Friedman-Kien AE, Saltzman BR. Clinical manifestations of classical,
endemic African, and epidemic AIDS-associated Kaposi's sarcoma. *J
Am Acad Dermatol.* 1990; 22(6 Pt 2):1237–1250.

Frisch M, Biggar RJ, Engels EA, et al.; AIDS–Cancer Match Registry
Study Group. Association of cancer with AIDS-related immunosuppression in adults. *JAMA.* 2001;285(13):1736–1745.

Frisch M, Biggar RJ, Goedert JJ. Human papillomavirus-associated
cancers in patients with human immunodeficiency virus infection
and acquired immunodeficiency syndrome. *J Nat Cancer Institute.*
2000a;92(18):1500–1510.

Frisch M, Goodman MT. Human papillomavirus-associated carcinomas
in Hawaii and the mainland U.S. *Cancer.* 2000b;88(6):1464–1469.

Fulco PP, Hynicka L, Rackley D. Raltegravir-based HAART regimen in a patient with large B-cell lymphoma. *Ann Pharmacother.*
2010;44(2):377–382.

Gabarre J, Azar N, Autran B, et al. High-dose therapy and autologous
haematopoietic stem-cell transplantation for HIV-1-associated lymphoma. *Lancet.* 2000;355(9209):1071–1072.

Gage JT, Vance EA, Hildenbrand PG, et al. Brain lesion and AIDS. *Proc
Baylor Univ Medical Center.* 2000;13(4):424–429.

Gaidano G, Dalla-Favera R. Molecular pathogenesis of AIDS-related
lymphomas. *Adv Cancer Res.* 1995;67:113–153.

Gaisa M, Ita-Nagy F, Sigel K, et al. High rates of anal high-grade squamous intraepitelial lesions in HIV-infected women who do not meet
screening guidelines. *Clin Infect Dis.* 2017;64(3)289–294.

Garon EB, Rizvi NA, Hui R, et al. Pembrolizumab for the treatment of
non-small-cell lung cancer. *N Engl J Med.* 2015;372:2018–2028.

Gates AE, Kaplan LD. Biology and management of AIDS-associated
non-Hodgkin's lymphoma. *Hematol Oncol Clin North Am.*
2003;17(3):821–841.

Gay CL, Bosch RJ, Ritz J, et al. Clinical trial of the anti-PD-L1 antibody
BMS-936559 in HIV-1 infected participants on suppressive antiretroviral therapy. *J Infect Dis.* June 1, 2017;215(11):1725–1733.

Gbabe OF, Okwundu CI: Dedicoat M, et al. Treatment of severe or progressive Kaposi's sarcoma in HIV-infected adults. *Cochrane Database
Syst Rev.* 2014;9:CD003256.

Gerard L, Meignin V, Galicier L, et al. Characteristics of non-Hodgkin
lymphoma arising in HIV-infected patients with suppressed HIV
replication. *AIDS.* 2009;23(17):2301–2308.

Gichangi P, De Vuyst H, Estambale B, et al. HIV and cervical cancer in
Kenya. *Intern J Gynaecol Obst.* 2002;76(1):55–63.

Gill ON, Weinberg JR, Fisher IS, et al. Meta-surveillance—safer cyber-
surveillance. *Lancet.* 1995;346(8977):776.

Gill PS, Akil B, Colletti P, et al. Pulmonary Kaposi's sarcoma: clinical
findings and results of therapy. *Am J Med.* 1989;87(1):57–61.

Gill PS, Wernz J, Scadden DT, et al. Randomized phase III trial
of liposomal daunorubicin vs. doxorubicin, bleomycin, and
vincristine in AIDS-related Kaposi's sarcoma. *J Clin Oncol.*
1996;14(8):2353–2364.

Goldstein JD, Dickson DW, Moser FG, et al. Primary central nervous
system lymphoma in acquired immune deficiency syndrome: a clinical and pathologic study with results of treatment with radiation.
Cancer. 1991;67(11):2756–2765.

Gopal S, Patel MR, Yanik EL, et al. Temporal trends in presentation and
survival for HIV-associated lymphoma in the antiretroviral therapy
era. *J Natl Cancer Inst.* 2013;105:1221–1229.

Gosselaar C, Roobol MJ, Roemeling S, et al. The role of the digital
rectal examination in subsequent screening visits in the European
Randomized Study of Screening for Prostate Cancer (ERSPC),
Rotterdam. *Eur Urol.* 2008;54:581–588.

Gosselaar C, Roobol MJ, van den Bergh RC, et al. Digital rectal examination and the diagnosis of prostate cancer—a study based on 8 years
and three screenings within the European Randomized Study of
Screening for Prostate Cancer (ERSPC), Rotterdam. *Eur Urol.*
2009;55(1):139–146.

Govindarajan A, Coburn NH, Kiss A, et al. Population-based assessment of the surgical management of locally advanced colorectal cancer. *J Natl Cancer Inst.* 2006;98(20):1474–1481.

Grew D, Bitterman D, Leichman CG, et al. HIV infection is associated with poor outcomes for patients with anal cancer in
the highly active antiretroviral therapy era. *Dis Colon Rectum.*
2015;58(12):1130–1136.

Grimm P, Billiet I, Bostwick D, et al. Comparative analysis of prostate
specific antigen free survival outcomes for patients with low, intermediate, and high risk prostate cancer treatment by radical therapy: results from the Prostate Cancer Results Study Group. *Br J Urol
Int.* 2012;109(Suppl 1):22–29.

Grover S, Desir F, Jing Y, et al. Reduced cancer survival among adults
with HIV and AIDS-defining illnesses despite no difference in cancer stage at diagnosis. *J AIDS.* 2018;79(4):421–429.

Grover S, Mehta P, Wang Q, et al. Association between CD4 count and
chemoradiation therapy outcomes among cervical cancer patients
with HIV. *J Acquir Immune Defic Syndr.* 2020;85(2):201–208.
http://doi:10.1097/QAI.0000000000002420

Gruffaz M, Vasan K, Tan B, et al. TLR4-mediated inflammation promotes KSHV-induced cellular transformation and tumorigenesis by activating the STAT3 pathway. *Cancer Res.* December 15,
2018;77(24):7094–7108.

Guerrero-Garcia TA, Mogollon RJ, Castillo JJ. Bortezomib in plasmablastic lymphoma: a glimpse of hope for a hard-to-treat disease. *Leuk
Res.* 2017;62:12–16.

Guiguet M, Boue F, Cadranel J, et al. Effect of immunodeficiency, HIV
viral load, and antiretroviral therapy on the risk of individual malignancies (FHDH-ANRS CO4): a prospective cohort study. *Lancet
Oncol.* 2009;10(12):1152–1159.

Guihot A, Marcelin, AG, Massiani MA, et al. Drastic decrease of the
HIV reservoir in a patient treated with nivolumab for lung cancer.
Ann Oncol. 2018;29(2):517–518.

Gulrich AE, Yueming L, McDonald A, et al. Rates of non-AIDS defining cancers in people with HIV infection before and after AIDS diagnoses. *AIDS.* 2002;16:1155–1161.

Gupta NK, Nolan A, Omuro A, et al. Long-term survival in AIDS-
related primary central nervous system lymphoma. *Neuro Oncol.*
2017;19:99–108.

Hamilton-Dutoit SJ, Pallesen G, Karkov J, et al. Identification of EBV-
DNA in tumour cells of AIDS-related lymphomas by in-situ hybridi-
sation. *Lancet.* 1989;1(8637):554–552.

Haq IU, Dalla Pria A, Papanastasopoulos P, et al. The clinical application of plasma Kaposi sarcoma herpesvirus viral load as a tumour biomarker: results from 704 patients. *HIV Med.* 2016;17:56–61.

Heard I, Etienney I, Potard V, et al. High prevalence of anal human
papillomavirus-associated cancer precursors in a contemporary
cohort of asymptomatic HIV-infected women. *Clin Infect Dis.*
2015;60(10):1559–1568.

Heard I, Pizot-Martin I, Potard V, et al. Prevalence of and risk factors
for anal oncogenic human papillomavirus infection among HIV-
infected women in France in the combination antiretroviral therapy
era. *J Infect Dis.* 2016;213(9):1455–1461.

Heidenreich A, Bastian PJ, Bellmunt J, et al. European Association of
Urology (EAU) guidelines on prostate cancer: part 1. Screening,
diagnosis, and local treatment with curative intent—update 2013.
Eur Urol. 2014;65(1):124–137.

Hengge UR, Ruzicka T, Tyring SK, et al. Update on Kaposi's sarcoma
and other HHV8 associated diseases: part 1. Epidemiology, environmental predispositions, clinical manifestations, and therapy. *Lancet
Infect Dis.* 2002;2(5):281–292.

Henrich TJ, Hanhauser E, Marty FM, et al. Antiretroviral-free HIV-1
remission and viral rebound after allogeneic stem cell transplantation: report of 2 cases. *Ann Intern Med.* 2014;161:319–327.

Heppt MV, Schlaak M, Eigenlter TK et al. Checkpoint blockade for metastatic melanoma and Merkel cell carcinoma in PLWH. *Ann Oncol*. 2017;28(12):3104–3106.

Herida M, Mary-Krause M, Kaphan R, et al. Incidence of non-AIDS defining cancers before and during the highly active antiretroviral therapy era in a cohort of human immunodeficiency virus-infected patients. *J Clin Oncol* 2003;21;3447–3453.

Hernández-Ramírez RU, Shiels MS, Dubrow R, et al. Cancer risk in HIV-infected people in the USA from 1996 to 2012: a population-based, registry-linkage study. *Lancet HIV*. 2017;4(11):e495–e504.

Hessol NA, Whittemore H, Vittinghoff E, et al. Incidence of first and second primary cancers diagnosed among people with HIV, 1985–2013: a population-based, registry linkage study. *Lancet HIV*. 2018;5(11):e647–e655.

Hill DR. The role of radiotherapy for epidemic Kaposi's sarcoma. *Semin Oncol*. 1987;14:1207.

Hirsch BE, McGowan JP, Fine SM, et al. *Screening for anal dysplasia and cancer in adults with HIV.* [Internet]. *New York State Department of Health AIDS Institute Clinical Guidelines.* Baltimore, MD: Johns Hopkins University; 2022.

Hladik W, Dollard SC, Mermin J, et al. Transmission of human herpesvirus 8 by blood transfusion. *N Engl J Med*. 2006;355(13):1331–1338.

Hoffmann C, Tabrizian S, Wolf E, et al. Survival of AIDS patients with primary central nervous system lymphoma is dramatically improved by HAART-induced immune recovery. *AIDS*. 2001;15(16):2119–2127.

Hoover DR, Black C, Jacobson LP, et al. Epidemiologic analysis of Kaposi's sarcoma as an early and later AIDS outcome in homosexual men. *Am J Epidemiol*. 1993;138(4):266–278.

Horner MJ, Shiels MS, Pfeiffer RM, et al. Deaths attributable to cancer in the United States HIV population during 2001–2015. *Clin Infect Dis*. 2021;72(9):e224–e231. http://doi:10.1093/cid/ciaa1016

Hosseinipour MC, Kang M, Krown SE, Bukuru A, et al. As-needed vs immediate etoposide NCT03094286chemotherapy in combination with antiretroviral therapy for mild-to-0moderate AIDS-associated Kaposi sarcoma in resource-limited settings: A5264/AMC-067 Randomized clinical trial. *Clin Infect Dis*. 2018;67(2):251–260.

Howlader N, Noone AM, Krapcho M, et al. *SEER statistics review, 1975–2012*. Bethesda, MD: National Cancer Institute; 2015. http://seer.cancer.gov/archive/csr/1975_2012

Hsiao W, Anastasia K, Hall J, et al. Association between HIV status and positive prostate biopsy in a study of US veterans. *Scientific World J*. 2009;9:102–108.

Huncharek M, Haddock KS, Reid R, et al. Smoking as a risk factor for prostate cancer: a meta-analysis of 24 prospective cohort studies. *Am J Pub Health*. 2010;100(4):693–701.

Hurst J, Hoffmann M, Pace M, et al. Immunological biomarkers predict HIV-1 viral rebound after treatment interruption. *Nat Commun*. 2015;6:8495.

Hutter G, Nowak D, Mossner M, et al. Long-term control of HIV by CCR5 Delta32/Delta32 stem-cell transplantation. *N Engl J Med*. 2009;360:692–698.

Impola U, Cuccuru MA, Masala MV, et al. Preliminary communication: matrix metalloproteinases in Kaposi's sarcoma. *Br J Dermatol*. 2003;149(4):905–907.

International Agency for Research on Cancer. *Human immunodeficiency viruses and human T-cell lymphotropic viruses*. Geneva: World Health Organization; 1996.

Iscovich J, Boffetta P, Franceschi S, et al. Classic Kaposi sarcoma: epidemiology and risk factors. *Cancer*. 2000;88(3):500–517.

Islami F, Moreira DM, Boffetta P, et al. A systematic review and meta-analysis of tobacco use and prostate cancer mortality and incidence in prospective cohort-studies. *Eur Urol*. 2014;66(6):1054–1064.

Jacobson LP, Jenkins FJ, Springer G, et al. Interaction of human immuno-deficiency virus type 1 and human herpesvirus type 8 infections on the incidence of Kaposi's sarcoma. *J Infect Dis*. 2000;181(6):1940–1949.

Jacomet C, Girard PM, Lebrette MG, et al. Intravenous methotrexate for primary central nervous system non-Hodgkin's lymphoma in AIDS. *AIDS*. 1997;11(14):1725–1730.

Jephcott CR, Paltiel C, Hay J. Quality of life after non-surgical treatment of anal carcinoma: a case–control study of long-term survivors. *Clin Oncol*. 2004;16(8):530–535.

Johnson LG, Madeleine MM, Newcomer LM, et al. Anal cancer incidence and survival: the surveillance, epidemiology, and end results experience, 1973–2000. *Cancer*. 2004;101(2):281–288.

Johnston C, Harrington R, Jain R, et al. Safety and efficacy of combination antiretroviral therapy in human immunodeficiency virus-infected adults undergoing autologous or allogeneic hematopoietic cell transplantation for hematologic malignancies. *Biol Blood Marrow Transplant*. 2016;22:149–156.

Joseph DA, King JB, Miller JW, et al. Prevalence of colorectal cancer screening among adults—behavioral risk factor surveillance system, United States, 2010. *MMWR*. 2012;61(2):51–56.

Kahn S, Jani A, Edelman S, et al. Matched cohort analysis of outcomes of definitive radiotherapy for prostate cancer in human immuno-deficiency virus-positive patients. *Int Radiat Oncol Biol Physics*. 2012;83(1):16–21.

Kaplan LD, Abrams DI, Feigal E, et al. AIDS-associated non-Hodgkin's lymphoma in San Francisco. *JAMA*. 1989;261(5):719–724.

Kaplan LD, Hopewell PC, Jaffe H, et al. Kaposi's sarcoma involving the lung in patients with the acquired immunodeficiency syndrome. *J AIDS*. 1988;1(1):23–30.

Kaplan LD, Straus DJ, Testa MA, et al. Low-dose compared with standard-dose m-BACOD chemotherapy for non-Hodgkin's lymphoma associated with human immunodeficiency virus infection. National Institute of Allergy and Infectious Diseases AIDS Clinical Trials Group. *N Engl J Med*. 1997;336(23):1641–1648.

Karp J, Profeta G, Marantz PR, et al. Lung cancer in patients with immunodeficiency syndrome. *Chest*. 1993;103(2):410–413.

Kelly H, Chikandiwa A, Vilches LA, et al. Association of antiretroviral therapy with anal high-risk human papillomavirus, anal intraepithelial neoplasia, and anal cancer in people living with HIV: a systematic review and meta-analysis. *Lancet HIV*. 2020;7(4):e262–e278. http://doi:10.1016/S2352-3018(19)30434-5

Kimani S, Painschab MS, Kaimila B, et al. Safety and efficacy of rituximab in patients with diffuse large B-cell lymphoma in Malawi: a prospective, single-arm, non-randomized phase ½ clinical trial. *Lancet Glob Health*. 2021;9(7):e1008–e1016.

Kirk GD, Merlo C, O'Driscoll P, et al. HIV infection is associated with an increased risk for lung cancer, independent of smoking. *Clin Infect Dis*. 2007;45(1):103–110.

Kiviat NB, Hawes S, Lampinen T, et al. The effect of HAART on detection of anal HPV and squamous intraepithelial lesions among HIV infected homosexual men. Paper presented at the 6th International Conference on Malignancies in AIDS and Other Immunodeficiencies. Bethesda, MD; 2002.

Klugman AD, Schaffner J. Colon adenocarcinoma in HIV infection: a case report and review. *Am J Gastroenterol*. 1994;89(2):254–256.

Knowles DM. Etiology and pathogenesis of AIDS-related non-Hodgkin's lymphoma. *Hematol Oncol Clin North Am*. 1996;10(5):1081–1109.

Knowles DM. *Neoplastic hematopathology*. Philadelphia: Lippincott Williams & Wilkins; 2001.

Knowles DM, Chamulak GA, Subar M, et al. Lymphoid neoplasia associated with the acquired immunodeficiency syndrome (AIDS): the New York University Medical Center experience with 105 patients (1981–1986). *Ann Intern Med*. 1988;108(5):744–753.

Kojic EM, Cu-Uvin S, Conley L, et al. Human papillomavirus infection and cytologic abnormalities of the anus and cervix among HIV-infected women in the study to understand the natural history of HIV/AIDS in the era of effective therapy (the SUN study). *Sex Transm Dis*. 2011;38(4):253–259.

Komanduri KV, Luce JA, McGrath MS, et al. The natural history and molecular heterogeneity of HIV-associated primary malignant lymphomatous effusions. *J AIDS*. 1996;13(3):215–224.

Kong CY, Sigel K, Criss SD, et al. Benefits and harms of lung cancer screening in HIV-infected individuals with CD4\+ cell count at least 500 cells/μl. *AIDS*. 2018;32(10):1333–1342.

Koon HB, Krown SE, Lee JY, et al. Phase II trial of imatinib in AIDS-associated Kaposi's sarcoma: AIDS Malignancy Consortium Protocol 042. *J Clin Oncol.* 2014;32(5):402–408.

Kowalkowski MA, Day RS, Chan W, et al. Cumulative HIV viremia and non-AIDs-defining malignancies among a sample of HIV-infected male veterans. *J AIDS.* 2014;62(2):204–211.

Krishnan A, Molina A, Zaia J, et al. Durable remissions with autologous stem cell transplantation for high-risk HIV-associated lymphomas. *Blood.* 2005;105(2):874–878.

Krown SE, Moser CB, MacPhail P, et al. Treatment of advanced AIDS-associated Kaposi sarcoma in resource-limited settings: a three-arm, open-label, randomised, non-inferiority trial. *Lancet.* 2020;395(10231):1195–1207. http://doi:10.1016/S0140-6736(19)33222-2

Krown SE, Roy D, Lee JY, et al. Rapamycin with antiretroviral therapy in AIDS-associated Kaposi sarcoma: an AIDS Malignancy Consortium study. *J AIDS.* 2012;59(5):447–454.

Krown SE, Testa MA, Huang J. AIDS-related Kaposi's sarcoma: prospective validation of the AIDS Clinical Trials Group staging classification. AIDS Clinical Trials Group Oncology Committee. *J Clin Oncol.* 1997;15(9):3085–3092.

La Ruche G, You B, Mensah-Ado I, et al. Human papillomavirus and human immunodeficiency virus infections: relation with cervical dysplasia–neoplasia in African women. *Int J Cancer.* 1998;76(4):480–486.

Lafrenie RM, Wahl LM, Epstein JS, et al. HIV-1-Tat modulates the function of monocytes and alters their interactions with microvessel endothelial cells: a mechanism of HIV pathogenesis. *J Immunol.* 1996;156(4):1638–1645.

Lavole A, Greillier L, Mazieres J, et al. First-Line carboplatin plus pemetrexed with pemetrexed maintenance in HIV+ patients with advanced non-squamous non-small cell lung cancer: the phase II IFCT-1001 CHIVA trial. *Eur Respir J.* 2020;56(2):1902066. http://doi:10.1183/13993003.02066-2019

Leapman MS, Stone K, Wadia R, et al. Prostate cancer screening and incidence among aging persons living with HIV. *J Urol.* 2022;207(2):324–332.

Lederman MM, Cannon PM, Currier JS, et al. A cure for HIV infection: "not in my lifetime" or "just around the corner"? *Pathog Immun.* 2016;1:154–164.

Lee JY, Lensing SY, Berry-Lawhorn JM, et al. Design of the Anal Cancer/HSIL Outcomes Research study (ANCHOR study): a randomized study to prevent anal cancer among persons living with HIV. *Contemp Clin Trials.* 2022;113:106679.

Le Garff G, Samri A, Lambert-Niclot S, et al. Transient HIV-specific T cells increase inflammation in an HIV-infected patient treated with nivolumab. *AIDS.* 2017;31(7):1048–1051.

Lehnert T, Methner M, Pollok A, et al. Multivisceral resection for locally advanced primary colon and rectal cancer: an analysis of prognostic factors in 201 patients. *Ann Surg.* 2002;235(2):217–225.

Leiker AJ, Wang CJ, Sanford NN, et al. Feasibility and outcome of routine use of concurrent chemoradiation in PLWH with squamous cell anal cancer. *Am J Clin Oncol.* 2020;43(10):701–708. http://doi:10.1097/COC.0000000000000736

Leport C, Rousseau F, Perronne C, et al. Bacterial prostatitis in patients infected with the human immunodeficiency virus. *J Urol.* 1989;141(2):334–336.

Letang E, Almeida J, Miró J, et al. Predictors of immune reconstitution inflammatory syndrome-associated with Kaposi sarcoma in Mozambique: a prospective study. *J AIDS.* 2010;53(5):589–597.

Levine AM, Seaberg EC, Hessol NA, et al. HIV as a risk factor for lung cancer in women: data from the Women's Interagency HIV study. *J Clin Oncol.* 2010;28(9):1514–1519.

Levine AM, Sullivan-Halley J, Pike MC, et al. Human immunodeficiency virus-related lymphoma: prognostic factors predictive of survival. *Cancer.* 1991;68(11):2466–2472.

Levine AM, Tulpule A. Clinical aspects and management of AIDS-related Kaposi's sarcoma. *Eur J Cancer.* 2001;37(10):1288–1295.

Lewden C, Salmon D, Morlat P, et al. Causes of death among human immunodeficiency virus (HIV)-infected adults in the era of potent antiretroviral therapy: emerging role of hepatitis and cancers, persistent role of AIDS. *Int J Epidemiol.* 2005;34(1):121–130.

Lewitschnig S, Gedela K, Toby M, et al. 18F-FDG PET/CT in HIV-related central nervous system pathology. *Eur J Nucl Mol Imaging.* 2013;40(9):1420–1427.

Licho R, Litofsky NS, Senitko M, et al. Inaccuracy of Tl-201 brain SPECT in distinguishing cerebral infections from lymphoma in patients with AIDS. *Clin Nuclear Med.* 2002;27(2):81–86.

Liebowitz D, Kieff E. Epstein–Barr virus latent membrane protein: induction of B-cell activation antigens and membrane patch formation does not require vimentin. *J Virol.* 1989;63(9):4051–4054.

Lillo FB, Ferrari D, Veglia F, et al. Human papillomavirus infection and associated cervical disease in human immunodeficiency virus-infected women: effect of highly active antiretroviral therapy. *J Infect Dis.* 2001;184(5):547–551.

Lim S-T, Karim R, Tulpule A, et al. Prognostic factors in HIV-related diffuse large-cell lymphoma: before versus after highly active antiretroviral therapy. *J Clin Oncol.* 2005;23(33):8477–8482.

Lin W, Chen S. Checkpoint kinase 1 is overexpressed during hPV16-induced cervical carcinogenesis. *Gynecol Obstet Invest.* 2018;83(3):2990395.

Lince-Deroche N, Phiri J, Michelow P, et al. Costs and cost effectiveness of three approaches for cervical cancer screening among HIV-positive women in Johannesburg, South Africa. *PLoS One.* 2015;10(11):e0141969.

Lister A, Abrey LE, Sandlund JT. Central nervous system lymphoma. *Am Soc Hematol. Educ Prog.* 2002:283–296.

Little RF, Pittaluga S, Grant N, et al. Highly effective treatment of acquired immunodeficiency syndrome-related lymphoma with dose-adjusted EPOCH: impact of antiretroviral therapy suspension and tumor biology. *Blood.* 2003;101(12):4653–4659.

Liu Y, Sigel KM, Westra W, et al. HIV-infected patients with anal cancer precursors: clinicopathological characteristics and human papillomavirus subtype distribution. *Dis Colon Rectum.* 2020;63(7):890–896.

Locker GY, Hamilton S, Harris J, et al. ASCO 2006 update of recommendations for the use of tumor markers in gastrointestinal cancer. *J Clin Oncol.* 2006:24(33):5313.

Loriot Y, Miler K, Sternberg CN, et al. Effect of enzalutamide on health-related quality of life, pain, and skeletal-related events in asymptomatic and minimally symptomatic, chemotherapy-naive patients with metastatic castration-resistant prostate cancer (PREVAIL): results from a randomised, phase 3 trial. *Lancet Oncol.* 2015;16(5):509–521.

Lowenthal DA, Straus DJ, Wise Campbell S, et al. AIDS-related lymphoid neoplasia: the Memorial Hospital experience. *Cancer.* 1988;61(11):2325–2337.

Luo Q, Johnson AS, Hall HI, et al. Kaposi sarcoma rates among persons living with human immunodeficiency virus in the United States: 2008–2016. *Clin Infect Dis.* 2021;73(7):e2226–e2233.

Luppi M, Barozzi P, Santagostino G, et al. Molecular evidence of organ-related transmission of Kaposi sarcoma-associated herpesvirus or human herpesvirus-8 in transplant patients. *Blood.* 2000;96(9):3279–3281.

Lurain K, Ramaswami R, Mangusan R, et al. Use of pembrolizumab with or without pomalidomide in HIV-associated non-Hodgkin's lymphoma. *J Immunother Cancer.* 2021 Feb;9(2):e002097. http://doi:10.1136/jitc-2020-002097

Lurain K, Uldrick TS, Ramaswami R, et al. Treatment of HIV-associated primary CNS lymphoma with antiretroviral therapy, rituximab, and high-dose methotrexate. *Blood.* 2020;136(19):2229–2232. http://doi:10.1182/blood.2020006048

Machalek DA, Poynten M, Jin F, et al. Anal human papillomavirus infection and associated neoplastic lesions in men who have sex with men: a systematic review and meta-analysis. *Lancet Oncol.* 2012;13(5):487–500.

MacMahon EM, Glass JD, Hayward SD, et al. Epstein–Barr virus in AIDS-related primary central nervous system lymphoma. *Lancet.* 1991;338(8773):969–973.

Mahale P, Engels EA, Coghill AE, et al. Cancer risk in older persons living with human immunodeficiency virus infection in the United States. *Clin Infect Dis.* 2018;67(1):50–57.

Mahale P, Ugoji C, Engles EA, et al. Cancer risk following lymphoid malignancies among HIV-infected people. *AIDS*. 2020;34(8):1237–1245. http://doi:10.1097/QAD.0000000000002528

Makinson A, Cheret A, Abgrall S, et al. *Early lung cancer diagnosis in HIV infected population with an important smoking history with low-dose Ct: a pilot study (EP48 HIV CHEST)*. Bethesda, MD: National Library of Medicine; 2015. https://www.clinicaltrials.gov/ct2/show/NCT01207986?term=NCT01207986&rank=1. NLM Identifier: NCT 01207986.

Mandelblatt JS, Kanetsky P, Eggert L, et al. Is HIV infection a cofactor for cervical squamous cell neoplasia? *Cancer Epidemiol*. 1999;8(1):97–106.

Mandell SP, Mack CD, Bulger EM. Motor vehicle mismatch: a national perspective. *Injury Prev*. 2010;16(5):309–314.

Marcus JL, Chao CR, Leyden WA, et al. Prostate cancer incidence and prostate-specific antigen testing among HIV-positive and HIV-negative men. *J AIDS*. 2014;66:495–502.

Marcus JL, Leyden WA, Chao CR, et al. Immunodeficiency, AIDS-related pneumonia, and risk of lung cancer among HIV-infected individuals. *AIDS*. 2017;31(7):989–993.

Mbulaiteye SM, Katabira ET, Wabinga H, et al. Spectrum of cancers among HIV-infected persons in Africa: the Uganda AIDS-Center Registry Match Study. *Int J Cancer*. 2006;118(4):985–990.

McGowan JP, Shah S. Long-term remission of AIDS-related primary central nervous system lymphoma associated with highly active antiretroviral therapy. *AIDS (London)*. 1998;12(8):952–954.

McNeil CJ, Lee JS, Cole SR, et al. Anal cancer incidence in men with HIV who have sex with men: are black men at higher risk? *AIDS*. 2022;36(5):657–664.

Mdodo R, Frazier EL, Dube SR, et al. Cigarette smoking prevalence among adults with HIV compared with the general adult population in the United States: cross-sectional surveys. *Ann Intern Med*. 2015;162(5):335–344.

Melbye M, Rabkin C, Frisch M, et al. Changing patterns of anal cancer incidence in the United States, 1940–1989. *Am J Epidemiol*. 1994;139(8):772–780.

Michaud JM, Zhang T, Shireman TI, et al. Hazard of cervical, oropharyngeal, and anal cancers in HIV-infected and HIV-uninfected Medicaid beneficiaries. *Cancer Epidemiol Biomarkers Prev*. 2020;29(7):1447–1457.

Minaar CA, Baeyens A, Akinwale Ayeni O, et al. Defining characteristics of nodal disease on PET/CT scans in patients with HIV-positive and -negative locally advanced cervical cancer in South Africa. *Tomography*. 2019;5(4):339–345.

Minkoff H, Ahdieh L, Massad, LS et al. The effect of highly active antiretroviral therapy on cervical cytologic changes associated with oncogenic HPV among HIV-infected women. *J AIDS*. 2001;15(16):2157–2164.

Minkoff H, Zhong Y, Burk RD, et al. Influence of adherent and effective antiretroviral therapy use on human papillomavirus infection and squamous intraepithelial lesions in human immunodeficiency virus-positive women. *J Infect Dis*. 2010;201(5):681–690.

Mitsuyasu RT, Groopman JE. Biology and therapy of Kaposi's sarcoma. *Semin Oncol*. 1984;11(1):53–59.

Monforte A, Abrams D, Pradier C, et al. HIV-induced immunodeficiency and mortality from AIDS-defining and non-AIDS-defining malignancies. *AIDS (London)*. 2008;22(16):2143–2153.

Monini P, de Lellis L, Fabris M, et al. Kaposi's sarcoma-associated herpesvirus DNA sequences in prostate tissue and human semen. *N Engl J Med*. 1996;334(18):1168–1172.

Montgomery JD, Jacobson LP, Dhir R, Jenkins FJ. Detection of human herpesvirus 8 (HHV-8) in normal prostates. *Prostate*. 2006;66(12):1302–1310.

Moore AL, Sabin CA, Madge S, et al. Highly active antiretroviral therapy and cervical intraepithelial neoplasia. *AIDS*. 2002;16(6):927–929.

Morlat P, Roussillon C, Henard S, et al. Causes of death among HIV-infected patients in France in 2010 (national survey): trends since 2000. *AIDS*. 2014;28(8):1181–1191.

Mosam A, Shaik F, Uldrick TS, et al. A randomized controlled trial of HAART versus HAART and chemotherapy in therapy-naive patients with HIV-associated Kaposi sarcoma in South Africa. *J AIDS*. 2012;60(2):150.

Mounier N, Spina M, Gabarre J, et al. AIDS-related non-Hodgkin lymphoma: final analysis of 485 patients treated with risk-adapted intensive chemotherapy. *Blood*. 2006;107(10):3832–3840.

Moyer VA. Screening for prostate cancer: US Preventive Services Task Force recommendation statement. *Ann Intern Med*. 2012;157(2):120–135.

Moyer VA. Screening for lung cancer. US Preventative Services Task Force recommendation statement. *Ann Intern Med*. 2014;160(5):330–338.

Munger K, Phelps WC, Bubb V, et al. The E6 and E7 genes of the human papillomavirus type 16 together are necessary and sufficient for transformation of primary human keratinocytes. *J Virol*. 1989;63(10):4417–4421.

Murthy N, Wodi AP, Bernstein H, et al. Advisory Committee on Immunization Practices Recommended Immunization Schedule for Adults Aged 19 Years or Older—United States, 2022. *MMWR Morb Mortal Wkly Rep*. 2022;71:229–233. http://dx.doi.org/10.15585/mmwr.mm7107a1

Myerson RJ, Kong F, Birnbaum EH, et al. Radiation therapy for epidermoid carcinoma of the anal canal: clinical and treatment factors associated with outcome. *Radiother Oncol*. 2001;61(1):15–22.

Nagata N, Shimbo T, Yazaki H, et al. Predictive clinical factors in the diagnosis of gastrointestinal Kaposi's sarcoma and its endoscopic severity. *PLoS One*. 2012;7(11):1–7.

Nasti G, Martellotta F, Berretta M, et al. Impact of highly active antiretroviral therapy on the presenting features and outcome of patients with acquired immunodeficiency syndrome-related Kaposi sarcoma. *Cancer*. 2003a;98(11):2440–2446.

Nasti G, Talamini R, Antinori A, et al. AIDS-related Kaposi's sarcoma: evaluation of potential new prognostic factors and assessment of the AIDS Clinical Trial Group Staging System in the HAART Era—the Italian Cooperative Group on AIDS and Tumors and the Italian Cohort of Patients Naive from Antiretrovirals. *J Clin Oncol*. 2003b;21(15):2876–2882.

National Comprehensive Cancer Network NCCN. NCCN clinical practice guidelines in oncology. Rectal cancer. Version 1.2016. https://www.nccn.org/professionals/physician_gls/pdf/rectal.pdf. Published November 4, 2015a. Accessed May 13, 2016.

NCCN. NCCN clinical practice guidelines in oncology. Non-small cell lung cancer, version 2.2016. https://www.nccn.org/professionals/physician_gls/pdf/nscl.pdf. Published November 23, 2015b. Accessed December 8, 2015.

NCCN. NCCN clinical practice guidelines in oncology. Colon cancer, version 2.2016. https://www.nccn.org/professionals/physician_gls/pdf/colon.pdf. Published November 23, 2015c. Accessed May 13, 2016.

NCCN. NCCN clinical practice guidelines in oncology. Cancer in people with HIV, version 1.2022. https://www.nccn.org/professionals/physician_gls/pdf/hiv.pdf. Published February 3, 2022a. Accessed October 8, 2022.

NCCN. NCCN clinical practice guidelines in oncology. Central nervous system cancers, version 2.2022. https://www.nccn.org/professionals/physician_gls/pdf/cns.pdf. Published September 29, 2022b. Accessed October 8, 2022.

National Lung Screening Trial Research Team. Reduced lung-cancer mortality with low-dose computed tomographic screening. *N Engl J Med*. 2011;365(5):395–409.

Navarro WH, Kaplan LD. AIDS-related lymphoproliferative disease. *Blood*. 2006;107(1):13–20.

Nayudu SK, Balar B. Colorectal cancer screening in human immunodeficiency virus populations: are they at average risk? *World J Gastrointestinal Oncol*. 2012;4(12):259–264.

NCT00006436. Clinicaltrials.gov. EPOCH and rituximab to treat non-Hodgkin's lymphoma in patients with HIV infection.

NCT00267865. Clinicaltrials.gov. Chemotherapy and HAART to treat AIDS-related primary brain lymphoma.

NCT01207986. Clinicaltrials.gov. Early lung cancer diagnosis in HIV infected population with an important smoking history with low dose CT: a pilot study.

NCT02135419. Clinicaltrials.gov. Topical or ablative treatment in preventing anal cancer in patients with HIV and anal high-grade squamous intraepithelial lesions.

NCT02408861. Clinicaltrials.gov. Nivolumab and ipilimumab in treating patients with a HIV associated relapsed or refractory classical Hodgkin lymphoma or solid tumors that are metastatic or cannot be removed by surgery.

NCT02595866. Clinicaltrials.gov. Testing the addition of an experimental medication MK-3475 (pembrolizumab) to usual antiretroviral medications in patients with HIV and cancer.

NCT02659930. Clinicaltrials.gov. Pomalidomide in combination with liposomal doxorubicin in people with advanced or refractory Kaposi sarcoma.

NCT02660710. Clinicaltrials.gov. Rituximab plus CHOP chemotherapy for diffuse large B-cell lymphoma.

NCT03094286. Clinicaltrials.gov. Durvalumab in solid tumors.

NCT03113942. Clinicaltrials.gov. Study of pomalidomide in anal cancer precursors.

NCT03202992. Clinicaltrals.gov. Study of topical ABI-1968 in subjects with precancerous anal lesions resulting from human papillomavirus (HPV) infection.

NCT03304093. Clinicaltrials.gov. Immunotherapy by nivolumab for HIV+ patients.

NCT03316274. Clinicaltrials.gov. Intra-lesional nivolumab therapy for limited cutaneous Kaposi sarcoma.

NCT03332069. Clinicaltrials.gov. Modulated electro-hyperthermia plus chemoradiation for locally advanced cervical cancer patients in South Africa.

NCT03354936. Clinicaltrials.gov. ANRS CO24 OncoVIHAC (onco VIH anti checkpoint).

NCT03617198. Clinicaltrials.gov. CD4 CAR+ ZFN-modified T cells in HIV therapy.

Neef H, Horth W, Makowiec F, et al. Outcome after resection of hepatic and pulmonary metastasis of colorectal cancer. *J Gastrointest Surg.* 2009;13(10):1813–1820.

Newton R, Ziegler J, Bourboulia D, et al. Infection with Kaposi's sarcoma-associated herpesvirus (KSHV) and human immunodeficiency virus (HIV) in relation to the risk and clinical presentation of Kaposi's sarcoma in Uganda. *Br J Cancer.* 2003;89(3):502–504.

Norden AD, Drappatz J, Wen PY, et al. Survival among patients with primary central nervous system lymphoma, 1973–2004. *J Neuro-Oncol.* 2011;101(3):487–493.

Northfelt DW, Dezube BJ, Thommes JA, et al. Pegylated-liposomal doxorubicin versus doxorubicin, bleomycin, and vincristine in the treatment of AIDS-related Kaposi's sarcoma: results of a randomized phase III clinical trial. *J Clin Oncol.* 1998;16(7):2445–2451.

Noy A. Update in Kaposi sarcoma. *Curr Opin Oncol.* 2003;15(5):379–381.

Noy A, Lee JY, Cesarman E, et al. AMC 048: modified CODOX-M/IVAC-rituximab is safe and effective for HIV-associated Burkitt lymphoma. *Blood.* 2015;126:160–166.

Ntekim A, Campbell O, Rothenbacher D. Optimal management of cervical cancer in PLWH: a systematic review. *Cancer Med.* 2015;4:1381–1393.

Nyitray AG, Hicks JT, Hwang LY, et al. A phase II clinical study to assess the feasibility of self and partner anal examinations to detect anal canal abnormalities including anal cancer. *Sex Transm Infect.* March 2018;94(2):124–130.

Oehler-Janne C, Huguet F, Provencher S, et al. HIV-specific differences in outcome of squamous cell carcinoma of the anal canal: a multicentric cohort study of PLWH receiving highly active antiretroviral therapy. *J Clin Oncol.* 2008;26(15):2550–2557.

Okotie OT, Roehl KA, Han M, et al. Characteristics of prostate cancer detected by digital rectal examination only. *Urology.* 2007;70(6):1117–1120.

Okuma Y, Hishima T, Kashima J, et al. High PD-L1 expression indicates poor prognosis of HIV-infected patients with non-small cell lung cancer. *Cancer Immunol Immunother.* March 2018;67(3):495–505.

Okuma Y, Hosomi Y, Imamura A. Lung cancer patients harboring epidermal growth factor receptor mutation among those infected by human immunodeficiency virus. *Onco Targets Ther.* 2014;31:111–115.

Olson JE, Janney CA, Rao RD, et al. The continuing increase in the incidence of primary central nervous system non-Hodgkin lymphoma: a surveillance, epidemiology, and end results analysis. *Cancer.* 2002;95(7):1504–1510.

Ong WL, Manohar P, Millar J, et al. Clinicopathological characteristics and management of prostate cancer in the human immunodeficiency virus (HIV)-positive population: experience in an Australian major HIV center. *Br J Urol Int.* 2015;116(Suppl 3):5–10.

Orlando G, Fasolo MM, Schiavini M, et al. Role of highly active antiretroviral therapy in human papillomavirus-induced genital dysplasia in HIV-1-infected patients. *AIDS (London).* 1999;13(3):424–425.

Palefsky JM. Human papillomavirus-associated anal and cervical cancers in HIV-infected individuals: incidence and prevention in the antiretroviral era. *Curr Opin HIV AIDS.* 2017;12(1):26–30.

Palefsky JM, Holly EA, Gonzales J, et al. Detection of human papillomavirus DNA in anal intraepithelial neoplasia and anal cancer. *Cancer Res.* 1991;51(3):1014–1019.

Palefsky JM, Holly EA, Ralston ML, et al. Effect of highly active antiretroviral therapy on the natural history of anal squamous intraepithelial lesions and anal human papillomavirus infection. *J AIDS.* 2001;28(5):422–428.

Palefsky JM, Lee JY, Jay N, et al. Treatment of anal high-grade squamous intraepithelial lesion to prevent anal cancer. *N Engl J Med.* 2022;386(24):227302282.

Pantanowitz L, Bohac G, Cooley T, et al. Human immunodeficiency virus-associated prostate cancer: clinicopathological findings and outcome in a multi-institutional study. *Br J Urol Int.* 2008;101:1519–1523.

Patel P, Hanson DL, Sullivan PS, et al. Incidence of types of cancer among HIV-infected persons compared with the general population in the United States, 1992–2003. *Ann Intern Med.* 2008;148(10):728–736.

Patil P, Elem B, Zumla A. Pattern of adult malignancies in Zambia (1980–1989) in light of the human immunodeficiency virus type 1 epidemic. *J Tropical Med Hygiene.* 1995;98(4):281–284.

Penn I. Kaposi's sarcoma in organ transplant recipients: report of 20 cases. *Transplantation.* 1979;27(1):8–11.

Persad GC, Little RF, Grady C. Including persons with HIV infection in cancer clinical trials. *J Clin Oncol.* 2008;26(7):1027–1032.

Petrovas C, Casazza JP, Brenchley JM, et al. PD-1 is a regulator of virus-specific CD8\+ T-cell survival in HIV infection. *J Exp Med.* 2006;203:2281–2292.

Piketty C, Seliger-Leneman H, Bouvier AM. Incidence of HIV-related anal cancer remains increased despite long-term combined antiretroviral treatment: results from the French Hospital Database on HIV. *J Clin Oncol.* 2012;30(35):4360–4366.

Piketty C, Selinger-Leneman H, Grabar S, et al. Marked increase in the incidence of invasive anal cancer among HIV-infected patients despite treatment with combination antiretroviral therapy. *AIDS.* 2008;22(10):1203–1211.

Plancoulaine S, Abel L, van Beveren M, et al. Human herpesvirus 8 transmission from mother to child and between siblings in an endemic population. *Lancet.* 2000;356(9235):1062–1065.

Pluda J, Broder S, Yarchoan R. Therapy of AIDS and AIDS-associated neoplasms. *Cancer Chemother Biol Response Modif.* 1992;13:404–439.

Polesel J, Clifford GM, Rickenbach M, et al. Non-Hodgkin lymphoma incidence in the Swiss HIV Cohort Study before and after highly active antiretroviral therapy. *AIDS (London).* 2008;22(2):301–306.

Polizzotto MN, Uldrick TS, Wyvill KM, et al. Pomalidomide for symptomatic Kaposi's sarcoma in people with and without HIV infection: a phase I/II study. *J Clin Oncol.* December 2016b;34(34):4125–4131.

Polizzotto MN, Uldrick TS, Wyvill KM, et al. Clinical features and outcomes of patients with symptomatic Kaposi sarcoma herpesvirus

(KSHV)-associated Inflammation: prospective characterization of KSHV inflammatory cytokine syndrome (KICS). *Clin Infect Dis.* 2016a;62(6):730–738. http://doi:10.1093/cid/civ996

Pourcher V, Desnoyer A, Assoumou L et al. Phase II trial of lenalidomide in HIV-infected patients with previously treated Kaposi's sarcoma: results of the ANRS 154 Lenakap Trial. *AIDS Res Hum Retroviruses.* 2017;33(1):1–10.

Powles T, Matthews G, Bower M. AIDS related systemic non-Hodgkin's lymphoma. *Sex Transm Infect.* 2000;76(5):335–341.

Powles T, Thirwell C, Newsom-Davis T, et al. Does HIV adversely influence the outcome in advanced non-small-cell lung cancer in the era of HAART? *Br J Cancer.* 2003;89:457–459.

Rahmanian S, Wewers ME, Koletar S, et al. Cigarette smoking in the HIV-infected population. *Proc Am Thorac Soc.* 2011;8(3):313–319.

Ramaswami R, Polizzotto MN, Lurain K, et al. Safety, activity, and long-term outcomes of pomalidomide in the treatment of Kaposi sarcoma among individuals with or without HIV infection. *Clin Cancer Res.* 2022;28(5):840–850.

Ramirez-Marrero FA, Smit E, de la Torre-Feliciano T, et al. Risk of cancer among Hispanics with AIDS compared with the general population in Puerto Rico: 1987–2003. *Puerto Rico Health Sci J.* 2010;29(3):256–264.

Rasmussen TA, Rajdev L, Rhodes A, et al. Impact of anti-PD-1 and anti-CTLA-4 on the human immunodeficiency virus (HIV) reservoir in people living with HIV with cancer on antiretroviral therapy: the AIDS Malignancy Consortium 095 study. *Clin Infect Dis.* 2021;73(7):e1973–e1981. http://doi:10.1093/cid/ciaa1530

Ratner L, Lee J, Tang S, et al. Chemotherapy for human immunodeficiency virus-associated non-Hodgkin's lymphoma in combination with highly active antiretroviral therapy. *J Clin Oncol.* 2001;19(8):2171–2178.

Ravalli S, Chabon A, Khan A. Gastrointestinal neoplasia in young HIV antibody-positive patients. *Am J Clin Pathol.* 1989;91:458–461.

Re A, Cattaneo C, Michieli M, et al. High-dose therapy and autologous peripheral-blood stem-cell transplantation as salvage treatment for HIV-associated lymphoma in patients receiving highly active antiretroviral therapy. *J Clin Oncol.* 2003;21(23):4423–4427.

Re A, Michieli M, Casari S, et al. High-dose therapy and autologous peripheral blood stem cell transplantation as salvage treatment for AIDS-related lymphoma: long-term results of the Italian Cooperative Group on AIDS and Tumors (GICAT) study with analysis of prognostic factors. *Blood.* 2009;114(7):1306–1313.

Reddy KP, Kong CY, Hyle EP, et al. Lung cancer mortality associated with smoking and smoking cessation among people living with HIV in the United States. *JAMA Intern Med.* November 1, 2017;177(11):1613–1621.

Reekie J, Kosa C, Engsig F, et al. Relationship between current level of immunodeficiency and non-acquired immunodeficiency syndrome-defining malignancies. *Cancer.* November 15, 2010;116(22):5306–5315.

Reid E, Suneja G, Ambinder RF, et al. Cancer in people living with HIV, Version 1.2018, NCCN clinical practice guidelines in oncology. *J Natl Compr Canc Netw.* 2018;16(8):986–1017.

Reinhold JP, Moon M, Tenner CT, et al. Colorectal cancer screening in HIV-infected patients 50 years of age and older: missed opportunities for prevention. *Am J Gastroenterol.* 2005;100:1805–1812.

Renwick N, Halaby T, Weverling GJ, et al. Seroconversion for human herpesvirus 8 during HIV infection is highly predictive of Kaposi's sarcoma. *AIDS.* 1998;12(18):2481–2488.

Richel O, de Vries HJ, van Noesel CJ, et al. Comparison of imiquimod, topical fluorouracil, and electrocautery for the treatment of anal intraepithelial neoplasia in HIV-positive men who have sex with men: an open-label, randomised controlled trial. *Lancet Oncol.* 2013;14:346–353.

Riedel DJ, Cox ER, Stafford KA, et al. Clinical presentation and outcomes of prostate cancer in an urban cohort of predominantly African American, human immunodeficiency virus-infected patients. *Urology.* 2015;85(2):415–421.

Riedel DJ, Rositch AF, Redfield RR. Patterns of HIV viremia and viral suppression before diagnosis of non-AIDS-defining cancers in HIV-infected individuals. *Infect Agent Cancer.* 2015b;38(10):1–7.

Riley RR, Duensing S, Brake T, et al. Dissection of human papillomavirus E6 and E7 function in transgenic mouse models of cervical carcinogenesis. *Cancer Res.* 2003;63(16):4862–4871.

Robbins HA, Pfeiffer RM, Shiels MS, et al. Excess cancers among HIV-infected people in the United States. *J Natl Cancer Inst.* 2015;107:pii: dju503.

Robert C, Ribas A, Wolchok JD, et al. Anti-programmed-death-receptor-1 treatment with pembrolizumab in ipilimumab-refractory advanced melanoma: a randomised dose-comparison cohort of a phase 1 trial. *Lancet.* 2014;384:1109–1117.

Rodrigo JA, Hicks LK, Cheung MC, et al. HIV-associated Burkitt lymphoma: good efficacy and tolerance of intensive chemotherapy including CODOX-M/IVAC with or without rituximab in the HAART era. *Adv Hematol.* 2012;2012:1–9.

Rohner E, Bütikofer L, Schmidlin K, et al. Cervical cancer risk in women living with HIV across four continents: A multicohort study. *Int J Cancer.* 2020;146(3):601–609. http://doi:10.1002/ijc.32260

Rohner E, Valeri F, Maskew M, et al. Incidence rate of Kaposi sarcoma in HIV-infected patients on antiretroviral therapy in southern Africa: a prospective multicohort study. *J AIDS.* 2014;67(5):547–554.

Ronit A, Kristensen T, Klitbo DM, et al. Incidental lung cancers and positive computed tomography images in people living with HIV. *AIDS.* 2017;31:1973–1977

Rosenblum ML, Levy RM, Bredesen DE, et al. Primary central nervous system lymphomas in patients with AIDS. *Ann Neurol.* 1988;23:S13–S16.

Royse K, El Chaer F, Amirian ES, et al. Disparities in Kaposi sarcoma incidence and survival in the United States: 2000–2013. *PLoS One.* 2017;12(8):e0182750.

Ruiz A, Ganz WI, Post MJ, et al. Use of thallium-201 brain SPECT to differentiate cerebral lymphoma from toxoplasma encephalitis in AIDS patients. *Am J Neuroradiol.* 1994;15(10):1885–1894.

Rust B, Kiem HP, and Uldrick T. CAR T-cell therapy for cancer and HIV through novel approaches to HIV-associated haematological malignancies. *Lancet Haematol.* 2020;7(9):e690–e696. http://doi:10.1016/S2352-3026(20)30142-3

Ryan CJ, Smith MR, Fizazi K, et al. Abiraterone acetate plus prednisone versus placebo plus prednisone in chemotherapy-naive men with metastatic castration-resistant prostate cancer (COU-AA-302): final overall survival analysis of a randomised, double-blind, placebo-controlled phase 3 study. *Lancet Oncol.* 2015;16(2):152–160.

Sacktor N, Lyles RH, Skolasky R, et al. HIV-associated neurologic disease incidence changes: Multicenter AIDS Cohort Study, 1990–1998. *Neurology.* 2001;56(2):257–260.

Safai B. Pathophysiology and epidemiology of epidemic Kaposi's sarcoma. *Semin Oncol.* 1987;2:7–12.

Sandler AS, Kaplan LD. Diagnosis and management of systemic non-Hodgkin's lymphoma in HIV disease. *Hematol Oncol Clin North Am.* 1996;10(5):1111–1124.

Santesso N, Mustafa RA, Schunemann HJ, et al. World Health Organization guidelines for treatment of cervical intraepithelial neoplasia 2-3 and screen-and-treat strategies to prevent cervical cancer. *Int J Gynaecol Obstet.* 2016;132:252–258

Sauer R, Liersch T, Merkel S, et al. Preoperative versus postoperative chemoradiotherapy for locally advanced rectal cancer: results of the German CAO/ARO/AIO-94 randomized phase III trial after a median follow-up of 11 years. *J Clin Oncol.* 2012;20(16):1926–1933.

Saville M, Lietzau J, Pluda J, et al. Activity of placlitaxel (Taxol) as therapy for HIV-associated Kaposi's sarcoma. *Lancet.* 1995;346:26–28.

Schiffman M, Kjaer SK. Natural history of anogenital human papillomavirus infection and neoplasia. *JNCI Monographs.* 2003;2003(31):14–19.

Schreiber D, Chhabra A, Rineer J, et al. Outcomes and tolerance of human immunodeficiency virus-positive veterans undergoing dose-escalated external beam radiotherapy for localized prostate cancer. *Clin Genitourinary Cancer.* 2014;12(2):94–99.

Sellers SA, Edmonds A, Ramirez C, et al. Optimal lung cancer screening criteria among persons living with HIV. *J Acquir Immune Defic Syndr*. 2022;90(2):184–192.

Serraino D, Boschini A, Carrieri P, et al. Cancer risk among men with, or at risk of, HIV infection in southern Europe. *AIDS*. 2000;14(5):553–559.

Sgadari C, Monini P, Barillari G, et al. Use of HIV protease inhibitors to block Kaposi's sarcoma and tumour growth. *Lancet Oncol*. 2003;4(9):537–547.

Shah NN, Singavi AK, Harrington A. Daratumumab in primary effusion lymphoma. *N Engl J Med*. 2018;379(7):689–690.

Shah R, Al-Sukhni W, Kim RD, et al. Resection of hepatic and pulmonary metastasis from colorectal carcinoma. *JACS*. 2006;202(3):468–475.

Shahani AJ, Gulsoy EB, Gibbs JW, et al. Integrated approach to the data processing of four-dimensional datasets from phase-contrast x-ray tomography. *Opt Express*. 2014;22(20):24606–24621.

Shebl FM, Engels EA, Goedert JJ, et al. Pulmonary infections and risk of lung cancer among persons with AIDS. *J AIDS*. 2010;55:375–379.

Shepherd FA, Crowley J, van Houtte P, et al.; the IASLC Lung Cancer Staging Project. Clinical staging of small cell lung cancer in the forthcoming (seventh) edition of the Tumor, Node, Metastasis Classification for Lung Cancer. *J Thoracic Oncol*. 2007;2(12):1067–1077.

Shepherd L, Ryom L, Law M, et al. Cessation of cigarette smoking and the impact on cancer incidence in HIV-positive persons: the D:A:D study. *Clin Infect Dis*. 2018;68(4):650–657. http://doi:10.1093/cid/ciy508

Shiels MS, Althoff KN, Pfeiffer RM, et al. HIV infection, immunosuppression, and age at diagnosis of non-AIDS-defining cancers. *Clin Infect Dis*. 2017;64(4):468–475.

Shiels, MS, Cole SR, Mehta SH, et al. Lung cancer incidence and mortality among HIV-infected and HIV-uninfected injection drug users. *J AIDS*. 2010a;55(4):510–515.

Shiels MS, Copeland G, Goodman M, et al. Cancer stage at diagnosis in patients infected with the human immunodeficiency virus and transplant recipients. *Cancer*. 2015;121(12):1063–2071.

Shiels MS, Goedert JJ, Moore RD, et al. Reduced risk of prostate cancer in US men with AIDS. *Cancer Epidemiol Biomarkers Prev*. 2010b;19(11):2910–2915.

Shiels MS, Pfeiffer RM, Engels EA. Age at cancer diagnosis among persons with AIDS in the United States. *Ann Intern Med*. 2010c;153(7):452–460.

Shiels MS, Pfeiffer RM, Gail MH, et al. Cancer burden in the HIV-infected population in the United States. *J Nat Cancer Institute*. 2011a;103:753–762.

Shiels MS, Pfeiffer RM, Hall HI, et al. Proportions of Kaposi sarcoma, selected non-Hodgkin lymphomas, and cervical cancer in the United States occurring in persons with AIDS, 1980–2007. *JAMA*. 2011b;305(14):1450–1459.

Shiels MS, Pfeiffer RM, Hildesheim A, et al. Circulating inflammation markers and prospective risk for lung cancer. *J Nat Cancer Inst*. 2013;105(24):1871–1880.

Siegel R, DeSantis C, Jemal A. Colorectal cancer statistics, 2014. *CA Cancer J Clinicians*. 2014;64(2):104–117.

Siegel R, Naishadham D, Jemal A. Cancer statistics, 2012. *CA Cancer J Clinicians*. 2012;62(1):10–29.

Sigel C, Cavalcanti MS, Daniel T, et al. Clinicopathologic features of colorectal carcinoma in PLWH. *Cancer Epidemiol Biomarkers Prev*. 2016;25:1098–1104.

Sigel K, Crothers K, Dubrow R, et al. Prognosis in HIV-infected patients with non-small cell lung cancer. *Br J Cancer*. 2013;109:1974–1980.

Sigel K, Wisnivesky J, Crothers K, et al. Immunological and infectious risk factors for lung cancer in US veterans with HIV: a longitudinal cohort study. *Lancet HIV*. 2017;4(2):e67–e73.

Sigel K, Wisnevesky J, Gordon K, et al. HIV as an independent risk factor for incident lung cancer. *AIDS*. 2012;26:1017–1025.

Sigel K, Wisnivesky J, Shahrir S, et al. Findings in asymptomatic HIV-infected patients undergoing chest computed tomography testing: implications for lung cancer screening. *AIDS*. 2014;28(7):1007–1014.

Silverberg MJ, Chao C, Leyden WA, et al. HIV infection, immunodeficiency, viral replication, and the risk of cancer. *Cancer Epidemiol Biomarkers Prev*. 2011;20(12):2551–2559.

Silverberg MJ, Lau B, Achenbach CJ, et al. Cumulative incidence of cancer among persons with HIV in North America. *Ann Intern Med*. 2015;163(7):507–518.

Silverberg MJ, Lau B, Justic AC, et al. Risk of anal cancer in HIV-infected and HIV-uninfected individuals in North America. *Clin Infect Dis*. 2012;54(17):1026–1034.

Silverberg MJ, Leyden W, Steven Gregorich S, et al. Is intensive cervical cancer screening justified in immunosuppressed women? [Abstract 162]. Paper presented at the Conference on Retroviruses and Opportunistic Infections (CROI). Boston, MA; February 22–25, 2016.

Simard EP, Pfeiffer RM, Engels EA. Spectrum of cancer risk late after AIDS onset in the United States. *Arch Intern Med*. 2010;170(15):1337–1345.

Simard EP, Pfeiffer RM, Engels EA. Cumulative incidence of cancer among individuals with acquired immunodeficiency syndrome in the United States. *Cancer*. 2011;117(5):1089–1096.

Skiest DJ, Crosby C. Survival is prolonged by highly active antiretroviral therapy in AIDS patients with primary central nervous system lymphoma. *AIDS*. 2003;17(12):1787–1793.

Smith AJB, Varma S, Rositch AF, et al. Gynecologic cancer in HIV-positive women: a systematic review and meta-analysis. *Am J Obstet Gynecol*. 2019;221(3):194–207. http://doi:10.1016/j.ajog.2019.02.022

Smith DM, Kingery JD, Wong JK, et al. The prostate as a reservoir for HIV-1. *AIDS*. 2004;18(11):1600–1602.

Smith JS, Sanusi B, Swarts A, et al. A randomized clinical trial comparing cervical dysplasia treatment with cryotherapy vs loop electrosurgical excision procedure in HIV-seropositive women from Johannesburg, South Africa. *Am J Obstet Gynecol*. 2017;217(2):183.e1–183.e11.

Smith RE, Colangelo L, Wieand HS, et al. Randomized trial of adjuvant therapy in colon carcinoma: 10-Year results of NSABP Protocol C-01. *J Natl Cancer Inst*. 2004;96(15):1128–1132.

Spano JP, Massiani MA, Bentata M, et al. Lung cancer in patients with HIV infection and review of the literature. *Med Oncol*. 2004;21:109–115.

Sparano JA, Lee S, Chen MG, et al. Phase II trial of infusional cyclophosphamide, doxorubicin, and etoposide in patients with HIV-associated non-Hodgkin's lymphoma: an Eastern Cooperative Oncology Group Trial (E1494). *J Clin Oncol*. 2004;22(8):1491–1500.

Sparano JA, Lee JY, Kaplan LD, et al. Rituximab plus concurrent infusional EPOCH chemotherapy is highly effective in HIV-associated B-cell non-Hodgkin lymphoma. *Blood*. 2010;115(15):3008–3016.

Stadler RF, Gregorcyk SG, Euhus DM, et al. Outcome of HIV-infected patients with invasive squamous-cell carcinoma of the anal canal in the era of highly active antiretroviral therapy. *Dis Colon Rectum*. 2004;47(8):1305–1309.

Stebbing J, Sanitt A, Nelson M, et al. A prognostic index for AIDS-associated Kaposi's sarcoma in the era of highly active antiretroviral therapy. *Lancet*. 2006;367(9521):1495–1502.

Stebbing J, Sanitt A, Teague A, et al. Prognostic significance of immune subset measurement in individuals with AIDS-associated Kaposi's sarcoma. *J Clin Oncol*. 2007;25(16):2230–2235.

Stelzle D, Tanaka LF, Lee KK, et al. Estimates of the global burden of cervical cancer associated with HIV. *Lancet Glob Health*. 2021;9(2):e161–e169. http://doi:10.1016/S2214-109X(20)30459-9

Stewart S, Jablonowski H, Goebel FD, et al. Randomized comparative trial of pegylated liposomal doxorubicin versus bleomycin and vincristine in the treatment of AIDS-related Kaposi's sarcoma: International Pegylated Liposomal Doxorubicin Study Group. *J Clin Oncol*. 1998;16(2):683–691.

Stier EA, Abbasi W, Agyemang AF, et al. Brief report: recurrence of anal high-grade squamous intraepithelial lesions among women living with HIV. *J Acquir Immune Defic Syndr*. 2020;84(1):66–69.

Stier EA, Sebring MC, Mendez AE, et al. Prevalence of anal human papillomavirus infection and anal HPV-related disorders in women: a systematic review. *Am J Ob Gyn*. 2015;213(3):278–309.

Straus DJ, Huang J, Testa MA, et al. Prognostic factors in the treatment of human immunodeficiency virus-associated non-Hodgkin's lymphoma: analysis of AIDS Clinical Trials Group protocol 142—low-dose versus standard-dose m-BACOD plus granulocyte-macrophage colony-stimulating factor; National Institute of Allergy and Infectious Diseases. *J Clin Oncol.* 1998;16(11):3601–3606.

Sugarman J, Lewin SR, Henrich TJ, et al. Ethics of ART interruption after stem-cell transplantation. *Lancet HIV.* 2016;3:e8–e10.

Sumner L, Kamitani E, Chase S, et al. A systematic review and meta-analysis of mortality in anal cancer patients by HIV status. *Cancer Epidemiol.* 2022;76:102069.

Sun D, Cao M, Li H, et al. Risk of prostate cancer in men with HIV/AIDS: a systematic review and meta-analysis. *Prostate Cancer Prostatic Dis.* 2021;24(1):24–34. http://doi:10.1038/s41391-020-00268-2

Sung H, Ferlay J, Siegel RL, et al. Global Cancer Statistics 2020: GLOBOCAN estimates of incidence and mortality worldwide for 36 cancers in 185 countries. *CA Cancer J Clin.* 2021;71(3):209–249. http://doi:10.3322/caac.21660

Suneja G, Shiels MS, Melville SK. Disparities in the treatment and outcomes of lung cancer among HIV-infected individuals. *AIDS.* 2013;27(3):459–468.

Susko M, Wang, CJ, Lazar AA, et al. Factors impacting differential outcomes in the definitive radiation treatment of anal cancer between HIV-positive and HIV-negative patients. *Oncologist.* 2020;25(9):772–779. http://doi:10.1634/theoncologist.2019-0824. Online ahead of print.

Taieb J, Tabernero J, Mini E, et al. Oxaliplatin, fluorouracil, and leucovorin with or without cetuximab in patients with resected stage III colon cancer (PETACC-8): an open-label, randomised phase III trial. *Lancet Oncol.* 2014;15(8):862–873.

Tam HK, Zhang Z-F, Jacobson LP, et al. Effect of highly active antiretroviral therapy on survival among HIV-infected men with Kaposi sarcoma or non-Hodgkin lymphoma. *Int J Cancer.* 2002;98(6):916–922.

Tesoiero JM, Gieryic SM, Carrascal A, et al. Smoking among HIV-positive New Yorkers: prevalence, frequency, and opportunities for cessation. *AIDS Behav.* 2010;14(4):824–835.

Tornesello ML, Buonaguro FM, Beth-Giraldo E, et al. Human immunodeficiency virus type 1 Tat gene enhances human papillomavirus early gene expression. *Intervirology.* 1993;36(2):57–64.

Trautmann L, Janbazian L, Chomont N, et al. Upregulation of PD-1 expression on HIV-specific CD8\+ T cells leads to reversible immune dysfunction. *Nat Med.* 2006;12:1198–1202.

Travi G, Ferreri A, Cinque P, et al. Long term remission of HIV-associated primary CNS lymphoma achieved with highly active antiretroviral therapy alone. *J Clin Oncol.* 2012;30(10):e119–e121.

Uldrick TS, Polizzotto MN, Yarchoan R. Recent advances in Kaposi sarcoma herpesvirus-associated multicentric Castleman disease. *Curr Opin Oncol.* 2012;24(5):495–505.

Uldrick TS, Gonçalves PH, Abdul-Hay M, et al. Assessment of the safety of pembrolizumab in patients with HIV and advanced cancer: a phase 1 study. *JAMA Oncol.* 2019;5(9):1332–1339. http://doi:10.1001/jamaoncol.2019.2244

US Department of Health and Human Services (DHHS) Panel on Antiretroviral Guidelines for Adults and Adolescents. Guidelines for the use of antiretroviral agents in adults and adolescents with HIV. http://www.aidsinfo.nih.gov/ContentFiles/AdultandAdolescentGL.pdf. Published 2022a. Accessed September 25, 2022.

US Department of Health and Human Services (US DHHS). Panel on Guidelines for the Prevention and Treatment of Opportunistic Infections in Adults and Adolescents with HIV. Guidelines for the prevention and treatment of opportunistic infections in HIV-infected adults and adolescents: recommendations from the Centers for Disease Control and Prevention, the National Institutes of Health, and the HIV Medicine Association of the Infectious Diseases Society of America. https://clinicalinfo.hiv.gov/en/guidelines/hiv-clinical-guidelines-adult-and-adolescent-opportunistic-infections/human-0. Published 2022b. Accessed October 8 2022.

Vallet-Pichard A, Pol S. Hepatitis viruses and human immunodeficiency virus co-infection: pathogenesis and treatment. *J Hepatol.* 2004;41(1):156–166.

Vernone SD, Hart CE, Reeves WC, et al. The HIV-1 Tat protein enhances E2-dependent human papillomavirus 16 transcription. *Virus Res.* 1993;27(2):133–145.

Volberding P, Kusick P, Feigal D. Effects of chemotherapy for HIV-associated Kaposi's sarcoma on long-term survival. *Proc Am Soc Clin Oncol.* 1989;3(9):abstract 11.

Walmsley S, Northfelt DW, Melosky B, et al. Treatment of AIDS-related cutaneous Kaposi's sarcoma with topical alitretinoin (9-cis-retinoic acid) gel: Panretin Gel North American Study Group. *J AIDS.* 1999;22(3):235–246.

Wang ES, Straus DJ, Teruya-Felstein J, et al. Intensive chemotherapy with cyclophosphamide, doxorubicine, high-dose methotrexate/ifosfamide, etoposide, and high-dose cytarabine (CODOX-M/IVAC) for human immunodeficiency virus-associated Burkett lymphoma. *Cancer.* 2003;98(3):1196–1205.

Wang Y, Wang Y, Gaisa MM, et al. Negative predictive value of human papillomavirus testing: implications for anal cancer screening in people living with HIV/AIDS. *J Oncol.* January 22, 2020;2020:6352315. http://doi:10.1155/2020/6352315. eCollection 2020

Wasserberg N, Nunoo-Mensah JW, Gonzalez Ruiz C, et al. Colorectal cancer in HIV-infected patients: a case control study. *Colorectal Dis.* 2007;22(10):1217–1221.

Welch K, Finkbeiner W, Alpers CE, et al. Autopsy findings in the acquired immune deficiency syndrome. *JAMA.* 1984;252(9):1152–1159.

Westwood TD, Hogan C, Julyan PJ, et al. Utility of FDG-PETCT and magnetic resonance spectroscopy in differentiating between cerebral lymphoma and non-malignant CNS lesions in HIV-infected patients. *Eur J Radiol.* 2013;82(8):e374–e379.

Whitlock EP, Lin JS, Liles E, et al. Screening for colorectal cancer: a targeted, updated systematic review for the US Preventive Services Task Force. *Ann Intern Med.* 2008;149(9):638–658.

Wightman F, Solomon A, Kumar SS, et al. Effect of ipilimumab on the HIV reservoir in an HIV-infected individual with metastatic melanoma. *AIDS.* 2015;29(4):504–506.

Wilkin TJ, Palmer S, Brudney KF, et al. Anal intraepithelial neoplasia in heterosexual and homosexual HIV-positive men with access to antiretroviral therapy. *J Infect Dis.* 2004;190(9):1685–1691.

Wilson WH, Sin-Ho J, Pitcher BN, et al. Phase III randomized study of R-CHOP versus DA-EPOCH-R and molecular analysis of untreated diffuse large B-cell lymphoma: CALGB/Alliance 50303. *Blood.* 2016;128:469.

Winstone, TA, Man SF, Hull M, et al. Epidemic of lung cancer in patients with HIV infection. *Chest.* 2013;143(2):305–314.

Wistuba IL, Behrens C, Milchgrub S, et al. Comparison of molecular changes in lung cancers in HIV-positive and HIV-indeterminate subjects. *JAMA.* 1998;279(19):1554–1559.

Wolf T, Brodt H-R, Fichtlscherer S, et al. Changing incidence and prognostic factors of survival in AIDS-related non-Hodgkin's lymphoma in the era of highly active antiretroviral therapy (HAART). *Leuk Lymphoma.* 2005;46(2):207–215.

Woolfrey AE, Malhotra U, Harrington RD, et al. Generation of HIV-1-specific CD8\+ cell responses following allogeneic hematopoietic cell transplantation. *Blood.* 2008;112(8):3484–3487.

Yegüez JF, Martinez SA, Sands DR, et al. Colorectal malignancies in PLWH. *Am Surg.* 2003;69(11):981–987.

Zanet E, Taborelli M, Rupolo M, et al. Postautologous stem cell transplantation long-term outcomes in 26 PLWH affected by relapsed/refractory lymphoma. *AIDS.* 2015;29(17): 2303–2308.

Zhang JY, Zhang Z, Wang X, et al. PD-1 up-regulation is correlated with HIV-specific memory CD8\+ T-cell exhaustion in typical progressors but not in long-term nonprogressors. *Blood.* 2007;109: 4671–4678.

Zheng J, Wang L, Cheng Z, et al. Molecular changes of lung malignancy in HIV infection. *Sci Rep.* 2018;8(1):13128.

Ziegler JL, Drew WL, Miner RC, et al. Outbreak of Burkitt's-like lymphoma in homosexual men. *Lancet.* 1982;2(8299):631–633.

Ziegler JL, Templeton AC, Vogel CL. Kaposi's sarcoma: a comparison of classical, endemic, and epidemic forms. *Semin Oncol.* 1984;11(1):47–52.

30.

DERMATOLOGIC COMPLICATIONS OF HIV

Kudakwashe Mutyambizi, Craig S. Weeks, and Philip Bolduc

OVERVIEW OF CUTANEOUS FINDINGS IN HIV INFECTION

LEARNING OBJECTIVE

Review the approach to skin findings in the context of acute and chronic HIV infection.

WHAT'S NEW?

Multiple biopsies increase diagnostic yield for identification of cutaneous complications of HIV.

KEY POINTS

- Dermatoses that are rare in the general population but common in HIV populations should prompt testing for HIV when there is no pre-existing diagnosis.

- Correct diagnosis and management of skin complaints can improve the quality of life of persons with HIV (PWH) who have increased longevity with antiretroviral therapy (ART).

- The appearance of AIDS-defining cutaneous illnesses in previously immune reconstituted patients on ART should prompt a reassessment of CD4$^+$ T-cell count and HIV RNA levels.

- In patients who have been on ART for less than 24 weeks, the appearance or worsening of dermatoses may be due to immune reconstitution inflammatory syndrome (IRIS).

The hallmark of HIV infection is immune dysregulation and immunosuppression. As the immune system deteriorates, inflammatory dermatoses, metabolic dysregulation, adverse drug reactions, opportunistic infections, and cutaneous malignancies become more common, atypical in presentation, and recalcitrant to therapy. Both acute and chronic skin complaints contribute significantly to reduced quality of life for HIV patients (Mirmirani et al., 2002).

The US Centers for Disease Control and Prevention (CDC) recommends that individuals between ages 13 and 64 years be tested for HIV at least once in their lifetime, with increased screening of high-risk individuals and testing based on symptoms. The presence of dermatoses uncommon in the general population but concentrated in the HIV population, or dermatoses strikingly recalcitrant to therapy, should warrant suspicion and testing for HIV. In patients with known HIV/AIDS, there is a correlation between CD4$^+$ T-cell count and the occurrence of characteristic dermatoses (Goldstein et al., 1997; Rigopoulos et al., 2004). Direct CD4$^+$ T-cell testing is the gold standard assessment of immune function; however, the World Health Organization's (WHO) clinical staging provides guidelines regarding skin findings that should raise suspicion for immune deterioration, thus prompting CD4$^+$ T-cell testing, and have significance in international settings in which CD4$^+$ T-cell testing is of limited availability (Baveewo et al., 2011; Weinberg et al., 2010). The occurrence of AIDS-defining illnesses such as Kaposi's sarcoma or acute systemic illnesses and infections in patients previously immunocompetent by CD4$^+$ T-cell count or previously well controlled on ART should prompt an assessment of CD4$^+$ T-cell count and HIV RNA levels to evaluate for immune deterioration. In patients who have been on ART for less than 24 weeks, acute systemic illnesses may be due to IRIS or treatment toxicity and, during this period, do not closely run parallel to the WHO clinical staging guidelines (Ratnam et al., 2006). With these caveats, the dermatoses discussed in this chapter are presented along with the corresponding CD4$^+$ T-cell count at which they typically occur (Zancanaro et al., 2006).

HIV practitioners can competently diagnose many of the dermatological conditions discussed in this chapter as well as perform diagnostic biopsies and minor cosmetic procedures. Clinics often maintain a supply of liquid nitrogen to treat warts and an electrocautery machine known as a hyfrecator to electrodessicate lesions such as molluscum contagiosum. Referral to a dermatologist is recommended when presented with diagnostic or management uncertainty, particularly in the acutely ill PWH, with common or chronic dermatoses recalcitrant to therapies familiar to the HIV practitioner, and for optimal tissue procurement when the clinician is uncertain of appropriate biopsy site or method.

It is important for HIV practitioners to be aware that several serious disseminated opportunistic infections, some of which may be fatal, may first manifest as an acute cutaneous eruption. Therefore, it is important for a skin biopsy to be performed in an acutely febrile PWH with a newly developed skin eruption. The biopsy should be accompanied with a request for urgent processing with special stains for bacteria, atypical mycobacteria, fungi, and viruses as appropriate. Tissue is placed in 10% formalin for routine processing, but a portion should be placed in normal saline so that cultures for microorganisms can be performed to aid in definitive diagnosis.

In general, when sampling a lesion, especially one that is papular or pustular, an early, new lesion that is not excoriated is most likely to yield tissue with changes that afford the dermatopathologist the best opportunity to make an accurate diagnosis (Altman et al., 2015). A notable exception in this population is biopsy of suspected Kaposi's sarcoma because early lesions can present a confusing picture histologically. An older, more mature lesion, if present, will have greater diagnostic yield (Maurer et al., 2005). When in doubt, one should consider taking multiple biopsies from the lesion in different stages of evolution and from different cutaneous sites. If the practitioner is not comfortable performing a good skin biopsy, dermatological referral for evaluation and biopsy determination should be made. Box 30.1 provides guidelines for referral.

RECOMMENDED READING

Altman K, Vanness E, Westergaard RP. Cutaneous manifestations of human immunodeficiency virus: a clinical update. *Curr Infect Dis Rep.* 2015;17(3):464.

Mirmirani P, Maurer TA, Berger TG, et al. Skin-related quality of life in HIV-infected patients on highly active antiretroviral therapy. *J Cutan Med Surg.* 2002;6(1):10–15.

INFLAMMATORY DERMATOSES AND HIV

LEARNING OBJECTIVE

Discuss the incidence, presentation, and management of inflammatory dermatoses in HIV.

WHAT'S NEW?

Traditional immunosuppressants and newer biologic therapies have both been used safely in controlled settings and for short courses in PWH with refractory psoriasis and debilitating psoriatic arthritis who are on concurrent ART.

KEY POINTS

- Initiation of ART, ultraviolet B (UVB), and oral retinoids are good initial therapies for PWH with psoriatic arthritis.

- Topical tacrolimus inhibitors and UV light have both been used safely in PWH.

- PWH receiving systemic biologics for debilitating psoriatic arthritis should be carefully selected and closely monitored.

- Papular pruritic eruption of AIDS and HIV-associated eosinophilic pustular folliculitis are HIV/AIDS-associated dermatologic illnesses and should prompt testing for HIV in a previously undiagnosed person.

SEBORRHEIC DERMATITIS

Seborrheic dermatitis is a common skin disorder, with a prevalence of approximately 5% in the general population. It was noted to be the most common dermatosis in PWH, with a prevalence of greater than 83% in HIV/AIDS populations in the pre-ART era (Sadick et al., 1990). Seborrheic dermatitis is seen at all clinical stages of disease. *Malassezia* species are the causative organisms. The typical presentation is of episodic variably pruritic, thin, erythematous plaques with branny (small, husk-like) or greasy yellow-white scale involving the scalp and central face, particularly the eyebrows and nasolabial folds. Scalp involvement ranges from light "dandruff" to crusted plaques. Involvement of the anterior chest and groin areas is common. HIV should be considered in rapid and exaggerated presentations with thick, extensive plaques and also in cases recalcitrant to advanced treatment regimens. The clinical differential for facial seborrheic dermatitis includes rosacea; an overlapping presentation with psoriasis called sebopsoriasis that is often more difficult to treat than standard seborrheic dermatitis; contact dermatitis; *tinea faciei*; and connective tissue disease. In *tinea faciei*, a potassium hydroxide (KOH) preparation can identify dermatophytes exhibiting characteristic hyphae. In contrast, seborrheic dermatitis is thought to be an inflammatory response to the commensal yeast *Malassezia* species (thus, KOH evaluation has no role), with the increased presentation in PWH thought to be due to a more vigorous inflammatory response as the yeast proliferate in the setting of $CD4^+$ T-cell lymphopenia (Oble et al., 2005; Pedrosa et al., 2014). Seborrheic dermatitis is a clinical diagnosis; thus, biopsy is infrequently performed. Histology reveals psoriasiform hyperplasia, neutrophilic spongiosis, perifollicular mound parakeratosis with necrotic keratinocytes, and plasma cells, which occasionally present in

HIV-associated seborrheic dermatitis (Soeprono et al., 1986). Treatment does not differ between PWH and HIV-negative persons; first-line therapy is with low- to mid-potency topical steroids for the face and trunk respectively, topical antifungals such as ketoconazole, or combinations thereof (Osborne et al., 2003). More refractory cases can be treated with oral itraconazole 200 mg once daily, although attention must be paid to interactions with ART agents. ART therapy improves seborrheic dermatitis occurring in the setting of HIV/AIDS; however, PWH typically continue to experience episodic flares.

PSORIASIS

Psoriasis also presents at all clinical stages of HIV, but more frequently at CD4[+] T-cell counts of less than 350 cells/mm[3] (Bartlett et al., 2007). Psoriasis has a prevalence of approximately 2% or 3% in the general population, with various series suggesting a similar or higher incidence in HIV populations (Mallon & Bunker, 2000; Obuch et al., 1992). The prevalence of psoriatic arthritis in the general population has previously been underestimated and is now thought to be approximately 11% in the US psoriasis population, and it is more concentrated in PWH (Dover et al., 1991; Gelfand et al., 2005). Psoriasis characteristically presents as variably pruritic, episodic, well-demarcated plaques with silvery white scale anywhere on the body but with a predilection for the scalp, elbows, lower back, gluteal folds, external genitalia, and acral sites. Preexisting psoriasis can worsen with HIV infection and immune deterioration, and psoriasis can develop de novo with HIV infection. *De novo* psoriasis in HIV often involves palmar-plantar locations with pustules, nail dystrophy, and psoriatic arthritis that can be debilitating. Inverse psoriasis (involving intertriginous areas), generalized pustular psoriasis, and erythrodermic psoriasis also occur more frequently in HIV (Obuch et al., 1992). Erythrodermic psoriasis can be difficult to distinguish from other causes of erythroderma, including atopic dermatitis, drug-induced erythroderma, pityriasis rubra pilaris, Sézary syndrome, and a paraneoplastic presentation or HIV presentation; thus, it typically warrants a biopsy. Histology reveals parakeratosis, collections of neutrophils in the stratum corneum and epidermis, and a diminished granular layer. Whereas increased defensins and canthelicidins in the skin of psoriatics in the general population have been associated with their relatively low frequency of bacterial superinfection compared to other chronic dermatoses that also result in a compromised skin barrier, such as atopic dermatitis, there is an increased frequency of bacterial superinfection in HIV psoriatics (Mallon & Bunker, 2000; Zheng et al., 2007). Theories regarding the increased incidence and severity of psoriasis in HIV include the fact that overexpression of tumor necrosis factor (TNF) occurs in both psoriasis and HIV. Furthermore, CD4[+] T-cell depletion in HIV skews the T-cell population to CD8[+] T-cells, the effector cells in psoriasis, and the HIV tat gene directly induces epidermal proliferation (Duvic, 1990; Kim et al., 1992).

In treating psoriasis, exacerbating medications should be discontinued. Of note, systemic steroids exacerbate psoriasis.

Topical treatments including topical steroids, vitamin D analogues, and topical calcineurin inhibitors such as tacrolimus are first-line therapies for mild to moderate plaque psoriasis. A black box warning on tacrolimus and malignancy risk has not identified a causal relationship, and studies have shown that topical calcineurin inhibitors can be safely used in the immunosuppressed HIV population (de Moraes et al., 2007; Toutous-Trellu et al., 2005). Randomized controlled studies have not been conducted to evaluate the efficacy and safety of systemic treatments for psoriasis in the HIV setting; thus, much of the following data are derived from case reports and case series.

Systemic therapies can be used in combination with each other and with topical treatments to optimize efficacy. ART can effectively treat both moderate to severe psoriasis and psoriatic arthritis, and it is a first-line treatment, as is UV light, for this severity category (Duvic et al., 1994; Menon et al., 2010; Meola et al., 1993). UVB is preferentially used over psoralens plus UVA (PUVA) given its more favorable side-effect profile. Although in vitro studies have shown that UVB light can activate latent HIV in chronically infected monocytes, it has not been associated with short-term changes in immune function in vivo or changes in HIV RNA levels in PWH receiving concomitant suppressive ART therapy (Breuer-McHam et al., 1999; Meola et al., 1993; Stanley et al., 1989). Oral retinoids, particularly acitretin, are an attractive second-line therapy because they are non-immunosuppressants with efficacy for moderate to severe psoriasis and psoriatic arthritis. Acitretin use is limited by hypertriglyceridemia; liver function test (LFT) elevation, particularly in combination with some antiretroviral medications; and an extended 3-year teratogenicity period in women of childbearing age due to re-esterification to etretinate (Dogra et al., 2014).

PWH with refractory or debilitating psoriatic arthritis are candidates for immunosuppressant therapies, including low-dose methotrexate and brief courses of cyclosporine and TNF-α inhibitors. In a case report, dramatic improvement of HIV-associated psoriatic arthritis was achieved, but frequent polymicrobial infections were experienced on etanercept (Aboulafia et al., 2000). In a 2018 Cochrane review of 25 reported cases of systemic immunosuppressives used to treat psoriatic disease in PWH, including methotrexate, cyclosporine, etanercept, adalimumab, infliximab, and ustekinumab, evidence suggests that these biologic therapies may be effective for refractory psoriasis and may actually have a positive effect on CD4[+] T-cell counts and HIV viral load when used in combination with ART (Nakamura et al., 2018). Rigorous patient selection, concomitant ART therapy, strict prophylaxis against opportunistic infections, monitoring of CD4[+] T-cell counts and HIV RNA levels and close clinical monitoring of are advised when treating HIV-associated psoriasis with immunosuppressant therapy.

ATOPIC DERMATITIS AND XEROSIS

The prevalence of eczema in the US adult population is estimated at 10.7%, with approximately 17% of the population experiencing at least one of four eczematous symptoms (Hanifin et al., 2007). An atopic dermatitis-like condition occurs frequently in HIV populations, often despite never having had a history of atopic dermatitis in childhood. One series reported that 29% of PWH who attended an urban HIV clinic in the pre-ART era had this condition (Lin et al., 1995). This atopic dermatitis-like condition is characterized by pruritus and a spectrum of generalized scaling from xerosis to ichthyosis, with variable plaques and lichenification involving extremities and flexural areas (Singh & Rudikoff, 2003). Often, this xerotic condition initially presents when the CD4 + T-cell count is still higher than 400 cells/mm^3 and is thus an early clinical sign of HIV/AIDS, typically preceding the other HIV-related papulosquamous disorders. The generalized ichthyotic form typically occurs with CD4 + T-cell counts less than 50 cells/mm^3 (Sadick et al., 1990). Decreased cellular immunity and a switch to the TH2-like cytokine profile resulting in polyclonal activation of B cells with increased IgE production are thought to contribute to the increase in atopic conditions in HIV (Nissen et al., 1999). In addition, nutritional deficits and autonomic nervous dysfunction causing alterations in sweating, sebaceous gland secretion, and reduction in natural moisturizing factor secretion are thought to contribute to xerosis and ichthyosis (Cockerell & Calame, 2013). Decreased lipids and increased water are found in the dermis of PWH compared to HIV-negative reference groups, as well as excessive levels of epidermal carotenoids, mainly lycopene, potentially leading to these adverse effects such and premature skin aging (Mischo et al., 2014). Biopsy, which is not regularly performed for this diagnosis, shows variable hyperkeratosis and parakeratosis, spongiosis, and superficial perivascular lymphocytic infiltrate. The clinical differential diagnosis includes scabies, psoriasis, and contact dermatitis. For erythematous plaques, topical steroid preparations, preferably ointments, and topical calcineurin inhibitors are appropriate first-line therapies. Topical keratolytics such as urea and lactic acid formulations are useful for areas of lichenification. Widespread flares may require short courses of systemic steroids, bridging to phototherapy for more sustained flares. Oral antihistamines and a dry skin care regimen of short lukewarm showers, frequent use of non-allergic emollients, and avoidance of allergens should be used in conjunction. Bacterial superinfection is common and should be managed with antibiotics.

PAPULAR PRURITIC ERUPTION OF AIDS

Papular pruritic eruption (PPE) is a markedly pruritic papulosquamous eruption characterized by symmetric crops of nonfollicular, often urticarial erythematous papules involving the extensor extremities. Excoriations and prurigo nodularis are frequently associated secondary changes because of marked pruritus in this condition. PPE is uncommon in the general adult population but has a prevalence in the HIV population of 11%–46%, thus the designation *PPE of AIDS* (Eisman, 2006). It has a greater prevalence in HIV/AIDS

cohorts in Sub-Saharan Africa than in the United States. Among other theories, PPE is hypothesized to be due to an exaggerated response to arthropod antigens that occurs in the setting of immune dysregulation (Resneck et al., 2004). PPE can develop well before other symptoms and serologic diagnosis of HIV is made; however, its occurrence has historically been correlated with lower CD4 + T-cell counts, particularly less than 100 cells/mm^3 (Boonchai et al., 1999; Cockerell & Calame, 2013). However, studies from India found otherwise; one-third of cases occurred in PWH with CD4 + T-cell counts above 350 (Farsani et al., 2013) and 86% above 200 (Mohammed et al., 2019). This difference is yet unexplained but highlights that PPE can be seen at any CD4 + count.

The clinical differential of PPE includes eosinophilic folliculitis, which, in contrast, affects the face and upper trunk, and prurigo nodularis, which also may also be pruritic. The diagnosis is typically made clinically based on the distribution of lesions. Early lesions without secondary changes carry the highest histologic diagnostic yield; they may show a dense perivascular and interstitial infiltrate of lymphocytes and some eosinophils and neutrophils, which may extend deeply around adnexa and vessels, although nonspecific findings occur (Calonje et al., 2012). The disease has a chronic waxing and waning course and is associated with decreased quality of life due to pruritus (Hevia et al., 1991; Liu et al., 2013). Given its association with low CD4+ T-cell counts, initiation of ART may improve the disease, although it can also flare with immune reconstitution. UVB has been shown to decrease both papules and pruritus, and it may have greater efficacy in regimens combining other modalities including oral antihistamines, pentoxifylline, topical steroids, topical tacrolimus, and topical anti-itch preparations (Bellavista et al., 2013). Reducing exposure to bites by wearing clothing that covers skin and application of insect repellant is also recommended.

HIV-ASSOCIATED EOSINOPHILIC PUSTULAR FOLLICULITIS

Eosinophilic pustular folliculitis (EPF, or Ofugi's disease) is rare in the general adult population but common in the HIV/AIDS population, particularly once the CD4 + T-cell count declines below 250 cells/mm^3. HIV-associated eosinophilic folliculitis is characterized by persistent, markedly pruritic erythematous, mostly follicular papules and occasional pustules on the face, trunk, and upper extremities. Urticarial plaques and nonfollicular erythematous papules are also described. Peripheral eosinophilia can also be common along with elevated IgE levels (Rosenthal et al., 1991). It is thought to be an exaggerated cutaneous reaction to *Malassezia* yeast or other microorganisms colonizing the follicular infundibulum and reflects TH1/2 immune dysregulation. CD163 + macrophages have been implicated in the pathogenesis (Okada et al., 2013). Additional theories include autoimmune activation against antigens in sebocytes in HIV-positive individuals (Fearfield et al., 1999). The clinical differential includes PPE as well as acne, molluscum, and drug reactions. Biopsy may be useful, with erythematous nonexcoriated follicular lesions carrying the highest diagnostic yield. Spongiosis involving the follicular epithelium and intra- and perifollicular mixed infiltrate is typically seen, with eosinophilic abscess formation in long-standing lesions. Treatment is often difficult, with pruritus contributing to reduced quality of life. Phototherapy (UVB or UVA), oral antihistamines, itraconazole, isotretinoin, and metronidazole are all reported treatments; however, no controlled clinical trials have been performed. Whereas classic EPF is preferentially treated with oral indomethacin, topical steroids are preferred for HIV-related EPF (Nomura et al., 2016), and other potential treatments include UVB phototherapy and oral antihistamines.

RECOMMENDED READING

Cockerell CC, Calame A. *Cutaneous manifestations of HIV disease.* London: Manson; 2013.

Toutous-Trellu L, Abraham S, Pechere M, et al. Topical tacrolimus for effective treatment of eosinophilic folliculitis associated with human immunodeficiency virus infection. *Arch Dermatol.* 2005;141(10):1203–1208.

HIV DRUG REACTIONS AND INTERACTIONS

LEARNING OBJECTIVE

Describe common and important cutaneous adverse drug reactions in PWH and pertinent factors in their management.

WHAT'S NEW?

In recent years, several adverse drug reactions to ART medications have been identified that were not observed or were underrepresented in preapproval trials.

KEY POINTS

- Nonnucleoside reverse transcriptase inhibitors (NNRTIs) are the most common antiretroviral drugs that cause morbilliform skin eruptions.

- Abacavir hypersensitivity reaction can be fatal, and predisposed individuals can be identified by testing for the HLA-B5701 allele prior to commencing abacavir therapy.

- The injectable fillers poly-l-lactic acid and calcium hydroxyapatite are approved for facial fat loss treatment in HIV.

- Ritonavir, a CYP34A inhibitor often used to boost other antiretroviral drugs, increases the levels of corticosteroids, which can result in hypothalamic–pituitary–adrenal (HPA) axis dysfunction and Cushing's syndrome.

Historically, the incidence of medication-related skin rashes in the HIV-positive population was approximately 50% (Davis & Shearer, 2008), although literature is lacking on the incidence with newer antiretrovirals. Drug hypersensitivity reactions are classified into two categories: those secondary to ART regimens and those secondary to other medications taken by PWH. Since its inception, ART has revolutionized the management of HIV/AIDS, with new drug classes and single-tablet combination formulations designed to decrease pill burden now available. However, antiretroviral drugs have been complicated by adverse drug reactions, including reactions that may not have been recognized or underrepresented in preapproval clinical trials (Introcaso et al., 2010). Thus, recognition of known and identification of previously unreported drug reactions are extremely important in the management of antiretroviral-related drug hypersensitivity reactions. It can be a particular challenge to differentiate between drug hypersensitivity reactions, IRIS, and worsening HIV infection when patients are commencing ART. Some of the adverse drug reactions are mediated through genetic and immunologic factors via the major histocompatibility complex (Chaponda et al., 2011). IgE levels increase with progression of HIV, and altered cytokine profiles are also believed to play a role (Davis & Shearer, 2008). Immune dysregulation in HIV is also thought to make HIV patients more susceptible to reactions to non-ART medications. In addition, antiretroviral drugs can result in alterations in metabolism of other medications, particularly through the cytochrome P450 pathway, thus increasing their toxicity.

NONNUCLEASE REVERSE TRANSCRIPTASE INHIBITORS

NNRTIs are the most common antiretroviral agents to cause morbilliform skin eruptions, which are usually distributed over the face, trunk, and extremities. Nevirapine is well known for its ability to cause rashes, particularly within the first 6 weeks of use. According to the manufacturer, 13% of patients taking nevirapine develop some degree of morbilliform eruption during early treatment; this has been reported to be as high as 28% in some populations (Introcaso et al., 2010). Many patients with mild or moderate rash can continue therapy with close monitoring, and the rash will spontaneously resolve. Severe rash is seen in at least 8% of patients, and development of concomitant hepatitis in the drug hypersensitivity syndrome is an indication for immediate discontinuation of nevirapine given the potential for fatal hepatitis. Risk factors for the development of morbilliform eruption with the use of nevirapine include higher CD4$^+$ T-cell count (>250 cells/mm^3 in women and >400 cells/mm^3 in men), lower HIV-1 RNA levels, Chinese ethnicity, and female gender (Davis & Shearer, 2008). In addition, nevirapine can cause the mucocutaneous Stevens–Johnson syndrome at a rate of 0.5%–1%, although patients with CD4$^+$ T-cell counts of less than 200 cells/mm^3 (i.e., with AIDS) have a higher risk (Warren et al., 1998). The incidence may be higher in Sub-Saharan Africa, where nevirapine is more commonly used in antiretroviral regimens. Stevens–Johnson syndrome is characterized by flat, atypical targets or pruritic papules that are widespread or distributed on the trunk first and then spread to the neck, face, and proximal upper extremities. The palms and soles may be early sites of involvement. Bullae developing on the conjunctivae and mucous membranes of the nares, mouth, anorectal junction, vulvovaginal region, and urethral meatus are characteristic, with toxic epidermal necrolysis diagnosed when there is more than 30% body surface area skin detachment (Bolognia et al., 2012). In several studies, the use of prednisone and/or a 2-week lead-in dose of nevirapine 200 mg once daily failed to decrease the occurrence of the nevirapine-associated rash (Knobel et al., 2001); nevertheless, a dose escalation protocol is recommended starting with nevirapine 200 mg/d for 2 weeks, followed by an increase to the standard 400 mg/d dose only if there is no rash or no worsening rash after the trial 2-week period (Anton et al., 1999).

NUCLEOSIDE REVERSE TRANSCRIPTASE INHIBITOR

Abacavir, a nucleoside reverse transcriptase inhibitor, can cause a well-documented, multiorgan, potentially life-threatening hypersensitivity reaction. This abacavir hypersensitivity reaction (AHR) is seen in 5%–8% of patients on treatment. Symptoms consist of fever, rash, malaise, fatigue, tachypnea, pharyngitis, cough, wheezing, nausea, vomiting, and diarrhea that commence 9–11 days after initiating therapy. Symptoms that become worse with each subsequent dose are a classic characteristic of AHR. Symptoms of AHR recur within 24 hours of rechallenge and can be fatal. Therefore, the use of abacavir in any person suspected to have AHR is contraindicated. Pre-ART genetic testing has shown that the absence of the HLA-B5701 allele dramatically decreases (by 99.9%) the likelihood of developing abacavir hypersensitivity (Mallal et al., 2008). For this reason, the ART guidelines of both the US Department of Health and Human Services and the International Antiviral Society USA recommend obtaining this test prior to initiation of any abacavir-containing regimen.

PROTEASE INHIBITORS

Protease inhibitors (PIs) are generally associated with lipodystrophy, encompassing peripheral lipoatrophy and central adiposity, which can be an indication for discontinuation. The injectable fillers poly-l-lactic acid and calcium hydroxyapatite are approved for facial fat loss treatment in HIV (Jagdeo et al., 2015). Indinavir has the greatest variety of cutaneous side effects among PIs, including acute porphyria, Stevens–Johnson syndrome, hypersensitivity syndrome, morbilliform drug eruptions, gynecomastia, alopecia, pyogenic granuloma-like lesions, and paronychia (Ward et al., 2002). Ritonavir is a CYP34A inhibitor, and, through this mechanism, it decreases clearance of corticosteroids, thus increasing their levels and the risk of hypothalamic–pituitary–adrenal axis dysfunction and Cushing's syndrome (Hyle, 2013). This should be considered when prescribing systemic steroids, inhaled corticosteroids such as fluticasone, or topical steroids when applied to a large body surface area.

OTHER ANTIRETROVIRAL THERAPIES

Few other antiretroviral drugs have a strong association with severe adverse drug reactions. Approximately 6% of persons taking atazanavir, a PI, have reported typically mild rash not requiring treatment cessation. Most patients on atazanavir develop benign unconjugated hyperbilirubinemia, in some patients high enough to cause visible jaundice. A hypersensitivity to the fusion inhibitor enfuvirtide has been seen in fewer than 1% of people taking it. However, 98% of users experience injection site reactions, which are frequently symptomatic (Ball et al., 2003). The enfuvirtide injection site reaction is characterized by tender erythema, induration, and nodule or cyst formation. On histology, a palisaded granulomatous response may be seen, with multinucleated cells aggregated around altered collagen, and surrounding eosinophils, histiocytes, lymphocytes, plasma cells, and variable fibrosis. The Package Insert for raltegravir, an integrase inhibitor, was updated to include dermatological side effects including Stevens–Johnson syndrome and toxic epidermal necrolysis following postmarketing case reports.

ANTIBIOTICS

Antibiotic drug reactions are seen at a higher rate in PWH than in the general population. Trimethoprim–sulfamethoxazole is a commonly used antibiotic in HIV, especially for the prophylaxis of *Pneumocystis jirovecii* pneumonia (PCP). Given its importance in the prevention of PCP pneumonia, a desensitization schedule has been developed for those patients who have had reactions in the past and would benefit from its use. Desensitization has been successful using the following dosing schedule: an initial dose of trimethoprim 0.4 mg and sulfamethoxazole 2 mg, followed by doubling the dose daily over days 2–9 and at 10 days administering the full-strength dose (trimethoprim 160 mg/sulfamethoxazole 800 mg) (Gompels et al., 1999).

RECOMMENDED READING

Hyle EP, Wood BR, Backman ES, et al. High frequency of hypothalamic–pituitary–adrenal axis dysfunction after local corticosteroid injection in HIV-infected patients on protease inhibitor therapy. *J AIDS*. 2013;63(5):602–608.

Introcaso CE, Hines JM, Kovarik CL. Cutaneous toxicities of antiretroviral therapy for HIV: part II. Nonnucleoside reverse transcriptase inhibitors, entry and fusion inhibitors, integrase inhibitors, and immune reconstitution syndrome. *J Am Acad Dermatol*. 2010;63(4):563–569;quiz 569–570.

CUTANEOUS OPPORTUNISTIC INFECTIONS

LEARNING OBJECTIVE

Discuss the diagnosis and management of viral, fungal, bacterial, and parasitic opportunistic infections occurring in HIV patients.

WHAT'S NEW?

In January 2022, the Advisory Committee on Immunization Practices (ACIP) updated recommendations for vaccination, now recommending two doses of recombinant Zoster vaccine (RZV) in immunocompromised individuals and PWH ≥19 years of age.

KEY POINTS

- Cutaneous *Cryptococcus* may manifest before systemic symptoms; therefore, prompt diagnosis and management can prevent fatal outcomes.

- Molluscum, histoplasmosis, and *Cryptococcus* may all present with umbilicated papulonodules; however, there is a central white core to the molluscum lesion, and patients are well as opposed to systemically ill with cryptococcal infection.

- Postherpetic neuralgia is very common in HIV patients who develop herpes zoster, and initiation of Neurontin along with antiviral therapy at diagnosis may mitigate neuralgia.

- The prozone effect may result in a false-negative syphilis test in HIV patients, and dilution of the assay should be requested when syphilis is suspected.

- The CDC recommends an intensive regimen for the management of crusted scabies as follows: ivermectin dosed at 200 µg/kg taken on days 1, 2, 8, 9, and 15, and, for severe disease, also days 22 and 29, in combination with topical permethrin daily for 7 days and then twice a week until cure.

ONYCHOMYCOSIS

Onychomycosis is reported to affect approximately 2%–13% of the general population (Rosen et al., 2015) and is very common in PWH. Dermatophytes *Trichophyton mentagrophytes* and *T. rubrum* are responsible for most infections. Proximal subungual onychomycosis is a pattern seen commonly in HIV-positive patients, especially those with a CD4 [+] T-cell count of less than 450 cells/mm[3], and although it is not considered an AIDS-defining condition, it should prompt testing for HIV infection if not already determined. *T. rubrum* is the offending dermatophyte, although it can also be caused by *T. megninii*. In the general population, superficial white onychomycosis is typically caused by *T. mentagrophytes,* whereas in PWH, *T. rubrum* is the causative agent. The clinical differential includes psoriasis, lichen planus, trauma, and periungual squamous cell carcinoma. Most topical antifungals do not penetrate the thick nail keratin and thus are ineffective. Efinaconazole is a topical triazole solution for the treatment of onychomycosis; it is applied daily for 48 weeks to affected nails. Localized dermatitis is a potential side effect. In preapproval trials, a modest 15.2%–17.8% of patients achieved complete cure of onychomycosis. Tavorabole, a boron-based agent that was FDA approved for onychomycosis in 2014, had even lower efficacy, with 6.5%–9.1% of patients achieving clearance (Zeichner, 2015). Terbinafine is considered first-line systemic therapy, dosed at 250 mg/day for 3 or 4 months for toenails and 6 weeks for fingernails (~50% cure rate). Itraconazole may

also be effective at 200 mg/day for 3 months for toenails and 6 weeks for fingernails or at 200 mg twice daily for 1 week per month for 3 months for toenails and 2 months for fingernails. The efficacy of fluconazole is lower than that of terbinafine and itraconazole. Patients with active liver disease should not receive terbinafine and testing of LFTs at baseline and every 4–6 weeks is recommended given the risk of hepatotoxicity. Congestive heart disease is a contraindication to itraconazole use. In addition, itraconazole interacts with more medications compared to terbinafine (de Berker, 2009), particularly with the ART boosting agents ritonavir and cobicistat. Finally, the causative agent may differ between the general population and PWH, which is relevant when selecting therapy. For example, nondermatophyte molds, such as *Scytalidium, Aspergillus,* and *Fusarium,* and yeast such as *Candida* are implicated in onychomycosis in HIV patients more often than in the general public. Much higher cure rates are achieved with itraconazole than with terbinafine for these organisms, whereas the reverse is true for dermatophytes (Cambuim et al., 2011; Warshaw et al., 2005). For these reasons, and given the potential side effects of systemic therapies, culture of nail clippings involved with onychomycosis is recommended before initiation of therapy by some dermatologists.

CANDIDIASIS

Angular cheilitis is typically caused by *Candida albicans* and presents as fissured white plaques at the angles of the lips. It occurs with some frequency in the elderly, but it may suggest HIV infection in young adults and may warrant testing if there is no other known reason for immunosuppression. Topical antifungal creams are effective and avoid systemic circulation for this focal disease. Associated burning and dysphagia suggest oral candidiasis, with atrophic or removable yellow-white pseudomembranous or hyperplastic plaques typically seen on the tongue or dorsal palate. Oral candidiasis is often a harbinger of immunologic failure in patients on ART, although it can also be caused by steroids and antibiotics (Cockerell & Calame, 2013). Nystatin or clotrimazole troches, and oral antifungals such as fluconazole or ketoconazole when there is associated odynophagia, are effective. Ketoconazole should be taken with food and avoided in the setting of malabsorption given the risk of treatment failure.

Candida intertrigo is common in HIV-infected populations, and it can appear as eroded glistening erythematous plaques or as pustules with scale over a macerated erythematous surface within and extending from skin folds. While smaller lesions may be treated with topical antifungals, oral fluconazole or ketoconazole, is recommended for larger or extensive plaques.

CUTANEOUS CRYPTOCOCCOSIS

Cryptococcus neoformans causes an AIDS-defining systemic infection, with skin lesions preceding the more common central nervous system and pulmonary involvement in only 10% of cases. The patient is typically febrile and very ill. Lesions can present as papules that may be umbilicated, nodules, pustules, ulcers, and plaques. A skin biopsy is necessary for diagnosis, revealing round yeast with narrow-based budding and a slimy capsule in a granulomatous or gelatinous background, highlighted by fungal stains. Culture is definitively diagnostic, and treatment is with amphotericin B or fluconazole; adjunctive flucytosine can also be used (Cockerell & Calame, 2013), with close monitoring of renal function for potential flucytosine dose adjustment. ART has decreased the incidence of cryptococcal infection; however, institution of ART in patients with cryptococcal infection can result in fatal IRIS (Lortholary et al., 2005), so ART should not be initiated until 2–10 weeks into antifungal therapy (DHHS, 2022b). Relapses are not uncommon, and secondary prophylaxis with fluconazole 200–400 mg/d for patients with CD4$^+$ T-cell counts of less than 200 cells/mm^3 is recommended.

CUTANEOUS HISTOPLASMOSIS

Histoplasmosis manifests with cutaneous lesions secondary to pulmonary or disseminated disease, as primary cutaneous manifestation is rare. The rash is nonspecific, characterized by diffuse erythematous macules, papules that may be umbilicated, pustules, crusted ulcers, or psoriasiform papules. The face is most often involved, followed by truncal and extremity involvement (Cockerell & Calame, 2013). The differential diagnosis includes molluscum contagiosum and cryptococcosis. HIV patients with cutaneous histoplasmosis may be well appearing on initial presentation; however, prompt diagnosis is important because they can rapidly and fatally decompensate with systemic involvement (Wheat et al., 1990). Diagnosis of cutaneous histoplasmosis requires tissue biopsy, which reveals spores with a pseudo-capsule (the fungal wall) parasitizing macrophages. Culture confirms the diagnosis. Mild infection in non-HIV patients is self-limiting and may not require treatment; however, treatment is required in PWH. Treating systemic disease also treats skin involvement and is typically done with itraconazole; amphotericin is reserved for meningitis or other disseminated infection (Hage et al., 2015). Similar to cryptococcosis, relapses can occur, and secondary prophylaxis with itraconazole in AIDS patients is advised.

MOLLUSCUM CONTAGIOSUM

Molluscum is a common viral infection in children and their caregivers, but it warrants testing for HIV in adults with limited exposure to children. Skin-colored discrete umbilicated papules are typical, although giant facial molluscum and extensive beard involvement occur with advanced immunosuppression. While many molluscum lesions will self-resolve with antiretroviral therapy, giant molluscum can persist even after immune reconstitution, is extremely difficult to treat and is stigmatizing. Molluscum is differentiated from cryptococcosis and histoplasmosis, which can also have umbilicated papules, by the presence of a central core in molluscum lesions. Also, patients appear well with molluscum infection, whereas they are systemically ill with cryptococcal and histoplasma infection. Treatment options include cryotherapy or pulsed dye therapy for smaller lesions and curettage and excision for larger lesions; immune-modulating agents such as topical imiquimod, interferon-alpha and cimetidine; chemical agents (e.g. cantharidin, potassium hydroxide, podophyllotoxin, benzoyl peroxide, tretinoin, trichloroacetic acid, lactic acid, glycolic acid, and salicylic acid); antivirals (cidofovir); and photodynamic therapy with 5-aminolevulinic acid—which have all shown efficacy in case reports (Drain et al., 2014; Foissac et al., 2014; Leung et al., 2017), although high-quality clinical trial data are lacking.

CONDYLOMA ACUMINATUM

Condyloma acuminatum (anogenital warts), which is caused by the human papillomavirus (HPV), is the most common sexually transmitted infection in the United States. Warts appear as flesh-colored to gray, rounded to pointy papules, frequently on a short peduncle. Podophyllin, trichloroacetic acid, and cryotherapy are three of the most commonly used treatments for genital warts. Cryotherapy and trichloroacetic acid yield a treatment success rate of 75%, whereas that of podophyllin is reported to be 20%–50% (Murray et al., 2015). Therapies for recalcitrant anogenital warts include topical 5-fluoracil, cidofovir, intralesional interferon-α and surgical excision (Nambudiri et al., 2013). Approximately 5% of MSM and 15% of MSM with HIV have a history of perianal warts. Anogenital warts are more common in women, and women with HIV are five-times more likely than their uninfected counterparts to have these warts (Hagensee et al., 2004). In addition, squamous epithelial lesions occur in 79% of women with HIV with anal HPV infection compared to 43% of women without HIV. The frequency of intraepithelial neoplasia within anogenital warts is higher than previously realized, warranting aggressive surveillance and treatment (McCloskey et al., 2007). To establish evidence-based management of high-grade anorectal lesions, The ANCHOR study enrolled PWH aged ≥35 years with biopsy-proven anal HSIL to receive either treatment or active monitoring of these high-grade lesions. The trial was halted ahead of schedule when an interim analysis showed significantly lower risk of anal cancer in the treatment group when compared to active monitoring (Palefsky et al., 2022). Recommendations for screening and management of lower-grade lesions remain unclear.

HERPES SIMPLEX

Herpes simplex virus (HSV) infection is caused by either HSV-1 or HSV-2 and is a common viral infection in the general population. It presents as grouped vesicles on an erythematous base. In PWH, the infections occur more frequently and are less likely to self-resolve. When CD4$^+$ T-cells decrease below 100 cells/mm^3, the incidence of HSV outbreaks reaches 27% (Severson & Tyring, 1999). Recommended treatment for a PWH with recurrent herpes infection is valacyclovir 1 g twice daily for 5–10 days or acyclovir 200 mg five times a day for the same period. Acyclovir-resistant HSV has become a problem in patients with AIDS; reported acyclovir resistance in PWH is 10-fold higher than that in immunocompetent counterparts—0.6% and 6%, respectively (Lolis et al., 2008).

Resistance to acyclovir also implies resistance to valacyclovir, and, in many cases, famciclovir is also not an effective treatment. Treatment of choice for acyclovir-resistant HSV is intravenous foscarnet or cidofovir. Topical cidofovir and foscarnet have been used as successful treatments as well (Strick et al., 2006).

HERPES ZOSTER

Herpes zoster, also known as shingles, is caused by the reactivation of varicella zoster virus (VZV), which also causes chickenpox. Ten to twenty percent of adults are affected by shingles. As T-cell immunity wanes, with age or immunosuppression, the incidence of infection increases. Therefore, herpes zoster is very common with HIV infection, and it may be the presenting manifestation. In immunocompetent patients, the infection is usually limited to one dermatome. Pain and constitutional symptoms of fever, malaise, and headache may precede the eruptive phase, which consists of clusters of vesicles on an erythematous base within a dermatome. Involvement of multiple dermatomes is common in PWH, and disseminated infection is frequent. Treatment is with acyclovir 800 mg/day for 7–10 days, valacyclovir 1 g three times a day, or acyclovir 10 mg/kg when intravenous treatment is warranted. Foscarnet 40 mg/kg three times a day is used for treatment of acyclovir-resistant VZV (Cockerell & Calame, 2013). Continual pain, referred to as postherpetic neuralgia (PHN), can occur and last months to years. Immunocompromised patients are at a higher risk of developing PHN, and effective, early treatment of pain with gabapentin and/or opioids at presentation along with antivirals can reduce the risk of PHN.

While no study has specifically evaluated vaccination in VZV-susceptible adolescents and adults with HIV, it is assumed to be safe and effective. The ACIP recommends vaccination for the prevention of primary varicella infection with the live-attenuated varicella vaccine (Varivax) in PWH provided they have a CD4 count greater than 200 cells/mm^3; it should be avoided in PWH with CD4$^+$ T-cell counts of less than 200 cells/mm^3 or CD4$^+$ T-cell 15% or less (CDC, 2022c). Two vaccines for the prevention of recurrent varicella disease have been approved, but as of June 2020, the live-attenuated Zostavax (ZVL) is no longer available in the United States. The newer RZV is more immunogenic than its predecessor. It is not a live virus vaccine and as such it may be safe to give to PWH regardless of CD4$^+$ T-cell count, but this has yet to be determined in clinical trials. In January 2022, the ACIP updated its recommendations for zoster vaccination, advising a two-dose RZV vaccination series in PWH aged 19 years and older without respect to CD4 count. PWH who already received ZVL should undergo revaccination with RZV (CDC, 2022c).

METHICILLIN-RESISTANT STAPHYLOCOCCUS AUREUS

Staphylococcus aureus has acquired the mecA gene, which makes it less sensitive to many of the antibiotics typically used to treat skin and soft-tissue infections. Methicillin-resistant

S. aureus (MRSA) grew to epidemic proportions during the 2000s, with a higher rate of MRSA infection in PWH. One study reported that the prevalence was 18-times higher in the HIV population compared to the general population (Crum-Cianflone et al., 2007). However, subsequent data suggest a reduction in MRSA-driven skin and soft-tissue infections in PWH from the late 2000s peak (Hemmige et al., 2020).

Incision and drainage is the most important component of treatment for localized skin infections. Many cutaneous MRSA infections are generally sensitive to the antibiotics trimethoprim–sulfamethoxazole, doxycycline, clindamycin, and linezolid. These antibiotics are generally effective against MRSA, and culture and sensitivity data are helpful in guiding treatment. Both skin and nasal colonization are potential reservoirs for reinfection. Studies have indicated that mupirocin can be used to eradicate nasal colonization, whereas chlorhexidine can be used for the skin (Kuehnert et al., 2006).

BACILLARY ANGIOMATOSIS

This infectious disease occurs rarely in PWH, but awareness of bacillary angiomatosis (BA) is important because it is a clinical mimicker of Kaposi's sarcoma (KS) that can be treated effectively with erythromycin 500 mg four times a day, yet it is potentially systemic and fatal if untreated. Clinically, purple "grape-like" papules to nodules are seen in a focal or widespread distribution. In contrast to KS, they rarely manifest as patches or plaques. BA can be distinguished from KS on histology, with a lobular capillary proliferation with an edematous stroma and clusters of neutrophils seen throughout the lesion (Cockerell & Calame, 2013). There is often an amorphous material that represents colonies of bacteria, and culture for *Bartonella* speciation has relevance given that *Bartonella quintana* is more frequently associated with neurologic sequelae compared to *B. henselae* (Gasquet et al., 1998).

SYPHILIS

Primary syphilis typically presents with an asymptomatic orogenital ulcer, whereas secondary syphilis is typically papulosquamous to psoriasiform but can mimic many other dermatoses. The color is characteristic, resembling a "clean-cut ham" or having a coppery tint. Palms and soles may present with classic coppery-colored scaly plaques. Temporal, irregular, "moth-eaten" alopecia of the beard, scalp, and eyebrows may occur. Of concern, syphilis has an accelerated rate of progression in HIV, with potential development of neurosyphilis, and can have atypical presentations including multiple chancres and syphilitic vasculitis. Diagnosis can be complicated by the prozone effect, in which a false-negative Rapid Plasma Reagin or Venereal Disease Research Laboratory test is achieved due to overwhelming antibody titers interfering with formation of an antigen-antibody lattice network in the test. Dilution of the assay overcomes this false-negative result, and this should be requested when syphilis is suspected and there is a negative result (Smith & Holman, 2004). Treatment is with penicillin formulations, and better response with decreased progression to neurosyphilis has been noted in PWH on ART (Ghanem et al., 2007).

SCABIES

Scabies is caused by an infestation of the skin by the *Sarcoptes scabiei* mite. The first symptom of scabies is usually pruritus, especially at night. Scabies is a very common infection, with an approximate prevalence of 200 million annual cases (Global Burden of Disease, 2015). Scabies mites cannot jump or fly and therefore require skin-to-skin contact for infection to occur. Scabies mites have not demonstrated the ability to transmit HIV. Diagnosis is made through clinical examination. Burrow scrapings can be examined under a microscope for scabies mites, eggs, and feces; however, the absence of these on microscopic evaluated does not eliminate the possibility of infection. Dermoscopy has been shown to be a valuable tool in the diagnosis of scabies, with a characteristic "delta wing jet" appearance of burrows identified on dermoscopy (Suh et al., 2014).

"Norwegian" or "crusted" scabies is a more florid infection leading to proliferation of heaped up, crusted burrows teeming with scabies mites. These crusted lesions typically occur in the web spaces of the hands and feet, over the elbows, and on the ears or temples. This typically occurs in highly immunocompromised patients, including PWH with low CD4 $^+$ T-cell counts. Norwegian scabies is highly infectious and can be easily spread to healthcare workers by skin-to-skin contact.

Per CDC guidelines, first-line treatment of scabies is either topical permethrin cream or oral ivermectin (Workowski, 2021). Permethrin cream is applied below the neck (and above the neck if lesions are evident) and washed off after 8–14 hours on days 1 and 14, or ivermectin 200 µg/kg is given on days 1 and 14. The CDC recommendation for treatment of crusted scabies to avoid treatment failure is an intensive regimen of ivermectin dosed at 200 µg/kg taken on days 1, 2, 8, 9, and 15, and, for severe disease, also on days 22 and 29, in combination with topical permethrin daily for 7 days and then twice a week until cure (Ortega-Loayza et al., 2013). Compliance may therefore be difficult.

AMOEBA

Naegleria fowleri, Balamuthia mandrillaris, and *Acanthamoeba* are free-living protozoa that cause a rapidly progressive fatal infection in the immunocompromised host. *Acanthamoeba* is a recognized pathogen in immunocompromised patients and has been cultured from the cornea, nasal and sinus cavities, ears, throat, lungs, and skin. *Acanthamoeba* can infect the skin directly or can spread to the skin by hematogenous dissemination from primary foci in the lungs or sinuses (Chandrasekar et al., 1997). More frequent sites of cutaneous involvement include the face, trunk, and extremities. The lesions typically present as nonspecific necrotic ulcers or nodules that may be quite tender or asymptomatic.

Evaluations should include biopsy with histology showing trophozoites and culture for speciation. The survival rate is poor. Optimal treatment has not been determined; thus, combination therapy is recommended with miltefosine, fluconazole, and pentamidine. Trimethoprim–sulfamethoxazole, metronidazole, and a macrolide can be added to this regime in patients failing therapy (Mayer et al., 2011).

MONKEY POX

LEARNING OBJECTIVE

Discuss the demographics, presentation, diagnosis, treatment, and prevention of monkeypox.

KEY POINTS

- On July 23, 2022, and August 4, 2022, the WHO and US DHHS, respectively, declared the monkeypox virus outbreak a public health emergency.

- Clinical disease is characterized by a viral prodrome followed by painful lesions, often anogenital, that can be severe and lead to disfiguring scarring.

- Vaccination with a two-dose series of modified vaccinia Ankara (MVA) vaccine (JYNNEOS) is currently recommended for PWH, as they are at risk for severe disease.

Monkeypox virus (MPV, MPX, MPXV) is one of the four *orthopoxvirus* known to cause human disease, along with *variola virus*, which causes smallpox, *cowpox virus*, and *vaccinia virus* (Bennett et al., 2020). MPV (has been an endemic zoonosis since the 1950s in parts of Africa, namely the Congo basin in central/western Africa; although sporadic outbreaks in nonendemic countries occur, sustained transmission had not been observed (Sklenovská & Van Ranst, 2018). In May 2022, a cluster of MPV first identified in the United Kingdom began to spread worldwide, leading the WHO to declare a public health emergency in July 2022, followed shortly thereafter by the DHHS in August 2022 (DHHS, 2022a). Initial cases were associated with high-risk sexual behavior including having multiple and/or anonymous sexual partners, often in the presence of other co-occurring sexually transmitted infections. Reports show an increased risk of MPV in gay, bisexual, and other MSM, though ongoing monitoring indicates any direct skin-to-skin contact can lead to transmission. Demographic data also show that while most cases have occurred in White persons, Black and Hispanic persons, who make up 34% of general population, account for more than one-half of MPV cases (Philpott et al., 2022). Further, 40% of those testing positive for MPV also have HIV. Whether this increased risk is due to viral, host, or other behavioral factors remains a subject of ongoing investigation (Tarín-Vincente, 2022). Regardless of the reasons for these findings, it continues to highlight healthcare disparities and the importance of health equity.

Clinically, MPV manifests with a 1–2-week incubation period, followed by a systemic illness and rash. Systemic symptoms include a prodrome of fever, myalgias, malaise, headaches, predominant lymphadenopathy, or chills occurring as first symptom, not accompanied by a rash. Unique to the 2022 MPV outbreak, a significant minority (42%) of those with MPV had a rash, typically anogenital and/or oral, as the first sign of illness; classic "prodromal" symptoms presented later in the disease course. The rash appears within 1 to 3 days of systemic illness, progressing through stages from maculopapular to vesicular to pustular over the course of 5 to 7 days. Lesions are characteristically painful and are generally but not always in the same stage of maturation; they can be few in number, first at the site of inoculation with subsequent spread more diffusely over time (Iñigo Martinez et al., 2022). Over the next 1–3 weeks, lesions scab over and heal. Individuals should be considered infectious until all lesions have scabbed over completely. Keeping lesions covered until this occurs can greatly reduce transmission (CDC, 2022a; Philpott et al., 2022; Tarín-Vincente et al., 2022).

Diagnostic testing for MPV is via PCR testing for orthopoxvirus DNA, by swabbing lesions with a synthetic/noncotton swab, submitted in viral transport medium. Lesions need not be unroofed to obtain adequate genetic material for testing (CDC, 2022b). After diagnostic confirmation, many individuals will have a mild, self-limiting disease course requiring only supportive care; severe disease is uncommon. When it occurs, severe disease most often manifests as severe pain or secondary bacterial cellulitis of lesions, though bronchopneumonia, sepsis, encephalitis, myocarditis, and ocular lesions have been observed (Thornhill et al., 2022).

Treatment with oral or intravenous tecovirimat, developed for smallpox, is available off-label for people who are at increased risk of severe disease and are exposed to monkeypox or diagnosed with MPV infection (DHHS, 2022b). Two vaccines may be used for the prevention of MPV disease: MVA vaccine (JYNNEOS) and ACAM2000. MVA vaccine is made from attenuated, nonreplicating vaccinia virus, suitable for use in immunocompromised individuals (including PWH) and people with skin disorders, given as two doses (either subcutaneous or intradermal) 4 weeks apart. ACAM2000 is a replication-competent smallpox vaccine that should be avoided in the immunocompromised and those with certain skin conditions (CDC, 2022c). The two-dose MPV vaccination is also indicated as postexposure prophylaxis for individuals that have known close contact within the last 14 days with someone who tested positive for MPV (CDC, 2022d).

RECOMMENDED READING

Drain PK, Mosam A, Gounder L, et al. Recurrent giant molluscum contagiosum immune reconstitution inflammatory syndrome (IRIS) after initiation of antiretroviral therapy in an HIV-infected man. *Int J STD AIDS*. 2014;25(3):235–238.

McCloskey JC, Metcalf C, French MA, et al. The frequency of high-grade intraepithelial neoplasia in anal/perianal warts is higher than previously recognized. *Int J STD AIDS*. 2007;18(8):538–542.

Smith G, Holman RP. The prozone phenomenon with syphilis and HIV-1 co-infection. *South Med J*. 2004;97(4):379–382.

CUTANEOUS MALIGNANCIES IN HIV

LEARNING OBJECTIVE

Review the status of cutaneous malignancies in PWH.

WHAT'S NEW?

As life expectancy of PWH has increased, cancers have become a more prevalent cause of morbidity and mortality.

KEY POINTS

- In the United States, first-line treatment for HIV-associated KS remains antiretroviral therapy, with chemotherapy indicated for progressive cutaneous disease or visceral involvement and radiation therapy for bulky obstructive tumors.

- There is an increased risk of metastatic disease in PWH with invasive melanoma, with worse outcomes associated with lower CD4$^+$ T-cell counts.

- There is a three- to fivefold increased risk of developing nonmelanoma skin cancer in HIV, and basal and squamous cell cancers are more aggressive in PWH.

KAPOSI'S SARCOMA

Prior to the HIV epidemic, KS was rare in the United States. It was seen mostly in elderly men from the Mediterranean or recipients of solid organ transplants. The increasing prevalence of KS in the early HIV years led to the discovery of human herpesvirus-8 (HHV-8), the causative agent of KS. Mucocutaneous violaceous patches, plaques, or nodules may be seen, with biopsy revealing a vascular proliferation on histology with confirmatory HHV-8 immunostaining. First-line treatment for HIV-associated KS is ART. IRIS can result in KS progression during the initiation of ART, and patients on ART can still develop KS (Krown et al., 2008). Chemotherapy is indicated for rapidly progressive cutaneous KS and when there is visceral involvement; radiation may be helpful when bulky plaques cause pain or lymphatic blockage (Murphy et al., 1997). There have been reports of HHV-8 reactivation and development of KS in patients exposed to topical and systemic steroids (Boudhir et al., 2013).

MELANOMA AND NONMELANOMA SKIN CANCERS

The non-AIDS-defining skin cancers in HIV include basal cell cancers, squamous cell cancers, and melanomas. Case reports suggest an increased incidence of melanoma in PWH (Wilkins et al., 2006). In addition, PWH are more likely to develop metastases with invasive melanoma, and lower CD4$^+$ T-cell count is predictive of worse prognosis (Rodrigues et al., 2002). In addition, there is a three- to fivefold increased risk of developing nonmelanoma skin cancer in HIV. Basal cell carcinomas are more common than squamous cell carcinomas (SCCs), as is the case in the general population but in contrast to immunocompromised transplant patients, in whom SCCs are more common. Both basal cell carcinomas and SCCs are more aggressive in the HIV population (Wilkins et al., 2006). Despite this, screening guidelines for melanoma, BCC and SCC are the same for PWH as those for the general population.

ACKNOWLEDGMENTS

The author acknowledges John M. Curtain, PA-C, MPH, the author of this chapter in the previous edition.

RECOMMENDED READING

Wilkins K, Turner R, Dolev JC, et al. Cutaneous malignancy and human immunodeficiency virus disease. *J Am Acad Dermatol.* 2006;54(2):189–206;quiz 207–110.

REFERENCES

Aboulafia D M, Bundow D, Wilske K, Ochs UI. Etanercept for the treatment of human immunodeficiency virus-associated psoriatic arthritis. *Mayo Clin Proc.* 2000;75(10):1093–1098.

Altman K, Vanness E, Westergaard RP. Cutaneous manifestations of human immunodeficiency virus: a clinical update. *Curr Infect Dis Rep.* 2015;17(3):464.

Anton P, Soriano V, Jimenez-Nacher I, et al. Incidence of rash and discontinuation of nevirapine using two different escalating initial doses. *AIDS.* 1999;13(4):524–525.

Ball RA, Kinchelow T; ISR Substudy Group. Injection site reactions with the HIV-1 fusion inhibitor enfuvirtide. *J Am Acad Dermatol.* 2003;49(5):826–831.

Bartlett BL, Khambaty M, Mendoza N, et al. Dermatological management of human immunodeficiency virus (HIV). *Skin Therapy Lett.* 2007;12(8):1–3.

Baveewo S, Ssali F, Karamagi C, et al. Validation of World Health Organisation HIV/AIDS clinical staging in predicting initiation of antiretroviral therapy and clinical predictors of low CD4\++ T cell count in Uganda. *PLoS One.* 2011;6(5):e19089.

Bellavista S, D'Antuono A, Infusino SD, et al. Pruritic papular eruption in HIV: a case successfully treated with NB-UVB. *Dermatol Ther.* 2013;26(2):173–175.

Bennett JE, Dolin R, Blaser MJ, et al. 132. In Mandell, Douglas, and Bennett's (eds.), *Principles and practice of infectious diseases, vol. 2,* New York: Elsevier; 2020:1809–1817.

Bolognia JL, Jorizzo JL, Schaffer J. *Dermatology.* 3rd ed. New York: Elsevier; 2012.

Boonchai W, Laohasrisakul R, Manonukul J, Kulthanan K. Pruritic papular eruption in HIV seropositive patients: a cutaneous marker for immunosuppression. *Int J Dermatol.* 1999;38(5):348–350.

Boudhir H, Mael-Ainin M, Senouci K, et al. Kaposi's disease: an unusual side-effect of topical corticosteroids. *Ann Dermatol Venereol.* 2013;140(6–7):459–461.

Breuer-McHam J, Marshall G, Adu-Oppong A, et al. Alterations in HIV expression in AIDS patients with psoriasis or pruritus treated with phototherapy. *J Am Acad Dermatol.* 1999;40(1):48–60.

Calonje E, Brenn T, Lazar A, Mckee P. *McKee's pathology of the skin.*4th ed. St. Louis, MO: Saunders; 2012:901.

Cambuim II, Macedo DP, Delgado M, et al. Clinical and mycological evaluation of onychomycosis among Brazilian HIV/AIDS patients [in Portuguese]. *Rev Soc Bras Med Trop.* 2011;44(1):40–42.

Centers for Disease Control and Prevention (CDC). Interim clinical considerations for use of JYNNEOS and ACAM2000 vaccines during the 2022 U.S. monkeypox outbreak. https://www.cdc.gov/poxvirus/monkeypox/health-departments/vaccine-considerations.html. Published 2022c. Accessed August 30, 2022.

CDC. Monkeypox: clinical recognition, https://www.cdc.gov/poxvirus/monkeypox/clinicians/clinical-recognition.html. Published 2022a. Accessed September 30, 2022.

CDC. Monkeypox: preparation and collection of specimens. https://www.cdc.gov/poxvirus/monkeypox/clinicians/prep-collection-specimens.html. Published 2022b. Accessed September 30, 2022.

CDC. Vaccination strategies. https://www.cdc.gov/poxvirus/monkeypox/interim-considerations/overview.html. Published 2022d. Accessed August 30, 2022.

Chandrasekar PH, Nandi PS, Fairfax MR, Crane LR. Cutaneous infections due to *Acanthamoeba* in patients with acquired immunodeficiency syndrome. *Arch Intern Med.* 1997;157(5):569–572.

Chaponda M, Pirmohamed M. Hypersensitivity reactions to HIV therapy. *Br J Clin Pharmacol.* 2011;71(5):659–671.

Cockerell C, Calame A. *Cutaneous manifestations of HIV disease.* London: Manson; 2013.

Crum-Cianflone NF, Burgi AA, Hale BR. Increasing rates of community-acquired methicillin-resistant *Staphylococcus aureus* infections among HIV-infected persons. *Int J STD AIDS.* 2007;18(8):521–526.

Davis CM, Shearer WT. Diagnosis and management of HIV drug hypersensitivity. *J Allergy Clin Immunol.* 2008;121(4):826–832, e825.

de Berker D. Clinical practice: fungal nail disease. *N Engl J Med.* 2009;360(20):2108–2116.

de Moraes AP, de Arruda EA, Vitoriano MA, et al. An open-label efficacy pilot study with pimecrolimus cream 1% in adults with facial seborrhoeic dermatitis infected with HIV. *J Eur Acad Dermatol Venereol.* 2007;21(5):596–601.

Department of Health and Human Services (DHHS), Administration for Strategic Preparedness & Response. Determination that a public health emergency exists. https://m.domesticpreparedness.com/updates/hhs-strengthens-countrys-preparedness-for-health-emergencies-announces-administration-for-strategic-preparedness-and-response/. Published 2022a. Accessed September 30, 2022.

DHHS, Panel on Guidelines for the Prevention and Treatment of Opportunistic Infections in Adults and Adolescents with HIV. Guidelines for the prevention and treatment of opportunistic infections in adults and adolescents with HIV. National Institutes of Health, Centers for Disease Control and Prevention, HIV Medicine Association, and Infectious Diseases Society of America. https://clinicalinfo.hiv.gov/en/guidelines/adult-and-adolescent-opportunistic-infection.Monkeypox. Published 2022b. Accessed September 30, 2022.

Dogra S, Yadav S. Acitretin in psoriasis: an evolving scenario. *Int J Dermatol.* 2014;53(5):525–538.

Dover JS, Johnson RA. Cutaneous manifestations of human immunodeficiency virus infection: part II. *Arch Dermatol.* 1991;127(10):1549–1558.

Drain PK, Mosam A, Gounder L, et al. Recurrent giant molluscum contagiosum immune reconstitution inflammatory syndrome (IRIS) after initiation of antiretroviral therapy in an HIV-infected man. *Int J STD AIDS.* 2014;25(3):235–238.

Duvic M. Immunology of AIDS related to psoriasis. *J Invest Dermatol.* 1990;95(5):38S–40S.

Duvic M, Crane MM, Conant M, et al. Zidovudine improves psoriasis in human immunodeficiency virus-positive males. *Arch Dermatol.* 1994;130(4):447–451.

Eisman S. Pruritic papular eruption in HIV. *Dermatol Clin.* 2006;24(4):449–457, vi.

Farsani TT, Kore S, Nadol P, et al Etiology and risk factors associated with a pruritic papular eruption in people living with HIV in India. *J Int AIDS Soc.* September 3, 2013;16(1):17325. http://doi:10.7448/IAS.16.1.17325. PMID: 24004854; PMCID: PMC3763046.

Fearfield LA, Rowe A, Francis N, et al. Itchy folliculitis and human immunodeficiency virus infection: clinicopathological and immunological features, pathogenesis and treatment. *Br J Dermatol.* 1999;141(1):3–11.

Foissac M, Goehringer F, Ranaivo IM, et al. Efficacy and safety of intravenous cidofovir in the treatment of giant molluscum contagiosum in an immunosuppressed patient [in French]. *Ann Dermatol Venereol.* 2014;141(10):620–622.

Gasquet S, Maurin M, Brouqui P, et al. Bacillary angiomatosis in immunocompromised patients. *AIDS.* 1998;12(14):1793–1803.

Gelfand JM, Gladman DD, Mease PJ, et al. Epidemiology of psoriatic arthritis in the population of the United States. *J Am Acad Dermatol.* 2005;53(4):573.

Ghanem KG, Erbelding EJ, Wiener ZS, Rompalo AM. Serological response to syphilis treatment in HIV-positive and HIV-negative patients attending sexually transmitted diseases clinics. *Sex Transm Infect.* 2007;83(2):97–101.

Global Burden of Disease 2015 Disease and Injury Incidence and Prevalence Collaborators. Global, regional, and national incidence, prevalence and years lived with disability for 310 diseases and injuries, 1990–2015; a systematic analysis for the Global Burden of Disease Study 2015. *Lancet.* 2016;388(10053):1545.

Goldstein B, Berman B, Sukenik E, Frankel SJ. Correlation of skin disorders with CD4$^+$ T cell lymphocyte counts in patients with HIV/AIDS. *J Am Acad Dermatol.* 1997;36(2 Pt 1):262–264.

Gompels MM, Simpson N, Snow M, et al. Desensitization to co-trimoxazole (trimethoprim-sulphamethoxazole) in HIV-infected patients: is patch testing a useful predictor of reaction? *J Infect.* 1999;38:111–115.

Hage CA, Azar MM, Bahr N, et al. Histoplasmosis: up-to-date evidence-based approach to diagnosis and management. *Semin Respir Crit Care Med.* 2015;36(5):729–745.

Hagensee ME, Cameron JE, Leigh JE, Clark RA. Human papillomavirus infection and disease in HIV-infected individuals. *Am J Med Sci.* 2004;328(1):57–63.

Hanifin JM, Reed ML, Eczema P, et al.; Impact Working Group. A population-based survey of eczema prevalence in the United States. *Dermatitis.* 2007;18(2):82–91.

Hemmige V, Arias CA, Pasalar S, Giordano TP. Skin and soft tissue infection in people living with human immunodeficiency virus in a large, urban, public healthcare system in Houston, Texas, 2009–2014. *Clin Infect Dis.* 2020;70(9):1985–1992. http://doi:10.1093/cid/ciz509

Hevia O, Jimenez-Acosta F, Ceballos PI, et al. Pruritic papular eruption of the acquired immunodeficiency syndrome: a clinicopathologic study. *J Am Acad Dermatol.* 1991;24(2 Pt 1):231–235.

Hyle EP, Wood BR, Backman ES, et al. High frequency of hypothalamic–pituitary–adrenal axis dysfunction after local corticosteroid injection in HIV-infected patients on protease inhibitor therapy. *J AIDS.* 2013;63(5):602–608.

Iñigo Martínez J. Gil Montalbán E, Jiménez Bueno S, et al. Monkeypox outbreak predominantly affecting men who have sex with men, Madrid, Spain, 26 April to 16 June 2022. *Euro Surveill.* 2022;27(27):200471. https://doi.org/10.2807/1560-7917.ES.2022.27.27.2200471

Introcaso CE, Hines JM, Kovarik CL. Cutaneous toxicities of antiretroviral therapy for HIV: part II. Nonnucleoside reverse transcriptase inhibitors, entry and fusion inhibitors, integrase inhibitors, and immune reconstitution syndrome. *J Am Acad Dermatol.* 2010;63(4):563–569; quiz 569–570.

Jagdeo J, Ho D, Lo A, Carruthers A. A systematic review of filler agents for aesthetic treatment of HIV facial lipoatrophy (FLA). *J Am Acad Dermatol.* 2015; 73(6):1040–1054, e1014.

Kim CM, Vogel J, Jay G, Rhim JS. The HIV tat gene transforms human keratinocytes. *Oncogene.* 1992;7(8):1525–1529.

Knobel H, Miro JM, Domingo P, et al. Failure of a short-term prednisone regimen to prevent nevirapine-associated rash: a double-blind placebo-controlled trial: the GESIDA 09/99 study. *J AIDS.* 2001;28(1):14–18.

Krown SE, Lee JY, Dittmer DP; AIDS Malignancy Consortium. More on HIV-associated Kaposi's sarcoma. *N Engl J Med.* 2008;358(5):535–536; author reply 536.

Kuehnert MJ, Kruszon-Moran D, Hill HA, et al. Prevalence of *Staphylococcus aureus* nasal colonization in the United States, 2001–2002. *J Infect Dis.* 2006;193(2):172–179.

Leung AKC, Barankin B, Hon KLE. Molluscum contagiosum: an update. *Recent Pat Inflamm Allergy Drug Discov.* 2017;11(1):22–31. http://doi:10.2174/1872213X11666170518114456

Lin RY, Lazarus TS. Asthma and related atopic disorders in outpatients attending an urban HIV clinic. *Ann Allergy Asthma Immunol.* 1995;74(6):510–515.

Liu Z, Xie Z, Zhang L, et al. Reliability and validity of dermatology life quality index: assessment of quality of life in human immunodeficiency virus/acquired immunodeficiency syndrome patients with pruritic papular eruption. *J Tradit Chin Med.* 2013;33(5):580–583.

Lolis MS, Gonzalez L, Cohen PJ, Schwartz RA. Drug-resistant herpes simplex virus in HIV infected patients. *Acta Dermatovenerol Croat.* 2008;16(4):204–208.

Lortholary O, Fontanet A, Memain N, et al.; Cryptococcosis Study Group. Incidence and risk factors of immune reconstitution inflammatory syndrome complicating HIV-associated cryptococcosis in France. *AIDS.* 2005;19(10):1043–1049.

Mallal S, Phillips E, Carosi G, et al. HLA-B*5701 screening for hypersensitivity to abacavir. *N Engl J Med.* 2008;358(6):568–579.

Mallon E, Bunker CB. HIV-associated psoriasis. *AIDS Patient Care STDS.* 2000;14(5):239–246.

Maurer TA. Dermatologic manifestations of HIV infection. *Top HIV Med.* 2005; 13(5):149–154.

Mayer PL, Larkin JA, Hennessy JM. Amebic encephalitis. *Surg Neurol Int.* 2011;2:50.

McCloskey JC, Metcalf C, French MA, et al. The frequency of high-grade intraepithelial neoplasia in anal/perianal warts is higher than previously recognized. *Int J STD AIDS.* 2007;18(8):538–542.

Menon K, Van Voorhees AS, Bebo BF, et al. Psoriasis in patients with HIV infection: from the medical board of the National Psoriasis Foundation. *J Am Acad Dermatol.* 2010;62(2):291–299.

Meola T, Soter NA, Ostreicher R, Sanchez M, Moy JA. The safety of UVB phototherapy in patients with HIV infection. *J Am Acad Dermatol.* 1993;29(2 Pt 1):216–220.

Mirmirani P, Maurer TA, Berger TG, et al. Skin-related quality of life in HIV-infected patients on highly active antiretroviral therapy. *J Cutan Med Surg.* 2002;6(1):10–15.

Mischo M, von Kobyletzki LB, Bründermann E, et al. Similar appearance, different mechanisms: xerosis in HIV, atopic dermatitis and ageing. *Exp Dermatol.* 2014;23(6):446–448. http://doi:10.1111/exd.12425. PMID: 24758518.

Mohammed S, Vellaisamy SG, Gopalan K, et al. Prevalence of pruritic papular eruption among HIV patients: a cross-sectional study. *Indian J Sex Transm Dis AIDS.* 2019;40(2):146–151. http://doi:10.4103/ijstd.IJSTD_69_18. PMID: 31922105; PMCID: PMC6896392.

Murphy M, Armstrong D, Sepkowitz KA, et al. Regression of AIDS-related Kaposi's sarcoma following treatment with an HIV-1 protease inhibitor. *AIDS.* 1997;11(2):261–262.

Murray H, Barber CJ, Foreman RM, et al.; GBD 2013 DALYs and HALE Collaborators. Global, regional, and national disability-adjusted life years (DALYs) for 306 diseases and injuries and healthy life expectancy (HALE) for 188 countries, 1990–2013: quantifying the epidemiological transition. *Lancet.* 2015;386:2145–2191.

Nakamura M, Abrouk M, Farahnik B, et al. Psoriasis treatment in HIV-positive patients: a systematic review of systemic immunosuppressive therapies. *Cutis.* 2018;101(1):38, 42, 56.

Nambudiri VE, Mutyambizi K, Walls AC, et al. Successful treatment of perianal giant condyloma acuminatum in an immunocompromised host with systemic interleukin 2 and topical cidofovir. *JAMA Dermatol.* 2013;149(9):1068–1070.

Nissen D, Nolte H, Permin H, et al. Evaluation of IgE-sensitization to fungi in HIV-positive patients with eczematous skin reactions. *Ann Allergy Asthma Immunol.* 1999;83(2):153–159.

Nomura T, Katoh M, Yamamoto Y, et al. Eosinophilic pustular folliculitis: A published work-based comprehensive analysis of therapeutic responsiveness. *J Dermatol.* 2016;43(8):919–927. http://doi:10.1111/1346-8138.13287

Oble DA, Collett E, Hsieh M, et al. A novel T cell receptor transgenic animal model of seborrheic dermatitis-like skin disease. *J Invest Dermatol.* 2005;124(1):151–159.

Obuch ML, Maurer TA, Becker B, Berger TG. Psoriasis and human immunodeficiency virus infection. *J Am Acad Dermatol.* 1992;27(5 Pt 1):667–673.

Okada S, Fujimura T, Furudate S, et al. Immunosuppression-associated eosinophilic pustular folliculitis (IS-EPF) developing after highly active anti-retroviral therapy (HAART): the possible mechanisms through CD163+ M2 macrophages. *Eur J Dermatol.* 2013;23(5):713–714.

Ortega-Loayza AG, McCall CO, Nunley JR. Crusted scabies and multiple dosages of ivermectin. *J Drugs Dermatol.* 2013;12(5):584–585.

Osborne GE, Taylor C, Fuller LC. The management of HIV-related skin disease. Part II: neoplasms and inflammatory disorders. *Int J STD AIDS.* 2003;14:235.

Palefsky JM, Lee JY, Jay N; ANCHOR Investigators Group. Treatment of anal high-grade squamous intraepithelial lesions to prevent anal cancer. *N Engl J Med.* 2022;386(24):2273–2282. https://doi.org/10.1056/NEJMoa2201048

Pedrosa AF, Lisboa C, Goncalves Rodrigues A. Malassezia infections: a medical conundrum. *J Am Acad Dermatol.* 2014;71(1):170–176.

Philpott D, Hughes CM, Alroy KA, et al. Epidemiologic and clinical characteristics of monkeypox cases—United States, May 17–July 22, 2022. *MMWR Morb Mortal Wkly Rep.* 2022;71:1018–1022. http://dx.doi.org/10.15585/mmwr.mm7132e3

Ratnam I, Chiu C, Kandala NB, Easterbrook PJ. Incidence and risk factors for immune reconstitution inflammatory syndrome in an ethnically diverse HIV type 1-infected cohort. *Clin Infect Dis.* 2006;42(3):418–427.

Resneck JS Jr, Van Beek M, Furmanski L, et al. Etiology of pruritic papular eruption with HIV infection in Uganda. *JAMA.* 2004;292(21):2614–2621.

Rigopoulos D, Paparizos V, Katsambas A. Cutaneous markers of HIV infection. *Clin Dermatol.* 2004;22(6):487–498.

Rodrigues LK, Klencke BJ, Vin-Christian K, et al. Altered clinical course of malignant melanoma in HIV-positive patients. *Arch Dermatol.* 2002;138(6):765–770.

Rosen T, Friedlander SF, Kircik L. Onychomycosis: epidemiology, diagnosis, and treatment in a changing landscape. *J Drugs Dermatol.* 2015;14(3):223–233.

Rosenthal D, LeBoit PE, Klumpp L, Berger TG. Human immunodeficiency virus-associated eosinophilic folliculitis. A unique dermatosis associated with advanced human immunodeficiency virus infection. *Arch Dermatol.* 1991;127(2):206–209.

Sadick NS, McNutt NS, Kaplan MH. Papulosquamous dermatoses of AIDS. *J Am Acad Dermatol.* 1990;22(6 Pt 2):1270–1277.

Severson JL, Tyring SK. Relation between herpes simplex viruses and human immunodeficiency virus infections. *Arch Dermatol.* 1999;135(11):1393–1397.

Singh F, Rudikoff D. HIV-associated pruritus: etiology and management. *Am J Clin Dermatol.* 2003;4(3):177–188.

Sklenovská N, Van Ranst M. Emergence of monkeypox as the most important orthopoxvirus infection in humans. *Front Public Health.* 2018;6:241. https://doi.org/10.3389/fpubh.2018.00241

Smith G, Holman RP. The prozone phenomenon with syphilis and HIV-1 co-infection. *South Med J.* 2004;97(4):379–382.

Soeprono FF, Schinella RA, Cockerell CJ, Comite SL. Seborrheic-like dermatitis of acquired immunodeficiency syndrome: a clinicopathologic study. *J Am Acad Dermatol.* 1986;14(2 Pt 1):242–248.

Stanley SK, Folks TM, Fauci AS. Induction of expression of human immunodeficiency virus in a chronically infected promonocytic cell line by ultraviolet irradiation. *AIDS Res Hum Retroviruses.* 1989;5(4):375–384.

Strick LB, Wald A, Celum C. Management of herpes simplex virus type 2 infection in HIV type 1-infected persons. *Clin Infect Dis.* 2006;43(3):347–356.

Suh KS, Han SH, Lee KH, et al. Mites and burrows are frequently found in nodular scabies by dermoscopy and histopathology. *J Am Acad Dermatol.* 2014; 71(5):1022–1023.

Tarín-Vicente EJ, Alemany A, Agud-Dios M, et al. Clinical presentation and virological assessment of confirmed human monkeypox virus cases in Spain: a prospective observational cohort study. *Lancet.* 2022;400(10353):661–669. https://doi.org/10.1016/S0140-6736(22)01436-2

Thornhill JP, Barkati S, Walmsley S, et al. Monkeypox virus infection in humans across 16 countries—April–June 2022. *N Engl J Med.* 2022;387(8):679–691. https://doi.org/10.1056/NEJMoa2207323

Toutous-Trellu L, Abraham S, Pechere M, et al. Topical tacrolimus for effective treatment of eosinophilic folliculitis associated with human immunodeficiency virus infection. *Arch Dermatol.* 2005;141(10):1203–1208.

Ward HA, Russo GG, Shrum J. Cutaneous manifestations of antiretroviral therapy. *J Am Acad Dermatol.* 2002;46(2):284–293.

Warren KJ, Boxwell DE, Kim NY, Drolet BA. Nevirapine-associated Stevens–Johnson syndrome. *Lancet.* 1998;351(9102):567.

Warshaw EM, Nelson D, Carver SM, et al. A pilot evaluation of pulse itraconazole vs. terbinafine for treatment of *Candida* toenail onychomycosis. *Int J Dermatol.* 2005;44(9):785–788.

Weinberg JL, Kovarik CL. The WHO clinical staging system for HIV/AIDS. *Virtual Mentor.* 2010;12(3):202–206.

Wheat LJ, Connolly-Stringfield PA, Baker RL, et al. Disseminated histoplasmosis in the acquired immune deficiency syndrome: clinical findings, diagnosis and treatment, and review of the literature. *Medicine.* 1990;69(6):361–374.

Wilkins K, Turner R, Dolev JC, et al. Cutaneous malignancy and human immunodeficiency virus disease. *J Am Acad Dermatol.* 2006;54(2):189–206; quiz 207–210.

Workowski KA, Backham LH, Chan PA, et al. Sexually transmitted diseases treatment guidelines, 2021. *MMWR Recomm Rep.* 2021;70(4):1–187.

Zancanaro PC, McGirt LY, Mamelak AJ, et al. Cutaneous manifestations of HIV in the era of highly active antiretroviral therapy: an institutional urban clinic experience. *J Am Acad Dermatol.* 2006;54(4):581–588.

Zeichner JA. New topical therapeutic options in the management of superficial fungal infections. *J Drugs Dermatol.* 2015;14(10):s35–s41.

Zheng Y, Niyonsaba F, Ushio H, et al. Cathelicidin LL-37 induces the generation of reactive oxygen species and release of human alpha-defensins from neutrophils. *Br J Dermatol.* 2007;157(6):1124–1131.

31.

ENDOCRINE AND METABOLIC DISORDERS

Rajagopal V. Sekhar

CHAPTER GOAL

Upon completion of this chapter, the reader should be able to:

- Understand the spectrum of endocrine and metabolic complications affecting people with HIV (PWH), and clinical management of these complications.

- Understand the mechanism and clinical management of endocrine and metabolic diseases in PWH.

- Understand the emerging knowledge that oxidative stress, glutathione deficiency, and aging hallmarks in PWH are potentially reversible and improve strength, cognition, body composition, and health.

INTRODUCTION

With the advent of effective antiretroviral (ARV) therapeutic regimens, HIV infection has become a chronic disease. PWH have a longer life expectancy, and we are now able to see the emergence of disorders in such people who live longer, and these include an increasing prevalence of endocrine and metabolic abnormalities. The underlying etiology of these disorders can be attributed to multiple factors, including the effects of HIV itself, antiretroviral therapies (ART), inflammation, endothelial and immune dysfunction, and mitochondrial dysfunction. Since endocrine disorders are often insidious in their development, clinical suspicion and appropriate dynamic testing are necessary for accurate diagnosis and management and should include the participation of an endocrinologist where possible. Since PWH are now living longer, we are witnessing the evolution of HIV as a chronic disease, with new emerging phenotypes that range from an increase in the incidence and prevalence of metabolic diseases such as central obesity, metabolic syndrome, and fatty liver disease. There are also reports of "premature or accelerated aging" affecting PWH, in which relatively younger PWH develop geriatric complications typically seen in HIV uninfected people who are 20–30 years older. These include physical decline, mitochondrial dysfunction, muscle weakness, inflammation, endothelial dysfunction, insulin resistance, and cognitive decline, but underlying mechanisms are not well understood, and effective interventions are either limited or lacking. This chapter will focus on the historical and the currently evolving perspectives of endocrine and metabolic disorders in HIV infection, and discuss mechanisms, endocrine disorders, emerging complications, and therapeutic strategies.

WHAT'S NEW?

- The emerging phenomenon of premature aging in PWH, and its potential reversibility with GlyNAC (combination of glycine and N-acetylcysteine).

- Fatty liver disease, abdominal obesity, and metabolic syndrome continue to play a role in PWH.

- Endocrine disorders in transgender PWH.

- Emerging novel role for glutathione to improve cellular nutrition and cellular health.

KEY POINTS

- The endocrine complications of HIV infection are changing, with newer phenomena emerging as PWH continue to live longer.

- Metabolic complications continue to affect an increasing number of PWH.

- HIV infection, ARVs, and other factors play a role in the development of endocrine disease.

- For endocrine disorders in HIV, early referral to an endocrinologist is suggested.

- Please note that this chapter presents a discussion of the many known and emerging endocrine and metabolic abnormalities associated seen in PWH. Chapter 32 will focus on the specifics of uniquely HIV-associated lipodystrophy. Its recognition as a new syndromic clinical finding began soon after the advent and wide-spread use of combination ART. This chapter will elucidate the current understanding of the etiology of this syndrome, its associations with specific ARVs, and the current understanding of current therapeutic interventions.

ENDOCRINE AND METABOLIC DISEASE IN HIV

Although HIV infection has been associated with endocrine and metabolic complications since the 1980s, these complications have been dynamically changing as a result of improvements in pharmacotherapy and increasing lifespan, and other unknown contributors. Of note has been an increase in cardiometabolic complications, premature/accelerated aging, fatty liver disease, and metabolic syndrome, but the underlying mechanisms for many of these disorders are still not completely understood. PWH also continue to have more conventional disorders affecting the endocrine systems involving diabetes, thyroid, adrenal pituitary, bone, and gonadal systems. This chapter will discuss both existing endocrine and metabolic disease in PWH, and emerging new phenomena.

Elevations in inflammation and abnormalities in immune function in PWH could be contributing in part to some of these disorders, and PWH have been described to have elevated proinflammatory cytokines and abnormalities in immune phenomena that affect endocrine function (Merrill et al., 1989; Salim et al., 1988; Tracey & Cerami, 1990). For example, interleukin-1 (IL-1) has been shown to increase adrenocorticotropic hormone (ACTH) in cultured pituitary cells (Meyer et al., 1987; Szebeni et al., 1991). Other pituitary hormones may also be affected; effects include prolactin elevations (Parra et al., 2004) and deficient growth hormone secretion (Koutkia et al., 2004). HIV-positive mononuclear cells can increase interferon-α (Grunfeld et al., 1992) and impair glucocorticoid receptor activity (Norbiato et al., 1996), and abnormalities in IL-1 and tumor necrosis factor (TNF) can affect gonadal function by inhibiting gonadal steroidogenesis (Calkins Et al., 1988; Hales, 1992; Xiong & Hales, 1993). Interestingly, results from a small pilot study showed that correcting deficiency of the endogenous antioxidant protein glutathione was associated with a striking decline in inflammation with significant decreases in hsCRP and TNF-α blood levels within 2 weeks (Sekhar, 2015), and further studies are needed to confirm and extend these findings.

Another contributor to HIV-related endocrine disease is opportunistic infections. For example, cytomegalovirus (CMV) infection predisposes to an increased risk of developing adrenalitis (Glasgow et al., 1985). Infections caused by mycobacterial pathogens may also affect adrenal function, whereas CMV, cryptococcal, and toxoplasma infections can affect central nervous system (CNS) function and cause retinitis, meningitis, and pituitary disease (Giampalmo et al., 1990). CMV infection has been reported in one instance to cause hypernatremia, likely through a reset osmostat (Keuneke et al., 1999). Thyroid function can be affected by opportunistic pathogens in HIV, including *Pneumocystis jiroveci*, which is a rare cause of thyroiditis (Drucker et al., 1990).

PWH are also experiencing an increase in the incidence and prevalence of metabolic disorders, including centripetal fat accumulation as in the metabolic syndrome, fatty liver disease, and mitochondrial dysfunction. The underlying mechanisms are not well understood, and effective interventions are lacking. There is an urgent need for exploratory studies to guide relevant clinical trials to facilitate identification of mechanisms and develop therapeutic strategies.

The development and clinical use of ART have led to significant benefits for PWH, including decreased early mortality, decreased opportunistic infection, and improved nutritional status. However, these benefits are associated with increases in the incidence and prevalence of endocrine and metabolic complications, most notably dyslipidemia, and changes in body morphology ranging from lipodystrophy (Carr et al.,

1998) to central obesity in the context of metabolic syndrome. The role of ARV drugs are discussed next.

PROTEASE INHIBITORS

The initial use of protease inhibitor (PI) drugs in PWH led to observations of abnormalities in total body fat distribution, most notably an increase in abdominal fat that was initially described by colorful names such as the "protease paunch" (Mishriki, 1998) or "Crixivan belly" (Huff, 1997–1998). Since then, the PI class of drugs has been linked to the development of abdominal obesity and biochemical abnormalities comprising severe hypertriglyceridemia, dyslipidemia, insulin resistance, and diabetes. Many PI drugs, including lopinavir/ritonavir, nelfinavir, amprenavir, and saquinavir, are metabolized by the hepatic cytochrome 450 CYP3A4 isoenzyme pathway. PI drugs have been shown to directly impact insulin resistance. For example, indinavir can inhibit GLUT4 activity and thus impair insulin-stimulated glucose uptake and predispose to hyperglycemia (Caron et al., 2001; Murata et al., 2000). In addition to their permissive role in metabolic and glycemic abnormalities, PI drugs have also been implicated in the development of prolactin abnormalities (Hutchinson et al., 2000) and in osteomalacia (Cozzolino et al., 2003).

NUCLEOSIDE REVERSE TRANSCRIPTASE INHIBITORS

Nucleoside reverse transcriptase inhibitors have also been described to induce changes in body morphology. For example, stavudine has been linked to the development of lipoatrophy in HIV (Saint-Marc et al., 1999). These drugs have also been linked to the development of mitochondrial dysfunction (Mallon et al., 2005), which could result in abnormalities of glucose and lipid metabolism (Sekhar et al., 2002; Shikuma et al., 2001).

NONNUCLEOSIDE REVERSE TRANSCRIPTASE INHIBITORS

Nonnucleoside reverse transcriptase inhibitors (NNRTIs) have been linked to dyslipidemia (Padmapriyadarsini et al., 2011) and fat depletion in 3T3-L1 cells (Minami et al., 2011).

INTEGRASE INHIBITORS

Integrase Inhibitors have been associated with significant weight gain. The NA-ACCORD, a large observational cohort study in the United States and Canada compared 22,972 adult, antiretroviral treatment-naive PWH initiated with integrase strand transfer inhibitor (INSTI), PI or NNRTI-based ART, and found that compared to PI and NNRTI drugs, the INSTI agents were associated with the highest amount of weight gain, with the highest weight gain being with dolutegravir (+7.2 kg), followed by raltegravir (+5.8 kg) and elvitegravir (+4.1 kg) (Bourgi et al., 2020a). This has also been reported in other studies in PWH on dolutegravir based regimens (Bourgi et al., 2020b).

ENDOCRINE DISORDERS IN HIV

Any endocrine or metabolic disorder can affect PWH, and these include diabetes; metabolic syndrome; disorders of adrenal, thyroid, pituitary, and gonadal function; and bone and dyslipidemia. Bone disorders and dyslipidemia are discussed elsewhere in other chapters.

DIABETES MELLITUS

The prevalence of diabetes mellitus (DM) is increasing in PWH worldwide (Tzur et al., 2015). Earlier reports such as the Multicenter AIDS Cohort Study (MACS) found that exposure to ART resulted in a 14% incidence of DM in men with HIV (Brown et al., 2005). However, more recent publications have estimated this to be as high as 15.1% with a relative risk of 2.4 compared to the general population (Duncan et al., 2018). Another study followed PWH for 10 years in Malawi, Africa, and found the prevalence of DM to be higher in every age group (from 30 to 60+ years)+) compared to controls (Mathabire Rücker et al., 2018). More recently, a study from India found that PWH with lower CD4$^+$ T-cell counts had significantly higher glycemia and insulin resistance (Bajaj et al., 2020). In addition, there are reports suggesting that glycosylated hemoglobin (HbA1c) may underestimate glycemia in PWH (Kim et al., 2009; Slama et al., 2014), which suggests that the magnitude of hyperglycemia in PWH may be even greater. One study examined HbA1c in 1,500 men without and 1,357 men with HIV in the MACS cohort over 13 years and found that HbA1c underestimates glycemia in men with HIV (Slama et al., 2014). Another study that compared 100 adults with HIV and type 2 diabetes to 200 adults without HIV and type 2 diabetic, found similar results, and linked it to use of abacavir and increased mean corpuscular volume (Kim et al., 2009). The reasons for this meteoric rise in the incidence of DM are likely to be multifactorial, but a recent meta-analysis implicated ART as potentially the single most consistent determinant of DM in PWH worldwide (Nduka et al., 2017). Another recent meta-analysis investigated gestational diabetes in pregnant women with HIV and found that the pooled prevalence of gestational diabetes among pregnant women with HIV was high (Biadgo et al., 2019). Collectively, these reports indicate an increase in the incidence and prevalence of DM among PWH and suggest that relying solely on HbA1c could lead to underdiagnosing and undertreating diabetes. The implications are that it is important to carefully screen for hyperglycemia and diabetes in PWH and to correlate HbA1c with other measures of glycemic control, including fasting and prandial home glucose monitoring, for a reliable assessment of glycemic status and control. The overall management of DM in PWH is similar to that in persons without HIV and requires the combined approach of a team comprising a diabetes educator, dietitian, physician, and diabetes nursing staff and careful attention to the triumvirate of exercise, diet, and pharmacotherapy. Early screening of pregnant women with HIV for gestational diabetes is vital to reduce its complications related to pregnancy. The long-term complications of DM include retinopathy, nephropathy, neuropathy, and coronary artery disease. Interestingly, PWH are at risk of retinitis due to opportunistic infections, to HIV-associated nephropathy, and to neuropathy, and have an increased risk of cardiovascular disease. The concurrence of these end organ complications from both HIV infection and DM theoretically suggests that PWH could be at higher risk from the twin burden of two chronic diseases, HIV and DM.

ADRENAL DISORDERS

HIV infection can involve adrenal dysfunction. The incidence of hypoadrenalism is reported to be 20% in PWH (González-González et al., 2001), and postmortem studies have shown that up to two-thirds of people with AIDS may have adrenal involvement (Bricaire et al., 1988). Presentation of adrenal dysfunction may be subtle and escape clinical scrutiny, and it is relatively common in hospitalized PWH (Membreno et al., 1987). The etiology of adrenal hypofunction can range from primary hypoadrenalism involving the adrenal gland, with elevations in adrenocorticotropic hormone (ACTH) levels (Villette et al., 1990) to secondary hypoadrenalism because of pituitary suppression attributable to inherent pituitary pathology or possibly suppression of the hypothalamo-pituitary-adrenal axis by exogenous steroid use (Danaher et al., 2009; Kaviani et al., 2011). PWH have also been described to develop hyperadrenalism with iatrogenic Cushing's syndrome when administered steroids via oral, inhaled, and parenteral routes (Gray et al., 2010; Johnson et al., 2006; Samaras et al., 2005; Yombi et al., 2008).

PWH may also have abnormalities in the mineralocorticoid axis (Stricker et al., 1999). Women with HIV and wasting syndrome may have significant shunting of adrenal steroid metabolism away from androgenic pathways and toward cortisol production (Grinspoon et al., 2001).

THYROID ABNORMALITIES

The clinical presentation of thyroid abnormalities in HIV infection ranges from asymptomatic hypo- or hyperthyroidism to clinically overt disease. The prevalence of thyroid dysfunction appears to be higher in PWH. Although earlier reports suggested that thyroid dysfunction in PWH is generally similar to that seen in the population without HIV (Hoffman & Brown, 2007), recent reports indicate that the prevalence of thyroid dysfunction may be much higher. A recent study evaluated thyroid function in 178 PWH and found that 33% of participants had evidence of thyroid dysfunction (Ji et al., 2016). Most of these abnormalities involve hypothyroidism, ranging from an increased prevalence of subclinical hypothyroidism (Madeddu et al., 2006; Silva et al., 2015) to clinical hypothyroidism (Beltran et al., 2003). Factors contributing to thyroid disorders in HIV infection include, but are not limited to, ARVs, infection, and immune factors.

ARVs could play a role in the development of thyroid abnormalities in PWH. For example, HIV-related nonautoimmune primary hypothyroidism and subclinical hypothyroidism have been linked to stavudine, decreased CD4$^+$ T-cell counts, and male gender (Calza et al., 2002; Madeddu et al., 2006; Quirino et al., 2004; Silva et al., 2015).

HIV-related immune system and other factors are also linked to the development of abnormal thyroid function tests. For example, CD4[+] T-cell counts have been inversely correlated with thyroid binding globulin (Bourdoux et al., 1991), and diminished levels of triiodothyronine (T3) and reverse T3 with increased thyroid binding globulin may be associated with HIV progression. Hyperthyroidism can also occur in PWH. Autoimmune Graves's disease is an anti-thyroid-stimulating hormone receptor antibody after the initiation of ART and after an increase in CD4[+] T-cell count (Jubault et al., 2000).

Infection as an etiological factor for thyroid disease was much more prevalent in the pre-ART era and was caused by a wide variety of infectious microorganisms. However, these can still be seen in people not on ART, those with ART drug resistance, or those who are nonadherent to medications.

Although the clinical presentation of thyroid abnormalities ranges from asymptomatic hypo- or hyperthyroidism to clinically overt disease, the diagnostic workup is similar to that in HIV-negative persons and should begin with evaluations of thyroxine and thyrotropin, with additional testing for thyroiditis antibodies where appropriate.

PARATHYROID DISORDERS

Hyperparathyroidism is a condition marked by elevated secretion of parathyroid hormone. Hyperparathyroidism can be primary due to abnormalities within the parathyroid gland itself, most often due to adenoma, and rarely due to cancer. Secondary causes of hyperparathyroidism are due to conditions such as renal impairment and vitamin D deficiency. The etiology of primary hyperparathyroidism in the population with HIV is similar to the general population and typically presents as hypercalcemia; this should be appropriately investigated with the final treatment being surgical removal of the parathyroid adenoma. However, vitamin D deficiency is reported to impact a third of PWH (Van den Bout-Van Den Beukel et al., 2008) and is a common cause for secondary hyperparathyroidism (Dao et al., 2011; Mueller et al., 2010) with referrals to endocrinologists. Antiretroviral drugs such as efavirenz have been implicated in the increased prevalence of vitamin D deficiency in the population with HIV (Nylén et al., 2016), but other factors such as low CD4[+] T-cell counts and advanced AIDS may also play a role (Theodorou et al., 2014). Other ARV drugs such as tenofovir disoproxil fumarate have also been linked to secondary hyperparathyroidism in PWH (Noe et al., 2018).

GONADAL DYSFUNCTION

Gonadal dysfunction is common in PWH (Crum et al., 2005; Rietschel et al., 2000). In male adults with HIV, decreased levels of testosterone may be associated with fatigue, muscle wasting and sarcopenia, decreased bone density, low libido, weight loss, decreased strength (Grinspoon et al., 1996; Wanke et al., 2000), and impotence (Mylonakis et al., 2001).

In a study of 300 PWH, 17% were found to be hypogonadal, and all PWH with low testosterone had secondary hypogonadism. Interestingly, there was no correlation between hypogonadism and erectile dysfunction, but increasing age and a higher body mass index were positively correlated with hypogonadism, whereas smoking was negatively correlated (Crum-Cianflone et al., 2007). Although underlying causes are not fully understood, elevated levels of prolactin have been implicated in the development of male hypogonadism (Collazos et al., 2009). Treatment of PWH with AIDS wasting syndrome with testosterone or placebo was associated with a sustained increase in lean mass only with testosterone after a 6-month period (Grinspoon et al., 1999). Testosterone therapy, especially in older PWH, should involve careful monitoring of prostate-specific antigen levels, liver profiles, and hematocrit levels.

Women with HIV have increased rates of oligomenorrhea and amenorrhea. HIV has been shown to infect the cervix, uterus, and fallopian tubes (Howell et al., 1997). In one study, 8% of women with HIV had evidence of early menopause and 48% had anovulatory cycles, whereas women who ovulated had higher CD4[+] T-cell counts (Chirgwin et al., 1996). In a recent study from Nigeria reporting abnormalities in premenopausal women with HIV, the mean serum levels of the FSH, LH, progesterone, and estradiol did not differ between the follicular and luteal phase of the menstrual cycle, suggesting loss of hormonal regulation, and the researchers linked these abnormalities to hypothyroidism, which could be corrected with treatment (Ukibe et al., 2017).

GYNECOMASTIA

Males with HIV have a 2.9% incidence of developing gynecomastia, which is not linked to progression of HIV disease (Biglia, 2004), but is linked to hypogonadism, lipoatrophy, hepatitis C (Manfredi et al., 2001), and lipodystrophy (Biglia et al., 2004). The role of ARVs in the development of gynecomastia is controversial, with no correlation found in some studies (Manfredi et al., 2001), whereas other studies have linked gynecomastia with PI-based ARV regimens (Manfredi et al., 2004; Peyriere et al., 1999; Toma & Therrien, 1998). When associated with PI therapy, gynecomastia does not resolve after cessation of ART, and underlying mechanisms are not clear. Treatment of gynecomastia includes removal of any identifiable cause and, in extreme cases, surgical removal.

PITUITARY DISEASE

The pituitary gland is located in the sella turcica and comprises the anterior pituitary (adenohypophysis) and posterior pituitary (neurohypophysis). The adenohypophyseal hormones are intimately involved in controlling thyroid, adrenal, and gonadal function; growth; and milk secretion. The neurohypophysis primarily controls water balance, acting via antidiuretic hormone. Many pituitary hormones are regulated by prohormones secreted by the hypothalamus and are delivered to the pituitary via a portal system through the pituitary stalk (e.g., corticotropin releasing hormone, growth hormone releasing hormone, thyrotropin releasing hormone, gonadotropin releasing hormone (GnRH), and vasopressin), with the sole exception being prolactin, which is under inhibitory control by dopamine. Therefore, pituitary disease can be caused by pathology at the level of the hypothalamus, pituitary stalk compression, or disease in the pituitary gland itself.

Growth Hormone Disorders

Disorders of growth hormone (GH) are reported in HIV infection. Adult HIV-associated lipodystrophy is described to have GH deficiency with reduced pulse and amplitude of GH secretion, which may be related to an increased somatostatin tone, decreased ghrelin, and increased circulatory free fatty-acid concentrations (Koutkia et al., 2004). Children with HIV and adults with AIDS wasting syndrome have low levels of insulin-like growth factor-1 (IGF-1) and IGF binding protein 3 and increased concentrations of GH, suggesting resistance to GH (Frost et al., 1996; Pinto et al., 2000; Ratner Kaufman et al., 1997; Rondanelli et al., 2002).

Pituitary Adrenal Disorders

Iatrogenic Cushing's syndrome, together with secondary hypoadrenalism, is a frequent observation in PWH who receive steroid therapy (Danaher et al., 2009; Gray et al., 2010; Johnson et al., 2006; Kaviani et al., 2011; Samaras et al., 2005; Yombi et al., 2008). This is likely caused by the effect of several ARV drugs (almost entirely ritonavir or cobicistat boosting) on the hepatic cytochrome P450 system, which prolongs the half-life of steroids. This drug interaction results in elevated levels of exogenously administered steroids and suppression of ACTH, and, thereby, of endogenous cortisol production, resulting in iatrogenic Cushing's syndrome together with endogenous adrenal insufficiency. Because sudden withdrawal of exogenous steroids in this situation could precipitate a catastrophic adrenal crisis, caution must be exercised while discontinuing steroids, and a gentle taper is recommended.

Prolactin Disorders

PWH have been reported to have disturbances in basal and rhythmic prolactin secretions associated with CD4 + T-lymphocytes (Parra et al., 2004). Elevation in serum prolactin is described in PWH (Collazos et al., 2002), and hyperprolactinemia in men with HIV has been linked to hypogonadism and gynecomastia (Collazos et al., 2009). Although the etiology of the hyperprolactinemia is unclear, use of PIs has been linked to elevations in prolactin (Ram et al., 2004).

Posterior Pituitary Disorders

Posterior pituitary disorders are caused by excess secretion of antidiuretic hormone (ADH), resulting in hyponatremia, or a paucity of ADH, resulting in diabetes insipidus. In one report, 33% of people with AIDS were found to have hyponatremia primarily owing to the syndrome of inappropriate ADH secretion (Agarwal et al., 1989). PWH may also develop hypernatremia caused by diabetes insipidus due to intracranial pathology—a recently published case report highlights the role of primary CNS lymphoma in a person with HIV who presented with diabetes insipidus (Tavares-Bello et al., 2017).

METABOLIC DISORDERS IN HIV

METABOLIC SYNDROME

With increased longevity in PWH, there is also an increasing risk of developing metabolic syndrome, with central obesity, insulin resistance, hypertriglyceridemia, and hypertension, which could predispose to an increase risk of cardiovascular disease (Hadigan et al., 2001). Whereas the prevalence of metabolic syndrome in people without HIV is 3%, PWH taking ART have a prevalence of 16%–18% (Samaras et al., 2007). Women with HIV appear to have an even higher burden of metabolic syndrome, with a 33% prevalence compared to 22% for women without HIV (Sobieszczyk et al., 2008).

Clinically, the previously discussed data translate into PWH having an increased incidence and prevalence of abdominal obesity, insulin resistance, dyslipidemia, and hypertension, all of which contribute to elevated cardiometabolic risk in this population. Treatment of these disorders involves a combination of patient education; adherence to dietary control; encouragement of physical activity and exercise, where possible; and appropriate pharmacotherapy targeting glycemic control, blood pressure, and lipids.

NONALCOHOLIC FATTY LIVER DISEASE

Liver disease is an important contributor to morbidity and mortality among PWH. Despite the success with therapeutic interventions to cure hepatitis C viral coinfection, there is an increase in the prevalence of nonalcoholic fatty liver disease (NAFLD), defined as liver fat accumulation (causing fatty liver) in the absence of other causes of liver disease such as excess alcohol consumption, viral hepatitis, or any other specific hepatic pathology. NAFLD ranges from simple hepatic steatosis at one end of the spectrum, to nonalcoholic steatohepatitis (NASH) and hepatic fibrosis, which progresses to cirrhosis and hepatocellular carcinoma on the other end. NASH is now the third most-common indication for liver transplantation in the United States. The prevalence of NAFLD and NASH is increasing in PWH. A study examining PWH with altered transaminases found the prevalence of NASH reported up to 55% (Morse et al., 2015). NAFLD in PWH may have a more aggressive progression to NASH: a recently published study examined the clinical and histological differences between HIV-associated NAFLD and primary NAFLD, and reported that HIV-associated NAFLD was associated with increased severity of liver disease and higher prevalence of NASH (Vodkin et al., 2015). Further, the presence of NAFLD is linked to the development of systemic inflammation, insulin resistance, diabetes, and cardiovascular disease. Conversely, NAFLD is a well-recognized complication of type 2 diabetes, with reported prevalence as high as 80%–85%, and, given the rising incidence and prevalence of type 2 diabetes in PWH, NAFLD and NASH could soon become the most significant metabolic complication of HIV infection. Thus, the combination of high prevalence of NAFLD/NASH in PWH with increased severity of NASH makes it an extremely urgent public health concern, especially since mechanisms are not well understood and effective interventions are lacking.

HIV, MITOCHONDRIAL IMPAIRMENT, AND CELLULAR HEALTH

PWH are well described to have an impairment in mitochondrial fat oxidation. Mitochondrial impairment is also well described in non-HIV-associated conditions which include type 2 diabetes, obesity, and aging, but underlying mechanisms are unclear and currently there are no viable or effective interventions to reverse mitochondrial dysfunction in any human condition. It is from this perspective that the results of two small pilot open-label trial in PWH which that investigated mechanisms and reported reversibility of mitochondrial impairment are relevant (Nguyen et al., 2014, Kumar et al., 2020). Based on their discoveries in rodents and older humans (Nguyen et al., 2013) that adequate availability of the endogenous antioxidant protein glutathione is critically necessary for optimal mitochondrial fatty-acid oxidation, these pilot trials evaluated and found that PWH with impaired mitochondrial fatty-acid oxidation and elevated oxidative stress had severe deficiency of intracellular glutathione. The glutathione deficiency was caused by deficient synthesis attributable to decreased availability of two of its precursor amino acids, glycine and cysteine, and diminished expression of the enzymes of glutathione synthesis. In the first pilot trial, PWH received supplementation with GlyNAC (combination of glycine and N-acetylcysteine, NAC, as a cysteine donor) were supplemented for a short duration of 2 weeks, and were found to correct their deficiency, normalize glutathione synthesis, increase glutathione concentrations, and lower oxidative stress. This was associated with a significant improvement of mitochondrial fuel oxidation in the fasted and fed states, together with a 31% decrease in insulin resistance, and decrease in total body fat, waist circumference (Nguyen et al., 2014), and inflammation (Sekhar et al., 2015), and improved quality of life (Sekhar, 2021). However, this pilot study lacked a matched HIV-negative control group and had a very short duration of supplementation. The same group conducted a second small open-label trial where PWH were matched to uninfected controls for age, gender and body mass index (Kumar et al., 2020). The trial again found that PWH had severely elevated oxidative stress, glutathione deficiency, mitochondrial dysfunction, and insulin resistance, but also had evidence of endothelial dysfunction, impaired mitophagy, impaired strength and exercise capacity, and cognitive impairment. PWH were supplemented with GlyNAC for 12-weeks and all parameters were found to improve but withdrawing GlyNAC for 8-weeks led to a loss of benefits. Novel observations in this small study were improvements in

the expression of PGC1α and PINK1, which are established regulators of mitochondrial biogenesis and mitophagy—these findings suggest that GlyNAC supplementation is associated with generation of new and healthy mitochondria (biogenesis) and removal of dysfunctional mitochondria (mitophagy). The multiple specific improvements of multiple cytokines, markers of genomic damage, intracellular glutathione, and regulators of energy metabolism suggest significant improvements in cellular health. These studies offer clues to the origins of multiple pathophysiological defects and clinical complications in PWH, and future randomized clinical trials are needed to definitively confirm these results. If confirmed in larger randomized clinical trials, this discovery could have profound implications for improving the metabolic health of PWH by using nutritional supplementation of oral GlyNAC.

PREMATURE AGING IN PWH

Effective antiretroviral therapy has improved the health and life expectancy of PWH (Palella et al., 2008; Mack et al., 2003). However, emerging evidence suggests that PWH are developing premature aging, where complications typically associated with a geriatric age range of 70 to 80 years are being reported in people 10–20 years earlier (Bhatia et al., 2012; Guaraldi, 2011; Jiminez et al., 2018; Onen, 2011). A recent report where 336 young PWH with a median age of 44 years were compared to age, sex and ethnicity-matched HIV-negative controls, found that PWH had significantly higher manifestation of geriatric conditions, with lower quality-of-life scores, a fivefold higher utilization of healthcare resources, and a fourfold increase in mortality (Rajasuriar et al., 2017). Premature aging in PWH has also been reported to be linked to comorbidities typically associated with a geriatric age including slower gait speed (Schrack et al., 2015), declining strength and physical function (Khoury et al., 2017), impaired cognition (Kuhn et al., 2019; Wang, 2017), mitochondrial aging (Nguyen et al., 2014; Payne, 2011), and elevated inflammation (McDonald et al., 2013; Monczor et al., 2018; Sekhar et al., 2015). These whole-body measures indicative of premature aging in PWH are also supported by cellular findings in corneal epithelial cells, monocyte and immune dysfunction, and the emergence of frailty at an earlier age (Rajasuriar, 2017; Jiménez, 2018) (PMID: 23746838).

Although premature aging in PWH is now being recognized as a new, significant public health challenge, there is limited knowledge about underlying causal mechanisms, and effective interventions are lacking. Hallmarks of aging refer to a discrete set of defects which are believe to contribute to geriatric aging in uninfected humans (López-Otín et al., 2013). A recent small human clinical trial investigated and found that compared to uninfected controls, PWH matched for age, gender, and body mass index had evidence of impaired strength, gait speed, exercise capacity, and cognition, together with multiple hallmarks of aging affecting mitochondrial dysfunction, nutrient sensing, insulin resistance, impaired mitophagy, inflammation, and genomic damage. Interestingly, these defects (including aging hallmarks) improved after 12-weeks of supplementation with GlyNAC, with many catching up to levels in matched, uninfected controls (Kumar et al., 2020). These findings have important implications for reversing premature aging, and promoting healthy aging in PWH, and they warrant additional studies, including randomized controlled clinical trials, to definitively confirm these emerging results.

ENDOCRINE AND METABOLIC COMPLICATIONS IN TRANSGENDER PWH

Although transgender PWH usually receive hormonal therapy and could develop endocrine and metabolic complications, carefully conducted studies are limited. A matched case-control study investigated metabolic syndrome and thyroid and adrenal function, comparing transgender women (cases) to cis-gender men with HIV (controls), and found no differences between the two groups in terms of metabolic syndrome, but a higher frequency of subclinical hypothyroidism (median TSH 1.6-fold higher) associated with a higher BMI and use of steroids as well as adrenal insufficiency (Pommier et al., 2019). A more recent study evaluating inflammation in cryopreserved peripheral blood monocytes from PWH found that estrogen elevated the TLR4 activation induced by lipopolysaccharide (LPS) in cis-gender men with HIV, with increased monocyte activation and inflammatory cytokine production (IL-6, TNF-α)—these findings could have implications for use of estrogens as feminizing hormone therapy in transgender women (Kettelhut et al., 2022), especially in relation to a higher risk of cardiovascular disease (Aranda et al., 2021). More studies are warranted to further investigate and understand endocrine and cardiometabolic risks and complications of gender affirming therapy in transgender PWH.

CONCLUSION

PWH can be affected by endocrine and metabolic abnormalities. Although the more common disorders are dyslipidemia, diabetes, metabolic syndrome, and insulin resistance, other disorders affecting bone, adrenal glands, pituitary, and thyroid function may also be present. For rapid diagnosis and treatment of endocrine disorders in PWH, early referral to an endocrinologist is highly recommended.

REFERENCES

Agarwal A, Soni A, Ciechanowsky M, et al. Hyponatremia in patients with the acquired immunodeficiency syndrome. *Nephron.* 1989;53:317–321.

Aranda G, Halperin I, Gomez-Gil E, et al. Cardiovascular risk associated with gender affirming hormone therapy in transgender population. *Front Endocrinol (Lausanne).* 2021;12:718200. http://doi: 10.3389/fendo.2021.718200

Bajaj S, Sonkar KK, Verma S et al. Assessment of glycemic status, insulin resistance and hypogonadism in HIV Infected male patients. *J Assoc Physicians India.* 2020;68(8):43–46.

Beltran S, Lescure FX, Desailloud R, et al. Increased prevalence of hypothyroidism among human immune deficiency virus-infected patients: a need for screening. *Clin Infect Dis.* 2003;37:579–583.

Bhatia R, Ryscavage P, Taiwo B. Accelerated aging and human immunodeficiency virus infection: emerging challenges of growing older in the era of successful antiretroviral therapy. *J. Neurovirol.* 2012;18(4):247–255.

Biadgo B, Ambachew S, Abebe M, et al. Gestational diabetes mellitus in HIV-infected pregnant women: a systematic review and meta-analysis. *Diabetes Res Clin Pract.* 2019;155:107800.

Biglia A, Blanco JL, Martínez E, et al. Gynecomastia among HIV-positive patients is associated with hypogonadism: a case–control study. *Clin Infect Dis.* 2004;39(10):1514–1519.

Bourdoux PP, De Wit SA, Servais GM, et al. Biochemical thyroid profile in patients infected with human immunodeficiency virus. *Thyroid.* 1991;1:147–149.

Bourgi K, Jenkins CA, Rebeiro PF, et al. Weight gain among treatment—naïve persons with HIV starting integrase inhibitors compared to non-nucleoside reverse transcriptase inhibitors or protease inhibitors in a large observational cohort in the United States and Canada. *J Int AIDS Soc.* April 2020a;23(4):325484.

Bourgi K, Rebeiro PF, Turner M, et al. Greater weight gain in treatment-naïve persons starting dolutegravir-based antiretroviral therapy. *Clin Infect Dis.* March 17, 2020b;70(7):1267–1274.

Bricaire F, Marche C, Zoubi D, et al. Adrenocortical lesions and AIDS. *Lancet.* 1988;1:881.

Brown TT, Cole SR, Li X, et al. Antiretroviral therapy and the prevalence and incidence of diabetes mellitus in the multicenter AIDS cohort study. *Arch Intern Med.* 2005;165:1179–1184.

Calkins JH, Siegel MM, Nankin HR, et al. Interleukin-1 inhibits Leydig cell steroidogenesis in primary cell culture. *J Clin Endocrinol Metab.* 1988;123:1605–1610.

Calza L, Manfredi R, Chiodo F. Subclinical hypothyroidism in HIV-positive patients receiving highly active antiretroviral therapy. *J AIDS.* 2002;31:361–363.

Caron M, Auclair M, Vigouroux C, et al. The HIV protease inhibitor indinavir impairs sterol regulatory element-binding protein-1 intranuclear localization, inhibits preadipocyte differentiation, and induces insulin resistance. *Diabetes.* 2001;50:1378–1388.

Carr A, Samaras K, Burton S, et al. A syndrome of peripheral lipodystrophy, hyperlipidaemia and insulin resistance in patients receiving HIV protease inhibitors. *AIDS.* 1998;12(7):F51–F58.

Chirgwin KD, Feldman J, Muneyyirci-Delale O, et al. Menstrual function in human immunodeficiency virus-infected women without acquired immunodeficiency syndrome. *J AIDS Hum Retrovirol.* 1996;12:489–494.

Collazos J, Esteban M. Has prolactin a role in the hypogonadal status of HIV-positive patients? *J Int Assoc Physicians AIDS Care (Chic).* 2009;8(1):43–46.

Collazos J, Ibarra S, Martinez E, et al. Serum prolactin concentrations in patients infected with HIV. *HIV Clin Trials.* 2002;3:133–138.

Cozzolino M, Vidal M, Arcidiacono MV, et al. HIV-protease inhibitors impair vitamin D bioactivation to 1,25-dihydroxyvitamin D. *AIDS.* 2003;17:513–520.

Crum NF, Furtek KJ, Olson PE, et al. A review of hypogonadism and erectile dysfunction among HIV-infected men during the pre- and post-HAART eras: diagnosis, pathogenesis, and management. *AIDS Patient Care STDS.* 2005;19(10):655–671.

Crum-Cianflone NF, Bavaro M, Hale B, et al. Erectile dysfunction and hypogonadism among men with HIV. *AIDS Patient Care STDS.* 2007;21:9–19.

Danaher PJ, Salsbury TL, Delmar JA. Metabolic derangement after injection of triamcinolone into the hip of an HIV-infected patient receiving ritonavir. *Orthopedics.* 2009;32(6):450.

Dao CN, Patel P, Overton ET, et al. Low vitamin D among HIV-infected adults: prevalence of and risk factors for low vitamin D Levels in a cohort of HIV-infected adults and comparison to prevalence among adults in the US general population. *Clin Infect Dis.* 2011;52:396.

Drucker DJ, Bailey D, Rotstein L. Thyroiditis as the presenting manifestation of disseminated extrapulmonary Pneumocystis carinii infection. *J Clin Endocrinol Metab*. 1990;71:1663–1665.

Duncan AD, Goff LM, Peters BS. Type 2 diabetes prevalence and its risk factors in HIV: a cross-sectional study, *PLoS One*. 2018;13(3):e0194199.

Frost RA, Fuhrer J, Steigbigel R. Wasting in the acquired immune deficiency syndrome is associated with multiple defects in the serum insulin-like growth factor system. *Clin Endocrinol*. 1996:44:501.

Giampalmo A, Buffa D, Quaglia AC. AIDS pathology: Various critical considerations (especially regarding the brain, the heart, the lungs, the hypophysis and the adrenal glands). *Pathologica*. 1990;82(1982):663–677.

Glasgow BJ, Steinsapir KD, Anders K, et al. Adrenal pathology in the acquired immune deficiency syndrome. *Am J Clin Pathol*. 1985;84:594–597.

González-González JG, de la Garza-Hernández NE, Garza-Morán RA, et al. Prevalence of abnormal adrenocortical function in human immunodeficiency virus infection by low-dose cosyntropin test. *Int J STD AIDS*. 2001;12(12):804–810.

Gray D, Roux P, Carrihill M, et al. Adrenal suppression and Cushing's syndrome secondary to ritonavir and budesonide. *S Afr Med J*. 2010;100(5):296–297

Grinspoon S, Corcoran C, Anderson E, et al. Sustained anabolic effects of long-term androgen administration in men with AIDS and wasting. *Clin Infect Dis*. 1999;28:634–636.

Grinspoon S, Corcoran C, Lee K, et al. Loss of lean body and muscle mass correlates with androgen levels in hypogonadal men with acquired immunodeficiency syndrome and wasting. *J Clin Endocrinol Metab*. 1996;81:4051–4058.

Grinspoon S, Corcoran C, Stanley T, et al. Mechanisms of androgen deficiency in human immunodeficiency virus-infected women with the wasting syndrome. *J Clin Endocrinol Metab*. 2001;86:4120–4126.

Grunfeld C, Pang M, Doerrler W, et al. Lipids, lipoproteins, triglyceride clearance, and cytokines in human immunodeficiency virus infection and the acquired immunodeficiency syndrome. *J Clin Endocrinol Metab*. 1992;74:1045–1052.

Guaraldi G, Orlando G, Zona S, et al. Premature age-related comorbidities among HIV-infected persons compared with the general population. *Clin Infect Dis*. 2011;53:1120–1126.

Hadigan C, Meigs JB, Corcoran C, et al. Metabolic abnormalities and cardiovascular disease risk factors in adults with human immunodeficiency virus infection and lipodystrophy. *Clin Infect Dis*. 2001. 32(1):130–139.

Hales DB. Interleukin1 inhibits Leydig cell steroidogenesis primarily by decreasing 17α-hydroxylase/C17–20 lyase cytochrome P450 expression. *Endocrinology*. 1992;131:2165–2172.

Hoffman CJ, Brown TT. Thyroid function abnormalities in HIV infected patients. *Clin Infect Dis*. 2007;45:488–494.

Howell AL, Edkins RD, Rier SE, et al. Human immunodeficiency virus type 1 infection of cells and tissues from the upper and lower human female reproductive tract. *J Virol*. 1997;71:3498–3506.

Huff A. Protease inhibitor side effects take people by surprise. *GMHC Treat Issues*. 1997–1998;12(1):25–27.

Hutchinson J, Murphy M, Harries R, et al. Galactorrhoea and hyper-prolactinoma associated with protease inhibitors. *Lancet*. 2000;356:1003–1004.

Ji S, Jin C, Hoxtermann S, et al. Prevalence and Influencing factors of thyroid dysfunction in HIV-positive patients. *Biomed Res Int*. 2016; 2016:3874257. doi: 10.1155/2016/3874257

Jiménez Z, Sánchez-Conde M, Brañas F. HIV infection as a cause of accelerated aging and frailty. *Rev Esp Geriat Gerontol*. 2018;53(2):105–110.

Johnson SR, Marion AA, Vrchoticky T, et al. Cushing syndrome with secondary adrenal insufficiency from concomitant therapy with ritonavir and fluticasone. *J Pediatr*. 2006;148(3):386–388.

Jubault V, Penformin F, Schillo F, et al. Sequential occurrence of thyroid autoantibodies and Grave's disease after immune restoration in severely immunocompromised human immuno-deficiency virus-1 infected patients. *J Clin Endocrinol Metab*. 2000;85:4254–4257.

Kaviani N, Bukberg P, Manessis A, et al. Iatrogenic osteoporosis, bilateral HIP osteonecrosis, and secondary adrenal suppression in an HIV-positive man receiving inhaled corticosteroids and ritonavir-boosted highly active antiretroviral therapy. *Endocr Pract*. 2011;17(1):74–78.

Keuneke C, Anders HJ, Schlöndorff D. Adipsic hypernatremia in two patients with AIDS and cytomegalovirus encephalitis. *Am J Kidney Dis*. 1999;33(2):379–382.

Kettelhut A, Bowman E, Gabriel J, et al. Estrogen may enhance Toll-like receptor 4-induced inflammatory pathways in people with HIV: implications for transgender women on hormone therapy. *Front Immunol*. 2022;13:879600. http://doi:10.3389/fimmu.2022.879600

Khoury AL, Morey MC, Wong TC, et al. Diminished physical function in older HIV-infected adults in the Southeastern U.S. despite successful antiretroviral therapy. *PLoS One*. 2017;12(6):e0179874.

Kim PS, Woods C, Georgoff P, et al. A1c underestimates glycemia in HIV infection. *Diabetes Care*. 2009;32(9):1591–1593.

Koutkia P, Meininger G, Canavan B, et al. Metabolic regulation of growth hormone by free fatty acids, somatostatin, and ghrelin in HIV-lipodystrophy. *Am J Physiol Endocrinol Metab*. 2004;286(2):E296–E303.

Kuhn T, Jin Y, Huang C, et al. The joint effect of aging and HIV infection on microstructure of white matter bundles. *Hum Brain Mapp*. 2019;40(15):4370–4380.

Kumar P, Liu C, Suliburk JW, et al. Supplementing glycine and N-acetylcysteine (GlyNAC) in aging HIV patients improves oxidative stress, mitochondrial dysfunction, inflammation, endothelial dysfunction, insulin resistance, genotoxicity, strength, and cognition: results of an open-label clinical trial. *Biomedi cines*. 2020;8(10):390. http://doi:10.3390/biomedicines8100390

López-Otín C, Blasco MA, Partridge L, Serrano M, Kroemer G. The hallmarks of aging. *Cell*. 2013;6;153(6):1194–217. http://doi:10.1016/j.cell.2013.05.039

Mack KA, Ory MG. AIDS and older Americans at the end of the twentieth century. *J Acquir Immune Defic. Syndr*. 2003;33(Suppl 2):S68–S75.

Madeddu G, Spanu A, Chessa F, et al. Thyroid function in human immunodeficiency virus patients treated with highly active antiretroviral therapy (HAART): a longitudinal study. *Clinical Endocrinology (Oxf)*. 2006;64(4):375–383.

Mallon PW, Unemori P, Sedwell R, et al. In vivo, nucleoside reverse-transcriptase inhibitors alter expression of both mitochondrial and lipid metabolism genes in the absence of depletion of mitochondrial DNA. *J Infect Dis*. 2005;191(10):1686–1696.

Manfredi R, Calza L, Chiodo F. Another emerging event occurring during HIV infection treated with any antiretroviral therapy: Frequency and role of gynecomastia. *Infez Med*. 2004;12(1):51–59.

Manfredi R, Calza L, Chiodo F. Gynecomastia associated with highly active antiretroviral therapy. *Ann Pharmacother*. 2001;35(4):438–439.

Mathabire Rücker SC, Tayea A, Bitilinyu-Bangoh J, et al. High rates of hypertension, diabetes, elevated low-density lipoprotein cholesterol, and cardiovascular disease risk factors in HIV-positive patients in Malawi. *AIDS*. 2018;32(2):253–260.

McDonald P, Moyo S, Gabaitiri L et al. Persistently elevated serum interleukin-6 predicts mortality among adults receiving combination antiretroviral therapy in Botswana: results from a clinical trial. *AIDS Res Hum Retroviruses*. 2013;29(7):993–999.

Membreno L, Irony I, Dere W, et al. Adrenocortical function in acquired immunodeficiency syndrome. *J Clin Endocrinol Metab*. 1987;65:482–487.

Merrill JE, Koyanagi Y, Chen ISY. Interleukin-1 and tumor necrosis factor α can be induced from mononuclear phagocytes by human immunodeficiency virus type 1 binding to the CD4 receptor. *J Virol*. 1989;63:4404–4408.

Meyer WJ, Smith EM, Richards GE, et al. In vivo immunoreactive adrenocorticotropin (ACTH) production by human mononuclear leukocytes from normal and ACTH-deficient individuals. *J Clin Endocrinol Metab*. 1987;64:98–105.

Minami R, Yamamoto M, Takahama S, et al. Comparison of the influence of four classes of HIV antiretrovirals on adipogenic differentiation: the minimal effect of raltegravir and atazanavir. *J Infect Chemother.* 2011;17(2):183–188.

Mishriki YY. A baffling case of bulging belly: protease paunch. *Postgrad Med.* 1998;104(3):45–46.

Monczor AN, Li X, Palella FJ Jr et al. Systemic inflammation characterizes lack of metabolic health in nonobese HIV-infected men. *Mediators Inflamm.* 2018;2018:5327361.

Morse CG, McLaughlin M, Matthews L, et al. Nonalcoholic steatohepatitis and hepatic fibrosis in HIV-1-monoinfected adults with elevated aminotransferase levels on antiretroviral therapy. *Clin Infect Dis.* 2015;60(10):1569–1578.

Mueller NJ, Fux CA, Ledergerber B, et al. High prevalence of severe vitamin D deficiency in combined antiretroviral therapy-naive and successfully treated Swiss HIV patients. *AIDS.* 2010;24:1127.

Murata H, Hruz PW, Mueckler M. The mechanism of insulin resistance caused by HIV protease inhibitor therapy. *J Biol Chem.* 2000;275:20251–20254.

Mylonakis E, Koutkia P, Grinspoon S. Diagnosis and treatment of androgen deficiency in human immunodeficiency virus-infected men and women. *Clin Infect Dis.* 2001;33:857–864.

Nduka CU, Stranges S, Kimani PK, et al. Is there sufficient evidence for a causal association between antiretroviral therapy and diabetes in HIV patients? A meta-analysis. *Diabetes Metab Res Rev.* 2017;33(6):e2902.

Nguyen D, Hsu JW, Jahoor F, et al. Effect of increasing glutathione with cysteine and glycine supplementation on mitochondrial fuel oxidation, insulin sensitivity, and body composition in older HIV-infected patients. *J Clin Endocrinol Metab.* 2014;99(1):169–177.

Nguyen D, Samson SL, Reddy VT, et al. Impaired mitochondrial fatty acid oxidation and insulin resistance in aging: a novel protective role of glutathione. *Aging Cell.* 2013;12(3):415–425.

Noe S, Oldenbuettel C, Heldwein S, et al. Secondary hyperparathyroidism in patients in Central Europe. *Horm Metab Res.* 2018;50(4):317–324.

Norbiato G, Bevilacqua M, Vago T, et al. Glucocorticoids and interferon-alpha in the acquired immunodeficiency syndrome. *J Clin Endocrinol Metab.* 1996;81:2601–2606.

Nylén H, Habtewold A, Makonnen E, et al. Prevalence and risk factors for efavirenz-based antiretroviral treatment-associated severe vitamin D deficiency: a prospective cohort study. *Medicine.* 2016;95(34):e4631.

Önen NF, Overton ET. A review of premature frailty in HIV-infected persons; another manifestation of HIV-related accelerated aging. *Curr Aging Sci.* 2011;4(1):33–41.

Padmapriyadarsini C, Ramesh Kumar S, et al. Dyslipidemia among HIV-infected patients with tuberculosis taking once-daily nonnucleoside reverse-transcriptase inhibitor-based antiretroviral therapy in India. *Clin Infect Dis.* 2011;52(4):540–546.

Palella FJ Jr, Delaney KM, Moorman AC, et al. Declining morbidity and mortality among patients with advanced human immunodeficiency virus infection HIV outpatient study investigators. *N Engl J Med.* 1998;338:853–860.

Parra A, Reyes-Terán G, Ramírez-Peredo J, et al. Differences in nocturnal basal and rhythmic prolactin secretion in untreated compared to treated HIV-infected men are associated with CD4⁺ T-lymphocytes. *Immunol Cell Biol.* 2004;82(1):24–31.

Payne BA, Wilson IJ, Hateley CA, et al. Mitochondrial aging is accelerated by anti-retroviral therapy through the clonal expansion of mtDNA mutations. *Nat Genet.* 2011;43(8):806–810.

Peyriere H, Mauboussin JM, Rouanet I, et al. Report of gynecomastia in five male patients during antiretroviral therapy for HIV infection. *AIDS.* 1999;13:2167–2169.

Pinto G, Blanche S, Thiriet I, et al. Growth hormone treatment of children with human immunodeficiency virus-associated growth failure. *Eur J Pediatr.* 2000;159:937–938.

Pommier JD, Laouenan C, Michard F, et al. Metabolic syndrome and endocrine status in HIV-infected transwomen. *AIDS.* 2019;33(5):855–865.

Quirino T, Bongiovanni M, Ricci E, et al. Hypothyroidism in HIV-infected patients who have or have not received HAART. *Clin Infect Dis.* 2004;38:596–597.

Rajasuriar R., Chong ML, Ahmad Bashah, NS, et al. Major health impact of accelerated aging in young HIV-infected individuals on antiretroviral therapy. *AIDS.* 2017:31(10):1393–1403. https://doi.org/10.1097/QAD.0000000000001475

Rajasuriar R, Chong ML, Ahmad Bashah NS, et al. Major health impact of accelerated aging in young HIV-infected individuals on antiretroviral therapy. *AIDS.* 2017;31(10):1393–1403.

Ram S, Acharya S, Fernando JJ, et al. Serum prolactin in HIV infection. *Clin Lab.* 2004;50:617–620.

Ratner Kaufman F, Gertner JM, Sleeper LA, et al. Growth hormone secretion in HIV-positive versus HIV-negative hemophilic males with abnormal growth and pubertal development. The Hemophilia Growth and Development Study. *J AIDS Hum Retrovirol.* 1997;15:137–144.

Rietschel P, Corcoran C, Stanley T, et al. Prevalence of hypogonadism among men with weight loss related to human immunodeficiency virus infection who were receiving highly active antiretroviral therapy. *Clin Infect Dis.* 2000;31:1240–1244.

Rondanelli M, Caselli D, Arico M, et al. Insulin-like growth factor 1 (IGF-1) and IGF-binding protein 3 response to growth hormone is impaired in HIV-infected children. *AIDS Res Hum Retroviruses.* 2002;18:331–339.

Saint-Marc T, Partisani M, Poizot-Martin I, et al. A syndrome of peripheral fat wasting (lipodystrophy) in patients receiving long-term nucleoside analogue therapy. *AIDS.* 1999;13(13):1659–1667.

Salim YS, Faber V, Wiik A, et al. Anticorticosteroid antibodies in AIDS patients. *APMIS.* 1988;96:889–894.

Samaras K, Pett S, Gowers A, et al. Iatrogenic Cushing's syndrome with osteoporosis and secondary adrenal failure in human immunodeficiency virus-infected patients receiving inhaled corticosteroids and ritonavir-boosted protease inhibitors: six cases. *J Clin Endocrinol Metab.* 2005;90(7):4394–4398.

Samaras K, Wand H, Law M, et al. Prevalence of metabolic syndrome in HIV infected using International Diabetes Foundation and Adult Treatment Panel III criteria: associations with insulin resistance, disturbed body fat compartmentalization, elevated C-reactive protein, and hypoadiponectinemia. *Diabetes Care.* 2007;30:113–119.

Schrack JA, Althoff KN, Jacobson LP, et al. Accelerated gait speed decline in HIV-infected men. *J Acquir Immune Defic Syndr.* 2015;70(4):370–376.

Sekhar RV, Jahoor F, White AC, et al. Metabolic basis of HIV-lipodystrophy syndrome. *Am J Physiol Endocrinol Metab.* 2002;283(2):E332–E337.

Sekhar RV. Supplementing glycine and N-acetylcysteine (GlyNAC) rapidly improves health-related quality of life and lowers perception of fatigue in patients with HIV. *AIDS.* July 15, 2021;35(9):1522–1524. http://doi:10.1097/QAD.0000000000002939

Sekhar RV, Liu CW, Rice S. Increasing glutathione concentrations with cysteine and glycine supplementation lowers inflammation in HIV patients. *AIDS.* 2015;29(14):1899–1900.

Shikuma CM, Hu N, Milne C, et al. Mitochondrial DNA decrease in subcutaneous adipose tissue of HIV-infected individuals with peripheral lipoatrophy. *AIDS.* 2001;15:1801–1809.

Silva GA, Andrade MC, Sugui Dde A, et al. Association between antiretrovirals and thyroid diseases: a cross-sectional study. *Arch Endocrinol Metab.* 2015;59(2):116–122.

Slama L, Palella FJ, Abraham AG, et al. Inaccuracy of haemoglobin A1c among HIV-infected men: effects of CD4 cell count, antiretroviral therapies and haematological parameters *J Antimicrob Chemother* 2014;69(12):2260–2267.

Sobieszczyk ME, Hoover DR, Anastos K, et al. Prevalence and predictors of metabolic syndrome among HIV-infected and HIV-uninfected women in the Women's Interagency HIV Study. *J AIDS.* 2008;48:272–280.

Stricker RB, Goldberg DA, Hu C, et al. A syndrome resembling primary aldosteronism (Conn syndrome) in untreated HIV disease. *AIDS*. 1999;13:1791–1792.

Szebeni J, Dieffenbach C, Wahl SM, et al. Induction of alpha interferon by human immunodeficiency virus type 1 in human monocyte–macrophage cultures. *J Virol*. 1991;65:6362–6364.

Tavares-Bello C, Sousa Santos F, Sequiera Duarte J, et al. Diabetes insipidus and hypopituitarism in HIV: an unexpected cause. *Endocrinol Diabetes Metab Case Rep*. 2017;17–24.

Theodorou M, Sersté T, Van Gossum M, et al. Factors associated with vitamin D deficiency in a population of 2044 HIV-infected patients. *Clin Nutr*. 2014;33(2):274–279.

Toma E, Therrien R. Gynecomastia during indinavir antiretroviral therapy in HIV infection. *AIDS*. 1998;12:681–682.

Tracey KJ, Cerami A. Metabolic responses to cachectin/TNF: a brief review. *Ann N Y Acad Sci*. 1990;587:325–331.

Tzur F, Chowers M, Agmon-Levin N, et al. Increased prevalence of diabetes mellitus in a non-obese adult population: HIV-infected Ethiopians. *Isr Med Assoc J*. 2015;17(10):620–623.

Ukibe NR, Ukibe SN, Emelumadu OF, et al. Impact of thyroid function abnormalities on reproductive hormones during menstrual cycle in premenopausal HIV infected females at NAUTH, Nnewi, Nigeria. *PLoS One*. 2017;12(7):e0176361.

Van den Bout-Van Den Beukel, C, Fievez L, Michels M, et al. Vitamin D deficiency among HIV type 1-infected individuals in the Netherlands: effects of antiretroviral therapy. *AIDS Res Hum Retrovir*. 2008;24:1375–1382.

Villette JM, Bourin P, Doinel C, et al. Circadian variations in plasma levels of hypophyseal, adrenocortical and testicular hormones in men infected with human immunodeficiency virus. *J Clin Endocrinol Metab*. 1990;70:572–577.

Vodkin I, Valasek MA, Bettencourt R, et al. Clinical, biochemical and histological differences between HIV-associated NAFLD and primary NAFLD: a case-control study. *Aliment Pharmacol Ther*. 2015;41(4):368–378.

Wang Y, Santerre M, Tempera I, et al. HIV-1 Vpr disrupts mitochondria axonal transport and accelerates neuronal aging. *Neuropharmacology*. 2017;117:364–375.

Wanke CA, Silva M, Knox TA, et al. Weight loss and wasting remain common complications in individuals infected with human immunodeficiency virus in the era of highly active antiretroviral therapy. *Clin Infect Dis*. 2000;31:803.

Xiong Y, Hales DB. The role of the tumor necrosis factor-alpha in the regulation of mouse Leydig cell steroidogenesis. *Endocrinology*. 1993;132:2438–2444.

Yombi JC, Maiter D, Belkhir L, et al. Iatrogenic Cushing's syndrome and secondary adrenal insufficiency after a single intra-articular administration of triamcinolone acetonide in HIV-infected patients treated with ritonavir. *Clin Rheumatol*. 2008;27(Suppl 2):S79–S82.

32.

HIV-ASSOCIATED LIPODYSTROPHY AND LIPOATROPHY

Rajagopal V. Sekhar

LEARNING OBJECTIVES

Upon completion of this chapter, the reader should be able to:

- Understand what is known about HIV-associated lipodystrophy (HAL).

- Understand the clinical implications of lipodystrophy in persons with HIV (PWH).

- Be aware of therapeutic interventions to treat and improve the health status of PWH with lipodystrophy.

WHAT'S NEW?

- The incidence of new-onset lipodystrophy has declined in recent years.

- Increased oxidative stress, inflammation, and mitochondrial dysfunction in HIV is discussed.

KEY POINTS

- HIV is associated with abnormal fat distribution, which is termed *lipodystrophy*.

- HIV lipodystrophy can manifest as fat loss (lipoatrophy), fat gain (lipohypertrophy), or a mixed pattern.

- Therapeutic options are limited, and treatment is challenging.

- HIV lipodystrophy is associated with increased risk of developing cardiovascular disease (CVD), fatty liver disease, and renal disease.

- HIV lipodystrophy is associated with a negative body image.

INTRODUCTION

The advent of combination antiretroviral therapy (ART) in the mid to late 1990s resulted in significant health benefits for people with HIV (PWH) by reducing AIDS-related mortality and increasing life expectancy. Additional collateral benefits were an improvement in nutritional status and a reduction in HIV-associated opportunistic infections.

In parallel with these benefits, PWH began to develop unusual changes in body habitus with variable combinations of loss of peripheral fat in the limbs, buttocks, and face (termed *lipoatrophy*) and central fat accumulation in the abdomen (termed *lipohypertrophy*). These changes afflicting these individuals were described as a lipodystrophic syndrome (Carr et al., 1998), and the condition was referred to as *HAL*.

Although the origins of HAL are unclear, its onset has been associated with several factors. Since improvements in ART regimens have increased the life span of PWH, it is possible that the HAL phenotype is simply a representation of HIV as a chronic disease. The specific effects of antiretroviral drugs have also been implicated. The initial usage of combination ART in the 1990s was accompanied by multiple reports of abnormalities in body fat distribution linked to the protease inhibitor (PI) and nucleoside reverse transcriptase inhibitor (NRTI) classes of drugs, with terminologies ranging from "protease paunch," "Crixivan belly," and "buffalo hump" to reporting breast enlargement in women and men (Carr et al., 1998; Herry et al., 1997; Lo et al., 1998; Massip et al., 1997; Miller et al., 2003; Vazquez, 1999). Factors other than ART implicated in the pathogenesis of HAL included immune phenomenon and effects mediated directly by HIV itself. However, despite more than 2 decades of intensive research to understand the mechanistic underpinnings of HIV lipodystrophy and lipoatrophy, the answers continue to remain elusive (Bacchetti et al., 2005a, 2005b; Sattler, 2003; Tien and & Grunfeld, 2004).

LIPODYSTROPHY, LIPOHYPERTROPHY, AND LIPOATROPHY

Lipodystrophy is a broad term that collectively describes a variable combination of accumulation of fat in several regions—including the abdomen (Engelson et al., 1999; Miller et al., 2003; Vigano et al., 2005; Yin & Glesby, 2005); interscapular dorsocervical region, termed the "buffalo hump" (Lo et al., 1998; Roth et al., 1998; Torres et al., 1999); and the submental region, where it was termed the "bull neck" (Meinrenken, 1998)—together with a simultaneous loss of fat from the limbs, face, and buttocks (Bacchetti, 2005a, 2005b; Lichenstein, et al., 2003; Martin & Mallon, 2005; Parruti & Toro, 2005). This "mixed" pattern of lipodystrophy includes a variable and simultaneous expression of both lipoatrophy (fat loss) and lipohypertrophy (fat gain) occurring concomitantly in the same person. These abnormalities in body habitus are often accompanied by distinct biochemical abnormalities, including dyslipidemia (mainly hypertriglyceridemia) and insulin resistance. In 2001, the US Cholesterol Education Program Adult Treatment Panel III (ATP III) defined *metabolic syndrome* to include three of the following five criteria: increased waist circumference (>102 cm men, >88 cm women), increased triglycerides (>150 ng/dL), reduced high-density lipoprotein cholesterol (HDL-C; < 40 mg/dL men, < 50 mg/dL women), high blood pressure (>130/ >85 mm Hg), and elevated fasting glucose (>110 mg/dL) (National Cholesterol Education Program, 2001). This remains the standard definition used by most epidemiologic studies of populations with this condition. A study that evaluated PWH reported a 14% prevalence of metabolic syndrome by the International Diabetes Federation criteria and 18% by ATP III criteria (Samaras et al., 2007). In effect, the changes associated with HAL, especially with the mixed pattern, resemble an accelerated form of metabolic syndrome.

DEFINITION AND PREVALENCE OF HAL

The initial description of HAL by Carr and colleagues in 1998 was followed by numerous reports of this condition by the HIV medical and scientific community. However, the prevalence varied widely due to the absence of a consensus case definition, leading to wide fluctuations in the clinical diagnosis of HAL (Carter et al., 2001). Since it became necessary to have a standard and uniformly accepted case definition for HAL, the HIV Lipodystrophy Case Definition Study Group developed a statistical model for the diagnosis of lipodystrophy (including age, sex, duration of HIV infection, HIV disease stage, waist-to-hip ratio (WHR), anion gap, serum HDL-C concentration, trunk-to-peripheral fat ratio, percentage leg fat, and intra- and extra-abdominal fat ratio as variables), with a quantitative scale for identification (Carr et al., 2003; Carr & Law, 2003). This model identified HIV lipodystrophy with a fair degree of accuracy, but it required multiple parameters whose measurement was not feasible or practical in a clinical outpatient setting. Thus, the field is still challenged by the lack of a simple, effective, practical, clinically applicable, and relevant case definition for HAL. The current practical approach to the PWH with mixed lipodystrophy is for the treating clinician to document objective evidence of central obesity and peripheral lipoatrophy, with evidence of dyslipidemia, insulin resistance, or both.

Despite these uncertainties, HIV infection was associated with an increased prevalence of lipodystrophy at the turn of the century, with multiple studies reporting peripheral fat wasting, increased central fat accumulation, or both in PWH (Bergersen et al., 2004; Bernasconi et al., 2002; Miller et al., 2003; Worm et al., 2002), with a higher association of lipoatrophy with the use of nucleoside analogue therapy, especially stavudine (Bernasconi et al., 2002; Chêne et al., 2002). When fat accumulation and fat loss were analyzed, it was found that the prevalence of fat accumulation was 56%, that of fat

loss was 24%, and the mixed form occurred in 83% of PWH (Safrin & Grunfeld, 1999). More stringent analyses of the relative prevalence of the individual components of lipodystrophy have reported on average 45% central obesity, up to 62% for any lipodystrophy, and 38% for peripheral lipoatrophy (Lichtenstein et al., 2004; Paparizos et al., 2000; Saves et al., 2002; Tien & Grunfeld, 2004). HAL has also been described to affect children. A study from India found that lipodystrophy was observed in 34% of children, with lipoatrophy being the most common subtype, followed by lipohypertrophy (Bhutia et al., 2014). These data confirm a significant presence of the lipodystrophic phenotype in the population with HIV. However, since the use of stavudine appeared to be closely linked to lipoatrophy, phasing out the use of this drug has lowered the incidence of new-onset lipoatrophy (Innes et al., 2018; Ribera et al., 2008). Alongside these changes, the risk of abdominal obesity in PWH appears to be rising for any given body mass index, and the excess odds of abdominal obesity is stronger with older age, hypertension, and hypertriglyceridemia (Gelpi et al., 2018). This is also the clinical experience of this author, where the incidence of de novo HAL with a mixed pattern of lipodystrophy has declined significantly over the past decade, with almost no persons presenting with lipoatrophy, although the proportion of PWH with abdominal obesity has substantially increased. These observed changes are likely due to the advent of improved and newer classes of ART agents, suggesting that older ART drugs may have played even a great contributory role in the pathogenesis of HAL than originally suspected. An alternate possibility is that when lipodystrophy was described in the 1990s, it could simply have been a coincidental juxtaposition of nucleoside analogue–induced lipoatrophy, abdominal obesity attributable to other causes, and a coincidental occurrence of both phenotypes in some PWH. This hypothesis provides the most parsimonious explanation to link the HAL phenotype from the 1990s to the current phenotype of abdominal obesity with its associated metabolic and cardiovascular risk profile. The lipoatrophic phenotype is rapidly disappearing, whereas the central obesity phenotype persists and is increasing in its prevalence. Additional studies are needed to understand the dynamic evolution of the HIV body phenotype. Despite these observations, since HAL is linked to an increased risk of metabolic complications, including CVD, diabetes, and liver fat accumulation, it is still important to understand the underlying contributory mechanisms.

DIAGNOSING HAL

The clinical diagnosis of HAL is based on multiple approaches, including self-reporting, use of questionnaires, clinical scales with scores, anthropometric formulas, and radiographic techniques. Standard anthropometric tests have the advantage of being readily available to clinicians (Schwenk, 2002; Schwenk et al., 2001). Computed tomography, magnetic resonance imaging, and dual-energy X-ray absorptiometry (DXA) scans provide quantifiable data on the location and mass of visceral fat, subcutaneous adipose tissue, and subcutaneous limb fat (Cavalcanti et al., 2005; Schambelan et al., 2002). However, the usefulness of these imaging modalities in the outpatient clinical setting is limited because of availability, expense, radiation exposure, and dependence on single-slice data instead of whole-body studies. Therefore, they are impractical for use in routine clinical practice. A study of 100 PWH on ART used DXA scan for anthropometric measures and proposed a fat mass ratio of 1.26, waist-to-thigh ratio of 1.74, and arm-to-trunk ratio of 2.08 to diagnose lipodystrophy (Beraldo et al., 2015). Routine measurement of body weight, waist circumference and/or WHR may be helpful and is recommended for all PWH, especially since the phenotype of central fat accumulation is more prevalent in this population.

MECHANISMS UNDERLYING THE DEVELOPMENT OF HAL

The notion of fat loss in some regions of the body concomitant with fat accumulation in other regions has led to questions of whether fat is reciprocally "redistributed" from one site to another. However, evidence to support this hypothesis is lacking. A large cross-sectional study of people with and without HIV did not find any correlation between changes in central and peripheral fat in men with HIV (Bacchetti et al., 2005a, 2005b). These data suggest that, in HIV, central fat accumulation and peripheral fat loss are independent of each other, which means that two distinctly separate phenomena are operating in these individuals—one to cause lipoatrophy and the other to cause abdominal obesity.

Several mechanistic studies using stable isotope tracer methodologies shed light on some of the fundamental biochemical defects underlying HIV (Reeds et al., 2003; Sekhar et al., 2002). It has been shown that HAL is associated with accelerated rates of adipocyte lipolysis. Although there is a significant increase in adipocyte re-esterification, most of the fatty acids released by adipocyte lipolysis are released into the plasma. Since oxidation of plasma fatty acids is blunted, they are available for increased re-esterification and accumulation in the liver and the central compartment, including the abdomen. These fundamental defects may account for the phenotypic appearance of lipodystrophy, where lipoatrophy may be accounted for by the increased lipolysis, and lipohypertrophy in selected sites may be the result of increased adipocyte re-esterification. In addition, the increased delivery of fatty acids to the liver raises the possibility of an increased risk of fatty liver disease, which is increasingly being described in PWH (Morrison et al., 2019). The factors contributing to these metabolic defects are unclear, but antiretroviral drugs, immune phenomena, adipokines, and HIV itself are involved.

Antiretroviral drugs have been implicated in the mechanistic origins of HAL. As noted earlier, one of the older drugs, stavudine, approved by the US Food and Drug Administration (FDA) in 1994, has been strongly linked to the development of lipoatrophy (Bernasconi et al., 2002; Chêne, 2002). The incidence of lipoatrophy receded significantly after discontinuing this NRTI as part of standard ART regimens, replacing it with abacavir or tenofovir (Innes et al., 2018; Ribera et al., 2008). PIs have also been linked to the development of lipohypertrophy. A study using a human preadipocyte cell line found that the PI ritonavir caused massive apoptosis, whereas atazanavir triggered both autophagy and mitophagy (Gibellini et al., 2012). A more recent study found that exposure of adipose tissue-derived stem cells to atazanavir resulted in marked regression of adipogenic differentiation by inducing apoptosis (Akita et al., 2021). An altered pattern of circulating microRNA has also been linked to adipocyte differentiation (Srinivasa et al., 2021). The fat redistribution in HAL could depend on the sensitivity of adipocytes to drug-induced mitochondrial toxicity, which result in both atrophy and metabolic complications (Mashiko et al., 2022). The progression of HAL has been a dynamic process with a high incidence and prevalence in the late 1990s and early 2000s, but that of decreasing lipoatrophy and increasing central obesity since that time. As PWH with HAL are living longer and there are improvements and changes in the use of ART, it is important to follow and monitor the natural progression of this condition in these individuals.

INCIDENCE OF NEW-ONSET HAL

The incidence of the mixed phenotype of HAL (especially new-onset lipoatrophy) has been declining over the past decade. Most of the descriptions of HAL span the 1995–2010 timeframe, but there are limited data regarding new-onset HAL in the 2010–2020 timeframe. The experience of this author in a busy HIV clinic is a sharply declined incidence of mixed and lipoatrophic phenotypes of HAL over the past decade, but the phenotypic features of those PWH who already had HAL have not resolved. Reasons for this decline in new-onset HAL are not well understood but could be related to the introduction and use of newer ART medications, while omitting PIs and the older nucleoside analogues such as stavudine and didanosine. In support of these observation, a recent study in children and adolescents reported a low prevalence of HAL in Senegalese children on long-term stavudine sparing regimen of ART medications (Cames et al., 2018).

CLINICAL IMPLICATIONS OF HAL

PWH with HAL may develop several clinical complications as a result of lipodystrophy. Abdominal obesity and peripheral lipoatrophy lead to the psychological discomfort of a potentially disfiguring condition (Persson, 2005; Peterson et al., 2008; Turner et al., 2006). Abdominal obesity may also produce physical discomfort from abdominal distension, along with the potential for umbilical herniation and gastroesophageal reflux disease (Miller et al., 2003). Visceral fat accumulation has also been linked to an elevated risk of developing insulin resistance, CVD, and fatty liver disease. In addition, visceral fat accumulation is a known predictor of all-cause mortality in non-HIV-infected people (Kuk et al., 2006).

DYSLIPIDEMIA

The increased association of HAL with dyslipidemia and its management are an important clinical consideration, especially in the context of an increasing incidence of HIV-associated cardiovascular disease. See Chapter 39 Cardiovascular Disease for a discussion regarding the management of hyperlipidemia in PWH.

INSULIN RESISTANCE

PWH with HAL have an increased predisposition to insulin resistance and diabetes mellitus. Factors contributing to this include antiretroviral drugs, lipotoxicity, immune cytokines, and hepatic steatosis. An estimated 30%–90% of persons receiving PIs may develop insulin resistance, although the incidence of diabetes mellitus is less than 10% (van der Valk et al., 2001). Lipodystrophy (peripheral lipoatrophy and/or lipohypertrophy) and the presence of the dorsocervical fat pad or "buffalo hump" have also been linked to hyperinsulinemia and insulin resistance (Balasubramanyam et al., 2004; Calza et al., 2004; Hadigan et al., 2006).

Antiretroviral drugs may also play a role in the development of insulin resistance in HIV. Drugs from the PI class predispose to insulin resistance by inhibiting the insulin-sensitive glucose transporter Glut4 (Mallon et al., 2005). Thirty-five percent of PWH in one study was reported to have developed insulin resistance while on a PI-containing regimen (Murata et al., 2002). PIs also predispose to impaired glucose tolerance and fasting hyperinsulinemia (Hadigan et al., 2001). NRTI drugs, especially the thymidine analogs, also promote insulin resistance in HIV, induce lipotoxicity by disrupting mitochondrial oxidative phosphorylation, and cause defective mitochondrial fatty acid oxidation.

Defective lipid kinetics together with impaired fat oxidation (Reeds et al., 2003; Sekhar et al., 2002, 2005) promote accumulation of ectopic fat in critical metabolic sites of insulin action (e.g., liver and skeletal muscle), resulting in insulin resistance (Gan et al., 2002; Sutinen et al., 2002). Studies in rodents and humans have reported that correcting the deficiency of the endogenous antioxidant glutathione (GSH) significantly improves insulin sensitivity. A pilot study using the gold standard "hyperinsulinemic–euglycemic clamp" to measure insulin sensitivity found that improving levels of GSH using oral supplementation with N-acetylcysteine and glycine in PWH increased insulin sensitivity by 32% within 2 weeks (Nguyen et al., 2014). HAL is associated with defects in adipocyte function that result in altered secretion of critical adipokines such as adiponectin. Deficiency of adiponectin is strongly linked to insulin resistance, and it also occurs in PWH with HAL (Addy et al., 2003; Kim et al., 2007; Samaras et al., 2007).

CARDIOVASCULAR RISKS

It has been known for many years that PWH are at increased risk for cardiovascular disease (CVD) (d'Arminio et al., 2004; Friis-Moller et al., 2003) and myocardial infarction (Beires et al., 2018; Friis-Moller et al., 2008; Glesby et al., 2018; Triant et al., 2008; Varriale, 2004). The mechanistic underpinnings of this increased risk are complex and likely include a combination of factors, including chronic inflammation, adipocyte dysfunction, excessive lipolysis, elevated

low-density lipoprotein cholesterol (LDL-C), and decreased HDL-C and proatherogenic lipoprotein particle sizes with small dense LDL-C, along with adipokine, and immune cytokines. Further impacting the prevalence of CVD in PWH are traditional Framingham risk factors including diabetes, hypertension, smoking, and family history.

RENAL COMPLICATIONS

HIV lipodystrophy may adversely affect renal function. Data from the LIPOKID study, a prospective cohort study of PWH in Switzerland published in 2018 suggests that HAL is independently associated with chronic kidney disease (CKD) (Bouatou et al., 2018). It is not clear whether this is unique to HAL since renal complications have also been described in PWH with generalized lipodystrophy (Akinci et al., 2018). Nonetheless, it is important to regularly monitor renal function in the clinical care of all PWH and perhaps more closely in those with features of lipodystrophy (see Chapter 40 Renal Complications).

SYSTEMIC STEATOSIS

There are reports of hepatic and intramyocellular fat accumulation in HAL. In HIV, fatty liver disease may be induced by a combination of factors, including coinfection with hepatitis B or C, chronic inflammation, and metabolic defects in lipid cycling as described previously (Ristig et al., 2005). Interestingly, in PWH with HAL, insulin resistance appears to be related to hepatic fat accumulation more than intra-abdominal fat accumulation (Sutinen et al., 2002). Excess circulating free fatty acids due to excessive lipolysis can be stored in other ectopic sites and contribute to systemic steatosis. An important site for fat deposition is skeletal muscle, and elevated levels of intramyocellular triglycerides have been reported in the soleus and tibialis anterior muscles (Luzi et al., 2003). An important consequence of increased myocellular fat is the development of insulin resistance in these persons. More recently the ART class of integrase strand transfer inhibitors (INSTIs) have been associated with significant weight gain in PWH. The NA-ACCORD, a large observational cohort study in the United States and Canada compared 22,972 adult, ARV-treatment naive PWH who were initiated with INSTI, PI or nonnucleoside reverse transcriptase inhibitor (NNRTI)-based ART. The study found that compared to PI and NNRTI drugs, the INSTI agents were most associated with weight gain, with the highest weight gain being with dolutegravir (+7.2 kg), followed by raltegravir (+5.8 kg) and elvitegravir (+4.1 kg) (Bourgi et al., 2020a). Similar findings have been reported in other studies in patients on dolutegravir-based regimens (Bourgi et al., 2020b). Although the mechanisms have not been determined, weight gain with INSTIs has become a growing concern, especially in women with HIV (Kerchberger et al., 2020). A recent pooled analysis of eight randomized controlled clinical trials involving over 5,000 ARV-treatment naive PWH who initiated ART between 2003 and 2015 found evidence of higher weight gain in those taking newer ARV drugs, especially the INSTIs

(Sax et al., 2020). Again, INSTIs were associated with higher weight gain than the PIs and NNRTIs. The study also identified other factors associated to weight gain such as lower baseline CD4+ T- cell count, higher HIV RNA levels, female gender, and Black race (Sax, 2020).

ECTOPIC FAT ACCUMULATION

In patients with HAL, ectopic fat accumulation occurs in the interscapular dorsocervical "buffalo hump" area and the submental "bull neck" area (Lo et al., 1998). Such patterns of ectopic fat accumulation predispose to other comorbidities, such as obstructive sleep apnea and limited neck motion, along with neck and back discomfort (Gold & Annino, 2005; Reynolds et al., 2006).

METABOLIC SYNDROME

The combination of the previously discussed defects has led to an increase in metabolic syndrome in many PWH. A study of Hispanic PWH found that the presence of lipodystrophy was associated with a higher prevalence of metabolic syndrome (69%) compared to nonlipodystrophic patients (39%) (Ramirez-Marrero et al., 2014). A more recent study of 1861 PWH in four Southern States (i.e., Texas, Mississippi, Florida, and Georgia) found a prevalence of metabolic syndrome of 34%. The participants were 55% Black; 72% male; 46% ≥50 years old; 69% had undetectable HIV RNA levels; and 98% were on ART (Sears et al., 2019).

OXIDATIVE STRESS, INFLAMMATION AND MITOCHONDRIAL DEFECTS

Elevations in oxidative stress and inflammation were found in a study of 243 participants with HIV, lipodystrophy and metabolic syndrome (González-Domenech et al., 2022) receiving three different ARV regimens, and these defects worsened despite ARV treatment for 6 months, especially with regimens containing PIs. Another study evaluating the microRNA profile on genes affecting adipose regulation in patients with HAL found a link to inflammation (Srinivasa et al., 2021), and this was also confirmed in a study of 110 patients with HAL who were found to have elevated inflammation and a high-risk profile for cardiovascular events (Sacilotto et al., 2021). A small pilot study found elevated oxidative stress, glutathione deficiency, mitochondrial dysfunction, and elevated inflammatory cytokines in PWH, and these defects improved after supplementation with GlyNAC for 12-weeks, but defects recurred after withdrawal of GlyNAC (Kumar et al., 2020). This small pilot study was notable for its reduction in several risk factors linked to cardiovascular and metabolic disease, including insulin resistance, waist circumference, C-reactive protein levels, endothelial dysfunction, and systemic inflammation. In particular, there is increased evidence of mitochondrial dysfunction in PWH, and it is reported that subcutaneous adipose tissue in PWH has decreased mitochondrial DNA and oxidative phosphorylation, but only PWH with lipoatrophy also had deficiency of adenosine triphosphate (ATP) (Gojanovich et al., 2019). Collectively, these defects attest to multiple metabolic perturbations at different levels, which collectively contribute to the metabolic and other complications associated with HIV and HAL.

BODY IMAGE PERCEPTION

Psychological evaluation of patients with HAL reveals an increased prevalence of mood, anxiety, pain, and eating disorders (Calabrò et al., 2020). Although abnormalities in body shape and appearance which underlie HAL are well known to negatively affect the self-image, more recent data suggest that these negative self-perceptions still persist and could affect medication adherence. A cross-section study in 227 adults found a negative impact of self-reported lipodystrophy on body image in both genders, but women were more critical (Soares et al., 2020). This is becoming increasingly relevant as women with HIV live longer lives. A recent study in 63 women with HIV found that 81% of women reported lipodystrophy, and this was associated with poor body image and anxiety after controlling for age and duration of infection (Raggio et al., 2020).

TREATMENT OF HAL AND RELATED COMPLICATIONS

There is no single therapy for all the clinical manifestations of HAL as described above. Treatments are generally directed to the individual components and complications of HAL. Medical management has included trials of underlying pathophysiological defects, including the use of thiazolidinedione drugs to increase fat deposition in lipodystrophic sites. Although data from clinical studies are conflicting (Carr et al., 2004; Hadigan et al., 2004; Sutinen et al., 2003), a small stable isotope-based study examining the interplay of kinetic factors of fat metabolism in the adipocytes suggested that rosiglitazone increased fat deposition in adipocytes. However, this benefit was offset by elevated rates of lipolysis which results in the inability of adipocytes to retain triglycerides (Sekhar et al., 2011).

Growth hormone (GH) has been used in an attempt to lower abdominal fat, but doses used in several clinical trials were supraphysiological. Using GH at a physiological dose resulted in some decrease in lipolysis (D'Amico et al., 2006). A more recent study evaluated the combination of rosiglitazone and human GH in 72 patients with HIV-associated abdominal obesity and insulin resistance (Leung et al., 2016). This study found beneficial effects on adiponectin concentrations with a combination of rosiglitazone and GH; however, GH alone did not demonstrate any significant impact on adiponectin levels despite reductions in visceral adipose tissue. More studies are needed to determine a role for GH in treatment of HAP in PWH.

The GH analog tesamorelin (Egrifta™) was approved by the FDA in 2010 and has been shown to have benefits in lowering central fat and improving dyslipidemia (Falutz et al., 2007; Stanley et al., 2014). Use of this product has been limited by the need for daily subcutaneous injections, and certainty regarding long-term benefits. It is also expensive with a monthly cost of about $3,000 (Pharmacoeconomic Review, 2016).

A recent study that used farnesyltransferase inhibitors (FTIs) tipifarnib and lonafarnib was successful in preventing lipodystrophy and metabolic syndrome induced by lopinavir/ritonavir in mice (Tanaka et al., 2018). The authors believe these data support FTIs as a possible strategy to prevent or treat PI-associated lipodystrophy and metabolic syndrome in PWH. Further human studies are needed to understand and clarify a therapeutic for role of FTIs.

Surgical treatment of excess fat accumulation has been done with liposuction, but long-term success is limited by the tendency of fat to reaccumulate (Hultman et al., 2007). A recent study comparing liposuction to excisional lipectomy in patients with HAL recommends the latter as the primary treatment (Barton et al., 2021). Facial lipoatrophy has been treated with lipofilling with autologous fat transfer (Uzzan et al., 2012) or polyalkylimide gel (De Santis et al., 2012). Other artificial fillers including silicone have been used with psychological improvement in body image perception (Mori et al., 2006). Patients should be evaluated for a negative self-image and offered counseling where necessary.

CONCLUSION

HIV infection and ART continue to be associated with HAL. Although these complications affected many patients in the mid to late 1990s and early 2000s, the relative incidences of lipoatrophy and lipohypertrophy are changing over time, with a decrease in the former and an increase in the latter, especially in the aging population with HIV. Nevertheless, these changes in body morphology are complicated by physical symptoms because of the nature of fat accumulation, psychological discomfort because of abnormal body image perception, and metabolic complications such as dyslipidemia and insulin resistance with an increased risk of CVD and fatty liver disease. Effective preventive therapies are needed for these complications as current treatment options are limited and often are just symptom or complication focused. In addition, there is a vital need for further research to understand the pathophysiologic mechanisms of HAL in PWH. These negative perceptions of body image associated with lipodystrophy in HIV patients could impact adherence to medication compliance. A recent study evaluating the effect of lipodystrophy on self-esteem and medication adherence in 250 patients with HIV found that lipodystrophy and low income adversely affected self-esteem, and were a barrier to medication adherence (Siqueira et al., 2021).

REFERENCES

Addy CL, Gavrila A, Tsiodras S, et al. Hypoadiponectinemia is associated with insulin resistance, hypertriglyceridemia, and fat redistribution in human immunodeficiency virus-infected patients treated with highly active antiretroviral therapy. *J Clin Endocrinol Metab.* 2003;88:627–636.

Akinci B, Unlu SM, Simsir IY, et al. Renal complications of lipodystrophy: a closer look at the natural history of kidney disease. *Clin Endocrinol.* 2018;89(1):65–75. http://doi:10.1111/cen.13732.

Akita S, Suzuki K, Yoshimoto H, et al. Cellular mechanism underlying highly-active or antiretroviral therapy-induced lipodystrophy: atazanavir, a protease inhibitor, compromises adipogenic conversion of adipose-derived stem/progenitor cells through accelerating ER stress-mediated cell death in differentiating adipocytes. *Int J Mol Sci.* 2021;22(4):2114. http://doi:10.3390/ijms22042114

Bacchetti P, Gripshover B, Grunfeld C, et al. Fat distribution in men with HIV infection. *J AIDS.* 2005b; 40:121–131.

Bacchetti P, Gripshover B, Grunfeld C, et al.; Study of Fat Redistribution and Metabolic Change in HIV Infection (FRAM). Fat distribution in men with HIV infection. *J AIDS.* 2005a;40(2):121–131.

Balasubramanyam A, Sekhar RV, Jahoor F, et al. Pathophysiology of dyslipidemia and increased cardiovascular risk in HIV lipodystrophy: a model of "systemic steatosis." *Curr Opin Lipidol.* 2004;15:59–67.

Barton N, Moore R, Prasad K, Evans G. Excisional lipectomy versus liposuction in HIV-associated lipodystrophy. *Arch Plast Surg.* 2021;48(6):685–690. http://doi:10.5999/aps.2020.02285

Beires MT, Silva-Pinto A, Santos AC, et al. Visceral adipose tissue and carotid intima-media thickness in HIV-infected patients undergoing cART: a prospective cohort study. *BMC Infect Dis.* 2018;18(1):32.

Beraldo RA, Vassimon HS, Aragon DC, et al. Proposed ratios and cutoffs for the assessment of lipodystrophy in HIV-seropositive individuals. *Eur J Clin Nutr.* 2015;69(2):274–278.

Bergersen BM, Sandvik L, Bruun JN. Body composition changes in 308 Norwegian HIV- positive patients. *Scand J Infect Dis.* 2004;36:186–191.

Bernasconi E, Boubaker K, Junghans C, et al. Abnormalities of body fat distribution in HIV- infected persons treated with antiretroviral drugs: the Swiss HIV Cohort Study. *J AIDS.* 2002;31:50–55.

Bhutia E, Hemal A, Yadav TP, et al. Lipodystrophy syndrome among HIV infected children on highly active antiretroviral therapy in northern India. *Afr Health Sci.* 2014;14(2):408–413.

Bouatou Y, Gayet Ageron A, Bernasconi E et al. Lipodystrophy increases the risk of CKD development in HIV positive patients in Switzerland: the LIPOKID study. *Kidney Int Rep.* 2018;3(5):1089–1099.

Bourgi K, Jenkins CA, Rebeiro PF et al. Weight gain among treatment—naïve persons with HIV starting integrase inhibitors compared to non-nucleoside reverse transcriptase inhibitors or protease inhibitors in a large observational cohort in the United States and Canada. *J Int AIDS Soc.* 2020a;23(4):325484.

Bourgi K, Rebeiro PF, Turner M, et al. Greater weight gain in treatment-naive persons starting dolutegravir- based antiretroviral therapy. *Clin Infect Dis.* 2020b;70(7):1267–1274.

Calabrò PF, Ceccarini G, Calderone A, et al. Psycho pathological and psychiatric evaluation of patients affected by lipodystrophy. *Eat Weight Disord.* 2020;25(4):991–998. http://doi:10.1007/s40 519-019-00716-6

Calza L, Manfredi R, Chiodo F. Insulin resistance and diabetes mellitus in HIV infected patients receiving antiretroviral therapy. *Metab Syndr Relat Disord.* 2004;2:241–250.

Cames C, Pascal L, Ba A, et al. Low prevalence of lipodystrophy in HIV-infected Senegalese children on long-term antiretroviral treatment: the ANRS 12279 MAGGSEN Pediatric Cohort Study. *BMC Infect Dis.* 2018;18:374.

Carr A, Emery S, Law M, et al. An objective case definition of lipodystrophy in HIV-infected adults: a case–control study. *Lancet.* 2003;361:726–735.

Carr A, Law M. An objective lipodystrophy severity grading scale derived from the lipodystrophy case definition score. *J AIDS.* 2003;33:571–576.

Carr A, Samaras K, Burton S, et al. A syndrome of peripheral lipodystrophy, hyperlipidemia and insulin resistance in patients receiving HIV protease inhibitors. *AIDS.* 1998;12:F51–F58.

Carr A, Workman C, Carey D, et al. No effect of rosiglitazone for treatment of HIV-1: randomized, double-blind, placebo-controlled trial. *Lancet.* 2004;363(9407):429–438.

Carter VM, Hoy JF, Bailey M et al. The prevalence of lipodystrophy in an ambulant HIV-infected population: it all depends on the definition. *HIV Med.* 2001;2(3):174–180.

Cavalcanti RB, Cheung AM, Raboud J, et al. Reproducibility of DXA estimations of body fat in HIV lipodystrophy: implications for clinical research. *J Clin Densitom.* 2005;8:293–297.

Chêne G, Angelini E, Cotte L, et al. Role of long-term nucleoside-analogue therapy in lipodystrophy and metabolic disorders in human immunodeficiency virus-infected patients. *Clin Infect Dis.* 2002;34(5):649–657.

D'Amico S, Shi J, Sekhar RV, et al. Physiologic growth hormone replacement improves fasting lipid kinetics in patients with HIV lipodystrophy syndrome. *Am J Clin Nutr.* 2006;84(1):204–211.

d'Arminio A, Sabin CA, Phillips AN, et al. Cardio- and cerebrovascular events in HIV-infected persons. *AIDS.* 2004;18(13):1811–1817.

De Santis G, Pignatti M, Baccarani A, et al. Long-term efficacy and safety of polyacrylamide hydrogel injection in the treatment of human immunodeficiency virus-related facial lipoatrophy: a 5-year follow-up. *Plastic Reconstruct Surg.* 2012;129(1):101–109.

Engelson ES, Kotler DP, Tan Y, et al. Fat distribution in HIV-infected patients reporting truncal enlargement quantified by whole-body magnetic resonance imaging. *Am J Clin Nutr.* 1999;69:1162–1169.

Falutz J, Allas S, Blot K, et al. Metabolic effects of a growth hormone-releasing factor in patients with HIV. *N Engl J Med.* 2007;357(23):2359–2370.

Friis-Moller N, Reiss P, Sabin CA, et al. Class of antiretroviral drugs and the risk of myocardial infarction. *N Engl J Med.* 2007;356:1723–1735.

Friis-Moller N, Weber R, Reiss P, et al. Cardiovascular disease risk factors in HIV patients—association with antiretroviral therapy. Results from the D:A:D study. *AIDS.* 2003;17(8):1179–1193.

Gan SK, Samaras K, Thompson CH, et al. Altered myocellular and abdominal fat partitioning predict disturbance in insulin action in HIV protease inhibitor-related lipodystrophy. *Diabetes.* 2002;51:3163–3169.

Gelpi M, Afzal S, Lundgren J, et al. Higher risk of abdominal obesity, elevated LDL cholesterol, hypertriglyceridemia, but not of hypertension in PLWH: results from the Copenhagen Comorbidity in HIV Infection (COCOMO) Study. *Clin Infect Dis.* 2018;67(4):579–586. http://doi.org/10.1093/cid/ciy146

Gibellini L, De Biasi S, Pinto M, et al. The protease inhibitor atazanavir triggers autophagy and mitochoagy in human preadipocytes. *AIDS.* 2012;26(16):2017–2026.

Glesby MJ, Hanna DB, Hoover DR, et al. Abdominal fat depots and subclinical carotid artery atherosclerosis in women with and without HIV Infection. *J AIDS.* 2018;77(3):308–316

Gojanovich GS, Shikuma CM, Milne C, et al. Subcutaneous adipocyte adenosine triphosphate levels in HIV infected patients. *AIDS Res Hum Retroviruses.* 2020;36(1):75–82. http://doi.org/10.1089/AID.2019.0121

Gold DR, Annino DJ Jr. HIV-associated cervicodorsal lipodystrophy: etiology and management. *Laryngoscope.* 2005;115:791–795.

González-Domenech CM, Plaza-Andrades IJ, Garrido-Sanchez L, Queipo-Ortuño MI. Synergic effect of meta bolic syndrome and lipodystrophy on oxidative stress and inflammation process in treated HIV-patients. *Enferm Infec Microbiol Clin.* 2022;40(6):310–316. http://doi:10.1016/j.eimce.2020.11.026. PMID: 35680349.

Hadigan C, Kamin D, Liebau J, et al. Depot-specific regulation of glucose uptake and insulin sensitivity in HIV-lipodystrophy. *Am J Physiol Endocrinol Metab.* 2006;290:E289–E298.

Hadigan C, Meigs JB, Corcoran C, et al. Metabolic abnormalities and cardiovascular disease risk factors in adults with human immunodeficiency virus infection and lipodystrophy. *Clin Infect Dis.* 2001;32:130–139.

Hadigan C, Yawetz S, Thomas A, et al. Metabolic effects of rosiglitazone in HIV lipodystrophy: a randomized, controlled trial. *Ann Intern Med.* 2004;140(10):786–794.

Herry I, Bernand L, de Truchis P, et al. Hypertrophy of the breasts in a patient treated with indinavir. *Clin Infect Dis.* 1997;25:937–938.

Hultman CS, McPhail LE, Donaldson JH, Wohl DA. Surgical management of HIV-associated lipodystrophy: role of ultrasonic-assisted liposuction and suction-assisted lipectomy in the treatment of lipohypertrophy. *Ann Plast Surg.* 2007;58(3):255–263.

Innes S, Harvery J, Collins IJ, et al. Lipoatrophy/lipohypertrophy outcomes after antiretroviral therapy switch in children in the UK/Ireland. *PLoS One.* 2018;13(4):e0194132.

Kerchberger AM, Sheth AN, Angert CD, et al. Weight gain associated with integrase stand transfer inhibitor use in women. *Clin Infect Dis.* 2020;71(3):593–600.

Kim RJ, Carlow DC, Rutstein JH, et al. Hypoadiponectinemia, dyslipidemia, and impaired growth in children with HIV-associated facial lipoatrophy. *J Pediatr Endocrinol Metab.* 2007;20:65–74.

Kuk JL, Katzmarzyk PT, Nichaman MZ, et al. Visceral fat is an independent predictor of all-cause mortality in men. *Obesity.* 2006;14:336–341.

Kumar P, Li C, Suliburk JW, et al. Supplementing glycine and N-acetylcysteine (GlyNAC) in aging HIV patients improves oxidative stress, mitochondrial dysfunction, inflammation, endothelial dysfunction, insulin resistance, genotoxicity, strength, and cognition: results of an open-label clinical trial. *Biomedicines.* 2020;8(10):390.

Leung V, Chiu YL, Kotler DP, et al. Effect of recombinant human growth hormone and rosiglitazone for HIV-associated abdominal fat accumulation on adiponectin and other markers of inflammation. *HIV Clin Trials.* 2016;17(2):55–62

Lichtenstein K, Wanke C, Henry K, et al. Estimated prevalence of HIV-associated adipose redistribution syndrome (HARS): abnormal abdominal fat accumulation in HIV-infected patients. *Antiviral Ther.* 2004;9: L33.

Lichtenstein KA, Delaney KM, Armon C, et al. Incidence of and risk factors for lipoatrophy (abnormal fat loss) in ambulatory HIV-1-infected patients. *J AIDS.* 2003; 32:48–56.

Lo JC, Mulligan K, Tai VW, et al. "Buffalo hump" in men with HIV-1 infection. *Lancet.* 1998;351:867–870.

Luzi L, Perseghin G, Tambussi G, et al. Intramyocellular lipid accumulation and reduced whole body lipid oxidation in HIV lipodystrophy. *Am J Physiol Endocrinol Metab.* 2003;284:E274–E280.

Mallon PW, Wand H, Law M, et al.; HIV Lipodystrophy Case Definition Study; Australian Lipodystrophy Prevalence Survey Investigators. Buffalo hump seen in HIV-associated lipodystrophy is associated with hyperinsulinemia but not dyslipidemia. *J AIDS.* 2005;38:156–162.

Martin A, Mallon PW. Therapeutic approaches to combating lipoatrophy: do they work? *J Antimicrob Chemother.* 2005;55:612–615.

Mashiko T, Tsukada K, Takada H, et al. Genetic and cytometric analyses of subcutaneous adipose tissue in patients with hemophilia and HIV-associated lipodystrophy. *AIDS Res Ther.* 2022;19(1):14. http://doi: 10.1186/s12981-022-00432-9

Massip P, Marchou B, Bonnet E, et al. Lipodystrophy with protease inhibitors in HIV patients. *Thérapie.* 1997; 52:615.

Meinrenken S. "Bull-neck" in HIV-positive patients: result of therapy? *Disch Med Wochenschr.* 1998;22:123(21):A9.

Miller J, Carr A, Emery S, et al. HIV lipodystrophy: prevalence, severity and correlates of risk in Australia. *HIV Med.* 2003;4:293–301.

Mori A, Lo Russo G, Agostini T, et al. Treatment of human immunodeficiency virus-associated facial lipoatrophy with lipofilling and submalar silicone implants. *J Plastic Reconstruct Aesthetic Surg.* 2006;59(11):1209–1216.

Morrison M, Hughes HY, Naggie S, Syn WK. Nonalcoholic fatty liver disease among individuals with HIV infection: a growing concern? *Dig Dis Sci.* 2019;64(12):3394–3401.

Murata H, Hruz PW, Mueckler M. Indinavir inhibits the glucose transporter isoform Glut4 at physiologic concentrations. *AIDS.* 2002;16:859–863.

National Cholesterol Education Program. Executive summary of the third report of the National Cholesterol Education Program (NCEP) Expert Panel on Detection, Evaluation, and Treatment of High Blood Cholesterol in Adults (Adult Treatment Panel III). *JAMA.* 2001;285:2486–2497.

Nguyen D, Hsu JW, Jahoor F, et al. Effect of increasing glutathione with cysteine and glycine supplementation on mitochondrial fuel oxidation, insulin sensitivity, and body composition in older HIV-infected patients. *J Clin Endocrinol Metab.* January 2014;99(1):169–177.

Paparizos VA, Kyriakis KP, Polydorou-Pfandl D, et al. Epidemiologic characteristics of Koebner's phenomenon in AIDS-related Kaposi's sarcoma. *J AIDS*. 2000;25:283–284.

Parruti G, Toro GM. Persistence of lipoatrophy after a four-year long interruption of antiretroviral therapy for HIV1 infection: case report. *BMC Infect Dis*. 2005;5:80.

Persson A. Facing HIV: body shape change and the (in) visibility of illness. *Med Anthropol*. 2005;24:237–264.

Peterson S, Martins CR, Cofranscesci J Jr. Lipodystrophy in the patient with HIV: social, psychological and treatment considerations. *Anesthet Surg J*. 2008;28(4):443–451.

Pharmacoeconomic Review. *Report: Tesamorelin (egrifta)* [Internet]. Ottawa, ON: Canadian Agency for Drugs and Technologies in Health. Executive summary; August 2016.

Raggio GA, Looby SE, Robbins GK, et al. Psychosocial correlates of body image and lipodystrophy in women aging with HIV. *J Assoc Nurses AIDS Care*. 2020;31(2):157–166. http://doi: 10.1097/JNC.00000 00000000139

Ramírez-Marrero FA, Santana-Bagur JL, Joyner MJ, et al. Metabolic syndrome in relation to cardiorespiratory fitness, active and sedentary behavior in HIV\+ Hispanics with and without lipodystrophy. *P R Health Sci J*. 2014;33(4):163–169.

Reeds DN, Middendorf B, Patterson BW, et al. Alterations in lipid kinetics in men with HIV-dyslipidemia. *Am J Physiol Endocrinol Metab*. 2003;285:E490–E497.

Reynolds NR, Neidig JL, Wu AW, et al. Balancing disfigurement and fear of disease progression: patient perceptions of HIV body fat redistribution. *AIDS Care*. 2006;18:663–673.

Ribera E, Paradineiro JC, Curran A, et al. Improvements in subcutaneous fat, lipid profile, and parameters of mitochondrial toxicity in patients with peripheral lipoatrophy when stavudine is switcher to tenofovir (LIPOTEST study). *HIV Clin Trials*. 2008;9(6):407–417.

Ristig M, Drechsler H, Powderly WG. Hepatic steatosis and HIV infection. *AIDS Patient Care STDs*. 2005; 19:356–365.

Roth VR, Kravcik S, Angel JB. Development of cervical fat pads following therapy with human immunodeficiency virus type 1 protease inhibitors. *Clin Infect Dis*. 1998;27:65–67.

Sacilotto LB, Papini SJ, Mendes AL, Gatto M, Pereira PCM, Corrente JE, da Silva JF. Relationship between lipodystrophy, body composition, metabolic profile, and serum levels of adipocytokines. *Front Nutr*. 2021;8:750721. http://doi:10.3389/fnut.2021.750721

Safrin S, Grunfeld G. Fat distribution and metabolic changes in patients with HIV infection. *AIDS*. 1999;13(18):2493–505.

Samaras K, Wand H, Law M, et al. Prevalence of metabolic syndrome in HIV-infected patients receiving highly active antiretroviral therapy using International Diabetes Foundation and Adult Treatment Panel III Criteria: associations with insulin resistance, disturbed body fat compartmentalization, elevated C-reactive peptide, and hypoadiponectinemia. *Diabetes Care*. 2007;30:113–119.

Sattler F. Body habitus changes related to lipodystrophy. *Clin Infect Dis*. 2003;36: S84–S90.

Saves M, Raffi F, Capeau J, et al. Factors related to lipodystrophy and metabolic alterations in patients with human immunodeficiency virus infection receiving highly active antiretroviral therapy. *Clin Infect Dis*. 2002;34:1396–1405.

Sax PE, Erlandson KM, Lake JE, et al. Weight gain following initiation of antiretroviral therapy: risk factors in randomized clinical trials. *Clin Infect Dis*. 2019;71:1380–1389.

Schambelan M, Benson CA, Carr A, et al. Management of metabolic complications associated with antiretroviral therapy for HIV-1 infection: recommendations of an International AIDS Society USA panel. *J AIDS*. 2002;31:257–275.

Schwenk A. Methods of assessing body shape and composition in HIV-associated lipodystrophy. *Curr Opin Infect Dis*. 2002;15:9–16.

Schwenk A, Breuer P, Kremer G, et al. Clinical assessment of HIV-associated lipodystrophy syndrome: bioelectrical impedance analysis, anthropometry and clinical scores. *Clin Nutr*. 2001;20:243–249.

Sears S, Buendia JR, Odem S, et al. Metabolic syndrome among people living with HIV receiving medical care in southern United States: prevalence and risk factors. *AIDS Behav*. 2019;23(11):2916–2925.

Sekhar RV, Jahoor F, Pownall HJ, et al. Severely dysregulated disposal of postprandial triacylglycerols exacerbates hypertriacylglycerolemia in HIV lipodystrophy syndrome. *Am J Clin Nutr*. 2005;81:1405–1410.

Sekhar RV, Jahoor F, White AC, et al. Metabolic basis of HIV lipodystrophy syndrome. *Am J Physiol Endocrinol Metab*. 2002;283:E332–E337.

Sekhar RV, Patel SG, D'Amico S, et al. Effects of rosiglitazone on abnormal lipid kinetics in HIV-associated dyslipidemic lipodystrophy: a stable isotope study. *Metabolism*. 2011;60(6):754–760.

Siqueira LR, Cunha GHD, Galvão MTG. Effect of lipodystrophy on self-esteem and adherence to antiretroviral therapy in people living with HIV. *AIDS Care*. 2021;4:1–10. http://doi:10.1080/09540 121.2021.1936442. Epub ahead of print.

Soares LR, Casseb JSDR, Chaba DCDS, et al. Self-reported lipodystrophy, nutritional, lipemic profile and its impact on the body image of HIV-1-infected persons, with and without antiretroviral therapy. *AIDS Care*. 2020;32(10):1317–1322. http://doi:10.1080/09540 121.2019.1687832

Srinivasa S, Garcia-Martin R, Torriani M. Altered pattern of circulating miRNAs in HIV lipodystrophy perturbs key adipose differentiation and inflammation pathways. *JCI Insight*. 2021;6(18):e150399. http://doi: 10.1172/jci.insight.150399. PMID: 34383714; PMCID: PMC8492307.

Stanley TL, Feldpausch MN, Oh J, et al. Effect of tesamorelin on visceral fat and liver fat in HIV-infected patients with abdominal fat accumulation: a randomized clinical trial. *JAMA*. 2014;312(4):380–389.

Sutinen J, Hakkinen AM, Westerbacka J, et al. Increased fat accumulation in the liver in HIV-infected patients with antiretroviral therapy-associated lipodystrophy. *AIDS*. 2002;16:2183–2193.

Sutinen J, Hakkinen AM, Westerbacka J, et al. Rosiglitazone in the treatment of HAART-associated lipodystrophy: a randomized double-blind placebo-controlled study. *Antiviral Ther*. 2003;8(3):199–207.

Tanaka T, Nakazawa H, Kuriyama N et al. Farnesyltransferase inhibitors prevent HIV protease inhibitor (lopinavir/ritonavir) induced lipodystrophy and metabolic syndrome in mice. *Exp Ther Med*. 2018;15(2):1314–1320.

Tien PC, Grunfeld C. What is HIV-associated lipodystrophy? Defining fat distribution changes in HIV infection. *Curr Opin Infect Dis*. 2004;17:27–32.

Torres RA, Unger KW, Cadman JA, et al. Recombinant human growth hormone improves truncal adiposity and "buffalo humps" in HIV-positive patients on HAART. *AIDS*. 1999;13:2479–2481.

Triant VA, Lee H, Hadigan C, et al. Increased acute myocardial infarction rates and cardiovascular risk factors among patients with HIV disease. *J Clin Endocrinol Metab*. 2007;92:2506–2512.

Turner R, Testa MA, Su M, et al. The impact of HIV-associated adipose redistribution syndrome (HARS) on health-related quality of life. *Antiviral Ther*. 2006;11:L25.

Uzzan C, Boccara D, Lacheré A, et al. Treatment of facial lipoatrophy by lipofilling in HIV infected patients: retrospective study on 317 patients on 9 years. *Ann Chir Plast Esthet*. 2012;57(3):210–216.

van der Valk M, Bisschop PH, Romijn JA. Lipodystrophy in HIV-1-positive patients is associated with insulin resistance in multiple metabolic pathways. *AIDS*. 2001;15:2093–2100.

Varriale P, Saravi G, Hernandez E, et al. Acute myocardial infarction in patients infected with human immunodeficiency virus. *Am Heart J*. 2004;147(1):55–59.

Vazquez E. Understanding and treating protease paunch. *Posit Aware*. 1999;10(4):59–63.

Vigano A, Mora S, Manzoni P, et al. Effects of recombinant growth hormone on visceral fat accumulation: pilot study in human immunodeficiency virus-infected adolescents. *J Clin Endocrinol Metab*. 2005;90:4075–4080.

Worm D, Kirk O, Anderson O, et al. Clinical lipoatrophy in HIV-1 patients on HAART is not associated with increased abdominal girth, hyperlipidemia or glucose intolerance. *HIV Med*. 2002;3(4):239–246.

Yin MT, Glesby MJ. Recombinant human growth hormone therapy in HIV-associated wasting and visceral adiposity. *Expert Rev Anti-Infect Ther*. 2005;3:727–738.

33.

NON-OPPORTUNISTIC INFECTIONS
RESPIRATORY COMPLICATIONS

Priyanka Chakrabarti

CHAPTER GOAL

Upon completion of this chapter, the reader should be able to:

- Demonstrate knowledge regarding the diagnosis and treatment of respiratory complications in people with HIV (PWH).

LEARNING OBJECTIVE

Review and characterize the respiratory complications related to HIV infection to provide early and accurate diagnosis and treatment.

KEY POINTS

NONSPECIFIC INTERSTITIAL PNEUMONITIS

- Nonspecific interstitial pneumonitis (NSIP) encompasses several lymphocytic pulmonary syndromes including follicular bronchiolitis, lymphocytic bronchiolitis, lymphocytic interstitial pneumonitis (LIP), and diffuse infiltrative CD8 $^+$ lymphocytosis syndrome (DILS).

- PWH may be asymptomatic or present with subacute dyspnea, nonproductive cough, and fever in a patient with CD4 $^+$ T-cell counts greater than 200 cells/mm^3. X-ray findings are nonspecific, but characteristically show bilateral reticulonodular "interstitial" infiltrates.

- The diagnosis of NSIP requires histologic confirmation by biopsy. The optimum treatment remains unclear.

LYMPHOCYTIC INTERSTITIAL PNEUMONITIS

- LIP is a common respiratory complication of HIV infection in children but a rare complication in adults with HIV.

- It presents with slowly progressive dyspnea and nonproductive cough. X-ray findings are nonspecific but characteristically show bilateral reticulonodular "interstitial" infiltrates with a basal lung predominance.

- The diagnosis requires histologic confirmation by biopsy. Antiretroviral therapy (ART) has been used successfully for treatment.

PULMONARY ARTERIAL HYPERTENSION

- The prevalence of pulmonary arterial hypertension (PAH) is higher in PWH compared to the general population.

- The clinical presentation is like that in the general population, with progressive dyspnea, nonproductive cough, chest pain, and sometimes syncope or presyncope. These symptoms should prompt an evaluation for early diagnosis.

- The diagnosis is first suggested by chest radiograph revealing prominent pulmonary arteries or by electrocardiogram. Right heart catheterization is the standard of diagnosis.

- Potential therapies for HIV-associated PAH include ART, oxygen, diuretics, and directed therapy. Prostanoids (epoprostenol, treprostinil, and iloprost), endothelin receptor antagonists (bosentan), and phosphodiesterase-5 inhibitors (sildenafil) are used in persons with HIV-associated PAH and have improved mortality.

NONSPECIFIC INTERSTITIAL PNEUMONITIS

The prevalence of NSIP is unknown. It was found in 48% of asymptomatic PWH in the 1980s (Ognibene et al., 1988) and in 38% of PWH and pulmonary symptoms or abnormal imaging studies (Suffredini et al., 1987). Different from LIP, it has been characterized only in adults and not in children.

The etiology of NSIP is unknown. Evidence suggests immune dysregulation may contribute, and thus the prevalence of NSIP has declined with the use of combination ART (Collins et al., 2019). NSIP was found in 7% of PWH admitted for interstitial lung disease since the introduction of ART (Wolff et al., 2001). NSIP encompasses several lymphocytic pulmonary syndromes in PWH: follicular bronchiolitis, lymphocytic bronchiolitis, LIP, and DILS. Histologically, it is characterized by the presence of perivascular and peribronchial interstitial lymphocytes, plasma cells, and macrophages; however, these are also found along the pleura and interlobar fibrous septate (Travis et al., 1992).

Clinical symptoms are minimal or nonexistent; subacute dyspnea, nonproductive cough, and fever have been reported (Suffredini et al., 1987). Physical exam may reveal crackles. Imaging studies may be normal or may show diffuse interstitial infiltrates (reticular, reticulonodular, or alveolar). Pleural effusions may also be seen. High-resolution computed tomography (CT) is also unspecific. Ground-glass pattern, consolidations, and honeycombing have been described. Similar to LIP, spirometry typically shows decreased diffusing capacity. Definitive diagnosis is made by histology of lung tissue. The treatment is unclear. It can remain stable for many years or regress on its own. Theoretically, ART may improve its symptoms, but there is no pathological evidence to support this theory.

HIV LYMPHOCYTIC INTERSTITIAL PNEUMONITIS

LIP is a rare histopathologic disease that accounts for 40% of lung diseases in children with AIDS but only 1% or 2% of lung diseases in adults with HIV (Anderson & Lee, 1988; Stover et al., 1985).

Histologically, LIP is characterized by diffuse infiltration with polyclonal lymphocytes and occasionally plasma cells and histiocytes into the alveolar septae and along lymphatic vessels (Halprin et al., 1972). Type II pneumocyte hyperplasia and germinal center within lymphoid follicles are commonly found. Biopsies show CD8+ and CD20+ cells predominance. Fibrosis may develop in advanced cases.

Although the etiology of LIP is not clear, it has been suggested that Epstein–Barr virus (EBV) may play a role. EBV DNA has been found in fragments of lung tissues taken from children with LIP (Reddy et al., 1988). Contrarily, other studies have not shown any difference in the frequency of EBV detection in lung biopsies when comparing adult PWH with LIP and control groups (van Zyl-Smit et al., 2015). HIV itself may play a role in the pathology of LIP, as has been demonstrated in a transgenic mouse model in which HIV induced a lymphoid interstitial pneumonitis syndrome (Hanna et al., 1998). HIV RNA copies have been amplified from lung biopsy samples of PWH and LIP, and HIV-specific IgG is frequently present in the bronchoalveolar lavage fluid (Resnick et al., 1987). A predominant CD8+ T-cell infiltrate was found on histology in PWH and LIP (van Zyl-Smit et al., 2015). Human T-lymphotropic virus type I (HTLV-I) has been linked to LIP in Japan (Setoguchi et al., 1991).

The clinical presentation of LIP is similar in adults and children. Cough is the predominant symptom associated with slowly progressive dyspnea. Symptoms are usually present for several months. Fever, chest pain, weight loss, and arthralgias have also been reported. Physical exam may be completely normal or may reveal crackles. Children may have clubbing, salivary gland enlargement, lymphadenopathy, and hepatosplenomegaly.

Chest X-rays are normal or show bilateral reticular or nodular opacities. Focal areas of confluent pulmonary opacifications have been described as well as pulmonary cysts and patchy consolidations, the latter being less common. Chest CT shows diffuse ground-glass opacities with small nodules (2–3 mm) in a peribronchovascular distribution (Pitcher et al., 2010). Like other diffuse interstitial lung diseases, spirometry typically shows decreased total lung capacity and decreased diffusing capacity.

There is no consensus regarding the optimal treatment for LIP in PWH. Corticosteroids at a dosage of 1 mg/kg/d are recommended. However, in several case reports, ART has been demonstrated to be effective by itself (Garcia Lujan et al., 2004; Innes et al., 2004; Ripamonti et al., 2003).

DIFFUSE INFILTRATIVE CD8+ LYMPHOCYTE SYNDROME

DILS is a rare multisystemic syndrome characterized by CD8+ T-cell lymphocytosis associated with a CD8+ T-cell infiltration of multiple organs. It is primarily characterized by parotid gland enlargement, xerophthalmia, xerostomia, and interstitial pneumonitis. Respiratory clinical manifestations include nonproductive cough and dyspnea. Diffuse lymphadenopathy, hepatosplenomegaly, lymphocytic gastritis, and seventh cranial nerve palsy have also been described.

Histologic examination demonstrates visceral lymphocytic infiltration that could be a direct consequence of the large amount of CD8+ T-cells. Lymphoid follicles with CD8+ germinal centers are seen in salivary and parotid glands biopsies. HIV has been detected in macrophages within the germinal center of lymphoid tissues; therefore, ART plays a major role in treatment. Immunosuppression with steroids is also recommended.

PULMONARY ARTERIAL HYPERTENSION

PAH has a higher prevalence among PWH compared to the general population. It was reported to be 0.5% in 1991 (Speich et al., 1991) and remains the same in the combination ART era (Opravil & Sereni, 2008; Sitbon et al., 2008; Zuber et al., 2004).

The occurrence of PAH in PWH is not related to the CD4+ T-cell count. No risk factors have been found. However, a small study reported that chronic hepatitis C, drug addiction, and female sex increased the risk of developing PAH by threefold (Quezada et al., 2012). In a series that compared PAH in PWH and PAH in participants without HIV, PWH were significantly younger and had milder disease (50% vs. 75% had New York Heart Association functional class III or IV, respectively) (Petipretz et al., 1994).

The clinical presentation of PWH and PAH is similar to that of patients without HIV. PWH experience symptoms related to right heart dysfunction, such as progressive shortness of breath, pedal edema, nonproductive cough, fatigue, syncope, and chest pain. Physical exam may reveal increased intensity of the pulmonary second heart sound, third and fourth sound gallop, tricuspid and pulmonary regurgitation murmurs, elevated jugular venous pressure, and peripheral edema.

Chest radiographs may show cardiomegaly and enlarged pulmonary artery, but clear lung fields. Transthoracic echocardiogram shows signs of right ventricle pressure overload, including systolic flattening of the interventricular septum, and hypertrophy of the ventricle wall. The tricuspid regurgitant jet velocity can be used to calculate an estimated pulmonary artery systolic pressure (ePASP) which is elevated in PAH.

Right heart catheterization is the standard for diagnosing PAH, assessing severity of PAH, and monitoring response to treatment. PAH is defined by an mPAP of 25 mm Hg or higher, a mean pulmonary capillary wedge pressure of 15 mm Hg or less, and a normal or reduced cardiac output (Galie et al., 2009). It is important to note that a thorough evaluation should be done to exclude other causes of pulmonary hypertension.

Treatment of HIV-associated PAH is similar to that of PAH in patients without HIV. Treatment is guided by the WHO functional classification for PAH which is based on symptomology and functional limitations. PWH should be counseled against smoking and pregnancy. PAH directed therapy includes endothelin receptor antagonists, phosphodiesterase inhibitors, and prostacyclin pathway agonists. Although there are no controlled clinical trials, prostanoids (epoprostenol, treprostinil, and iloprost), endothelin receptor antagonists (bosentan), and phosphodiesterase-5 inhibitors (sildenafil) have been used in HIV-associated PAH and have been shown to improve symptoms and hemodynamic parameters. Caution should be taken with the use of these medications because of possible severe drug interactions, particularly with protease inhibitors and cobicistat.

Oxygen is recommended if arterial blood partial pressure of oxygen (PaO2) is 60 mm Hg or less. Diuretics reduce the right ventricular preload and are recommended in PWH with right heart failure. The role of digoxin is controversial; however, it has been shown to improve cardiac output in PWH with acute right ventricular dysfunction attributable to PAH. Anticoagulation is not routinely recommended in PWH as there are no direct data of its benefit. Calcium channel blockers are not recommended in HIV-associated PAH. Observational data shows efficacy of vasoreactivity in only a small number of patients with HIV and PAH and very limited long-term response. Although there is no conclusive evidence of the effect of ART on the progression of HIV-associated PAH, it is recommended to start ART in all PWH with PAH regardless of the CD4[+] T-cell count. ART has been demonstrated to cause improvements in pressure gradient over time and to significantly reduce the risk of death in PWH and PAH.

PAH is an independent risk factor for death among PWH (Opravil & Sereni, 2008). However, with the advent of ART and the new treatment modalities, the overall survival rate at 1 year is 88% and 72% at 3 years (Degano et al., 2010).

REFERENCES

Anderson V, Lee H. Lymphocytic interstitial pneumonitis in pediatric AIDS. *Pediatr Pathol*. 1988;8:417–421.

Collins B, Mulhall P, Travaline J. Nonspecific interstitial pneumonia in a patient with HIV. *SN Comprehensive Clinical Medicine*. 2019;1:203–204.

Degano B, Guillaume M, Savale L, Montani D, et al. HIV-associated pulmonary arterial hypertension: survival and prognostic factors in the modern therapeutic era. *AIDS*. 2010;24:67–75.

Galie N, Hoeper M, Humbert M. Guidelines for the diagnosis and treatment of pulmonary hypertension. *Eur Heart J*. 2009;30:2493–2537.

Garcia Lujan R, Echave-Sustaeta J, Garcia Quero C, et al. Lymphoid interstitial pneumonia resolved through antiretroviral therapy in an adult infected by human immunodeficiency virus. *Arch Bronconeumol*. 2004;40:537–539.

Halprin G, Ramirez J, Pratt O. Lymphoid interstitial pneumonia. *Chest*. 1972;62:418–423.

Hanna Z, Kay DG, Cool M et al. Transgenic mice expressing human immunodeficiency virus type 1 in immune cells develop a severe AIDS-like disease. *J Virol*. 1998;72:121–132.

Innes A, Huang L, Nishimura S. Resolution of lymphocytic interstitial pneumonitis in an HIV infected adult after treatment with HAART. *Sex Transm Infect*. 2004;80:417–418.

Ognibene F, Masur H, Rogers P, et al. Nonspecific interstitial pneumonitis without evidence of Pneumocysitis carinii in asymptomatic patients infected with human immunodeficiency virus (HIV). *Ann Intern Med*. 1988;109:874–879.

Opravil M, Sereni D. Natural history of HIV-associated pulmonary arterial hypertension: trends in the HAART era. *AIDS*. 2008;22:35–40.

Petipretz P, Brenot F, Azarian R. Pulmonary hypertension in patients with human immunodeficiency virus infection: comparison with primary pulmonary hypertension. *Circulation*. 1994;89:2722–2727.

Pitcher R, Beningfield S, Zar H. Chest radiographic features of lymphocytic pneumonitis in HIV-infected children. *Clin Radiol*. 2010;65:150–154.

Quezada M, Martin-Carbonero L, Soriano V, et al. Prevalence and risk factors associated with pulmonary hypertension in HIV-infected patients on regular follow-up. *AIDS*. 2012;26:1387–1392.

Reddy A, Lyall E, Crawford D. Epstein–Barr virus and lymphoid interstitial pneumonitis: an association revisited. *Pediatr Infect Dis J*. 1998;17:82–83.

Resnick L, Pitchenik A, Fisher E, et al. Detection of HTLVIII/LAV specific IgG and antigen in bronchoalveolar lavage fluid from two patients with lymphocytic interstitial pneumonitis associated with AIDS related complex. *Am J Med*. 1987;82:553–556.

Ripamonti D, Rizzi M, Maggiolo F, et al. Resolution of lymphocytic interstitial pneumonia in a human immunodeficiency virus infected adult following the start of highly antiretroviral therapy. *Scand J Infect Dis*. 2003;35:348–351.

Setoguchi Y, Takahashi S, Nukiwa T, et al. Detection of human T-cell lymphotropic virus type I-related antibodies in patients with lymphocytic interstitial pneumonia. *Am Rev Respir Dis*. 1991;144:1361–1365.

Sitbon O, Lascoux-Combe C, Delfraissy JF, et al. Prevalence of HIV-related pulmonary arterial hypertension in the current antiretroviral therapy era. *Am J Respir Crit Care Med*. 2008;177:108–113.

Speich R, Jenni R, Opravil M, et al. Primary pulmonary hypertension in HIV infection. *Chest*. 1991;100:1268–1271.

Stover D, White D, Romano P, et al. Spectrum of pulmonary diseases associated with the acquired immune deficiency syndrome. *Am J Med*. 1985;78:429–437.

Suffredini A, Ognibene F, Lack E, et al. Nonspecific interstitial pneumonitis: a common cause of pulmonary disease in the acquired immunodeficiency syndrome. *Ann Intern Med.* 1987;107:7–13.

Travis W, Fox C, Devaney K. Lymphoid pneumonitis in 50 adult patients infected with the human immunodeficiency virus: lymphocytic interstitial pneumonitis versus nonspecific interstitial pneumonitis. *Hum Pathol.* 1992;23:529–541.

van Zyl-Smit RN, Naidoo J, Wainwright H, et al. HIV associated lymphocytic interstitial pneumonia: a clinical, histological and radiographic study from an HIV endemic resource-poor setting. *BMC Pulm Med.* 2015;15:38–44.

Wolff AJ, O'Donnell AE. Pulmonary manifestations of HIV infection in the era of highly active antiretroviral therapy. *Chest.* 2001;120(6):1888–1893. http://doi:10.1378/chest.120.6.1888. PMID: 11742918.

Zuber J, Calmy A, Evison J. Pulmonary arterial hypertension related to HIV infection improved hemodynamics and survival associated with antiretroviral therapy. *Clin Infect Dis.* 2004;38:1178–1185.

34.

PSYCHIATRIC ILLNESS AND TREATMENT IN HIV POPULATIONS

Richa Vijayvargiya and Elizabeth H. David

CHAPTER GOAL

Upon completion of this chapter, the reader should be able to:

- Discuss the psychiatric concomitants of HIV illness and the role of psychiatric care in the overall treatment of persons living with HIV (PWH).

LEARNING OBJECTIVES

- Discuss the bidirectional relationship between HIV infection and psychiatric illnesses and /symptoms.

- Recognize symptoms suggesting the presence of a psychiatric component to the clinical picture.

- Describe general principles of treatment and identify when specific intervention by mental health professionals is advised.

WHAT'S NEW?

- This chapter has been updated to reflect terminology from the *Diagnostic and statistical manual of mental disorders text revision* (*DSM-5 TR*) (American Psychiatric Association, 2022), and has been updated with relevant new citations. The section discussing the impact on PWH from the COVID-19 pandemic has been updated with new statistics.

KEY POINTS

- Mental illness is both a risk factor for acquiring HIV and a consequence of HIV infection.

- Careful diagnosis of psychiatric disorders among PWH is essential given their impact on mental wellbeing and health outcomes, including adherence to antiretroviral medication, disease progression, and mortality.

- Referral to a psychiatrist may be an important step in ensuring an accurate mental diagnosis and an appropriate treatment plan in patients experiencing psychiatric symptoms.

- It is important to consider cultural factors when conceptualizing the risk and nature of mental illness in PWH.

- The COVID-19 pandemic has presented specific challenges that have influenced the mental health of PWH.

INTRODUCTION

From the earliest recognized AIDS deaths in 1981 to the commencement of combination antiretroviral therapy (ART) in the mid-1990s and the simpler combination ART regimens now available, HIV has remained a disease and an epidemic in constant evolution. For many years a near-certain death sentence, it has become a treatable chronic condition, with issues of HIV-associated dementia and rapid death by opportunistic infection generally replaced by treatment of "premature" aging and slow neurological decline and questions of maximizing adherence to treatment. Issues that have not changed include the tremendous psychosocial burden to the individual and family and the economic cost to the PWH and society, as well as factors of stigmatization and marginalization of HIV populations. Many PWH were already stigmatized before contracting this illness. The prevalence of HIV infection is much higher in gay/bi/transgender populations, in people of color, in substance users, in prison populations, in the homeless, in individuals with histories of physical and emotional trauma, and in people with mental illness (Whetten et al., 2008). HIV infection then adds to the burden through the psychological manifestations it causes (e.g., demoralization, depression, mania, anxiety, insomnia, and neurocognitive deficits), through disturbances in appearance (e.g., wasting, lipodystrophy, and Kaposi's sarcoma) and function (e.g., kidney disease, diabetes, sexual dysfunction, and chronic pain), and through tremendous losses (e.g., people, independence, health, employment, and sense of control). From the earliest days of the epidemic, it has been recognized that mental illness and HIV infection are closely related (Hoffman, 1984), with some estimates of comorbidity as high as 50%–70% (Blashill et al., 2011; Gaynes et al., 2008). Psychiatric illnesses are in and of themselves potentially lethal conditions, with increased rates of suicide and increased rates of illness and death from other conditions, including cancer, diabetes, and cardiovascular and cerebrovascular disease. They are associated with tremendous costs in terms of quality of life, lost productivity, and treatment. In combination with HIV-related illness, these issues are magnified.

Addressing these complex mental health issues is central to prevention, diagnosis, and treatment of HIV-related illness. Psychiatric illness is both a risk factor for disease and a barrier to adequate treatment. Substance abuse and "triple diagnosis" individuals (i.e., HIV, substance abuse, and mental illness) have been particularly problematic (see Chapter 26). The chronically mentally ill are both overrepresented in this population and more difficult to reach and treat owing to homelessness, distrust, and the unstructured nature of their lives. Survivors of physical and emotional trauma are a group increasingly recognized as both vulnerable to HIV infection and difficult to treat. They are prone to risky behaviors but slow to establish trusting relationships with treaters. In addition to these issues of primary mental illness is the factor of secondary mental health problems—those caused by the virus and/or its treatment.

MENTAL ILLNESS AND HIV INFECTION

The interaction between HIV and mental illness is complex. According to a population-based study in 2022, PWH have been found to have a significantly increased risk of experiencing mental disorders compared to people without HIV, with an adjusted hazard ratio of 1.63. Specifically, depression, anxiety, and serious mental illness among PWH were associated with respective adjusted hazard ratios of 1.94, 1.38, and 2.18 (Gooden et al., 2022). For many individuals, the psychiatric condition is a pre-existing one, predisposing to HIV infection through behavioral factors and risk environment (Meade et al., 2012; Prince et al., 2012; Rhodes, 2002). The risk factors for HIV are well established and involve blood/bodily fluid contact with infected individuals through unprotected sexual behaviors, needle sharing, multiple sexual partners, and fetal/natal exposure. Individuals with pre-existing psychiatric illness often engage in risky behaviors with little thought or fear of consequences. This relates to increased emotional immaturity and impulsivity (as in bipolar disorder, personality disorders, anxiety conditions, and posttraumatic stress disorder (PTSD)), poor contact with reality (as in schizophrenia and other psychotic conditions), denial and disinhibition (as in substance use disorders), cognitive dysfunction (as in major neurocognitive disorders and dementia), active thoughts of self-harm (as in depression), and victimization or impaired judgment (Kent & Blumenfield, 2011; Owe-Larssom et al., 2009). Barriers to treatment, such as distrust of authority (including fear of legal consequences), poor communication skills, limited access (including financial and transportation), lack of motivation, and unstructured lifestyle, all result in poor overall health care and delayed diagnosis of all health issues. Diagnosis of mental health issues is frequently challenging, and adherence to treatment is frequently impacted by these same factors.

Even for PWH without psychiatric illness, the diagnosis of serious medical illness is a significant emotional blow. Freud (1910) stated that emotional health involves the ability to integrate and balance aspects of love, work, and play. What could more thoroughly disrupt this balance and integration than an illness such as HIV, with so many devastating consequences, such a lifelong treatment, and so many far-reaching biological, psychological, and social consequences? Every day, every pill, every medical visit, and every secret kept from family, friends, and coworkers is a reminder that one is compromised, vulnerable, damaged, not normal. PWH are subject to harmful stigma which may exacerbate stress and contribute to mental disorders. In a study of 201 PWH in the United States, over one-third had experienced verbal stigma because of HIV in the prior 3 months (Reif et al., 2021). In her landmark work, Kubler-Ross (1969) discussed this trauma and the individual's response to it through repetitive processes of denial, anger, bargaining, and depression before (ideally) reaching a degree of acceptance. Treaters see the negative aspect of this emotional upheaval in its behavioral correlates: unrealistic anger at medical staff, equally unrealistic expectations of outcomes, guilt, fear, increased substance use, demoralization/hopelessness/amotivation, poor adherence to treatment, suicidal thoughts/suicide, and helplessness/neediness. We can help through building a positive and supportive treatment alliance that facilitates communication, acknowledges the huge cost to the individual, tolerates some of the stress behaviors, and does not take these behaviors personally but also sets limits of appropriateness. Timely referral to a psychiatrist or a psychotherapist is essential when stress becomes distress and behavior goes beyond those limits of appropriateness or when persons become dangerous to themselves or others.

HIV enters the central nervous system (CNS) very early in the course of systemic infection, and the brain becomes an important site of damage in PWH (Ho et al., 1985). This causes many of those infected to develop neurological and psychological symptoms with etiology posited to relate to functional disturbances in inflammatory processes. Activated circulating monocytes introduce the virus across the blood–brain barrier, and CNS macrophages, microglia, and astrocytes each become infected, releasing cytokines and chemokines that lead to neuronal cell damage (Williams et al., 2014). Evidence also suggests a disturbance in glutamate functioning within the CNS, with increased extracellular glutamate leading to excitotoxicity (Vazquez-Santiago et al., 2014). Accelerated aging from HIV infection and HIV treatments, damage caused by opportunistic infections or comorbid medical conditions (e.g., hepatitis C virus), and concomitant use of drugs of abuse (Gannon et al., 2011) also play important roles. AIDS mania and a continuum of neurocognitive deficits from very subtle to frank and debilitating dementia are well-defined psychiatric syndromes directly related to the presence of virus, but depression, insomnia, and anxiety are also among the mental health symptoms that result from the infection itself. This part of disease progression seems to be less amenable to ART compared to the more peripheral manifestations (Heaton et al., 2010), although antiretrovirals with higher levels of CNS penetration may promote improvement in some functions (Cysique et al., 2004). Unfortunately, those agents capable of crossing the blood–brain barrier are also the medications most likely to have psychiatric symptomatology as a side effect of use—a Pyrrhic victory in many ways.

Regardless of etiology, the presence of psychiatric symptoms and substance abuse is associated with poorer outcomes in HIV illness—lower levels of treatment adherence, slower virologic suppression, less subjective quality of life, increased morbidity and mortality, and increased utilization of medical services (Blashill et al., 2011; Carrico et al., 2011; Leserman, 2008; Nel & Kagee, 2011; Pence et al., 2007). Adequate treatment of the psychiatric illness, however, improves outcome across all categories (Cook et al., 2006; Horberg et al., 2008; Mellins et al., 2009; Walkup et al., 2008). In fact, among a population of men who have sex with men in Taiwan, PWH who receive treatment with antidepressant medication were shown to have a similar rate of adherence to antiretroviral medication as nondepressed PWH (Yen et al., 2022). Although most of the literature cited in this chapter relates to adult PWH, the diagnostic descriptions and treatments can, for the most part, be applied to adolescents and children (Benton, 2010; Rao et al., 2007).

PSYCHIATRIC DISORDERS AND TREATMENT

Careful diagnosis is essential given the complex interaction between psychiatric illness, HIV infection, substance abuse, comorbid medical conditions, and side effects of medications. Psychiatric illness cannot be diagnosed if these other medical factors play the primary role in causing symptoms (i.e., delirium), and psychiatric medications will seldom be of benefit in those cases. The following brief descriptions are based on the criteria from DSM-5 TR (American Psychiatric Association, 2022). The context of HIV infection results in no appreciable changes from the usual clinical manifestations of psychiatric disorders, with the possible exception of AIDS mania. Equally, pharmacological and nonpharmacological approaches to the treatment of psychiatric illness in the context of HIV illness are not radically different from those in HIV-negative populations. PWH do seem to have some increased sensitivity to the side effects of antipsychotic drugs, even absent of antiretroviral treatment (Hriso et al., 1991; Kelly et al., 2002; Ramachandran et al., 1997). Because many psychopharmacologic agents are metabolized by the same elements of the cytochrome P450 isoenzyme system that metabolize protease inhibitors (PIs) and nonnucleoside/nucleotide reverse transcriptase inhibitors (NNRTIs), there were many fears early on that they could not be used concomitantly. In fact, however, there are surprisingly few clinically significant interactions except as specifically noted in the following sections. As in all clinical situations, however, a "start low and go slow" philosophy is warranted, and the relative risks and benefits of treatment must be carefully weighed.

STRESS AND ADJUSTMENT DISORDERS

There are multiple stressors associated with living with a serious and debilitating illness. Some kinds of emotional and behavioral reactions to this stress are normal, short-lived, and do not require treatment beyond support, reassurance, education, and therapeutic optimism. Assistance with access to resources and support networks or with informing family or significant others of the diagnosis can be "curative." Such reactions typically occur immediately after diagnosis and at periods of acute change in the illness (opportunistic infections, deteriorating CD4$^+$ T-cell count/HIV RNA levels, initiation of ART, and onset of other comorbid medical complications) or in social circumstances (loss and financial problems). Typically, individuals with these acute stress reactions are able to attribute the onset and nature of their symptoms to specific life events. They can also be distracted from their emotions and symptoms and are capable of feeling pleasure and interest in other things. *Adjustment reactions* (normal responses to stressful circumstances) are typically treated with supportive counseling and psychotherapy. It is only when stress reactions—anger, worry, guilt, sadness, and insomnia—are sustained for months, reach a point that they interfere with normal life functioning, or actually threaten survival (substance abuse, high-risk activities, and self-destructive thoughts/behaviors) that they require intervention. *Adjustment disorders* may also respond to support and psychotherapy, but they may necessitate psychiatric medications and/or hospital admission. The specific medication used depends on the symptoms being manifested. A complex of sadness, guilt, and insomnia frequently responds to use of antidepressants, particularly the more sedating ones (sertraline and mirtazapine). Symptoms on the anxiety continuum may benefit from use of almost any medication with a sedating side effect. Low-dose trazodone or antihistamine (hydroxyzine or diphenhydramine are commonly used) can be helpful, although caution must be used because these agents tend to cause drying of mucous membranes, which can exacerbate oral thrush. Antihistamines should be used in caution in elderly PWH and those with dementia as these medications can increase the risk of delirium in these populations. The use of benzodiazepines is rarely indicated (see later discussion). Because of the known relationship between stress and compromised immune function, early appropriate intervention is important (Leserman, 2008).

ANXIETY DISORDERS AND PTSD

This group of illnesses includes generalized anxiety disorder (i.e., persistent feelings of anxiety), the phobias (i.e., irrational fear of a particular thing or behavior), panic disorder (i.e., spontaneous attacks of intense anxiety), and obsessive–compulsive disorder (i.e., intrusive anxiety-provoking thoughts that compel ritualized behaviors thought to alleviate that anxiety). PTSD (i.e., anxiety-related thoughts and behaviors connected to memories of past traumatic life experiences) was formerly included in this group, but it has been separated into its own category in DMS-5. All involve activation of the sympathetic nervous system (i.e., psychological and physiological fight–flight–freeze responses) in situationally inappropriate circumstances because there is no current emergency. Careful diagnosis requires that endocrine disorders (especially thyroid-related), substance use (including caffeine, steroids, and psychostimulants), agitated depression, dementia, and delirium be eliminated as primary etiological factors. PWH have rates of anxiety disorders greater than those of the general population (Gaynes et al., 2008; Klinkenberg et al., 2004; Martinez et al., 2002), as well as an increased incidence of past traumatic experiences (Pence, 2009). Treatment ideally consists of a combination of psychotherapy, as well as an increased incidence of past traumatic experiences (supportive, interpersonal, mindfulness, cognitive–behavioral, biofeedback, exposure and response prevention, and flooding) and psychopharmacotherapy with antidepressants and/or antianxiety agents. Because therapeutic benefit with antidepressant is delayed in onset, it may be useful to supplement early treatment with low-dose benzodiazepine—lorazepam or other short-acting agent for panic disorder or phobias (used as needed at onset of panic attack or exposure to phobic object, but no more than three or four times a day) and clonazepam or other long-acting medication for generalized anxiety. Benzodiazepines are rarely the regimen of choice for more than the first 2–4 weeks, however, and should be discontinued at the earliest time practical. Some alternative treatments have also been shown to be effective, including relaxation/meditation, breath training, acupuncture, and guided imagery. All of the antidepressants except bupropion have efficacy in anxiety disorders, and selection of a specific medication should be based on safety (the serotonin and serotonin/norepinephrine reuptake inhibitors (SNRIs) are overall much safer than tricyclics or monoamine oxidase inhibitors), side-effect profile (e.g., relative sedation vs. excitation; potential for gastric symptoms; appetite stimulation vs. suppression; anticholinergic effects; concerns for liver function; assistance with pain control), and past response to medications in the PWH or a family member. The selective serotonin reuptake inhibitors (SSRIs) can increase dream and flashback symptoms in individuals with past traumatic experiences, although small doses of prazosin can mitigate this effect. As noted previously, antianxiety agents include benzodiazepines, antihistamines, buspirone, and small doses of antidepressants (e.g., trazodone) or atypical antipsychotics (e.g., Seroquel—an off-label use). All except buspirone work by sedating the individual, and they can be taken at the onset of anxiety symptoms. (Buspirone, like the antidepressants, must be taken on a regular basis to be effective.) The benzodiazepines also disinhibit behaviors, cause various degrees of cognitive impairment including amnesia and motor slowing/incoordination (a serious issue in a population already at risk for neurocognitive impairment), increase the risk of falls, and can trigger relapse or increased substance use in individuals with substance abuse problems. They are meant for temporary use only and can usually be discontinued when the antidepressants have become effective (2–4 weeks). A consensus survey of psychiatrists treating PWH revealed clonazepam to be the most frequently used benzodiazepine, followed by lorazepam (Freudenreich et al., 2010). Alprazolam, midazolam, and triazolam should be avoided because of their high potential for addiction and their adverse interactions with antiretrovirals (ARVs). Again, the byword for concomitant use of any psychopharmacologic agent with an ARV is "Start low. Go slow."

AFFECTIVE DISORDERS

Disorders of mood, particularly depression, are the most common psychiatric manifestations of HIV disease, with rates much higher in PWH than in the general population (Berger-Greenstein et al., 2007; Gaynes et al., 2011; Treisman & Angelinno, 2007) and increasing frequency with advancing disease (Atkinson et al., 2008). Depression hinders treatment of PWH, thus increasing risk of disease progression and spread (Benton, 2008; Villes et al., 2007), and it may have direct effects on immune responses (Alciati et al., 2007). PWH are at greater risk to die by suicide compared to the general population, with about 21% reporting suicidal ideation, and 5% attempting suicide in the past year. Completed suicide is estimated to occur in about 1%–2% of PWH. Psychiatric disorders and substance use disorders both increase the risk for suicide in PWH (Brown et al., 2021). Adequate treatment, however, reverses all these trends for both depression (Horberg et al., 2008; Mellins et al., 2009; Walkup et al., 2008) and bipolar disorder (Walkup et al., 2011).

Major depression consists of a constellation of symptoms related to persistent low mood (including crying spells, guilt, low self-esteem, negative ruminations, social isolation, and loss of pleasure and interest), mental slowing (including poor attention, concentration, memory, and energy; loss of libido; and motor retardation), and changes in behavior (e.g., increased or decreased sleep or appetite). Those with severe illness may also have psychotic symptoms (i.e., hallucinations and delusions) usually with depressive content. Careful diagnosis is essential because many of these symptoms might also be caused by serious medical illness, major neurocognitive impairment (e.g., dementia and delirium), side effects of medications, substance abuse, or grief and loss. Unlike adjustment disorders, individuals with major depression generally cannot cite a precipitating event nor be distracted from their negative emotions. It is the relentless nature of the symptoms that results in a sense of hopelessness and despair, with a progressive narrowing of emotional focus until it may seem that death (i.e., suicide) is the only way out. Treatment ideally consists of combined psychotherapy and psychopharmacology with antidepressant medications, sometimes adding augmenting agents (a second antidepressant from another class, lithium, testosterone, thyroid medications, psychostimulants, and mood stabilizers). Low doses of antipsychotics are indicated on a temporary basis if psychotic features are present. Ketamine in very low doses is being used in some centers, but it must be used with extreme caution in PWH on ART. Replicated evidence has shown psychotherapeutic interventions (e.g., cognitive–behavioral therapy, stress management interventions, and supportive therapy) have moderate antidepressant effects on PWH (van Luenen et al., 2018). Alternative treatments including exercise, meditation/relaxation, acupuncture, and herbal medications have been found to be helpful. Individuals on St. John's wort should be cautioned, however, because this popular herbal antidepressant has significant adverse clinical interactions with multiple ARVs, anticancer drugs, anti-inflammatory agents, antibiotics, psychopharmacologic agents, cardiovascular drugs, antihypoglycemics, oral contraceptives, proton pump inhibitors, statins, and antiasthmatic medications (Nicolussi et al., 2019). All of the normal antidepressant drugs show efficacy in the population with HIV, and choice of a particular medication should be based on safety (Watkins et al., 2011), side-effect profile, and past response to medications in the PWH or a family member. A consensus study revealed that the SSRIs are the most common first-line drugs, with citalopram the number one choice (Freudenreich et al., 2010), although this may be changing with newer US Food and Drug Administration warnings about QT prolongation caused by this medication in higher doses. The SSRIs do have an anticoagulant effect, and used long term, they can result in significant decreases in bone density. They can also cause bruxism and extrapyramidal side effects as well as sexual dysfunction. Switching drugs within a pharmacologic class is of benefit if individuals find specific side effects intolerable. If a medication in any given class of antidepressants fails to show therapeutic benefit (8- to 12-week trial of adequate doses), a switch to another class of drugs is advised because agents within any given class have similar efficacy (Warden & Rush, 2007), so a switch to an SNRI (venlafaxine and duloxetine) and then to bupropion is a useful algorithm when there is treatment failure (Freudenreich et al., 2010). Particular caution is suggested in using bupropion (either as an antidepressant or in smoking cessation) in combination with the PIs (especially saquinavir or indinavir) or NNRTIs (especially efavirenz) because metabolism of bupropion can be inhibited, thus increasing the risk of seizures. Lopinavir/ritonavir, on the other hand, increases metabolism of bupropion, so bupropion doses must be increased when used with this antiretroviral combination (Hogeland et al., 2007). Mirtazapine can be particularly useful for those with chronic pain, weight loss, nausea, and vomiting (especially from chemotherapy regimens). Monoamine oxidase inhibitors (MAOIs) are not generally used in this population, and they are contraindicated for concomitant use with other antidepressants and most antipsychotics. Of note, the antibiotic linezolid is also an MAOI. All antidepressant regimens take several weeks to have therapeutic benefit, and the symptoms may not all resolve simultaneously. For this reason, particular caution and close observation are warranted in the early weeks of treatment: if energy, motivation, and a sense of agency return before suicidal thoughts and impulses disappear, a person who has had suicidal thoughts but insufficient energy to act on them may suddenly find the energy to act. The use of antidepressants in children and younger adolescents is particularly fraught with danger of suicide, and most antidepressant medications now carry a black box warning for this population. Inpatient psychiatric treatment is necessary if there are questions of safety, and this is obviously a situation in which it is best to err on the side of caution. Duration of treatment is a significant question. In the general population, an individual with a single episode of depression is generally treated for 4–6 months, whereas individuals with more than two episodes receive protracted therapy with antidepressants.

Because of concurrent medical illnesses, stress, and the propensity for HIV virus to cause/exacerbate affective symptoms, long-term use of antidepressants is frequently necessary.

Bipolar disorder is defined by intermittent episodes of low (i.e., depressive) and high (i.e., hypomanic or manic) moods, each lasting days, weeks, or months and in a continuum of severity from mild to disabling. These mood swings are not a reaction to life events. The lows are identical to the depressive episodes described previously. The high episodes consist of persistent elevated mood tone (e.g., euphoric or irritable), increased energy (e.g., racing thoughts that bounce from topic to topic, little need for sleep, rapid speech, and increased libido), and an inflated sense of self-worth, and they often lead to engaging in risky behaviors. In mania, there can be frank psychosis, with delusions (usually grandiose), disorganized thinking, and hallucinations leading to severe impairment in functioning and judgment. Bipolar disorder occurs at higher rates among PWH than in the general population (DeSousa Gurgel et al., 2013). HIV prevalence is about 1% among patients with bipolar disorder, with bipolar disorder preceding the diagnosis of HIV in 65% of patients. The rates of adherence to antiretroviral medication as well as psychopharmacologic medication are lower among PWH with bipolar disorder (Yalin et al., 2021).

Psychopharmacologic treatment in bipolar disorder consists of mood stabilizer medications (e.g., lithium, valproic acid, carbamazepine, lamotrigine, and "second-generation" antipsychotic medications), with antidepressants and antipsychotics added if these symptoms are prominent. Some clinicians believe that long-acting benzodiazepine can be helpful in the first days of treatment for active mania, but these agents can further disinhibit and should be used only on a short-term basis. All of these medications are effective and reasonably safe in HIV populations. Lithium has a very narrow window of safety, and it is eliminated by the kidney. Particular caution is necessary in individuals with kidney dysfunction, diarrhea, electrolyte disturbances, or cognitive impairment, but there are no specific interactions with ARVs. Lithium can cause or exacerbate thyroid dysfunction, tremor, acne, and psoriasis. Valproic acid appears to have few clinically significant drug interactions with ARVs. However, it is metabolized by the liver, and it can increase liver enzymes and cause hyperammonemia. In addition, there is risk of severe hepatitis, weight gain, thrombocytopenia, nystagmus, and tremor. The use of carbamazepine is more complicated: it is metabolized by the cytochrome P450 system, and it induces its own metabolism. There have been reports of clinically significant carbamazepine toxicity when used in combination with ritonavir and other potent CYP3A4 inhibitors and also of virologic failure caused by enzyme induction (Liedtke et al., 2004). In addition, carbamazepine causes a significant risk for bone marrow suppression. Lamotrigine is effective particularly for depressive symptoms and appears to be safe when used in combination with ART. Initiation and discontinuation of this agent must be managed very carefully because of the risk of life-threatening Stevens–Johnson syndrome. It should be remembered that use of antidepressants without a mood stabilizer in a bipolar person can trigger a manic episode.

AIDS mania is a specific manifestation of late-stage HIV infection, rarely seen in the combination ART era. The mood is more likely to be irritable, sullen, and withdrawn than euphoric and hyper talkative, and there is frequently no prior personal or family history of psychiatric illness. Otherwise, the symptoms are typical of mania. Episodes, however, tend to be protracted, frequently with a prodrome of progressive cognitive decline. Symptoms do not usually respond to the usual psychopharmacological approaches, nor is there spontaneous remission if the condition is left untreated. The treatment of choice is initiation of aggressive ART.

PSYCHOTIC DISORDERS

Psychotic disorders are defined by loss of contact with reality (i.e., hallucinations and delusions) as well as by varying degrees of disorganized thinking and behavior. Insight and judgment are often compromised, and it is frequently difficult to communicate clearly with these individuals because they can seem lost in their own, sometimes quite bizarre, world. Symptoms can be present on a temporary/episodic basis (e.g., brief psychotic episode and schizophreniform disorder) or may be more chronic (as in schizophrenia). Although disruption of thinking and behavior are most typical, any psychotic illnesses may involve some affective symptoms, even if only because the person recognizes that they are somehow different from others. When symptoms of an emotional nature (depression or excitation) are a prominent and invariant part of the psychosis, schizoaffective disorder must be considered. Differential diagnosis includes affective disorder with psychotic features, medical illness (psychosis secondary to a medical condition such as HIV), side effects of medications, delirium/dementia, and substance abuse. Initial medical work-up of anyone with a new-onset psychosis should probably include a urine drug screen (although many of the newer synthetic substances do not appear on standard tests), serology, endocrine screen, liver function tests, and computed tomography and/or magnetic resonance imaging of the brain. Visual hallucinations are rare in primary psychiatric illness, and they should also prompt a more complete medical evaluation. The chronically mentally ill are at increased risk of exposure to HIV owing to factors such as homelessness, poor insight/judgment, lack of knowledge, victimization, and increased rates of substance abuse and other high-risk behaviors (Prince et al., 2012). Without adequate psychiatric treatment, their psychosis is a serious barrier to medical treatment because of poor adherence, difficulties communicating with providers, and unstable lifestyle (Carrico et al., 2011). Treatment consists of control of symptoms with medications along with psychosocial support. All the antipsychotic medications work in PWH. As previously noted, PWH, even without ARV treatment, seem to be somewhat more sensitive to the dopamine-mediated extrapyramidal side effects of these drugs. These side effects are most common with the high-potency first-generation antipsychotics (i.e., haloperidol and fluphenazine). Both the first-generation and newer antipsychotics have significant risk for metabolic, cardiac (prolonged QT intervals), and endocrine side effects, and all are metabolized by the liver. They do not seem to have clinically significant interactions with ARV

treatments, with the possible exception of lurasidone, but the issue of QT prolongation should be closely monitored because some of the ARVs also have this side effect. In the consensus survey, quetiapine was the most used agent for psychosis, perhaps because it is also useful in mood stabilization and sedation (Freudenreich et al., 2010). A recent meta-analysis also revealed that quetiapine is the safest of the antipsychotic drugs to use for psychosis and behavioral control in individuals with dementia (Kales et al., 2012). Clozapine and the low-potency first-generation medications (e.g., chlorpromazine and thioridazine) are seldom used (Freudenreich et al., 2010), although certainly not contraindicated. Use of depo injections tends to result in fewer side effects than seen with daily oral formulations and can be particularly useful in individuals for whom compliance with antipsychotic medication is problematic. It is safest, however, to initiate treatment with oral medication and then switch to the long-acting forms later.

PERSONALITY DISORDERS AND THE DIFFICULT-TO-TREAT PWH

Personality can be thought of as enduring patterns of behavior, and this is partly what we refer to when we say we "know" a person—the person has somewhat predictable responses to given circumstances, a familiar emotional tone, consistent belief systems, and a well-formed sense of identity and agency. When these patterns are stable and healthy, one's responses to adversity (coping techniques) help to mitigate stress, and one can modulate emotional responses to fit the circumstances, thus maintaining a stable sense of self and other and control over one's world. In personality disorders, an individual is stuck in repetitive patterns that do not work: coping techniques that actually escalate stressful situations, relationship paradigms that result in little perceived support and an increasing sense of frustration by and with others, spiraling loss of emotional control, and, ultimately, the fearful recognition that one is out of control of both internal and external worlds. Borderline and antisocial personality disorders are common in populations with HIV because these individuals tend to engage in high-risk behaviors that expose them to contracting the virus. The presence of these character pathologies also complicates treatment adherence (Hansen et al., 2009; Gilchrist et al., 2011). They tend to be easily frustrated, to expect immediate gratification, to want sure-fire/magical interventions, and to demand "special" treatment from everybody. They also challenge authority and have limited ability to structure their own lives adequately and consistently. As difficult and challenging as it can be to work with these individuals, it is important to remember that their behavior is not intentional—it is their best effort to adjust to and control their chaotic world (Groves et al., 1978). Frequently, the emotions they engender in others are only reflections of the emotional turmoil within themselves. These are individuals for whom referral to psychotherapy and the presence of a strong, consistent treatment team with a clearly delineated treatment contract are essential to preserve coherent participation in medical care. Because their psychological symptoms tend to be so reactive to events in the environment, switching rapidly and wildly, caution should be used in initiating medications. Although consistent use of an SSRI or a mood stabilizer may be useful, chasing symptoms with medications is contraindicated. It is generally much more useful to help these individuals understand that their problems may be related to their own patterns of response and poor behavioral choices than to teach them that medication is going to provide them with internal peace or a sense of purpose, meaning, security, and attachment.

SUBSTANCE USE DISORDERS

For a full discussion of this topic, see Chapter 26. Suffice it to say here that concurrent substance abuse complicates diagnosis and treatment of all other psychiatric conditions as well as HIV-related illnesses. These complications, as well as problems with adherence to treatment and overall morbidity and mortality, are additive in nature. It is essential to the good treatment of HIV illness that clinicians screen for substance abuse and address it consistently and aggressively.

MAJOR NEUROCOGNITIVE DISORDERS (DELIRIUM AND DEMENTIA)

HIV infection is associated with a number of CNS complications that may be temporary (i.e., delirium) or permanent (i.e., the continuum of neurocognitive deficits from asymptomatic to frank dementia). Dementia is a common manifestation of HIV illness, and it is discussed in Chapter 35. Delirium is a potentially life-threatening medical condition, generally of sudden and rapid onset and pursuing a waxing and waning course. Also referred to as *encephalopathy*, delirium is the most common neuropsychiatric diagnosis in hospitalized or critically ill PWH, with an estimated frequency of 40%–65% (Gallago et al., 2011). It can manifest with any psychiatric symptom (e.g., anxiety, depression, mania, and psychosis) but most frequently includes disturbances in orientation, awareness/alertness, reality testing (e.g., hallucinations, including visual—which are very unusual in primary psychiatric conditions), communication (e.g., mumbled, incoherent speech), and motor behavior (e.g., lethargy, agitation, and picking at skin/clothing/intravenous lines). Several screening tools are used to diagnose delirium, of which the Cognitive Assessment Measurement Scale (CAMS and CAMS-ICU) is probably the most thoroughly researched. Definitive treatment involves correction of the underlying medical condition (e.g., infection, electrolyte disturbance, medication side effect, endocrine imbalance, and intoxication). *Temporary* use of low-dose antipsychotic medications can be helpful, but they should be tapered and discontinued as the delirium resolves. Avoid the use of any anticholinergic agents (particularly diphenhydramine and other antihistamines) and of antipsychotics with high anticholinergic side effects (Thorazine and thioridazine). Olanzapine, a sedating antipsychotic, may help with agitation but has been reported to cause, exacerbate, and/or prolong delirium in some cases. Use of benzodiazepines is also generally counterproductive, with the obvious exception of delirium caused by alcohol or benzodiazepine withdrawal. Measures that improve the individual's connection with reality can be very helpful. These include constant soft lighting (shadows are often misperceived), quiet and soothing background noise, a visible clock and/or calendar in the room, a written list of names of nursing staff and others, and repeated self-introduction of caregivers and visitors.

SEXUAL DYSFUNCTION

Sexual dysfunctions are very common in HIV illness. Disorders of desire (e.g., hypoactive sexual desire disorder) may be almost universal in PWH and erectile dysfunction is very common in men with AIDS (Shindel et al., 2011). Although certainly related to stress, depression, and uncertainties about spreading the disease to sexual partners, it also seems that the virus itself, the myriad comorbid conditions (including hypogonadism, diabetes, and peripheral neuropathy), and the multiple medications used to treat all these conditions play a role (Collazos, 2007; Huntingdon et al., 2019; Moreno-Perez et al., 2010; Scanavino, 2011). Treatment, therefore, is obviously complex. To the degree that these disorders are due to secondary issues, efforts can be made to change those conditions. Depression, stress, and comorbid conditions can be treated, and sometimes medications can be changed, or doses modified to minimize sexual side effects. Sexual counseling and therapy are helpful in teaching the PWH that sexual behavior and loving are not always about intercourse. Medications for erectile dysfunction (e.g., sildenafil, vardenafil, and tadalafil) can be used in this population, but doses must be reduced when given in the context of ART because metabolism is delayed. This obviously increases the probability of adverse side effects from the erectile dysfunction drugs, including visual changes, priapism, hypotension, and myocardial infarct. As with all medications, risks and benefits must be carefully weighed by the PWH and the clinician.

SLEEP DISTURBANCE

Insomnia is defined as difficulty initiating and/or maintaining sleep or overall nonrestful sleep. It tends to impair daytime function, and it is even more common in PWH than in the general population. This condition has been linked to poor quality of life and nonadherence to treatment (Saberi et al., 2011). Stress and depression play a role in etiology, and some ARVs disrupt sleep continuity. Efavirenz, a medication from the NNRTI class, is most consistently associated with sleep disturbances, including delayed sleep initiation, impaired sleep maintenance, and vivid nightmares. However, it appears that insomnia may be a primary symptom of viral presence, with changes in sleep architecture and decreased sleep efficiency noted even prior to onset of any symptoms of HIV/AIDS (Norman et al., 1992). Pharmacological treatment of insomnia includes the use of benzodiazepines, nonbenzodiazepine hypnotics, antihistamines, antidepressants, and antipsychotics. Of the benzodiazepines, clonazepam, lorazepam, oxazepam, and temazepam are relatively safe, although, as previously noted, their use in individuals with current or past substance abuse is problematic. Use of alprazolam, flurazepam, quazepam, and triazolam is contraindicated with ARVs and ketoconazole and also in those with kidney or hepatic disease. Sustained use of benzodiazepine medications is rarely, if ever, indicated. All of the nonbenzodiazepine hypnotics (eszopiclone, zaleplon, and zolpidem) are relatively safe in HIV populations, although dosages of zolpidem should be reduced if used with PIs, even in boosting dosages. Dosages of all nonbenzodiazepine hypnotics should also be reduced in those with hepatic disease. Antihistamines (especially diphenhydramine and hydroxyzine) are typically effective, and they are safe in PWH. However, it should be remembered that some individuals have paradoxical excitatory responses to these medications. Sleep induction is an off-label use for any antidepressant or antipsychotic. Nonetheless, low-dose tricyclics (especially doxepin and amitriptyline) and mirtazapine can be very useful in this regard. They can also help with control of neuropathic pain, which can improve sleep quality. In higher doses, all are associated with weight gain, which can be beneficial in some cases. Trazodone is frequently used to induce and maintain sleep in normal populations, but its use in PWH on ART is problematic because final metabolism of the trazodone is slowed, and untoward side effects (e.g., sleep disruption, vivid dreams, increased sedation, anxiety, and hypotension) occur. Of the antipsychotics, quetiapine and olanzapine are frequently used, although again, this is an off-label usage. As previously noted, PWH are much more sensitive to the extrapyramidal side effects of these medications. They also cause endocrine disturbances (prolactinemia) and metabolic side effects that may be cumulative with those of ART, such as lipodystrophy, hyperlipidemia, and insulin resistance (Omonuwa et al., 2009). Brief behavioral treatment for insomnia, a psychological treatment modality, has also been shown to improve the sleep outcomes of PWH and insomnia (Buchanan et al., 2016).

PSYCHIATRIC EFFECTS OF ANTIRETROVIRAL THERAPY

Many of the ARV agents have prominent psychiatric side effects that have been discussed previously. The most prominent of these psychiatric symptoms is vivid dreams and nightmares (Abers et al., 2014). Unfortunately, these issues seem to be more common, problematic, and sustained in individuals who are already vulnerable or experiencing psychiatric symptoms—that is, those with chronic mental illness. The vivid dreams and nightmares can be especially troubling for individuals with PTSD or past traumatic experiences. Although psychiatric diagnoses should not be a contraindication for use of these agents when indicated, special caution and close follow-up are certainly warranted. As with PTSD, low-dose prazosin can sometimes ameliorate the sleep disturbance experienced.

USE OF PSYCHIATRIC CONSULTATION

Mental health issues in PWH are very common (Bing et al., 2001; Robertson et al., 2014). In an ideal world, mental health professionals would be integrated into every HIV treatment setting, and individuals suspected of having significant illness

or distress could be seen rapidly and frequently after referral. In reality, this is rarely the case, and even when psychiatrists and other mental health providers are on-site, visits are commonly delayed because of the sheer number of those needing care. So, when is referral most warranted and useful? First and foremost, the individual must be aware of and agree to mental health evaluation. Exceptions to this relate to those individuals who are incapable of understanding the need for assessment and treatment, who are imminently dangerous to self or other, or who are systematically destroying themselves and their treatment/treatment team by their behavior. Beyond that, the first part of a decision for referral rests on the primary problem and referring to the correct person. Certain individuals will benefit most from referral to support groups of like-minded people with similar problems, and many actually prefer this form of treatment. Although there are certainly exceptions, most psychiatrists are not the primary resource for either substance abuse counseling or for individual/marital/group psychotherapy. The first task is handled, in general, by specific substance abuse counselors and by self-help groups (e.g., Alcoholics Anonymous, Narcotics Anonymous). Psychotherapy is also more frequently done by behavioral specialists other than psychiatrists (e.g., psychologists, social workers, and licensed counselors). Pain management and medical management of substance detox and sobriety are also frequently handled by other caregivers. In most settings, it is possible to refer directly to these providers, who can then screen for cases requiring specific psychiatric intervention. Psychologists are specifically trained in diagnostic processes (including psychological and neuropsychological testing and screening) and in psychotherapeutic interventions. Psychiatrists, although trained in behavioral interventions and therapy techniques, are medical doctors, and they are the first-line resource for evaluation of individuals with complex psychiatric/medical issues, those who will probably require psychotropic medications, and those who have not responded to conventional psychotropic medications. Although psychiatrists can be helpful in diagnosing delirium and can assist in behavioral management of symptoms, the presence of these major neurocognitive disorders (including acute intoxication) generally makes it impossible to ascertain if there is true psychiatric illness underlying the current medical process. The final caveat is this: When in doubt, consult. Most psychiatrists would rather be included when they are not needed than absent when they could be of help.

CULTURAL CONSIDERATIONS IN TREATING COMORBID HIV AND PSYCHIATRIC ILLNESS

The stigma associated with HIV is very well known, as is the stigma associated with psychiatric illness, but when the two are combined the consequences can be multiplicative and mutually reinforcing. Often it is fear of marginalization and/or discrimination that causes individuals to avoid HIV and mental health screenings and to be poorly adherent to treatment once diagnoses are made. These obstacles are further magnified when the individuals impacted by comorbid HIV and psychiatric illness belong to historically marginalized demographic groups. Whether it is because of their gender, ethnicity, or sexual orientation, individuals may encounter challenges in both navigating the healthcare system and receiving care that is uniquely suited to their needs. For instance, African and Caribbean Black women have been found to experience higher rates of HIV-related stigma and are more likely to report being marginalized or discriminated against based on racist and sexist stereotypes (Loutfy et al., 2012). This finding is of particular concern and importance in the United States, as African American women continue to be disproportionately represented among new HIV cases (CDC, 2020). Despite these statistics and the best efforts of public health clinicians, many HIV/mental health interventions lack sufficient cultural sensitivity and are therefore less likely to be effective across different demographic groups. A 2016 cohort study of 31,000 individuals with HIV found that while 47% of respondents had an indication for antidepressant treatment, Black non-Hispanics, Hispanics, and other non-White ethnicities were significantly less likely to initiate antidepressant treatment than their White non-Hispanic peers (Bengtson et al., 2016). These findings suggest a strong cultural component to acceptance of mental health treatment, one that may be mediated by historical mistrust of the healthcare system and/or a reliance on alternative methods of emotional support. In 2016, respondents in a qualitative study of primary care providers who treat African American PWH reported that their patients were more likely to seek emotional support from family or their spiritual community rather than seeking formal mental health treatment (Le et al., 2016). Accordingly, interventions aimed at identifying and preventing adverse HIV and mental health outcomes in these vulnerable groups should be tailored to address these pervasive cultural stigmas and norms. Neither HIV treatment nor mental health treatment are a one-size-fits-all endeavor, and clinicians should continue to enlist the input of PWH, families, and spiritual and community leaders to develop programs that suit the diversity and cultural sensitivities of the people they seek to help and heal.

PSYCHOSOCIAL CONSIDERTATION DURING THE COVID-19 PANDEMIC

The emergence of the novel coronavirus disease known as COVID-19 and subsequent declaration of a pandemic with Centers for Disease Control (CDC) recommendations for physical distancing and social isolation may disproportionally impact the psychological health of PWH. Older PWH are known to experience increased rates of loneliness and social isolation (Halkiti et al., 2017). This fact compounded with public health recommendations to reduce risk of transmission of COVID-19 are likely leading to a unique experience of stress in PWH.

In a study examining changes in mental health among PWH during the COVID-19 pandemic, 31% reported worsened mental health; 8% reported an improvement; and 61% were unchanged. Common concerns among PWH included

worry about acquiring COVID-19 because of possible increased vulnerability to infection owing to HIV. PWH also were concerned about the impact of the pandemic on financial stability and isolation related to physical distancing (Parisi et al., 2022). For PWH who lived through the 1980s and 1990s, prior to the development and FDA approval of combination ART, the COVID-19 pandemic may also represent a disturbing reminder of the early HIV pandemic. These reoccurring themes of large-scale infectious diseases can retrigger memories of death, fear, and uncertainty.

Given the above, PWH represent a population that is uniquely impacted by the COVID-19 pandemic, whether they contract the coronavirus or not. As such, all providers should strive to pay particular attention to their patients with HIV as we move through the COVID-19 pandemic.

CONCLUSION

From the earliest days of the AIDS epidemic, it has been apparent that large numbers of PWH also have psychiatric illness. This, of course, raises the question of the direction of relatedness: Is psychiatric illness a risk factor for HIV infection, or does the HIV virus cause or predispose to psychiatric symptoms? The answer seems to be "yes"—the association goes both ways. Individuals with psychiatric illness (including depression, bipolar disorders, anxiety disorders, PTSD, schizophrenia, dementia, and substance use disorders) tend to engage in behaviors that place them at increased risk for exposure to the HIV virus. Contracting HIV infection results in numerous psychosocial stressors that trigger or exacerbate expression of psychological symptoms in vulnerable individuals. The virus itself precipitates changes in the CNS that cause psychiatric manifestations. Finally, treatment with certain of the current ARV agents can result in psychiatric/behavioral symptoms. In turn, the presence of these psychiatric symptoms creates additional problems with diagnosis and treatment of HIV-related illnesses. All PWH should be screened for the presence of psychiatric illness. Fortunately, PWH respond well to traditional psychopharmacological and psychotherapeutic approaches to mental distress and illness, and, with adequate psychiatric treatment, they have good adherence and response to HIV treatment. Psychiatric illness alone is no longer considered to be a contraindication to full treatment of HIV or AIDS.

REFERENCES

Abers MS, Shandera WX, Kass JS. Neurological and psychiatric adverse effects of antiretroviral drugs. *CNS Drugs*. 2014;28(2):131–145.

Alciati A, Gallo L, Monforte AD, et al. Major depression-related immunological changes and combination antiretroviral therapy in HIV-seropositive patients. *Hum Psychopharmacol*. 2007;22(1):33–40.

American Psychiatric Association. *Diagnostic and statistical manual of mental disorders*. 5th ed. Arlington, VA: American Psychiatric Publishing; 2022.

Atkinson JH, Heaeton RK, Patterson TL, et al. Two-year prospective study of major depressive disorder in HIV-positive men. *J Affect Disord*. 2008;108:225–233.

Bengtson AM, Pence BW, Crane HM, et al. Disparities in depressive symptoms and antidepressant treatment by gender and race/ethnicity among people living with HIV in the United States. *PLoS One.* 2016;11(8):e0160738.

Benton TD. Depression and HIV/AIDS. *Curr Psychiatry Rep.* 2008;10(3):280–285.

Benton TD. Psychiatric considerations in children and adolescents with HIV/AIDS. Child Adolesc Psychiatr *Clin North Am.* 2010;19(2):387–400.

Berger-Greenstein JA, Cuevas CA, Brady SM, et al. Major depression in patients with HIV/AIDS and substance abuse. *AIDS Patient Care STDS.* 2007;21:942–949.

Bing EG, Burnam MA, Longshore D, et al. Psychiatric disorders and drug use among human immunodeficiency virus-infected adults in the United States. *Arch Gen Psychiatry.* 2001;58:721–728.

Blashill AJ, Perry N, Safren SA. Mental health: a focus on stress, coping, and mental illness as it relates to treatment retention, adherence, and other health outcomes. *Curr HIV/AIDS Rep.* 2011;8(4):215–222.

Brown LA, Majeed I, Mu W, et al. Suicide risk among persons living with HIV. *AIDS Care.* 2021; 33(5):616–622.

Buchanan DT, McCurry SM, Eilers K, et al. Brief behavioral treatment for insomnia in persons living with HIV, *Behav Sleep Med.* 2018;16(3):244-258. http://doi:10.1080/15402 002.2016.1188392

Carrico AW, Bangsberg DR, Weisner SD, et al. Psychiatric correlates of HAART utilization and viral load among HIV-positive impoverished persons. *AIDS.* 2011; 25(8):1113–1118.

Centers for Disease Control (CDC). HIV among African Americans online 2020. http://www.cdc.gov/hiv/group/racialethnic/africanam ericans/index.html. Published . Accessed.

Collazos J. Sexual dysfunction in the highly active antiretroviral therapy era. *AIDS Rev.* 2007; 9:237–245.

Cook JA, Burke-Miller J, Anastos K, et al. Effects of treated and untreated depressive symptoms on highly active antiretroviral therapy use in a US multi-site cohort of HIV-positive women. *AIDS Care.* 2006;18(2):3–100.

Cysique LA, Maruff P, Brew BJ. Prevalence and pattern of neuropsychological impairment in human immunodeficiency virus-infected/acquired immunodeficiency syndrome (HIV/AIDS) patients across pre- and post-highly active antiretroviral therapy eras: a combined study of two cohorts. *J Neurovirol.* 2004;10(6):350–357.

de Sousa Gurgel W, da Silva Carneiro AH, Barreto Rebouças D, et al. Affective disorders study group (GETA): prevalence of bipolar disorder in a HIV-infected outpatient population. *AIDS Care.* 2013;25(12):1499–1503.

Freud S. Five lectures on psycho-analysis. *Am J Psychol.* 1910;21.

Freudenreich O, Goforth HW, Cozza KL, et al. Psychiatric treatment of persons with HIV/AIDS: an HIV psychiatry consensus survey of current practices. *Psychosomatics.* 2010;51:480–488.

Gallego L, Barreiro P, Lopez-Ibor JJ. Diagnosis and clinical features of major neuropsychiatric disorders in HIV infection. *AIDS Rev.* 2011;13:171–179.

Gannon P, Khan MZ, Kolson DL. Current understanding of HIV-associated neurocognitive disorders pathogenesis. *Curr Opin Neurol.* 2011;24(3):275–283.

Gaynes BN, Farley JF, Dusetzina SB, et al. Does the presence of accompanying symptom clusters differentiate the comparative effectiveness of second-line medication strategies for treating depression? *Depress Anxiety.* 2011;28(11):989–998.

Gaynes BN, Pence BW, Eron JJ Jr, et al. Prevalence and comorbidity of psychiatric diagnoses based on reference standard in an HIV\+ population. *Psychosom Med.* 2008;70:505–511.

Gilchrist G, Blazquez A, Torrens M. Psychiatric, behavioral and social risk factors for HIV infection among female drug users. *AIDS Behav.* 2011;15(8):1834–1843.

Gooden TE, Gardner M, Wang J, et al. The risk of mental illness in people living with HIV in the UK: a propensity score-matched cohort study. *Lancet HIV.* 2022;9(3):172–181.

Groves, JE. Taking care of the hateful patient. *N Engl J Med.* 1978;298:883–887.

Halkitis PN, Krause KD, Vieira DL. Mental health, psychosocial challenges and resilience in older adults living with HIV. *Interdiscip Top Gerontol Geriatr.* 2017;42:187–203.

Hansen N, Vaughan E, Cavanaugh C, et al. Health-related quality of life in bereaved HIV-positive adults: relationships between HIV symptoms, grief, social support, and axis II indication. *Health Psychol.* 2009;28:249–257.

Heaton RK, Clifford DB, Franklin DR, et al. HIV-associated neurocognitive disorders persist in the era of potent antiretroviral therapy: CHARTER study. *Neurology.* 2010;75(23):2087–2096.

Ho D, Tota TR, Schooley RT, et al. Isolation of HTV-III from cerebrospinal fluid and neural tissues of patients with neurologic syndromes relate to the acquired immunodeficiency syndrome. *N Engl J Med.* 1985;313(24):1493–1497.

Hoffman, RS. Neuropsychiatric complications of AIDS. *Psychosomatics.* 1984;25:393–395.

Hogeland GW, Swindells S, McNabb JC, et al. Lopinavir/ritonavir reduces bupropion plasma concentrations in healthy subjects. *Clin Pharmacol Ther.* 2007;81(1):69–75.

Horberg MA, Silverberg MJ, Hurley LB, et al. Effects of depression and selective serotonin reuptake inhibitor use on adherence to highly active antiretroviral therapy and on clinical outcomes in HIV-positive patients. *J Acquir Immune Defic Syndr.* 2008;7(3):384–390.

Hriso E, Kuhn T, Masdeu JC, Grundman M. Extrapyramidal symptoms due to dopamine- blocking agents in patients with AIDS encephalopathy. *J Psychiatry.* 1991;148(11):1558–1561.

Huntingdon B, Muscat DM, de Wit J, et al. Factors associated with general sexual functioning and sexual satisfaction among people living with HIV: a systematic review. *J of Sex Res.* 2019. http://doi: 10.1080/00224499.2019.1689379

Kales HC, Kim HM, Zivin K, et al. Risk of mortality among individual antipsychotics in patients with dementia. 2012;169:71–79.

Kelly DV, Beique LC, Bowmer MI. Extrapyramidal symptoms with ritonavir/indinavir plus risperdone. *Ann Pharmacother.* 2002;36(5):827–830.

Kent LK, Blumenfield M. Psychodynamic psychiatry in the general medical setting. *J Am Acad Psychoanal Dyn Psychiatry.* 2011;9(1):41–62.

Klinkenberg WD, Dacks SL; HIV/AIDS Treatment Adherence, Health Outcomes and Cost Study Group. Mental disorders and drug abuse in persons living with HIV/AIDS. *AIDS Care.* 2004;16(Suppl 1):S22–S42.

Kubler-Ross E. *On death and dying.* New York: Macmillan; 1969.

Le H-N, Hipolito MMS, Lambert S, et al. Culturally sensitive approaches to identification and treatment of depression among HIV infected African American adults: a qualitative study of primary care providers' perspectives. *J Depress Anxiety.* 2016;5(2):223.

Leserman J. Role of depression, stress and trauma in HIV disease progression in HIV. *Psychosom Med.* 2008;70:539–545.

Liedtke MD, Lockhart SM, Rathbun RC. Anticonvulsant and antiretroviral interactions. *Ann Pharmacother.* 2004;38(3):482–489. http://doi:10.1345/aph.1D309

Loutfy MR, Logie CH, Zhang Y, et al. Gender and ethnicity differences in HIV-related stigma experienced by people living with HIV in Ontario, Canada. *PLoS One.* 2012;7(12):e48168.

Martinez A, Israelski BS, Walker C, et al. Posttraumatic stress disorder in women attending human immunodeficiency virus outpatient clinics. *AIDS Patient Care STDs.* 2002;98:9–17.

Meade CS, Bevilacqua LA, Key MD. Bipolar disorder is associated with HIV transmission risk behavior among patients in treatment for HIV. *AIDS Behav.* 2012;16(8):2267-2271.

Mellins CA, Havens JF, McDonnell C, et al. Adherence to antiretroviral medications and medical care in HIV-positive adults diagnosed with mental and substance abuse disorders. *AIDS Care.* 2009;21(2):168–177.

Moreno-Pérez, O, Escoín, C, Serna-Candel C. Risk factors for sexual and erectile dysfunction in HIV-infected men: the role or protease inhibitors. *AIDS.* 2010;24:255–264.

Nel A, Kagee A. Common mental health problems and antiretroviral therapy adherence. *AIDS Care.* 2011;23(11):1360–1365.

Nicolussi S, Drewe J, Butterweck V et al. Clinical relevance of St. John's wort drug interactions revisited. *Br J Pharm.* 2019;177(6):1212–1226.

Norman SE, Cheick AD, Freeman C, et al. Sleep disturbances in men with asymptomatic human immunodeficiency (HIV) infection. *Sleep.* 1992;15:150–155.

Omonuwa TS, Goforth HW, Preud'homme X, et al. The pharmacologic management of insomnia in patients with HIV. *J Clin Sleep Med.* 2009;5(3):251–262.

Owe-Larssom B, Sall, L, Allgulander C. HIV infection and psychiatric illness. *Afr J Psychiatry.* 2009;115–128.

Parsi CE, Varma DS, Wang Y, et al. Changes in mental health among people with HIV during the COVID-10 pandemic: qualitative and quantitative perspectives. *AIDS and Behav.* 2022;26(6):1980–1991.

Pence BW. The impact of mental health and traumatic life experiences on antiretroviral treatment outcomes for people living with HIV/AIDS. *J Antimicrob Chemother.* 2009;63(4):636–640.

Pence BW, Miller WC, Gaynes BN, et al. Psychiatric illness and virologic response in patients initiating highly active antiretroviral therapy. *J Acquir Immune Defic Syndr.* 2007;44(2):159–165.

Prince JD, Walkup J, Akincigil A, et al. Serious mental illness and risk of new HIV/AIDS diagnosis: an analysis of Medicaid beneficiaries in eight states. *Psych Serv.* 2012;63(10):1032-1038.

Ramachandran G, Glickman L, Levenson J, et al. Incidence of extrapyramidal syndromes in AIDS patients and a comparison group of medically ill inpatients. *J Neuropsych Clin Neurosci* 1997;9:579-83.

Rao R, Sagar R, Kabra SK, et al. Psychiatric morbidity in HIV-positive children. *AIDS Care.* 2007;19(6):828–833.

Reif S, Wilson E, McAllaster C, et al. The relationship between social support and experienced and internalized HIV-related stigma among people living with HIV in the Deep South. *Stigma and Health.* 2021;6(3):363–369.

Rhodes T. The "risk environment": a framework for understanding and reducing drug-related harm. *Int J Drug Policy.* 2002;13:85–94.

Robertson K, Bayon C, Molina JM, et al. Screening for neurocognitive impairment, depression, and anxiety in HIV-infected patients in Western Europe and Canada. *AIDS Care.* 2014;26(12):1555–1561

Saberi P, Neilands TB, Johnson MO. Quality of sleep: associations with antiretroviral nonadherence. *AIDS Patient Care STDS.* 2011;26(9):517–524.

Scanavino M de T. Sexual dysfunctions of HIV-positive men: associated factors, pathophysiology issues, and clinical management. *Adv Urol.* 2011;2011:854792–854792.

Shindel A, Horberg M, Smith J, et al. Sexual dysfunction, HIV, and AIDS in men who have sex with men. *AIDS Patient Care STD.* 2011;25:41–49.

Treisman G, Angelinno A. Interrelation between psychiatric disorders and the prevention and treatment of HIV infection. *Clin Infect Dis.* 2007;45(Suppl 4):S313–S317.

van Luenen S, Garnefski N, Spinhoven P, et al. The benefits of psychosocial interventions for mental health in people living with HIV: a systemic review and meta-analysis. *AIDS and Behav.* 2018;22:9–42.

Vazquez-Santiago FJ, Noel RJ Jr, Prter JT, et al. Glutamate metabolism and HIV-associated neurocognitive disorders. *J Neurovirol.* 2014;20(4):31–331.

Villes V, Spire B, Lewden C, et al. The effect of depressive symptoms at ART initiation on HIV clinical progression and mortality: implications in clinical practice. *Antivir Ther.* 2007;12:1067–1071.

Walkup J, Wei W, Sambamoorthi U, et al. Antidepressant treatment and adherence to combination antiretroviral therapy among patients with AIDS and diagnosed depression. *Psychiatr Q.* 2008;79(1):43.

Walkup JT, Akincigil A, Chakravarty S, et al. Bipolar medication use and adherence to antiretroviral therapy among patients with HIV-AIDS and bipolar disorder. *Psychiatr Serv.* 2011;62(3):313–316.

Warden D, Rush AJ. The STAR*D project results: a comprehensive review of findings. *Curr Psychiatry Rep.* 2007;9(6):449–459.

Watkins CC, Pieper AA, Treisman GJ. Safety considerations in drug treatment of depression in HIV-positive patients: an updated review. *Drug Saf.* 2011;34(8):623–639.

Whetten K, Reif S, Whetten R, et al. Trauma, mental health, distrust and stigma among HIV-positive persons: implications for effective care. *Psychosom Med.* 2008;70(5):531–538.

Williams DW, Veenstra M, Gaskill PJ, et al. Monocyte mediated HIV neuropathogenesis: mechanisms that contribute to HIV associated neurocognitive disorders. *Curr HIV Res.* 2014;12(2):85096.

Yalin N, Conti I, Bagchi S, et al. Clinical characteristics and impacts of HIV infection in people with bipolar disorders. *J Affect Dis.* 2021;294:794–801.

Yen Y, Lai H, Kuo Y, et al. Association of depression and antidepressant therapy with antiretroviral therapy adherence and health-related quality of life in men who have sex with men. *PLoS One.* 2022;17(2):0264503.

35.

NEUROLOGICAL EFFECTS OF HIV INFECTION

Rodrigo Hasbun and Joseph S. Kass

LEARNING OBJECTIVE

Discuss the clinical features, differential diagnosis, and management of HIV-associated neurocognitive disorders (HAND).

HIV-ASSOCIATED NEUROCOGNITIVE DISORDER

RODRIGO HASBUN

WHAT'S NEW?

- CD8 [+] T- cell encephalitis has been described as a severe form of HAND in patients receiving antiretroviral therapy (ART).

- The central nervous system (CNS) penetration-effectiveness score has been correlated with cerebrospinal fluid (CSF) viral escape.

- CSF viral escape occurred in 7.2% of 1,063 patients, with the most important predictor being a regimen composed of protease inhibitors (PIs) (especially atazanavir) and nucleoside reverse transcriptase inhibitors (NRTIs).

- Neurocognitive impairment has been associated with lack of retention-in-care in older adults, with virologic failure, and, when coupled with frailty, it is associated with greater risk for falls, disability, and death.

- CNS-targeted ART on HAND has shown no benefit in eight clinical trials.

KEY POINTS

- There is a high prevalence of HAND in ART-naive patients and in patients treated with ART with virologic suppression.

- Rapid screening tools such as the Montreal Cognitive Assessment test and the Frontal Assessment Battery test have been evaluated for their use in diagnosing HAND in the clinic.

- HAND is associated with significant cognitive, behavioral, and motor abnormalities that can impact ART adherence, retention-in-care in older individuals, virologic success, and quality of life.

- A recent meta-analysis of eight clinical trials of CNS-targeted ART has not shown benefit in HAND (Webb et al., 2022), while corticosteroids should be considered in patients with CD8 [+] T-cell encephalitis (Lucas et al., 2021).

Despite the use of combination ART with suppressed viremia, up to 39% of PWH currently have neurocognitive impairment (Métral et al., 2020), and up to 42% of patients have at least 1 copy/mL of HIV-1 RNA in the CSF (Anderson et al., 2017). It is unclear if inadequate CSF penetration by some of the ARVs accounts for this high prevalence and whether CNS-active ART improves cognitive impairment. However, higher CSF penetration scores have been correlated with a lower probability of detectable CSF HIV RNA levels (Anderson, 2017). A recent study documented that CSF viral escaped occurred in 7.2% of 1,063 patients with the most important predictor being a regimen composed of PIs (especially atazanavir) and NRTIs (Mukerji et al., 2018). CSF viral escape may be either symptomatic or asymptomatic (Patel et al., 2018). Integrase inhibitors such as bictegravir attain adequate CSF levels and could account for the paucity of symptomatic CSF viral escape cases that are currently being reported (Tiraboshi et al., 2019).

Recently, it has been proposed to divide HAND into four distinct biotypes based on viral and immune pathogenesis (Johnson & Nath, 2022):

1) **Macrophage-mediated HIV encephalitis**: HIV causes a chronic form of encephalitis (HIVE) that is clinically characterized by either dementia or mild neurocognitive impairment. Since the introduction of combination ART in 1996, the incidence of HIV dementia has decreased by 50% (McArthur et al., 2005), but the prevalence of mild neurocognitive disorder (MND) has increased up to 39% (Robertson et al., 2007). HIVE is the result of direct microglial infection, interruption of trophic factors, or caused by inflammatory cytokines (Boisse et al., 2008). HIV enters the brain primarily by the "Trojan horse mechanism": it is carried by monocytes and lymphocytes that cross the blood–brain barrier. HIV has a predilection for the basal ganglia, deep white matter, and hippocampus, resulting in subcortical dementia. Brain computed tomography (CT) scanning or magnetic resonance imaging (MRI) typically show cerebral atrophy

and symmetrical white matter lesions. HIV dementia is a diagnosis of exclusion; other coinfections (e.g., JC virus-associated progressive multifocal leukoencephalopathy (PML), hepatitis C, neurosyphilis, and cryptococcal meningitis), cerebrovascular disease, malnutrition, and drug abuse should be ruled out before making the diagnosis.

2) **CNS viral escape**: PWH receiving ART regimens with low CNS penetration, complicated by their own poor medication adherence or drug-resistant viral mutations can have detectable CSF HIV RNA levels despite virological suppression in the blood. These patients may complain of headaches, tremors, memory impairment, or even focal neurological deficits or seizures. MRI of the brain can show white matter changes in the deep brain nuclei. Even though unproven, consideration to change ART regimens to enhance CNS penetration should be considered. This entity is now seen less frequently in clinical practice as integrase inhibitors have excellent CNS penetration in contrast to PIs.

3) **T-cell-mediated HIV encephalitis**: A severe manifestation of symptomatic CSF viral escape called CD8 [+] T- cell encephalitis has been described in PWH receiving ART with good immunological response (Lescure et al., 2013). Patients can present with neurocognitive impairment, headache, focal neurological deficits, and seizures, with MRI of the brain showing bilateral white matter lesions. CSF usually shows a lymphocytic pleocytosis with CD8 \+ T-cells greater than 65%. A brain biopsy, if performed, shows pronounced CD8 [+] T- cell infiltration with the presence of scant HIV antigens (Figure 35.1) (Johnson et al., 2013) Patients improve dramatically with corticosteroids and with improved CNS penetration of their ART regimen. In the largest case series to date, use of corticosteroids decrease mortality from 69% to 30% in patients with CD8 [+] T-cell encephalitis (Lucas et al., 2021). The optimal dose and duration of corticosteroids are currently unknown.

4) **HIV protein-associated encephalopathy**: This encephalopathy is observed in PWH on ART with undetectable plasma and CSF HIV RNA levels but with detectable HIV proteins such as Tat in the CSF. The HIV viral proteins Tat, Nef, gp120, Vpr, and Gag have been associated with slowly progressive cognitive and psychomotor impairments with neuroimaging findings of cerebral atrophy. If patient undergoes brain biopsy or autopsy, neuronal loss Aβ and Tau are found. Unfortunately, there are no known treatments at this time.

Neuropsychological impairment is a surrogate marker for the presence of HIVE on autopsy (Cherner et al., 2002). Cognitive impairment has also been associated with ART nonadherence (Maggiolo et al., 2007), lack of retention-in-care in older adults (Jacks et al., 2015), and a negative impact on quality of life. In the pre-ART era, it was shown to be an independent predictor of death (Ellis et al., 1997). Further, CSF HIV RNA levels are increased in persons with HIV with neurocognitive impairment, as are several CSF biomarker levels, such as tumor necrosis-α, neurofilament light, neopterin, β2 microglobulin, and monocyte chemotactic protein-1 (Boisse et al., 2008). A recent clinical model identified the following variables as associated with detectable CSF viral load: detectable serum HIV-1 RNA on polymerase chain reaction (PCR), a CNS penetration score lower than 9, non-Caucasian race, less than 95% ART adherence, depression, and less than 36 months of ART duration (Hammond et al., 2014).

CLINICAL MANIFESTATIONS OF HAND

The clinical manifestations of HAND are related to the involvement of HIV in the subcortical structures. The following can occur: slowing of neurocognitive processing speed, motor and psychomotor abnormalities, and executive, planning, or multitasking dysfunction (Valcour, 2011c). HAND affects the following three areas:

- Cognitive: memory, concentration, mental processing speed, and comprehension.

- Behavioral: apathy, depression, agitation, and sometimes mania.

- Motor function: unsteady gait, poor coordination, abnormal tone, and tremors.

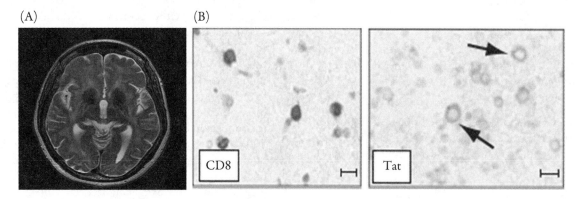

(A)   (B)

Figure 35.1 (A) Magnetic resonance imaging of a PWH with virological suppression for 4 years with biopsy-proven CD8[+] T-cell encephalitis. (B) The presence of CD8[+] T-cells and HIV Tat antigens on brain biopsy and arrows point to stained HIV Tat antigens. SOURCE: Johnson TP, et al. Induction of IL-17 and nonclassical T-cell activation by HIV_TAT protein. *PNAS*. 2013.13;110(33):13588–13593.

In addition, patients with CD8 [\+] T-cell encephalitis can also manifest with new-onset seizures, *status epilepticus*, and altered mental status. Further, HAND is associated with virologic failure (Shahani et al., 2018), and, when combined with frailty, it is associated with greater risk for falls, disability, and death (Erlandson et al., 2018).

RISK FACTORS

Several studies have documented host genetic factors (polymorphisms in apolipoprotein E4, chemokine receptor CCR2, and monocyte chemoattractant protein-1), HIV-specific disease factors (history of AIDS-defining illness or low CD4 [+] T-cell nadir, particular HIV variants, HIV RNA levels in CSF, duration of HIV infection, and older age at seroconversion), age >50 years old, and comorbidities (e.g., anemia, vascular disease, metabolic abnormalities, and hepatitis C coinfection) associated with HAND (Alfahad et al., 2013).

SCREENING TOOLS FOR COGNITIVE IMPAIRMENT

Despite the high prevalence of HAND in HIV clinics, it has not become routine to screen patients for cognitive impairment or to consider more CNS-active ART for those affected, even though there are now recommendations from an international consortium to do so (Mind Exchange Working Group, 2013). Screening tools under evaluation in HAND include several versions of the HIV dementia scale, the Mini Mental Status Exam (MMSE), standardized questionnaires that assess symptoms such as the Medical Outcomes survey, and the Montreal Cognitive Assessment (MoCA) and Frontal Assessment Battery test. The dementia scales are reliable but only in severe cases of HAND, the MMSE is not sensitive enough to detect HAND, and the subjective reporting of cognitive symptoms will miss patients because of poor insight or mood disturbances (Valcour, 2011a, 2011b). The MMSE is now proprietary. Studies have shown that the MoCA is a rapid, reliable, and sensitive test to detect cognitive impairment in PWH (Hasbun et al., 2012, Rosca et al., 2019). A recent large study comparing different screening tools for HAND showed the Frontal Assessment Battery test had the highest correct classification rate (Triunfo et al., 2018).

DEFINITIONS OF NEUROCOGNITIVE DISORDERS

In 2007, the diagnostic criteria for HAND were revised (Antinori, 2007). Three classifications of HANDs were defined using these new criteria: asymptomatic neurocognitive impairment (ANI), MND, and HIV-associated dementia (HAD). *ANI* was defined as having a combination of the following: (1) an acquired mild-to-moderate impairment in cognitive function documented by a score of at least one standard deviation below demographically corrected norms on tests on at least two different cognitive domains, (2) the functional impairment has been seen for more than 1 month, (3) the impairment does not meet criteria for delirium or dementia, and (4) the cognitive impairment is not fully explained by comorbid conditions. The definition of *MND* is identical to that of ANI, but it also includes interference with activities of daily living. The diagnosis of HAD includes a marked impairment of cognitive impairment. Another approach to define neurocognitive impairment is the utilization of the Global Deficit Score (Jacks, 2015) that considers both the number and severity of the individual's performance on the battery of standardized tests. More recently, experts in the field have proposed to modify the 2007 HAND definition to exclude ANI (Nightingale et al., 2021). They propose a new framework that relies more heavily on clinical observations than neurocognitive testing.

CEREBROSPINAL FLUID ACTIVITY OF ANTIRETROVIRALS

There are currently more than 30 US Food and Drug Administration (FDA)-approved ARVs or combinations in six mechanistic classes for treatment of HIV infection, but only some have adequate CSF penetration (US Department of Health and Human Services (USDHHS), 2022a). The CNS penetration-effectiveness (CPE) score has been designed to classify the different ARVs on the basis of their capability of lowering CSF RNA levels (Letendre, 2011). ARVs were assigned a score of from 1 to 4 based on their chemical properties, CSF penetration, and/or effectiveness in CNS studies (Table 35.1). A higher CNS penetration score was associated with higher virologic suppression in the CSF (Letendre, 2010). Further, a study showed that 10% of patients with virologic suppression in the serum had viral escape (detectable CSF RNA levels) (Edén, 2010). In addition, a higher CSF penetration score is associated with a lower rate of neurocognitive impairment (Carvalhal, 2016).

Eight randomized studies in the current era have evaluated the impact of CNS-active ARVs in HAND. A meta-analysis of 3,303 PWH with 13,103 person-year follow-up showed no benefit of ART with high CNS penetration on HIV-related cognitive impairment (Webb et al., 2022).

RECOMMENDED READING

Webb AJ, Borrelli EP, Vyas A, Taylor LE, Buchanan AL. The effect of antiretroviral therapy with high central nervous system penetration on HIV-related cognitive impairment: a systematic review and meta-analysis. *AIDS Care.* July18, 2022:1–12. doi:1080/09540121.20222098231.

Johnson TP, Nath A. Biotypes of HIV-associated neurocognitive disorders based on viral and immune pathogenesis. *Curr Opin Infect Dis.* June 12, 2022;35(3):223–230.

Nightingale S, Dreyer AJ, Saylor D, Gisslén M, Winston A, Joska JA. Moving on from HAND: why we need new criteria for cognitive impairment in persons living with human immunodeficiency virus and a proposed way forward. *Clin Infect Dis.* September 15, 2021;73(6):1113–1118.

Table 35.1 CNS PENETRATION-EFFECTIVENESS (CPE) SCORE OF DIFFERENT ARVS

DRUG CLASS	4	3	2	1
NRTIs	Zidovudine	Abacavir Emtricitabine	Didanosine Lamivudine Stavudine	Tenofovir Zalcitabine
NNRTIs	Nevirapine	Delavirdine Efavirenz	Etravirine	
Protease inhibitors	Indinavir	Darunavir/r Fosamprenavir/r Indinavir Lopinavir/r	Atazanavir Atazanavir/r Fosamprenavir	Nelfinavir Ritonavir Saquinavir Saquinavir/r
Entry/fusion inhibitors		Maraviroc		Enfuvirtide
Integrase inhibitors		Raltegravir Dolutegravir		

NRTI, nucleoside reverse transcriptase inhibitor; NNRTI, nonnucleoside reverse transcriptase inhibitor.

Adapted from Letendre et al. *Top Antivir Med.* 2011;19(4):137–142.

MENINGITIS

Rodrigo Hasbun

LEARNING OBJECTIVE

Review the differential diagnosis and clinical management of meningitis in people with HIV (PWH).

WHAT'S NEW?

- ART initiation should be deferred in cryptococcal meningitis.

- A recent clinical trial showed that one dose of liposomal amphotericin B in combination with oral flucytosine and oral fluconazole in patients with cryptococcal meningitis in Africa was as effective as the standard of care (Jarvis et al., 2022). This new regimen is now advocated by the World Health Organization (WHO) as the first-line therapy.

- HIV testing is done in only 50% of CNS infections even though the US Centers for Disease Control and Prevention recommends universal testing.

- Meningococcal A vaccine has decreased the burden of meningococcal meningitis serogroup A in Africa but outbreaks remain with non-A serogroup meningococcal or nonmeningococcal meningitis isolates.

KEY POINTS

- The differential diagnosis of meningitis in PWH is broad (e.g., viral, bacterial, fungal, mycobacterial, and lymphomatous) (Table 35.2).

- All adults with meningitis should be tested for HIV.

- Meningitis in PWH is usually treatable, and a cause should be investigated.

- A meta-analysis of studies of meningitis in PWH in Africa documented that the three most common causes were *C. neoformans*, *M. tuberculosis*, and bacterial meningitis.

NEUROLOGIC EVENTS IN EARLY-STAGE HIV INFECTION

Acute HIV infection may manifest as an "aseptic meningitis" presentation, but this is most likely underdiagnosed as < 50% of adults with meningitis are tested for HIV, and only 1% are

Table 35.2 CAUSES OF MENINGITIS IN PWH

Viral	Acute HIV seroconversion, CD8[+] T-cell encephalitis, enterovirus, herpes simplex virus, arboviruses (West Nile virus, St. Louis encephalitis), cytomegalovirus, varicella zoster virus, influenza virus, Epstein–Barr virus, lymphocytic choriomeningitis virus, mumps
Bacterial	Bacterial meningitis, endocarditis, parameningeal focus (e.g., epidural abscess and mastoiditis), syphilis, Lyme disease, *Mycoplasma pneumoniae*, *Bartonella henselae*, Brucella species, *Ehrlichia*, *Rickettsia*, leptospirosis, *Mycobacterium tuberculosis*
Fungal	*Cryptococcus neoformans*, *Coccidioides immitis*, *Histoplasma capsulatum*, Aspergillus species, zygomycosis
Parasitic	*Naegleria/Acanthamoeba*, *Taenia solium*, *Angiostrongylus cantonensis*, *Toxoplasma gondii*
Noninfectious	Medications (e.g., antibiotics and nonsteroidal anti-inflammatory drugs), meningeal carcinomatosis (lymphoma and leukemia), vasculitis, chemical meningitis (intrathecal injections and spinal anesthesia), seizures

tested for HIV RNA levels to rule out HIV seroconversion syndrome (Ma et al., 2020). Individuals with HIV exposure and infection may present with severe headache, stiff neck, diffuse macular rash, photophobia, and a lymphocytic pleocytosis in the CSF. Patients typically have positive plasma HIV RNA levels and/or a positive HIV p24 antigen.

Approximately one-third of PWH who present with meningitis do so during the early stages of the HIV disease (i.e., CD4$^+$ T-cell count >200 cells/mm^3) (Vigil et al., 2018). The most common causes of meningitis in these patients are herpes simplex type 2, varicella zoster virus (VZV), and arboviruses (e.g., West Nile, St. Louis encephalitis). Herpes simplex type 2 can present with the initial genital outbreak of herpes or in patients with recurrent episodes of aseptic meningitis (Mollaret's meningitis). Arboviruses should be suspected in the summer and fall in patients with fever and recent mosquito bites. Unfortunately, viral PCR and arboviral serologies are obtained in the minority of patients with meningitis (Nesher et al., 2016; Shukla et al., 2017). Other less common causes of meningitis in PWH include VZV, syphilis, and bacterial meningitis. VZV can present with a dermatomal vesicular rash and an aseptic meningitis presentation, and the diagnosis of VZV meningitis should prompt screening for HIV. In more advanced stages of HIV infection, VZV can present as disseminated disease. It can also present without a rash (zoster sine herpete), with the Ramsay–Hunt syndrome, or with stroke, myelopathy, retinitis, or encephalitis.

The diagnosis is made by a CSF VZV PCR or by a CSF anti-VZV antibody or presumptively from a VZV PCR of a vesicular lesion in patient presenting with a CNS infection. CSF VZV PCR has a specificity of greater than 95% but a sensitivity of only 30%. A positive VZV PCR confirms the diagnosis, but a negative test does not rule out the diagnosis. CSF anti-VZV antibody is the more sensitive test, with a 98% sensitivity (Aberle et al., 2005; DeBiasi & Tyler, 2004; Nagel, 2007; Osiro & Salomon, 2017). Treatment is with high-dose intravenous acyclovir.

Syphilis can also present as an aseptic meningitis syndrome in patients with a diffuse rash that involves the palms and soles. A serum rapid plasma reagin of *greater than 1:32* and a CD4$^+$ T-cell count of less than 350 cells/mm^3 are associated with neurosyphilis and should prompt the performance of a lumbar puncture (Marra et al., 2004). Bacterial meningitis represents a diagnostic consideration in all stages of HIV, but its incidence has decreased with the advent of the conjugate vaccines (Lopez Castelblanco et al., 2014). If bacterial meningitis is suspected, intravenous dexamethasone and antibiotic therapy with vancomycin, ceftriaxone, and ampicillin should be initiated to cover for *Streptococcus pneumoniae*, *Neisseria meningitides*, and *Listeria monocytogenes* until CSF cultures are negative (Tunkel et al., 2004). If the patient has *Listeria monocytogenes* or *Cryptococcus neoformans* meningitis, dexamethasone should be discontinued as its use has been associated with higher mortality or morbidity, respectively (Beardsley, et al., 2016; Charlier et al., 2017). Further, delayed cerebral injury has been documented in 4% of patients with bacterial meningitis with an association with the use of steroids (Gallegos et al., 2018). Despite this, dexamethasone

should continue to be used in pneumococcal meningitis where it is associated with a decrease in mortality (Hasbun et al., 2017).

NEUROLOGIC EVENTS IN LATE-STAGE HIV INFECTION (CD4$^+$ T-CELL COUNT < 200 CELLS/MM^3)

The most common cause of meningitis in patients with advanced immunosuppression is *Cryptococcus neoformans*, TB, CMV, and toxoplasmosis. In cryptococcal meningitis, the CSF examination typically shows a lymphocytic pleocytosis, but inflammation may be absent. CSF India ink examination is positive in up to 50% of cases, and the CSF cryptococcal antigen test is positive in approximately 90% of cases. The film array multiplex meningitis encephalitis PCR panel that includes *Cryptococcus neoformans or gattii* can be falsely negative in up to 50% of cryptococcal isolates, and testing should be combined with a cryptococcal antigen (Leisman et al., 2018). An opening pressure should be documented since elevated opening pressure is associated with higher CSF fungal burden and higher neurological morbidity and mortality (Gambarin & Hamill, 2002). The preferred therapy for cryptococcal meningitis is a combination of intravenous amphotericin B deoxycholate at 0.7–1 mg/kg/d plus flucytosine 100 mg/kg/d divided in four doses for 2 weeks, followed by fluconazole 400 mg/d PO. Daily CSF drainage is necessary to decrease the intracranial hypertension (i.e., >25 cm of H$_2$O) by either repeat lumbar punctures. Temporary percutaneous lumbar drains or ventriculostomy may be required if persistent elevations in intracranial pressure occur, as measured by lumbar puncture (Perfect et al., 2012). If flucytosine is not available or the patient experiences drug toxicity, the treatment regimen can be switched to a combination of amphotericin B with fluconazole either 400 mg or 800 mg once daily for 14 days. A repeat lumbar puncture should be done at the end of the 2-week period to document a negative CSF fungal culture. Intravenous amphotericin B should be continued if the patient has persistently positive CSF cultures, is clinically deteriorating or comatose, or has persistently elevated and symptomatic intracranial pressures (Perfect et al., 2012). A therapeutic lumbar puncture to decrease intracranial pressure was associated with a reduced risk of death in a study performed in Africa (Rolfes et al., 2014). The same study also documented that ART should be delayed until 5 weeks after initial presentation to avoid an increase in mortality (Boulware et al., 2014). In underdeveloped countries, the treatment advocated by the WHO is different with the recommendation of one week of intravenous amphotericin B followed by 7 days of oral flucytosine and 7 days of oral fluconazole. A recent clinical trial showed that one dose of liposomal amphotericin B in combination with oral flucytosine and oral fluconazole in patients with cryptococcal meningitis in Africa was as effective as the standard of care (Jarvis et al., 2022). This new regimen of one single IV dose of liposomal amphotericin B is now advocated by the WHO as the first-line therapy as of April 2022.

CMV can cause meningitis, ventriculitis, polyradiculitis, polyradiculomyelopathy, retinitis, esophagitis, and colitis in patients with advanced HIV disease (CD4 $^+$ T-cell count < 50 cells/mm^3). CMV infection of the nervous system accounts for fewer than 1% of CMV infections in PWH (McCutchan, 1995) and often develops concurrently with other, more common CMV extraneural disease such as retinitis or gastrointestinal involvement even while individuals are on treatment with ganciclovir for extra-CNS disease (Bermann & Kim, 1994). CMV encephalitis is the most common manifestation of CNS infection owing to CMV. The CSF typically show low or absent pleocytosis in up to 22% of patients with CSF protein levels < 100 mg/ml in 60% of patients. CMV encephalitis can have typical MRI findings of periventricular enhancement in up to one-third of patients. CMV is seen more commonly in patients with AIDS and is associated with adverse clinical outcomes in approximately two-thirds of the patients (Handley et al., 2021). Clinically, infection can present as diffuse encephalitis, ventriculoencephalitis, or focal encephalitis. Diffuse encephalitis develops over several weeks and thus presents subacutely with memory loss, attention and concentration difficulties, and delirium. Focal neurological deficits may also be seen. Pathologically, microglial nodules may be found in the cortex, brainstem, cerebellum, and basal ganglia, occurring most commonly in gray matter (Morgello et al., 1987). On neuroimaging, MRI may show a variety of patterns. The brain may appear normal, or it may show hyperintense T2 lesions in the areas described previously and nodular lesions with or without enhancement on T1 postcontrast images (Maschke et al., 2002).

Ventriculoencephalitis presents with lethargy, confusion, cranial nerve deficits, ataxia, and focal neurological deficits, and it sometimes occurs concomitantly with CMV polyradiculitis. Ventriculoencephalitis may be more insidious in onset and have a poorer prognosis (Maschke et al., 2002). Pathologically, necrotizing lesions are seen in the ventricular system, and imaging shows periventricular enhancement with or without ventriculomegaly. The third and less common type of CMV encephalitis, focal encephalitis, presents with focal neurological deficits corresponding to a cerebral mass lesion. MRI will show ring-enhancing lesions with surrounding edema.

CSF PCR for CMV DNA confirms the diagnosis of CMV encephalitis. The detection of other viruses often confounds the diagnosis; thus, the index of suspicion must be based on the presentation and imaging findings in the context of profound immunosuppression. The differential diagnosis for CMV encephalitis must include HIV encephalitis, PML, and neurosyphilis. When CMV encephalitis presents as a ring-enhancing lesion, the differential diagnosis expands to other etiologies known to present similarly, such as toxoplasmosis, primary CNS lymphoma, and tuberculous meningitis with tuberculomas (Offiah & Turnbull, 2006).

CMV is treated initially with intravenous ganciclovir 5 mg/kg every 12 hours, and then switched to oral valganciclovir when the patient is stable (USDHHS, 2022b). Sometimes in severe encephalitis cases, combination treatment with both ganciclovir and foscarnet has been used (Portegies et al., 2004;

Silva et al., 2010). Cidofovir can be used as an alternate treatment option. Empiric treatment of CMV infection is often advised because CSF results may be delayed.

Mycobacterial TB can occur at any stage of the HIV illness, but extrapulmonary disease (e.g., meningitis, lymphadenitis, pleuritis, and pericarditis) occurs more frequently in patients with CD4 $^+$ T-cell counts of less than 200 cells/mm^3. The incidence of TB has declined in the United States, and there are fewer than 1,000 cases of coinfection reported annually (USDHHS, 2022b). TB and HIV must be treated together rather than sequentially, particularly in patients with CD4 $^+$ T-cell counts less than 50 cells/mm^3. Tuberculous meningitis usually has a subacute to chronic presentation, lymphocytic pleocytosis, a low CSF glucose, and basilar involvement with cranial nerve palsies and altered mental status. A Thwaites's diagnostic score less than 4 (which covers five parameters: age, duration of illness, white blood cell count, total CSF white blood cell count, and percentage of CSF neutrophils) or a Lancet consensus score of greater than 6 (including 20 parameters divided in four categories: clinical, CSF, CNS imaging, and evidence of TB elsewhere) indicate possible TB meningitis, and patients with these scores should be considered for empiric therapy. The CSF acid-fast bacilli smear is insensitive, and CSF cultures are positive in only 38–88% of cases (Thwaites, 2012). Caution should be used as neurobrucellosis and patient with fungal meningitis may also have high scores for TB meningitis (Erdem et al., 2015, Sulaiman et al., 2020). A CSF *M. tuberculosis* PCR and an adenosine deaminase level can also aid in the diagnosis. Duration of treatment is 1 year. The mortality is higher for PWH than those without HIV and TB meningitis (51.3% vs. 23%) (Thao et al., 2013). Prognostic factors for death in HIV coinfected patients include severity of illness, lower CSF pleocytosis, lower weight, lower CD4 $^+$ T-cell counts, and abnormal sodium levels (Thao et al., 2018).

Finally, toxoplasmosis may also present with a meningitis/encephalitis presentation in patients with advanced AIDS (Opintan et al., 2017). Toxoplasmosis classically presents with fever, focal neurological signs, seizures, and headaches, with MRI of the brain showing multiple ring-enhancing lesions. Toxoplasmosis is a very unlikely cause of disease if the serum *Toxoplasma* IgG is negative (Rosenow & Hirschfield, 2007). If the serology is negative or the neuroimaging is not suggestive of toxoplasmosis, an early brain biopsy is advocated (Rosenow & Hirschfield, 2007).

MENINGITIS IN PWH VERSUS PERSONS WITHOUT HIV

A recent study of 549 adults with community-acquired meningitis who were tested for HIV revealed that 25% were infected (Vigi et al., 2018). PWH presented with less meningeal symptoms (e.g., headache, neck stiffness, and Kernig's sign), but with higher rates of hypoglycorrhachia, elevated CSF protein, and abnormal cranial imaging. PWH also were more likely to have cryptococcal meningitis, neurosyphilis, and VZV than those without HIV. PWH were also more likely to have a pathogen identified (57%) than those without HIV (31%). An adverse clinical outcome was seen in approximately 25% of patients with abnormal neurological exam and hypoglycorrhachia being identified as predictors. HIV coinfection was not associated with an adverse outcome.

IMMUNE RECONSTITUTION SYNDROME IN HIV

immune reconstitution inflammatory syndrome (IRIS) occurs after the initiation of combination ART and either "unmasks" a previous subclinical infection or worsens a known infection despite appropriate therapy (paradoxical reaction). In the CNS, IRIS can develop with many opportunistic processes, most commonly cryptococcal meningitis, TB meningitis, and PML (Huis in't Veld et al., 2012). The two most common and serious CNS IRIS events are cryptococcal and tuberculous meningitis. TB IRIS usually presents between a few weeks to 3 months after the initiation of ART, and it can present with meningitis or tuberculomas or both. Risk factors include low $CD4^+$ T-cell counts, disseminated TB, and extrapulmonary TB. Treatment should consist of adjunctive steroids. CSF acid-fast bacilli cultures are typically negative. Cryptococcal IRIS can develop between 1 and 10 months after initiating ART and can present as culture-negative meningitis, cryptococcomas, pneumonitis, and/or lymphadenopathy. Adjunctive steroids should be considered. Additionally, $CD8^+$ T-cell encephalitis syndrome has been described in patients receiving ART with low or undetectable serum HIV RNA levels (Lucas et al., 2021). These patients usually have a low $CD4^+$ T-cell count nadir and a history of opportunistic infections, and they usually present with high $CD4^+$ T-cell counts. They can present with memory disturbances, headaches, diplopia, ataxia, and, sometimes, seizures. MRI of the brain shows bilateral white matter lesions, and CSF shows lymphocytic pleocytosis with detectable CSF HIV RNA. The treatment is corticosteroids as it can decrease mortality from 68% to 30% and consider optimizing the CNS penetration of ART.

MENINGITIS IN RESOURCE-LIMITED COUNTRIES

The majority of patients with meningitis in Africa have unknown etiologies. A recent study of 1,501 patients with meningitis in Mozambique showed that only ~10% had an etiologic diagnosis (61% bacterial meningitis and 39% cryptococcal meningitis) (Nhantumbo et al., 2022). A review of 1,303 episodes of meningitis with confirmed etiologies among PWH in Sub-Saharan Africa showed that 52% had cryptococcal meningitis; 19.6% had TB; 14.2% had bacterial meningitis; and 14.2% had other etiologies (Veltman et al., 2014). Mortality rates were high, ranging from 25% to 68% in the different studies. A recent clinical trial done in Africa concluded that a one dose of liposomal amphotericin B plus 2 weeks of oral flucytosine and oral fluconazole as was effective in cryptococcal meningitis as the WHO recommended treatment (1 week of amphotericin B plus oral flucytosine for 7 days, followed by oral fluconazole for 7 days) (Jarvis et al.,

2022). The WHO has updated their recommendation and is now advocating the single dose of liposomal amphotericin B plus oral flucytosine and fluconazole as the preferred regimen.

MYELOPATHY

Joseph S. Kass

LEARNING OBJECTIVE

Discuss the clinical presentation, differential diagnosis, and management of HIV-associated vacuolar myelopathy in PWH.

WHAT'S NEW?

The incidence of HIV-associated vacuolar myelopathy (VM) has been reduced significantly. It remains a cause of disability in end-stage HIV and has a poor prognosis.

KEY POINTS

- VM is an uncommon complication that tends to occur in the late stages of HIV infection.

- Acute transverse myelitis and inflammatory CSF are unlikely to be VM.

- Human T-cell lymphotropic virus type 1 (HTLV-1) infection is another infectious cause of myelopathy, and it should be considered in endemic geographic areas and in cases of coinfection with HIV.

- Both HIV and HTLV-1 can cause chronic myelopathy involving dorsal and lateral columns.

- The work-up for a myelopathic patient includes MRI of the spine with and without contrast and may include CSF analysis and investigations for nutritional deficiencies and toxic agents.

HIV-ASSOCIATED VACUOLAR MYELOPATHY

PWH may develop *myelopathy* for many reasons. At the time of seroconversion, an acute transverse myelitis may develop, whereas severe immunosuppression puts individuals at risk of developing HIV-associated VM as well as opportunistic processes that either invade or compress the spinal cord. PWH may also develop myelopathy from causes typical of the general population without HIV, such as spondylosis with spinal stenosis.

Primary HIV-associated acute transverse myelitis is a rare inflammatory myelopathy resulting from immune activation, and typically develops within days to weeks of acute HIV seroconversion. Individuals present with an acute myelopathy in the thoracic region, experiencing lower extremity weakness, a thoracic sensory level with numbness below the sensory level, sphincter dysfunction, and eventually hyperreflexia and spasticity. CSF is typically inflammatory with a lymphocytic pleocytosis. This acute transverse myelitis tends to respond well to steroids, intravenous immunoglobulin (IVIG), and ART (Hamada et al., 2011).

In contrast, VM is a chronic myelopathy seen in the late stages of HIV infection and affects 10%–15% of untreated people with AIDS. VM unfolds as a slow, painless progression of neurologic symptoms over several months, most commonly lower extremity weakness and spasticity (Di Rocco, 1999). Patients typically complain of progressive weakness or clumsiness in the lower extremities, as well as leg cramps and difficulty walking. Urinary symptoms such as frequency and urgency, along with erectile dysfunction, are also common. Sensation in the legs, particularly proprioception and vibratory sense, is usually impaired, but a clear sensory level on the trunk is unusual. Arms are typically spared until advanced-stage disease. Localized back pain is not a common feature. Individuals are also typically hyperreflexic in the lower extremities (hyperreflexia may spread to the upper extremities if the cervical cord is involved) and exhibit extensor plantar responses. There is no effective treatment for VM. Patients with VM often have coexisting HAD and peripheral neuropathy. Rehabilitation is helpful to maximize physical capacity. ART does not appear to alter the natural history of the disease (Banks et al., 2002). Antispasmodic agents such as baclofen, tizanidine, or botulinum toxin can be used for symptomatic relief of spasticity.

VM is the result of a chronic inflammatory degeneration with vacuolization and myelin pallor of the lateral and posterior tracts, typically affecting the thoracic cord most severely. On histologic examination, the lateral and dorsal columns demonstrate axonal injury and macrophage infiltration with lipid-laden macrophages and microglia infected with HIV (Dal Pan et al., 1997; Petito et al., 1994; Tyor et al., 1993). As many as 20%–50% of individuals with AIDS may have pathological evidence of VM at autopsy (Dal Pan et al., 1994; Di Rocco & Simpson, 1998; McArthur et al., 2005), yet only 6.5% to 10% of individuals with AIDS manifest clinical VM (Cho & Vaitkevicius, 2012). MRI of the spinal cord in VM lacks pathognomonic features to differentiate it from non–HIV-related spinal cord disease. Although the spinal cord may appear normal, most affected spinal cords appear atrophic with or without hyperintensities on T_2-weighted images (Chong et al., 1999; Yousem & Grossman, 2010).

The differential diagnosis for myelopathy in a PWH is broad and includes the following categories: (1) infections, including HTLV-1-associated myelopathy/tropical spastic paraparesis (HAM/TSP; discussed later), tuberculosis (TB) spondylitis or meningomyelitis, cytomegalovirus (CMV) radiculomyelitis, varicella zoster myelitis, *Toxoplasma* myelopathy, neurosyphilis with tabes dorsalis, and bacterial epidural abscess (particularly among people who inject drugs); (2) neoplastic diseases, especially lymphoma and spinal metastases from systemic neoplasms; (3) nutritional deficiencies such as B12, folate, copper, thiamine (presenting as beriberi), and vitamin E; and (4) toxic etiologies such as lathyrism (Di Rocco & Simpson, 1998). Thus, an MRI of the spinal cord with and without contrast, lumbar puncture

with CSF analysis, and serum analysis for vitamin and mineral deficiencies will be needed to evaluate for these etiologies (Chong et al., 1999).

Clinicians should consider common infectious causes initially. One study from Cape Town, Africa—an area known for a high prevalence of TB and HIV—reviewed 216 cases of myelopathy and cauda equina syndrome in patients with HIV (median CD4$^+$ count 185 cell/mm^3). Investigators found that 68% of myelopathy cases were due to TB (Candy et al., 2014). This large number of TB-related myelopathy cases in patients with HIV has also been seen in other small studies in Africa (Bhigjee et al., 2001; Modi et al., 2011). TB spondylitis could be diagnosed radiographically with a high degree of certainty using MRI, and the diagnosis was confirmed with either CSF analysis or open biopsy.

MRI IN HIV-ASSOCIATED VACUOLAR MYELOPATHY

MRI of the spinal cord in VM is nonspecific and thus lacks pathognomonic features to differentiate it from non-HIV-related spinal cord disease. The spinal cord may appear normal, but the most affected spinal cords appear atrophic with or without hyperintensities on T2-weighted images (Chong et al., 1999; Yousem & Grossman, 2010).

HTLV-1-ASSOCIATED MYELOPATHY (HAM)/ TROPICAL SPASTIC PARAPARESIS (TSP)

HTLV-1 is a retrovirus that is T-cell tropic and causes a proliferation of T-cells (Manns et al., 1999). Although its full disease spectrum remains unknown, this virus is associated with adult T-cell leukemia/lymphoma, uveitis, and HAM, which is also referred to as TSP. The prevalence of HTLV-1 infection increases with age, and it is more common in women than in men. It is also geographically clustered, with high rates in southern Japan, the Caribbean, areas of Africa, the Middle East, South America, the Pacific Melanesian Islands, and Papua New Guinea. Among low-risk groups in the United States and Europe, seroprevalence is approximately 1%, with the majority of these individuals remaining asymptomatic. Approximately 1% of HTLV-1-positive individuals develop a myelopathy (Pillat et al., 2011). Given the overlapping risk factors for both HIV and HTLV-1 infection, HIV and HTLV-1 coinfection should be considered in PWH presenting with a slowly progressive myelopathy.

Patients with HAM present with progressive muscle weakness in the legs, hyperreflexia, clonus, extensor plantar responses, sensory disturbances, urinary incontinence, and lower back pain. HTLV-1 antibodies are present in both plasma and the CSF, as well as in brain and spinal cord tissue. The diagnostic approach to HAM/TSP is like that outlined previously for VM, including MRI of the spine with and without contrast, lumbar puncture, and an investigation for nutritional deficiencies and toxic exposures. Definitive diagnosis requires an assay to detect HTLV-1 antibodies in plasma and CSF, including an assay capable of distinguishing between HTLV-1 and HTLV-2.

HAM/TSP is thought to arise from chronic inflammation of the spinal cord attributable to a brisk activation of cytotoxic T lymphocytes against HTLV-1 within the CNS (Yamauchi et al., 2021). No antiretroviral or immune-modulating therapy has proven curative. INF-α is the only medication that has been tested for the treatment of HAM/TSP in a randomized controlled trial, and it demonstrated improved neurological symptoms after four weeks of therapy (Izumo et al., 1996). Corticosteroids remain the most commonly used disease modifying agent despite observational studies that offer conflicting data about benefit in the treatment of HTLV-1 myelopathy. Research is under way to develop new therapies in addition to preventive and therapeutic vaccines for HTLV-1 (Martin & Taylor, 2011), but currently prevention education, particularly regarding breastfeeding and sexual behavior, is the only known method of reducing incidence.

RECOMMENDED READING

Di Rocco A. Diseases of the spinal cord in human immunodeficiency virus infection. *Semin Neurol.* 1999;19:151–155.

Izumo S, Goto I, Itoyama Y, et al. Interferon-alpha is effective in HTLV-I-associated myelopathy: a multicenter, randomized, double-blind, controlled trial. *Neurology.* 1996;46:1016–1021.

Manns A, Hisada M, La Grenade L. Human T-lymphotropic virus type I infection. *Lancet.* 1999;353:1951–1958.

Yamauchi J, Araya N, Yagishita N, et al. An update on human T-cell leukemia virus type I (HTLV-1)-associated myelopathy/tropical spastic paraparesis (HAM/TSP) focusing on clinical and laboratory biomarkers. *Pharmacol Ther.* 2021;218:107669.

DISTAL SYMMETRICAL POLYNEUROPATHY

Joseph S. Kass

WHAT'S NEW?

Use of a high-concentration capsaicin dermal patch has shown efficacy in patients with painful HIV distal symmetric polyneuropathy (SDPN), and in one, it study produced a sustained reduction in pain over 12 weeks.

KEY POINTS

- DSPN is the most common neurologic complication of HIV infection, occurring in 30%–60% of patients.

- Antiretroviral (ARV) toxic neuropathy is associated with use of older NRTI therapy, especially for didanosine and stavudine.

- Treatment includes removal of neurotoxins and management of pain and discomfort.

Distal Symmetrical polyneuropathy (DSPN) occurs in 30%–60% of patients with HIV (Ellis et al., 2010; Evans et al., 2011), making it the most common neurologic complication in HIV disease. Its incidence increases to as high as 62% in advanced HIV (Schifitto et al., 2002; Simpson et al., 2006). DSPN may develop at any time after the onset of HIV infection, with a mean time to developing neuropathy of 9.5 years after HIV diagnosis (Robinson-Papp & Simpson, 2009b). However, a smaller study suggested that signs of neuropathy may be detected in as many as 35% of PWH with a median of only 3.5 months after HIV transmission (Wang et al., 2014). Although the etiology of DSPN is still under investigation, it is most likely an indirect result of HIV infection, probably through immune-mediated mechanisms (Pardo et al., 2001).

Advanced immunosuppression was the major risk factor for developing DSPN before the advent of ART (Childs et al., 1999); it remains a risk factor for untreated individuals (Vecchio et al., 2020). Risk factors for developing DSPN among ARV-treated individuals include older age, Caucasian race, lower hemoglobin levels, hypertriglyceridemia, lower $CD4^+$ cell count nadir, current combination ART use, and past use of the dideoxynucleoside drugs (didanosine, stavudine, and zalcitabine) (Banerjee et al., 2011; Ellis et al., 2010; Simpson et al., 2006; Tagliati et al., 1999). Although the prevalence of DSPN appears to decline with ART initiation (Vecchio et al., 2020; Ellis et al., 2010), ART-treated individuals with undetectable viral loads and higher $CD4^+$ cell counts may still develop DSPN (Verma et al., 2004). Virologically suppressed individuals who initiate ART after $CD4^+$ T-cell counts fall below 350/μL appear to be at increased risk of DSPN compared to those who never achieve that degree of immunosuppression. This correlation holds true even after adjusting for age, duration of HIV infection, and use of dideoxynucleoside drugs (didanosine, stavudine, and zalcitabine) (D-drugs). It also suggests that earlier initiation of ART may help reduce the risk of DSPN, but the elevated risk of DSPN in individuals who experience a low CD4 nadir is independent of the eventual success of ART in achieving virologic suppression (Ellis et al., 2010).

Neuropathy associated with D-drugs (especially didanosine, stavudine, and zalcitabine NRTIs) is the only neurologic complication of HIV that has increased since the introduction of ART (Keswani et al., 2002). The risk of ARV toxic neuropathy (ATN) appears to be substantially higher when didanosine and stavudine were used together, especially when combined with hydroxyurea (Moore et al., 2000). DSPN and ATN are clinically very similar, although ATN often has a more acute onset with more rapid progression (Pardo et al., 2001; Price et al., 1999). A current hypothesis is that mitochondrial dysfunction mediates NRTI toxicity (Kallianpur & Hulgan, 2009).

Typical DSPN symptoms include symmetric spontaneous and evoked tingling, numbness, stabbing sensations, and burning predominantly in the feet and progressing to the upper extremities (Figure 35.2) (Cornblath & McArthur, 1988; DeVivo et al., 2000; Price et al., 1999; Wulff & Simpson, 1999a). In research cohorts, DPSN may be detected in the absence of clinical symptoms if one of the following signs manifests bilaterally: diminished ability to recognize vibration and reduced sharp-dull discrimination in the feet and toes or reduced ankle reflexes. Not all DSPN patients experience neuropathic pain. Although 57% of the over 1,500

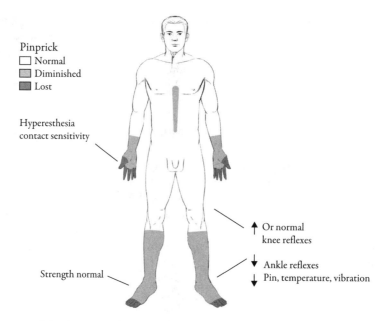

Pinprick
☐ Normal
▨ Diminished
▩ Lost

Hyperesthesia
contact sensitivity

↑ Or normal
knee reflexes

↓ Ankle reflexes
↓ Pin, temperature, vibration

Strength normal

Figure 35.2 Typical signs and symptoms of distal sensory polyneuropathy

CHARTER cohort subjects were diagnosed with DSPN, only 38% reported neuropathic symptoms (Ellis et al., 2010). Risk factors for neuropathic pain differed from risk factors for DSPN itself and included past D-drug use and higher rather than lower CD4[+] T-cell nadir (Ellis et al., 2010).

DSPN is the result of damage to and loss of both large- and small-caliber sensory nerve fibers, with macrophage infiltration in the dorsal root ganglia and along the nerve trunks (Keswani et al., 2002). Activation of macrophages and the production of proinflammatory cytokines appear to play significant roles in the neuropathogenesis of DSPN (Pardo et al., 2001). Secreted viral proteins such as the envelope glycoprotein gp120 may also contribute to HIV-induced neurotoxicity (Keswani et al., 2003). DNA damage in the mitochondria of distal axons may add to the distal degeneration of sensory nerve fibers (Lehmann et al., 2011). Sural nerve biopsies obtained from patients with ATN have shown severe axonal destruction, prominent in unmyelinated fibers (Dalakas & Cupler, 1996). Prominent mitochondrial abnormalities have more significantly been noted in association with NRTIs, supporting the suggestion that neuronal mitochondrial damage underlies ATN (Chen et al., 1991). Further support for this concept is derived from in vitro observations of graded inhibition of γ-DNA polymerase by different NRTIs (Martin et al., 1994). The D-drugs are the most potent inhibitors of this enzyme in vitro (Martin et al., 1994), whereas zidovudine, lamivudine, abacavir, emtricitabine, and tenofovir have only minimal effects. Mitochondrial DNA content in lymphocytes, however, does not correlate with the presence of ATN (Simpson et al., 2006).

The differential diagnosis of DSPN/ATN includes other toxic neuropathies caused by other medications commonly used in patients with HIV such as metronidazole, dapsone, vincristine, isoniazid (DeVivo et al., 2000), and fluoroquinolones (Cohen, 2001), as well as diabetes mellitus, vitamin B12 deficiency, diffuse infiltrative lymphocytosis syndrome,

alcohol abuse, hepatitis C, and uremia (DeVivo et al., 2000; Williams et al., 2002).

Both DSPN and ATN are usually diagnosed on clinical grounds. On study reported that a brief screening examination performed at a single center by trained nonphysicians correlated well with the diagnosis of DSPN made by an experienced neurologist (Marra et al., 1998). In a multicenter study, however, nonphysician neurological findings were less reliable (Simpson et al., 2006). Nerve conduction studies can be useful, typically showing axonal neuropathy with absent or reduced sensory nerve action potentials, although they might be normal in either mild cases or when the neuropathy is restricted to small fibers (DeVivo et al., 2000). Punch skin biopsies have been used to identify reduced densities of unmyelinated nerve fibers in HIV-associated sensory neuropathies. Skin biopsy analysis is now available in some settings, and it is particularly helpful either when symptoms of burning pain are more prominent than actual neurologic signs or when a nonorganic cause of sensory symptoms is suspected (Polydefkis et al., 2002). Quantitative sudomotor axon reflex test may also be performed to document small-fiber neuropathy. In a study of 102 patients with HIV, autonomic dysfunction was present in 62% of participants (Robinson-Papp et al., 2013). Sural nerve biopsy is rarely indicated except when mononeuritis multiplex is suspected, because this entity raises the specter of vasculitis.

Diagnosis of neurotoxic neuropathy can be confirmed by withdrawal of the suspected neurotoxin and monitoring for attenuation of symptoms. Symptoms typically improve or resolve over 2–10 weeks in approximately two-thirds of patients (Blum et al., 1996). When ARV alternatives are not available, one can "treat through" by maintaining the ARV regimen and adding adjuvant pain-modifying agents. Symptoms may not always subside upon stopping the offending agent, and even if they do, recovery may be only partial (Price et al., 1999; Wulff & Simpson, 1999a).

Treatment of HIV sensory neuropathies focuses on removing neurotoxins and managing pain and discomfort. One study showed that 40% of patients with HIV have severe pain, with a numeric pain rating scale of 5 or greater out of 10, and 90% experience some pain (Smyth et al., 2007). Experiencing neuropathic pain appears to increase the risk of unemployment and experiencing dependence in instrumental activities of daily living (Ellis et al., 2010). In addition, neuropathic pain itself, but not the severity of neuropathic pain, is associated with current major depressive disorder and greater severity of depressive symptoms (Ellis et al., 2010).

Although there is no FDA-approved treatment for the pain HIV-associated DSPN, various pain-modifying agents have been used for HIV sensory neuropathies, including antidepressants, anticonvulsants, and narcotics. In mild neuropathies, over-the-counter treatments such as acetaminophen can be helpful (DeVivo et al., 2000; Wulff & Simpson, 1999a). One randomized control study demonstrated evidence of efficacy for topical capsaicin 8% (Simpson et al., 2008). One randomized control study demonstrated evidence of efficacy for topical capsaicin 8% (Simpson et al., 2008). Night splints may also be useful in the management of neuropathic pain with improvement of sleep (Sandoval et al., 2010). Pain-modifying anticonvulsants and antidepressants have been useful clinically (DeVivo et al., 2000; Wulff & Simpson, 1999a) and can improve quality of life and function for many patients with HIV-associated sensory neuropathies (Simpson, 2003). However, placebo-controlled trials for the treatment of neuropathic pain have shown no significant benefit from amitriptyline, low-dose topical capsaicin, pregabalin, gabapentin, subcutaneous recombinant human nerve growth factor, subcutaneous prosapeptide, intranasal peptide T, or lamotrigine (Phillips et al., 2010). Lamotrigine did show some superiority to placebo in the neurotoxic ARV-exposed stratum as a secondary outcome measure of the study. Although placebo-controlled trials have been negative, tricyclic antidepressants (e.g., desipramine and amitriptyline) occasionally can be useful. Sedation is common with some, particularly amitriptyline, so these agents are more useful for control of nighttime neuropathic pain. Daytime sedation can generally be avoided by using small doses and escalating slowly. Use of opiate medication must be approached with caution because of the prevalence of risk factors for aberrant prescription opiate use often found in this population (Chou et al., 2009). Alternative treatments include acupuncture and hypnosis (Dorfman et al., 2013). Further management details are provided by Verma, and colleagues (2004).

CONSIDERATIONS FOR RESOURCE-LIMITED SETTINGS

A recent study of DSPN in seven resource-limited settings estimated DSPN incidence in PWH who were ART-naive and had a CD4 $^+$ T-cell count < 300 cells/mm^3 compared to people without HIV and in PWH virally suppressed on 1 of 3 ARV regimens. A total of 860 PWH were enrolled from Brazil, India, Malawi, Peru, South Africa, Thailand, and Zimbabwe. Before initiating combination ART, 21.3% of PWH had DSPN compared with 8.5% of people without HIV. PWH with DSPN were more likely to report inability to work and depression than PWH without DSPN. Overall prevalence of DSPN among those virally suppressed on ART decreased from 20.3% at week 48 to 15.3% at week 144, and finally to 10.3%, at week 192. Incident DSPN was seen in 127 PWH. Longitudinally, DSPN was more likely in older individuals and PWH with less education ($P = .03$). There was no significant association between ART regimen and DSPN (Vecchio et al., 2020).

INFLAMMATORY DEMYELINATING POLYNEUROPATHY

Joseph S. Kass

LEARNING OBJECTIVE

Discuss the clinical features, differential diagnosis, and management of acute and chronic inflammatory demyelinating polyneuropathy in patients with HIV.

WHAT'S NEW?

The differential diagnosis of acute inflammatory demyelinating polyneuropathy (AIDP) includes disorders of the spinal cord, such as transverse myelitis, acute spinal cord compression, and acute infarction of the spinal cord; disorders affecting anterior horn cells, including poliomyelitis and West Nile virus; acute peripheral neuropathies such as tick paralysis, porphyria, Lyme disease, and lead or arsenic poisoning; and neuromuscular junction disorders such as botulism, myasthenia gravis, or Lambert–Eaton myasthenic syndrome.

KEY POINTS

- AIDP and chronic inflammatory demyelinating polyneuropathies (CIDP) are not common HIV-associated peripheral neuropathies. Their cause is autoimmune-induced inflammation and breakdown of peripheral nerve myelin.

- AIDP has rapid onset and progression and often develops during HIV seroconversion or before immunosuppression has evolved.

- AIDP/CIDP in PWH is not associated with the classic CSF albuminocytological dissociation expected in people without HIV. PWH often have a CSF lymphocytic pleocytosis.

- AIDP is treated with either plasmapheresis or intravenous immunoglobulin and with ganciclovir/foscarnet/cidofovir if CMV is detected as a causative agent.

- CIDP is treated with corticosteroids or intermittent courses of either plasmapheresis or intravenous immunoglobulin that may be continued long term until therapeutic response.

Peripheral neuropathy is the most common neurologic manifestation in PWH and can manifest in a number of ways: distal symmetric polyneuropathy, inflammatory polyneuropathy (AIDP/CIDP), mononeuritis multiplex, autonomic neuropathy, and progressive polyradiculopathy (Wulff & Simpson, 1999b, 2000). Whereas distal symmetric polyneuropathy (DSPN) is the most common presentation and can occur secondary to direct HIV infection or as a side effect of NRTIs (Parry et al., 1997; Wulff et al., 2000), inflammatory demyelinating neuropathies in patients with HIV are much less common (Leger et al., 1989).

Inflammatory demyelinating polyradiculoneuropathies are classified as either acute or chronic based on the duration of symptom progression. AIDP, also known as Guillain–Barré syndrome (GBS), is defined as progressive, usually ascending weakness with hyporeflexia or areflexia and with symptoms nadiring by 4 weeks. In contrast, CIDP is classified by progressive proximal and distal weakness and sensory loss with symptom progression for longer than 8 weeks.

The association between inflammatory polyneuropathies and HIV was first reported in 1985 by Lipkin et al. (Lipkin et al., 1985). AIDP typically occurs in the early stages of HIV infection during the seroconversion stage or during early HIV infection before seroconversion has evolved (Markarian et al., 1998; Mishra et al., 1985; Wulff & Simpson, 1999b). In patients with relatively intact immune function, AIDP may be the first clinical manifestation of HIV infection (Parry et al., 1997). The Miller–Fisher variant of GBS, characterized by ataxia, ophthalmoplegia, and areflexia, has been reported in advanced AIDS, with elevated anti-GQ1b antibody titer despite severe immunosuppression (Hiraga et al., 2007). GBS has also been reported as a manifestation of immune reconstitution syndrome in patients treated with combination ART who experience a dramatic increase in CD4[+] T-cell counts (Piliero et al., 2003; Rauschkaa et al., 2003). CIDP generally occurs later during the advanced stage of HIV infection (Verma & Bradley, 2000, Verma, 2001).

PATHOGENESIS

Both AIDP and CIDP are thought to be due to an underlying autoimmune inflammatory response against peripheral nerve myelin-associated antigens, resulting in breakdown of peripheral nerve myelin (Radziwill et al., 2002). Rarely, HIV infection has been reported in association with an acute axonal motor neuropathy, where the pathology is thought to be associated with an immune response against the peripheral nerve axon (Dardis, 2015; Goldstein et al., 2013; Jadhav et al., 2014; Wagner et al., 2007).

CLINICAL FEATURES

AIDP is frequently associated with a preceding illness, such as upper respiratory infection or acute enterocolitis. AIDP commonly presents with paresthesias, followed by back pain, ascending symmetric weakness, and decreased or absent reflexes. Frank numbness is not common but neuropathic pain is very common. Patients may also experience facial weakness, ophthalmoplegia, and autonomic dysfunction (commonly labile blood pressures and tachycardia).

CIDP can present with progressive or relapsing proximal and distal weakness, sensory loss, and absent reflexes. Pain is a less common presentation (Dimachkie & Barohn, 2014).

CEREBROSPINAL FLUID ANALYSIS

CSF is characteristically acellular in AIDP in PWH. Protein levels may be normal during the first week of the illness but will increase within 2 or 3 weeks of symptom onset. Elevated CSF protein has been associated mainly with increased permeability of the blood–CSF barrier (Winer, 2001). On the other hand, AIDP seen with HIV infection may be associated with lymphocytic pleocytosis. In a study of 10 patients with HIV-associated AIDP, CSF white blood cell count ranged from 2 to 17 cells/mm³ (Brannagan, 2003). The presence of increased protein in the CSF is useful for the diagnosis, and a lymphocytic CSF pleocytosis (10–50 cells/mm³) distinguishes HIV-associated inflammatory demyelinating neuropathies from those without HIV infection (Wulff & Simpson, 1999b). However, the absence of CSF pleocytosis does not rule out HIV infection and hence warrants testing for HIV in all patients with AIDP (Brannagan, 2003). In addition, either elevated CSF protein or elevated white blood cell counts may be found in PWH even in the absence of an autoimmune neuropathy (Marshall et al., 1988). Generally, CSF pleocytosis is suggestive of either inflammatory/infectious etiology or underlying malignancy. Markedly elevated cell counts or the presence of CSF polymorphonuclear granulocytes in a patient whose clinical presentation appears typical of either AIDP or CIDP should alert the physician to consider alternative diagnoses (Hughes, 1991). Enterovirus myelitis, West Nile myelitis, European tick-borne encephalitis virus, and herpes virus infection (CMV, VZV, EBV, and HSV-1 and -2) may show an initial polymorphonuclear pleocytosis. Lyme disease and HIV infection need to be considered with a lymphocytic pleocytosis (Rauschkaa et al., 2003).

Researchers reported that the mean CD4[+] T-cell count was 367 cells/mm³ (range, 55–800 cells/mm³) in a series of 10 patients with HIV and GBS. An acute polyradiculoneuropathy in patients with CD4[+] T-cell count of less than 50 cells/mm³ may be secondary to CMV infection, and empiric ganciclovir may be indicated (Brannagan & Zhour, 2003).

ELECTROPHYSIOLOGY

Diagnosis is aided by nerve conduction studies showing features of demyelination—that is, slowing of nerve conduction velocities, prolonged distal latencies, temporal dispersion, conduction block, and prolonged F-wave latencies.

BIOPSY

Nerve biopsies are rarely performed to diagnose either AIDP or CIDP, but biopsy may be considered if the clinical or physiologic picture is atypical. Pathology includes macrophage-mediated segmental demyelination and an inflammatory infiltrate (Cornblath et al., 1987).

DIFFERENTIAL DIAGNOSIS

The differential diagnosis of AIDP includes disorders of the spinal cord such as transverse myelitis, acute spinal cord compression, and acute infarction of the spinal cord (which in the initial phases may present with flaccid areflexia below the level of the lesion because of spinal shock); disorders affecting anterior horn cells, including poliomyelitis and West Nile virus; acute peripheral neuropathies such as tick paralysis, porphyria, Lyme disease, and lead or arsenic poisoning; and neuromuscular junction disorders such as botulism, myasthenia gravis, or Lambert–Eaton myasthenic syndrome (Wakerly & Yuki, 2015). TB, toxoplasmosis, and HSV-2, syphilis, and lymphoma can also present with signs and symptoms of polyradiculitis.

In individuals with subacute/chronic neuropathy and HIV with CD4 $^+$ T-cell counts of less than 50 cells/mm^3, mononeuritis multiplex, distal symmetric polyneuropathy (DSPN), and CMV-related polyradiculomyelitis or polyradiculitis need to be considered in the differential diagnosis. CMV polyradiculitis (or polyradiculomyelitis if the infection involves not only the nerve roots but also the spinal cord) typically presents as an ascending weakness beginning in the lower extremities with areflexia, sensory loss, and weakness. Patients typically experience urinary retention and decreased anal sphincter tone. MRI of the spine with contrast demonstrates enhancement of the nerve roots, typically involving the cauda equina. Nerve conduction studies will show low compound muscle action potentials and mildly slowed conduction velocity corresponding to axonal involvement. Electromyography will show acute denervation with spontaneous activity and decreased recruitment. CSF studies in CMV polyradiculitis usually reveal a polymorphonuclear-predominant pleocytosis, elevated protein, and decreased glucose levels. CSF PCR for CMV DNA can confirm the diagnosis.

CMV infection of the peripheral nervous system may also manifest as an asymmetric multifocal neuropathy, observed in patients with HIV and low CD4 $^+$ T-cell counts. Infection affects individual peripheral nerves, with the radial, ulnar, peroneal, and lateral cutaneous nerves of the thigh being the most commonly involved nerves (Anders & Goebel, 1999). Rapid progression has been reported and can become confluent (Robinson-Papp, 2009b), mimicking an acute or subacute polyneuropathy. Electrodiagnostic studies of the nerves show multifocal sensory and motor nerve dysfunction in an axonal pattern with acute denervation. CSF studies may or may not be positive for CMV DNA PCR, and nerve biopsy may also fail to reveal CMV. Empiric treatment is warranted when clinical suspicion is high, especially in the setting of concomitant CMV infection affecting other organs. Treatment is also with either ganciclovir or foscarnet as the first-line option. The differential diagnosis should include mononeuritis multiplex in PWH with high CD4 $^+$ T-cell counts, hepatitis C with cryoglobulinemia, mononeuritis multiplex owing to vasculitis in association with B-cell lymphoma, and distal sensory polyneuropathy associated with either HIV or ART with D-drugs.

TREATMENT

AIDP is treated with either high-dose IVIG therapy or plasmapheresis. These treatments enhance recovery and arrest clinical progression (Cornblath et al., 1987; Hadden et al., 1998; Plasma Exchange/Sandoglobulin Guillain–Barré Syndrome Trial Group, 1997). IVIG and plasma exchange have been shown to be equally effective in treating AIDP in patients without HIV (Plasma Exchange/Sandoglobulin Guillain–Barré Trial Group, 1997; van der Meche et al., 1992). In 2015, researchers reported improvement in CD4 $^+$ and CD8 $^+$ T-cell counts and HIV-1 RNA levels in their patient treated with IVIG for HIV-associated GBS (Rosca et al., 2015). Because of the possibility of CMV polyradiculomyelitis or polyradiculitis, patients with severe immunosuppression (CD4 $^+$ T-cell counts < 50 cells/mm^3) should be treated with intravenous ganciclovir, foscarnet, or cidofovir or a combination of these, in addition to the standard treatment. CIDP is treated with oral prednisone, pulse intravenous high-dose methylprednisolone or dexamethasone, or intermittent courses of plasmapheresis or IVIG. A randomized controlled study confirmed the benefit of prednisone in HIV-related CIDP, although this treatment approach may worsen immunosuppression (Lindenbaum et al., 2001). Acute relapses in CIDP are treated with either IVIG or plasmapheresis.

PROGNOSIS

Initial clinical course and response to pharmacological treatment in AIDP is similar in patients with or without HIV (Verma, 2001). Schreiber and colleagues (2011) reported on a patient with GBS as the initial presentation of HIV infection who recovered fully using IVIG and rehabilitation without initiation of ART, suggesting that patients with GBS early in the course of HIV infection may behave like those with GBS without HIV. Compared to patients without HIVs, patient with HIV-associated GBS may experience relapses and may be more likely to develop CIDP (Brannagan, 2003). With CIDP, although treatment can halt the progression of the disease and remyelination of the peripheral nerves can take place, there is evidence that unrecoverable secondary axonal damage can occur in some cases (Hughes, 1991).

NEUROLOGICAL COMPLICATIONS OF PWH WITH CMV INFECTION

Joseph S. Kass

LEARNING OBJECTIVE

Discuss the clinical syndromes, differential diagnosis, and management of neurological complications of CMV infection in patients with HIV.

KEY POINTS

- CMV CNS disease occurs late in the course of HIV, and it may involve different parts of the CNS.

- Diagnosis is based on the clinical findings, results of imaging, and virologic markers.

- The treatment should be started empirically while awaiting the CSF CMV DNA PCR results.

CMV, a member of the herpesvirus family, is a frequent opportunistic viral infection in PWH and occurs when the CD4 + T-cell count is less than 100 cells/mm³ attributable to reactivation of latent infection. CMV infection of the nervous system accounts for fewer than 1% of CMV infections in patients with HIV (McCutchan, 1995) and often develops concurrently with other, more common CMV extraneural disease such as retinitis or gastrointestinal involvement. Clinical syndromes of CMV infection in the nervous system include encephalitis, polyradiculomyelitis, polyradiculitis, and multifocal neuropathy (Anders & Goebel, 1999). Although these syndromes are uncommon, recognition, treatment with antivirals, and restoring immune response are paramount to reduce the risk of death.

CMV encephalitis is the most common manifestation of CNS infection owing to CMV. Clinically, infection can present as diffuse encephalitis, ventriculoencephalitis, or focal encephalitis. Diffuse encephalitis develops over several weeks and thus presents subacutely with memory loss, attention and concentration difficulties, and delirium. Focal neurological deficits may also be seen. Pathologically, microglial nodules may be found in the cortex, brainstem, cerebellum, and basal ganglia, but occur most commonly in gray matter (Morgello et al., 1987). On neuroimaging, MRI may show a variety of patterns. The brain may appear normal, or it may show hyperintense T2 lesions in the areas described previously and nodular lesions with or without enhancement on T1 postcontrast images (Maschke et al., 2002).

Ventriculoencephalitis presents with lethargy, confusion, cranial nerve deficits, ataxia, and focal neurological deficits, and it sometimes occurs concomitantly with CMV polyradiculitis. Ventriculoencephalitis may be more insidious in onset and have a poorer prognosis (Maschke et al., 2002). CMV encephalitis has been reported to occur even while patients are on treatment with ganciclovir for extra-CNS disease (Bermann & Kim, 1994). Pathologically, necrotizing lesions are seen in the ventricular system, and imaging shows periventricular enhancement with or without ventriculomegaly. The third and less common type of CMV encephalitis is focal encephalitis, and it presents with focal neurological deficits corresponding to a cerebral mass lesion. MRI will show ring-enhancing lesions with surrounding edema.

CSF PCR for CMV DNA confirms the diagnosis of CMV encephalitis. The CSF may also show pleocytosis with either a polymorphonuclear or a mononuclear predominance, along with elevated protein and decreased glucose levels. Viral culture is rarely positive. The detection of other viruses often confounds the diagnosis; thus, the index of suspicion must be

based on the presentation and imaging findings in the context of profound immunosuppression. The differential diagnosis for CMV encephalitis must include HIV encephalitis, PML, and neurosyphilis. When CMV encephalitis presents as a ring-enhancing lesion, the differential diagnosis expands to other etiologies known to present similarly, such as toxoplasmosis, primary CNS lymphoma, and tuberculous meningitis with tuberculomas (Offiah & Turnbull, 2006).

CMV polyradiculitis (or polyradiculomyelitis if the infection involves not only the nerve roots but also the spinal cord) typically presents as an ascending weakness beginning in the lower extremities with areflexia, sensory loss, and weakness. Patients typically experience urinary retention and decreased anal sphincter tone. MRI of the spine with contrast demonstrates enhancement of the nerve roots, typically involving the cauda equina. Nerve conduction studies will show low compound muscle action potentials and mildly slowed conduction velocity corresponding to axonal involvement. Electromyography will show acute denervation with spontaneous activity and decreased recruitment. CSF studies in CMV polyradiculitis usually reveal a polymorphonuclear-predominant pleocytosis, elevated protein, and decreased glucose levels. CSF PCR for CMV DNA can confirm the diagnosis.

The differential diagnosis of CMV polyradiculitis includes GBS, which may be clinically indistinguishable and only differentiated on nerve conduction studies showing a more demyelinating pattern (Corral et al., 1997). Other opportunistic infections, including TB, toxoplasmosis, and HSV-2, can present in a similar manner. Syphilis and lymphoma can also cause polyradiculitis.

Treatment for both CMV encephalitis and CMV polyradiculitis/polyradiculomyelitis is similar. Induction treatment with either intravenous ganciclovir or foscarnet is the usual first-line treatment option. Sometimes in severe encephalitis cases, combination treatment with both ganciclovir and foscarnet has been used (Portegies et al., 2004; Silva et al., 2010). Cidofovir can be used as an alternate treatment option. Empiric treatment of CMV infection is often advised because CSF results may be delayed. Maintenance treatment with ganciclovir has been recommended, but the duration of treatment has not been well studied. Of note, patients with CMV polyradiculitis/polyradiculomyelitis have been shown to be more responsive to treatment compared to patients with CMV encephalitis (Cinque et al., 1998).

The best described CMV infection of the peripheral nervous system is an asymmetric multifocal neuropathy, observed in patient with HIV and low CD4 + counts. Infection affects individual peripheral nerves, with the radial, ulnar, peroneal, and lateral femoral cutaneous nerve of the thigh most commonly involved (Anders, 1999). Rapid progression has been reported and can become confluent (Robinson-Papp, 2009a), mimicking a polyneuropathy. Electrodiagnostic studies of the nerves show multifocal sensory and motor nerve dysfunction in an axonal pattern with acute denervation. CSF studies may or may not be positive for CMV DNA PCR, and nerve biopsy may also fail to reveal CMV. Empiric treatment is warranted when clinical suspicion is high, especially in the setting of concomitant CMV infection affecting other organs. Treatment is also with either ganciclovir or foscarnet as the first-line option. The differential diagnosis should include mononeuropathy multiplex in patients with HIV and high $CD4^+$ T-cell counts, hepatitis C with cryoglobulinemia, mononeuropathy multiplex owing to vasculitis in association with B-cell lymphoma, and distal sensory polyneuropathy (DSPN) associated with either HIV or ARV treatment (ATN) with dideoxynucleoside reverse transcriptase inhibitors (NRTIs).

INTRACRANIAL LESIONS

Joseph S. Kass

LEARNING OBJECTIVE

Discuss the clinical presentation, differential diagnosis, and treatment of intracranial lesions in patients with HIV.

WHAT'S NEW?

Because of concern for drug–drug interactions, particularly in patients receiving ART, most clinicians favor levetiracetam as the first-line for managing seizures. In the setting of status epilepticus, fosphenytoin, levetiracetam, and valproate appear to have equal efficacy. Enzyme-inducing antiepileptic drugs should be avoided in people on ART that include PIs or nonnucleoside reverse transcriptase inhibitors.

KEY POINTS

- HIV-related focal intracranial lesions generally occur in PWH with $CD4^+$ T-cell counts less than 200 cell/mm^3.

- The most common focal mass lesion is toxoplasmosis. The use of prophylactic agents such as trimethoprim–sulfamethoxazole can decrease the incidence of toxoplasmosis.

- Primary CNS lymphoma (PCNSL) is the most common HIV-related brain neoplasm seen in PWH. On imaging studies, it is usually a solitary intracranial mass lesion in the setting of a negative toxoplasmosis serology.

- PML on neuroimaging is a nonenhancing lesion of the white matter involving the subcortical U-fibers without edema or mass effect.

- PWH may also develop mass lesions typical of people without HIV, so the differential diagnosis of focal intracranial lesion in PWH should include both HIV-related and non-HIV-related pathologies.

Intracranial mass lesions are common neurologic findings and account for as much as half of the neurologic disorders seen in PWH. Although intracranial mass lesions typically occur in PWH with advanced immunosuppression (CD^+ counts < 200 cells/mm^3), an intracranial lesion can occasionally be the initial presenting symptom of AIDS. Intracranial lesions in PWH can be broadly categorized into three groups: opportunistic infections, neoplasms, and cerebrovascular disease (American Academy of Neurology (AAN), 1998).

The clinical presentation of intracranial lesions varies depending on the underlying etiology. Typical presenting clinical symptoms include alteration in level of awareness or consciousness as well as focal neurologic deficits. In developed countries such as the United States, the most common etiologies include toxoplasmosis, PCNSL, bacterial and fungal abscesses, and PML. Additional differential diagnosis includes primary brain tumor, brain metastasis from systemic cancer, tuberculoma, and lesions of fungal origin. Differentiating among this large differential diagnosis of intracranial lesions can be challenging. In patients with large lesions with mass effect and impending herniation, open biopsy with decompression is recommended. Achieving the correct diagnosis is paramount to managing the causal pathogen in a timely manner. Achieving this goal requires a knowledge-based diagnostic algorithm that accounts for the relative frequency of various types of intracranial lesions. Figure 35.3 provides a useful process of differential considerations based on level of immunosuppression, typical clinical and radiographic presentations, management options, and prognosis with or without empirical treatment (AAN, 1998).

Cerebral toxoplasmosis is the most common cause of space-occupying intracranial focal mass lesions in PWH and typically results from reactivation of latent infection of *Toxoplasma gondii*, an obligate intracellular parasite (AAN, 2000a). In the United States, the incidence of cerebral toxoplasmosis has declined with widespread use of prophylaxis agents such as trimethoprim–sulfamethoxazole and ART in PWH (AAN, 1998).

Toxoplasmosis often presents with subacute changes in level of consciousness, fever, headaches, seizures, and focal neurologic deficit. It should be suspected in any patient with HIV and an intracranial mass lesion, especially if the patient has a CD^+ T-cell count of less than 100 cells/mm^3, is not receiving toxoplasmosis prophylaxis, and has immunoglobulin G antibodies to *T. gondii* (AAN, 2000a). Investigative studies such as CSF analysis, *Toxoplasma* serology, or imaging studies do not always provide a definitive diagnosis. In this patient population, performing a lumbar puncture is often contraindicated because mass effect from the lesion increases the risk of herniation. In cases in which CSF is obtained, analysis frequently shows a nonspecific mild mononuclear pleocytosis with elevated protein. CSF PCR can detect *T. gondii* with high specificity (100%) but variable sensitivity (30%–50%) (AAN, 2002). Consequently, whereas a positive *Toxoplasma* PCR result is highly suggestive of the diagnosis, a negative result does not exclude it.

Imaging studies can also provide supportive information. MRI with and without contrast has greater sensitivity than contrast-enhanced CT, especially for detecting multiple lesions, subcortical lesions, and posterior fossa involvement. However, neither imaging modality alone is sufficient to make a diagnosis because there is no pathognomonic radiographically distinguishing feature of toxoplasmosis compared to PCNSL. Toxoplasmosis typically presents as multiple,

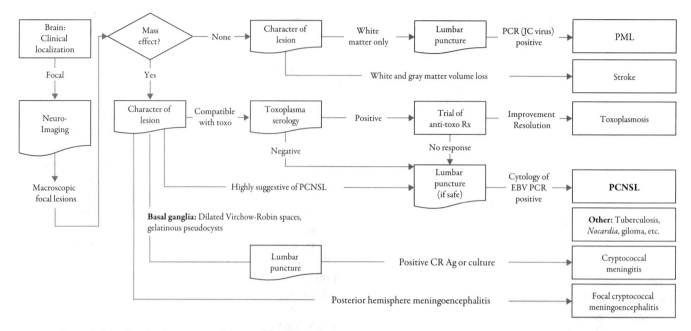

Figure 35.3 General algorithm for diagnostic evaluation of focal brain disease   SOURCE: Adapted from American Academy of Neurology (AAN). Evaluation and management of intracranial mass lesions in AIDS. Report of the Quality Standards Subcommittee of the American Academy of Neurology. *Neurology.* 1998;50:21–26.

homogeneous, ring-enhancing lesions with cerebral edema and mass effect. It has a predilection for the basal ganglia and corticomedullary junction, with involvement of both white and gray matter (AAN, 2000a). Although a solitary mass lesion with edema is often observed in PCNSL, it can also be seen in toxoplasmosis (AAN, 2000a). Thallium single-photon emission computed tomography (SPECT) and positron emission tomography (PET) can be useful in distinguishing toxoplasmosis from lymphoma. Lymphoma has increased thallium uptake on SPECT and hypermetabolism of glucose and methionine on PET. Toxoplasma is hypometabolic on PET and does not show uptake of thallium (AAN, 2000a). As a result of the limitations of these investigative modalities, diagnosis of toxoplasmosis is often presumptive. Individuals with typical clinical presentations and radiographic findings are treated empirically for toxoplasmosis for two weeks, and a positive clinical and radiographic response indicates the diagnosis. Open or stereotactic brain biopsy can yield a definitive diagnosis; however, this approach of treating empirically and assessing for response eliminates the morbidity and rare mortality risk of the procedure. However, biopsy should not be delayed in patients who do not improve with empirical management, have large mass effect with impending herniation, and require a rapid definitive diagnosis.

First-line anti-*Toxoplasma* treatment includes sulfadiazine, pyrimethamine, and folinic acid (leucovorin) (AAN, 2000a). Folinic acid must be given to counteract myelosuppression from pyrimethamine. Duration of acute therapy is at least 6 weeks before beginning secondary prophylaxis (chronic suppressive therapy) with pyrimethamine, leucovorin, and a sulfadiazine. Recrudescence occurs in up to 30% of patients, typically in patients with poor adherence to secondary prophylaxis but occasionally in individuals with good treatment adherence (AAN, 2000a). In patients with sulfa allergy or intolerance, clindamycin is a reasonable alternative

to sulfadiazine, although clindamycin use is associated with a slightly increased incidence of recrudescence. If the patient is intolerant to both sulfadiazine and clindamycin, alternatives include high-dosed trimethoprim–sulfamethoxazole, azithromycin, and atovaquone. Atovaquone is less tolerated because of gastrointestinal side effects. Clinical improvement should occur within the first 10–14 days of treatment. Clinical improvement occurs prior to radiographic evidence of improvement, which may be noted within 2 or 3 weeks of treatment initiation. Lack of improvement within the first 2 weeks should raise suspicion for an alternative diagnosis.

The use of adjunctive corticosteroids, such as dexamethasone, should be brief, and implemented only in very particular circumstances, such as when there is radiographic evidence of midline shift or impending herniation, signs of critically elevated intracranial pressure, or clinical deterioration within the first 48 hours of therapy. Under these circumstances, the benefits of steroids outweigh the many risks of steroid administration. Steroids may also serve to confound the diagnosis for several reasons. Steroids can improve clinical presentation, making it difficult to distinguish between the anti-inflammatory effects of the steroids and the therapeutic effectiveness of empiric anti-toxoplasmosis treatment. In addition, steroid's anti-inflammatory actions affect the radiographic presentation by decreasing the intensity of contrast enhancement and surrounding edema, thus interfering with reliable comparative interpretation of subsequent radiographic images. Steroids can also complicate the pathological diagnosis of PCNSL if a biopsy is needed, rendering the biopsy falsely negative for the presence of lymphoma. Aside from more acute steroid complications such as avascular necrosis, hyperglycemia, and psychiatric symptoms, the prolonged use of steroids may also render the patient susceptible to other opportunistic infections.

An important differential diagnosis is PCNS, which along the systemic non-Hodgkin's lymphoma, Kaposi's sarcoma, and invasive cervical carcinoma, is one of the four AIDS-defining neoplasms. PCNSL is commonly seen in PWH with CD4 [+] T-cell counts of less than 50 cells/mm^3 and is rarely the initial presenting symptom of AIDS. AIDS-related PCNSL pathogenesis is strongly related to reactivation of latent Epstein–Barr virus (EBV) infection. The clinical presentation is very similar to cerebral toxoplasmosis, with patients presenting with symptoms such as encephalopathy, impaired cognitive function, seizures, and focal neurologic deficits such as aphasia and hemiparesis. Investigative studies such as CSF analysis and imaging are often utilized. As with cerebral toxoplasmosis, lumbar puncture is at times contraindicated because of a heightened risk of hernation owing to mass effect from the lesion. CSF analysis, particularly cytology, can be helpful, but it has a very low sensitivity. PCR assay of CSF for EBV DNA can be diagnostic. PCR for EBV DNA has a sensitivity greater than 80% and a specificity greater than 95%. As with toxoplasmosis, MRI often provides higher diagnostic yield than CT scan, but CT with contrast remains useful particularly in patients who have contraindication to MRI. PCNSL can present with single or multiple well-defined ring or patchy enhancing lesions with edema and mass effect. It often involves supratentorial regions such as the corpus callosum and periventricular or periependymal areas (PCNSL in AIDS) (AAN, 2000b). As previously mentioned, SPECT and PET can be useful in differentiating lymphoma from other etiologies, including toxoplasmosis. Although PET and SPECT have limited sensitivity, they have high specificity. A diagnosis is often made using a combination of CSF cytology, toxoplasmosis serologic testing, failure of trial of empirical antibiotics usually for treatment of toxoplasmosis, and positive CSF PCR for EBV DNA; if necessary, a brain biopsy may be obtained (AAN, 2000b). Open or stereotactic brain biopsy is typically required prior to whole-brain irradiation, which is the current mainstay treatment for PCNSL. Whole-brain radiation appears to be able to prevent further neurologic progression or produce reversal of deficits. However, the treatment plan is based on the patient's overall health status. There can be spread of lymphoma with involvement of the eyes; therefore, a complete ophthalmologic examination including a slit-lamp examination should be performed (AAN, 2000b).

Other etiologies of intracranial mass lesions include other neoplasms, cerebrovascular disease, and opportunistic infections. Kaposi's sarcoma may rarely manifest as an intracranial lesion. PWH may also develop brain lesions unrelated to immunocompromised status, such as glioma or metastatic disease.

In addition to toxoplasmosis, PWH may develop parasitic, fungal, or bacterial infections that present as a mass lesion. Most of these opportunistic infections present with meningitis and focal neurological signs and symptoms related to the presence of a mass lesion. Although neurocysticercosis (NCC) is not more common in patients with HIV, the incidence of HIV infection is significant in countries where NCC is endemic. Coinfection has been rarely reported, but reports of concomitant infection with HIV, NCC, and an additional pathogen have been reported. Furthermore, in the setting of immunocompromise, interpretation of imaging findings may be particularly difficult. On imaging studies, the appearance of NCC varies depending on the stage of infection. MRI is favored over CT scan, especially for evaluation of intraventricular and cisternal/subarachnoid cysts as well as cystic degeneration and pericystic inflammatory reaction (Serpa et al., 2007).

Common bacterial mass lesions include abscess from *Mycobacterium tuberculosis*, *Nocardia*, *Listeria monocytogenes*, and *Treponema pallidum*. In developing countries, particularly in highly endemic areas such as Southeast Asia and Africa, tuberculous meningitis is common. Because of its proclivity for the basal meninges, tuberculous meningitis often presents clinically with multiple cranial neuropathies and hydrocephalus (AAN, 2000a). Neuroimaging may show masses, which are often tuberculomas. Intracranial tuberculomas can be seen on MRI as hypointense or isointense with gadolinium contrast enhancement owing to varying amounts of caseous necrosis. This variable appearance of intracranial tuberculoma is attributed to the changing nature of the granulomatous lesion (Park & Song, 2008). The diagnosis of tuberculous meningitis can be challenging and requires a combination of CSF analysis including culture for TB, acid-fast bacilli stain, and TB PCR along with a clinical evaluation for systemic TB.

Common etiologies of fungal abscesses include *Cryptococcus neoformans*, *Candida albicans*, aspergillosis, mucormycosis histoplasmosis, and coccidioidomycosis. Of these fungi, cryptococcosis is the most common opportunistic fungal infection in PWH and arises from an acquired infection from *C. neoformans*, an encapsulated yeast. Neuroimaging, usually a contrast-enhanced brain MRI, may show cryptococcomas—multiple enhancing lesions of various sizes most often seen within perivascular spaces. These lesions usually resolve with treatment. A definitive diagnosis is made by a positive CSF culture for *C. neoformans*, a positive CSF India ink stain, or a reactive CSF cryptococcal antigen test. For additional information, see Chapter 28.

PML is characterized by multifocal areas of demyelination often in subcortical and periventricular areas and arises because of reactivation of JC virus infecting oligodendroglia in the setting of advanced immunosuppression. On imaging studies, the lesions do not typically enhance with contrast and do not produce edema or mass effect. The subcortical U-fibers are involved. However, in the setting of IRIS, PML can present with contrast enhancement, focal edema, and mass effect on MRI with contrast (Tan et al., 2009).

PWH with intracranial lesions are at heightened risk of developing seizures. Antiepileptic drugs (AEDs) should not be given for routine prophylaxis to patients with a CNS mass lesion because not all individuals with CNS lesions will develop seizures. However, once the patient experiences a seizure, chronic AED administration is appropriate. In 2012, the AAN issued an evidence-based guideline for clinicians about AED selection for PWH (Birbeck et al., 2012). The guideline describes the strength of evidence for each of its recommendations based on the quality of evidence available from clinical investigations. Most of the recommendations in this guideline were rated as having weak evidence.

The AAN guideline states that it may be important to avoid enzyme-inducing AEDs (EI-AEDs) in people on ART that include PI or nonnucleotide reverse transcriptase inhibitors (NNRTIs) because pharmacokinetic interactions may result in virologic failure (Birbeck et al., 2012). Phenobarbital, phenytoin, and carbamazepine are commonly used EI-AEDs, and phenobarbital, although rarely used in high-resource countries, is the mainstay of seizure management in low-resource countries where HIV is highly prevalent. The guideline identifies circumstances in which specific dose adjustments to the ART should be made when certain AEDs are used concomitantly. For example, those concurrently on phenytoin and lopinavir/ritonavir may need a 50% dosage increase in lopinavir/ritonavir to maintain adequate serum levels of the PI to ensure virologic control. Patients coadministered atazanavir/ritonavir and lamotrigine may require a 50% increase in lamotrigine dose to maintain adequate serum levels of the AED and achieve seizure control. Patients taking both zidovudine and the P450 inhibitor valproic acid may require a zidovudine dose reduction to maintain unchanged zidovudine levels (Birbeck et al., 2012). Although not specifically recommended in the guideline, AEDs that bypass hepatic metabolism and are renally excreted such as levetiracetam are often favored for patients on ART given their lack of drug–drug interactions. Although previously either intravenous phenytoin or fosphenytoin was the recommended treatment for status epilepticus, a recent study comparing three intravenous AEDs—levetiracetam (60 mg/kg), fosphenytoin (20 mg/kg), and valproic acid (40 mg/kg) for the treatment of benzodiazepine-refractory status epilepticus in both children and adults determined that each medication had similar efficacy (Kapur et al., 2019). Although this study was not specific for PWH, etiologies of status epilepticus varied, and the results of this study should be applicable to PWH presenting with a mass lesion causing status epilepticus.

Using the approach discussed in this chapter, common etiologies of intracranial mass lesion can be systemically evaluated in order to make a diagnosis and institute therapy. In settings with limited resources where sophisticated neuroimaging, CSF PCR, and biopsy are unavailable, clinical findings on history and physical examination combined with the prevalence of infectious etiologies should guide the diagnosis and subsequent empiric therapeutic intervention.

REFERENCES

Aberle SW, Aberle JH, Steininger C, et al. Quantitative real time PCR detection of varicella-zoster virus DNA in cerebrospinal fluid in patients with neurological disease. *Med Microbiol Immunol*. 2005;194:7–12.

Alfahad T, Nath A. Update on HIV-associated neurocognitive disorders. *Curr Neurol Neurosci Rep*. 2013;13:387.

American Academy of Neurology (AAN). Evaluation and management of intracranial mass lesions in AIDS: report of the Quality Standards Subcommittee of the American Academy of Neurology. *Neurology*. 1998;50:21–26.

AAN. Opportunistic and fungal infections of the central nervous system. *Neurol Continuum*. 2002;8(3):125.

AAN. Opportunistic infections: toxoplasmosis. The Neurologic complications of AIDS. *Neurol Continuum*. 2000a;6(5):128–149.

AAN. Primary central nervous system lymphoma in AIDS: the neurologic complications of AIDS. *Neurol Continuum*. 2000b;6(5):177–185.

Anders HJ, Goebel FD. Neurological manifestations of cytomegalovirus infection in the acquired immunodeficiency syndrome. *Int J STD AIDS*. 1999;10:151–161.

Anderson AM, Muñoz-Moreno JA, McClernon DR, et al. Prevalence and correlates of persistent HIV-1 RNA in cerebrospinal fluid during antiretroviral therapy. *J Infect Dis*. 2017;215(1):105–113.

Antinori A, Arendt G, Becker JT, et al. Updated research nosology for HIV-associated neurocognitive disorders. *Neurology*. 2007;69(18):1789–1799.

Banerjee S, McCutchan JA, Ances BM, et al. Hypertriglyceridemia in combination antiretroviral-treated HIV-positive individuals: potential impact on HIV sensory polyneuropathy. *AIDS*. 2011;25(2):F1–F6.

Banks LT, Geraci A, Liu M, et al. A natural history of HIV myelopathy in the HAART era. *Neurology*. 2002;58:A441.

Beardsley J, Wolbers M, Kibengo FM, et al. Adjunctive dexamethasone in HIV-associated *Cryptococcal mengitis*. *N Engl J Med*. 2016;374(6):542–54.

Bermann SM, Kim RC. The development of cytomegalovirus encephalitis in AIDS patients receiving ganciclovir. *Am J Med*. 1994;96:415–419.

Bhigjee AI, Madurai S, Bill PL, et al. Spectrum of myelopathies in HIV seropositive South African patients. *Neurology*. 2001;57:348–351.

Birbeck G, French J, Perucca E, et al. Evidence-based guideline: antiepileptic drug selection for people with HIV/AIDS: report of the Quality Standards Subcommittee of the American Academy of Neurology and the Ad Hoc Task Force of the Commission on Therapeutic Strategies of the International League Against Epilepsy. *Neurology*. 2012;78(2):139–145.

Blum AS, Dal Pan GJ, Feinberg J, et al. Low-dose zalcitabine-related toxic neuropathy: frequency, natural history, and risk factors. *Neurology*. 1996;46(4):999–1003.

Boisse L, Gill MJ, Power C. HIV infection of the central nervous system: clinical features and neuropathogenesis. *Neurol Clin*. 2008;26:799–819.

Boulware DR, Meya DB, Muzoora C, et al. Timing of antiretroviral therapy after diagnosis of cryptococcal meningitis. *N Engl J Med*. 2014;370:2487–2498.

Brannagan TH 3rd, Zhou Y. HIV associated Guillain–Barré syndrome. *J Neurol Sci*. 2003;208(1–2):39–42.

Candy S, Chang G, Andronikous S. Acute myelopathy or cauda equine syndrome in HIV positive adults in a tuberculosis endemic setting: MRI, clinical, and pathologic findings. *AJNR*. 2014;35(8):1634–1641.

Carvalhal A, Gill MJ, Letendre SL, et al. Central nervous system penetration effectiveness of antiretroviral drugs and neuropsychological impairment in the Ontario HIV Treatment Network Cohort Study. *J Neuroviral*. 2016;22(3):349–357.

Charlier C, Perrodeau E, Leclercq A, et al. Clinical features and prognostic factors of listeriosis: the MONALISA national prospective cohort study. *Lancet Infect Dis*. 2017;17(5):510–519.

Chen CH, Vazquez-Padua M, Cheng YC. Effect of anti-human immunodeficiency virus nucleoside analogs on mitochondrial DNA and its implication for delayed toxicity. *Mol Pharmacol*. 1991;39(5):625–628.

Cherner M, Masliah E, Ellis RJ, et al. Neurocognitive dysfunction predicts postmortem findings of HIV encephalitis. *Neurology*. 2002;59(10):1563–1567.

Childs E, Lyles R, Selnes OA et al. Plasma viral load and CD4+ lymphocytes predict HIV-associated dementia and senory neurology. *Neurology*. 1999;52:607–613.

Cho T, Vaitkevicius H. Infectious myelopathies. *Continuum*. 2012;18(6):1351–1373.

Chong J, Di Rocco A, Tagliati M, et al. MR findings in AIDS-associated myelopathy. *Am J Neuroradiol*. 1999;20(8):1412–1416.

Chou R, Fanciullo GJ, Fine PG, et al. Opioids for chronic noncancer pain: prediction and identification of aberrant drug-related behaviors: a review of the evidence for an American Pain Society and American Academy of Pain Medicine clinical practice guideline. *J Pain*. 2009;10(2):131–146.

Cinque P, Cleator GM, Weber T, et al. Clinical review diagnosis and clinical management of neurological disorders caused by cytomegalovirus in AIDS patients. *J Neuro Virol*. 1998;4:120–132.

Cohen JS. Peripheral neuropathy associated with fluoroquinolones. *Ann Pharmocother*. 2001;35(12):1540–1547.

Cornblath DR, McArthur JC. Predominantly sensory neuropathy in patients with AIDS and AIDS-related complex. *Neurology*. 1988;38(5):794–796.

Cornblath DR, McArthur JC, Kennedy PGE, et al. Inflammatory demyelinating peripheral neuropathies associated with human T-cell lymphotropic virus type III infection. *Ann Neurol*. 1987;21:32040.

Corral I, Quereda C, Casado JL, et al. Acute polyradiculopathies in HIV-positive patients. *J Neurol*. 1997;244:499–504.

Dalakas MC, Cupler EJ. Neuropathies in HIV infection. *Baillieres Clin Neurol*. 1996;5(1):199–218.

Dal Pan GJ, Berger JR. Spinal cord disease in human immunodeficiency virus infection. In Berger JR, Levy RM, eds. *AIDS and the nervous system*. 2nd ed. Philadelphia: Lippincott-Raven; 1997:173–187.

Dal Pan GJ, Glass JD, McArthur JC. Clinicopathologic correlations of HIV-1-associated vacuolar myelopathy: an autopsy-based case–control study. *Neurology*. 1994;44(11):2159–2164.

Dardis C. Acute motor axonal neuropathy in a patient with prolonged CD4 depletion due to HIV: a local variant of macrophage activation syndrome? *Oxford Med Case Rep*. 2015;2:200–2002.

DeBiasi RL, Tyler KL. Molecular methods diagnosis of viral encephalitis. *Clin Microbiol Rev*. 2004;17(4):903–925.

DeVivo DC, Percy AK, Chiriboga CA, et al. Neuromuscular disorders in HIV-1 infection. *Continuum*. 2000;6:73–76.

Dimachkie MM, Barohn RJ. Distal myopathies. *Neurol Clin*. 2014;32(3):817–842.

Di Rocco A. Diseases of the spinal cord in human immunodeficiency virus infection. *Semin Neurol*. 1999;19:151–155.

Di Rocco A, Simpson DM. AIDS-associated vacuolar myelopathy. *AIDS Patient Care STDs*. 1998;12(6):457–461.

Dorfman D, George MC, Schnur J, et al. Hypnosis for treatment of HIV neuropathic pain: a preliminary report. *Pain Med*. 2013;14:1048–1056.

Edén A, Fuchs D, Hagberg L, et al. HIV-1 viral escape in cerebralspinal fluid of subjects on suppressive treatment. *J Infect Dis*. 2010;202(12):1819–1825.

Ellis R, Deutsch R, Heaton RK, et al. Neurocognitive impairment is an independent risk factor for death in HIV infection: San Diego HIV Neurobehavioral Research Center Group. *Arch Neurol*. 1997;54(4):416–424.

Ellis RJ, Rosario D, Clifford DB, et al. Continued high prevalence and adverse clinical impact of human immunodeficiency virus-associated sensory neuropathy in the era of combination antiretroviral therapy: the CHARTER Study. *Arch Neurol*. 2010;67(5):552–558.

Erdem H, Senbayrak S, Gencer S, et al. Tuberculosis and brucellosis meningitis differential diagnosis. *Travel Med Infect Dis*. 2015;13(2):185–191.

Erlandson KM, Perez J, Abdo M, et al. Frailty, neurocognitive impairment, or both in predicting poor health outcomes among adults living with human immunodeficiency virus. *Clin Infect Dis*. 2019;68(1):131–138.

Evans SR, Ellis RJ, Chen H, et al. Peripheral neuropathy in HIV: prevalence and risk factors. *AIDS*. 2011;25(7):919–928.

Gallegos C, Tobolowsky F, Nigo M, Hasbun R. Delayed cerebral thrombosis in adults with bacterial meningitis: a novel complication of adjunctive steroids? *Crit Care Med*. 2018;46(8):e 811–e814.

Gambarin KH, Hamill RJ. Management of increased intracranial pressure in cryptococcal meningitis. *Curr Infect Dis Rep*. 2002;4(4):332–338.

Goldstein JM, Azizi SA, Booss J, et al. Human immunodeficiency virus-associated motor axonal polyradiculoneuropathy. *Arch Neurol*. 1993;50:1316–1319.

Hadden RD, Cornblath DR, Hughes RA, et al.; Plasma Exchange/Sandoglobulin Guillain–Barré Syndrome Trial Group. Electrophysiological classification of Guillain–Barré syndrome: clinical associations and outcome. *Ann Neurol*. 1998;44(5):780–788.

Hamada Y, Watanabe K, Aoki T, et al. Primary HIV infection with acute transverse myelitis. *Intern Med*. 2011;50:1615–1617.

Hammond ER, Crum RM, Treisman GJ, et al. The cerebrospinal fluid HIV risk score for assessing central nervous system activity in persons with HIV. *Am J Epidemiol*. 2014;180(3):297–307.

Handley G, Pankow S, Dien Bard J, et al. Distinguishing cytomegalovirus meningoencephalitis from other viral central nervous system infections. *J Clin Virol*. 2021;142:104936.

Hasbun R, Eraso J, Ramireddy S, et al. Screening for neurocognitive impairment in HIV individuals: the utility of the Montreal Cognitive Assessment Test. *J AIDS Clinic Res*. 2012;3:10.

Hasbun R, Rosenthal N, Balada-Llasat JM, et al. Epidemiology of meningitis and encephalitis in the United States, 2011–2014. *Clin Infect Dis*. 2017;65(3):359–363.

Hiraga A, Kuwabara S, Nakamura A, et al. Fisher/Guillain–Barré overlap syndrome in advanced AIDS. *J Neurol Sci*. 2007;258(1–2):148–150.

Hughes RA. Inflammatory neuropathy: sixth meeting of the Peripheral Neuropathy Association. St. Catherine's College, Oxford, England, August 14–18, 1990. *Neurology*. 1991;41(5):758–759.

Huis in't Veld D, Sun HY, Hung CC, Colebunders R. The immune reconstitution inflammatory syndrome related to HIV co-infections: a review. *Eur J Clin Microbiol Infect Dis*. 2012;31(6): 919–927.

Jacks A, Wainwright D, Salazar L, et al. Neurocognitive deficits increase lack of retention-in-care among older adults with newly diagnosed HIV infection. *AIDS*. 2015;29(13):1711–1714.

Jadhav S, Agrawal M, Rathi S. Acute motor axonal neuropathy in HIV infection. *Indian J Pediatr*. 2014;81:193.

Jarvis JN, Lawrence DS, Meya DB, et al. Single-dose liposomal amphotericin B treatment for cryptococcal meningitis. *N Engl J Med*. 2022;386(12):1109–1120.

Johnson TP, Nath A. Biotypes of HIV-associated neurocognitive disorders based on viral and immune pathogenesis. *Curr Opin Infect Dis*. 2022;35(3):223–230.

Johnson TP, Patel K, Johnson KR, et al. Induction of IL-17 and nonclassical T-cell activation by HIV-Tat protein. *Proc Natl Acad Sci USA*. 2013;110:13588–13593.

Kallianpur AR, Hulgan T. Pharmacogenetics of nucleoside reversetranscriptase inhibitor-associated peripheral neuropathy. *Pharmacogenomics*. 2009;10(4):623–637.

Kapur J, Elm J, Chamberlain JM, et al. Randomized trial of three anticonvulsant medications for status epilepticus. *N Engl J Med*. 2019;381:2103–2113.

Keswani SC, Pardo CA, Cherry CL, et al. HIV-associated sensory neuropathies. *AIDS*. 2002;16(16):2105–2117.

Keswani SC, Polley M, Pardo CA, et al. Schwann cell chemokine receptors mediate HIV-1 gp120 toxicity to sensory neurons. *Arch Neurol*. 2003;54(3):287–296.

Leger JM, Bouche P, Bolgert F, et al. The spectrum of polyneuropathies in patients infected with HIV. *J Neurol Neurosurg Psychiatry*. 1989;52(12):1369–1374.

Lehmann HC, Chen W, Borzan J, et al. Mitochondrial dysfunction in distal axons contributes to human immunodeficiency virus sensory neuropathy. *Arch Neurol*. 2011;69(1):100–110.

Leisman RM, Strasburg AP, Heitman, AK. et al. Evaluation of a commercial multiplex molecular panel for diagnosis of infectious meningitis and encephalitis. *J Clin Microb*. 2018;56(4):1927–1917.

Lescure FX, Moulignier A, Savatovsky J, et al. CD8 encephalitis in HIV-positive patients receiving cART: a treatable entity. *Clin Infect Dis*. 2013;57(1):101–108.

Letendre S. Central nervous system complications in HIV disease: HIV-associated neurocognitive disorder. *Top Antivir Med*. 2011;19(4):137–142.

Letendre S, Fitzsimons C, Ellis R, et al. Correlates of CSF viral loads in 1221 volunteers of the CHARTER Cohort. [Abstract 172]. Paper presented at the 17th Conference on Retrovirus and Opportunistic Infections. San Francisco, CA; February 16–19, 2010.

Lindenbaum Y, Kissel JT, Mendell JR. Treatment approaches for Guillain–Barré syndrome and chronic inflammatory demyelinating polyradiculopathy. *Neurol Clin.* 2001;19(1):187–204.

Lipkin WI, Parry G, Kiprov D, et al. Inflammatory neuropathy in homosexual men with lymphadenopathy. *Neurology.* 1985;35(10):1479–1483.

Lopez Castelblanco R, Lee M, Hasbun R. Epidemiology of bacterial meningitis in the US: a population-based study. *Lancet Infect Dis.* 2014;14:813–819.

Lucas SB, Wong KT, Nightingale S, Miller RF. HIV-associated CD8 encephalitis: A UK case series and review of histopathologically confirmed cases. *Front Neurol.* 2021;12:628296.

Ma B, Vigil K, Hasbun R. HIV testing in adults presenting with CNS infections. *Open Forum Infect Dis.* June 2020;7(6):ofaa217.

Maggiolo F, Airoldi M, Kleinloog HD, et al. Effect of adherence to HAART on virologic outcome and on the selection of resistance-conferring mutations in NNRTI- or PI-treated patients. *HIV Clin Trials.* 2007;8(5):282–292.

Manns A, Hisada M, La Grenade L. Human T-lymphotropic virus type I infection. *Lancet.* 1999;353(9168):1951–1958.

Markarian Y, Wulff EA, Simpson DM. Peripheral neuropathy in HIV disease. *AIDS Clin Care.* 1998;10(12):89–91, 93, 98.

Marra C, Maxwell CL, Smith SL, et al. Cerebrospinal fluid abnormalities in patients with syphilis: association with clinical and laboratory features. *J Infect Dis.* 2004;189(3):369–376.

Marra CM, Boutin P, Collier AC. Screening for distal sensory peripheral neuropathy in HIV-positive persons in research and clinical settings. *Neurology.* 1998;51(6):1678–1681.

Marshall DW, Brey RL, Cahill WT, et al. Spectrum of cerebrospinal fluid findings in various stages of human immunodeficiency virus infection. *Arch Neurol.* 1988;45:954–958.

Martin JL, Brown CE, Matthews-Davis N, et al. Effects of antiviral nucleoside analogs on human DNA polymerases and mitochondrial DNA synthesis. *Antimicrob Agents Chemother.* 1994;38(12):2743–2749.

Martin F, Taylor GP. Prospects for the management of human T-cell lymphotropic virus type 1-associated myelopathy. *AIDS Rev.* 2011;13(3):161–170.

Maschke M, Kastrup O, Diener HC. CNS manifestations of cytomegalovirus infections diagnosis and treatment. *CNS Drugs.* 2002;16(5):303–315.

McArthur JC, Brew BJ, Nath A. Neurological complications of HIV infection. *Lancet Neurol.* 2005;4(9):543–555.

McCutchan JA. Cytomegalovirus infections of the nervous system in patients with AIDS. *Clin Infect Dis.* 1995;20(4):747–754.

Métral M, Darling K, Locatelli I, et al. The Neurocognitive Assessment in the Metabolic and Aging Cohort (NAMACO) study: baseline participant profile. *HIV Med.* 2020;21(1):30–42

Mind Exchange Working Group. Assessment, diagnosis, and treatment of HIV-associated neurocognitive disorder: a consensus report of the Mind Exchange Program. *Clin Infect Dis.* 2013;56(7):1004–1017.

Mishra BB, Sommers W, Koski CL, et al. Acute inflammatory demyelinating polyneuropathy in the acquired immune deficiency syndrome. *Ann Neurol.* 1985;18:131–132.

Modi G, Ranchhod J, Hari K, et al. Non-traumatic myelopathy at the Chris Hani Baragwanath Hospital, South Africa—the influence of HIV. *Q JM.* 2011;104:697–703.

Moore RD, Wong WM, Keruly JC, et al. Incidence of neuropathy in HIV-positive patients on monotherapy versus those on combination therapy with didanosine, stavudine and hydroxyurea. *AIDS.* 2000;14(3):273–278.

Morgello S, Cho ES, Nielsen S, et al. Cytomegalovirus encephalitis in patients with acquired immunodeficiency syndrome: an autopsy study of 30 cases and a review of the literature. *Hum Pathol.* 1987;18:289–297.

Mukerji SS, Misra V, Lorenz D, et al. Impact of antiretroviral regimens on cerebrospinal fluid viral escape in a prospective multicohort study of antiretroviral therapy-experience Human immunodeficiency virus-1- infected adults in the United States. *Clin Infect Dis.* 2018;67(8):1182–1190.

Nagel MA, Forghani B, Mahalingam R, et al. The value of detecting anti-VZV IgG antibody in CSF to diagnose VZV vasculopathy. *Neurology.* 2007;68(13):1069–1073.

Nesher L, Hadi CM, Salazar L, et al. Epidemiology of meningitis with a negative CSF Gram-stain: underutilization of available diagnostic tests. *Epidemiol Infect.* 2016;144(1):189–197.

Nhantumbo AA, Comé CE, Maholela PI, et al. Etiology of meningitis among adults in three quaternary hospitals in Mozambique, 2016–2017: The role of HIV. *PLoS One.* 2022;17(5):e0267949.

Offiah CE, Turnbull IW. The imaging appearances of intracranial CNS infections in adult HIV and AIDS patients. *Clin Radiol.* 2006;61:393–401.

Opintan JA, Awadzi BK, Biney IJK, et al. High rates of cerebral toxoplasmosis in HIV patients presenting with meningitis in Accra, Ghana. *Trans R Soc Trop Med Hyg.* 2017;111(10):464–471.

Osiro S, Salomon N. Varicella-zoster (VZV) multifocal vasculopathy in a patient with systemic lupus erythematosus—a diagnostic and treatment dilemma. *IDCases.* 2007;81–83.

Pardo CA, McArthur JC, Griffin JW. HIV neuropathy: insights in the pathology of HIV peripheral nerve disease. *J Peripheral Nerv Syst.* 2001;6(1):21–27.

Park H, Song Y. Multiple tuberculoma involving the brain and spinal cord in a patient with miliary pulmonary tuberculosis. *J Korean Neurosurg Soc.* 2008;44(1):36–39.

Parry O, Mielke J, Latif AS, et al. Peripheral neuropathy in individuals with HIV infection in Zimbabwe. *Acta Neurol Scand.* 1997;96(4):218–222.

Patel AK, Patel KK, Gohel S, et al. Incidence of symptomatic CSF viral escape in HIV infected patients receiving atazanavir/ritonavir-containing ART: a tertiary care cohort in western India. *J Neurovirol* 2018:24(4):498–505.

Perfect JR, Dismukes WE, Dromer F, et al. Clinical practice guidelines for the treatment of cryptococcal disease: 2010 update from the Infectious Diseases Society of America. *Clin Infect Dis.* 2012;50:291–322.

Petito CK, Vecchio D, Chen YT. HIV antigen and DNA in AIDS spinal cords correlate with macrophage infiltration but not with vacuolar myelopathy. *J Neuropathol Exp Neurol.* 1994;53(1):86–94.

Phillips TJ, Cherry CL, Cox S, et al. Pharmacological treatment of painful HIV-associated sensory neuropathy: a systematic review and meta-analysis of randomised controlled trials. *PLoS One.* 2010;5(12):e14433.

Piliero PJ, Fish DG, Preston S, et al. Guillain–Barré syndrome associated with immune reconstitution. *Clin Infect Dis.* 2003;36(9): e111–e114.

Pillat MM, Bauer ME, de Oliveira AC, et al. HTLV-1-associated myelopathy/tropical spastic paraparesis (HAM/TSP): still an obscure disease. *Cent Nerv Syst Agents Med Chem.* 2011;11(4):239–245.

Plasma Exchange/Sandoglobulin Guillain–Barré Syndrome Trial Group. Randomised trial of plasma exchange, intravenous immunoglobulin, and combined treatments in Guillain–Barré syndrome. *Lancet.* 1997;349:225–230.

Polydefkis M, Yiannoutsos CT, Cohen BA, et al. Reduced intraepidermal nerve fiber density in HIV-associated sensory neuropathy. *Neurology.* 2002;58(1):115–119.

Portegies P, Solod L, Cinque P, et al. EFNS Task Force guidelines for the diagnosis and management of neurological complications of HIV infection. *Eur J Neurol.* 2004;11:297–304.

Price RW, Yiannoutsos CT, Clifford DB, et al. Neurological outcomes in late HIV infection: adverse impact of neurological impairment on survival and protective effect of antiviral therapy. AIDS Clinical Trial Group and Neurological AIDS Research Consortium Study Team. *AIDS.* 1999;13(13):1677–1685.

Radziwill AJ, Kuntzer T, Steck AJ. Immunopathology and treatments of Guillain–Barré syndrome and of chronic inflammatory demyelinating polyneuropathy. *Rev Neurol (Paris).* 2002;158(3):301–310.

Rauschkaa H, Jellingerb K, Lassmannc H, et al. Guillain–Barré syndrome with marked pleocytosis or a significant proportion of polymorphonuclear granulocytes in the cerebrospinal fluid: neuropathological investigation of five cases and review of differential diagnoses. *Eur J Neurol.* 2003;10:479–486.

Robertson KR, Smurzynski M, Parsons TD, et al. The prevalence and incidence of neurocognitive impairment in the HAART era. *AIDS.* 2007;21:1915–1921.

Robinson-Papp J, Gonzalez-Duarte A, Simpson DM, et al. The roles of ethnicity and antiretrovirals in HIV-associated polyneuropathy: a pilot study. *J Acquir Immune Defic Syndr.* 2009a;51(5):569–573.

Robinson-Papp J, Sharma S, Simpson DM, et al. Autonomic dysfunction is common in HIV and associated with distal symmetric polyneuropathy. *J Neurovirol.* 2013;19:172–180.

Robinson-Papp J, Simpson DM. Neuromuscular diseases associated with HIV-1 infection. *Muscle Nerve.* 2009b;40(6):1043–1053.

Rolfes MA, Hullsiek KH, Rhein J, et al. The effect of therapeutic lumbar punctures on acute mortality from cryptococcal meningitis. *Clin Infect Dis.* 2014;59(11):1607–1614.

Rosca EC, Albarqouni L, Simu M. Montreal cognitive assessment (MoCA) for HIV-associated neurocognitive disorders. *Neuropsychol Rev.* 2019: 29(3):313–327.

Rosca EC, Rosca O, Simu M. Intravenous immunoglobulin treatment in a HIV-1 positive patient with Guillain–Barré syndrome. *Int Immunopharmacol.* 2015;29(2):964–965.

Rosenow JM, Hirschfeld A. Utility of brain biopsy in patient with acquired immunodeficiency syndrome before and after introduction of highly active antiretroviral therapy. *Neurosurgery.* 2007;61(1):130–141.

Sandoval R, Runft B, Roddey T. Pilot study: does lower extremity night splinting assist in the management of painful peripheral neuropathy in the HIV/AIDS population? *J Int Assoc Phys AIDS Care (Chic).* 2010;9(6):368–381.

Schifitto G, McDermott MP, McArthur JC, et al.; Dana Consortium on the Therapy of HIV Dementia and Related Cognitive Disorders. Incidence of and risk factors for HIV-associated distal sensory polyneuropathy. *Neurology.* 2002;58(12):1764–1768.

Schreiber AL, Norbury JW, DeSousa EA. Functional recovery of untreated human immunodeficiency virus-associated Guillain–Barré syndrome: a case report. *Ann Phys Rehabil Med.* 2011;54:519–524.

Serpa JA, Moran A, Goodman JC, Giordano TP, White AC. Neurocysticercosis in the HIV era: a case report and review of the literature. *Am J Trop Med Hyg.* 2007;77(1):113–117.

Shahani L, Salazar L, Woods SP, Hasbun R. Baseline neurocognitive functioning predicts viral load suppression at 1-year follow-up among newly diagnosed HIV infected patients. *AIDS Behav.* 2018;22(10):3209–3213.

Shukla B, Aguilera EA, Salazar L, Wootton SH, Kaewpoowat Q, Hasbun R. Aseptic meningitis in adults and children: diagnostic and management challenges. *J Clin Virol.* 2017;94:110–114.

Silva CA, Penalva de Oliveira AC, Vilas-Boas L, et al. Neurologic cytomegalovirus complications in patients with AIDS: retrospective review of 13 cases and review of the literature. *Rev Inst Med Trop Sao Paulo.* 2010;52(6):305–310.

Simpson DM, Brown S, Tobias J; NGX-4010 C107 Study Group. Controlled trial of high-concentration capsaicin patch for treatment of painful HIV neuropathy. *Neurology.* 2008;70:2305–2313.

Simpson JK 3rd. Chronic neuropathic pain. *N Engl J Med.* 2003;348(26):2688–2689.

Smyth K, Affandi JS, McArthur JC, et al. Prevalence of and risk factors for HIV-associated neuropathy in Melbourne, Australia 1993–2006. *HIV Med.* 2007;8:367–373.

Sulaiman T, Medi S, Erdam H, et al. The diagnostic utility of the "Thwaites' system" and "lancet consensus scoring system" in tuberculosis vs. non-tuberculosis subacute and chronic meningitis: multicenter analysis of 395 adult patients. *BMC Infect Dis.* 2020;20(1):788.

Tagliati M, Grinnell J, Godbold J, et al. Peripheral nerve function in HIV infection: clinical, electrophysiologic, and laboratory findings. *Arch Neurol.* 1999;56(1):84–89.

Tan K, Roda R, Ostrow L, McArthur J, Nath A. PML-IRIS in patients with HIV infection: clinical manifestations and treatment with steroids. *Neurology.* 2009;72(17):1458–1464.

Thao LTP, Heemskerk AD, Geskus RB, et al. Prognostic models for 9-month mortality in tuberculous meningitis. *Clin Infect Dis.* 2018;66(4):523–532.

Thwaites GE. The management of suspected encephalitis. *BMJ.* 2012;344:e3489. doi:10.1136/bmj.e3489

Tirbaboshi J, Arkaitz I, Saye H, et al. Total and unbound bictegravir concentrations and viral suppression in cerebrospinal fluid of human immunodeficiency virus-infected patients. *J Infect Dis* 2019;221(9):1425–1428.

Triunfo M, Vai D, Montrucchio C, et al. Diagnostic accuracy of new and old cognitive screening tools for HIV-associated neurocognitive disorders. *HIV Med.* 2018;19:455–464.

Tunkel AR, Glaser CA, Bloch KC, et al. The management of encephalitis: clinical practice guidelines by the Infectious Diseases Society of America. *Clin Infect Dis.* 2004;47(3):303–327.

Tyor WR, Glass JD, Baumrind N, et al. Cytokine expression of macrophages in HIV-1-associated vacuolar myelopathy. *Neurology.* 1993;43(5):1002–1009.

US Department of Health and Human Services (DHHS) Panel on Antiretroviral Guidelines for Adults and Adolescents. Guidelines for the use of antiretroviral agents in adults and adolescents with HIV. http://www.aidsinfo.nih.gov/ContentFiles/AdultandAdolescentGL.pdf. Published 2022a. Accessed September 25, 2022.

US Department of Health and Human Services (DHHS), Panel on Guidelines for the Prevention and Treatment of Opportunistic Infections in Adults and Adolescents with HIV. Guidelines for the prevention and treatment of opportunistic infections in adults and adolescents with HIV. National Institutes of Health, Centers for Disease Control and Prevention, HIV Medicine Association, and Infectious Diseases Society of America. https://clinicalinfo.hiv.gov/en/guidelines/adult-and-adolescent-opportunistic-infection. Monkeypox. Published 2022b. Accessed September 30, 2022.

Valcour VG. Evaluating cognitive impairment in the clinical setting: practical screening and assessment tools. *Top Antivir Med.* 2011c;19(5):175–180.

Valcour V, Paul R, Chiao S, et al. Screening for cognitive impairment in human immunodeficiency virus. *Clin Infect Dis.* 2011a;53(8):836–842.

Valcour V, Sithinamsuwan P, Letendre S, et al. Pathogenesis of HIV in the central nervous system. *Curr HIV/AIDS Rep.* 2011b;8(1):54–61.

Van der Meche FG, Schitz PI; Dutch Guillain–Barré Study Group. A randomized trial comparing intravenous immune globulin and plasma exchange in Guillain–Barré syndrome. *N Engl J Med.* 1992;326(17):1123–1129.

Vecchio AC, Marra CM, Schouten J, et al. Distal sensory peripheral neurology in human immunodeficiency virus type1-positive individuals before and after antiretroviral therapy initiative in diverse resource-limited settings. *Clin Infect Dis.* 2020;71(1):158–165.

Veltman JA, Bristow CC, Klausner JD. Meningitis in HIV-positive patients in sub-Saharan Africa: a review. *J Int AIDS Soc.* 2014;17:19184.

Verma A. Epidemiology and clinical features HIV-1 associated neuropathies. *J Peripheral Nerv Syst.* 2001;6(1):8–13.

Verma A, Bradley WG. HIV-1 associated neuropathies. *CNS Spectrums.* 2000;5(5):66–67.

Verma S, Estanislao L, Mintz L, et al. Controlling neuropathic pain in HIV. *Curr HIV/AIDS Rep.* 2004;1(3):136–141.

Vigil KJ, Salazar L, Hasbun R. Community-Acquired Meningitis in HIV-infected Patients in the United States. *AIDS Patient Care STDS.* 2018;32(2):42–47.

Wagner JC, Bromber MB. HIV infection presenting with motor axonal variant of Guillain–Barré syndrome. *J Clin Neuromusc Disord.* 2007;9:303–305.

Wakerly BR, Yuki N. Mimics and chameleons in Guillain–Barré and Miller–Fisher syndromes. *Practical Neurol.* 2015;15:90–99.

Wang SX, Ho EL, Grill M, et al. Peripheral neuropathy in primary HIV infection associates with systemic and CNS immune activation. *J Acquir Immune Defic Syndr*. 2014;66(3):303–310.

Webb AJ, Borrelli EP, Vyas A, et al. The effect of antiretroviral therapy with high central nervous system penetration on HIV-related cognitive impairment: a systematic review and meta-analysis. *AIDS Care*. 2022;18:1–12.

Williams D, Geraci A, Simpson DM. AIDS and AIDS-treatment neuropathies. *Curr Headache Rep*. 2002;6(2):125–130.

Winer JB. Guillain–Barré syndrome. *J Clin Pathol*. 2001;54:381–385.

Wulff EA, Simpson DM. Neuromuscular complications of the human immunodeficiency virus type 1 infection. *Semin Neurol*. 1999a;19(2):157–164.

Wulff EA, Simpson DM. Neuromuscular complications of HIV-1 infection. *Curr Infect Dis Rep*. 1999b;1(2):192–197.

Wulff EA, Wang AK, Simpson DM. HIV-associated peripheral neuropathy: epidemiology, pathophysiology and treatment. *Drugs*. 2000;59(6):1251–1260.

Yousem DM, Grossman RI. *The requisites: neuroradiology*. 3rd ed. Philadelphia: Mosby; 2010:209.

36.

HIV AND HEPATITIS COINFECTION

Karen J. Vigil

> **CHAPTER GOALS**
>
> Upon completion of this chapter, the reader should be able to:
>
> - Discuss the epidemiology, clinical presentation, diagnosis, treatment, and complications of hepatitis B and hepatitis C in people with HIV (PWH).

INTRODUCTION

Hepatitis B virus (HBV) and hepatitis C virus (HCV) are the leading causes of cirrhosis and hepatocellular carcinoma worldwide. They are transmitted perinatally or through early childhood exposure, sexual contact, and injection drug use. Approximately 10% of PWH also have chronic HBV infection, and up to 30% have coinfection with HCV.

HIV AND HEPATITIS B COINFECTION

LEARNING OBJECTIVE

Discuss the clinical presentation, diagnosis, treatment, and treatment complications of HBV in PWH.

WHAT'S NEW?

- Heplisav-B® is a 5'-C-phosphate-G-3' (CpG) conjugated hepatitis B vaccine that only requires two doses (0 and 1 month).

- A tenofovir alafenamide (TAF) antiretroviral regimen has been demonstrated to be noninferior than a tenofovir disoproxil fumarate (TDF) combination among PWH and chronic HBV infection.

KEY POINTS

- PWH should have a complete evaluation for HBV infection.

- All PWH without evidence of prior immunity or current HBV infection should be vaccinated against HBV.

- PWH and HBV-coinfection should receive treatment for both viruses, regardless of CD4⁺ T-cell count or independent need for HBV treatment.

- HBV treatment in persons HIV/HBV-coinfection should include two active agents against HBV, in the context of fully suppressive antiretroviral therapy (ART) against HIV.

CLINICAL PRESENTATION

Acute hepatitis B occurs 1 to 4 months after exposure. Approximately 30% of persons will present with icteric hepatitis and symptoms of fatigue, fever, right upper quadrant pain, and nausea; while the majority will have a subclinical presentation. Fulminant hepatitis is uncommon and develops in < 0.5% of people.

Around 20% of PWH will progress to chronic HBV, compared to < 10% in people without HIV. Of those, 15%–40% will progress to end-stage liver disease or hepatocellular carcinoma (HCC), and 25% will died because of complications of HBV.

DIAGNOSIS AND EVALUATION

Initial testing for HBV should include serologic testing for surface antigen (HBsAg), core antibody (anti-HBc total), and surface antibody (anti-HBs). HBsAg can usually be detected approximately 4 weeks after exposure. Resolution of acute HBV is characterized by negative HBsAg and the presence of anti-HBs and anti-HBc, but reactivation may occur following severe immunosuppression. Chronic HBV is defined as the presence of HBsAg detected on two occasions at least 6 months apart. Occult HBV infection, defined as the presence of anti-HBc alone with HBV DNA viremia in the absence of HBsAg, has been found in approximately 10% of PWH in the United States. Other possible causes of isolated anti-HBc are the preseroconversion "window phase" of acute HBV infection (between loss of HBsAg and emergence of anti-HBs), resolved hepatitis B infection with anti-HBs loss, or a false positive test. Individuals with occult HBV are also at increased risk of HBV reactivation, cirrhosis, and of HCC (Shire et al., 2004).

Persons with chronic HBV should be tested for HBe-antigen (HBeAg), HBe-antibody (anti-HBe), and HBV DNA. Individuals with HBeAg usually have high HBV DNA and elevated alanine aminotransferase (ALT) levels and are at high risk of future liver complications. Seroconversion from positive HBeAg to anti-HBe-antibody can imply a transition from active disease to an inactive carrier state, but this occurs less commonly in people coinfected with HIV and HBV. This inactive carrier state is also characterized by HBV DNA levels less than 2000 IU/mL and normal ALT. These persons do remain at risk for HBV reactivation and liver disease progression, but at a lower rate than that of individuals with active disease. Finally, there also exists a state of HBeAg-negative active hepatitis, which is a result of mutations in the precore and core promoter regions. These individuals are at significant risk of progressive liver disease, and HBV DNA levels should be monitored regularly, with treatment instituted as recommended (Hadziyannis & Papatheodoridis, 2006).

Elevations of hepatic transaminases are suggestive of inflammation, and hepatic synthetic function is measured by serum albumin and coagulation factors. An assessment of the degree of liver fibrosis is important, and options for this include liver biopsy or noninvasive testing such as transient elastography or an increasing array of serum biomarker tests. Persons with cirrhosis should have HCC screening by ultrasound every 6–12 months, and all persons with cirrhosis should be comanaged with a hepatologist (Lok & McMahon, 2009).

Current HIV guidelines recommend antiretroviral treatment of all PWH, persons with HIV/HBV-coinfection should be a priority group for HIV treatment. ART must include two drugs with activity against HBV, such as tenofovir alafenamide (TAF) or TDF plus emtricitabine or lamivudine, regardless of the stage of HBV or degree of liver fibrosis (Terrault et al., 2018).

HIV/HBV-COINFECTION CONSIDERATIONS

In general terms, the presence of HIV/HBV-coinfection worsens outcomes related to HBV. PWH are less likely to resolve acute HBV exposure and have higher levels of HBV DNA compared to those without HIV (Colin, 1999). HIV/HBV-coinfection is associated with more rapid progression of HBV-related cirrhosis, HCC, and fatal hepatic failure (Thio et al., 2002). Indeed, HBV infection was associated with a relative risk of 3.73 for liver-related deaths in HIV/HBV-coinfected participants in the Data Collection on Adverse Events of Anti-HIV Drugs (D:A:D) study (Weber et al., 2006).

Because the immune response plays a key role in both HBV clearance and the immune damage associated with chronic HBV infection, HIV/HBV-coinfection impacts the course of HBV infection. HIV-induced immunosuppression increases the risk of reactivation of quiescent HBV, and initiation of ART may result in exacerbation of HBV liver disease (hepatitis flares) or fulminant hepatitis (Sulkowski et al., 2001).

Stopping antiretroviral agents with activity against HBV (lamivudine, emtricitabine, and TDF or TAF) may lead to HBV rebound, sometimes accompanied by a severe flare and hepatocellular damage (Dore et al., 2010). Thus, when persons with HIV/HBV-coinfection change ARV regimens, it is crucial to maintain agents with anti-HBV activity. If anti-HBV treatment is discontinued, serum transaminase levels should be monitored regularly; if a hepatic flare occurs, then HBV therapy should be restarted immediately because this could be life-saving (US Department of Health and Human Services (DHHS), Panel on Opportunistic Infections, 2022b).

HBV PREVENTION

People with HIV should be counseled about transmission risks for HBV, including sexual transmission, sharing of needles and syringes, and tattooing or body piercing. People at risk for HBV should be advised to avoid these behaviors associated with transmission (DHHS, 2022b).

HBV vaccination is the most effective way to prevent HBV infection. If there is no evidence of chronic infection or previous vaccination (anti-HBs < 10 IU/mL), then a hepatitis B vaccination series should be administered (DHHS, 2022b). Individuals who are positive for anti-HBs and anti-HBc have a resolved infection and do not require vaccination. Individuals with "isolated anti-HBc" (see previous description) who have an undetectable HBV DNA should receive a complete HBV vaccine series.

Unfortunately, the preventive HBV vaccination is less effective in PWH, with efficacy rates in this population of approximately 65%, and those with a CD4 $^+$ T-cell count less than 350 cells/mm^3 have even lower response rates. HBV vaccination of all nonimmune PWH is currently recommended regardless of CD4 $^+$ T-cell count, and vaccination should not be deferred in persons with CD4 $^+$ T-cell counts of less than 350 cells/mm^3 (DHHS, 2022b). Various revaccination strategies are available for persons who do not respond to an initial series. A repeat three-dose vaccination series or a double dose of vaccine is recommended in PWH not responding to a complete vaccination (Terrault et al., 2018). A new two-dose recombinant hepatitis B vaccine, Heplisav-B®, was approved by the FDA in 2017. Heplisav-B® is a vaccine conjugated with the Toll-like receptor 9 agonist adjuvant CpG and has the advantage that only requires two doses given at 0 and 1 months. Randomized clinical studies have demonstrated higher seroprotection response when compared to Engerix-B® including in people with diabetes mellitus and chronic kidney disease. Studies in PWH are undergoing.

GOALS OF TREATMENT

The goals of treatment for HBV infection are to achieve sustained suppression of viral replication to below detectable levels and to improve or stabilize the degree of liver disease in order to prevent cirrhosis, hepatic failure, and HCC. Measurements of response to therapy include the decline in HBV DNA to undetectable levels, loss of HBeAg or gain of anti-HBe-antibody (termed seroconversion), normalization of serum ALT, and improvement in liver histology. Functional cure is represented by an undetectable HBsAg, which may reduce progression to cirrhosis and liver cancer (Sherman, 2015).

HIV TREATMENT RECOMMENDATIONS IN THE SETTING OF HBV-COINFECTION

Because coinfection with HIV is associated with more rapid progression of HBV-related liver disease and there is evidence that earlier treatment of HIV may slow the development of liver disease by improving immune function and reducing

HIV-related inflammation and immune activation, current HIV treatment guidelines recommend that all persons with HIV/HBV-coinfection to start ART and that the ART regimen include two drugs with activity against HBV (DHHS, 2022a).

The Panel on Opportunistic Infections makes the following recommendations for persons with HIV/HBV (DHHS, 2022b; American Association for the Study of Liver Disease/ Infectious Diseases Society of America; Terrault et al., 2018):

- Regardless of CD4$^+$ T-cell count or the need for HBV treatment, ART that includes agents active against both HIV and HBV is recommended for all persons with HIV and HBV.

- ART must include two drugs active against HBV, preferably TDF or TAF and emtricitabine or lamivudine, regardless of the level of HBV DNA.

- If the individual refuses HIV treatment, then there are few options available to treat HBV because entecavir given without suppressive ART may result in HIV resistance, and telbivudine and adefovir are not recommended. A 48-week course of pegylated interferon-α-2a can be considered in such circumstances (Terrault et al., 2018).

- In circumstances in which tenofovir use is not acceptable as part of the ART regimen, the alternate recommendation is to use entecavir in addition to a fully suppressive ART.

- Chronic use of lamivudine or emtricitabine as the single active agent against HBV should be avoided because of the high rate of subsequent HBV resistance.

Individuals being treated for HBV should have HBV DNA measured every 12–24 weeks. If the HBV DNA is greater than 1,000 IU/mL after 1 year, then adherence to medication should be assessed and HBV resistance testing considered. Viral failure and resistance are more common in PWH with HBV, especially when lamivudine is used alone for treatment. The risk of resistance has declined with the use of more potent drugs such as tenofovir and entecavir (Luetkemeyer et al., 2011). Unfortunately, even with long-term suppression of HBV DNA, the loss of HBsAg (functional cure) of HBV is not common in PWH coinfection (Sherman, 2015), and indefinite treatment is usually recommended.

SPECIAL CONSIDERATIONS

Immune Reconstitution Inflammatory Syndrome

Immune reconstitution during the course of HIV/HBV treatment can lead to a severe flare of chronic HBV infection, with significant increases in hepatic transaminases, perhaps because of enhanced host immune responses against HBV. HBV-associated immune reconstitution inflammatory syndrome (IRIS) is most likely to occur during the first few weeks after starting ART and can present as acute hepatitis. Careful monitoring of hepatic transaminases after the initiation of ART is helpful (Audsley et al., 2011). Development of signs of hepatic synthetic dysfunction, such as elevated prothrombin time or low albumin, should prompt evaluation by a hepatologist. Distinguishing between HBV-related IRIS and drug-induced liver toxicity can be challenging and may require examination of liver histology and consultation with a hepatologist. Very little information is available regarding the best treatment for HBV-related IRIS, and the decision regarding whether to continue, modify, or interrupt therapy should be individualized based on the severity of hepatic injury.

Treatment Interruptions

Because of the overlap in anti-HIV and HBV activity of emtricitabine, lamivudine, and tenofovir, interruption of treatment should be avoided in HIV/HBV-coinfection to avoid potentially severe flares of HBV with hepatic inflammation and necrosis. In particular, when there is a need to discontinue one of the HBV-active drugs in the HIV treatment regimen, careful follow-up of liver function tests (LFTs) is required, and addition of a second agent with anti-HBV activity should be considered. If there is a need to change ART because of HIV resistance and HBV suppression is maintained despite HIV treatment failure, the antiretrovirals with activity against HBV should be continued for HBV treatment in addition to other appropriate antiretroviral agents.

TREATMENT OPTIONS FOR HEPATITIS B INFECTION

It is currently recommended to start all PWH on ART. The preferred treatment regimen for people with HIV/ HBV-coinfection is an antiretroviral treatment with the backbone regimen of TAF or TDF with lamivudine or emtricitabine. Both TDF and TAF have a high genetic barrier of resistance. Monotherapy with lamivudine or emtricitabine is not recommended because of the increased possibility to develop resistance. Treatment is recommended lifelong. Discontinuation of treatment has been associated with hepatitis flares. Treatment of HBV alone is not recommended.

SUMMARY

Hepatitis B infection is a common and potentially severe comorbidity for PWH. Screening for HBV infection, vaccination, and careful assessment of chronic HBV infection are important components of HIV care. Consideration of chronic HBV status when selecting HIV treatment regimens is essential in optimizing management of both infections. Monitoring for response to treatment for HBV and screening for complications such as cirrhosis or HCC are part of the ongoing care of persons with HIV/HBV-coinfection.

HIV AND HEPATITIS C COINFECTION

LEARNING OBJECTIVE

Discuss the clinical presentation, diagnosis, and treatment of HCV in PWH.

WHAT'S NEW?

- Direct acting antivirals (DAAs) achieve a cure of greater than 90% in PWH and chronic HCV infections.

- To decrease the incidence of new cases in the general population, individuals that develop acute HCV should be treated immediately and not wait for spontaneous resolution.

- HCV RNA should be obtained at 12 weeks posttreatment to determine cure (SVR12). Monitoring of HCV RNA during treatment is not recommended.

KEY POINTS

- HCV-treatment regimens are now simpler and efficacious. Therefore, all PWH with HCV should be offered treatment. Drug–drug interactions, disease severity, and, especially, cost considerations remain.

EPIDEMIOLOGY

As ART continues to extend the life span of PWH by decades, HIV/HCV coinfection has become an increasingly important cause of both morbidity and mortality. Liver disease has emerged as the leading cause of non-AIDS-related deaths in PWH with HCV or HBV (Centers for Disease Control and Prevention (CDC), 2020). HIV/HCV coinfection places a growing burden on the HIV healthcare delivery system, as evidenced by an analysis conducted by the AIDS Clinical Trials Group (ACTG) Longitudinal Linked Randomized Trials (ALLRT) cohort. When controlling for age, race, sex, history of AIDS-defining events, and current CD4$^+$ T-cell count and HIV RNA levels, the relative risk of hospitalization, emergency department visits, and disability days for persons with HIV/HCV versus HIV mono-infected participants was 1.8 (95% confidence interval (CI): 1.3–2.5), 1.7 (95% CI: 1.4–2.1), and 1.6 (95% CI: 1.3–1.9), respectively. Based on the ACTG's study findings, programs serving persons with HIV/HCV coinfection can expect to experience an almost 70% higher rate of utilization for this group (Linas et al., 2011). A study from the New York City Department of Health and Mental Hygiene using death certificate data, showed persons with HIV/HCV coinfection to be at exceptionally high risk for premature death (median age, 52.0 years) compared to those with HCV alone (median age, 60.0 years) or those with neither virus (median age, 78.0 years). Decedents had an odds ratio of 2.2 for death from liver cancer and 3.1 for drug-related causes, with 53.6% of deaths attributed to HIV/AIDS and 94% occurring prematurely (defined as younger than age 65 years) (Pinchoff et al., 2014).

HCV is a single-stranded RNA virus transmitted primarily through blood exposure and, less commonly, through sexual or vertical transmission. Because HIV and HCV share similar routes of transmission, approximately one-fifth of all PWH in the United States are also infected with HCV. This percentage increases to 80% for people who inject drugs (PWID) (CDC, 2020). Heterosexual transmission risk is low and generally quoted as less than 1% per year, although high-risk sex practices such as aggressive anal intercourse and multiple sex partners increase transmission risk. Vertical transmission is possible, with pregnant women with HIV/HCV coinfection having a 15%–20% chance of passing HCV to their infants compared to the 5%–15% rate in infants born to HCV-mono-infected mothers (Bevilacqua et al., 2009; Mast et al., 2005). Most studies to date do not support elective cesarean delivery for HCV-positive women. Breastfeeding is not known to transmit HCV, but because breastfeeding may transmit HIV, it is contraindicated for mothers with HIV/HCV coinfection in the United States.

In recent years, HIV/HCV coinfection has been a changing epidemic, as evidenced by data from the Swiss HIV Cohort Study. What was once a disease of PWID and hemophiliacs has become a sexually transmitted disease of MSM. The 4.1 cases per 100 person-years seen in MSM in 2011 in the Swiss Cohort Study represented an 18-fold increase from 1998, with HCV seen in association with a history of unsafe anal sex, a past syphilis history, and chronic HBV (Wandeler et al., 2012). In 2011, a report was published that included 5-year data from 74 MSM with HIV who had no history of injection drug use (IDU) and had newly elevated ALT levels with a positive HCV antibody test (Fierer et al., 2012). This matched case–control study was conducted beginning in July 2007 and examined men who were within 12 months of the clinical onset of HIV infection and who had no IDU history. MSM with HIV newly infected with HCV were significantly more likely to have had receptive anal intercourse (mOR 24.87) or insertive anal intercourse (matched odds ratio (mOR) 2.62) with no condom use and with ejaculation, engaged in group sex (mOR 19.2), engaged in sex while high on drugs (mOR 11.37), previously had syphilis (mOR 8.8), and/or had sex while using crystal methamphetamine (mOR 26.8). HIV/HCV coinfection results in increased HCV RNA levels, which are thought to increase the infectiousness of HCV acquired through sexual contact. People with HIV should be counseled that unprotected sex can transmit other infections, including HCV.

The connection between prescription narcotic abuse, HIV, and HCV was highlighted by a community outbreak of HIV linked to IDU of oxymorphone in a rural county of Indiana. Prior to this investigation, only five HIV cases per year were reported. As of April 21, 2015, 135 persons had confirmed or probable HIV infection in a community of 4,200 persons. Mean age was 35 years, with 54.8% being males, 80% reporting IDU, and 17% who had not yet been interviewed. All reported their drug of choice was injectable crushed oxymorphone, sometimes with other illicit drugs. Of these, 7.4% were female commercial sex workers. Strikingly, coinfection with HCV was found in 84.4% of individuals (Conrad et al.,

2015). Those interviewed reported an average of nine syringe-sharing or sex partners and social contacts who may be at risk. Of the 230 contacts tested, 109 (47.4%) were positive for HIV. Injectable drug use in this community is multigenerational, with the crushed oxymorphone (40 mg tablets are not designed to resist crushing) dissolved in nonsterile water and injected via insulin syringes with the syringes often shared. This outbreak highlights the vulnerability of many resource-poor rural communities that traditionally have low rates of HIV and HCV and the need for community interventions at multiple levels. This is a reminder of how often concomitant transmission of the two viruses continues to occur, particularly in vulnerable PWID and MSM.

CLINICAL COURSE

The most striking feature of HCV when acquired by a person with HIV is its ability to cause chronic hepatitis in as much as 90% of persons within 6 months. This occurs because of the lack of CD4 $^+$ T-cell responses and significantly reduced IFN-γ ELISpot responses against HCV (Elliott et al., 2006). Between 60% and 70% of chronically infected persons will have fluctuating serum ALT levels because this is the enzyme most associated with liver cell injury in HCV. Less than 20% have nonspecific symptoms, including fatigue and generalized weakness. There are significant similarities and differences between HIV and HCV. Both are RNA viruses with rapid replication rates (10 trillion HCV virions vs. 10 billion HIV virions produced daily). Both are prone to frequent mutations and exist as heterogeneous quasispecies to avoid the immune system. Both viruses incite abundant but ineffective antibody responses. Although both have many reservoirs in the human body, HCV exists primarily in the cytoplasm of hepatocytes and can be eradicated from the body. HIV is integrated into the nuclei of CD4 $^+$ T lymphocytes and long-lived memory T-cell reservoirs and therefore cannot be eradicated with current ART. HCV RNA levels are only broadly predictive of long-term prognosis, whereas HIV RNA is very predictive of clinical events in untreated persons.

There are six different HCV genotypes (1–6) at various prevalence rates throughout the world. In the United States, genotype (GT) 1 accounts for two-thirds of cases, with GTs 2–4 occurring less commonly.

DIAGNOSIS

HCV may be diagnosed earlier in asymptomatic PWH with elevated ALT/AST levels because of greater frequency of lab monitoring (Mohsen & Easterbrook, 2003). Coinfection with HIV greatly impacts the natural history of HCV infection. Individuals with HIV/HCV coinfection are less likely to spontaneously clear HCV, have increased HCV RNA, and progress more rapidly to cirrhosis and end-stage liver disease (ESLD) (Asselah et al., 2006). Predictors of severe liver fibrosis include age older than 40 years at time of infection, alcohol consumption of more than 50 g/d, daily marijuana use, high body mass index, male gender, postmenopausal status, and longer duration of infection (Poynard et al., 1997). Although ART may slow this rate, it continues to exceed that seen in persons with HCV mono-infection. Low CD4 $^+$ T-cell counts also appear to magnify the progression. A meta-analysis of eight studies that examined the role of HIV with HCV found that persons with HIV/HCV coinfection had approximately two times the risk of cirrhosis on liver biopsy and six times the risk of decompensated liver disease with ascites, varices, or encephalopathy compared to HCV-mono-infected individuals (Poynard et al., 1997). A Veterans Health Administration study examined 4,820 persons with HIV/HCV coinfection and 6,079 persons with HCV in care from 1997 to 2010. All had detectable HCV RNA levels and were HCV-treatment naive. Hepatic decompensation was significantly greater at 10 years in the HIV/HCV group (7.4% vs. 4.8%; $p < 0.001$) (Lo et al., 2014). Approximately one-third of persons with chronic HCV will progress to cirrhosis at a median time of less than 20 years (Thomas et al., 2000). Once cirrhosis has developed, 50% will decompensate within the first 5 years, with ascites being the usual first sign. Approximately 1%–4% of cirrhotic individuals per year will develop HCC. Median survival time is 35 months versus 65 months for those without HIV (Beretta et al., 2011).

Although the average time from infection to fibrosis is shortened from 35 to 25 years in persons with HIV/HCV, Fierer's group at Mt. Sinai School of Medicine (New York City) found that MSM with HIV who developed HCV had a much more rapid onset of fibrosis. In a 2008 analysis, 9 of 11 (82%) men had stage 2 (moderate) fibrosis at a median of only 4 months after diagnosis (Fierer et al., 2012). In 2013, researchers reported on four individuals who developed decompensated cirrhosis and death within 2–8 years post-HCV infection (Fierer et al., 2013). The authors noted that the order in which the infections are acquired is important. When HCV is acquired after HIV, there is accelerated progression to fibrosis that may be proportional to the degree of immunosuppression. However, not all studies have seen such rapid progression. The European NEAT cohort evaluated fibrosis rates in 41 PWH who subsequently developed HCV. Most were MSM on ART with a mean CD4 $^+$ T-cell count of 500 cells/mm^3. FibroScan transient elastometry (used to assess liver stiffness) over a maximum follow-up of 8 years found no significant hepatic changes (Boesecke et al., 2014).

Deferring HCV treatment in the age of DAAs may lead to increased rates of HCC and death. Data from the SHCS and published HCV data were used for mathematical modeling to predict the decrease in progression to cirrhosis, HCC, and death in person with HIV/HCV. If therapy was initiated during stages F0 or F1, the percentage of liver-related-deaths was 2%. However, if treatment was deferred until F3 or F4 stage, mortality increased to 7% and 22%, respectively. If individuals are not treated immediately, they remain infectious. Important from a public health perspective, those treated between 1 month and 1 year after diagnosis remained infectious from a HCV standpoint for approximately 5 years, compared to 12 years for stage 2,

15 years for stage 3, and nearly 20 years for stage 4 (Zahnd et al., 2016).

DECISION TO TREAT

All PWH should be screened for HCV with antibody testing upon entry into care and annually thereafter for those at risk and whenever HCV infection is suspected (Thompson et al., 2021). HCV RNA levels should be tested in all those with a positive antibody test to assess for active disease because antibodies persist for a lifetime even in persons who have cleared the virus. Infants born to mothers with HIV/HCV coinfection should also have antibody testing performed. HCV transmission may be facilitated by the presence of genital erosions related to sexually transmitted diseases. Reinfection with HCV can occur, necessitating that individuals be aware that high-risk behaviors put them at risk for reinfection (Danta & Dusheiko, 2008). Persons with HCV/HIV coinfection should be advised to avoid alcohol consumption and to avoid sharing razors, toothbrushes, syringes, and so on to prevent spread of infection to others. Those who are susceptible to hepatitis A or hepatitis B should be vaccinated against these viruses because dual or triple infections are typically more severe (Low et al., 2008).

PWH should be treated similarly as HCV-mono-infected patients. The efficacy and safety of current direct acting agents is similar in PWH. However, drug–drug interaction should be reviewed carefully. If CD4$^+$ T-cell count is less than 200 cells/mm^3, HIV treatment to improve the immune status could take precedence. Initial ART regimens for people with HIV/HCV coinfection are similar to PWH without HCV infection. However, drug–drug interactions between antiretroviral drugs and direct-acting antivirals (DDA) should be considered when choosing the initial therapy or when switching a suppressive antiretroviral regimen in order to start treatment for HCV.

Testing for HCV RNA levels by polymerase chain reaction is the only reliable way to diagnose acute HCV infection because approximately 30% of individuals do not have detectable antibodies at the onset of symptoms. A positive HCV antibody test with history of a prior negative HCV antibody test is also indicative of recent seroconversion. More than 90% will have antibodies by 3 months postexposure, with less than 5% of persons with HIV/HCV (usually those with advanced immunosuppression) failing to produce detectable HCV antibodies. Acute HCV is asymptomatic in 70%–80% of cases, but cure rates are significantly higher with acute disease. It is therefore important to routinely screen at-risk individuals and promptly investigate elevated hepatic transaminase levels. Acutely infected HCV persons who are symptomatic have a higher likelihood of spontaneous viral clearance. However, because of the high efficacy and safety of DAA, experts recommend treating these people rather than monitoring them. Acute HCV infection may present with flu-like symptoms, nausea, abdominal pain, and jaundice. Infrequently, severe hepatic dysfunction with transaminases up to 10 times normal is seen, but fulminant hepatitis is rare (DHHS, 2022b).

Prior to initiating HCV treatment in persons with HIV/HCV coinfection, specific baseline lab tests should be conducted. These include a complete blood count (CBC) with platelets, hepatic function panel including ALT, AST, alkaline phosphatase, albumin, and total bilirubin, prothrombin time/international normalized ratio (PT/INR), calculated glomerular filtration rate (eGFR), HIV, and HCV RNA levels. If a nonpangenotypic DAA will be prescribed, then HCV genotype is recommended. A pregnancy test is recommended for all females of childbearing potential if ribavirin (RBV) use is planned because of its known teratogenicity. Counseling against alcohol consumption is key because this can rapidly worsen fibrosis. HBV and hepatitis A virus vaccination should be offered to all people without evidence of exposure to these infections.

Liver fibrosis should be assessed prior to start treatment. Because of the risks associated with biopsy, alternatives such as FibroScan and FibroSURE have rapidly risen in popularity and acceptance in clinical practice. FibroScan utilizes a mild-amplitude, low-frequency vibration transmitted through the liver to measure tissue "stiffness." This noninvasive and less expensive monitoring tool has been used in Europe for more than a decade and has been approved in the United States since 2013 for clinical use. FibroSURE uses six blood serum tests (α_2-macroglobulin, haptoglobin, apolipoprotein A1, γ-glutamyl transferase, ALT, and total bilirubin) along with age and gender to generate a score that correlates with degree of liver disease. Other noninvasive biomarker formulas, such as APRI, which incorporates platelet counts with tests of coagulation and transaminases, and fibrosis-4 (FIB-4) may also be used to evaluate degree of fibrosis. APRI and FibroSURE have been validated in HIV/HCV coinfection and predict no disease versus cirrhosis accurately but are not as accurate in the mid-range of the disease spectrum (Rallon et al., 2011; Schneider & Sarrazin, 2014).

Several formulas are used to assess the degree of cirrhosis. The Child–Turcotte–Pugh score uses encephalopathy, ascites, bilirubin, albumin, and PT or INR to classify severity of cirrhosis (class A, 5–6 points; class B, 7–9 points; and class C, 10–15 points). The Model for End-stage Liver Disease (MELD) score uses serum creatinine, bilirubin, and INR and two or more dialysis sessions within the previous week to predict probability of survival for persons with ESLD. This is the formula currently used for liver allocation by the United Network of Organ Sharing and predicts the 3-month mortality rate. A MELD calculator is provided on the Mayo Clinic website (http://www.mayoclinic.org/medical-professionals/model-end-stage-liver-disease/meld-model). The HALT-C formula for predicting cirrhosis uses platelet count, INR, AST, and ALT to predict the probability of a biopsy demonstrating cirrhosis (Lok & McMahon, 2009).

THERAPEUTIC MODALITIES

Multiple, all-oral combinations of DAAs are now available as the recommended regimens for treatment (Table 36.1).

Table 36.1 CURRENT DIRECT ANTIVIRAL AGENTS FOR HEPATITIS C

DIRECT ANTIVIRAL AGENT	GENOTYPES TREATED	CLASS	GFR	COMMENTS
Elbasvir/grazoprevir Zepatier®	1 and 4	NS5A inhibitor ± NS3/4A protease inhibitor	No dose adjustment in patients with renal impairment including those on hemodialysis	NS5A testing is required in patients with GT 1a
Ledipasvir/sofosbuvir Harvoni®	1 to 6	NS5A inhibitor ± nucleotide polymerase inhibitor (NS5B)	No dosage recommendation for patients with glomerular filtration rate less than 30 mL/min/1.73 m²	First fixed oral combination
Sofosbuvir/ velpatasvir Epclusa®	1 to 6	Nucleotide polymerase inhibitor (NS5B) ± NS5A inhibitor	No dosage recommendation for patients with glomerular filtration rate less than 30 mL/min/1.73 m²	
Sofosbuvir/ velpatasvir/ voxilapresvir Vosevi®	1 to 6	Nucleotide polymerase inhibitor (NS5B) ± NS5A inhibitor ± NS3/4A protease inhibitor	No dosage recommendation for patients with glomerular filtration rate less than 30 mL/min/1.73 m²	For patients who have failed therapy with a NS5A inhibitor–containing regimen
Glecaprevir/ pibrentasvir Mavyret®	1 to 6	HCV NS3/4A protease inhibitor ± HCV NS5A inhibitor	No dose adjustment in patients with renal impairment including those on hemodialysis	
Daclatasvir (Daklinza)® ± Sofosbuvir (Sovaldi®) (alternative regimen)	1 and 3	NS5A inhibitor ± nucleotide polymerase inhibitor (NS5B)	No dosage adjustment is required for patients with any degree of renal impairment	Several drug interactions with antiretroviral treatments

Evidence supports treating all people with HCV unless their life expectancy is less than 12 months because of a non-liver-related condition. As such, current guidelines places PWH in the "high priority" for treatment category given the increased risk of fibrosis and HCC. Treatment response is similar in persons with HIV/HCV coinfection and persons with HCV-mono-infection. Peg-IFN-α-2a or -2b and RBV had a cure rate of approximately 50% and had severe side effects. Therefore, guidelines no longer recommend their use.

Monitoring of HCV RNA levels during treatment is not recommended. There are no data to support discontinuing treatment if the person is viremic. HCV RNA levels should be obtained at 12 weeks posttreatment to determine cure (SVR12).

Drug–drug interactions increase the complexity of treating HCV in PWH on ART, as does the issue of renal function. Based on current evidence, the preferred treatment for persons with chronic kidney disease (CKD) stage 4 or 5 (eGFR < 30 mL/min or end-stage renal disease) is either sofosbuvir (400 mg)/velpatasvir (100 mg100mg) or glecaprevir (300 mg)/pibrentasvir (120 mg). ART switches may need to occur prior to treatment for HCV. Individuals may return to their prior regimen after treatment is completed. Although choosing a regimen to avoid drug interactions may seem daunting, interrupting ART while on HCV treatment is not recommended. Treatment interruption is associated with increased cardiovascular events as well as fibrosis progression and liver-related events. Because this area is in constant flux, see "Guidelines for the Use of Antiretroviral Agents in HIV-1-Infected Adults and Adolescents" (DHHS, 2022a) under the HIV/HCV coinfection section (updated 2021) and "AASLD/IDSA 2021 HCV Guidance: Recommendations for Testing, Managing and Treating Hepatitis C" under the Management of Unique Populations section, for current advice on ART for HIV when treating HCV.

The standard of care for hepatitis C now are the oral DDAs. They are engineered to work at multiple HCV-specific sites, such as the protease and polymerase enzymes (Figure 36.1). The first generation, boceprevir and telaprevir, were NS3/4A protease inhibitors (PIs). Although briefly state-of-the-art between their licensure in 2010 and 2012, they are no longer recommended in the United States because more-efficacious and less-toxic drugs have been developed. The second wave of HCV therapies have simple rules for use, shorter duration of therapy, and fewer drug–drug interactions and side effects and are highly effective in both HCV-mono-infected and HIV/HCV-coinfected people.

DIRECT ACTING AGENTS

The HCV genome encodes 10 polyproteins, seven nonstructural proteins, and three structural proteins (NS3/4A, NS5A, NS5B) that play an important role in HCV replication and

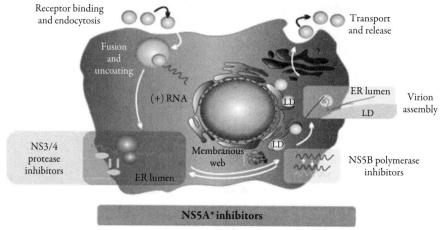

Figure 36.1 HCV life-cycle and antiviral therapy for people with HCV   ER = endoplasmic reticulum; LD = luminal domain.

are the target of current DAA (Figure 36.2). Sofosbuvir (SOF) and simeprevir (SIM) were the initial second-generation DAA approved in the United States. SIM was discontinued in May 2018 because of decreased utilization. However, SOF has become the cornerstone of most of the current combination treatments for HCV.

NS5B Polymerase Inhibitor(s)

NS5B polymerase is required for viral replication, acting as a chain terminator. SOF is a nucleotide analog inhibitor of this enzyme. The NS5B site is highly conserved among all genotypes; SOF is pangenotypic. It is given as 400 mg once daily. It is not metabolized by the CYP450 enzyme complex and thus is an ideal candidate for use in people with HIV/HCV coinfection.

The nonnucleoside polymerase inhibitors, dasavuvir was coformulated with ombitasvir, paritaprevir, and ritonavir

(RTV) as a fixed-dose combination. It had lower genetic barrier of resistance and is no longer available in the market.

NS3/4A Protease Inhibitors

Glecaprevir, grazoprevir, paritaprevir, and voxileprevir are the current DAAs available in this class. They are noncovalent inhibitors of the NS3/4A serine protease of HCV.

NS5A Inhibitors

The exact mechanism of action of the NS5A inhibitors is not completely understood. However, some studies showed that they bind to the N-terminal domain of NS5A, causing structural distortion and inhibiting both viral RNA replication and virion assembly at an early stage. Daclatasvir, elbasvir, ledipasvir, ombitasvir, pibrentasvir, and velpastavir are antivirals in this class. Daclatasvir has been discontinued

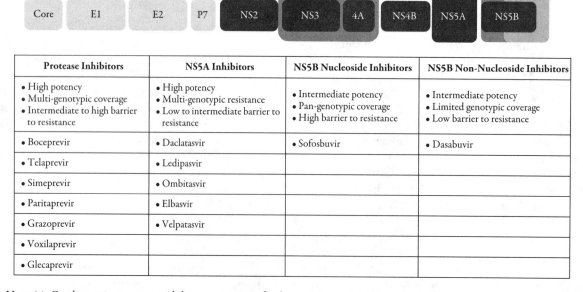

Protease Inhibitors	NS5A Inhibitors	NS5B Nucleoside Inhibitors	NS5B Non-Nucleoside Inhibitors
• High potency • Multi-genotypic coverage • Intermediate to high barrier to resistance	• High potency • Multi-genotypic resistance • Low to intermediate barrier to resistance	• Intermediate potency • Pan-genotypic coverage • High barrier to resistance	• Intermediate potency • Limited genotypic coverage • Low barrier to resistance
• Boceprevir	• Daclatasvir	• Sofosbuvir	• Dasabuvir
• Telaprevir	• Ledipasvir		
• Simeprevir	• Ombitasvir		
• Paritaprevir	• Elbasvir		
• Grazoprevir	• Velpatasvir		
• Voxilaprevir			
• Glecaprevir			

Figure 36.2 Hepatitis C polyprotein structure and therapeutic targets for direct-acting antiviral drug development   SOURCE: Adapted from Poordad F, Chee GM. *Curr Gastroenterol Rep.* Interferon free-hepatitis C treatment regimens: the beginning of another era. 2012;14(1):74–77.

from the marker. All others are coformulated in fixed-dose combinations.

FIXED-DOSE COMBINATIONS

Ledipasvir/Sofosbuvir

Ledipasvir 90 mg and sofosbuvir 400 mg (LDV/SOF, trade name Harvoni*) was the first interferon- and ribavirin-free once-daily, single-tablet regimen for HCV approved by the FDA (on October 14, 2014).

The ION-4 study was a phase 3, multicenter, open-label trial of 335 persons with HIV/HCV. Enrolled participants had GT 1 and 4 (75% GT 1a, 23% GT 1b, and 2% GT 4), 20% had compensated cirrhosis, and 55% were treatment experienced. Based on drug–drug interaction data available at the beginning of the trial, ARTs allowed in study were emtricitabine (FTC)/TDF with efavirenz (EFV), rilpivirine (RPV), or raltegravir (RAL). The primary end point was SVR12 post-treatment, with SVR24 as the secondary end point.

No difference in response rates at week 12 of treatment was seen with GT 1a versus GT 1b based on sex, treatment history, concomitant ART, or cirrhosis status. Thirteen individuals (4%) did not achieve SVR. One person died at week 4 of treatment; two had breakthrough on treatment that was believed by treating physicians to likely be related to poor adherence; and ten relapsed after treatment. All 10 relapsers were Black, with 7 having the TT allele in the gene encoding IL28B (which confers an increased risk of failure with IFN-containing regimens). The combination of Black race and the presence of the TT allele was found to have a significant association in the univariate analysis. Black race alone in the multivariate analysis was significantly associated with relapse. The association of lower SVR with Black race, which comprised 34% of the study population, was not seen in the studies of LDV/SOB in HCV-mono-infected persons and was not related to the CYP2B6 polymorphism, which is more common in Black persons and results in increased EFV levels (Naggie et al., 2015).

LDV/SOF increases exposure to TDF by approximately 40%. Individuals on RTV-containing regimens may experience a relative increase of 30%–60% in TDF exposure and so were excluded from the trial along with those on cobicistat-containing combinations. Although 77% of persons had an adverse event, these were usually mild to moderate and resulted in no premature study discontinuations. Headache (25%), fatigue (21%), and diarrhea (11%) were the most common adverse events. Eight individuals experienced 15 serious adverse events, with HCC in two persons and portal vein thrombosis in two persons—all being reported in participants with cirrhosis. Three persons experienced serious infections. Grade 3 laboratory abnormalities occurred in 9%, and grade 4 laboratory abnormalities in 2% of individuals, with elevations in lipase, creatinine phosphokinase, and serum glucose being the most common.

Elbasvir/Grazoprevir

Elbasvir 50 mg and grazoprevir 100 mg (ELB/GRZ, trade name Zepatier*) is a fixed-dose combination taken once a day with or without food for the treatment of chronic HCV GT 1 or 4 infection in adults. Treatment is typically 12 weeks. RBV is added and treatment extended to 16 weeks if baseline NS5A polymorphisms are found in a GT 1a person. RBV may be added in GT 1a or 1b person who are Peg/RBV/PI-experienced. GT 4 persons who are Peg/IFN/RBV-experienced also receive 16 weeks of treatment. RBV is given as two daily doses depending on baseline NS5A polymorphisms and treatment experience. No dosage adjustment for ELB/GRZ is needed for renal impairment, including those on hemodialysis, although the RBV may need adjustment per guidelines. It is contraindicated in those with Child–Pugh B or C disease. ELB/GRZ is contraindicated with OATP1B1/3 inhibitors and strong CYP3A inducers such as EFV. Other contraindicated drugs include phenytoin and carbamazepine, rifampin, and St. John's wort. Coadministration with nafcillin, ketoconazole, bosentan, modafinil, entecavir (ETV), and cobicistat-containing compounds is not recommended. The risk of ALT elevations may be elevated with zidovudine (ATZ), darunavir (DRV), lopinavir (LPV), and cyclosporine. Statins also interact with ELB/GRZ. Thus, atorvastatin should not exceed 20 mg; rosuvastatin should not exceed 10 mg; and the lowest possible dose of fluvastatin, lovastatin, and simvastatin should be used. Tacrolimus levels may be increased by ELB/GRZ.

ELB/GRZ was approved for the treatment of GT 1 and 4 only based on results from the C-EDGE study. A total of 299 participants were enrolled with GT 1, 4, and 6. The SVR 12 was only 92% in persons with GT 1a, but 99% in persons with GT 1b and 100% in GT 4. Further analysis demonstrated lower SVR 12 rates in persons with baseline NS5A resistance associated variants (at positions 28, 30, 31, and 93) associated with more than fivefold loss in elbasvir susceptibility. Therefore, a baselines resistance test is recommended in people with GT 1a. If baselines resistance mutations are found, treatment should be extended for 16 weeks and RBV should be added.

In the C-EDGE Coinfection trial—a phase 3, open-label trial involving 218 HCV treatment-naive HCV/HIV coinfected individuals who received ELB/GRZ one tablet daily for 12 weeks—95.0% of individuals achieved a cure, with six relapses and one reinfection. The drug worked equally well in GT 1a or 1b and GT 4. In the study, 7% reported fatigue; 7% headache; 5% nausea; 5% insomnia; and 5% diarrhea. No serious adverse events occurred (Rockstroh et al., 2015).

It should be noted that the FDA has issued a black box warning that ELB/GRZ could cause LFT elevations of more than five times the upper limit of normal. Therefore, it is recommended to monitor LFTs while on treatment.

Sofosbuvir/Velpatasvir

The Sofobuvir 400 mg and velpatasvir 100 mg (SOF/VEL, trade name Epclusa*) fixed-dose combination tablet is a pangenotypic regimen approved on June 28, 2016, to be given as a once-daily for 12 weeks in persons without cirrhosis or with compensated cirrhosis. In individuals with decompensated cirrhosis, it must be used with RBV. Velpatasvir is a HCV NS5A inhibitor required for viral replication.

The ASTRAL-1 study was a randomized, double-blinded, placebo-controlled study that evaluated 12 weeks of treatment with SOF/VEL compared to placebo in treatment-naive and Peg-IFN treatment-experienced individuals without cirrhosis or with compensated cirrhosis. Persons with all genotypes were included. Of 328 persons with GT 1, 98% achieved SVR12. Rates were similar in persons with compensated cirrhosis. Even in previously treatment-experienced persons with IFN-based regimens and first-generation PIs, this combination achieved more than 96% efficacy (Pianko et al., 2015).

In the ASTRAL-5 study, velpatasvir/sofosbuvir was given to 106 people with HIV/HCV coinfection, virally suppressed on ART containing raltegravir, rilpivirine, or ritonavir boosted PIs either with tenofovir or abacavir. Genotypes 1 to 4 were included; 18% of participants had compensated cirrhosis. SVR 12 was achieved in 95% of the individuals and was well tolerated. The most commonly reported side effects were fatigue, headaches, nausea, and insomnia.

Glecaprevir/Pibrentasvir

Glecaprevir 100 mg and pibrentasvir 40 mg per tablet (GLE/PIB, trade name Mavyret*) is a fixed-dose combination tablet (with three tablets taken once a day). This combination has several advantages compared to others. It is not only pangenotypic, but it could also be used in persons with chronic kidney disease and is approved for 8 weeks in treatment-naive individuals with no cirrhosis based on data from ENDURANCE-1 and ENDURANCE-3 studies.

In ENDURANCE-1 and ENDURANCE-3, out of 1,208 persons with GT 1 and 3 treated for 8 weeks, 99.1% (95% CI: 98–100) of people with GT 1 and 95% (95% CI: 91–98; 149 of 157 persons) of persons with GT 3 achieved SVR 12 (Zeuzem et al., 2018). It is also approved for use in treatment-experienced persons for a total of 8–16 weeks based on cirrhosis stage and previously used DAA. Of note, this combination is contraindicated in individuals with advanced cirrhosis (Child–Pugh B or C). The EXPEDITION-2 study evaluated the 8 weeks of GLE/PIB in persons with HIV/HCV. Overall SVR 12 rate was 98%.

Sofosbuvir/Velpatasvir/Voxilaprevir

Sofosbuvir 400 mg, velpatasvir 100 mg, and voxileprevir 100 mg (SOF/VEL/VOX, trade name Vosevi*) is a pangenotypic, single-tablet, fixed-dose combination indicated for 12 weeks in persons with HCV GT 1a who have failed therapy with a NS5A inhibitor–containing regimen. Voxileprevir is a reversible potent inhibitor of the NS3/4A protease required for the cleavage of the HCV encoded polyprotein. It is administered once daily with food. Persons with advanced liver disease (Child–Pugh B and C) should not take this regimen.

POLARIS-1 and POLARIS-4 assessed the efficacy and safety of SOF/VEL/VOX for 12 weeks in persons with HCV infection and who had previously received unsuccessful treatment with DAA-based regimens. All HCV genotypes were included; 46% of individuals had cirrhosis. The most common NS5A inhibitors used in previous unsuccessful treatment were ledipasvir (55% of persons), daclatasvir (23%), and ombitasvir (13%) in POLARIS-1 while in POLARIS-4, it was sofosbuvir (85%). SVR rates were achieved by 96% and 100% of participants with GT 1a ($n = 101$) and 1b ($n = 45$), respectively. In POLARIS-1 and POLARIS-4, 83% and 49% of participants, respectively, had baseline viral substitutions associated with resistance to NS3 inhibitors or NS5A inhibitors. SVR 12 was achieved in 97% (199 of 205) of participants in POLARIS-1 and 100% (83 of 83) in POLARIS-4.

In a phase 2, open-label study, 49 persons with HCV GT 1 infection who previously failed to achieve sustained virologic response on a DAA-based regimen were randomized to receive SOF/VEL/VOX with or without RBV for 12 weeks. The primary efficacy endpoint was the proportion of participants who achieved SVR 12. SVR12 was achieved by 24 of 24 persons (100%; 95% CI: 86–100) receiving sofosbuvir/velpatasvir/voxilaprevir alone and 24 of 25 (96%; 95% CI: 80–100) receiving the same treatment with RBV. Virological response was achieved by 13 of 13 (100%) persons without baseline resistance associated substitutions (RASs) and by 34 of 35 (97%) with baseline RASs. No large, randomized control studies in persons with HIV/HCV coinfection have been done.

TREATMENT FAILURES

For those who fail HCV treatment, assessment for disease progression should be done every 6–12 months with a hepatic function panel, CBC, and INR. If they have cirrhosis, HCC surveillance every 6 months with ultrasound is advised and they should be referred to a hepatologist and have endoscopic evaluation for varices. Retreatment depends on genotype, initial treatment and reason for failure and is not in the scope of this chapter.

Liver transplantation is a possibility in persons in whom HCV therapy is contraindicated owing to decompensated cirrhosis. As long as the CD4 + T-cell count is greater than 100 cells/mm^3 and HIV RNA levels are less than 400 copies/mL and without other contraindications (e.g., metastatic disease, ongoing alcohol or drug abuse, and active opportunistic infection), PWH may be appropriate for referral to a transplant center for evaluation. Studies have shown higher rates of wait-list mortality and posttransplant mortality, as well as more severe recurrent HCV disease (Terrault et al., 2012). Data from a prospective multicenter trial showed lower 3-year survival (60% vs. 79%; $p < 0.001$) in persons with HIV/HCV coinfection versus those with only HCV, as well as lower graft survival (53% vs. 74%; $p < 0.001$). Graft rejection was more common in people with HIV/HCV coinfection (35% vs. 18%), likely related to the difficulties of managing immunosuppressive drugs in this population (Zahnd et al., 2015). New DAA drug therapy in HCV-mono-infected and people with HIV/HCV coinfection has shown pretransplant and posttransplant virologic responses of 70%–93% in some trials.

SUMMARY

The world of HIV/HCV coinfection is in rapid flux. Similar to HIV treatment, a combination of oral agents that disrupt the HCV virus at various sites of the life cycle has the best chance for decreasing viral replication long-term and curing infection. Questions regarding optimal combination as well as drug access and costs will need to be addressed in the next several years if the majority of persons with HIV/HCV coinfection are to be effectively treated.

ACKNOWLEDGMENTS

The authors acknowledge Aimee Wilkin, MD, MPH, the author of the first section of this chapter in the previous edition.

REFERENCES

AASLD-IDSA. Recommendations for testing, managing, and treating hepatitis C. http://www.hcvguidelines.org. Published 2022. Accessed September 2022.

Anderson JP, Tchetgen EJ, Lo R, et al. Antiretroviral therapy reduces the rate of hepatic decompensation among HIV and hepatitis C virus-coinfected veterans. *Clin Infect Dis.* 2014;58(5):719–727.

Asselah T, Rubbia-Brandt L, Marcellin P, et al. Steatosis in chronic hepatitis C: why does it really matter? *Gut.* 2006;55(1):123–130.

Audsley J, Seaberg E, Sasadeusz J, et al. Factors associated with elevated ALT in an international HIV/HBV coinfected cohort on long-term HAART. *PLoS One.* 2011;6(11):e26482.

Beretta M, Garlassi E, Cacopardo B, et al. Hepatocellular carcinoma in HIV-infected patients: check early, treat hard. *Oncologist.* 2011;16(9):1258–1269.

Bevilacqua E, Fabris A, Floreano P, et al. Genetic factors in mother-to-child transmission of HCV infection. *Virology.* 2009;390(1):64–70.

Boesecke C, Ingiliz P, Mandoerfer M, et al.; The NEAT Study Group. Is there long-term evidence of advanced liver fibrosis after acute hepatitis C in HIV coinfection? [Abstract 644]. Paper presented at the 21st Conference on Retroviruses and Opportunistic Infections. Boston, MA; March 3–6, 2014.

Centers for Disease Control and Prevention (CDC). HIV/AIDS and viral hepatitis fact sheet. http://www.cdc.gov/hepatitis/populations/hiv.htm. Published 2020. Accessed September 17, 2022.

Colin J, Cazals-Hatem D, Loriot M, et al. Influence of human immunodeficiency virus infection on chronic hepatitis B in homosexual men. *Hepatology.* 1999;29(4):1306–1310.

Conrad C, Bradley H, Broz D, et al. Community outbreak of HIV infection linked to injection drug use of oxymorphone—Indiana, 2015. *MMWR.* 2015;64(16):443–444.

Danta M, Dusheiko GM. Acute HCV in HIV-positive individuals—a review. *Curr Pharm Des.* 2008;14(17):1690–1697.

Department of Health and Human Services (DHHS), Panel on Antiretroviral Guidelines for Adults and Adolescents. Guidelines for the use of antiretroviral agents in adults and adolescents with HIV. https:// clinicalinfo.hiv.gov/en/guidelines/hiv-clinical-guide-lines-adult-and-adolescent-arv/whats-new-guidelines. Published September 1, 2022a. . Accessed September 11, 2022.

DHHS, Panel on Guidelines for the Prevention and Treatment of Opportunistic Infections in Adults and Adolescents with HIV. Guidelines for the prevention and treatment of opportunistic infections in HIV-infected adults and adolescents: recommendations from the Centers for Disease Control and Prevention, the National Institutes of Health, and the HIV Medicine Association of the Infectious Diseases Society of America. https://clinicalinfo.hiv.gov/en/guidelines/hiv-clinical-guidelines-adult-and-adolescent-opportunistic-infections/whats-new. Published September 7, 2022b. Accessed September 11, 2022.

Dore G, Soriano V, Rockstroh J, et al. Frequent hepatitis B virus rebound among HIV-hepatitis B virus coinfected patients following antiretroviral therapy interruption. *AIDS.* 2010;24(6):857–865.

Elliott LN, Lloyd A, Ziegler JB, et al. Protective immunity against hepatitis C virus infection. *Immunol Cell Biol.* 2006;84:239–249.

Fierer DS, Dieterich DT, Fiel MI, et al. Rapid progression to decompensated cirrhosis, liver transplant, and death in HIV-infected men after primary hepatitis C virus infection. *Clin Infect Dis.* 2013;56(7):1038–1043.

Fierer DS, Mullen MP, Dieterich DT, et al. Early-onset liver fibrosis due to primary hepatitis C virus infection is higher over time in HIV-infected men. *Clin Infect Dis.* 2012;55(6):887–888;author reply, 888–889.

Hadziyannis S, Papatheodoridis G. Hepatitis B e antigen-negative chronic hepatitis B: natural history and treatment. *Semin Liver Dis.* 2006;26:130–141.

Heuft M, Houba S, van den Berk G, et al. Protective effect of hepatitis B virus-active antiretroviral therapy against primary hepatitis B virus infection. *AIDS.* 2014;28(7):999–1005.

Launay O, Van der Vliet D, Rosenberg A, et al. Safety and immunogenicity of 4 intramuscular double doses and 4 intradermal low doses vs. standard hepatitis B vaccine regimen in adults with HIV-1: a randomized controlled trial. *JAMA.* 2011;305(14):1432–1440.

Linas BP, Wang B, Smurzynski M, et al. The impact of HIV/HCV coinfection on health care utilization and disability: results of the ACTG Longitudinal Linked Randomized Trials (ALLRT) Cohort. *J Viral Hepat.* 2011;18(7):506–512.

Lo Re III V, Kallan M, Tate J, et al. Hepatic decompensation in antiretroviral-treated patients coinfected with HIV and hepatitis C virus compared with hepatitis C virus-monoinfected patients: a cohort study. *Ann Intern Med.* 2014;160(6):369–379.

Lok AS, McMahon BJ. Chronic hepatitis B: update 2009. *Hepatology.* 2009;50(3):661–662.

Low E, Vogel M, Rockstroh J, et al. Acute hepatitis C in HIV-positive individuals. *AIDS Rev.* 2008;10(4):245–253.

Luetkemeyer A, Charlebois E, Hare C, et al. Resistance patterns and response to entecavir intensification among HIV–HBV-coinfected adults with persistent HBV viremia. *J AIDS.* 2011;58(3):e96–e99.

Mast EE, Hwang LY, Seto DS, et al. Risk factors for perinatal transmission of hepatitis C virus (HCV) and the natural history of HCV infection acquired in infancy. *J Infect Dis.* 2005;192(11):1880–1889.

Mohsen AH, Easterbrook P. Hepatitis C testing in HIV infected patients. *Sex Transm Infect.* 2003;79(1):76.

Naggie S, Cooper C, Saag M, et al. Ledipasvir and sofosbuvir for HCV in patients coinfected with HIV-1. *N Engl J Med.* 2015;373(8):705–713.

Pianko S, Flamm SL, Shiffman ML, et al. Sofosbuvir plus velpatasvir combination therapy for treatment-experienced patients with genotype 1 or 3 hepatitis C virus infection: a randomized trial. *Ann Intern Med.* 2015;163(11):809–817.

Pinchoff J, Drobnik A, Bornschlegel K, et al. Deaths among people with hepatitis C in New York City, 2000–2011. *Clin Infect Dis.* 2014;58(8):1047–1054.

Poynard T, Bedossa P, Opolon P. Natural history of liver fibrosis progression in patients with chronic hepatitis C. The OBSVIRC, METAVIR, CLINIVIR, and DOSVIRC groups. *Lancet.* 1997;349(9055):825–832.

Rallon NI, Soriano V, Naggie S, et al. IL28B gene polymorphism and viral kinetics in HIV. HCV coinfected patients treated with pegylated interferon and ribavirin. *AIDS.* 2011;25(8):1025–1033.

Rockstroh JK, Nelson M, Katlama C, et al. Efficacy and safety of grazoprevir (MK-5172) and elbasvir (MK-8742) in patients with hepatitis C virus and HIV coinfection (C-EDGE COINFECTION): a non-randomised, open-label trial. *Lancet HIV.* 2015;2(8):e319–e327.

Schneider MD, Sarrazin C. Commentary: antiviral therapy of hepatitis C in 2014: do we need resistance testing? *Antivir Res.* 2014;105:64–71.

Sherman K. Management of the hepatitis B virus/HIV-coinfected patient. *Top Antivir Med.* 2015;23(3):111–114.

Shire N, Rouster S, Rajicic N, et al. Occult hepatitis B in HIV-infected patients. *J AIDS.* 2004;36(3):869–875.

Sulkowski MS, Mast EE, Seeff LB, et al. Hepatitis C virus infection as an opportunistic disease in persons infected with human immunodeficiency virus [review]. *Clin Infect Dis.* 2000;30(Suppl 1):S77–S84.

Sulkowski M, Thomas D, Chaisson R, et al. Reactivation of hepatitis B virus replication accompanied by acute hepatitis in patients receiving highly active antiretroviral therapy. *Clin Infect Dis.* 2001;32(1):144–148.

Terrault N, Lok A, McMahon B, et al. Update on prevention, diagnosis, and treatment of chronic hepatitis B: AASLD 2018 hepatitis B guidance. *Hepatology.* 2018;67:1560–1599.

Thio C, Seaberg E, Skolasky R Jr, et al. HIV-1, hepatitis B virus, and risk of liver-related mortality in the Multicenter Cohort Study (MACS). *Lancet.* 2002;360(9349):1921–1926.

Thomas DL, Strathdee SA, Vlahov D. Long-term prognosis of hepatitis C virus Infection. *JAMA.* 2000;284(20):2592.

Thompson MA, Horberg MA, Agwu AL, et al. Primary care guidance for persons with human immunodeficiency virus: 2020 update by the HV Medicine Association of the Infectious Diseases Society of America. *Clin Infect Dis.* 2020;73(11)e3572–e3605.

Wandeler G, Gsponer T, Bregenzer A, et al. Hepatitis C virus infections in the Swiss HIV Cohort Study: a rapidly evolving epidemic. Clin Infect Dis. November 15, 2012;55(10):1408–1416.

Weber R, Sabin CA, Friis-Moller N, et al. Liver-related deaths in persons infected with the human immunodeficiency virus: the D:A:D study. *Arch Intern Med.* 2006;166(15):1632–1641.

Zahnd C, Salazar-Vizcaya L, Dufour JF, et al. Modelling the impact of deferring HCV treatment on liver-related complications in HIV coinfected men who have sex with men. *J Hepatol.* 2016;65(1):26–32.

Zeuzem S, Foster GR, Wwang S, et al. Glecaprevir–pibrentasvir for 8 or 12 weeks in HCV genotype 1 or 3 infection. *N Engl J Med.* 2018;378(4):354.

37.

THE COVID-19 PANDEMIC AND HIV

Richard C. Prokesch

LEARNING OBJECTIVES

- Provide a brief overview of the COVID-19 pandemic and how it impacts persons with HIV.

- Briefly summarize the current state of COVID-19 treatment and prevention interventions, with special attention to HIV-specific considerations.

KEY POINTS

- SARS-CoV-2 infection has been rampant around the world and especially the United States; the pandemic has impacted the overall global economy as well as activities of daily living and stressed health care systems.

- HIV does not appear to be an independent risk factor for developing COVID-19; people living with HIV (PWH) on effective antiretroviral therapy (ART) have no greater risk of contracting or developing severe COVID-19 compared to individuals without HIV. However, approximately half of the US population of PWH is aged 50 years or older (with many experiencing multiple comorbidities), and older PWH are at increased risk of serious COVID-19 disease.

- Available therapies for COVID-19 are safe and relatively well-tolerated among PWH; special attention should be paid to drug–drug interactions between antivirals and ART.

- Similarly, vaccines for COVID-19 are safe and effective for PWH.

INTRODUCTION

On New Year's Eve 2019, the World Health Organization (WHO) China Country Office was notified about cases of pneumonia with unknown etiology in Wuhan City, Hubei Province of central China (WHO, 2020). Over the next few weeks, the number of cases rapidly increased, and the etiology was eventually determined to be a novel coronavirus, SARS-CoV-2; the disease syndrome became known as COVID-19. The virus likely was a zoonotic transmission from bats to an intermediate host thought to be a pangolin (a type of nocturnal anteater) and then to humans. Since it was a novel virus, the global population had little underlying immunity and thus it spread prolifically, with devastating worldwide consequences.

Most people with COVID-19 infection are asymptomatic or only have mild symptoms, and, thus, "silent" transmission has been a major contributor to the growth and persistence of the pandemic. As of September 2022, WHO surveillance data (available at: covid19.who.int) indicate there have been over 608,000,000 confirmed COVID-19 cases worldwide and over 6,500,000 reported deaths. Further, the United States has thus far had the most cases: over 94,000,000 confirmed cases and over 1,000,000 deaths. The infection has also disproportionally affected Black, Indigenous, people of color communities and populations in congregate settings (e.g., nursing homes, correctional facilities, and shelters). As is true with most viruses, SARS-CoV-2 evolves over time, and several mutated strains have arisen with subsequent changes in presenting symptoms as well as contagiousness.

CLINICAL PRESENTATION

Many individuals with COVID-19 have no or mild symptoms. Those who became symptomatic with the initial SARS-CoV-2 virus often had a flu-like prodrome with fevers, myalgias, and fatigue, followed by respiratory symptoms including shortness of breath, dyspnea on exertion, nonproductive cough, and hypoxemia. Some people lost the sensations of smell and taste. Gastrointestinal symptoms including diarrhea and abdominal pain were also relatively common. Individuals requiring hospitalization sometimes progressed to severe respiratory failure and "cytokine storm" ensuing from an overzealous and unregulated immune response, leading to acute respiratory distress syndrome, renal failure, thromboembolic events, and death.

As the virus has mutated, it has generally become less virulent and more contagious, and symptoms have changed to some extent—especially among vaccinated persons. However, newer mutations have evaded infection-induced and vaccine-induced humoral immunity to a greater extent than previous variants. For instance, the Omicron BA.1 variant commonly causes little or no symptoms; however, those who are symptomatic tend to have sore throats and upper respiratory symptoms with less frequent pneumonias and respiratory distress compared to people infected with the initial strain. There is a higher rate of reinfection with BA.1 and the newer strains.

HIV/COVID-19 COINFECTION

It is still not completely clear whether PWH are at greater risk for acquiring SARS-CoV-2 infection. Various European and US studies early in the pandemic of hospitalized PWH suggested that PWH have similar infection rates compared to individuals without HIV infection with similar clinical, radiographic and laboratory features (Del Amo et al., 2020; Park et al., 2020; Vizcarra et al., 2020). A multicenter research network study in the United States found no difference in mortality by HIV status (Hadi et al., 2020). More recent studies suggest worse outcomes for PWH with COVID-19 infection, with higher mortality rates observed in the United States, South Africa, and the United Kingdom (Brown et al., 2021; Dong et al., 2021; Hippisley-Cox et al., 2021). Coinfection with HIV was associated with a higher rate of severe and critical COVID-19 infection in a large study from the WHO that included data from 24 countries (Bertagnolio et al., 2021). Several US studies showed increased hospitalizations, ICU admissions, mechanical ventilation requirement, and death in PWH with COVID-19 who had low CD4$^+$ counts (< 200 cells/mm^3 in one study and < 350 cells/mm^3 in another) (Dandachi et al., 2021; Flannery et al., 2021; Sun et al., 2021).

In general, serious COVID-19 disease is seen more frequently in older persons, especially those over 60 years of age (CDC, 2020). Importantly, approximately half of all PWH in the United States are aged 50 years and older. Further, underlying medical conditions that have been shown to increase the risk of severe illness from COVID-19 include hypertension, obesity, chronic kidney disease, type 2 diabetes, cancer, receipt of solid organ or hematologic transplants, serious heart conditions, liver disease (especially cirrhosis), and chronic obstructive pulmonary disease (Chen et al., 2020; Fung & Babik, 2020; Lighter et al., 2020; Lippi & Henry, 2020; Petrilli et al., 2020; Richardson et al., 2020; Yang et al., 2020). Therefore, PWH—and especially older PWH—who have any of these comorbidities are at increased risk for severe COVID-19. It is therefore critical that all PWH receive effective ART and adhere to medications and achieve and maintain HIV viral load suppression and immune competence.

COVID-19 TREATMENT

Treatment options for COVID-19 are the same for persons with HIV and persons without HIV (Tables 37.1 and 37.2). It is imperative to look for possible drug–drug interactions between COVID-19 therapeutics and ART, plus any other comedications PWH might be taking.

Hospitalized Patients

Numerous data show that length of stay and outcomes are improved for people hospitalized with hypoxemia who receive daily dexamethasone (by mouth or intravenously) for 5 days. Remdesivir is also widely used in hypoxemic hospitalized patients, with some mixed data on its efficacy. For the most part, studies show that remdesivir shortens hospital stay; – however, its use does not change overall survival. Tocilizumab

Table 37.1 THERAPEUTIC MANAGEMENT OF NONHOSPITALIZED ADULTS WITH COVID-19

PATIENT DISPOSITION	RECOMMENDATIONS
Does not require hospitalization or supplemental oxygen	All patients should be offered symptomatic management. Dexamethasone or other systemic corticosteroids should not be used in the absence of another indication. For patients at high risk of progressing to severe COVID-19, preferred therapies include (listed in order of preference): ritonavir-boosted nirmatrelvir or remdesivir. Alternative therapies which may be used when neither of the preferred therapies are available, feasible to use, or clinically appropriate include (listed alphabetically): bebtelovimab or molnupiravir.
Discharged from hospital inpatient setting in stable condition and does not require supplemental oxygen	Panel recommends against continuing the use of remdesivir, dexamethasone, or baricitinib after hospital discharge.
Discharged from hospital inpatient setting and requires supplemental oxygen	There is insufficient evidence to recommend either for or against the continued use of remdesivir or dexamethasone.
Discharged from emergency department despite new or increasing need for supplemental oxygen (when hospital resources are limited, inpatient admission is not possible, and close follow-up is ensured)	Panel recommends using dexamethasone (6 mg by mouth once daily) for the duration of supplemental oxygen with careful monitoring for adverse events; dexamethasone use should not exceed 10 days. Because remdesivir is recommended for patients with similar oxygen needs who are hospitalized, clinicians may consider using it in this setting. As remdesivir requires IV infusions for up to 5 consecutive days, there may be logistical constraints to administering remdesivir in the outpatient setting.

SOURCE: Adapted from NIH COVID-19 treatment guidelines. https://www.covid19treatmentguidelines.nih.gov/management/clinical-management-of-adults/nonhospitalized-adults--therapeutic-management/.

Table 37.2 THERAPEUTIC MANAGEMENT OF HOSPITALIZED ADULTS WITH COVID-19: RECOMMENDATIONS FOR ANTIVIRAL OR IMMUNOMODULATOR THERAPY

DISEASE SEVERITY	RECOMMENDATIONS FOR ANTIVIRAL OR IMMUNOMODULATOR THERAPY	
	CLINICAL SCENARIO	RECOMMENDATION
Hospitalized for reasons other than COVID-19	Patients with mild-to-moderate COVID-19 who are at high risk of progressing to severe COVID-19	See Table 37.1.
Hospitalized but does not require oxygen supplementation	All patients	Panel recommends against the use of dexamethasone or other systemic corticosteroids for the treatment of COVID-19.
	Patients who are at high risk of progressing to COVID-19	Remdesivir.
Hospitalized and requires conventional oxygen	Patients who require minimal conventional oxygen	Remdesivir.
	Most patients	Use dexamethasone plus remdesivir; if remdesivir cannot be obtained, use dexamethasone.
	Patients who are receiving dexamethasone and who have rapidly increasing oxygen needs and systemic inflammation	Add oral baricitinib or intravenous tocilizumab to one of the options above.
Hospitalized and requires high-flow nasal cannula oxygen or noninvasive ventilation	Most patients	Promptly start one of the following, if not already initiated: dexamethasone plus oral baricitinib; or dexamethasone plus intravenous tocilizumab. If baricitinib, tofacitinib, tocilizumab, or sarilumab cannot be obtained, start dexamethasone. Add remdesivir to one of the options above in certain patients (refer to NIH Guidelines for additional details).
Hospitalized and requires mechanical ventilation or extracorporeal membrane oxygenation	Most patients	Promptly start one of the following, if not already initiated: dexamethasone plus oral baricitinib; or dexamethasone plus intravenous tocilizumab. If baricitinib, tofacitinib, tocilizumab, or sarilumab cannot be obtained, start dexamethasone.

SOURCE: Adapted from NIH COVID-19 treatment guidelines. https://www.covid19treatmentguidelines.nih.gov/tables/therapeutic-management-of-hospitalized-adults/.

and baricitinib have been shown to improve survival in critically ill patients with COVID-19 experiencing a cytokine storm-like picture, with multiorgan systems failure requiring mechanical ventilator support and often other life-saving interventions. Although antibiotics are often prescribed, the incidence of bacterial superinfection is relatively low in hospitalized COVID-19 patients.

Outpatient Therapies

Coformulated nirmatrelvir-ritonavir (Paxlovid™) is available for treatment of mild-moderate COVID-19 for individuals aged 12 years and older who are at increased risk for severe disease. It has been shown to reduce duration of the illness and to reduce hospitalizations. Medications should be started within 5 days after COVID-19 symptoms appear. According to the CDC, PWH may be at increased risk for severe outcomes from COVID-19 infection and thus should be considered for treatment. Coformulated nirmatrelvir-ritonavir may be given with ARVs, including those boosted with either ritonavir or cobicistat, and PWH should not interrupt their HIV

treatment while taking nirmatrelvir-ritonavir. PWH should be carefully monitored for potential increased nirmatrelvir-ritonavir exposure or protease inhibitor-associated adverse events, but dosing does not need to be changed in the event of concurrent use. With the short duration of nirmatrelvir-ritonavir therapy (i.e., 5 days), the potential for development of HIV drug resistance is low. Molnupiravir is an alternative to nirmatrelvir-ritonavir for mild-moderate disease, with studies indicating it is less effective. Additionally, it has not been approved for use in children and adolescents < 18 years of age because it may affect bone and cartilage growth.

Monoclonal antibodies and multiple other medications have and continue to be studied, in the hopes of identifying additional options and more effective therapeutic interventions. Ivermectin, which was widely politicized and touted earlier in the epidemic, is ineffective in treating COVID-19. However, despite evidence demonstrating lack of efficacy, it is still prescribed by some clinicians. Remdesivir therapy is recommended by some for outpatient treatment of patients who are at high risk for progression to severe disease, but data on its benefits in this context are inconclusive.

COVID-19 Vaccines

Several types of vaccines have been developed for the prevention of COVID-19. Messenger RNA (mRNA) vaccines (Pfizer-BioNTech and Moderna) contain synthetic vaccine antigens encapsulated within nanoparticles, which deliver mRNA directly into the cytoplasm where it will induce an immune response. Viral vector vaccines (Johnson & Johnson/Janssen and Oxford-AstraZeneca) use plasmids or killed organisms that act as vaccine antigens. Recombinant subunit vaccines (Novavax) use nanometer-sized particles to deliver the vaccine antigen.

Newer mutations have been more resistant to available vaccines, but their use still reduces severity of COVID-19 infection and hospitalization rates in most persons. Newer vaccines with improved activity against recent strains are in development. When vaccines were initially released, availability was limited, and they were only administered to healthcare workers and high-risk patients. However, with increased vaccine access, they are now widely available to most of the population, including children. Whereas PWH are at higher risk for severe infection, many PWH have been hesitant about receiving vaccines—therefore, it is important for HIV providers to explain the significant benefits of vaccination as well as the basic mechanism of their actions (as some people believe the vaccine will cause infection). Studies to date show that PWH have the same antibody levels and cellular response to COVID-19 vaccines as persons without HIV infection. However, there are some data suggesting that PWH with CD4 < 200 cells/mm^3 or poor immunosuppression have a reduced immune response to vaccines.

COVID-19 AND HIV CARE

The COVID-19 pandemic has greatly impacted and complicated many aspects of care for PWH. Fortunately, a supply chain shortage of most ART medications has not been observed to date, although some other medication-related factors have affected access to ART for some patients (e.g., changes in insurance status, modified pharmacy hours, and delays in communications regarding refills). Early in the pandemic, many clinical practices were shuttered, and hospital systems quickly became overwhelmed. Over subsequent months to years, remote ("virtual") visits became increasingly utilized by providers and patients who had access to secure telehealth platforms. However, for some practices that were already facing challenges with ensuring high levels of ongoing engagement and retention in care and ART adherence, such changes in service delivery created new stressors.

Modifications in care spurred by the pandemic include increasing prescription quantities to 90 days or longer to reduce frequency of travel to pharmacies (sometimes this practice was also extended to patients who had not attended a recent medical appointment); less frequent HIV-related laboratory monitoring for clinically stable patients (to reduce travel for separate phlebotomy services); and extended enrollment periods or flexibilities with regard to medical insurance coverage. Some of these practices continue to be observed, based on patient and provider experiences and preferences. For many clinical practices that were able to resume in-person care, personal protective equipment and mask requirements were instituted along with physical/social distancing and pre-visit screening measures.

Overall, health care utilization for non-COVID-19-related illnesses has been greatly affected by the pandemic (Lange et al., 2020). Some PWH are hesitant to seek medical care or might delay seeking care due to fears of exposure in clinical settings. Further, as many providers' attentions have been largely diverted to COVID-19 responses and recognition (especially in acute care settings), other important diagnoses with similar presentation, such as *P. jirovecii* pneumonia, may be overlooked (Coleman et al., 2020). Importantly, providers should ensure that PWH are up to date with immunizations, including seasonal influenza and pneumococcal vaccines.

ART provision and monitoring of PWH are not the only aspects of HIV care that have been affected by the pandemic. HIV prevention services including pre-exposure prophylaxis (PrEP) and HIV/sexually transmitted infection screening have also been markedly interrupted. Some individuals on PrEP have discontinued medications and/or have been unable to undergo regular lab monitoring because of decreased access to providers (Stephenson et al., 2021). As with HIV treatment, new telehealth programs have been developed to ensure continuous access to key prevention interventions such as PrEP.

REFERENCES

Bertagnolio S, Thwin SS, Silva R, et al. Clinical features of, and risk factors for, severe or fatal COVID-19 among people living with HIV admitted to hospital: analysis of data from the WHO Global Clinical Platform of COVID-19. *Lancet HIV*. 2022;9(7):e486–e495.

Brown LB, Spinelli MA, Gandhi M. The interplay between HIV and COVID-19: summary of the data and responses to date. *Curr Opin HIV AIDS*. 2021;16(1):63–73.

Centers for Disease Control (CDC) COVID-19 Response Team. Severe outcomes among patients with coronavirus disease 2019 (COVID-19)—United States. February 12–March 16, 2020. *MMWR Morb Mortal Wkly Rep*. 2020;69:343–346.

Chen R, Liang W, Jiang M, et al. Risk factors of fatal outcome in hospitalized subjects with Coronavirus Disease 2019 from a nationwide analysis in China. *Chest*. July 2020;158(1):97–105.

Coleman H, Snell LB, Simons R, Douthwaite ST, Lee MJ. Coronavirus disease 2019 and *Pneumocystis jirovecii* pneumonia: a diagnostic dilemma in HIV. *AIDS*. July 1, 2020;34(8):1258–1260.

Dandachi D, Geiger G, Montgomery MW, et al; HIV-COVID-19 Consortium. Characteristics, comorbidities, and outcomes in a multicenter registry of patients with human immunodeficiency virus and coronavirus disease 2019. *Clin Infect Dis*. 2021;73(7):e1964–e1972.

Del Amo J, Polo R, Moreno S, et al. Incidence and severity of COVID-19 in HIV-positive persons receiving antiretroviral therapy: a cohort study. *Ann Intern Med*. June 26, 2020; 73(7):536–541. http://doi:10.7326/M20-3689

Dong Y, Li Z, Ding S, et al. HIV infection and risk of COVID-19 mortality: a meta-analysis. *Medicine (Baltimore)*. 2021;100(26):e26573.

Flannery S, Schwartz R, Rasul R, et al. A comparison of COVID-19 inpatients by HIV status. *Int J STD AIDS*. 2021;32(12):1149–1156.

Fung M, Babik JM. COVID-19 in immunocompromised hosts: what we know so far. *Clin Infect Dis*. June 27, 2020;72(2):340–350. http://doi:10.1093/cid/ciaa863

Hadi YB, Naqvi SFZ, Kupec JT, Sarawari AR. Characteristics and outcomes of COVID-19 in patients with HIV: a multi-center research network study. *AIDS*. 2020;34(13):F3–F8. http://doi:10.1097/QAD.0000000000002666

Hippisley-Cox J, Coupland CA, Mehta N, et al. Risk prediction of COVID-19 related death and hospital admission in adults after COVID-19 vaccination: national prospective cohort study. *BMJ*. 2021;374:n2244.

Lange SJ, Ritchey MD, Goodman AB, et al. Potential indirect effects of the COVID-19 pandemic on use of emergency departments for acute life-threatening conditions—United States, January-May 2020. *MMWR Morb Mortal Wkly Rep*. June 26, 2020;69(25):795–800. http://doi:10.15585/mmwr.mm6925e2

Lighter J, Phillips M, Hochman S, et al. Obesity in patients younger than 60 years is a risk factor for COVID-19 hospital admission. *Clin Infect Dis*. July 28, 2020;71(15):896–897.

Lippi G, Henry BM. Chronic obstructive pulmonary disease is associated with severe coronavirus disease 2019 (COVID-19). *Respir Med*. June 2020;167:105941.

Park LS, Rentsch CT, Sigel K, et al. COVID-19 in the largest US HIV cohort. [Abstract LBPEC23]. *AIDS2020: 23rd International AIDS Conference*. Virtual; July 6–10, 2020. International AIDS Society. Geneva, Switzerland.

Petrilli CM, Jones SA, Yang J, et al. Factors associated with hospital admission and critical illness among 5279 people with coronavirus disease 2019 in New York City: prospective cohort study. *BMJ*. May 22, 2020;369:m1966. http://doi:10.1136/bmj.m1966

Richardson S, Hirsch JS, Narasimhan M, et al. Presenting characteristics, comorbidities, and outcomes among 5700 patients hospitalized with COVID-19 in the New York City area. *JAMA*. May 26, 2020;323(20):2052–2059.

Stephenson R, Chavanduka TMD, Rosso MT, et al. Sex in the time of COVID-19: results of an online survey of gay, bisexual and other men who have sex with men's experience of sex and HIV prevention during the US COVID-19 epidemic. *AIDS Behav*. 2021;25(1):40–48.

Sun J, Patel RC, Zheng Q, et al. COVID-10 disease severity among people with HIV infection or solid organ transplant in the United States: a nationally-representative, multicenter, observational cohort study. *medRxiv*. 2021;2021.07.26.21261028. http://doi: 10.1101/2021.07.26.21261028. Preprint.

Vizcarra P, Perez-Elias MJ, Quereda C, et al. Description of COVID-19 in HIV-infected individuals: a single-centre, prospective cohort. *Lancet HIV*. August 2020;7(8):e554–3564.

World Health Organization (WHO). World Health Organization situation report—1 (January 21, 2020): novel coronavirus (2018-nCoV). https://www.who.int/docs/default-source/coronaviruse/situation-reports/20200121-sitrep-1-2019-ncov.pdf. Published 2020. Accessed September 27, 2020.

Yang J, Zheng Y, Gou X, et al. Prevalence of comorbidities and its effects in patients infected with SARS-CoV-2: a systematic review and meta-analysis. *Int J Infect Dis*. May 2020;94:91–95.

38.

SEXUALLY TRANSMITTED DISEASES

Karen J. Vigil

LEARNING OBJECTIVE

Upon completion of this chapter, the reader should be able to demonstrate knowledge about established and evolving science regarding the diagnosis and treatment of the most prevalent sexual transmitted infections (STIs) in people with HIV (PWH), in order to decrease rate of transmission.

STIs are common in PWH. Education and counseling on changes in sexual behaviors of patients with STIs and their sexual partners, identification of asymptomatically infection, and effective diagnosis and treatment are the cornerstones for prevention.

GENITAL ULCERS

In the United States, most young, sexually active patients who have genital, anal, or perianal ulcers have either genital herpes or syphilis, with herpes being the most prevalent. Less common causes include chancroid and donovanosis.

SYPHILIS

WHAT'S NEW?

Since 2000, the incidence of syphilis continues to increase including a rise in cases of congenital syphilis. PWH and men who have sex with men (MSM) are the most affected groups.

KEY POINTS

- Syphilis incidence continues to increase and is more prevalent in PWH and MSM.

- Clinical manifestations are similar to the general population, but complications may be more common in PWH.

- Special attention to neurologic site involvement is required, as neurosyphilis may be more common among PWH.

- Although cerebrospinal fluid (CSF) abnormalities are more likely in PWH with CD4$^+$ cell count $\leq$ 350 cells/mm^3

and rapid plasma regain (RPR) $\geq$1:32, lumbar puncture is only recommended if there any sign or symptom of neurologic involvement.

- Penicillin is the treatment of choice for syphilis; alternatives have not been well studied in PWH.

Syphilis is a systemic disease caused by *Treponema pallidum*. In 2020, there were 133,945 reported cases of syphilis, a 52% increase since 2016. MSM accounted for 41.6% of cases (Center of Disease Control and Prevention (CDC), 2022). Coinfection with HIV has been reported in as much as 50%–70% of MSM with a high HIV-seroconversion rate in patients with primary and secondary syphilis (Su & Weinstock, 2011).

PRIMARY SYPHILIS

Primary syphilis refers to the chancre: a single, painless lesion with a clean base and indurated, raised borders. Chancres appears 1 week to 1 month after exposure. They are usually in the genital area but can occur anywhere on the body, including the oral cavity.

SECONDARY SYPHILIS

Secondary syphilis is characterized by a maculopapular erythematous rash that may involve the palms and soles. It typically occurs 3 weeks to 3 months after exposure. In PWH, rash could present with other several forms, including papulosquamous, vesicular, and pustular forms. Condyloma lata (broad-based, fleshy wart-like lesions that occur in moist, warm body areas) and lues maligna (pustular ulceronodular syphilides) are complications of secondary syphilis and are more frequent in PWH.

LATENT SYPHILIS

Latent syphilis is defined by positive serological test in the absence of any clinical signs or symptoms of syphilis. *Early latent syphilis* is defined as the one acquired within the preceding year. All other forms are either late latent syphilis or latent syphilis of unknown duration. The importance of this classification is secondary to transmission, being possible in any stages until early latent syphilis.

Neurosyphilis

Central nervous system involvement may occur at any stage of syphilis. Cerebrospinal fluid (CSF) laboratory abnormalities are common in persons with early syphilis, even in the absence of neurologic signs or symptoms. No evidence exists to support variation from recommended treatment for early syphilis for patients found to have such abnormalities. A CSF examination should be performed if clinical evidence of neurologic involvement is observed.

Neurosyphilis can take any of several other forms, including uveitis, retinitis, sensorineural hearing loss (otosyphilis), or central nervous system vasculitis. A lumbar puncture and CSF examination is recommended in these patients.

The 2021 Centers for Disease Control and Prevention (CDC) treatment guidelines (Workowski, 2021) recommend CSF examination:

- If there is evidence of neurologic symptoms.

- If there are ophthalmologic or auditory signs or symptoms.

- In patients with clinical presentation of tertiary syphilis (e.g.eg, aortitis or gumma).

- In patients with treatment failure.

CSF abnormalities are most likely in PWH with syphilis of any stage when CD4 $^+$ cell count is ≤ 350 cells/mm^3 and a serum rapid plasma reagin titer is >1:32 (Libois et al., 2007; Marra et al., 2004). However, CSF examination has not been associated with improved clinical outcomes in the absence of neurologic signs and symptoms.

Other presentations of tertiary syphilis include cardiovascular syphilis and gummatous syphilis. Cases of rapid progression after initial infection have been reported with both entities (Maharajan & Sampath Kumaar, 2005; Weinert et al., 2008).

DIAGNOSIS

Primary chancre could be diagnosed by visualization of spirochetes under darkfield microscopic examination. This applies to genital lesions and not oral lesions, because of the presence of nonpathogenic spirochetes in the mouth.

Nontreponemal antigen tests (VDRL and RPR) detect antibodies to nonspecific antigens in the host after infection by *T. pallidum*. They become positive 4–6 weeks after infection or 1–3 weeks after the appearance of a primary lesion. Treponemal tests (TPHA, TPPA, and FTA-ABS) detect antibodies that react with *T. pallidum* antigens. They are confirmatory for syphilis.

The diagnosis of neurosyphilis in PWH is difficult since HIV itself cause CSF abnormalities. Classic CSF findings in neurosyphilis are lymphocytic pleocytosis, total protein elevation, and a positive VDRL test. CSF VDRL may be false negative in 30%–70% of cases of neurosyphilis.

TREATMENT

PWH who have early syphilis might be at increased risk for neurologic complications (Lee, 2007) and might have higher rates of serologic treatment failure with currently recommended regimens than people without HIV. No treatment regimens for syphilis have been demonstrated to be more effective in preventing neurosyphilis in PWH than the syphilis regimens recommended for people without HIV (Rolfs et al., 1997). Careful follow-up after therapy is essential. The recommended and alternative treatment regimens for syphilis in PWH are summarized in Table 38.1.

FOLLOW-UP

PWH should be evaluated clinically and serologically for treatment failure at 6 and 12 months after therapy. If the patient meets the criteria for treatment failure (signs or symptoms that persist or recur or persons who have a sustained fourfold increase in nontreponemal test titer), a lumbar puncture with CSF examination should be performed and new treatment should be initiated. CSF examination and retreatment should be strongly considered for PWH whose nontreponemal test titers do not decrease fourfold within 6–12 months of therapy. If CSF examination is normal, treatment with benzathine penicillin G administered as 2.4 million units IM each at weekly intervals for 3 weeks is recommended.

Table 38.1 RECOMMENDED AND ALTERNATIVE TREATMENT REGIMENS FOR SYPHILIS IN PWH

TYPE OF SYPHILIS	RECOMMENDED REGIMEN	ALTERNATIVE REGIMEN
Primary, secondary, and early latent syphilis	Benzathine penicillin G, 2.4 MU IM in a single dose	–
Late latent syphilis or syphilis of unknown duration	Benzathine penicillin G, at weekly doses of 2.4 MU for 3 weeks	–
Neurosyphilis	Aqueous crystalline penicillin G 18–24 MU/day, administered as 3–4 MU IV every 4 hours or continuous infusion, for 10–14 days	Procaine penicillin 2.4 MU IM once daily *PLUS* Probenecid 500 mg orally four times a day, both for 10–14 days

MU, million units; IM, intramuscularly; IV, intravenously.

GONORRHEA

WHAT'S NEW?

The current recommended treatment for uncomplicated gonococcal infection is a single dose of intramuscular ceftriaxone 500 mg for people weighting < 150 kg. Dual therapy with azithromycin is no longer recommended unless there is need to treat concomitantly for other STI.

KEY POINTS

- Gonococcal infection remains an important cause of urethritis, cervicitis, pharyngitis, and proctitis, in sexually active PWH.

- Asymptomatic infection with gonorrhea is common at the female cervical site and male pharyngeal and rectal sites, such that routine, periodic screening for this STI is required to detect such cases.

- Nucleic-acid-based testing offers high sensitivity and ease of sample collection. Patient-collected samples could be used if instructions have been provided.

- Emergence of resistance to fluoroquinolone, azithromycin, and cephalosporins has been reported.

Gonorrhea is caused by *Neisseria gonorrhoeae*. In 2020, 677,769 cases of gonorrhea were reported to the CDC (2022)—that was a 45% increased rate from 2016. PWH are significantly more likely to have gonorrhea than people without HIV (Kent et al., 2005).

CLINICAL PRESENTATION

Acute urethritis is the main manifestation of gonorrhea. In men, urethral discharge—initially scant and later purulent—and dysuria are the major symptoms. The incubation period ranges from 1 to 10 days. Local complications include acute epididymitis, penile edema, penile lymphangitis, periurethral abscess, acute prostatitis, proctitis, seminal vesiculitis, infections of Tyson's and Cowper's glands, and pharyngitis. In women, gonorrhea presents as cervicitis and/or asymptomatic urethritis. Physical examination may show purulent or mucopurulent cervical, penile, or rectal exudates.

Disseminated gonococcal infection results from hematogenous dissemination of *Neisseria gonorrhoeae*. It can cause arthritis that primarily involves an asymmetric distribution in the knees, elbows, and more distal joints. A dermatitis picture with multiple discrete papules and pustules, often with a hemorrhagic component, could be present in approximately 75% of patients.

DIAGNOSIS

Gram stain of urethral discharge reveals gram negative diplococci during the first week after onset in men. In women this is less common. Although cultures are the gold standard for diagnosis, nucleic acid amplification tests (NAAT) in cervical swab, urethral swab, or urine have excellent sensitivity and specificity.

TREATMENT

Quinolone-resistant *N. gonorrhoeae* strains are widely disseminated throughout the United States and the world. Treatment failure to oral cephalosporins has been reported in Asia, Europe, Africa, and Canada (Lewis, et al., 2013; Unemo et al., 2012). Therefore, quinolones and oral cephalosporins are no longer recommended regimens for the treatment of gonorrhea in the United States. The recommended treatment regimens for gonorrhea infection in PWH are summarized in Table 38.2. There are limited data on alternative treatment for people with cephalosporin or IgE-mediated penicillin allergy. Gentamicin 240 mg IM plus azithromycin 2 grams orally is the current recommended treatment. However, there are no data on the efficacy of this regimen to treat rectal or pharyngeal infections. Consultation with an infectious disease specialist is recommended (Kirkaldy et al., 2014).

FOLLOW-UP

If failure to ceftriaxone is suspected, culture and antimicrobial susceptibility is recommended to guide next treatments.

Table 38.2 RECOMMENDED TREATMENT REGIMENS FOR GONORRHEA INFECTION IN PWH

TYPE OF GONORRHEA INFECTION	RECOMMENDED REGIMEN	ALTERNATIVE REGIMEN
Uncomplicated gonococcal infections of the pharynx, cervix, urethra, and rectum	Ceftriaxone 500 mg IM in a single dose (for persons with weight< 150kg) Ceftriaxone 1 gram IM in a single dose (for person weighing 150 kg or more)	If cephalosporin allergy: Gentamicin 240 mg IM *PLUS* azithromycin 2grams PO If ceftriaxone is not available: Cefixime 800 mg PO single dose
Disseminated gonococcal infection	Ceftriaxone 1gram IM or IV daily	–
Gonococcal meningitis and endocarditis	Ceftriaxone 1–2 grams IV every 12 hours for 10–14 days for meningitis and for at least 4 weeks for endocarditis	–

IM, intramuscularly; IV, intravenously; PO, orally.

CHLAMYDIA INFECTIONS

WHAT'S NEW?

The treatment of choice for chlamydial infections is doxycycline 100 mg orally two times daily for 7 days. In patients with proctitis accompanied by bloody discharge, perianal or mucosal ulcers, and/or tenesmus, the treatment could be extended for 21 days.

KEY POINTS

- Most *Chlamydia trachomatis* (CT) infections are asymptomatic and, thus, detected only by routine, periodic screening. Routine, periodic screening for CT is recommended for all sexually active PWH at exposed anatomic sites, at initial evaluation and every 12 months thereafter, or more frequently as indicated by risk.

- Nucleic-acid-based testing offers high sensitivity, ease of sample collection, and use of noninvasively acquired specimens. Self-collected vaginal, meatal, and rectal swabs have comparable performance as provider collected samples.

- Rectal CT infection is especially common among MSM; in this population, the CT subtypes that cause lymphogranuloma venereum (LGV) should be included in the differential diagnosis of those with severe symptoms of proctitis, especially when CT is found to be the cause.

Chlamydia is the most commonly reported STI in the United States in men and women. In 2020, a total of 1.6 million cases of chlamydia were reported to the CDC (2022). However, underreporting might be substantial as the disease may be asymptomatic. Chlamydia infection is more frequent in younger age groups, racial/ethnic minorities, MSM, and incarcerated populations (Burstein et al., 1998; Rietmeijer et al., 2008; Satterwhite et al., 2008). Genital and ocular chlamydial infection are cause by serotypes D to K, while serotypes L1, L2, and L3 cause lymphogranuloma venereum.

CLINICAL PRESENTATION

Chlamydia genital infection secondary to serotypes D to K could be asymptomatic or present as pharyngitis, urethritis, cervicitis, epididymitis, prostatitis, or proctitis. Pelvic inflammatory disease, perihepatitis, and infertility are long-term complications.

Serovars L1-L3 cause lymphogranuloma venereum (LGV). LGV is not endemic in the United States. Southeast Asia, the Caribbean, Latin America, and Africa are areas of more prevalence. It presents as one or more genital ulcers or papules, followed by the development of unilateral or bilateral fluctuant inguinal lymphadenopathy called buboes. Since 2003, there have been reports of outbreaks in Western Europe and in the United States of Chlamydia L2 serotype proctitis particularly in MSM.

DIAGNOSIS

NAAT for chlamydia genital infections (by polymerase chain reaction assay or transcription-mediated amplification) have great sensitivity and specificity and can be performed on first catch urine (without the requirement of a urethral swab) and vaginal and rectal swabs. All sexually active women aged < 25 years should be screened for chlamydia annually. Men and women who reported anal sex should also have anal swabs every year. Routine oropharyngeal screening is not recommended, but it is usually performed when screening for gonorrhea. If chlamydia is present, it should be treated similar to other presentations.

The diagnosis of LGV is challenging. Cell culture is the only diagnostic test approved by the US Food and Drug Administration. Serology helps in the diagnosis, as titers are typically elevated at the time of presentation. Diagnosis of LGV proctitis is even more difficult. NAAT may be used if a local laboratory has validated them. The CDC recommends that where LGV is suspected, the provider should collect a specimen and send the sample to the state health department for referral to the CDC. If this is not possible, an antibiotic regimen effective against LGV should be included in empiric treatment for proctitis.

TREATMENT

The treatment of choice for chlamydia infection is doxycycline 100 mg twice a day for 7 days and for 21 days for LGV. If symptoms include proctitis with bloody discharge, perianal or mucosal ulcers, or tenesmus, the treatment should be extended to 21 days.

HUMAN PAPILLOMA VIRUS (HPV)

WHAT'S NEW?

Gardasil-9, a nine-valent vaccine that targets HPV types 6, 11, 16, 18, 31, 33, 45, 52, and 58, is currently the only HPV vaccine distributed in the United States. A complete three-dose series is recommended to people through age 26. PWH between ages of 27 and 45 years might benefit from HPV vaccination and should discuss it with their providers.

KEY POINTS

- HPV is the most common STI in the United States. There are more than 100 HPV types; however, certain strains are associated with genital warts, and others with intraepithelial lesions and high-grade neoplasia.

- PWH have higher rates of HPV related lesions; genital warts can be more aggressive and difficult to eradicate.

HPV is a double-stranded DNA virus that may infect the genital tract. There are more than 200 types of HPV; more than 40 may infect the genital area. HPV may cause two major clinical syndromes: genital warts (condyloma acuminata) associated mainly to types 6 and 11, and epithelial cervical or anal neoplasia linked to serotypes 16 and 18 (for more information on cervical and anal neoplasia, refer to Chapter 29 Malignancies in HIV).

HPV detection is significantly more common among PWH (Mbulawa et al., 2009). Several studies have demonstrated that HPV increases the risk of HIV acquisition (Smith et al., 2010).

CLINICAL PRESENTATION

In most cases, HPV infection is transient and has no clinical manifestation or sequel and is self-limited. Genital warts typically present as single or multiple soft, fleshy, papillary or sessile, painless keratinized growths in the vulvovaginal area, penis, anus, urethra, or perineum. Women living with HIV have higher prevalence of genital warts, which may progress more rapidly in the presence of a declining immune status. Additionally, there are higher rates of Pap smear–detected abnormalities, dysplasia, and progression to cervical cancer relative to uninfected women.

DIAGNOSIS

Diagnosis of warts is made clinically; laboratory confirmation is not needed. PWH, especially MSM, have a significantly increased risk of anal cancer due to oncogenic human papillomavirus types; therefore, routine anal Pap screening in HIV care settings is recommended. Treatment of high-grade anal squamous intraepithelial lesions rather than active monitoring has been found to lower the risk of developing anal cancer (Palefsky et al., 2022).

TREATMENT

The main indications for treatment of vulvovaginal warts are bothersome symptoms and/or psychological distress. Vulvar biopsy to exclude precancerous or cancerous lesions is indicated when warts are identified in immunocompromised or postmenopausal women, when the lesions are visually atypical, or when warts fail to respond to standard therapy. The recommended treatment regimens for HPV in PWH are summarized in Table 38.3.

PREVENTION OR PROPHYLAXIS

There are three types of HPV vaccines: a bivalent vaccine that targets HPV types 16 and 18 (Cervarix™); a quadrivalent HPV vaccine that targets HPV types 6, 11, 16, and 18 (Gardasil); and a nine-valent vaccine that prevents infection with HPV types 6, 11, 16, 18, 31, 33, 45, 52, and 58. Only Gardasil-9 is currently available in the United States.

Routine vaccination is recommended for boys and girls at aged 11–12 years old and catch-up vaccination for adults until the age of 26 years (Meites et al., 2019). -9 is approved until age 45 years. Although people older than 26 years may have prior exposure to different HPV types, some might be at continuous risk of new HPV and might benefit from immunization.

Table 38.3 RECOMMENDED TREATMENT REGIMENS FOR HPV/WARTS IN PWH

External genital warts, patient-applied	Podofilox 0.5% solution or gel OR Imiquimod 5% cream OR Sinecatechins 15% ointment
External genital warts, provider-administered	Cryotherapy with liquid nitrogen or cryoprobe. Repeat applications every 1–2 weeks OR Trichloroacetic acid (TCA) or Bichloroacetic acid (BCA) 80%–90% OR Surgical removal either by tangential scissor excision, tangential shave excision, curettage, or electrosurgery
Vaginal warts	Cryotherapy with liquid nitrogen OR TCA or BCA 80%–90% applied to warts OR surgical removal
Urethral meatus warts	Cryotherapy with liquid nitrogen OR Surgical removal
Anal warts	Cryotherapy with liquid nitrogen OR TCA or BCA 80%–90% applied to warts OR Surgical removal

Therefore, for people aged 27 through 45 years, the decision to vaccinate should be made on an individual basis.

REFERENCES

Burstein GR, Waterfield G, Joffe A, Zenilman JM, Quinn TC, CA G. Screening for gonorrhea and chlamydia by DNA amplification in adolescents attending middle school health centers. Opportunity for early intervention. *Sex Transm Dis.* 1998;25:395.

Center for Disease Control and Prevention (CDC). Sexual transmitted diseases surveillance, 2020. https://www.cdc.gov/std/statistics/2020/default.htm. Published April 2022. Accessed September 30, 2022.

Kent CK, Chaw JK, Wong W, et al. Prevalence of rectal, urethral, and pharyngeal chlamydia and gonorrhea detected in 2 clinical settings among men who have sex with men: San Francisco, California, 2003. *Clin Infect Dis.* 2005;41:67–74.

Kirkcaldy RD, Weinstock HS, Moore PC, et al. The efficacy and safety of gentamicin plus azithromycin and gemifloxacin plus azithromycin as treatment of uncomplicated gonorrhea. *Clin Infect Dis.* 2014;59:1083–1091.

Lee M, Aynalem G, Kerndt P, et al. Symptomatic early neurosyphilis among HIV-positive men who have sex with men: four cities, United States, January 2002–June 2004. *MMWR Morb Mortal Wkly Rep.* 2007;56:625–628.

Lewis DA, Sriruttan C, Muller EE, et al. Phenotypic and genetic characterization of the first two cases of extended-spectrum- cephalosporin-resistant Neisseria gonorrhoeae infection in South Africa and association with cefixime treatment failure. *J Antimicrob Chemother.* 2013;68:1267–1270.

Libois A, De Wit S, Poll B, et al. HIV and syphilis: when to perform a lumbar puncture. *Sex Transm Dis.* 2007;34:141–144.

Maharajan M, GS K. Cardiovascular syphilis in HIV infection: a case-control study at the Institute of Sexually Transmitted Diseases, Chennai, India. *Sex Transm Infect.* 2005;81:361.

Marra CM, Maxwell CL, Smith SL, et al. Cerebrospinal fluid abnormalities in patients with syphilis: association with clinical and laboratory features. *J Infect Dis.* 2004;189:369–376.

Mbulawa ZZ, Coetzee D, Marais DJ, et al. Genital human papillomavirus prevalence and human papillomavirus concordance in heterosexual couples are positively associated with human immunodeficiency virus coinfection. *J Infect Dis.* 2009;199:1514.

Meites E, Szilagyi PG, Chesson HW, et al. Human papillomavirus vaccination for adults: updated recommendations of the Advisory Committee on Immunization Practices. *MMWR Morb Mortal Wkly Rep.* 2019;68:698–702.

Palefsky JM, Lee JY, Jay N, et al. Treatment of Anal High-Grade Squamous Intraepithelial Lesions to Prevent Anal Cancer. *N Engl J Med.* 2022;386:2273–2282.

Rietmeijer CA, Hopkins E, Geisler WM, Orr DP, Kent CK. Chlamydia trachomatis positivity rates among men tested in selected venues in the United States: a review of the recent literature. *Sex Transm Dis.* 2008;35:S8.

Rolfs RT, Joesoef MR, Hendershot EF, et al. A randomized trial of enhanced therapy for early syphilis in patients with and without human immunodeficiency virus infection. The Syphilis and HIV Study Group. *N Engl J Med.* 1997;337:307–314.

Satterwhite CL, Joesoef MR, Datta SD, Weinstock H. Estimates of Chlamydia trachomatis infections among men: United States. *Sex Transm Dis.* 2008;35:S3.

Smith JS, Moses S, Hudgens MG, et al. Increased risk of HIV acquisition among Kenyan men with human papillomavirus infection. *J Infect Dis.* 2010;201:1677.

Su JR, Weinstock H. Epidemiology of co-infection with HIV and syphilis in 34 states, United States—2009. In: Proceedings of the 2011 National HIV Prevention Conference. Atlanta, GA; August 13–17, 2011.

Unemo M, Golparian D, Nicholas R, et al. High-level cefixime- and ceftriaxone-resistant Neisseria gonorrhoeae in France: novel penA mosaic allele in a successful international clone causes treatment failure. *Antimicrob Agents Chemother.* 2012;56:1273–1280.

Weinert LS, Scheffel RS, Zoratto G, et al. Cerebral syphilitic gumma in HIV-infected patients: case report and review. *Int J STD AIDS.* 2008;19:62.

Workowski KA, Bachman LH, Chan PA. Sexually transmitted infections treatment guidelines, 2021. *MMWR Recomm Rep.* 2021;70:1–187.

39.

CARDIOVASCULAR DISEASE

Jarrett K. Sell and Jonathan J. Nunez

LEARNING OBJECTIVES

- Discuss the pathophysiology of cardiovascular disease (CVD) and myocardial infarction (MI) in persons living with HIV (PWH).

- Describe the associations between chronic HIV infection as it relates to an increased risk of CVD, MI, stroke, peripheral arterial disease, and sudden cardiac death (SCD).

- Discuss the association of specific antiretroviral therapies (ART) and cardiovascular risk.

- Assess CVD risk in PWH by application of the American Heart Association/American College of Cardiology (AHA/ACC) atherosclerotic cardiovascular disease (ASCVD) 10-year risk calculator.

- List medical therapies, including statins and non-statins, to lower the risk of CVD and MI in PWH.

- Discuss lifestyle interventions, including diet, exercise, weight loss and smoking cessation, to lower the risk of CVD and MI in PWH.

WHAT'S NEW?

- Persistent, systemic inflammation has been proposed as a mechanism of action for increased CVD risk in PWH; however, a recent (2021), randomized, controlled trial of colchicine a potent anti-inflammatory agent, did <u>not</u> show improved coronary artery endothelial function, a predictor of CVD, in PWH and no history of coronary artery disease (CAD).

- A recent prospective multicenter study has shown integrase strand inhibitors (INSTI) were associated with an early onset, excess incidence of cardiovascular disease in the first 2 years of exposure, after accounting for known CVD risk factors.

- Statin therapy is a pharmacotherapeutic intervention for secondary prevention of major adverse cardiovascular events in patients with ASCVD risk; however, a recent analysis of Veteran Administration (VA) medical centers found suboptimal and variable statin prescribing among veterans living with HIV and known ASCVD risk.

- The BEIJERINCK Study, a randomized controlled trial comparing monthly evolocumab, a PCSK9 inhibitor, to placebo in 464 PWH and dyslipidemia on maximally tolerated statin therapy, found a 57% reduction in LDL levels.

- The current evidence suggests that the net benefit of aspirin for primary prevention is small and may be considered only in those aged 40–59 years with a 10% or greater 10-year CVD risk and a low risk of bleeding.

KEY POINTS

- PWH are at increased risk for CVD, including MI, stroke, heart failure (HF), and SCD.

- The excess risk of CVD has been linked to the double burden of a high prevalence of traditional risk factors (e.g., DM, HTN, and smoking) and HIV-specific risk factors (e.g., inflammation, immune activation, immune suppression, and viremia).

- Some ART is thought to increase CVD risk through elevation of lipids levels and other mechanisms, although this is less commonly seen in the modern treatment era.

- PWH should be screened regularly for known CVD risk factors, including hypertension (HTN), diabetes mellitus, dyslipidemia, and cigarette smoking.

- Changing ART to improve lipid profiles in PWH should be considered but should not compromise virologic or immunologic control.

- PWH should be assessed for their 10-year CVD risk by using the ACC/AHA risk calculator.

- Statin therapies are recommended for primary and secondary prevention of CVD, and additional cholesterol-lowering medications may be indicated for select high-risk patients. Proven interventions to lower the risk of CVD and MI include diet, exercise, smoking cessation, and the use of lipid-lowering agents and antihypertensive medications.

- Prevalence of smoking for PWH is >33%, and treatment for tobacco dependence should routinely be offered to all candidates.

- Gains in life expectancy for PWH owing to successful ART will be lost if management of CVD is not optimized.

INTRODUCTION

There is considerable evidence that PWH are at increased risk for CVD, including MI and stroke. Epidemiological studies published through the years have consistently found higher rates of CVD, especially MI and stroke, among PWH compared to HIV-negative persons (Freiberg et al., 2013; Kovacs et al., 2022; Rao et al., 2019). Despite access to life-preserving ART, further studies in the United States and globally continue to highlight the greater burden of coronary artery disease in PWH, even when accounting for viral suppression (Hsue & Waters, 2019; Metkus et al., 2015; Post et al., 2014; Shah et al., 2018).

Most of these studies acknowledge a higher prevalence of known traditional risk factors for CVD among PWH and typically adjust for confounding variables. Cigarette smoking, in particular, is several-fold greater in PWH compared to the general population. After accounting for such traditional risks, significant differences between PWH and those without HIV generally persist—although the more factors added to these models, the greater the attenuation between HIV infection and CVD (Post et al., 2014; Rao et al., 2019).

Other factors, including poor diet, sedentary lifestyle, substance abuse, and even stress and mental illness, can increase the risk of CVD and may account for the excess CVD burden among PWH. However, data on these confounders are not typically collected (Khambaty et al., 2016; White et al., 2015).

There are now biologically plausible explanations for higher CVD risk accompanying HIV infection. Findings of higher levels of markers of immune activation and inflammation among infected patients with suppressed viremia compared to uninfected controls and a correlation between such markers and adverse events suggest infection-related pathogenic mechanisms for CVD in PWH (Deeks et al., 2013; Hunt, 2012; Scherzer et al., 2018). In addition, the increased risk of cardiovascular disease in those who are virally suppressed could be associated with reservoirs of HIV-infected cells. ART prevents HIV from spreading and infecting new cells but does not eliminate cells already infected with the HIV virus, and the virus continues to persist (McLaughlin et al., 2020). Moreover, although ART has been found to consistently reduce surrogate markers for inflammation, endothelial dysfunction, and immune activation, there has been evidence from observational studies that some ART contribute to CVD. It remains unclear if such associations are affected by co-confounding variables and, if truly contributing, what the mechanisms are that lead to CVD. The heightened risk for CVD in PWH, regardless of etiology, requires healthcare providers to be diligent in assessing CVD risk and intervening, when appropriate. Newer information has made it increasingly clear that the care for PWH requires not only chronic viral suppression, but also early recognition and management of CVD risk factors (Rao et al., 2019). More research are greatly needed to elucidate the mechanisms of HIV-associated CVD and therapeutic strategies to mitigate these risks.

EVIDENCE OF EXCESS RISK FOR CARDIOVASCULAR DISEASE IN HIV

One of the largest epidemiological studies examining differential rates of CVD among PWH and HIV-negative persons was conducted within a registry of patients receiving care in Boston that included 3,851 PWH and 1,044,589 HIV-negative patients (Triant et al., 2007). The difference in acute MI rates between HIV and non-HIV persons was significant, with a relative risk (RR) of 1.75 (95% confidence interval (CI): 1.51–2.02; $p < 0.0001$), adjusting for age, gender, race, hypertension (HTN), diabetes, and dyslipidemia (Triant et al., 2007).

Similar studies of the incidence of MI and stroke were conducted by the Kaiser Permanente system in California (Klein et al., 2014, 2015). Rates of both conditions were historically higher for PWH compared to HIV-negative members. However, a convergence over time was observed in the rates of MI and stroke experienced by PWH compared to HIV-negative patients. Improved detection and the management of CVD risk factors plus better treatment of HIV infection is hypothesized to account for the decline in CVD rates in this cohort of patients. Similar declines in the rates of CVD over the past decade were reported from cohorts in Europe and British Columbia (Cheung et al., 2016; Hatleberg et al., 2016).

A paper from the Veterans Aging Cohort Study (VACS) that included 81,000 participants (33% HIV-positive) found that PWH veterans had twice the risk of acute MI compared to those who were HIV-negative (Paisible et al., 2015). However, it also found a low prevalence of optimization of cardiac health in this high-risk VA population, including blood pressure control, treatment of hyperlipidemia, and smoking cessation. This alone may account for the increased risk of MI, and not HIV infection.

A 2018 systematic review by Shah included data from 80 longitudinal studies of 793,635 PWH and a total follow-up of 3.5 million person-years. The authors of this study reported a 2.16 RR of MI and stroke in PWH compared to HIV-negative individuals (Shah et al., 2018). This is comparable to a RR of 2.48 with HTN and 2.95 with smoking found in the multinational INTERHART study (Yusuf et al., 2004). A 2021 observational, longitudinal cohort of veterans from the VACS showed that HIV infection was associated with increased SCD risk (hazard ratio (HR) 1.14; 95% CI: 1.04–1.25), adjusting for possible confounders, and this risk was greatest for those with CD4 counts < 200 cells/mm^3 or viral load >500 copies/mL (Freiberg et al., 2021). Despite some variance in data from observational cohorts, the preponderance of these studies from the United States., Europe, and Sub-Saharan Africa support the fact that PWH indeed have an excess risk of CVD, including MI, stroke, HF, and SCD.

Beyond cohort studies, pathophysiological evidence of excess CVD accompanying HIV infection has been found. Relatively high levels of inflammation within the aorta, possibly mediated by monocyte activation, were demonstrated by fluorodeoxyglucose positron emission tomography (FDG-PET) scanning in a small study of ART-receiving

PWH without known CVD compared to uninfected controls with similar CVD risks. These data were later correlated with vulnerable coronary plaques (Subramanian et al., 2012; Tawakol et al., 2014). Similarly, a larger cross-sectional study, the Multicenter AIDS Cohort Study (MACS), examined coronary calcium scores and coronary plaque morphology in PWH and HIV-negative MSM and found that plaque was highly prevalent in both groups (Post et al., 2014). After adjustment for major confounders, there remained a higher prevalence of plaque in male PWH (prevalence ratio (PR) 1.13; 95% CI: 1.04–1.23), who were also more likely to have noncalcified plaques (the most vulnerable to rupture) (PR 1.25; 95% CI: 1.10–1.43). Older age was associated with noncalcified plaque in PWH but not in HIV-negative men. This factor seemed to drive the overall differences between these groups. Adjustment for additional confounders reduced the association between HIV infection and noncalcified plaques.

In 2020, there was a cohort study of patients from San Francisco looking at the association between cell-associated HIV RNA and DNA and the development of carotid plaque over time (McLaughlin et al., 2020). The latent HIV reservoir is a group of immune cells infected with HIV but are not actively producing new virus. As they are not producing new copies of virus, ART have no effect on them. In this study, 152 PWH were on ART and virally suppressed. Levels of HIV RNA and DNA were checked with blood samples, and ultrasound was performed to monitor carotid intima-media thickness (CIMT). The median age of patients was 47 years old, and they were living with HIV, on average, for 13 years. During follow-up, there was an association between CIMT and levels of HIV RNA ($p = 0.47$) and HIV DNA ($p = 0.042$). However, when taking into account traditional risk factors, the association was not statistically significant. Yet, when looking at the formation of new carotid artery plaques, there was a statistically significant relationship with HIV RNA and HIV DNA levels ($p = 0.008$ and $p = 0.02$). Their results suggest that decreasing the HIV reservoir size, which can occur with a prompt ART in persons newly infected with HIV, may decrease inflammation and reduce atherosclerosis.

The concept of HIV causing "accelerated" aging with CVD and other conditions (e.g., bone disease, frailty) possibly occurring earlier in PWH has been countered by data from the US Veterans Administration Aging Cohort and a large HIV case-control study in PWH from Denmark (Althoff, 2015 et al., 2015; Rasmussen et al., 2015). In both groups, excess risk of CVD with HIV infection was observed. However, this was detected at similar ages in HIV-positive and HIV-negative persons, and, over time, there was no observed increase in overall risk for those with HIV. In the North American NA-ACCORD cohort, the attributable risk of type 1 MI was much greater for PWH who smoked, had HTN, or elevated lipid levels as opposed to lower CD4 + T-cell counts, elevated plasma HIV RNA level, or a diagnosis of AIDS (Althoff et al., 2017). Consequently, modeling studies have found that interventions that target the management of blood pressure, glucose, and lipid levels, as well as smoking cessation, may have a much greater clinical impact than earlier initiation of HIV therapy or avoidance of ART that has been associated with risk of CVD (Smit et al., 2018).

In recent years it has become apparent that HF is more common in PWH. In the HIV-Heart Study being conducted within the Kaiser Permanente healthcare system, the rate of incident HF was compared between 39,000 PWH and more than 387,000 matched control (1:10) patients without HIV infection. Incident HF was higher among PWH (4% vs. 3%) with a hazard ratio indicating a 66% greater risk in the fully adjusted model that accounted for coronary syndrome events, suggesting an independent mechanism independent of atherosclerosis (Go et al., 2018). A recent study found that women with HIV had a higher incidence of myocardial fibrosis and subsequent reduced diastolic function also referred to as HF with reduced ejection fraction (Zanni et al., 2020). In addition, a retrospective cohort study evaluated HIV infection and variation in HF risk by age, sex, and ethnicity, and key findings noted the adjusted risk of HF in PWHs seemed stronger in younger patients (aged 21 to 41 years), women, and Asian/Pacific Islander adults (Go et al., 2022).

PROPOSED MECHANISMS

While traditional and non-HIV-related factors appear to be driving much of the CVD events that PWH experience, factors related to HIV infection and treatment may play a role. Overall, the pathogenesis of atherosclerosis in the setting of HIV infection is likely more complex than the current level of understanding. Numerous mechanistic studies have examined the association between CVD (i.e., plaque, coronary calcium, arterial inflammation, and endothelial dysfunction) and markers of inflammation, immune activation, and microbial translocation across the gut (Deeks et al., 2013; Hunt, 2012). In the FDG-PET study, aortic wall inflammation was significantly correlated with markers of monocyte and macrophage activation, suggesting that these cell lines play a role in the observed changes. The monocyte activation marker soluble CD163 was also correlated with a noncalcified coronary plaque in men and women with HIV and well-controlled viral loads. In the MACS coronary imaging study, as in most other cohorts, smoking rates were higher among those who were HIV-positive. That smoking interacts with HIV and aging to accelerate CVD was observed by an examination of CIMT, suggesting HIV infection modifies the effect of smoking and age on cardiovascular health (Fitch et al., 2013). In a related report, smoking and obesity were each significantly associated with levels of inflammatory markers including interleukin-6 (IL-6), sCD14, and sTNFR-I and -II (Krishnan et al., 2014). Similar findings linking smoking and inflammation were seen in the SUN cohort of PWH (Cioe et al., 2015). In that study, heavy alcohol intake was also associated with elevations of the coagulation marker D-dimer.

Data from another study suggest that T-cell activation and inflammation contribute to the development of vascular disease (Hsue et al., 2010). They have also suggested that HIV proteins, including transactivator of transcription (TaT) and negative factor (Nef), may induce inflammation and endothelial dysfunction (Hsue et al., 2019). Residual immune activation secondary to incomplete control of HIV infection (despite undetectable viremia), coinfections (e.g., cytomegalovirus and hepatitis C virus), and irreversible translocation of microbial products across an altered gut lumen occur in PWH. They are thought to promote a proinflammatory milieu that is proatherogenic (Deeks, et al., 2013; Hsue et al., 2019). However, a 2021 randomized controlled trial of colchicine, which is an anti-inflammatory agent, did not show improved coronary endothelial function, which is a predictor of CVD, in PWH and no history of coronary artery disease (CAD) (Hays et al., 2021).

A number of studies have also shown that the risk of CVD among PWH is likely influenced by immunodeficiency—specifically, nadir CD4+ T-cell count or low CD4+ T-cell counts (Drozd et al., 2015). Nadir CD4+ T-cell count has been linked to CIMT and arterial stiffness (Hsue et al., 2019). Two cohort studies found that low CD4+ T-cell counts were associated with incident MI (Hsue et al., 2019). In the NA-ACCORD observational cohort, lower current CD4+ T-cells, as well as a history of AIDS and detectable plasma HIV RNA levels, were predictors of primary MI. Collectively, it appears that markers of immune damage and viremia are predictive of or related to CVD clinical events. However, the mechanisms linking damage to the immune system from HIV to atherosclerosis remain to be elucidated (Figure 39.1).

The pathogenesis of HF in the setting of HIV infection remains unclear. One hypothesis is that HIV acts directly on the myocardium, as well as indirectly via inflammation and autoimmunity (Remick et al., 2014). Some antiretroviral drugs, including nucleoside reverse transcriptase inhibitors (NRTIs), in this theoretical model may contribute to pathogenesis. Preliminary data from the REPREIVE trial found that PWH who underwent cardiac MRI had an increased prevalence of myocardial steatosis (i.e., increased myocardial triglyceride content), which predisposes to diastolic dysfunction and HF risk (Nelian et al., 2020). It was also found that for PWH in this study, advanced age, low nadir CD4+ T-cell count, and body mass index (BMI) ≥25 kg/m² were all associated with HF.

THE EFFECT OF ART ON CVD

Multiple retrospective studies and several prospective studies have evaluated the impact of ART on CVD, and as in the epidemiological studies, these are often challenged by factors that confound analyses and/or lack an appropriate control group. The most obvious reason that ART may increase CVD risk is thought to be due to negative effects on lipid levels, especially LDL-C and triglycerides, which were more commonly seen with the older ritonavir-boosted protease inhibitors.

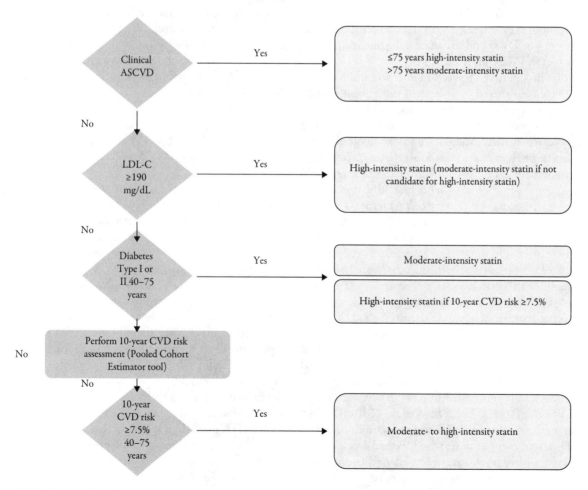

Figure 39.1 ACC/AHA statin benefit groups   SOURCE: Adapted from Stone et al. (2014) and Grundy et al. (2018).

The most persuasive data on the issue of ART-related CVD risk comes from the D:A:D cohort. This is a large, ongoing, prospective, observational study of tens of thousands of PWH, the majority from Europe but also the United States and Australia. In 2003, D:A:D investigators first reported the incidence of MI to be increased significantly with prolonged exposure to combination ART (Friis-Moller et al., 2003). The adjusted risk rate per year of exposure to ART ranged from 0.32 for no ART use to 2.93 for at least 6 years of ART use. Although there was a significant RR of MI with ART, the absolute risk of MI was low (over a period of 36,199 person-years, only 126 patients had an MI). The initial association between ART and MI was mainly driven by protease inhibitor (PI) therapy—specifically lopinavir-ritonavir and indinavir (D:A:D Study Group, 2007; Sabin et al., 2014). More recent data from D:A:D reported in 2018 found that ritonavir-boosted darunavir was associated with a 51% relative increased risk of MI and 49% increased risk of stroke over a 5-year period (Ryom et al., 2018). However, a more recent study from the French Hospital Database found no significant association between MI and exposure to darunavir or atazanavir (Costagliola et al., 2020). Another study also found that the boosted PI atazanavir was not associated with an increased MI risk. This may be due to the indirect hyperbilirubinemia that occurs with atazanavir as other studies found a cardio-protective effect of higher bilirubin levels in the blood. This is further corroborated by a retrospective analysis from the VA cohort, which found that veterans with and without HIV infection with elevated bilirubin levels had lower rates of CVD and HF after adjustment for traditional risk factors (Marconi et al., 2018).

An earlier link between the NRTI abacavir and MI from the D:A:D cohort ushered in a series of subsequent investigations that have reached mixed conclusion. Possible biomolecular mechanisms for this association have been sought and include increased platelet reactivity and/or endothelial cell and leukocyte interactions induced by abacavir, but these mechanisms remain to be proved (Baum et al., 2011; De Pablo et al., 2012). Another study of patients switching from abacavir to tenofovir alafenamide fumarate (TAF), found changes in platelet reactivity and collagen interaction, again suggesting abacavir causes platelet dysfunction. The investigators believe this could explain the findings of an association between abacavir and CVD (Mallon et al., 2018). A 2021 analysis of an administrative health plan data set looked at CVD risk associated with 14 different ART combinations and found that persons taking abacavir-lamivudine-darunavir had the highest incidence rate (IR 11/1000; 95% CI: 7.4–16.0) of acute MI (Dorjee et al., 2021). Per the latest US Department of Health and Human Services (USDHHS) and International Antiretroviral Association (IAS)-USA HIV treatment guidelines, abacavir should be avoided in patients with or at high risk for CVD (USDHHS, 2022; Saag et al., 2020). The IAS guidelines also note that in PWH at moderate to high risk for a CVD-related event or those who have had an event (MI or stroke), switching from abacavir-based or PI-containing regimens (except atazanavir) is recommended (Saag et al., 2020). As HIV therapy evolves and exposure to new agents

accumulate, the D:A:D investigators and other cohorts will regularly reexamine the risks associated with CVD events.

Recently there have been emerging data investigating whether INSTI use is associated with increased incidence of cardiovascular disease. The RESPOND cohort is a multicenter prospective study that included more than 32,000 PWH from Europe, Argentina, and Australia. Participants were followed to the first cardiovascular event, including: MI, stroke, or an invasive cardiovascular procedure (e.g., stenting or angioplasty). After controlling for underlying cardiovascular risk factors, such as HTN, dyslipidemia, diabetes, and chronic kidney disease, the findings suggested the risk of a cardiovascular event almost double during the first 6 months of starting a regimen with an INSTI (Neesgaard et al., 2022). This risk continued in the first 2 years of exposure but was not seen in those with more than 2 years of treatment. Contrary to these findings, no other randomized clinical trials have reported an increase in the incidence of cardiovascular disease in persons starting an INSTI. Thus, more studies are needed to confirm if there is a risk and if that risk is applicable to other populations around the world.

Further, there are other proposed mechanisms whereby ART may increase CVD risk in PWH. Recently there has been growing concern for weight gain in INSTI and tenofovir alafenamide regimens. Although more studies are needed to understand the mechanisms of excessive weight gain, the promotion of weight gain may lead to more insulin resistance and dyslipidemia (Lake & Trevillyan, 2021). Also worth noting is the risk of drug–drug interactions that could contribute to QT prolongation, which is associated with SCD. At least one study found that PWH have a four-times higher risk of SCD compared to those without HIV (Tseng & Foisy, 2012) (Table 39.1).

SCREENING AND ASSESSING CARDIOVASCULAR RISK

Given the higher risk of CVD among PWH, the standard of HIV care should include baseline screening for traditional risk factors and appropriate attention to management. This includes blood pressure measurement and weight with calculation of BMI. Baseline laboratory parameters recommended are a lipid panel (total cholesterol (TC), high-density lipoprotein (HDL)-C, LDL-C, and triglycerides (TG)) and fasting blood glucose level or hemoglobin A1C. Baseline renal and hepatic function should be measured as well. After a patient is started on ART, they should have a lipid profile repeated approximately 3 months after they stabilized on therapy. If the baseline and subsequent values are normal, then repeating a lipid panel yearly is recommended (Aberg et al., 2014; Thompson et al., 2021). Risks for CVD and dyslipidemias should generally be managed according to the most recent ACC/AHA guidelines (Grundy et al., 2018; Reiter-Brennan et al., 2020). An abundance of evidence suggests that the effects of cigarette smoking on CVD are magnified in those with HIV infection. Therefore, there is particular urgency for HIV care providers to ask patients about smoking and

Table 39.1 ACC/AHA GUIDELINES FOR DIAGNOSIS AND MANAGEMENT OF HYPERTENSION

BP CATEGORY	SYSTOLIC BP		DIASTOLIC BP	TREATMENT OR FOLLOW-UP
Normal	< 120 mm Hg	and	< 80 mm Hg	Evaluate yearly; encourage healthy lifestyle changes to maintain normal BP
Elevated	120–129 mm Hg	and	< 80 mm Hg	Recommend healthy lifestyle changes and reassess in 3–6 months
Hypertension stage 1	130–139 mm Hg	or	80–89 mm Hg	Assess the 10-year risk for heart disease and stroke using the atherosclerotic cardiovascular disease (ASCVD risk calculator) • If risk is < 10%, start with healthy lifestyle recommendations and reassess in 3–6 months • If risk is >10% or the patient has known clinical CVD, diabetes mellitus, chronic kidney disease, recommend lifestyle changes, and BP-lowering medication (one medication); reassess in 1 month for effectiveness of medication therapy • If goal is met after 1 month, reassess in 3–6 months • If goal is not met after 1 month, consider different medication or titration and continue monthly follow-up until control is achieved
Hypertension stage 2	≥140 mm Hg	or	≥90 mm Hg	Recommend healthy lifestyle changes and BP-lowering medication (two medications of different classes); reassess in 1 month for effectiveness • If goal is met in 1 month; reassess in 3–6 months • If goal is not met after 1 month, consider different medications or titration and continue follow-up until control is achieved

incorporate evidence-based interventions to facilitate cessation of smoking into their practice (see later discussion).

In the past, CVD risk for patients was usually assessed via the Framingham (MA) heart study risk calculator. Older studies have used this in PWH and found it generally performed well in assessing the 10-year risk of CVD. However, in retrospect, Framingham likely underestimated the actual CVD risk compared to use in HIV-negative patients (Law et al., 2006). The newer 10-year CVD risk AHA/ACC risk calculator has become the standard of care in the United States (Grundy et al., 2018) (Box 39.1). However, similar to the Framingham risk calculator, the ACC/AHA calculator appears to underestimate the risk of CVD in PWH (Regan et al., 2015; Thompson-Paul et al., 2015; Triant et al., 2018). More prospective data to validate these guidelines in PWH are needed to develop a risk calculator that includes HIV-specific factors, traditional CVD risk factors, and the ability to stratify patients based on sex.

Several inflammatory biomarkers of coagulation and inflammation have been studied for their potential role in predicting CVD events in PWH. Some of these markers include the highly sensitive C-reactive protein (hsCRP), D-dimer, IL-6, and fibrinogen. Combined data from three cohorts of PWH found that IL-6 and D-dimer were independently associated with the risk of serious non-AIDS events or death. Another study found that biomarkers in PWH can be clustered into a "cardiac phenotype" to risk-stratify these patients (Sherzer et al., 2018). Patients with high levels of CRP, IL-6, and D-dimer had a higher prevalence of pulmonary HTN and a threefold increase in mortality over approximately 7 years of follow-up. However, a study of the association between hypertension (HTN) and the inflammatory biomarkers IL-6 and hsCRP in PWH

without CVD and CD4 counts >500 cells/mm^3 found that traditional risk factors (i.e., race, age, gender, BMI, diabetes, and smoking) and not baseline levels of IL6 or hsCRP were associated with the prevalence and incidence of HTN (Ghazi et al., 2020). Other biomarkers under investigation are adiponectin and GlycA. Adiponectin, increases insulin sensitivity, and, in PWH lower adiponectin levels were found in ART-associated lipodystrophy and associated with subclinical CAD (McGettrick & Mallon, 2021). GlycA, although not currently measurable in most clinical labs, may be a more accurate biomarker of several biomarkers. Increased levels of GlycA were associated with other subclinical markers of CVD such as presence of coronary artery calcium, coronary stenosis, and plaque burden (Tibuakuu et al., 2019). It is hopeful that clustering of these biomarkers and help identify at-risk patients and target appropriate therapies to prevent or limit cardiovascular events.

INTERVENTIONS AND MANAGEMENT

There is currently no robust evidence to determine if the management of CVD risks in PWH should differ from that in the general population. Modifiable risk factors, including diabetes mellitus, dyslipidemia, HTN, obesity, and cigarette smoking, are important in PWH, likely more so than for the general population. As noted previously, the ACC/AHA risk calculator may underestimate the risk of heart disease in PWH persons (Triant et al., 2018). Some experts believe the clinicians should adjust the calculated risk upward by 1.5 to 2 times on the basis of this underestimation (So-Amah et al., 2020). Regardless, risk-based assessment for CVD in persons with HIV disease remains a rational starting point to

Box 39.1 KEY RECOMMENDATION FOR REDUCING THE RISK OF ATHEROSCLEROTIC CARDIOVASCULAR DISEASE (ASCVD) THROUGH CHOLESTEROL MANAGEMENT

- In all patients, regardless of age, emphasize a heart-healthy lifestyle to reduce ASCVD risk. In young adults 20–39 years of age, an assessment of lifetime risk facilitates the clinician–patient risk discussion.

- In patients with clinical ASCVD, the goal is to reduce low-density lipoprotein cholesterol (LDL-C) by >50% with high-intensity statin therapy or maximally tolerated statin therapy.

- In very-high-risk patients (history of multiple major ASCVD events or one event and multiple risk factors), with an LDL-C of >70 mg/dL on maximal statin therapy, consider adding ezetimibe. In patients whose LDL-C remains ≥70 mg/dL on maximally tolerated statin and ezetimibe, adding a PCSK9 inhibitor is reasonable following a clinician–patient discussion about the net benefit, safety, and cost.

- In patients with severe primary hypercholesterolemia (LDL-C level ≥190 mg/dL), begin high-intensity statin therapy without calculating 10-year ASCVD risk. If the LDL-C level remains ≥100 mg/dL, adding ezetimibe is reasonable. If the LDL-C on statin plus ezetimibe remains ≥100 mg/dL and the patient has multiple factors that increase the risk of ASCVD events, a PCSK9 inhibitor may be considered.

- In patients 40–75 years of age *with* diabetes mellitus and LDL-C ≥70 mg/dL, start moderate-intensity statin therapy without calculating 10-year ASCVD risk.

- In adults 40–75 years of age *without* diabetes mellitus with LDL-C ≥70 mg/dL and a 10-year ASCVD risk of ≥7.5%, start moderate-intensity statin if a discussion of treatment options favors statin therapy. If risk status is uncertain, consider using coronary artery calcium (CAC) to improve specificity. If CAC is zero, treatment with statin therapy may be withheld (except in cigarette smokers, diabetes mellitus, or strong family history of premature ASCVD). A CAC score of 1 to 99 favors statin therapy, especially in those ≥55 years of age. If the CAC score is ≥100 Agatston units, statin therapy is indicated unless deferred by clinician–patient risk discussion.

- In adults 40–75 years of age *without* diabetes mellitus and 10-year risk of 7.5%–19.9% risk-enhancing factors (family hx, LDL-C >160 mg/dL, metabolic syndrome, chronic kidney disease, premature menopause) favors statin therapy. The presence of inflammatory disorders **including HIV** with other risk-enhancing factors may favor statin therapy in patients at 10-year risk of only 5%–7.5%.

- Assess adherence and response to lifestyle changes and cholesterol-lowering medications with repeat lipid measurement 4–12 weeks after statin initiation repeated every 3–12 months.

SOURCE: Adapted from Reiter-Brennan (2020); Grundy (2018).

guide lifestyle counseling, medical therapy (mainly statins), and other potential risk-reduction interventions (Grundy et al., 2019).

Aggressively treating HIV infection with ART to attain full viral suppression should remain the primary objective, even in the presence of CVD risk factors or established CAD. Data from the SMART study (Lundgren et al., 2015), as well as the ATHENA cohort (Van Lelyveld et al., 2010), found that ongoing viremia and incomplete immune recovery increase the risk of cardiovascular events. In addition, a National Institutes of Health (NIH)-sponsored study of 6,517 patients, of whom 273 sustained an acute MI, found immunologic control was the most important HIV-related factor associated with acute MI (Triant et al., 2010).

Because of their potential effects on cholesterol (and thus CVD risk), the choice of ART should take into consideration a patient's individual CVD risk factors. Some combination ART regimens, such as ritonavir-boosted PIs, may increase lipid subsets, including LDL-C and triglycerides. The pharmacological booster cobicistat appears to increase LDL-C, similar to ritonavir, but with a smaller impact on triglycerides. The NRTI abacavir increases LDL-C and triglycerides, whereas tenofovir disoproxil fumarate (TDF) has been observed to lower LDL-C (Tungsiripat et al., 2010). As noted earlier, in some studies, including D:A:D and SMART, abacavir has been associated with an increased risk of CVD and MI (Dorjee et al., 2018; Dorjee et al., 2021; SMART, 2008). In clinical trials, the NRTI TAF produced increases in fasting lipid parameters (TC, HDL, direct LDL, and TGs) compared to TDF and has been associated with weight gain. (Sax et al., 2019). The more widely used INSTI raltegravir, dolutegravir, elvitegravir, and bictegravir have not been found to significantly effect lipid levels when assessed in multiple clinical trials (Dorjee et al., 2018).

In patients with moderate to severe dyslipidemia and increased CVD risk, switching ART to a regimen with less effect on cholesterol and/or triglycerides is recommended by the DHHS and IAS-USA treatment guidelines. However, this should not be done at the expense of compromising virologic control. In the SPRIAL study, patients with stable HIV disease were switched from a ritonavir-boosted PI-based regimen to raltegravir, leading to significant improvement in lipid profiles (Martinez et al., 2010). In the SPIRIT study, changing from a ritonavir-boosted PI plus dual nucleoside regimen to rilpivirine plus TDF/emtricitabine led to significant reductions in LDL cholesterol (Palella et al., 2014). In the MARCH study, patients switched from a boosted PI to maraviroc had significant reductions in mean TC over 96 weeks (Pett et al., 2018). Lastly, in the NEAT 022 study, all patients over the age of 50 years and those over 18 with a 10-year CVD risk score of >10% were switched from a ritonavir-boosted PI to dolutegravir (DTG). At 48 weeks, patients switched to DTG had significant improvements in TC and other lipid fractions and viral suppression was maintained by 93% in the DTG group and 95% in the PI-ritonavir group (Gatell et al., 2017).

Management of lipid disorders in PWH should follow guidelines established for the general population. Attention should be paid to the potential for drug–drug interactions between lipid-lowering and ART. There are several published cholesterol guidelines, but most practitioners in the United States follow those of AHA/ACC (Figure 39.2, Figure 39.3, and Box 39.2). The most recent US recommendations for the management of cholesterol are based on several factors, including 10-year risk of ASCVD, presence of diabetes mellitus, baseline LDL-C levels, and chronic inflammatory conditions, including HIV infection (Grundy et al., 2018). The AHA/ACC guidelines note that if ASCVD risk is uncertain, coronary artery calcium (CAC) may be used to determine indication for statin therapy (Grundy et al., 2018). These guidelines consider HIV to be a "risk-enhancing" factor which may influence starting medical therapy at a 10-year risk threshold below 7.5%. Depending on individual risk and the presence of risk-enhancing factors, this may include "high-intensity" or "moderate-intensity" dosing with statin therapy and the use of additional lipid-lowering agents (see discussion below).

STATIN THERAPY

The recommended therapy for CVD risk reduction in most patients is a 3-hydroxy-3-methylglutaryl coenzyme A reductase inhibitor or statin. These agents are very effective in lowering TC and LDL-C but vary in potency and drug interactions. There are a multitude of clinical trials supporting the role of statins for primary and secondary prevention of ASCVD (Grundy et al., 2018). Intensity of therapy should be determined by baseline risk and comorbidities (see Table 39.2). Preferred statins for PWH include pravastatin, fluvastatin, atorvastatin, rosuvastatin, and pitavastatin. Of note, simvastatin and lovastatin should not be used in patients taking PIs because of drug interactions. They are metabolized by the cytochrome P3A4 isoenzyme, and inhibition of this enzyme system results in elevated statin levels with an increased risk of rhabdomyolysis and hepatic toxicity. Conversely, the nonnucleoside reverse transcriptase inhibitor (NNRTI) efavirenz reduces the level of simvastatin and lovastatin and thus decreases efficacy of these drugs.

Prior studies have shown that PWH and ASCVD risk were less likely to be prescribed a statin (Blackman et al., 2020), making it important to assess for statin hesitancy or intolerance. Secondary effects that may result in statin intolerance include fatigue, myalgias, and myopathy, which can result in elevation of creatinine kinase (CK). Myalgias are reported by about 15% of persons taking statins, but most do not have elevations in CK (Guyton et al., 2014). In patients who report myalgias, it may be prudent to rule out other causes of muscle-related symptoms such as hypothyroidism, vitamin B_{12}, or other inflammatory musculoskeletal disorders. Re-challenging a statin-intolerant patient with a different agent or alternative dosing strategy (e.g. once a week dosing) can also be considered (Backes et al., 2017).

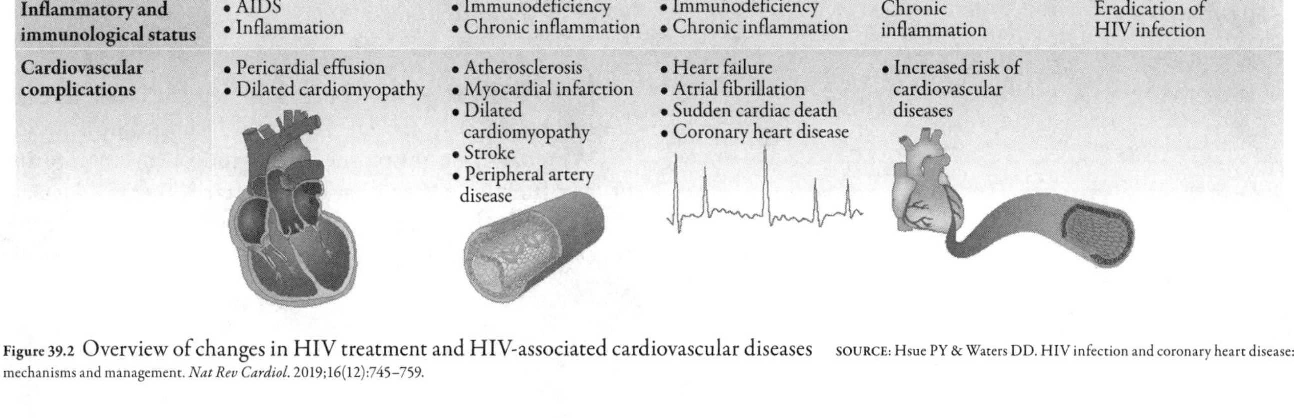

	Pre-ART	First-generation ART regimens	Contemporary ART regimens	Future	
				Optimized ART regimens	Curative therapies
HIV treatment	No HIV-specific therapy	• PI • NRTI • NNRTI	• PI • NRTI • NNRTI • CCR5 antagonist • Integrase inhibitor	• Early ART inhibition • Two-drug regimens • Injectable medications • New therapeutic targets	• Stem-cell-based therapies • Strategies to eliminate latency • Genome editing • Broadly neutralizing antibodies
Inflammatory and immunological status	• AIDS • Inflammation	• Immunodeficiency • Chronic inflammation	• Immunodeficiency • Chronic inflammation	Chronic inflammation	Eradication of HIV infection
Cardiovascular complications	• Pericardial effusion • Dilated cardiomyopathy	• Atherosclerosis • Myocardial infarction • Dilated cardiomyopathy • Stroke • Peripheral artery disease	• Heart failure • Atrial fibrillation • Sudden cardiac death • Coronary heart disease	• Increased risk of cardiovascular diseases	

Figure 39.2 Overview of changes in HIV treatment and HIV-associated cardiovascular diseases SOURCE: Hsue PY & Waters DD. HIV infection and coronary heart disease: mechanisms and management. *Nat Rev Cardiol.* 2019;16(12):745–759.

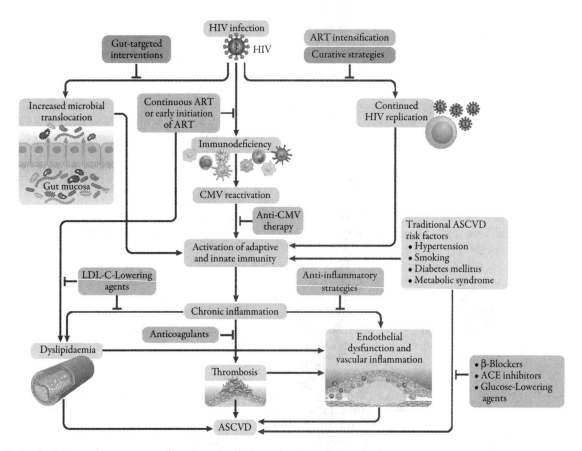

Figure 39.3 Pathophysiology and management of HIV-associated atherosclerotic cardiovascular disease SOURCE: Hsue PY & Waters DD. HIV infection and coronary
heart disease: mechanisms and management. *Nat Rev Cardiol.* 2019;16(12):745–759.

Box 39.2 FACTORS INCLUDED IN THE AHA/ACA RISK CALCULATOR

10-Year ASCVD Risk: Pooled Cohort Equation

Demographics
- Age (40–79 years)
- Gender
- Race

History
- Hypertension
- Diabetes mellitus
- Tobacco

Measurements
- TC
- High-density lipoprotein (HDL)
- Systolic blood pressure
- Diastolic blood pressure

Adapted from http://www.cvriskcalculator.com/.

Table 39.2 HIGH- AND MODERATE-INTENSITY STATIN THERAPY

HIGH-INTENSITY STATIN THERAPY	MODERATE-INTENSITY STATIN THERAPY
Lowers LDL-C *by* ~ ≥50%	Lowers LDL-C *by* ~30%–49%
Atorvastatin 40–80 mg	Atorvastatin 10–20 mg
Rosuvastatin 20–40 mg	Fluvastatin 40 mg bid
	Fluvastatin XL 80 mg
	Lovastatin 40 mg[a]
	Pitavastatin 1–4 mg
	Pravastatin 40 mg (80 g)
	Rosuvastatin (5 mg) 10 mg
	Simvastatin 20–40 mg[a]

LDL-C, low-density lipoprotein cholesterol.

[a] Should not be used with protease inhibitors.

SOURCE: Adapted from Grundy (2018).

Historically, there was concern for hepatoxicity with early
statins, but in 2012 the US Food and Drug Administration
(FDA) removed the recommendation for routine monitoring
of liver function tests in patients on statin therapy. Hepatic
transaminase levels can be checked at baseline to exclude
other hepatic pathology, and then repeated only as clinically

indicated thereafter. For PWH with chronic hepatitis B virus (HBV) or hepatitis C virus (HCV) it is prudent to monitor hepatic transaminases at least biannually.

The Randomized Trial to Prevent Vascular Events in HIV (REPRIEVE) trial was initiated by the NIH in 2015. This study is evaluating the use of pitavastatin versus placebo in 7,500 PWH adults aged 40–75 years at 100 clinical sites globally (https://clinicaltrials.gov/ct2/show/NCT02344290). Numerous primary outcomes will be measured, including the time to the first event of a composite major cardiovascular event, which includes atherosclerotic or other CVD death, nonfatal MI, unstable angina hospitalization, coronary arterial revascularization, nonfatal stroke, or transient ischemic attack (TIA). Secondary outcomes, such as change in lipid levels, inflammatory biomarkers, and all-cause mortality, are also being evaluated. In cohort of 755 study participants with low-to-moderate atherosclerotic cardiovascular (ASCVD) risk and well-controlled HIV, participants underwent coronary computed tomography angiography and were found to have higher than expected rates of coronary plaques, supporting the theory that HIV is an independent risk factor for coronary artery disease (Hoffmann et al., 2021). This study is now fully enrolled, and there should be preliminary data forthcoming (Fitch et al., 2020; Grinspoon et al., 2020).

FIBRIC ACID DERIVATIVES

In PWH who have *hypertriglyceridemia*, which is defined as a fasting serum level of >150mg/dL, lifestyle management, including weight loss and exercise, is initially recommended. Historically, elevated triglyceride levels were seen in PWH taking boosted protease inhibitors, but the incidence has declined in recent years with diminished use of PIs. In PWH who are intolerant to statins or continue to have elevated triglycerides on a statin, fibric acid derivatives, including gemfibrozil, or fenofibrate, remain a consideration for primary prevention of CVD in patients with high triglyceride levels (150 to 499 mg/dL) and borderline (5% to 7.4%) or intermediate (7.5% to 19.9%) risk. They are generally recommended in patients with severe triglyceride levels (≥500 mg/dL) (Oh et al., 2020). These drugs effectively lower triglycerides but have little impact on other lipid parameters, including HDL-C, LDL-C, and apolipoprotein B (apo-B). Data from D:A:D suggests a very minor association between elevated triglycerides and MI after adjusting for other lipid and nonlipid risk factors. Therefore, the D:A:D: study group concluded that use of fibrates alone to lower triglycerides is unlikely to have a major impact on the incidence of MI (D:A:D, 2011).

The current ACC/AHA treatment guidelines do not recommend fibrates for dyslipidemia (Grundy et al., 2018). They cite a lack of data supporting an effect on CVD outcomes and note that fibrates role in the primary prevention of CVD is less clear as it relates to a reduction in triglyceride levels. They note in adults with fasting triglycerides of 500 mg/dL or greater, and especially fasting triglycerides of 1,000 mg/dL or more, it is important to identify and address causes of hypertriglyceridemia. If triglycerides are persistently elevated or increasing, a very-low-fat diet, avoidance of refined carbohydrates

and alcohol, consumption of food rich in omega-3 fatty acids are recommended. Fibrates are recommended as first-line treatment for management of patients who are at risk for triglyceride-induced pancreatitis, which includes those with a prior history of pancreatitis or triglycerides >1,000 mg/dL (Berglund et al., 2015; Grundy et al., 2018). A Cochrane review from 2016 concluded that there is "moderate-quality" evidence suggesting fibrates lower the risk of CVD and coronary events in primary prevention, but the absolute risk reduction was less than 1% (Jakob et al., 2016). The ACC/AHA guidelines state that the combination of gemfibrozil with a statin should be avoided because of an increased risk for myopathy (Grundy et al., 2018).

EZETIMIBE

Ezetimibe is a drug that selectively inhibits gastrointestinal cholesterol absorption within the small intestine. Overall, this drug is safe, usually well tolerated, and effective in reducing LDL-C by an additional 12%–19% when taken with a statin therapy. Ezetimibe is neither a cytochrome P450 inhibitor nor a cytochrome P450 inducer, so metabolism with other drugs, including ART, is not a concern (Sizar et al., 2020). However, ezetimibe should not be used in patients with moderate or severe hepatic impairment.

Studies with ezetimibe have been performed in PWH. They have examined ezetimibe as both monotherapy and adjunctive therapy for lipid management but did not specifically assess CVD outcomes in PWH (Grandi et al., 2014; Leyes et al., 2014; Nirmala et al., 2022; Saeedi et al., 2015, Wohl et al., 2008). A study from Thailand that included PWH on a PI plus a statin for at least 6 months found the addition of 10 mg/day of ezetimibe produced a significant decline in mean serum TC, LDL, and TGs (Boonthos et al., 2018). Moreover, there were no adverse events or abnormal lab parameters noted in study participants. The IMPROVE-IT trial demonstrated that ezetimibe significantly reduces the risk of major cardiovascular events in a group of high-risk patients without HIV who had known CVD and already low LDL-C levels. In this trial, there was an absolute risk reduction of 2% in the cardiovascular event rate (32.7% vs. 34.7%) with the addition of ezetimibe in patients on simvastatin compared to those on simvastatin monotherapy (Cannon et al., 2015; Hammersley & Signy, 2017).

The 2018 ACC/AHA guidelines as well as the National Institute for Care Excellence (NICE) guidelines from the UK only recommend ezetimibe monotherapy for primary hyperlipidemia in patients for whom a statin is contraindicated or if they cannot tolerate statin therapy (NICE, 2016; Grundy et al., 2018). This is based on the lack of CVD outcome trials of ezetimibe monotherapy. A 2017 US update on non-statin therapies suggests the addition of 10 mg/d of ezetimibe in patients for whom additional lowering of LDL-C is desired (Lloyd-Jones et al., 2017). The current US guidelines note that it is "reasonable" to add ezetimibe in very high-risk patients with an LDL-C of greater than 70 mg/dL despite maximal statin therapy (Grundy et al., 2018). In a similar manner, the NICE guidelines from the UK and the European Society of

Cardiology support ezetimibe as add-on therapy in "high or very high-risk patients" who fail to meet specific LDL targets. A randomized trial in 2022 showed that a moderate-intensity statin plus ezetimide was noninferior to a high-intensity statin for reducing the combination of cardiovascular death, major cardiovascular events, or nonfatal stroke (Kim et al., 2022).

OMEGA-3 FATTY ACIDS

Three to five grams per day of omega-3 fatty acids (DHA/EPA or "fish oil") generally produce a 30% to 50% reduction in triglyceride levels. Their low cost, good tolerability, and lack of drug–drug interactions have made these agents historically attractive for use in the general population, including in PWH. In December 2019, the FDA approved the omega-3 drug icosapent ethyl (Vascepa®) as adjunctive therapy to reduce the risk of CVD in adults with triglycerides >150 mg/dL. It is recommended that patients considering icosapent ethyl should have either established CVD disease or diabetes and two or more additional CVD risk factors. It is the first approved drug of this class to reduce CVD risk among patients with elevated triglycerides but as an add-on to maximally tolerated statin therapy (Oh et al., 2020). It is also considerably more expensive than OTC generic omega-3 fatty acid formulations.

There are data, including a recent meta-analysis of nine clinical trials ($n = 578$), evaluating the effect of omega-3 fatty acids on lipid patterns in PHW who were taking ART (Fogacci et al., 2020). The conclusion from this meta-analysis was that omega-3s significantly reduced triglycerides and increased HDL cholesterol without affecting LDL or TC levels. They also noted the lack of adverse events with omega-3s. Another systematic review and meta-analysis of patients with baseline TG levels of greater than 200 mg/dL found the average combined reduction in TGs in patients taking omega-3 fatty acids was −114 mg/dL (Vieira & Silveira, 2017). Several other studies have looked at the use of fish oil supplements in HIV patients to assess their effect on inflammatory biomarkers and oxidative stress—both with potential relationships to CVD but found either no change or no clinical benefit (Amador-Licona et al., 2016, Oliveira et al., 2015; Swanson et al., 2018).

The relationship between circulating TG levels and atherosclerosis is still unclear. Current US cholesterol guidelines cite a lack of any randomized controlled trials evaluating this class of drugs and with no proof of beneficial CVD outcomes. They may prevent pancreatitis in patients with severe triglyceride elevations (>1,000 mg/dL) but have been associated with some adverse events, including gastrointestinal upset and infrequently skin conditions (rash and pruritus). Data from the British ASCEND trial found that 1 g of omega-3 fatty acid daily did not reduce nonfatal MI or stroke, TIA, or CVD death compared to an olive-oil placebo (8.9% vs. 9.2%) (Bowman et al., 2018). Two recent Cochrane reviews addressed the benefits of omega-3 fatty acids, including fish and plant-based sources (Abdelhamid et al., 2018; Abdelhamid et al., 2020). These extensive reviews note that increasing the intake of these compounds "probably slightly reduces the risk of coronary heart disease and CVD events but has little or no effect on all-cause CVD mortality." Several studies of omega-3 fatty acids and icosapent ethyl have shown an increased risk of atrial fibrillation (Gaba et al., 2022; Kalstad et al., 2021; Nicholls et al., 2020). Therefore, omega-3 fatty acids may be considered only for select patients primarily with elevated triglycerides and high cardiovascular risk after discussion of the known risks and benefits.

PCSK9 INHIBITORS

There are currently two FDA-approved PCSK inhibitors, alirocumab and evolocumab, which are specifically indicated for the treatment of high LDL cholesterol. These medications are humanized monoclonal antibodies that inactivate proprotein convertase subtilisin-kexin type 9 (PCSK9) (Shahreyar et al., 2018). This inactivation results in decreased LDL-receptor degradation, increased recirculation of the receptor to the surface of hepatocytes, and consequent lowering of LDL cholesterol levels in the bloodstream (Everett et al., 2015). These drugs have been shown to lower LDL cholesterol by approximately 60% in patients on statin therapy and are generally safe and well tolerated. They are administered as a subcutaneous injection either every 2 weeks or once a month.

There are several studies providing evidence that PCKS9 inhibitors reduce CVD events when added to statin therapy (Giugliano et al., 2017; Sabatine et al., 2017). A 2017 Cochrane study showed that PCSK9 inhibitors may slightly reduce risk of CVD events in patients with a history of CVD (Schmidt et al., 2017). However, these agents, which originally came on the market at $14,000 per year, have been reduced in price to about $6,000 per patient/year. The use of PCSK9 inhibitors remains limited to high-risk ASCVD patients—those with familial hypercholesterolemia or with known ASCVD who need further lowering of LDL despite maximal statin and ezetimibe therapy (Grundy et al., 2018; Lloyd-Jones et al., 2017). Of note, PSCK9 levels are elevated in HIV-positive persons, and in ART-naive patients, are positively associated with immunodeficiency and severity of HIV disease (Boccara et al., 2017). However, the role of PSCK9 inhibitor treatment on HIV prognosis remains unknown. In a small study of 19 PWH treated with evolocumab, an improvement in coronary blood flow was found (Leucker et al., 2020). The BEIJERINCK Study, a randomized controlled trial comparing monthly evolocumab to placebo in 464 PWH and dyslipidemia who are on maximally tolerated statin therapy, found a 57% reduction in LDL levels (Boccara et al., 2020a, 2020b).

BEMPEDOIC ACID

Bempedoic acid (Nexletol®) was approved by the FDA in 2020 for use in combination therapy. This drug lowers LDL cholesterol through inhibition of ATP citrate lyase. Bempedoic acid may increase serum uric acid levels and risk of tendon rupture, with about 11% of patients discontinuing use because of adverse effects, which can include muscle spasms, arthralgias, and diarrhea, and with tolerability that is comparable to ezetimibe (Ballantyne et al., 2020). It has been shown to lower LDL cholesterol by about 17% in clinical trials when combined with a moderate or high-intensity statin (Ray et al., 2019). A randomized trial of 301 patients at high risk of CVD showed that a combination of bempedoic acid and ezetimibe when added to maximally tolerated statins significantly lowered LDL levels by 38% when compared with placebo (Ballantyne et al., 2020). Pending further data this drug is mainly recommended as add-on therapy for patients who need further LDL-C lowering despite optimal use of a statin and ezetimibe. An advantage over the PCSK9 inhibitors is that it can be given orally and is less expensive than PCSK9 inhibitors. There are currently no data on the use of bempedoic acid in PWH.

ASPIRIN

Aspirin (acetylsalicylic acid or ASA) has been recommended by healthcare providers for the prevention of CVD and associated clinical events, including MI and stroke. Recent surveillance data from the CDC found that 27% of US adults were taking aspirin for primary prevention, and 74.9% for secondary CVD prevention (Wall et al., 2018). While the benefit of aspirin has been clearly demonstrated for people with established CVD, this risk-benefit equation is more complex in primary prevention of CVD and related clinical outcomes such as MI. Aspirin irreversibly inhibits cyclooxygenase-1 (COX-1) and blocks the formation and release of thromboxane A2, a strong platelet activator. The COX-1 enzyme is also responsible for producing prostaglandins that protect gastric mucosa, thus patients who take aspirin may be susceptible to gastrointestinal bleeding. Risk factors for GI bleeding with aspirin include higher dose and longer duration of use, history of gastrointestinal ulcers, bleeding disorders, renal failure, advanced liver disease, and thrombocytopenia. Other factors that increase the risk for bleeding with low-dose aspirin use include concurrent anticoagulation with warfarin, direct-acting anticoagulants (DOACs) or the use of nonsteroidal anti-inflammatory drugs (NSAIDs).

The evidence for aspirin in the *primary prevention* of CVD, MI, or stroke remains limited with very little published data on its use in PWH (O'Brien et al., 2013; Suchindran et al., 2014). With the last update in 2022, the US Preventive Services Task Force (USPSTF) downgraded aspirin for primary prevention to a "C" grade recommendation (see Box 39.3) (Davidson et al., 2022). The current evidence suggests that the net benefit of aspirin for primary prevention is small and may be considered in those aged 40–59 years with a 10% or greater 10-year CVD risk (http://tools.acc.org/ASCVD-Risk-Estimator) and a low risk of bleeding. The USPSTF recommends against starting aspirin for primary prevention in those over 60 years of age, giving this a "D" grade recommendation. However, the guidelines do not clearly provide guidance on continuation or discontinuation of aspirin for primary prevention in those that already taking aspirin. The optimal dose of aspirin is not known, but 75–100 mg is the dose most commonly recommended.

There are several recently completed primary prevention trials with aspirin that provide updated guidance regarding

---

Box 39.3 US PREVENTIVE SERVICES TASK FORCE (USPSTF) RECOMMENDATIONS FOR ASPIRIN THERAPY

ADULTS aged 40–59 years with a ≥10% 10-year CVD risk
The USPSTF suggests that the net benefit of aspirin for primary prevention is small and may be considered in those 40–59 years of age with a 10% or greater 10-year CVD risk and a low risk of bleeding (level of evidence = C).

ADULTS aged 60 years and older
The USPSTF recommends against starting aspirin for primary prevention of CVD in adults aged 60 years and older (level of evidence = D).

CVD = cardiovascular disease.
SOURCE: Adapted from Davidson et al. (2022).

---

the use of aspirin. The Aspirin in Reducing Events in the Elderly trial included 19,000 patients aged 70 years and older from Australia and the United States who took 100 mg of aspirin daily or placebo (McNeil et al., 2018). During almost 5 years of follow-up, the use of low-dose aspirin resulted in a significantly higher risk of major hemorrhage and did not result in a significantly lower risk of cardiovascular disease when compared to placebo. In addition, all-cause mortality was higher in the ASA group. The Aspirin to Reduce Risk of Initial Vascular Events (ARRIVE) trial from Europe randomly assigned more than 12,500 adults with presumed moderate CVD risk to aspirin 100 mg/d or placebo. During 5 years of follow-up there was no reduction in CVD events by intent-to-treat analysis (Gaziano et al., 2018). There was a 19% relative reduction in the composite endpoint of CVD events in patients who took ASA but also a doubling in the rate of GI bleeding (0.5% in absolute terms). The ASCEND trial, conducted in the United Kingdom, included 15,480 patients aged ≥40 years old with diabetes mellitus and without CVD were randomized to aspirin 100 mg daily or placebo. After a mean follow-up of 7.4 years, the frequency of the primary endpoint (composite of nonfatal MI, nonfatal stroke, TIA, or death from any vascular cause) was 8.5% with aspirin and 9.6% with placebo. The minor benefit of aspirin came at the expense of more major bleeding events (Bowman et al., 2018). A recent systemic review in 2022 also found that low-dose aspirin (< 100mg/day) was associated with a small decrease in major cardiovascular events (odds ratio (OR) 0.90; 95% CI: 0.85–0.95) and a small increase in major bleeding (OR 1.44; 95% CI: 1.32–1.57) (Guirguis-Blake et al., 2022).

The AHA/ACC guidelines note that low-dose aspirin may be considered among select adults aged 40 to 70 years who are at higher ASCVD risk but not at increased bleeding risk. They additionally note that aspirin should not be administered for the primary prevention of ASCVD among adults of any age who are at increased risk of bleeding (Arnett et al., 2019).

For *secondary prevention*, numerous studies have evaluated the role of aspirin in acute treatment of cardiac events and secondary prevention of CVD (Jones, 2018). There are strong data demonstrating that low-dose aspirin (75–100 mg/day) effectively reduces the risk of recurrence of vascular events in patients with a history of a previous MI, stroke, or TIA by approximately 20%. There has been FDA-approved labeling for this indication since the 1980s (Paikin & Eikelboom, 2012). Because of this consistently reported benefit, which has been found to outweigh the risk of major bleeding, aspirin therapy for secondary prevention is part of standard clinical practice.

BLOOD PRESSURE CONTROL

HTN has become more prevalent as the HIV population ages. It is one of the most important CVD risk factors and is strongly associated with CAD, stroke, HF, and renal disease. The prevalence varies with different HIV cohorts but is estimated to range from 10% to 50% (Boccara, 2017). Data from the CDC's Medical Monitoring Project found that 42% of PWH had HTN ($N = 8.631$), but only 49% had their blood pressure controlled (Olaiya et al., 2018). In a recent US study of Medicaid patients ($n = 3456$), the prevalence of comorbidities increased from the fourth year to the first year of entry into care; these included cardiovascular disease (28%–40%), HTN (24%–37%), and hyperlipidemia (12%–17%) (DerSarkissian et al., 2020). The global incidence of adult PWH with HTN is estimated to be 35% compared to 30% of HIV-negative adults (Fahme et al., 2018).

Factors associated with elevated blood pressure in PWH appear similar to those of the general population and include older age; male sex; African American, African, and Caribbean ethnicities; higher BMI; diabetes; and chronic kidney disease. Although less commonly seen than in the past, lipodystrophy and metabolic syndrome have also been associated with HTN in PWH adults (Fahme et al., 2018). Older studies of blood pressure changes in the D:A:D study and a US cohort found no evidence that ART increased the risk of HTN (Medina-Torne et al., 2012; Thiebault et al., 2005). Conversely, other studies have implicated both PIs and duration of ART as being associated with HTN (Boccara, 2017). Some researchers also believe that immune activation and chronic inflammation contribute to the pathophysiology of HTN in persons with HIV disease (van Zoest et al., 2017).

It Is appropriate to screen and manage HTN in adult PWH per the current national guidelines (Elton et al., 2018). It should be noted, however, that current ACC/AHA US HTN guidelines (Whelton et al., 2018) have been controversial and not collectively endorsed by all professional societies. The 2017 recommendation is for a diagnosis of "hypertension" rather than "prehypertension" for adults with a systolic BP of 130 mm Hg or greater. They also recommend drug treatment for "high-risk" people with HTN. These include those with existing CVD or a calculated 10-year CVD risk of 10% or greater, or another high-risk condition such as chronic kidney disease or diabetes (Whelton et al., 2018). Some feel that by following the new ACC/AHA guidelines a large number of people will be subject to medical treatment with little or no benefit in terms of CVD risk reduction and mortality (Bell, 2018; Brunstrom & Carlberg, 2018). They

believe the threshold for treating HTN should remain at 140 mm Hg. Regardless, for those for whom medical therapy is deemed necessary, it is important to be aware of potential drug–drug interactions with ART and antihypertensive agents. Moreover, management strategies should consider degree of frailty, comorbidities, and psychosocial factors and ideally should be individualized (Oliveros et al., 2020). Nonpharmacologic therapies including the DASH diet, restriction of sodium intake, and regular exercise all play a role for some patients. Unfortunately, there have not been any large-scale studies of specific blood pressure–lowering medications in PWH adults. However, there are small studies of renin-angiotensin antagonists showing very favorable results, and many adult PWH will likely need two or more medications to reach recommended blood pressure goals (Fahme et al., 2018).

Knowing that medication adherence is very important for PWH, it is worth noting that a recent study from Spain found that patients who took their blood pressure medications at bedtime had a significant decrease in CVD events compared to morning dosing (Hermida et al., 2020). Better outcomes were seen for MI, coronary revascularization, and stroke over a 6-year follow-up of 1,752 patients. In addition, there were no differences in adverse events including hypotension and sleep disturbances between the two groups.

SMOKING CESSATION

Smoking prevalence is remarkably high in many PWH cohorts, usually much higher than in the general population (Johnston et al., 2021), with 33.6 % of PWH being current smokers in 2014 (Frazier et al., 2018). Therefore, smoking cessation for PWH remains a very important part of CVD risk reduction. There is also an increased risk of lung cancer in PWH, which is directly influenced by smoking as well as immunosuppressive and inflammatory aspects of HIV (Sigel et al., 2017). The D:A:D study found that smoking cessation in PWH decreased the incident RR for MI from 3.73 in the first year of smoking cessation to 2.07 after 3 years of not smoking (Petoumunos et al., 2011). Another study from 2017 estimated that smoking cessation in PWH could prevent 38% of acute MIs (Althoff et al., 2017).

Getting patients to stop smoking may significantly reduce their AHA/ACA risk scores by 50% or greater. Counseling, including the "5 A strategy" (ask, advise, assess, assist, arrange follow-up), has proved successful (DeSocio et al., 2020). In addition, pharmacologic interventions including nicotine replacement, bupropion, and varenicline are all effective therapies (https://account.ncbi.nlm.nih.gov/?back_url=https%3A//pubmed.ncbi.nlm.nih.gov/%3Fterm%3Dremick%2B2014%23open-saved-search-panelapies) to assist patients with smoking cessation (see Box 39.4). The USPSTF recommends a combination of behavioral interventions and pharmacotherapy for all smokers (Patnode et al., 2021). New guidelines now recommend varenicline over a nicotine patch or bupropion and for most tobacco-dependent patients in whom treatment is initiated (Krist et al., 2021). They actually recommend dual therapy with varenicline plus a nicotine patch, although the evidence for combination treatment is limited (Leone et al., 2020). The new guidelines also recommend extended duration of these therapies (beyond the traditional 12 weeks) if clinically indicated.

A large multinational study of more than 8,000 adult smokers evaluated the safety of varenicline, bupropion, and 21 mg nicotine patches in regard to adverse cardiovascular effects. There was a very low incidence of cardiovascular events (< 0.5%) during 12 weeks of treatment and after 12 additional weeks of follow-up (Benowitz et al., 2018). These data support these therapies by themselves or in combination to help patients stop smoking.

Regarding specifically PWH, a study from France found varenicline significantly more effective than placebo in helping maintain continuous abstinence at 48 weeks (Mercie et al., 2018). A Cochrane review of 12 studies assessing the effectiveness of interventions (behavioral and pharmacotherapy) to motivate and assist tobacco use cessation in PWH found moderate evidence that combined interventions were effective for long-term abstinence (Pool et al., 2016). The Cochrane authors concluded that tobacco cessation should be offered to all PWH as even nonsustained periods of abstinence are beneficial. In addition, office-based interventions that include focus groups, dedicated time to address smoking cessation as part of the clinic visit, and periodic phone follow-up have shown efficacy in helping PWH stop smoking (Cropsey et al., 2019; Pacek et al., 2021).

NONPHARMACOLOGICAL INTERVENTIONS (DIET AND EXERCISE)

The process of atherosclerosis is thought to begin at a young age and progress over many decades before clinical CVD (e.g., acute coronary syndromes, stable or unstable angina, and MI) becomes evident. As noted earlier, this progression appears to be accelerated in PWH due to chronic infection, inflammation, and some ART-related factors. Lifestyle modifications including a healthy diet, regular physical activity, maintaining a normal BMI, limited alcohol use, and not smoking have been associated with improvements in CVD risk (Ozemek et al., 2020).

Regarding physical activity, the ACC/AHA guidelines for both cholesterol and HTN both recommend that adults should be advised to engage in aerobic physical activity 3–4 sessions per week, lasting on average 40 minutes per session and involving moderate-to-vigorous-intensity physical activity (Grundy et al., 2018; Whelton et al., 2018). These behaviors can lead to improvements in TC, LDL-C, HDL-C, blood glucose, and blood pressure—and ultimately lower 10-year and lifetime risk of CVD and subsequent clinical events.

Several published studies have found variable results in terms of exercise in PWH. One systematic review found that a low level of physical activity in PWH was consistently associated with older age, lower educational level, lower CD4 count, exposure to ART, and the presence of lipodystrophy. Other important barriers were the presence of bodily pain and depression (Vancampfort et al., 2018). A more recent and encouraging study found 12–24 weeks of cardiovascular and resistance exercise significantly reduced total and visceral fat in PWH 50–75 years old (Jankowski et al., 2020). As PWH are living longer, it is important for providers to encourage engagement in multiple aspects of a healthy lifestyle, including regular physical activity.

ACKNOWLEDGMENTS

The authors would like to acknowledge the contributions to previous editions of this chapter by David Wohl, MD, and Jeffery Kirschner, MD.

REFERENCES

Abdelhamid AS, Brown TJ, Brainard JS, et al. Omega-3 fatty acids for the primary and secondary prevention of cardiovascular disease. *Cochrane Database of Systematic Reviews.* 2020;3:CD003177. http//:doi:10.1002/14651858.CD003177.pub5

Aberg JA, Gallant JE, Ghanem KG, et al. Primary care guidelines for the management of persons infected with HIV: 2013 update by the HIV Medicine Association of the Infectious Diseases Society of America. *Clin Infect Dis.* 2014;58(1):1–34.

Althoff KN, McGinnis KA, Wyatt CM, et al. Comparison of risk and age at diagnosis of myocardial infarction, end-stage renal disease, and non-AIDS defining cancer in PWH versus uninfected adults. *Clin Infect Dis.* 2015;60:627–638.

Althoff KN, Palella FJ, Gebo K, et al. Impact of smoking, hypertension and cholesterol on myocardial infarction in HIV+ adults. [Abstract 130]. CROI 2017. Boston, MA; 2017.

Amador-Licona N, Díaz-Murillo TA, Gabriel-Ortiz G et al. Omega 3 fatty acids supplementation and oxidative stress in HIV-seropositive patients: a clinical trial. *PLoS One.* 2016;11(3):e0151637.

Arnett DK, Blumenthal RS, Albert MA, et al. ACC/AHA guideline on the primary prevention of cardiovascular disease: a report of the American College of Cardiology/American Heart Association Task Force on Clinical Practice Guidelines. *Circulation.* 2019;140(11):e596–e646.

Backes JM, Russinger JF, Gibson CA, Moriarity PM. Statin-associated muscle symptoms—managing the highly intolerant. *J Clin Lipidol.* 2017;11(1):24–33.

Ballantyne CM, Laufs U, Ray KK, et al. Bempedoic acid plus ezetimibe fixed-dose combination in patients with hypercholesterolemia and high CVD risk treated with maximally tolerated statin therapy. *Eur J Prev Cardiol.* 2020;27(6):593–603.

Baum PD, Sullam PM, Stoddart CA, et al. Abacavir increases platelet reactivity via competitive inhibition of soluble guanylyl cyclase. *AIDS.* 2011;25(18):2243–2248.

Bell KJ. Incremental benefits and harms of the 2017 American College of Cardiology American Heart Association High Blood Pressure Guideline. *JAMA Intern Med.* 2018;178(6):755–757.

Benowitz NL, Pipe A, West R et al. Cardiovascular safety of varenicline, bupropion, and nicotine patches in smokers: a randomized controlled trial. *JAMA Intern Med.* 2018;178(5):622–631.

Berglund L, Brunzell JD, Goldberg AC, et al. Evaluation and treatment of hypertriglyceridemia: an Endocrine Society clinical practice guideline. *J Clin Endocrinol Metab.* 2012;97(9):2969–2989.

Blackman AL, Pandit NS, Pincus KJ. Comparing rates of statin therapy in eligible patients living with HIV compared to uninfected patients. *HIV Med.* 2020;21(3):135–141.

Boccara F. Cardiovascular health in an aging HIV population. *AIDS.* 2017;31(Suppl 2):S157–S163.

Boccara F, Ghislain M, Meyer L, et al. Impact of protease inhibitors on circulating PCSK9 levels in PWH antiretroviral-naïve patients from an ongoing prospective cohort. ANRS-COPANA Study Group. *AIDS.* 2017;31(17):2367–2376.

Boccara F, Kumar P, Caramelli B, et al. Evolocumab treatment in patients with HIV and hypercholesterolemia/mixed dyslipidemia: BEIJERNICK study design and baseline characteristics. *Am Heart J.* 2020a; 220:203–212.

Boccara F, Kumar PN, Caramelli B, et al. Evolocumab in HIV-Infected patients with dyslipidemia: primary results of the randomized, double-blind BEIJERINCK study. *J Am Coll Cardiol.* May 26, 2020;75(20):2570–2584. http://doi:10.1016/j.jacc.2020.03.025

Boonthos K, Puttilerpong C, Penssuparp T. Short-term efficacy and safety of adding ezetimibe to current regimen of lipid-lowering drugs in PWH Thai patients treated with protease inhibitors. *Japan J Infect Dis.* 2018;71:220–224.

Bowman L, Marion Mafham M, Wallendszus K, et al. Effects of aspirin for primary prevention in persons with diabetes mellitus: the ASCEND Study Collaborative Group. *N Engl J Med.* 2018;379:1529–1539.

Brunstrom M, Carlberg B. Association of blood pressure lowering with mortality and cardiovascular disease across blood pressure levels: a systematic review and meta-analysis. *JAMA Intern Med.* 2018;178(1):28–36.

Cannon C, Blazing M, Giugliano R, et al. Ezetimibe added to statin therapy after acute coronary syndromes. *N Engl J Med.* 2015;372:2387–2397.

Cheung CC, Ding E, Sereda P, et al. Reductions in all-cause and cause-specific mortality among PWH individuals receiving antiretroviral therapy in British Columbia, Canada: 2001–2012. *HIV Med.* 2016; 17(9):694–701.

Cioe PA, Baker J, Kojic EM, et al. Elevated soluble CD14 and lower D-dimer are associated with cigarette smoking and heavy episodic alcohol use in persons living with PWH. *J Acquir Immune Defic Syndr.* 2015;70(4):400–405.

Costagliola D, Potard V, Lang S, et al. Is the risk of myocardial infarction in people with HIV associated with atazanavir or darunavir? A nested case-control study within the French hospital database on HIV. *J Infect Dis.* 2020;221(4):516–522.

Cropsey KL, Bean MC, Haynes L et al. Delivery and implementation of an algorithm for smoking cessation treatment for people with HIV and AIDS. *AIDS Care Psych Soc Aspect of AIDS/HIV.* 2019;2:223–229.

Data Collection on Adverse Events of Anti-HIV Drugs (D:A:D) Study Group. Class of antiretroviral drugs and the risk of myocardial infarction. *N Engl J Med.* 2007;356:1723–1735.

D:A:D Study Group. The impact of fasting on the interpretation of triglyceride levels for predicting myocardial infarction risk in HIV-positive individuals: the D:A:D study. *J Infect Dis.* 2011;204(4):521–525.

Davidson KW, Barry MJ, Mangione CM, et al. Aspirin use to prevent cardiovascular disease: US Preventive Services Task Force recommendation statement. *JAMA.* 2022;327(16):1577–1584.

De Pablo C, Orden S, Calatayud S, et al. Differential effects of tenofovir/emtricitabine and abacavir/lamivudine on human leukocyte recruitment. *Antivir Ther.* 2012;17(8):1615–1619.

Deeks S, Lewin SR, Havlir DA. The end of AIDS: HIV infection as a chronic disease. *Lancet.* 2013; 283(9903):1525–1533.

DerSarkissian M, Bhak RH, Oglesby A, et al. Retrospective analysis of comorbidities and treatment burden among patients with HIV infection in a US Medicaid population. *Curr Med Res Opin.* 2020;36(5):781–788.

DeSocio GV, Ricci E, Maggi P, et al. Is it feasible to impact on smoking habits in PWH patients? *J Acquir Immune Defic Syndr.* 2020;83(5):496–503.

Dorjee K, Choden T, Baxi SM, et al. Risk of cardiovascular disease associated with exposure to abacavir among individuals with HIV: a systematic review and meta-analyses of results from seventeen epidemiologic studies. *Int J Antimicrob Agents.* 2018;52(5):541–553.

Dorjee K, Desai M, Choden T, et al. Acute myocardial infarction associated with abacavir and tenofovir based antiretroviral drug combinations in the United States. *AIDS Res Ther.* 2021;18(1):57.

Drozd DR, Kitahata MM, Althoff KN, et al. Incidence and risk of myocardial infarction (MI) by type in the NA-ACCORD. [Abstract 748]. CROI 2015. Seattle, WA; 2015.

Elton PK, Carey RM, Aronow WS, et al.; ACC/AHA/AAAP/ABC/ACPM/AGS/ASH/ASPC/NMA/PCNA. Guideline for the prevention, detection, and management of high blood pressure in adults. *Hypertension.* 2018;71:e13–e115.

Everett BM, Smith RJ, Hiatt WR. Reducing LDL with PCSK9 inhibitors—the clinical benefit of lipid drugs. *N Engl J Med.* 2015;373:1588–1591.

Fahme SA, Bloomfield GS, Peck R. Hypertension and PWH adults: novel pathophysiologic mechanisms. *Hypertension* 2018;72:44–55.

Fitch KV, Kileel EM, Looby SE, et al.; REPRIEVE Investigators. Successful recruitment of a multi-site international randomized placebo-controlled trial in people with HIV with attention to diversity of race and ethnicity: critical role of central coordination. *HIV Res Clin Pract.* 2020;21(1):11–23.

Fitch KV, Looby SE, Rope A, et al. Effects of aging and smoking on carotid intima-media thickness in HIV-infection. *AIDS.* 2013;27(1):49–57.

Fogacci F, Strocchi E, Veronesi M, et al. Effect of omega-3 polyunsaturated fatty acids treatment on lipid pattern of HIV patients: a meta-analysis of randomized clinical trials. *Mar Drugs.* 2020;18(6):292.

Frazier EL, Sutton MY, Brooks JT, et al. Trends in cigarette smoking among adults with HIV compared with the general adult population, United States: 2009–2014. *Prev Med.* 2018;111:231–234.

Freiberg MS, Chang CC, Koller LH, et al. HIV infection and the risk of acute myocardial infarction. *JAMA Intern Med.* 2013;173(8):614–622.

Freiberg MS, Duncan MS, Alcorn C. HIV Infection and the risk of World Health Organization-defined sudden cardiac death. *J Am Heart Assoc.* 2021;10(18):e021268.

Friis-Moller N, Sabin CA, Weber R, et al. The Data Collection on Adverse Events of Anti-HIV Drugs (D:A:D) Study Group. Combination antiretroviral therapy and the risk of myocardial infarction. *N Engl J Med.* 2003;349:1993–2003.

Gaba P, Bhatt DL, Steg PG, et al. Prevention of cardiovascular events and mortality with icosapent ethyl in patients with prior myocardial infarction. *J Am Coll Cardiol.* 2022;79(17):1660–1671.

Gatell JM, Assoumou L, Moyle G, et al. Switching from a ritonavir-boosted protease inhibitor to a dolutegravir-based regimen for maintenance of viral suppression in patients with high cardiovascular risk. *AIDS.* 2017;31:2503–2514.

Gaziano JM, Brotons C, Coppolecchia R. Use of aspirin to reduce the risk of initial vascular events in patients at moderate risk of cardiovascular disease. (ARRIVE): a randomized double-blind placebo-controlled trial. *Lancet.* 2018;392:1035–1046.

Ghazi L, Baker JV, Sharma S, et al. Role of inflammatory biomarkers in the prevalence and incidence of hypertension among HIV-positive participants in the START trial. *Am J Hypertens.* 2020;33(1):43–52.

Giugliano RP, Keech A, Murphy SA. Clinical efficacy and safety of evolocumab in high-risk patients receiving a statin: secondary analysis of patients with Low LDL cholesterol levels and in those already receiving a maximal-potency statin in a randomized clinical trial. *JAMA* 2017;2(12):1385–1391.

Go AS, Horberg M, Reynolds K, et al. HIV infection independently increases the risk of developing heart failure: the HIV HEART study. [Abstract THAB0103]. AIDS 2018: 22nd International AIDS Conference. Amsterdam, Netherlands; July 23–27, 2018.

Go AS, Reynolds K, Avula HR, et al. Human immunodeficiency virus infection and variation in heart failure risk by age, sex, and ethnicity: the HIV HEART Study. *Mayo Clin Proc.* 2022;97(3):465–479.

Grandi AM, Nicolini E, Rizzi L, et al. Dyslipidemia in HIV-positive patients: a randomized, controlled, prospective study on ezetimibe \+ fenofibrate versus pravastatin monotherapy. *J Int AIDS Soc.* 2014;17:19004.

Grinspoon SK, Douglas PS, Hoffman U, et al. Leveraging a landmark trial of primary cardiovascular disease prevention in human immunodeficiency virus: introduction from the REPRIEVE Coprincipal Investigators. *J Infect Dis.* 2020;222:S1–S7.

Grundy SM, Stone NJ, Bailey AL, et al. 2018 AHA/ACC/AACVPR/AAPA/ABC/ACPM/ADA/AGS/APhA/ASPC/NLAPCNA Guideline on the management of blood cholesterol: Executive Summary: A report of the American College of Cardiology/American Heart Association Task Force on Clinical Practice Guidelines. *Circulation.* 2019;139(25):e1046–e1081. Epub 2018 Nov 10.

Guirguis-Blake JM, Evans CV, Perdue LA, Bean SI, Senger CA. Aspirin use to prevent cardiovascular disease and colorectal cancer: updated evidence report and systematic review for the US Preventive Services Task Force. *JAMA.* 2022;327(16):1585–1597.

Guyton JR, Bays HE, Grundy SM, et al. An assessment of the Statin Intolerance Panel: 2014 update. *J Clin Lipidol.* 2014;8(3 Suppl):S72–S81.

Hammersley D, Signy M. Ezetimibe: an update on its clinical usefulness in specific patient groups. *Ther Adv Chronic Dis.* 2017;8(1):4–11.

Hatleberg CI, Ryom L, El-Sadr W, et al. Improvements over time in short-term mortality following myocardial infarction in HIV-positive individuals. *AIDS.* 2016;30(10):1583–1596.

Hays AG, Schär M, Barditch-Crovo P, et al., A randomized, placebo-controlled, double-blinded clinical trial of colchicine to improve vascular health in people living with HIV. *AIDS.* 2021;35(7):1041–1050.

Hermida RC, Crespo JJ, Domingues-Sardina M, et al. Bedtime hypertension treatment improves cardiovascular risk reduction: the Hygia Chronotherapy Trial. *Eur Heart J.* 2020;41(48):4565–4576.

Hoffmann U, Lu MT, Foldyna B, et al. Assessment of coronary artery disease with computed tomography angiography and inflammatory and immune activation biomarkers among adults with HIV eligible for primary cardiovascular prevention. *JAMA Netw Open.* 2021;4(6):e2114923.

Hsue P, Hunt P, Schnell A., et al. Inflammation is associated with endothelial dysfunction among individuals with treated and suppressed HIV infection. [Abstract 708]. CROI 2010, San Francisco, CA; 2010.

Hsue PY, Waters DD. HIV infection and coronary heart disease: mechanisms and management. *Nat Rev Cardiol.* 2019;16(12):745–759.

Hunt PW. HIV and inflammation: mechanisms and consequences. *Curr HIV/AIDS Rep.* 2012;9(2):139–147.

Jakob T, Nordmann AJ, Schandelmaier S, et al. Fibrates for primary prevention of cardiovascular disease events. *Cochrane Database Syst Rev.* 2016;11(11):CD009753.

Jankowski CM, Mawhinney S, Wilson MP, et al. Body composition changes in response to moderate or high-intensity exercise among older adults with or without HIV infection. *JAIDS.* 2020;85(3):340–345.

Johnston PI, Wright SW, Orr M, et al. Worldwide relative smoking prevalence among people living with and without HIV. *AIDS.* 2021;35(6):957–970.

Jones R, Arps K, Davis DM. Clinician guide to the ABCs of primary and secondary prevention of atherosclerotic cardiovascular disease. https://www.acc.org/latest-in-cardiology/articles/2018/03/30/18/34/clinician-guide-to-the-abcs. Published April 2018. Accessed September 3, 2022.

Kalstad AA, Myhre PL, Laake K, et al. Effects of n-3 fatty acid supplements in elderly patients after myocardial infarction: a randomized, controlled trial. *Circulation.* 2021;143(6):528–539.

Khambaty T, Stewart JC, Gupta SK, et al. Association between depressive disorders and incident acute myocardial infarction in human immunodeficiency virus-infected adults: Veterans Aging Cohort Study. *JAMA Cardiol.* 2016;1(8):929–937.

Kim BK, Hong SJ, Lee YJ, et al. Long-term efficacy and safety of moderate-intensity statin with ezetimibe combination therapy versus high-intensity statin monotherapy in patients with atherosclerotic cardiovascular disease (RACING): A randomized, open-label, non-inferiority trial. *Lancet.* 2022;400:380.

Klein DB, Leyden WA, Chao CR. No difference in the incidence of myocardial infarction for HIV\+ and HIV– individuals in recent years. *Clin Infect Dis.* 2015;60(8):1278–1285.

Klein DB, Marcus JL, Leyden WA, et al. Infection and immunodeficiency as risk factors for ischemic stroke. [Abstract 741]. CROI 2014. Boston, MA; 2014.

Kovacs L, Kress TC, Belin de Chantemèle EJ. HIV, combination antiretroviral therapy, and vascular diseases in men and women. *JACC Basic Transl Sci.* 2022;7(4):410–421.

Krishnan S, Bosch RJ, Rodriguez B, et al. Correlates of inflammatory biomarkers one year after suppressive ART. [Abstract 757]. CROI 2014. Boston, MA; 2014.

Krist AH, Davidson KW, Mangione CM, et al. Interventions for tobacco smoking cessation in adults, including pregnant persons: US Preventive Services Task Force recommendation statement. *JAMA.* 2021;325(3): 265–279.

Lake JE, Trevillyan J. Impact of Integrase inhibitors and tenofovir alafenamide on weight gain in people with HIV. *Curr Opin HIV AIDS.* 2021;16(3):148–151.

Law M, Friis-Moller N, El-Sadr WA, et al. The use of the Framingham equation to predict myocardial infarctions in PWH patients: Comparison with observed events in the D:A:D study. *HIV Med.* 2006;7:218–230.

Leone FT, Zhang Y, Evers-Casey S, et al. Initiating pharmacologic treatment in tobacco-dependent adults: an official American Thoracic Society Clinical Practice guideline. *Am J Respir Crit Care Med.* 2020;202(2):5–31.

Leucker TM, Gerstenblith G, Schär M. Evolocumab, a PCSK9 monoclonal antibody, rapidly reverses coronary artery endothelial dysfunction in people living with HIV and people with dyslipidemia. *J Am Heart Assoc.* 2020;9(14):e016263.

Leyes P, Martinez E, Larrousse M, et al. Effects of ezetimibe on cho-lesterol metabolism in PWH patients with protease inhibitor-associated dyslipidemia: a single-arm intervention trial. *BMC Infect Dis*. 2014;11(14):497.

Lloyd-Jones DM, Morris PB, Ballantyne CM, et al. Focused update of the 2016 ACC expert consensus decision pathway on the role of non-statin therapies for LDL-cholesterol lowering in the manage-ment of atherosclerotic cardiovascular disease. *J Amer Coll Cardiol*. 2017;70(14):1785–1822.

Lundgren JD, Babiker AG, Gordin F, et al. Initiation of antiretrovi-ral therapy in early asymptomatic HIV Infection. *N Engl J Med*. 2015;373(9):795–807.

Mallon P, Winston A, Post F, et al. Platelet function upon switching to TAF vs continuing ABC: a randomized sub study. [Abstract 80]. CROI 2018. Boston, MA; 2018.

Marconi VC, Duncan MS, So-Armah K, et al. Bilirubin is inversely asso-ciated with cardiovascular disease among HIV-positive and HIV-negative individuals in VACS (Veterans Aging Cohort Study). *J Am Heart Assoc*. 2018;7(10):e007792.

Martinez E, Larrousse M, Llibre JM, et al. Substitution of raltegravir for ritonavir-boosted protease inhibitors in PWH patients: the SPIRAL study. *AIDS*. 2010;24(11):1697–1707.

McGettrick P, Mallon PWG. Biomarkers to predict cardiovas-cular disease in people living with HIV. *Curr Opin Infect Dis*. 2022;35(1):15–20.

McLaughlin MM, Ma Y, Scherzer R, et al. Association of viral persis-tence and atherosclerosis in adults with treated HIV infection. *JAMA Netw Open*. 2020;3(10):e2018099.

McNeil JJ, Nelson MR, Woods RL, et al. Effect of aspirin on all-cause mor-tality in the healthy elderly. *N Engl J Med*. 2018;379(16):1519–1528.

Medina-Torne S, Ganesan A, Barahona I, et al. Hypertension is common among PWH persons, but not associated with HAART. *J Int Assoc Physicians AIDS Care (Chic)*. 2012;11(1):20–25.

Mercie P, Arsandaux J, Katalama C, et al. Efficacy and safety of var-enicline for smoking cessation in people living with HIV I France. (ANRS 144 Inter-ACTIV): a randomized controlled phase 3 clinical trial. *Lancet HIV*. 2018;5(3):126–135.

Metkus TS, Brown T, Budoff M, et al. HIV infection is associated with an increased prevalence of coronary noncalcified plaque among par-ticipants with a coronary artery calcium score of zero: Multicenter AIDS Cohort Study (MACS). *HIV Med*. 2015;16(10):635–639.

Neesgaard B, Greenberg L, Miró JM, et al. Associations between integrase strand-transfer inhibitors and cardiovascular disease in people living with HIV: a multicentre prospective study from the RESPOND cohort consortium. *Lancet HIV*. 2022;9(7):e474–e485.

Neilan TG, Nguyen KL, Zaha VG, et al. Myocardial steatosis among antiretroviral therapy treated people with HIV participating in the REPRIEVE Trial. *J Infect Dis*. 2020;222(Suppl 1):S63–S69.

NICE. Ezetimibe for treating primary heterozygous familial and non-familial hypercholesterolemia. Guide TA385. http://nice.org.uk/guidance. Published 2016. Accessed September 15, 2022.

Nicholls SJ, Lincoff AM, Garcia M, et al. Effect of high-dose omega-3 fatty acids vs corn oil on major adverse cardiovascular events in patients at high cardiovascular risk: the STRENGTH randomized clinical trial. *JAMA*. 2020;324(22):2268–2280.

Nirmala N, Avendano EE, Morin RA. Effectiveness of ezetimibe in human immunodeficiency virus patients treated for hyperlipi-daemia: a systematic review and meta-analysis. *Infect Dis (Lond)*. 2022;54(2):99–109.

O'Brien S, Montenont E, Hu L, et al. Aspirin attenuates platelet acti-vation and immune activation in HIV-1-infected subjects on anti-retroviral therapy: a pilot study. *J Acquir Immune Defic Syndr*. 2013;63(3):280–288.

Oh RC, Trivette ET, Westerfield, KL. Management of hypertri-glyceridemia: common questions and answers. *Am Fam Phys*. 2020;102(6):347–354.

Olaiya O, Weiser J, Zhou W, et al. Hypertension among persons living with HIV in medical care in the United States—Medical Monitoring Project 2013–2014. *Open Forum Infect Dis*. 2018;5(3):ofy028.

Oliveira JM, Rondo PH, Lima LR, et al. Effects of low dose fish oil on inflammatory markers of Brazilian PWH adults on antiretroviral therapy: a randomized parallel, placebo-controlled trial. *Nutrients* 2015;7(8):6520–6528.

Oliveros E, Patel H, Kyung S, et al. Hypertension in older adults: assessment, management and challenges. *Clin Cardiol*. 2020;43(2):999–107.

Ozemek C, Erlandson KM, Jankowski CM. Physical activity and exer-cise to improve cardiovascular health for adults living with HIV. *Prog Cardiovasc Dis*. 2020;63(2):178–183.

Pacek LR, Holloway AD, Cropsey KL, et al. Cigarette smoking and cessation-related interactions with health care providers in the con-text of living with HIV: focus group study findings. *J Assoc Nurses AIDS Care*. 2021;32(2):e14–e19.

Paikin JS, Eikelboom JW. Cardiology patient page: aspirin. *Circulation*. 2012;125(10):e439–e442.

Paisible AL, Chang CH, So-Armah KA, et al. HIV infection, cardiovas-cular disease risk factor profile, and risk for acute myocardial infarc-tion. *J AIDS*. 2015;68:209–216.

Palella FJ Jr, Fisher M, Tebas P, et al. Simplification to rilpivirine/emtric-itabine/tenofovir disoproxil fumarate from ritonavir-boosted prote-ase inhibitor antiretroviral therapy in a randomized trial of HIV-1 RNA-suppressed participants. *AIDS*. 2014;28(3):335–344.

Patnode CD, Henderson JT, Coppola EL, et al. Interventions for tobacco cessation in adults, including pregnant persons: updated evidence report and systematic review for the US Preventive Services Task Force. *JAMA*. 2021;325(3):280–298. http://doi:10.1001/jama.2020.23541

Petoumenos K, Worm S, Reiss P, et al.; D:A:D Study Group. Rates of cardiovascular disease following smoking cessation in patients with HIV infection: results from the D:A:D study. *HIV Med*. 2011;12(7):412–421.

Pett SL, Amin J, Horban A, et al. Week 96 results of the randomized, multicenter Maraviroc Switch (MARCH) Study. *HIV Medicine*. 2018;19:65–71.

Pool ER, Dogar O, Lindsay RP, et al. Interventions for tobacco use ces-sation in people living with HIV and IADS. *Cochrane Database Syst Rev*. 2016;13(6):CD011120.

Post WS, Budoff M, Kingsley L, et al. Associations between HIV infec-tion and subclinical coronary atherosclerosis. *Ann Intern Med*. 2014;160:458–467.

Rao SG, Galaviz KI, Hawkins GC, et al. Factors associated with excess myocardial infarction risk in PWH adults: a systemic review and meta-analysis. *J Acquir Imune Defic Syndr*. 2019;81(2):224–230.

Rasmussen LD, May MT, Kronborg G, et al. Time trends for risk of severe age-related diseases in individuals with and without HIV infection in Denmark: a nationwide population-based cohort study. *Lancet HIV*. 2015;2(7):e288–e298.

Ray KK, Bays HE, Catapano AL, et al.; CLEAR Harmony Trial. Safety and efficacy of bempedoic acid to reduce LDL cholesterol. *N Engl J Med*. 2019;380(11):1022–1032.

Regan S, Meigs JB, Massaro J, et al. Evaluation of the ACC/AHA CVD risk prediction algorithm among PWH patients. [Abstract 751]. CROI 2015. Seattle, WA; 2015.

Reiter-Brennan C, Osei AD, Iftekhar Uddin SM, et al. ACC/AHA lipid guidelines: personalized care to prevent cardiovascular disease. *Cleve Clin J Med*. 2020;87(4):231–239.

Remick J, Georgiopoulou V, Marti C, et al. Heart failure in patients with human immunodeficiency virus infection: epidemiology, pathophysiology, treatment, and future research. *Circulation*. 2014;129(17):1781–1789.

Ryom L. Lundgren JD, El-Sadr W, et al. Cardiovascular disease and use of contemporary protease inhibitors: the D:A:D international pro-spective multicohort study. *Lancet HIV*. 2018;6:e291–e300.

Saag MS, Gandhi RT, Hoy JF, et al. Antiretroviral drugs for treatment and prevention of HIV infection in adults 2020 recommendations of the International Antiviral Society–USA Panel. *JAMA.* 2020;324(16):1651–1669.

Sabatine MS, Giugliano RP, Keech AC, et al. Evolocumab and clinical outcomes in patients with cardiovascular disease. *N Engl J Med.* 2017;376:1713–1722.

Sabin C, Reiss P, Ryom L, et al. Is there continued evidence for an association between abacavir and myocardial infarction risk? [Abstract 747]. CROI 2014. Boston, MA; 2014.

Saeedi R, Johns K, Frohlich J, et al. Lipid-lowering efficacy and safety of ezetimibe combined with rosuvastatin compared with titrating rosuvastatin monotherapy in HIV-positive patients. *Lipids Health Dis.* 2015;14:57.

Sax PC. Zolopa A, Eleon R. Tenofovir alafenamide vs. tenofovir disoproxil fumarate in single tablet regimens for initial HIV-1 therapy: a randomized phase 2 study. *J Acquir Immune Defic Syndr.* 2014;67(1):52–58.

Schmidt AF, Pearce LS, Wilkins JT, et al. PCSK9 monoclonal antibodies for the primary and secondary prevention of cardiovascular disease. *Cochrane Database of Systematic Reviews.* 2017;10(10):CD011748.

Shah ASV, Stelze D, Lee KK, et al. Global burden of atherosclerotic vascular disease in people living with HIV: systematic review and meta-analysis. *Circulation.* 2018;138:1100–1112.

Shahreyar M, Salem SA, Nayyar M. Hyperlipidemia: management with proprotein convertase subtilisin/kexin type 9 (PCSK9) inhibitors. *J Am Board Fam Med.* 2018;31(4):628–634.

Scherzer R, Shah SJ, Secemsky E, et al. Association of biomarker clusters with cardiac phenotypes and mortality in patients with HIV infection. *Circ Heart Fail.* 2018;11(4):e004312.

Sigel K, Makinson A, Thaler J. Lung cancer in persons with HV. *Curr Opin HIV AIDS.* 2017;12(1):31–38.

Sizar O, Nassereddin A, Talati R. Ezetimibe. StatPearls. 2020.

Smit M, van Zoest RA, Nichols BE, et al. Cardiovascular disease prevention policy in human immunodeficiency virus: recommendations from a modeling study. *Clin Infect Dis.* 2018;66(5):743–750.

So-Armah K, Benjamin LA, Bloomfield GS, et al. HIV and cardiovascular disease. *Lancet HIV.* 2020;7:e279–e293.

Strategies for Management of Antiretroviral Therapy (SMART)/INSIGHT/D:A:D Study Groups. Use of nucleoside reverse transcriptase inhibitors and risk of myocardial infarction in PWH patients. *AIDS.* 2008;22: F17–F24.

Stone NJ, Robinson JG, Lichenstein AH, et al. 2013 ACC/AHA guideline on the treatment of blood cholesterol to reduce atherosclerotic cardiovascular risk in adults: a report of the American College of Cardiology/American Heart Association Task Force on Practice Guidelines. *J Am Coll Cardiol.* 2014;63(25 Pt B):2889–2934.

Subramanian S, Tawakol A, Burdo TH, et al. Arterial inflammation in patients with HIV. *JAMA.* 2012;308:379–386.

Suchindran S, Regan S, Meigs JB, et al. Aspirin use for primary and secondary prevention in human immunodeficiency virus (HIV)-infected and HIV-uninfected patients. *Open Forum Infect Dis.* 2014;1(3):ofu076.

Swanson B, Keithley J, Baum L, et al. Effects of fish oil on HIV-related inflammation and markers of immunosenescence: a randomized clinical trial. *J Altern Complement Med.* 2018;24(7):709–716.

Tawakol A, Lo J, Zanni MV, et al. Increased arterial inflammation relates to high-risk coronary plaque morphology in PWH patients. *J Acquir Immune Defic Syndr.* 2014;66(2):164–171.

Thiebaut R, El-Sadr W, Friis-Moller N, et al.; D:A:D Study Group. Predictors of hypertension and changes in blood pressure in PWH patients. *Antiviral Ther.* 2005;10:811–823.

Thompson MA, Horberg MA, Agwu AL, et al. Primary care guidance for persons with human immunodeficiency virus: 2020 update by the HIV Medicine Association of the Infectious Diseases Society of America. *Clin Infect Dis.* December 6, 2021;73(11):e3572–e3605.

Thompson-Paul A, Buchacz K, Wei S, et al. Evaluation of the ACC/AHA CVD risk prediction algorithm among PWH patients. [Abstract 747]. CROI 2015. Seattle, WA; 2015.

Tibuakuu M, Fashanu OE, Zhao D, et al. Glyc A, a novel inflammatory marker, is associated with subclinical coronary disease. *AIDS.* 2019;33(3):547–557.

Triant V, Lee H, Hadigan C, et al. Increased acute myocardial infarction rates and cardiovascular risk factors among patients with human immunodeficiency virus disease. *J Clin Metab.* 2007;92(7):2506–2512.

Triant V, Perez J, Regan S, et al. Cardiovascular risk prediction functions underestimate risk in HIV infection. *Circulation.* 2018;137(21):2203–2214.

Triant V, Regan S, Lee H, et al. Association of immunologic and virologic factors with myocardial infarction rates in the U.S. health care system. *J Acquir Immune Defic Syndr.* 2010;55(5):615–619.

Tseng A, Foisy M. Important drug–drug interactions in PWH persons on antiretroviral therapy: an update on new interactions between HIV and non-HIV drugs. *Curr Infect Dis Rep.* 2012;14(1):67–82.

Tungsiripat M, Kitch D, Glesby MJ, et al. A pilot study to determine the impact on dyslipidemia of adding tenofovir to stable background antiretroviral therapy: ACTG 5206. *AIDS.* 2010;24(11):1781–1784.

US Department of Health and Human Services (DHHS). Panel on Antiretroviral Guidelines for Adults and Adolescents. Department of Health and Human Services. Guidelines for the use of antiretroviral agents in adults and adolescents living with HIV. https://clinicalinfo.hiv.gov/sites/default/files/guidelines/documents/adult-adolescent-arv/guidelines-adult-adolescent-arv.pdf. Updated January 20, 2022. Accessed September 3, 2022.

Vancampfort D, Mugisha J, Richards J, et al. Physical activity correlates in people living with HIV/AIDS: systematic review of 45 studies. *Disabil Rehabil.* 2018;40(14):1618–1629.

Van Lelyveld SF, Gras L, Kesselring A, et al. ATHENA national observational cohort study: Long-term complications in patients with poor immunological recovery despite virological successful HAART in Dutch ATHENA cohort. *AIDS.* 2012;26(4):465–474.

van Zoest RA, van den Born BH, Reiss P. Hypertension in people living with HIV. *Curr Opin HIV AIDS.* 2017; 12(6):513–522.

Vieira AD, Silveira GR. Effectiveness of n-3 fatty acids in the treatment of hypertriglyceridemia in HIV/AIDS patients: a meta-analysis. *Cien Saude Colet.* 2017;22(8):2659–2669.

Wall HK, Ritchey MD, Gillespie C, et al. *Vital Signs*: prevalence of key cardiovascular disease risk factors for million hearts 2022—United States, 2011–2016. *MMWR Morb Mortal Wkly Rep.* 2018;67:983–991.

Whelton PK, Carey RM, Aronow WS, et al. 2017 ACC/AHA/AAPA/ABC/ACPM/AGS/APhA/ASH/ASPC/NMA/PCNA guideline for the prevention, detection, evaluation, and management of high blood pressure in adults: executive summary: a report of the American College of Cardiology/American Heart Association Task Force on Clinical Practice Guidelines. *Circulation.* 2018;138(17):e426–e483.

White JR, Chang CC, So-Armah KA, et al. Depression and HIV infection are risk factors for incident heart failure among veterans: VACS. *Circulation.* 2015;132(17):1630–1638.

Wohl D, Waters D, Simpson R, et al. Ezetimibe alone reduces low-density lipoprotein cholesterol in PWH patients receiving combination antiretroviral therapy. *Clin Infect Dis.* 2008;47:1105–1108.

Yusuf S, Hawken S, Ounpuu S, et al. Effect of potentially modifiable risk factors associated with myocardial infarction in 52 countries (The INTERHEART Study): case-control study. *Lancet.* 2004;364:937–952.

Zanni MV, Awadalla M, Toibio M, et al. Immune correlates of diffuse myocardial fibrosis and diastolic dysfunction among aging women with human immunodeficiency virus. *J Infect Dis.* 2020; 221:1315–1320.

40.

RENAL COMPLICATIONS

Patricia Carr Reese and Umar Farooq

LEARNING OBJECTIVES

- Describe the broad pathologic spectrum of renal disease in persons living with HIV (PWH), including medication-induced renal injury.

- Explain the importance of screening and monitoring PWH for chronic kidney disease, along with the indications for nephrology referral and renal biopsy.

- Select appropriate ART regimens based on a patient's renal function and comorbidities.

- Describe the treatment options for PWH with end-stage renal disease (ESRD), including dialysis and solid organ transplant.

WHAT'S NEW?

- In 2021, the National Kidney Foundation (NKF) and the American Society of Nephrology (ASN) task force recommended use of the chronic kidney disease (CKD)-EPI creatinine equation refit without the race variable in all laboratories in the United States; in acknowledgment, that race as used in the eGFR equation, is a social and not biologic construct.

- The most common causes of CKD in PWH are noninfectious comorbidities (NICM), specifically hypertension, vascular disease, and diabetes.

- As a results of the HIV Organ Policy Equity (HOPE) Act, early outcomes from a multicenter pilot program following 75 PWH who received a kidney from deceased HIV-positive donors have been excellent with 100% patient survival and 92% graft survival, no differences in 1-year mean eGFR, HIV breakthrough, infectious hospitalizations, or opportunistic infections.

- Data gathered from the Observational Pharmaco-Epidemiological Research and Analysis (OPERA) cohort now support expanded use of full-dose, 300 mg daily, lamivudine in PWH and an eGFR between 30 and 49 mL/min per 1.73 m².

KEY POINTS

- PWH continue to have an increased risk of developing CKD. Because of ART availability, the most common etiologies of kidney disease have changed over the course of the epidemic from HIV-associated nephropathy (HIVAN) to renal complications from NICM such as diabetes, hypertension, hepatitis infection, tobacco use, and aging in general. Consistent evidence demonstrates preservation of renal function with ART in PWH.

- PWH are eligible for both renal dialysis and renal transplant.

- Tenofovir disoproxil fumarate (TDF) can impair renal function and should be changed to an alternative regimen when possible. INSTIs can increase serum creatinine because of inhibition of renal organic cation transporter 2 (OCT2), but do not cause direct nephrotoxicity.

- All PWH should be monitored on a regular basis for CKD. Screening yearly for proteinuria and eGFR is recommended for those who are clinically stable and virologically suppressed on ART.

EPIDEMIOLOGY OF RENAL DISEASE IN PERSONS WITH HIV

Although the incidence of HIVAN has greatly declined since the beginning of the HIV epidemic, the overall prevalence of kidney disease in PWH has increased as a result of improved survival. With improved life expectancy and increased age-related metabolic abnormalities, CKD is a significant comorbidity in PWH. The change in the spectrum of kidney disease is being driven by traditional risk factors including obesity, diabetes, hypertension, smoking, the use of nephrotoxic medications, and aging of the HIV population (Heron et al., 2020a; Waheed & Atta, 2014).

Despite widespread use of ART, PWH remain at a higher risk of renal insufficiency, cardiovascular disease, and overall mortality than matched cohorts of HIV-negative people (Kalayjian, 2011; Mallipattu et al., 2014). Up to 30% of PWH are at risk of developing proteinuria—a key marker of kidney disease. Moreover, cross-sectional cohorts from Europe, Asia, and North America have demonstrated high rates of CKD in PWH, with about 6% of PWH having stages 3–5 CKD (Post & Holt, 2009). Based on another large sample of US veterans, the incidence rate of end-stage renal disease (ESRD) in Black PWH is even higher than that of patients with diabetes (incidence rates per 1,000 person-years (py): 71.1 for HIV, 59.9 for diabetes mellitus, and 27.9 for individuals with neither HIV nor diabetes) (Choi et al., 2007). Compared to the general population, PWH have a 16-fold higher risk of requiring renal replacement therapy.

PATHOGENESIS

The *ApoL1* gene, which encodes a factor to lyse the parasite *Trypanosoma brucei*, is the key susceptibility allele in HIVAN and other kidney diseases in the APOL1 nephropathy spectrum. HIV-RNA localizes to podocytes and tubular epithelial cells in the kidney suggesting a direct role of the virus in kidney disease. Further, the role of viral proteins is supported by animal studies. The HIV regulatory protein *nef* and HIV accessory protein *vpr* are overexpressed in mice reproducing the HIVAN phenotype.

Kidney disease is a major cause of mortality from non-AIDS-related conditions in PWH, along with malignancies, cardiovascular disease, and liver disease (Ryom, 2019a). Renal pathology in PWH was originally reported in 1984 and was called "acquired immune deficiency syndrome (AIDS) nephropathy" (Rao et al., 1984). The histopathology on kidney biopsy of these persons showed a collapsing type of focal and segmental glomerulosclerosis, and the clinical presentation was that of proteinuria, usually nephrotic, and rapid progression to ESRD. Subsequently, HIVAN became more commonly recognized as a major cause of kidney disease in PWH. In the United States, the incidence of HIVAN peaked in the mid-1990s and dropped significantly after the introduction of highly active antiretroviral therapy (HAART) by the late 1990s (Ross & Klotman, 2002). More recent data show the annual incidence of ESRD in PWH in the United States is now about 800–900 cases per year (Cohen et al., 2017).

RISK FACTORS FOR NEPHROPATHY

Risk factors for the development of kidney disease in PWH include Black race, diabetes mellitus, hypertension, hepatitis C coinfection, cardiovascular disease, and family history of CKD (Mocroft et al., 2015; Naicker & Fabian, 2010). In addition, individuals with advanced undiagnosed and/or untreated HIV infection with CD4+ T-cell counts of less than 200 cells/mm³ and active viral replication are at high risk for developing HIVAN (Bige et al., 2012; Lescure et al., 2012).

GENETIC PREDISPOSITION

The major genetic risk factor for developing HIVAN and non-HIVAN focal segmental glomerulosclerosis (FSGS) in persons of African descent is the presence of polymorphisms in the apolipoprotein 1 (*APOL1*) gene, which is located on chromosome 22 (Genovese et al., 2010; Lescure et al., 2012;

Tzur et al., 2010). *APOL1* encodes a serum factor that lyses *Trypanosoma brucei*. Thus, selective mutations in Africans to counter an endemic parasite may have contributed to the current rates of HIVAN and FSGS in Black populations. Two *APOL1* risk alleles, G1 and G2, are associated with the increased susceptibility for the development of HIVAN and other types of kidney disease collectively termed *APOL1* nephropathy (Friedmam & Pollak, 2021; Genovese et al., 2010; Papeta et al., 2011). It is hypothesized that *APOL1* risk variants create pores in cell membranes within the kidney much like they do in trypanosomal organelles, but other studies suggest overexpression of risk variants lead to mitochondrial dysfunction and injury. There is still no consensus on the molecular mechanism of *APOL1* nephropathy (Friedman & Pollak, 2021). In PWH who carry the two *APOL1* risk alleles, this alone can explain 35% of cases of HIVAN and 18% of FSGS cases (Kopp et al., 2011). Two risk variants confer an odds ratio of approximately 7–10 for hypertension associated ESRD, 17 for FSGS, 29 for HIVAN in the United States, and 89 for HIVAN in Africa. These data suggest that these diseases have some overlapping mechanism of pathogenesis (Friedman & Pollak, 2021). *APOL1* homozygosity, present in 13% of the general Black American population, was noted in more than 60% of Black Americans with HIVAN and non-HIVAN FSGS (Kopp et al., 2011).

In animal models, HIV gene expression within kidney cells is required for the development of HIVAN (Bruggeman et al., 1997). Even in HIVAN persons with undetectable plasma HIV-RNA levels, proviral DNA can be found in the renal tissue of all PWH (Izzedine et al., 2011). This implies that the kidney acts as a separate compartment from blood, allowing HIV to replicate in the kidney even in PWH who achieve viral suppression in their plasma with treatment (Medapalli et al., 2011). HIV-RNA localizes to podocytes and tubular epithelial cells in the kidney. HIV regulatory protein *nef* and HIV accessory protein *vpr* are overexpressed in mice reproducing the HIVAN phenotype (Cohen et al., 2017). HIV induces apoptosis of cells in addition to causing cytopathic effects. These effects, in combination with cytokine release, are thought to play a role in the development of HIVAN. See Box 40.1.

MARKERS OF KIDNEY INJURY

Markers of kidney injury include an elevated serum creatinine, proteinuria, glycosuria, and an increased fractional excretion of uric acid (Makris & Spanou, 2016). Risk factors for proteinuria include older age, Black race, insulin resistance, hypertension, and a low CD4+ T-cell count (Heron et al., 2020a). The presence of albuminuria and overt proteinuria is also associated with increased cardiovascular morbidity and mortality in women initiating ART (Wyatt et al., 2011).

ASSESSMENT OF KIDNEY FUNCTION

Like the general population, kidney damage in PWH is assessed by using creatinine-based estimates of glomerular filtration rate (eGFR) with the Cockroft–Gault

equation, Modification of Diet in Renal Disease, and CKD
Epidemiology Collaboration (CKD-EPI) equation, but none
of these estimates has been systematically validated in PWH.

In 2021, the NKF and the ASN task force recommended
use of the CKD-epi creatinine equation refit without the race
variable in all laboratories in the United States; in acknowledgment, that race as used in the eGFR equation is a social
and not biologic construct (Delgado et al., 2021). They also
recommended higher utilization of the CKD-epi egfr-cystatin c
(eGFRcys) and eGFR creatinine-cystatin c (eGFRcr-cys_r)
refit without race for improved accuracy of diagnosis and
clinical decision making (Inker et al., 2021). Cystatin C
is an alternative marker of eGFR that does not depend on
muscle mass and is more sensitive for kidney damage than
creatinine-based formulas. Its role in diagnosis and as a prognostic marker in PWH remains to be defined. Dragović and
colleagues (2018) found that cystatin c may be elevated in
PWH with metabolic syndrome. Out of 89 PWH, the 33

individuals with metabolic syndrome had a statistically significantly higher cystatin c level compared to those without
notably, there were no significant differences with respect to
CD4[+] level, time on art, smoking status, or HBV/HCV status. Another study found that cystatin c may assist in clarifying the clinical significance of plasma creatinine fluctuations
after dolutegravir initiation, particularly in high-risk renal
PWH (Palich et al., 2018).

PATHOLOGIC SPECTRUM OF KIDNEY DISEASE

PWH can develop multiple forms of renal disease, including
acute kidney injury (AKI), HIVAN, HIV immune complex
kidney disease (HIVICK), thrombotic microangiopathy
(TMA), and medication-induced nephrotoxicity. However,
kidney disease in PWH has been evolving over time with
increased ART usage, viral suppression, and longer life expectancy in PWH. This has increased the prevalence of traditional
CKD risk factors in PWH, broadening the spectrum of renal
disease etiologies (see Box 40.2) (Swanepoel et al., 2018). In a
large academic center, renal biopsies from 437 PWH (80% on
ART) were re-evaluated to reassess spectrum of disease. This
cohort of biopsies from 2010–2018 showed the most common
pathology to be immune complex glomerulonephritis (17%),
follow by diabetic nephropathy (16%), HIVAN (14%), tenofovir nephrotoxicity (13%), FSGS-NOS (12%), and global
glomerulosclerosis-NOS (9%). Regarding the trends seen during this 9-year timeframe, tenofovir nephrotoxicity decreased
while FSGS-NOS and diabetic nephropathy increased. In
contrast, the same institution in 1987 reported HIVAN made
up for 76% of kidney biopsies in PWH, followed by ICGN
(9%) and interstitial nephritis (6%). In this study, researchers also showed that serologies and clinical syndromes, except
Fanconi syndrome, which is associated with tenofovir toxicity, were not predictive of biopsy findings (Kudose et al.,
2020). Therefore, renal biopsy remains an important diagnostic strategy for in most PWH with kidney disease to determine the underlying renal pathology as treatment strategies
often differ based on histopathologic findings.

ACUTE KIDNEY INJURY

Poor nutritional state of patients, dehydration, polypharmacy,
and less commonly, opportunistic infections, in PWH predispose to development of AKI, with incidence rates of 2.7 to
6.9 per 100 person years (py) (Campos et al., 2016). Higher
incidence of AKI is also associated with advanced age, diabetes mellitus, CKD, acute or chronic liver failure, CD4[+]
T-cell counts of less than 200 cells/mm³, HIV-1 RNA levels
of more than 10,000 copies/mL, and hepatitis coinfection
(Wyatt et al., 2006). Common causes of AKI in PWH are
similar to those in people without HIV, with pre-renal states
and acute tubular necrosis accounting for about one-third of
cases. Less common causes of AKI in PWH include obstruction from lymphadenopathy related to malignancy, tumor
lysis syndrome, and polyoma virus-induced renal dysfunction.
Regardless of the etiology, short- and long-term mortality is

Box 40.2 HIV-RELATED KIDNEY DISEASES

I. Glomerular dominant

   a. Immune complex-mediated glomerular disease (ICGN)
     i. IgA nephropathy
     ii. Lupus nephritis
     iii. Membranous nephropathy
     iv. Membranoproliferative pattern glomerulonephritis
     v. Bacterial infection-related glomerulonephritis
     vi. ICGN with no etiology other than HIV
     vii. Other immune complex diseases in the setting of HIV
   b. Podocytopathies
     i. Classic HIVAN
     ii. FSGS-NOS in the setting of HIV
     iii. Minimal-change disease in the setting of HIV
     iv. Other podocytopathy in the setting of HIV
   c. Other glomerular diseases
     i. Diabetic nephropathy
     ii. AA amyloidosis
     iii. Pauci-immune GN

II. Tubulointerstitial dominant

   a. Tenofovir toxicity
   b. Tubulointerstitial injury in the setting of classic HIVAN
   c. Acute tubular injury or acute tubular necrosis (associated with ART vs. other drugs)
   d. Tubulointerstitial nephritis (associated with ART vs. other drugs)
   e. Renal parenchymal infection by bacterial, viral, or fungal pathogens
   f. Immunologic dysfunction-related tubulointerstitial inflammation
     i. DILS
     ii. IRIS
   g. Other tubulointerstitial inflammation in the setting of HIV

III. Vascular dominant

   a. Thrombotic microangiopathy in the setting of HIV
   b. Arteriosclerosis and/or cholesterol emboli
   c. Infarction

IV. Other, in the setting of HIV infection

   a. Diabetic nephropathy
   b. Age-related nephrosclerosis

SOURCE: Adapted from Swanepoel CR et al. Kidney disease in the setting of HIV infection: conclusions from A Kidney Disease: Improving Global Outcomes (KDIGO) Controversies Conference. *Kidney International.* 2018;22(6):84–100.

increased in AKI in PWH by as much as fivefold. In one study from Portugal of 489 HIV hospitalized PWH, mortality was 27.3% in AKI versus 8% for non-AKI persons (Campos, 2016). In a study of 433 PWH who were hospitalized, at 1, 2, and 5 years of follow-up, the cumulative probability of death in those with AKI was 21%, 25%, and 31%, respectively compared to 10%, 13%, and 16.5% in patients without AKI (Lopes et al., 2016).

HIV-ASSOCIATED NEPHROPATHY

HIVAN is the most aggressive form of kidney disease associated with HIV infection and generally presents in patients with advanced HIV infection who exhibit rapidly declining GFR and significant proteinuria. The incidence of HIVAN significantly declined after the widespread use of ART, but it remains a cause of ESRD, most often seen in young Black patients. HIVAN is pathologically characterized by a collapsing form of focal and segmental sclerosis, prominent tubular microcysts, and tubulointerstitial inflammation (D'Agati et al., 1989).

FSGS-NOS has become a more common finding in renal biopsies in the ART era (Kudose et al., 2020). A subset of these patients with FSGS-NOS are believed to have an attenuated form of HIVAN given similar median severity of tubular atrophy, interstitial fibrosis, and inflammation to HIVAN cases. Additionally, many of these samples had presence of tubuloreticular inclusions, tubular microcysts, and moderate foot-process effacement seen in HIVAN. Differentiation between FSGS-NOS and attenuated HIVAN is difficult to evaluate without molecular studies addressing viral infection of renal epithelia, infiltrating leukocytes phenotype and dysregulation of host-signaling pathways. However, patients with FSGS-NOS tend to be older, hypertensive with cardiovascular disease, and usually on ART (Kudose et al., 2020).

IMMUNE COMPLEX GLOMERULONEPHRITIS AND HIV IMMUNE COMPLEX DISEASE OF THE KIDNEY

Various immune complex kidney diseases have been reported in patients with HIV-1 infection, such as postinfectious glomerulonephritis, membranoproliferative glomerulonephritis, membranous nephropathy, immunoglobulin A nephropathy, and lupus-like glomerulonephritis, and they were previously referred to collectively as HIV immune complex disease of the kidney (HIVICK) (Balow, 2005; Kalayjian, 2011). However, in 2017, KDIGO replaced HIVICK in favor of a more descriptive pattern of immune complex disease because of lack of certainty of HIV causality in most cases. The previously eluted glomerular immune deposits with specific anti-HIV antibodies in previous HIVICK cases were found in the research setting and not replicable in routine pathology laboratories. The transition away from collectively naming all immune complex disease as HIVICK was to encourage workup of secondary and possibly treatable causes of immune complex deposition (Swanepoel et al., 2018). In a review of renal biopsies in patient with HIV, immune complex glomerulonephritis (ICGN) was the most prevalent finding (Kudose et al., 2020). Further, in those 75 cases of ICGN, 79% had an identifiable etiology other than HIV infection. Of the remaining 21%, two-thirds of them were not on ART raising suspicion for true HIVICK in those cases.

TUBULOINTERSTITIAL DISEASE

Renal tubulointerstitial disease can include HIVAN, which has a tubulointerstitial component in addition to a glomerular component. Tenofovir and protease inhibitor toxicity can also play a role and will be discussed later in this chapter. PWH are also at risk for tubular injury by the same etiologies seen in the general population such as toxic, ischemic, septic, and hypovolemic insults. Antibiotics, proton pump inhibitors, and other medications can cause tubulointerstitial nephritis in the general and HIV population as well. However, two rare, but notable causes of tubulointerstitial injury that involve immune dysfunction from HIV and are characterized by prominent CD8[+] T-cell infiltrates (Swanepoel, 2018). Diffuse infiltrative lymphocytosis syndrome (DILS) effects the kidneys 10% of the time as a result of a hyperimmune reaction against HIV. Immune reconstitution inflammatory syndrome (IRIS) rarely involves the kidney but may occur in patients with advanced HIV infection after ART initiation unmasking a subclinical infectious process.

NONINFECTIOUS COMORBIDITIES

The most common causes of CKD in PWH are noninfectious comorbidities (NICM), specifically hypertension, vascular disease, and diabetes (Heron et al., 2020a). Hypertension can independently cause secondary FSGS but may also compound glomerular disease caused by HIV itself. Two primary drivers of comorbid hypertension are tobacco use and obesity. Both risk factors are relevant, as the prevalence of tobacco use among PWH is two to three times that of the general US population (Park et al., 2017), and although exact causal mechanisms are unknown, TAF and INSTIs, especially dolutegravir and bictegravir, have been found to lead to weight gain in multiple studies (Sax et al., 2020).

Progressive vascular disease may occur in PWH from a direct effect of HIV on renal vasculature but is also associated with dyslipidemia and chronic inflammation (Heron, 2020a). Thrombotic microangiopathy (TMA) is a rare complication of HIV-1 infection, with an incidence of isolated renal TMA of 0.3% (Becker et al., 2004). It manifests as thrombocytopenia and microangiopathic hemolytic anemia, with or without fever and neurological deficits. Opportunistic infections, high plasma HIV viral load, low CD4[+] counts, and various drugs used in advanced HIV disease can all contribute to development of TMA. In the post–combination ART era, atherosclerotic disease has become the dominant vascular causes of kidney disease in PWH with management focused on modifiable risk factors, including lifestyle management, smoking cessation, lipid lowering agents, and ART (Swanepoel et al., 2018).

Diabetes is four times more prevalent and associated with worse treatment outcomes in PWH compared to the general population (Heron et al., 2020a). Multiple studies, including the 31,072-participant Veterans Aging Cohort Study, have demonstrated a synergistic effect between HIV and diabetes, leading to more rapid CKD progression in PWH and diabetes compared to persons with either condition alone (Feng et al., 2021; Medapalli et al., 2012).

Taken together NICMs are a substantial contributor to CKD among PWH, and their importance will only grow as the cohort of PWH ages. This is further complicated by the polypharmacy required to treat these comorbid conditions, and the drug–drug interactions that ensue, especially among individuals requiring regimens that include boosted PIs.

TREATMENTS

Specific recommendations regarding therapy of the conditions noted above are limited because of the lack of prospective randomized controlled trials. Most of the treatment options, including supportive care, ART, inhibition of renin–angiotensin–aldosterone system, and corticosteroids, are based on retrospective studies and nonrandomized trials.

ANTIRETROVIRAL THERAPY (ART)

Multiple observational studies have supported the benefit of ART in slowing the progression or reversing renal disease in persons with HIVAN. In an older Johns Hopkins Clinic cohort of 4,000 PWH, ART was associated with a 60% risk reduction for HIVAN, with 6.8 and 26.4 episodes per 1,000 py in PWH who did or did not receive ART, respectively (Lucas et al., 2004). In addition, no persons in the Hopkins cohort developed HIVAN when ART was initiated before the development of AIDS.

Consistent evidence demonstrates preservation of renal function with ART in HIV populations. In the Strategies for Management of Antiretroviral Therapy (SMART) group study, continuous therapy versus episodic use of ART was evaluated in 5,472 PWH with CD4[+] T-cell counts of more than 350 cells/μL. In the continuous use group, fewer persons developed renal disease compared to the episodic use group (0.2 vs. 0.1 events/100 py) (SMART, 2006). In addition, in a prospective, multicenter cohort involving 1,776 PWH, ART intervention in persons with CKD stage 2 or greater and low CD4[+] T-cell counts led to an average increase of 9.2 mL/min in GFR at a median follow-up of 160 weeks. These results were magnified in those with a lower baseline GFR and greater decreases in viral load (Longenecker et al., 2009).

ANGIOTENSIN-CONVERTING-ENZYME INHIBITOR AND ANGIOTENSIN II BLOCKADE

Multiple randomized controlled trials in patients with CKD from the general population have demonstrated the efficacy of angiotensin-converting-enzyme (ACE) inhibitors and angiotensin receptor blockers (ARBs) in decreasing proteinuria, slowing the progression of kidney disease, and reducing the incidence of cardiovascular disease and death. However, data regarding their use in PWH are limited. An older study of 18 PWH with biopsy-proven HIVAN, of whom 9 persons were treated with captopril, had an enhanced renal survival compared to controls (mean renal survival, 156 ± 71 vs. 37 ± 5 days) (Kimmel et al., 1996). In another study of 44 patients with biopsy-proven HIVAN, patients treated with ACE inhibition had significantly less progression to ESRD compared to those without therapy (14% vs. 100% at 5 years) (Wei et al., 2003). Based on these results and data from non-HIV populations, ACE inhibitors or ARBs are recommended for PWH with CKD and glomerular diseases in the absence of contraindications to these medications (Swanepoel et al., 2018).

CORTICOSTEROIDS

In patients with HIVAN, older studies found that tubulointerstitial inflammation improves after treatment with steroids (Briggs et al., 1996). However, there are no randomized trials to support steroid use in this population. In a retrospective cohort study of 21 patients, of which 13 received corticosteroids, the relative risk for progressive renal failure with corticosteroid treatment at 3 months was 0.20 ($p < 0.05$) (Eustace et al., 2000). This association remained significant despite adjustment in logistical regression analyses for baseline creatinine; 24-hour proteinuria; CD4$^+$ count; history of intravenous drug use, hepatitis B, and hepatitis C coinfection (Eustace et al., 2000). However, there were 18 infections in corticosteroid-treated patients compared to 8 in the noncorticosteroid-treated group. Larger studies are needed to further clarify the value of steroids in patients with HIV-related kidney disease but, in the post-ART era, are unlikely to be performed. Based on older data noted above, some experts would still recommend a short course of corticosteroid therapy in those with a new diagnosis of HIVAN (Atta et al., 2008; Fine et al., 2008). Risks of adverse effects, including glucose intolerance, bone disease, and further immunosuppression, must always be weighed against the benefits when steroids are use in PWH.

NOVEL MEDICAL THERAPIES

Sodium-glucose cotransporter 2 inhibitors have been shown to reduce the risk of adverse renal outcomes, including dialysis, transplantation, and death, through multiple studies. This class of drugs has also been shown to have an additive effect to RAS blockade in patients with diabetes and albuminuric kidney disease (Neuen et al., 2019). They are likely to confer similar benefits for PWH, although no specific analyses have been published.

Direct-acting antivirals (DAA) for treatment of hepatitis C (HCV) have been available since 2011; however, their use has dramatically increased in recent years. Both hepatitis B and C are highly associated with CKD, can independently cause glomerulonephritis, as well as potentiate the impacts of HIV on the kidney (Heron et al., 2020a). Regression of kidney disease in HCV/HIV infected patients can be seen with successful management of both conditions. Worldwide, 25%–30% of PWH are coinfected with HCV, so increased use of highly effective DAAs could have a significant impact on CKD among PWH (Kupin, 2017).

RENAL REPLACEMENT THERAPY (DIALYSIS)

Compared to the general population, PWH disease have a two- to twenty-fold higher incidence of requiring renal replacement therapy (Campos et al., 2016). This number varies depending on patient populations and geographic location. Overall survival of HIV patients on dialysis historically was worse compared to that of the general ESRD population, mainly because of increased risk of infections (Atta et al., 2007). Older age, lower serum albumin level, lower CD4$^+$ T-cell count, and lack of ART have all been associated with poor survival in PWH undergoing hemodialysis or peritoneal dialysis. It appears that the incidence of ESRD has plateaued, but the prevalence of PWH undergoing dialysis in the United States has increased, likely because of the aging of the HIV population (Cohen et al., 2017). Survival among these patients receiving dialysis is now similar to persons without HIV disease (Campos et al., 2016; Razzak et al., 2015). Peritoneal dialysis is also an option for some PWH. In one study of 70 PWH on continuous peritoneal dialysis, there was no increase in technique failure rates or catheter patency compared to non-HIV patients at 1 year, although the rate of hospital admission and all-cause mortality was higher in the HIV group (Ndlovu & Assounga, 2017).

RENAL TRANSPLANTATION

Renal transplantation was previously contraindicated in PWH because of the concern of immunosuppressive agents in persons with an impaired immune system. However, data now show that renal transplantation is both safe and effective in PWH (Blumberg & Rogers, 2019; Locke et al., 2015; Zheng et al., 2019). Initially, renal transplantation in HIV patients was performed without induction therapy. However, the use of antithymocyte globulin as induction therapy is associated with a 2.6-fold lower risk of rejection, as shown in a study of 516 PWH (Locke et al., 2014). Many of the agents used in post transplantation immunosuppression have antiretroviral properties. Mycophenolate mofetil has virostatic properties through depletion of guanosine nucleosides necessary for the viral life cycle. Calcineurin inhibitors (tacrolimus and cyclosporine) selectively inhibit infected cell growth, and sirolimus disrupts infective viral replication through suppression of antigen-presenting cell function.

Currently undergoing investigation is *APOL1* status of the donor and reports suggesting increased rates of kidney failure after donation from high-risk *APOL1* genotypes. Recipient *APOL1* status does not appear to affect graft survival, which suggests that renal *APOL1*, and not circulating *APOL1* derived from the liver, is the main driver of *APOL1* kidney disease (Freedman et al., 2015). There is limited data from large prospectively designed trials, but the *APOL1* Long-term Kidney Transplantation Outcomes Network (APOLLO) study is currently underway (Freedman et al., 2019). Additional evaluation of these patients is needed to determine causality to the *APOL1* donor kidney. This would help donor and recipient education as they weigh risk and benefit of *APOL1* high-risk kidney donation against remaining on dialysis. A more comprehensive analysis is needed to change allocation and outcomes of kidney transplantation (Friedman & Pollak, 2021).

PWH considered eligible for renal transplant should have a CD4[+] T-cell count greater than 200 /mm[3] and an undetectable viral load while on a stable ART regimen. There is concern for drug–drug interactions between some antiretroviral drugs and immunosuppressive agents. This is especially true for ritonavir or cobicistat-boosted protease inhibitors (PI) that are metabolized through the cytochrome P450 system. Thus, although kidney transplantation is effective in PWH, it requires close monitoring of drug levels and rejection risk.

The HOPE Act was signed into law in November 2013 and implemented in 2015. This legislation allows for the transplantation of kidneys and other organs from donors with HIV to HIV-positive recipients to increase the donor pool, shorten wait time, and make transplantation a viable option for a greater number of patients with ESRD (Cohen et al., 2017). Early outcomes from a multicenter pilot program following 75 PWH who received a kidney from deceased HIV-positive donors have been excellent with 100% patient survival and 92% graft survival, no differences in 1-year mean eGFR, HIV breakthrough, infectious hospitalizations, or opportunistic infections (Durand et al., 2021; Klitenic et al., 2021).

RECOMMENDED READING

Heron JE, Bagnis CI, Gracey DM. Contemporary issues and new challenges in chronic kidney disease amongst people living with HIV. *AIDS Res Ther*. 2020;17(1):11.
Wojciechowski D, Ghandi RT, Rosales IA. Case 11-2019: a 49-year-old man with HIV infection and chronic kidney disease. *N Engl J Med*. 2019; 380:1464–1472.

ANTIRETROVIRAL THERAPY-RELATED KIDNEY COMPLICATIONS

ART been known for many years to cause both acute and chronic injury. This was seen early in the epidemic with several of the PI, particularly indinavir sulfate. Later it was found that TDF could cause AKI and proximal, sometimes irreversible tubular dysfunction. Other agents, as will be discussed below, are not inherently nephrotoxic but can increase serum creatinine levels by blocking tubular secretion. Lastly, with the aging of the HIV population and associated comorbidities, polypharmacy related to ART and medications for other comorbid conditions can increase the risk of acute and CKD in PWH.

NUCLEOS(T)IDE REVERSE TRANSCRIPTASE INHIBITORS

TDF is a nucleotide reverse transcriptase inhibitor that is used in PWH and has been associated with CKD. It is cleared by the kidneys via active proximal tubular secretion and glomerular filtration. Because of high renal toxicity rates of its acyclic nucleotide predecessors adefovir and cidofovir, both of which cause AKI and proximal tubular toxicity, there was initial concern regarding the potential renal toxicity of TDF. Early studies did not reveal significant toxicity related to TDF, but

after FDA approval, case reports emerged of Fanconi syndrome, kidney injury, and diabetes insipidus (Gaspar et al., 2004; Karras et al., 2003). The active ingredient of TDF is tenofovir (TFV) and nephrotoxicity is proportional to plasma TFV concentrations. TFV undergoes glomerular filtration and active secretion by the renal proximal tubule cells (PTC) via the organic anion transporter pathway. As it accumulates in the renal PTC, TFV alters DNA expression of endothelial nitric oxide synthase, the sodium-phosphorous cotransporter, sodium/hydrogen exchanger 3, and aquaporin 2. TFV toxicity is manifested as intense renal vasoconstriction, phosphaturia, proximal tubular acidosis, polyuria, and impaired urine concentrating ability (Novick et al., 2017). Proximal tubular dysfunction, which may manifest as a Fanconi syndrome or a limited defect, is the most common manifestation of mitochondrial disease and supports the hypothesis that tenofovir exposure causes mitochondrial dysfunction (Kalyesubula & Perazella, 2011). Fanconi syndrome is characterized by proximal tubular kidney dysfunction, with decreased tubular reabsorption and urinary wasting of phosphate, glucose, amino acids, bicarbonate, and sodium. This solute loss leads to acidosis, bone disease, and electrolyte abnormalities. Most patients do not develop full Fanconi syndrome but instead manifest primarily with urinary phosphate wasting and, hence, hypophosphatemia in most cases (Waheed & Atta, 2014). This may occur in isolation or in conjunction with AKI. Urinary phosphate wasting is a more sensitive marker of TDF-induced nephrotoxicity because hypophosphatemia is not present in all cases.

Of patients on TDF, 1%–2% will need to stop treatment because of tubulopathy (Hamzah et al., 2017). Risk of development of TDF-induced nephrotoxicity is cumulative and patients with low CD4[+] T-cell counts, advanced age, lower body weight, higher baseline serum creatinine, and those on a PI are most at risk (Heron et al., 2020a; Mocroft et al., 2016).

A long-term follow-up of 23,905 PWH in the Data Collection on Adverse Events of Anti-HIV Drugs (D:A:D) study cohort who initiated antiretrovirals with normal eGFR (>90 mL/min/1.73 m²) showed a significant increase in the development of CKD with exposure to tenofovir, ritonavir-boosted atazanavir, and ritonavir-boosted lopinavir, but not to other ritonavir-boosted PIs nor abacavir (Mocroft et al., 2015). These findings are consistent with previous studies in the cohort and add to the expanding literature on the long-term effects of antiretroviral agents on the kidney.

Tenofovir alafenamide (TAF) is a prodrug of TDF which has potent anti-HIV-1 activity and higher intracellular concentration in peripheral blood mononuclear cells compared to TDF while maintaining lower plasma concentration (Markowitz et al., 2014). TAF has an increased stability and mean 91% lower plasma concentration of TFV compared to TDF. Additionally, TFV released from TDF undergoes active renal secretion via organic anion transporters (OAT1 and OAT3), leading to higher exposure of renal proximal tubules to TFV and a potential for toxicity. Unlike TDF, TAF does not interact with renal transporters OAT1 and OAT3, and, therefore, it may be safer (Bam et al., 2014). An integrated analysis of 26 clinical trials confirmed these differences change clinical outcomes, as there were no episodes of proximal tubular nephropathy among patients taking TAF, compared to 10 cases among patients taking TDF ($P < 0.001$) and fewer discontinuations because of renal side effects among those on TAF compared to TDF (3/6360 vs. 14/2962, $P < 0.001$) (Gupta et al., 2019).

In a randomized controlled trial of PWH who had achieved virologic suppression (viral load < 50 mL/min) on a TDF-based regimen with a GFR of 50 mL/min or higher, patients were randomly assigned to continue the same ART or were switched to a TAF-based regimen (in combination with elvitegravir, cobicistat, and emtricitabine). The TAF-containing regimen led to continued viral suppression with improvement in bone mineral density and renal function (Mills et al., 2016). Other "switch" studies have also found that laboratory markers of moderately/severely increased proteinuria improved after patients were changed from TDF-to-TAF-based ART (Schwarze-Zande et al., 2020). Pilkington and colleagues (2020) completed a meta-analysis of 14 trials evaluating TAF and TDF safety and efficacy when boosted or not boosted. They found that TAF, when boosted by ritonavir or cobicistat and appropriately dose-reduced because of the "boosting" effect these agents have on it, provided a statistically significant improvement in efficacy over dose-unadjusted TDF as part of a boosted ART regimen ($P = 0.0004$). Of note, this was due almost entirely to increased levels of TFV in the blood resulting in increased renal side effects occurring with dose-unadjusted TDF given with ritonavir or cobicistat. Virologic efficacy and adverse effects of TAF compared to TDF as part of unboosted ART regimens demonstrated no significant differences in efficacy or adverse effects. Although uncommon, two case reports show that accumulation of TFV from TAF can still be sufficient to cause mitochondrial dysfunction (Bahr & Yarlagadda, 2019; Novick et al., 2017). A more recent case report describes the development of acute proximal renal tubulopathy (PRT) in a patient previously stable on TAF with the addition of gentamycin. This highlights the potential for expected drug–drug interactions that may be observed now that TAF is used more widely (Heron et al., 2020b).

Based on current knowledge of TDF toxicities, there is no absolute consensus regarding the monitoring of kidney function in patients on tenofovir-based ART regimens. Most experts recommend the combination of an every-3-month urine dipstick for glycosuria and proteinuria (the earliest clinical signs of PRT) along with an every-3-months eGFR-based approach. Some advocate for periodic monitoring of additional markers of renal function in all patients on tenofovir regardless of GFR (Fine & Gallant, 2013; Holt et al., 2014). Although the renal toxicity of TDF is mostly reversible with the cessation of this drug, patients often do not achieve their pre-TDF CrCl levels (Waheed & Atta, 2014). The safety of TAF use after TDF-induced PRT is supported by a prospective study in which 31 individuals with TDF-induced PRT and eGFR >30 mL/min/1.73 m^2 were switched to TAF and followed for 96 weeks (Campbell et al., 2021). At the end of observation, all individuals remained on TAF, and none had recurrence of glycosuria or PRT. With the increased

availability of single-table ART regimens that contain TAF, the use of TDF in the United States has significantly declined. Clinicians should be vigilant regarding monitoring patients for renal toxicity, with early change in regimen when toxicity is identified.

PROTEASE INHIBITORS

Currently, PIs are used less frequently with the availability of newer and safer antiretroviral drugs but still have a role for some patients, especially those with high-level drug resistance. Two of these agents, indinavir and atazanavir can cause urolithiasis. This was most frequently seen with indinavir, one of the first PIs approved by the FDA in 1996, but this has also been observed with other PIs (Huynh et al., 2011; Rockwood et al., 2011). With expanded use, indinavir was also associated with progression of CKD. This drug is rarely used in the United States, so its toxicity has become more of historical importance (McLaughlin et al., 2018).

Several studies found nephrotoxicity associated with atazanavir use after its approval in 2003. The largest included 22,603 D:A:D cohort participants with normal baseline kidney function (eGFR >90 mL/min) (Mocroft et al., 2010). The decline in eGFR by more than 20 mL/min to less than 70 mL/min was associated with the use of tenofovir with ritonavir-boosted atazanavir. An earlier study of the EuroSIDA cohort (a subset of the D:A:D cohort) found similar results in a smaller study of PWH. In a study of a large Veterans Health Administration population, Scherzer and colleagues (2012) showed an association between atazanavir use and rapid GFR decline. The formation of kidney stones with atazanavir use has been well-described in the literature (Chan-Tack et al., 2007). Therefore, a plausible mechanism for the potential toxicity may be related to the predilection for atazanavir to crystallize in renal interstitial tissues and urine. With many studies confirming an association of nephrotoxicity with atazanavir, close monitoring of renal function in patients taking this PI is recommended. If a decline in GFR or other evidence of nephrotoxicity is noted, it should be discontinued. If a PI is needed to maintain viral suppression, switching to darunavir is recommended (McLaughlin et al., 2018). Additional analyses from the D:A:D cohort, demonstrated that DRV/r was not associated with an increased risk of CKD (Ryom et al., 2019b). This is likely to be the case for DRV/c as well but was not specifically analyzed.

INTEGRASE STRAND TRANSFER INHIBITORS

Integrase strand transfer inhibitors have become the most used class of drugs to treat HIV disease because of their efficacy, safety, and tolerability. Raltegravir (RAL), was the first FDA-approved integrase strand transfer inhibitor (INSTI), and several published studies assessed the effect of this drug on renal function. In a retrospective study of 29 PWH started on RAL there was noted a small but nonsignificant increase in serum creatinine (Lindeman et al., 2016). The authors concluded there was no evidence of direct nephrotoxicity, but the increases were likely due to inhibition of renal OCT2.

In a similar fashion, it was subsequently found that another INSTI, dolutegravir, inhibits the tubular secretion of creatinine through the OCT2 at the basolateral membrane of the proximal tubular cells (Rathbun et al., 2014). This raises serum creatinine concentration without affecting the actual GFR. A phase 1 study included 34 healthy individuals who received 50 mg of dolutegravir twice daily or placebo for 14 days (Koteff et al., 2013). Participants received iohexol, which is freely filtered, and para-aminohippurate (PAH) on days 1, 7, and 14, to see if dolutegravir impacted GFR or renal blood flow. Additional tubular function biomarkers including albumin, cystatin C, and total protein were also measured. The authors determined that dolutegravir reversibly increased serum creatinine levels by 10%–14% but did not impact renal blood flow or glomerular filtration. This is also seen with bictegravir. As this low-level and transient rise in serum creatinine is due to the temporary effect of membrane transporter inhibition, it is generally not considered to be renal toxicity.

In the SPRING-1 and SPRING-2 HIV clinical trials that enrolled treatment-naive patients, a noticeable rise in serum creatinine was noted in patients who received dolutegravir without any significant clinically adverse effects (Raffi et al., 2013; Stellbrink et al., 2013). The rise in creatinine was typically seen in the first week of therapy then stabilized thereafter. In the VIKING Trial, a similar pattern was noted for PWH who had developed resistance to RAL and switched to dolutegravir (Eron et al., 2013).

Elvitegravir, another INSTI, is primarily metabolized by the liver into two metabolites. A very small amount is excreted unchanged in the urine (McLaughlin et al., 2018). It is therefore not felt to present any risk of nephrotoxicity. However, it is coadministered with cobicistat, so small increases in serum creatinine in patients taking this drug have also been reported (Imaz & Podzamczer, 2017).

Bictegravir is a second-generation INSTI that is currently widely used in the United States and other developing countries in both treatment-naive and experienced patients. This drug has been evaluated in several large phase 3 clinical trials, with in vitro studies showing relatively higher barrier to resistance compared to other antiretroviral agents. Coformulated bictegravir, emtricitabine, and tenofovir alafenamide was compared to dolutegravir-based combination ART in two noninferiority trials (Gallant et al., 2017; Sax et al., 2017). In these studies, the estimated GFR declined by −7.0 mL/min in the bictegravir arm and −11.3 mL/min in the dolutegravir arm at week 48, but there were no patient discontinuations because of kidney-related adverse events and no cases of tubulopathy.

Several subsequent studies evaluated the efficacy and safety of switching to a bictegravir-based regimen from either a dolutegravir-based or PI-based regimen (Daar et al., 2018; Molina et al., 2018). There were no discontinuations of therapy due to renal adverse effects. Changes in serum creatinine, serum eGFR, and urinary markers such as albumin-to-creatinine ratio, were also not significant.

Cabotegravir is a potent INSTI that is FDA-approved for pre-exposure prophylaxis or in combination with rilpivirine in a long-acting injectable formulation (Jaeger et al., 2021; Landovitz et al., 2021; Orkin et al., 2021). Monthly dosing of long-acting cabotegravir and rilpivirine was approved by the FDA in 2021. The FLAIR study, a randomized, open-label, multicenter and multicountry, phase 3 study demonstrated noninferiority between daily dolutegravir, abacavir, and lamivudine and every 4-week injectable cabotegravir and rilpivirine at maintaining viral suppression after 48 and then 96 weeks of study (Orkin et al., 2021). The ATLAS-2M trial demonstrated noninferiority with cabotegravir and rilpivirine administered at 8-week intervals compared to 4-week intervals (Jaeger et al., 2021). A phase 1 study demonstrated that oral administration of cabotegravir did not impact plasma concentrations of cabotegravir even in patients with severe renal impairment (Parasrampuria et al., 2019; ViiV Healthcare, 2022). Therefore, no dose adjustment is needed based on renal impairment for those patients not on renal replacement. Although not included in the study, dialysis is unlikely to affect plasma concentrations given the high degree of protein binding.

PHARMACOKINETIC ENHANCER

Several antiretrovirals are coformulated with cobicistat, a potent inhibitor of cytochrome 3A. Cobicistat increases serum levels of specific antiretroviral agents and allows once-daily dosing of these drugs (Johnson & Saravolatz, 2014). Although cobicistat has no inherent nephrotoxicity, it inhibits the cationic renal transporter MATE1 (multidrug and toxin extrusion protein-efflux) at the apical membrane of the proximal tubular cells, which blocks tubular secretion of creatinine (see Figure 40.1) (Lepist et al., 2011). This leads

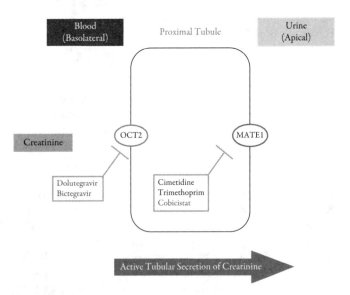

Figure 40.1 Effect of drugs on creatinine secretion   Inhibition of creatinine transporter by drugs shown will result in increase in serum creatinine without GFR effects; model for effect of tested drugs on creatinine secretion. BCRP, breast cancer resistance protein; MATE, multidrug and toxin extrusion protein; MRP, multidrug resistance protein; OCT, organic cation transporter; OCTN, organic cation/ergothioneine transporter; Pgp, P-glycoprotein. **SOURCE:** From Lepist I, et al., ICAAC 2011, Chicago. Poster A1-1724.

to an increase in plasma creatinine concentration without any effect on the actual GFR. This finding was evaluated in a study of 36 patients in which cobicistat use was associated with an increase in serum creatinine and an approximately 10 mL/min decrease in eGFR. The decrease in eGFR was reversible upon discontinuation of the medication, thus highlighting that this drug has no adverse effect on the actual GFR (German et al., 2010). The timing of the increase in creatinine and subsequent resolution after discontinuation of cobicistat was consistent with altered proximal tubular creatinine secretion.

DOSE ADJUSTMENT OF ART IN RENAL INSUFFICIENCY

Most nonnucleoside reverse transcriptase inhibitors (NNRTIs), integrase inhibitors, and PIs do not require dose modification in CKD or ESRD and can therefore be safely used. TDF alone or coformulated with other antiretroviral agents should be avoided in PWH with a CrCl level of less than 50 mL/min and stopped in those with declining eGFR. There may be instances in which other options are not available, and dose adjustments with TDF, including giving this drug three times weekly, can be considered. In general, the availability of TAF makes this less of a clinical issue for most patients taking tenofovir as part of their ART regimen.

Patient who are taking combination single-tablet regimens often will require separation of the component drugs for individual dosing if they have a decline in renal function. However, a small study ($n = 55$) found that once-daily single-tablet, E/C/F/TAF was effective in maintaining virologic suppression in PWH on chronic hemodialysis over 96 weeks of follow-up (Eron et al., 2019). It was well tolerated and associated with improved patient satisfaction.

Data gathered from the OPERA cohort now support expanded use of full-dose, 300 mg daily, lamivudine in PWH and an eGFR between 30 and 49 mL/min per 1.73 m^2 (Mounzer et al., 2021). Per manufacturer recommendations, patients with this eGFR should receive a dose adjustment to 150 mg daily. Patients receiving full-dose versus adjusted-dose lamivudine experienced more gastrointestinal symptoms and moderate lab abnormalities. However, there were no significant differences in the incidence of lactic acidosis, paresthesia, peripheral neuropathy, pancreatitis, rhabdomyolysis, anemia, neutropenia, thrombocytopenia, nausea, or severe laboratory abnormalities by lamivudine dose (full-dose 300 mg vs. adjusted-dose 150 mg daily, IRR 1.51; 95% CI: 0.59–3.92). Reduced doses of lamivudine are not available in single-tablet regimens, so continued use of full-dose lamivudine at a lower eGFR has a direct impact on pill burden and subsequently, medication compliance. Clinicians should monitor for side effects if continuing full-dose lamivudine at lower eGFRs, but this is a viable and patient centered option.

CKD SCREENING AND MONITORING IN PERSONS WITH HIV

Chronic kidney disease may have a prolonged asymptomatic period; therefore, all PWH should be monitored on a regular basis for CKD. Appropriate diagnosis and management of other risk factors for CK including diabetes and hypertension should also be part of routine care of PWH. In 2017, The Kidney Disease: Improving Global Outcomes (KDIGO) made specific recommendations regarding screening and monitoring for renal dysfunction in PWH (Swanepoel, 2018). They noted that kidney disease risk stratification should be considered when choosing an ART regimen for PWH. This document states that: "Standard ART" as recommended by treatment guidelines may be used in those with "low risk" for CKD (eGFR >90 mL/min, uPCR< 200 mg/g, < 50 years of age). Avoidance of potentially nephrotoxic ART agents (e.g., TDF, indinavir, atazanavir, and lopinavir) is recommend in those with "high risk" for CKD (eGFR< 70 mL/min/1.73 m^2, uPCR >500 mg/g, >60 years of age, HCV coinfection, DM, uncontrolled HTN, or CVD). Yearly screening of PWH for proteinuria and eGFR is recommended for those who are clinically stable and virologically suppressed on ART. Proteinuria can be quantified by a urine albumin: creatinine ratio or urine protein: creatinine ratio. Those at higher risk should have assessment of eGFR screening for proteinuria at least twice per year. All PWH should have renal function reassessed at baseline, then at 1 month after ART modification. Those on TDF with a ritonavir or cobicistat-boosted PI, should be assessed two to four times per year with eGFR, proteinuria, serum phosphorus, urinalysis, and fractional excretion of phosphate (Swanepoel et al., 2018).

RECOMMENDED READING

Wearne N, Davidson B, Blockman M, Swart A, Jones ES. HIV, drugs and the kidney. *Drugs Context*. 2020; 9:2019-11-1. http://doi:10.7573/dic.2019-11-

REFERENCES

Atta MG, Fine DM, Kirk GD, et al. Survival during renal replacement therapy among African Americans infected with HIV type 1 in urban Baltimore, Maryland. *Clin Infect Dis*. 2007;45(12):1625–1632.

Atta MG, Lucas GM, Fine DM. HIV-associated nephropathy: epidemiology, pathogenesis, diagnosis and management. *Expert Rev Anti Infect Ther*. 2008;6(3):365–371.

Bahr NC, Yarlagadda SG. Fanconi syndrome and tenofovir alafenamide: a case report. *Ann Intern Med*. 2019;170(11):814–815.

Balow JE. Nephropathy in the context of HIV infection. *Kidney Int*. 2005;67(4):1632–1633.

Bam RA, Birkus G, Babusis D, et al. Metabolism and antiretroviral activity of tenofovir alafenamide in CD4\+ T-cells and macrophages from demographically diverse donors. *Antivir Ther*. 2014;19(7):669–677.

Becker S, Fusco G, Fusco J, et al. HIV-associated thrombotic microangiopathy in the era of highly active antiretroviral therapy: an observational study. *Clin Infect Dis*. 2004;39(Suppl 5):S267–S275.

Bige N, Lanternier F, Viard JP, et al. Presentation of HIV-associated nephropathy and outcome in HAART-treated patients. *Nephrol Dial Transplant*. 2012. 27(3):1114–1121.

Blumberg EA, Rogers CC; American Society of Transplantation Infectious Diseases Community of Practice. Solid organ transplantation in the HIV-infected patient: guidelines from the American Society of Transplantation Infectious Diseases Community of Practice. *Clin Transplant*. 2019;33(9):e13499.

Briggs WA, Tanawattanacharoen S, Choi MJ, et al. Clinicopathologic correlates of prednisone treatment of human immunodeficiency virus-associated nephropathy. *Am J Kidney Dis*. 1996;28(4):618–621.

Bruggeman LA, Dikman S, Meng C, et al. Nephropathy in human immunodeficiency virus-1 transgenic mice is due to renal transgene expression. *J Clin Invest*. 1997;100(1):84–92.

Campbell L, Barbini B, Burling K, et al. Safety of tenofovir alafenamide in people with HIV who experienced proximal renal tubulopathy on tenofovir disoproxil fumarate. *J Acquir Immune Defic Syndr*. 2021;88(2):214–219.

Campos P, Ortiz A, Soto K. HIV and kidney diseases: 35 years of history and consequences. *Clin Kidney J*. 2016;9(6):772–781.

Chan-Tack KM, Truffa MM, Struble KA, et al. Atazanavir-associated nephrolithiasis: cases from the US Food and Drug Administration's Adverse Event Reporting System. *AIDS*. 2007;21(9):1215–1218.

Choi AI, Rodriguez RA, Bacchetti P, et al. The impact of HIV on chronic kidney disease outcomes. *Kidney Int*. 2007;72(11):1380–1387.

Cohen SD, Kopp JB, Kimmel PL. Kidney diseases associated with human immunodeficiency virus infection. *N Engl J Med*. 2017;377(24):2363–2375.

Daar ES, DeJesus E, Ruane P, et al. Efficacy and safety of switching to fixed-dose bictegravir, emtricitabine, and tenofovir alafenamide from boosted protease inhibitor-based regimens in virologically suppressed adults with HIV-1: 48-week results of a randomised, open-label, multi-center, phase 3, non-inferiority trial. *Lancet HIV*. 2018;5(7):347–356.

D'Agati V, Suh J, Carbone L, et al. Pathology of HIV-associated nephropathy: a detailed morphologic and comparative study. *Kidney Int*. 1989;35(6):1358–1370.

Delgado C, Baweja M, Crews DC, et al. A unifying approach for gfr estimation: recommendations of the NKF-ASN Task Force on reassessing the inclusion of race in diagnosing kidney disease [published online ahead of print, September 23, 2021]. *J Am Soc Nephrol*. 2021;32(12):2994–3015.

Dragović G, Srdić D, Al Musalhi K, et al. Higher levels of cystatin C in HIV/AIDS patients with metabolic syndrome. *Basic Clin Pharmacol Toxicol*. 2018;122:396–401.

Durand CM, Zhang W, Brown DM, et al. A prospective multicenter pilot study of HIV-positive deceased donor to HIV-positive recipient kidney transplantation: HOPE in action. *Am J Transplant*. 2021;21(5):1754–1764.

Eron JJ, Clotet B, Katlama C, et al. Safety and efficacy of dolutegravir in treatment-experienced subjects with ratlegravir-resistant HIV type 1 infection: 24-week results of the VIKING study. *J Infect Dis*. 2013;207(5):740–748.

Eron JJ, Lelievre JD, Kalayjian R. Longer-term safety and efficacy of elvitegravir/cobicistat/emtricitabine/ tenofovir alafenamide in virologically suppressed adults living with HIV and ESRD on chronic hemodialysis. *Open Forum Infectious Diseases*, 2019;6(S-2):864.

Eustace JA, Nuermberger E, Choi M, et al. Cohort study of the treatment of severe HIV-associated nephropathy with corticosteroids. *Kidney Int*. 2000;58(3):1253–1260.

Feng J, Bao L, Wang X, et al. Low expression of HIV genes in podocytes accelerates the progression of diabetic kidney disease in mice. *Kidney Int*. 2021;99(4):914–925.

Fine DM, Gallant JE. Nephrotoxicity of antiretroviral agents: is the list getting longer? *J Infect Dis*. 2013;207(9):1349–1351.

Fine DM, Perazella MA, Lucas GM, et al. Kidney biopsy in HIV: beyond HIV-associated nephropathy. *Am J Kidney Dis*. 2008;51(3):504–514.

Freedman BI, Julian BA, Pastan SO, et al. Apolipoprotein L1 gene variants in deceased organ donors are associated with renal allograft failure. *Am J Transplant*. 2015;15(6):1615–1622.

Freedman BI, Moxey-Mims MM, Alexander AA, et al. *APOL1* Long-Term Kidney Transplantation Outcomes Network (APOLLO): design and rationale. *Kidney Int Rep*. 2019;5(3):278–288.

Friedman DJ, Pollak MR. APOL1 nephropathy: from genetics to clinical applications. *Clini J Am Soc Nephrol*. 2021;16(2):294–303.

Gallant JE, Lazzarin A, Mills A, et al. Bictegravir, emtricitabine, and tenofovir alafenamide versus dolutegravir, abacavir, and lamivudine for initial treatment of HIV-1 infection (GS-US-380-1489): a double-blind, multicentre, phase 3, randomised controlled non-inferiority trial. *Lancet*. 2017;390(10107):2063–2072.

Gaspar G, Monereo A, Garcia-Reyne A, et al. Fanconi syndrome and acute renal failure in a patient treated with tenofovir: a call for caution. *AIDS*. 2004;18:351–352.

Genovese G, Friedman DJ, Ross MD, et al. Association of trypanolytic ApoL1 variants with kidney disease in African Americans. *Science*. 2010;329(5993):841–845.

German P, Warren D, West S, et al. Pharmacokinetics and bioavailability of an integrase and novel pharmacoenhancer-containing single-tablet fixed-dose combination regimen for the treatment of HIV. *J AIDS*. 2010;55(3):323–329.

Gupta SK, Post FA, Arribas JR, et al. Renal safety of tenofovir alafenamide vs. tenofovir disoproxil fumarate: a pooled analysis of 26 clinical trials. *AIDS*. 2019;33(9):1455–1465.

Hamzah L, Jose S, Booth JW, et al. Treatment-limiting renal tubulopathy in patients treated with tenofovir disoproxil fumarate. *J Infect*. 2017;74(5):492–500.

Heron JE, Bagnis CI, Gracey DM. Contemporary issues and new challenges in chronic kidney disease amongst people living with HIV. *AIDS Res Ther*. 2020a;17(1):11.

Heron JE, Bloch M, Vanguru V, et al. Renal proximal tubulopathy in an HIV-infected patient treated with tenofovir alafenamide and gentamicin: a case report. *BMC Nephrol*. 2020b;21(1):339.

Holt SG, Gracey DM, Levy MT, et al. A consensus statement on the renal monitoring of Australian patients receiving tenofovir based antiviral therapy for HIV/HBV infection. *AIDS Res Ther*. 2014;11:35.

Huynh J, Hever A, Tom T, et al. Indinavir-induced nephrolithiasis three and one-half years after cessation of indinavir therapy. *Int Urol Nephrol*. 2011;43(2):571–573.

Imaz A, Podzamczer D. Tenofovir alafenamide, emtricitabine, elvitegravir and cobicistat combination therapy for the treatment of HIV. *Expert Rev Anti Infect Ther*. 2017;15(3):195–209.

Inker LA, Eneanya ND, Coresh J, et al. New creatinine- and cystatin c-based equations to estimate GFR without race. *N Engl J Med*. 2021;385(19):1737–1749.

Izzedine H, Acharya V, Wirden M, et al. Role of HIV-1 DNA levels as clinical marker of HIV-1-associated nephropathies. *Nephrol Dial Transplant*. 2011;26(2):580–583.

Jaeger H, Overton ET, Richmond G, et al. Long-acting cabotegravir and rilpivirine dosed every 2 months in adults with HIV-1 infection (ATLAS-2M), 96-week results: a randomised, multicentre, open-label, phase 3b, non-inferiority study. *Lancet HIV*. 2021;8(11):e679–e689.

Johnson LB, Saravolatz LD. The quad pill, a once-daily combination therapy for HIV infection. *Clin Infect Dis*. 2014;58(1):93–98.

Kalayjian RC. Renal issues in HIV infection. *Curr HIV AIDS Rep*. 2011;8(3):164–171.

Kalyesubula R, Perazella MA. Nephrotoxicity of HAART. *AIDS Res Treat*. 2011;2011:562790.

Karras A, Lafaurie M, Furco A, et al. Tenofovir-related nephrotoxicity in human immunodeficiency virus-infected patients: three cases of renal failure, Fanconi syndrome, and nephrogenic diabetes insipidus. *Clin Infect Dis*. 2003;36:1070–1073.

Kimmel PL, Mishkin GJ, Umana WO. Captopril and renal survival in patients with human immunodeficiency virus nephropathy. *Am J Kidney Dis*. 1996;28(2):202–208.

Klitenic SB, Levan ML, Van Pilsum Rasmussen SE, Durand CM. Science over stigma: lessons and future direction of HIV-to-HIV transplantation. *Curr Transplant Rep*. 2021;8(4):314–323.

Kopp JB, Nelson GW, Sampath K, et al. Genetic variants in focal segmental glomerulosclerosis and HIV-associated nephropathy. *J Am Soc Nephrol*. 2011;22(11):2129–2137.

Koteff J, Borland J, Chen S, et al. A phase 1 study to evaluate the effect of dolutegravir on renal function via measured iohexol and PAH clearance in healthy subjects. *Br J Clin Pharmacol*. 2013;75:990–996.

Kudose S, Santoriello, Bomback AS, et al. The spectrum of kidney biopsy findings in HIV-infected patients in the modern era. *Kidney Int*. 2020;97(5):1006–1016.

Kupin WL. Viral-associated GN: hepatitis C and HIV. *Clin J Am Soc Nephrol*. 2017;12(8):1337–1342. http://doi:10.2215/CJN.04320416

Landovitz RJ, Donnell D, Clement ME, et al. Cabotegravir for HIV prevention in cisgender men and transgender women. *N Engl J Med*. 2021;385(7):595–608.

Lepist EI, Murray BP, Tong L, et al. Effect of cobicistat and ritonavir on proximal renal tubular cell uptake and efflux transporters. [Abstract A1-1724]. Presented at the 51st Interscience Conference on Antimicrobial Agents and Chemotherapy (ICAAC). Chicago, IL; September 17–20, 2011.

Lescure FX, Flateau C, Pacanowski J, et al. HIV-associated kidney glomerular diseases: changes with time and HAART. *Nephrol Dial Transplant*. 2012;27:2349–2355.

Lindeman TA, Dugan JM, Sahloff EG. Evaluation of serum creatinine changes with integrase inhibitor use in HIV-1 infected adults. *Open Forum Infect Dis*. 2016;3(2):1–3.

Locke JE, James NT, Mannon RB, et al. Immunosuppression regimen and the risk of acute rejection in HIV-infected kidney transplant recipients. *Transplantation*. 2014;97(4):446–450.

Locke JE, Mehta S, Reed RD, et al. l A national study of outcomes among HIV-infected kidney transplant recipients. *J Am Soc Nephrol*. 2015;26(9):2222–2229

Longenecker CT, Scherzer R, Bacchetti P, et al. HIV viremia and changes in kidney function. *AIDS*. 2009;23(9):1089–1096.

Lopes JA, Melo MJ, Raimundo M, et al. Long-term risk of mortality for acute kidney injury in HIV-infected patients: a cohort analysis. *BMC Nephrol*. 2013;14:32.

Lucas GM, Eustace JA, Sozio S, et al. Highly active antiretroviral therapy and the incidence of HIV-1-associted nephropathy: a 12-year cohort study. *AIDS*. 2004;18(3):541–546.

Makris K, Spanou L. Acute kidney injury: definition, pathophysiology, and clinical phenotypes. *Clin Biochem Review*. 2016;37(2):85–98.

Mallipattu SK, Salem F, Wyatt CM. The changing epidemiology of HIV-related chronic kidney disease in the era of antiretroviral therapy. *Kidney Int*. 2014;86(2):259–265.

Markowitz M, Zolopa A, Squires K, et al. Phase I/II study of the pharmacokinetics, safety and antiretroviral activity of tenofovir alafenamide, a new prodrug of the HIV reverse transcriptase inhibitor tenofovir, in HIV-infected adults. *J Antimicrob Chemother*. 2014;69(5):1362–1369.

McLaughlin MM, Guerrero AJ, Merker A. Renal effects of nontenofovir antiretroviral therapy in patients living with HIV. *Drugs Context*. 2018;7:1–15.

Medapalli RK, He JC, Klotman JP. HIV-associated nephropathy: pathogenesis. *Curr Opin Nephrol Hypertens*. 2011;20(3):306–311.

Medapalli RK, Parikh CR, Gordon K, et al. Comorbid diabetes and the risk of progressive chronic kidney disease in HIV-infected adults: data from the Veterans Aging Cohort Study. *J Acquir Immune Defic Syndr*. 2012;60(4):393–399.

Mills A, Arribas JR, Andrade-Villanueva J, et al. Switching from tenofovir disoproxil fumarate to tenofovir alafenamide in antiretroviral regimens for virologically suppressed adults with HIV-1 infection: a randomised, active-controlled, multicentre, open-label, phase 3, non-inferiority study. *Lancet Infect Dis*. 2016;16(1):43–52.

Mocroft A, Kirk O, Reiss P, et al. Estimated glomerular filtration rate, chronic kidney disease and antiretroviral drug use in HIV-positive patients. *AIDS*. 2010;24(11):1667–1678.

Mocroft A, Lundgren JD, Ross M, et al. Cumulative and current exposure to potentially nephrotoxic antiretrovirals and development of chronic kidney disease in HIV-positive individuals with a normal baseline estimated glomerular filtration rate: a prospective international cohort study. *Lancet HIV*. 2016;3(1):e23–e32.

Mocroft A, Lundgren JD, Ross M, et al.; D:A:D Study Group Royal Free Hospital Clinic Cohort, Insight Study Group, Smart Study Group and Espirit Study Group. Development and validation of a risk score for chronic kidney disease in HIV infection using protective cohort data from the D:A:D study. *PLoS Med*. 2015;12(3):e1001809.

Molina JM, Ward D, Brar I, et al. Switching to fixed-dose bictegravir, emtricitabine, and tenofovir alafenamide from dolutegravir plus abacavir and lamivudine in virologically suppressed adults with HIV-1: 48-week results of a randomised, double-blind, multicentre, active-controlled, phase 3, non-inferiority trial. *Lancet HIV*. 2018;5(7):357–365.

Mounzer K, Brunet L, Wyatt CM, et al. To dose-adjust or not to dose-adjust: lamivudine dose in kidney impairment. *AIDS*. 2021;35(8):1201–1208.

Naicker S, Fabian J. Risk factors for the development of chronic kidney disease with HIV/AIDS. *Clin Nephrol*. 2010;74(Suppl 1):S51–S56.

Ndlovu KCZ, Assounga A. Continuous ambulatory peritoneal dialysis in patients with HIV and end-stage renal failure. *Perit Dial Int*. 2017;37(3):321–330.

Neuen BL, Young T, Heerspink HJL, et al. SGLT2 inhibitors for the prevention of kidney failure in patients with type 2 diabetes: a systematic review and meta-analysis. *Lancet Diabetes Endocrinol*. 2019;7(11):845–854.

NovickT K, Choi MJ, Rosenberg AZ, et al. Tenofovir alafenamide nephrotoxicity in an HIV-positive patient. *Medicine*. 2017;96(36):e8046.

Orkin C, Oka S, Philibert P, et al. Long-acting cabotegravir plus rilpivirine for treatment in adults with HIV-1 infection: 96-week results of the randomised, open-label, phase 3 FLAIR study [published correction appears in *Lancet HIV*. December 2021;8(12):e734]. *Lancet HIV*. 2021;8(4):e185–e196.

Palich R, Tubiana R, Abdi B, et al. Plasma cystatin C as a marker for estimated glomerular filtration rate assessment in HIV-1-infected patients treated with dolutegravir-based ART. *J Antimicrob Chemother*. 2018;73(7):1935–1939.

Papeta N, Kiryluk K, Patel A, et al. APOL1 variants increase risk for FSGS and HIVAN but not IgA nephropathy. *J Am Soc Nephrol*. 2011;22(11):1991–1996.

Parasrampuria R, Ford SL, Lou Y, et al. A phase I study to evaluate the pharmacokinetics and safety of cabotegravir in adults with severe renal impairment and healthy matched control participants. *Clin Pharmacol Drug Dev*. 2019;8(5):674–681.

Park LS, Hernández-Ramírez RU, Silverberg MJ, Crothers K, Dubrow R. Prevalence of non-HIV cancer risk factors in persons living with HIV/AIDS: a meta-analysis. *AIDS*. 2016;30(2):273–291.

Pilkington V, Hughes SL, Pepperrell T, et al. Tenofovir alafenamide vs. tenofovir disoproxil fumarate: an updated meta-analysis of 14 894 patients across 14 trials. *AIDS*. 2020;34(15):2259–2268.

Post FA, Holt SG. Recent developments in HIV and the kidney. *Curr Opin Infect Dis*. 2009;22(1):43–48.

Raffi F, Rachlis A Stellbrink HJ, et al. Once-daily dolutegravir versus raltegravir in antiretroviral-naïve adults with HIV-1 infection: 48-week results from the randomized, double-blind, non-inferiority SPRING-2 Study. *Lancet*. 2013;381(9868):735–743.

Rao TK, Filippone EJ, Nicastri AD, et al. Associated focal and segmental glomerulosclerosis in the acquired immunodeficiency syndrome. *N Engl J Med*. 1984;310(11):669–673.

Rathbun RC, Lockhart SM, Miller MM, et al. Dolutegravir, a second-generation integrase inhibitor for the treatment of HIV-1 infection. *Ann Pharmacother*. 2014;48(3):395–403.

Razzak CS, Workeneh BT, Montez-Rath ME, et al. Trends in the out-comes of end-stage renal disease secondary to HIV-associated nephropathy. *Nephrol Dial Transplant*. 2015;30:1734–1740.

Rockwood N, Mandalia S, Bower M, et al. Ritonavir-boosted atazanavir exposure is associated with an increased rate of renal stones compared with efavirenz, ritonavir-boosted lopinavir and ritonavir-boosted darunavir. *AIDS*. 2011;25(13):1671–1673.

Ross MJ, Klotman PE. Recent progress in HIV-associated nephropathy. *J Am Soc Nephrol.* 2002;13(12):2997–3004.

Ryom L, Lundgren JD, Law M, et al. Serious clinical events in HIV-positive persons with chronic kidney disease. *AIDS.* 2019a;33(14):2173–2188.

Ryom L, Dilling Lundgren J, Reiss P, et al. Use of contemporary protease inhibitors and risk of incident chronic kidney disease in persons with human immunodeficiency virus: the Data Collection on Adverse Events of Anti-HIV Drugs (D:A:D) study. *J Infect Dis.* 2019b;220(10):1629–1634.

Sax PE, Erlandson KM, Lake JE, et al. Weight gain following initiation of antiretroviral therapy: risk factors in randomized comparative clinical trials. *Clin Infect Dis.* 2020;71(6):1379–1389.

Sax PE, Pozniak A, Montes ML, et al. Co-formulated bictegravir, emtricitabine, and tenofovir alafenamide versus dolutegravir with emtricitabine and tenofovir alafenamide, for initial treatment of HIV-1 infection (GS-US-380-1490): a randomised, double-blind, multicentre, phase 3, non-inferiority trial. *Lancet.* 2017;390(10107):2073–2082.

Scherzer R, Estrella M, Li Y, et al. Association of tenofovir exposure with kidney disease risk in HIV infection. *AIDS.* 2012;26(7):867–875.

Schwarze-Zander C, Piduhn H, Boesecke C, et al. Switching tenofovir disoproxil fumarate to tenofovir alafenamide in a real-life setting: what are the implications? *HIV Med.* 2020;21(6):378–385.

Stellbrink HJ, Reynes J, Lazzarin A, et al. Dolutegravir in antiretroviral-naive adults with HIV-1: 96-week results from a randomized dose-ranging study. *AIDS.* 2013;27(11):1771–1778.

Strategies for Management of Antiretroviral Therapy (SMART) Study Group. CD4\+ count-guided interruption of antiretroviral treatment. *N Engl J Med.* 2006;355(22):2283–2296.

Swanepoel CR, Atta MG, D'Agati, et al. Kidney disease in the setting of HIV INFECTION: CONCLUSIONS from A Kidney Disease: Improving Global Outcomes (Kdigo) Patient Controversies Conference. *Kidney Int.* 2018;22(6):84–100.

Tzur S, Rosset S, Shemer R, et al. Missense mutations in the APOL1 gene are highly associated with end stage kidney disease risk previously attributed to the MYH9 gene. *Hum Genet.* 2010;128(3):345–350.

ViiV Healthcare. Cabotegravir package insert. https://viivhcmedinfo.com/search-medical-scientific-information/viiv-document-viewer?cmd=GSKMedicalInformation&token=23108-86586 58d-fc8a-4281-ac8a-3e811bf65d33&dns=gsk-medcomms.veevavault.com&medcommid=REF--US-000964&product=Cabotegravir+and+Rilpivirine. Published 2022. Accessed September 30, 2022.

Waheed S, Atta MG. Predictors of HIV-associated nephropathy. *Expert Rev Anti-Infect Ther.* 2014;12(5):555–563.

Wei A, Burns G, Williams CM, et al. Long-term renal survival in HIV-associated nephropathy with angiotensin-converting enzyme inhibition. *Kidney Int.* 2003;64(4):1462–1471.

Wyatt CM, Hoover DR, Shi Q, et al. Pre-existing albuminuria predicts AIDS and non-AIDS mortality in women initiating antiretroviral therapy. *Antiviral Ther.* 2011;16(4):591–596.

Zheng X, Gong L, Xue W, et al. Kidney transplant outcomes in HIV-positive patients: a systematic review and meta-analysis. *AIDS Res Ther.* 2019;16(1):37

41.

HIV AND BONE HEALTH

Roger Bedimo

LEARNING OBJECTIVES

- Discuss the prevalence of low bone mineral density (BMD) and fractures in persons living with HIV (PWH).

- Describe the risk factors associated with diminished BMD and fractures in PWH.

- Discuss the potential pathogenic mechanisms of decreased bone health and increased fracture risk in PWH.

- List the screening indications and diagnostic tests used to identify bone disease and fracture risk in PWH.

- Discuss current treatment strategies for PWH found to have low BMD or who have sustained bone fractures.

WHAT'S NEW?

- With the increased survival of PWH (now approaching that of HIV-negative persons), the burden of comorbidity is significantly increasing; these include increased fracture risk.

- Persistent excess mortality in PWH in the modern antiretroviral therapy (ART) era is driven by noncommunicable diseases including fracture risk.

- PWH have lower lumbar spine and hip BMD than uninfected controls.

- A meta-analysis confirmed that HIV confers a 1.51-times increased risk of fragility fracture and a 4.05-times increased risk of hip fracture. The increased risk is not completely explained by differences in BMD alone, indicating there may be differences because of quality of bone or other HIV-related factors contributing to the marked fracture risk. More studies confirm that PWH have an increased risk of not only osteoporotic fractures, but all fracture.

- Incident fracture is associated with almost 50% greater risk of all-cause death among PWH in the United States. Postfracture, age- and sex-adjusted all-cause mortality rates per 100 person years (py) decreased significantly in the past couple of decades (Battalora et al., 2021), likely reflecting advances in HIV care.

- HIV itself impacts bone development in children, but initiation of antiretroviral therapy (ART) is associated with further decline in BMD and increased fracture risk.

- HIV infection and menopausal stage were independent predictors of lower BMD and had an additive effect on lumbar spine and total hip BMD Hepatitis C coinfection is associated with a significantly higher risk of fracture among PWH, despite the fact that HIV/hepatitis C virus (HCV) coinfection has not been associated more so with BMD than HIV or HCV alone in all studies.

KEY POINTS

- Multiple cohort studies have found a higher-than-expected prevalence of low BMD in populations of adults living with HIV.

- Fracture prevalence is greater in PWH compared to the general population. Incident fracture rates among PWH in the HIV Outpatient Study (HOPS) were increased nearly threefold compared to those for the US general population.

- Asymptomatic vertebral fractures are highly prevalent among PWH aged 50 years and older.

- More studies confirm that PWH have an increased risk of not only osteoporotic fractures, but all fractures.

- Cohort studies suggest that, in addition to traditional factors (e.g., age, smoking, and HCV coinfection, frailty, prolonged amenorrhea, and proteinuria), HIV disease-associated factors and ART factors are predictive indicators of fracture risk in PWH.

- ART initiation is associated with a BMD decrease of 2%–6%, with the largest decrease occurring in the first 6–12 months of treatment and then stabilizing.

- Greater BMD losses occur with initiation of zidovudine, tenofovir disoproxil fumarate (TDF), and protease inhibitors.

- Bisphosphonates can safely be administered to PWH with evidence supporting durable gains in BMD, including among youth with HIV.

- Incident fracture is associated with significantly increased all-cause mortality in PWH. However, postfracture mortality rates per 100 py decreased significantly in the past couple of decades, likely reflecting advances in HIV care.

- There are limited HIV-specific evidence-based recommendations regarding screening for bone disease, although extrapolation of screening recommendations from the general population is reasonable. Several organizations recommend using dual-energy X-ray absorptiometry (DXA) and/or the Fracture Risk Assessment Tool (FRAX) for screening of PWH aged 50 years and older.

- If the FRAX 10-year probability exceeds 20% for major osteoporotic fractures or 3% risk for hip fracture, Bone Health and Osteoporosis Foundation (BHOF) guidelines recommend initiating drug treatment.

INTRODUCTION

With improved long-term survival among persons living with HIV (PWH), age-related comorbidities, including osteoporosis and fragility fractures, have become more prevalent (Pramukti et al., 2020; Kim et al., 2021; Jespersen et al., 2021). There is increasing evidence that cardiovascular, renal, and bone disease and neurocognitive deficits are more common among long-term PWH with negative interactions between these comorbidities. Data from cohort and prospective randomized studies suggest that, for a multitude of reasons, PWH are at increased risk of metabolic bone disease and related fractures (Chang et al., 2021; Zhang et al., 2022).

BONE MINERALIZATION ABNORMALITIES

The World Health Organization (WHO) defines two categories of bone abnormalities based on comparison with the mean BMD of young healthy women (*T*-score): (1) osteoporosis, low bone mass and microarchitectural deterioration of bone tissue, BMD value more than 2.5 standard deviations below the mean BMD of young adult women (BMD *T*-score < −2.5), and (2) osteopenia, low bone mass, BMD value between 1 and 2.5 standard deviations below the mean BMD of young adult women (−2.5 < BMD *T*-score < −1) (WHO, 1994; Woolf & Pfleger, 2003). Osteomalacia is a third type of bone mineralization abnormality and refers to softening of bones because of impaired bone mineralization typically resulting from severe vitamin D deficiency (McComsey et al., 2010; WHO, 2002). Osteonecrosis or avascular necrosis is another bone abnormality resulting from interrupted blood supply to a bone or part of a bone, commonly occurring as a complication of trauma or fracture and typically located at the articular end of a bone (WHO, 2002).

HIV itself impacts bone development in children (Rukuni et al., 2021), but initiation of ART is associated with further decline in BMD and increased fracture risk (Guo et al., 2021). The long-term metabolic consequences of HIV and ART need further evaluation. Additional data highlight significant differences between men and women living with HIV.

Bone strength is a function of bone density and bone quality. Bone quality refers to rate of remodeling, microarchitecture, size, shape, amount of mineralization in the bone, and matrix quality (Yin et al., 2012a). Rate of remodeling is measured from serum levels of the bone turnover markers osteocalcin (OCN; a formation marker) and N-terminal telopeptide (NTX; a resorption marker). Microarchitecture is observed with computed tomography (CT) imaging. Mineralization quantity and matrix quality can be determined by biopsy, but this is rarely indicated. The importance of considering the microarchitecture or quality of bone was highlighted in a recent study from the Women's Interagency HIV Study (WIHS) (Sharma et al., 2018). In this analysis including 319 women with HIV and 118 without HIV, loss of BMD by DXA was similar between the two groups. However, the bone microarchitecture or quality of bone was significantly worse in the women with HIV. The effects of HIV on bone health are more complex than mere quantification by DXA alone.

PREVALENCE OF LOW BONE MINERAL DENSITY IN PWH

Multiple cohort studies have found a higher-than-expected prevalence of low BMD in populations of adults living with HIV (Brown & Qaqish, 2006). Notably, these studies represent diverse populations of PWH, including ART-naive and ART-experienced patients (Bedimo et al., 2012; Escota et al., 2016; McComsey et al., 2011). A meta-analysis of 29 studies of BMD in PWH confirmed the preceding information (Goh et al., 2018). The prevalence of osteopenia and osteoporosis was 2.4–3.4 times higher in PWH compared to HIV-uninfected adults depending on site (lumbar spine and hip). Traditional risk factors (i.e., low BMI, history of fracture, older age, being Hispanic or Caucasian, low testosterone levels, smoking, low CD4 $^+$ T-cell counts, low lean and fat mass, and lipodystrophy) were associated with low BMD. Persons treated with TDF as part of their ART regimen were also more likely to have low BMD compared to nonusers (53% vs. 43%), but the difference was not statistically significant.

Using data from the Study to Understand the Natural History of HIV and AIDS in the Era of Effective Therapy (SUN Study)—a prospective, observational cohort study funded by the Centers for Disease Control and Prevention (CDC)—researchers determined that low BMD at the hip and femoral neck was significantly more prevalent in PWH than in matched controls from NHANES (47% vs. 29%; $p < 0.001$). In this cohort of 653 participants (77% male, median age 41 years, median CD4 $^+$ T-cell count 464; 89% with HIV RNA levels < 400 copies/mL), 51% of participants had osteopenia and 10% had osteoporosis at baseline (Escota et al., 2015).

There are some data from resource-limited settings regarding low BMD in PWH. In one South African cohort of 444 PWH (median age, 35 years; 77% women), low BMD (Z-score < –2 standard deviations (SD)) was found in 17% of participants at the lumbar spine and 5% at the hip (Dave, 2015). This study found that median total hip and femoral neck BMD were lower among those receiving ART than in ART-naive participants. Similarly, femoral neck BMD was lower among ART-receiving compared to ART-naive participants. In addition, vitamin D deficiency was found in 15% of cohort participants and associated with efavirenz use. In multivariate analysis, exposure to efavirenz- or lopinavir/ritonavir-based ART was associated with lower total hip BMD. Having a higher weight, being male, and increased vitamin D levels were associated with higher total hip BMD. Additional factors independently associated with lower lumbar spine BMD included advanced age, weight, sex, and efavirenz use (Dave et al., 2015).

BONE HEALTH IN POSTMENOPAUAL WOMEN WITH HIV

Postmenopausal women with HIV demonstrate a greater decline in BMD. In a longitudinal study of bone loss in this specific population, higher rates of bone decline at the spine and forearm were observed compared to HIV-negative women (Yin & Overton, et al., 2011). Thus, higher rates of bone loss at the spine and forearm of women described in this study coupled with increased fracture prevalence among PWH suggest that an increased rate of fractures in postmenopausal women with HIV is concerning (Triant et al., 2008). Similarly, an older study found higher rates of bone loss in men with HIV older than age 50 years (Orwoll & Klein, 1995). However, there are still little data on bone loss for PWH aged older than 65 years, the period in which fractures are most prevalent in the general population.

In a recent cohort analysis, compared to HIV-negative women, women with HIV had 5%–9% lower BMD at all sites (including the lumbar spine, femoral neck, and wrist). The prevalence of osteoporosis was significantly higher among women with HIV. In fully adjusted models, HIV independently predicted reduced BMD. HIV infection and menopausal stage were independent predictors of lower BMD and had an additive effect on lumbar spine and total hip BMD (Sharma et al., 2022). The investigators concluded that additional research was needed to better understand underlying mechanisms by which HIV impacts BMD mitigate osteoporosis and fracture risk in aging populations.

TRAJECTORIES OF BONE MINERAL DENSITY IN PWH—ROLE OF ART

In the general population, BMD peaks at approximately 22–35 years of age (Orwoll & Klein, 1995). BMD appears to decrease by 2%–6% during the first 1–2 years of ART (Brown et al., 2009). Until recently, it was believed that PWH subsequently experienced relative stability regarding BMD although a recent longitudinal study contradicts this belief.

Grant and colleagues (2016) followed 97 PWH for a median of 7.5 years after ART initiation and compared their BMD data to that from 614 HIV-negative controls. While the rate of BMD loss after week 96 slowed in the cohort of PWH, the decline in lumbar spine BMD (but not at the total hip) remained significantly greater than that seen in the HIV-negative cohort. These data suggest ongoing metabolic bone disease despite HIV suppression with ART.

Conversely, an analysis of 384 participants of the European UPBEAT cohort found that while there was no difference in the rate of lumbar spine BMD change between HIV-positive and HIV-negative participants ($p = 0.51$), there was a trend toward greater decline in femoral neck BMD ($p = 0.08$) (Tinago et al., 2017). However, this study population was very young (median age 39), and those aged older than 30 years had a greater BMD decline. An analysis of incidence and predictors of fracture in 4640 HIV-positive participants from ACTG trials followed for a median of 5 years showed higher osteoporotic fracture rates within the first 2 years after ART initiation. Continuation of ART was not associated with increased fracture rates (Yin, 2012b). Again, the study population was relatively young (median age of 39 years).

Hoy (2015) reported results from the Strategic Timing of Antiretroviral Treatment (START) BMD substudy (INSIGHT START Study Group, 2015). The primary START study enrollment consisted of 4,685 adult PWH from 35 countries with CD4 $^+$ T- cell counts of greater than 500 cells/mm^3; the median age was 36 years, and 27% were female. Participants were randomly assigned to start ART at study entry or delay therapy until CD4 $^+$ T-cell count fell below 350 cells/mm^3 or development of AIDS or another condition that dictated the use of ART (deferred-initiation group). In the BMD substudy of this trial, 193 participants were randomly assigned to the early ART group and 204 to the deferred ART group (Hoy et al., 2015). Substudy participants underwent DXA scans of the lumbar spine, total hip, and femoral neck at baseline and annually thereafter. Mean follow-up time was 2.2 years. Hoy reported significantly greater loss of BMD at both the hip and the spine in participants randomly assigned to early ART. There was difference in the development of osteoporosis between groups or incident fractures in the main START study (Hoy et al., 2015). More data are needed on the change in BMD among persons who initiate ART with a high/normal CD4 $^+$ T-cell count, as in the START trial.

HIGHER PREVALENCE AND INCIDENCE OF FRACTURES IN PWH

Numerous studies have concluded that PWH are at greater risk of bone fractures. Triant and colleagues (2008) presented findings that fracture prevalence was greater in women and men who are HIV-positive compared to the general population. Based on an analysis of more than 11 years of data from a large US single healthcare database, she determined that PWH had a higher number of vertebral, hip, wrist, and combined fractures compared with HIV-negative participants. These findings were consistent across age, race, and sex categories, but no correlations were made as to specific risk factors because of lack of data. A recent review article highlighted that the heterogeneity and small sample size of studies of fractures among PWH make this a challenging topic to study (Premaor & Compston, 2018). However, despite a wide range of incident fractures among PWH, ranging from 0.1/1,000 py to 11.3 fractures/1,000 py, HIV is consistently associated with an approximately twofold increased risk of fracture (Pramukti et al., 2020).

Several large observational studies published findings correlating fracture incidence in PWH compared to control groups. Differences in population, controls, and fracture definitions (i.e., fracture and fragility fracture definitions) were unique to each study. The WIHS reported fracture incidence in 1,728 positive and 663 HIV-negative premenopausal women (Yin et al., 2010). Rates of fracture were not increased in women with HIV compared to HIV-negative women. However, in the women with HIV, having a history of an AIDS-defining illness was a more predictive indicator of fracture than being on ART.

Incident fractures rates among PWH in the HOPS study were increased nearly threefold compared to rates in the US general population between 2000 and 2006 (Young et al., 2011). Rates of first fractures at any anatomic site were analyzed in 5,826 participants (median baseline age of 40 years, 79% male, and 73% ART). Later analysis of the HOPS study, from 2000–2017, showed incident fracture is associated with almost 50% greater risk of all-cause death among PWH in the United States (Battalora et a., 2021). Postfracture, age- and sex-adjusted all-cause mortality rates per 100 py decreased significantly in the past couple of decades, likely reflecting advances in HIV care. Rates of fracture were indirectly standardized to the general population by age and sex using data from patients in the National Hospital Ambulatory Medical Care Survey (NHAMCS-OPD). Greater proportions of fractures were located at the hip, wrist, or spine in PWH. In this cohort, fractures were associated with lower CD4[+] T-cell count nadir, longer duration of HIV diagnosis, and HIV/HCV coinfection. The study suggested that younger PWH, particularly those between ages 25 and 54 years, are at an increased risk of bone fracture compared to the general population. On the basis of these data, the authors recommended regular assessment of PWH for fracture risk and particularly those with low nadir CD4[+] T-cell counts and other recognized fracture risk factors.

In the all-male Veterans Aging Cohort Study Virtual Cohort (VACS-VC) study, researchers reported that men with HIV were at greater risk for fragility fracture compared to HIV-negative counterparts (Womack et al., 2011). In this study of 119,318 men—of whom 33% were HIV-positive, 34% of this group were 50 years or older at baseline, and 55% were black or Hispanic. Fracture risk factors included age, race, alcohol dependency, liver disease, tobacco smoking, or current use of corticosteroids or proton pump inhibitors.

Hansen and colleagues (2012) studied the incidence of fragility fractures in HIV-infected individuals not being treatment with ART and PWH on ART in the Danish HIV Cohort. This was a comparative, sex- and age-matched study involving 5,306 PWH and a general population cohort of 26,530 HIV-negative participants. The PWH had an increased overall rate of fractures, an increased risk of low-energy fractures but not high-energy fractures. There was a moderate increased risk of low-energy fracture in PWH undergoing ART when controlled for traditional osteoporosis risk factors of age and cigarette smoking.

In the AIDS Clinical Trials Group A5224s, a substudy of ACTG A5202, McComsey and colleagues (2011) concluded that fracture rates increased in 269 participants during the first 2 years of ART initiated during the clinical trial compared to additional years of therapy. Although differences in BMD change were observed between patients who initiated different ART regimens, no significant differences in fracture rate were reported, although the cohort was young and follow-up was limited (Yin & Overton, 2011).

Osteoporotic fractures were associated with cumulative exposure to TDF and other ART in a large retrospective cohort study (56,600 patients) with a mean age of 45 years (Bedimo et al., 2012). However, 95% of this cohort was male, limiting the ability to generalize the conclusion to females.

Another publication highlighted an underappreciated fracture: asymptomatic vertebral fractures (Llop et al., 2018). In this cohort of 93 male and 35 females (mean age of 57 years), with more than 70% having low BMD at both hip and spine by DXA, 20% were found to have an asymptomatic vertebral fracture. Factors associated with these fractures included older age, longer time since HIV diagnosis, and renal insufficiency. The authors concluded that routine spinal imaging with plain X-rays should be considered in the aging HIV population.

Starup-Linde and colleagues (2020) performed a meta-analysis that included 84 papers focused on bone health and fracture risk in the setting of HIV. They concluded that HIV infection is associated with a significant increase in incident fragility fracture (HR 1.51) and a marked increased risk of hip fracture (HR 4.05). The increased risk was not explained by the differences in BMD alone, thus indicating a difference in quality of bone or other factors related to HIV disease.

Findings from several cohort studies have contributed to the developing field of fracture incidence in PWH. Among 1,006 participants from two CDC-funded cohorts (median age, 43 years; 83% male; median CD4[+] T-cell count 461 cells/mm³) osteopenia was found in 36% of participants and osteoporosis in 4%. A prior fracture was documented in 67 participants. During 4,068 patient years of observation after DXA scanning, 85 incident fractures occurred. These were predominantly rib/sternum ($n = 18$), hand ($n = 14$), foot ($n = 13$), and wrist ($n = 11$). Low BMD (osteopenia and/or osteoporosis) was diagnosed in nearly 40% of the participants. Associated risk factors for fractures included older age, lower nadir CD4[+] T-cell count, male–male sex HIV transmission risk, and prior history of fracture. Fourfold higher fracture rates were observed in PWH with osteoporosis compared to PWH with normal BMD. In multivariable analyses, osteoporosis and current/prior tobacco use were associated with incident fracture (Battalora et al., 2016).

In addition to traditional risk factors such as older age and smoking, HIV-associated factors (CD4 $^+$ T-cell count nadir) and ART factors are important predictive indicators of fracture risk in HIV-infected individuals (Yin, 2012a). In the 2022 *Clinician's Guide to Prevention and Treatment of Osteoporosis*, the BHOF included AIDS/HIV as disease risk factors for osteoporosis and fragility fractures (Battalora et al., 2014; LeBoff et al., 2022).

It is therefore abundantly documented that the incidence of osteoporotic fractures (OF) is also higher among PWH than age-matched uninfected participants (Triant et al., 2008; Womack et al., 2011; Young et al., 2011). Recent research has identified additional mediators of fracture risk in the setting of HIV.

About 15%–30% of PWH are coinfected with hepatitis C (HCV), which further increases OF risk (Bedimo et al., 2012; Hansen et al., 2012; Lo Re et al., 2012). HIV/HCV-coinfected patients have a threefold higher fracture incidence compared to uninfected individuals (Dong et al., 2014; Hansen et al., 2012), and up to twice the fracture risk of HIV-monoinfected participants (Hansen et al., 2012; Lo Re et al., 2012; Maalouf et al., 2013). Despite being consistently associated with higher OF risk in several reports (Hansen et al., 2012; Maalouf et al., 2013; Yin et al., 2010, 2012; Young et al., 2011), HCV coinfection has only been associated with further reductions in BMD among PWH in some (Anastos et al., 2007; Lawson-Ayayi et al., 2013), but not all studies (Bedimo et al., 2016; Lo Re et al., 2009). These findings raise the possibility that the higher fracture risk observed in patients with chronic HCV infection might not be due to low BMD alone but could involve other mechanism(s). In a large cohort of HIV-positive US Veterans, HCV coinfection remained a strong independent OF predictor, even after controlling for the presence of cirrhosis (Hazard ratio (HR): 1.31; 95% confidence interval (CI): 1.12–1.52; $p < 0.001$) (Maalouf et al., 2013). Therefore, severity of liver disease only partly explains the HCV-associated increased risk of OF (El-Maouche et al., 2011). Also, HIV/HCV coinfection is not associated with significantly lower femoral neck or lumbar spine BMD than HIV mono-infection (Bedimo et al., 2016).

Frailty, a phenotype generally seen in geriatric populations, has been recognized to occur at earlier age among PWH. Sharma and colleagues (2019), from the WIHS Cohort, reported that frailty was not only more common among women with HIV than their HIV-negative counterparts, but it was also independently associated to time to first fracture as well as second fracture. Sarcopenia, or the gradual loss of muscle mass, is a key component of frailty and has long been recognized as a complication of HIV infection. It is not surprising that frailty is linked to fracture risk.

From the MACS cohort, researchers have also linked proteinuria to fragility fractures. In this cohort of both HIV-negative men and men living with HIV, the presence of proteinuria, which was more common among men with HIV, conferred a 230% increase risk of fragility fracture (Gonciulea et al., 2019). These data highlight how chronic comorbidities often cluster in PWH and can significantly complicate long-term management beyond the use of ART.

PATHOPHYSIOLOGY AND RISK FACTORS

Bone loss in PWH is likely multifactorial, involving three common elements: the host, the virus, and ART. Lower bone density in PWH is attributable to host risks, including smoking, alcohol consumption, exposure to glucocorticoids, decreased activity, lipodystrophy, HCV coinfection, vitamin D deficiency, weight loss, hypogonadism, and chronic kidney disease.

At least one genetic marker or HLA supertype, specifically HLA-DQ3, has been associated with bone density status in one cohort study of PWH (Haskelberg et al., 2014). HIV may directly affect bone cells by viral protein induction of osteoclastogenesis or by causing osteoblast apoptosis (Raynaud-Messina et al., 2018). Recent data highlight that the effects of HIV proteins on bone loss may not be a direct effect but rather an indirect or bystander effect through mitochondrial toxicity, oxidative stress, or effects on other cell processes (Agidigi & Kim, 2019; Liu et al., 2017). Moreover, T-cell and B-cell activation during HIV infection results in increased circulating cytokines, including tumor necrosis factor-α, interleukin-6 (IL-6), and RANKL, which appear to induce osteoclast bone resorption (Titanji, 2017). In one, elevated levels of IL-6 were associated with risk of progression to osteoporosis among PWH (Hileman et al., 2014). Similar increases in cytokine levels have been reported in other chronic inflammatory diseases (e.g., rheumatoid arthritis).

Worth noting, ART initiation has been associated with a BMD decrease of 2%–6%, with the largest decrease occurring in the first 6–12 months of treatment and then stabilizing (Brown et al., 2009). Greater BMD loss was also seen with the older nucleoside agent zidovudine or AZT (van Vonderen et al., 2009) and is well documented with the use of TDF (McComsey et al., 2011; Yin & Overton, 2011). In addition, protease inhibitors (PIs) contribute to bone loss in the setting of HIV infection, which appears to be a class effect observed with all PIs that have been studied (McComsey et al., 2011; Moran et al., 2016). Fracture rates, both fragility and non-fragility, as noted previously, are higher in PWH and associated with HCV coinfection and possibly ART (Bedimo et al., 2012; Maalouf et al., 2013). Currently, the pooled estimate of fracture incidence is noted to be 11.3 per 1,000 py, which will likely increase as the population of PWH ages (Pramukti et al., 2020).

EFFECT OF ANTIRETROVIRALS ON BONE FRAGILITY AMONG PWH

The initiation of ART in HIV patients produces a universal decrease in BMD. However changes in BMD are more pronounced with exposure to TDF than to other antiretroviral agents in treatment-naive (McComsey et al., 2011; Stellbrink et al., 2010) or experienced patients (Cotter et al., 2013; Martin et al., 2009), and are likely mediated by increases in bone turnover.

In a randomized clinical trial, we found that the TDF-sparing regimen raltegravir + darunavir/ritonavir (RAL + DRV/RTV) and the traditional regimen tenofovir/

emtricitabine + darunavir/ritonavir (TDF/FTC + DRV/RTV) led to similar reductions in inflammatory markers (tumor necrosis factor-α), but, unlike TDF/FTC, RAL-based therapy was not associated with any increase in bone turnover markers (BTMs) or decline in BMD (Bedimo et al., 2014). In that study, we also showed that early changes in BTMs at week 16 predicted change in BMD by week 48: R = −0.39, p = 0.003 for C-telopeptide of type 1 collagen (CTX bone resorption marker); and R = −0.48, p < 0.001 for procollagen type 1 N-terminal propeptide (P1NP, bone formation marker). These findings suggest that early evaluation of BTMs might be used in trials or clinical practice to predict bone loss on ART. Our findings were confirmed in large randomized trials recently completed in Europe (NEAT001/ANRS143) (Raffi et al., 2014) and the United States (ACTG 5360s) (Brown et al., 2015). Finally, in a large cohort of HIV-positive US Veterans (56,660 HIV patients; 98.1% male; 31.2% HCV coinfected; mean age: 45.0 years) (Bedimo et al., 2012), we showed that cumulative exposure to TDF (HR 1.12; 95% CI: 1.03–1.21, P = 0.011) and, among protease inhibitors, lopinavir/ritonavir (which is associated with increases in tenofovir concentrations) was predictive of increased OF in the modern ART era. These findings were corroborated by another analysis we have carried out showing that Veterans receiving efavirenz/TDF/FTC had a lower OF risk than receiving other TDF-containing regimens (a), probably because of lower serum levels of tenofovir (LaFleur et al., 2016).

Elevated markers of inflammation and immune activation in patients on long-term suppressive ART (including interleukin-6, TNF-α and c-reactive protein) have been associated with increased risk of non-AIDS complications and mortality (Kuller et al., 2008; Sandler et al., 2011; Tenorio et al., 2014). In a large cohort in the Veterans Health Administration, those initiating TDF-based regimens containing efavirenz (EFV) had lower rates of osteoporotic fractures than those on TDF-based regimens containing protease inhibitors of integrase inhibitors (HR 0.56; 95% CI: 0.42–0.73) (LaFleur et al., 2016).

CLINICAL MANAGEMENT

GENERAL POPULATION SCREENING FOR BONE DISEASE

There are limited evidence-based recommendations for PWH regarding screening for bone disease, although extrapolation of recommendations from the general population is, at a minimum, reasonable.

The International Osteoporosis Foundation and BHOF, formerly the National Osteoporosis Foundation (NOF), in 2022 updated recommendations for clinicians for postmenopausal women and men aged 50 years and older (LeBoff et al., 2022). The reader is advised to consult the complete list of recommendations in the BHOF *The Clinician's Guide to Prevention and Treatment of*

Osteoporosis. A brief listing of the BHOF major recommendations is provided here:

- Counsel patients on risk of osteoporosis and related fractures.

- Advise patient on adequate intake of calcium (at least 1,200 mg/d for women >50 years and men >71 years; 1,000 mg/d for men 50–70 years) and vitamin D (800–1,000 IU/d), including supplements, if necessary, for individuals aged 50 years or older.

- Maintain serum vitamin D sufficiency (≥30 ng/mL but below ≤ 50 ng/mL).

- Recommend regular weight-bearing and muscle-strengthening exercise to reduce risk of falls and fractures.

- Advise against tobacco smoking and excessive alcohol consumption.

- Recommend BMD testing in:
  - Women aged 65 years and older and men aged 70 years or older.
  - Postmenopausal women and men 50–69 years, based on risk (which includes HIV).
  - Postmenopausal women and men >50 years with history of adult-age fracture.

- Assess secondary causes of osteoporosis when identified.

- Initiate medical therapies for patients with hip or vertebral (clinical or morphometric) fractures.

- Initiate therapy in patients with BMD *T*-scores of −2.5 or less at the femoral neck or spine by DXA, after appropriate evaluation.

- Initiate treatment in postmenopausal women and men aged 50 years and older with low bone mass (*T*-score between −1.0 and −2.5, osteopenia) at the femoral neck or spine and a 10-year hip fracture probability 3% or greater or a 10-year major osteoporosis-related fracture probability of 20% or greater based on the US-adapted WHO absolute fracture risk model FRAX.

- Patients taking FDA-approved medications for low BMD should have laboratory and bone density reevaluation after 2 years or more frequently when medically appropriate (LeBoff, 2022).

SCREENING FOR BONE DISEASE IN PWH

The Infectious Disease Society of America Primary Care Guidelines in 2020 recommended "baseline bone densitometry (DXA) screening for osteoporosis should be performed in postmenopausal women and men aged ≥50 years. There is insufficient evidence to guide recommendations for bone density testing in transgender or nonbinary individuals" (Thompson et al., 2021).

The European HIV guidelines (EACS) recommends DXA screening for any patient with one or more of the following conditions, preferably prior to initiation of ART (EACS, 2021):

- Postmenopausal women
- Men aged 50 years and older
- History of low-impact fracture or high risk for falls
- Clinical hypogonadism
- Oral glucocorticoid use
- Those aged between 40 and 50 years with high fracture risk.

The adherence to and the effectiveness of recommended measures in preventing fractures in the HIV population have not been evaluated. Among a national cohort of nearly 5 million male US veterans, there were only 11.5 primary prevention screenings per 1,000 py, a rate far below even the rate of fragility fractures in the same population (15.6 events/1,000 py) (Lafleur et al., 2016). In PWH, bisphosphonate therapy results in significant improvements in BMD (McComsey et al., 2007; Mondy et al., 2005), but the efficacy of these measures in reducing OF incidence needs further evaluation.

REPEAT SCREENING FOR BONE DISEASE

Of those patients that have been appropriately screened, the ideal interval for repeat screening is not clearly defined. In a study of 4,957 women over 67 years of age that were followed prospectively for up to 15 years, the ideal BMD testing interval was defined as the time for 10% of women to develop osteoporosis before having a hip or clinical vertebral fracture (Gourlay et al., 2012). This study found that those initially evaluated with normal BMD had an estimated BMD testing interval of 16.8 years, those with initial mild osteopenia (T-score −1.01 to −1.49) had an estimated BMD testing interval of 17.3 years, those with baseline moderate osteopenia (T-score −1.50 to −1.99) had an estimated BMD testing interval of 4.7 years, and those with severe osteopenia (T-score −2.00 to −2.49) had an estimated BDM testing interval of 1.1 years. This study would suggest that repeat BMD testing may not change significantly in 15 years in patients with normal baseline BMD and in 5 years in those with baseline mild to moderate osteopenia. The importance in avoiding short interval repeat DXA testing was further supported by another cohort study of 310 men and 492 women with a mean age of 74.8 that had two measurements of femoral neck BMD and were not on treatment for osteoporosis (Berry et al., 2013). In this cohort, a second BMD measurement after 4 years did not significantly improve the prediction of hip or major osteoporotic fracture. An additional 2022 prospective cohort study, specifically in 3,651 men, also demonstrated that repeating BMD measurement after 7 years did not improve fracture prediction in community-dwelling older men without HIV (Ensrud et al., 2022).

The lack of benefit of short interval repeat DXA testing for individuals with initial normal or mild osteopenia was also found in a study of 391 PWH who at baseline 28.6% had normal BMD, 49.6% osteopenia, and 21.7% osteoporosis (Negredo et al., 2012). In those with baseline normal BMD, 35.7% progressed to osteopenia, with a median progression time of 6.7 years. Of those with baseline osteopenia, 23.7% progressed to osteoporosis, with a median progression time of >8.5 years. Based on this data, the authors suggest that repeat testing under 6 years may not be necessary in those patients with baseline normal or mildly to moderately osteopenic ranges in PWH.

SCREENING FOR VITAMIN D INSUFFICIENCY

Vitamin D testing and supplementation remains an area of debate among clinicians. Various groups and institutions have published guidance regarding vitamin D deficiency although none are specific for PWH. The National Academy of Medicine, formerly the Institute of Medicine (IOM), 1ublished dietary reference intakes for calcium and vitamin D but did not provide screening recommendations or specific reference intakes for PWH (IOM, 2011). The EACS recommended screening at-risk patients and those on ART and having risk factors for low vitamin D or fracture risks (EACS, 2021). The US Preventive Services Task Force (USPSTF) (2021) and the American Academy of Family Physicians have concluded that the current evidence is insufficient to assess the balance of benefits and harms of screening for vitamin D deficiency in asymptomatic adults (LeFevre & LeFevre, 2018). The USPSTF also recommends against daily supplementation with 400 IU or less of vitamin D and 1,000 mg or less of calcium for the primary prevention of fractures in community-dwelling, postmenopausal women (grade "D" recommendation), while finding the evidence insufficient to assess the risk and harms of vitamin D and calcium supplementation for the primary prevention of fractures in men and premenopausal women (USPSTF et al., 2018). A 2022 report on the Vitamin D and Omega-3 Trial (VITAL) included 25,871 participants who were generally health and aged older than 50 years and found that 2,000 IU daily of vitamin D3 per day did not significantly lower fracture risk (LeBoff et al., 2022). While participants were not specifically selected for vitamin D deficiency, low bone mass, nor osteoporosis, this brings into question the benefits of routine vitamin D supplementation for primary prevention. Additional analysis also did not show fracture reduction in those with low 25-hydroxy vitamin D levels. There are limited data on vitamin D supplementation in PWH although several studies have demonstrated benefit for BMD and reduction in PTH and bone turnover markers (Havens et al., 2018a; Overton, 2015).

SCREENING FOR FALL RISK

Fall risk assessment tools are used to determine the probability of future falls. Typical categories of the assessment tools include fall risk factors (e.g., recent falls, medications, psychological, cognitive status, vision, mobility, transfer, behaviors, activities of daily living, environment, nutrition, continence, and other risk factors). Screening for frailty in the office setting is reasonable and may help identify PWH at heightened risk for falls and fragility fractures.

SCREENING FOR FRACTURE RISK

FRAX

FRAX was developed by the WHO Metabolic Bone Disease Group to assess fractures with more optimal predictors of fracture risk compared to *T*-scores (van den Bergh et al., 2010; WHO Metabolic Bone Disease Group, 2008). This assessment tool is not HIV-specific. FRAX provides the 10-year probability of hip fracture and the 10-year probability of a major osteoporotic fracture (hip, spine, shoulder, or forearm). Probability is estimated based on clinical risk factors and BMD values from the femoral neck (WHO Metabolic Bone Disease Group, 2008). Models have been developed based on location (i.e., Asia, Europe, Middle East and Africa, North America, Latin America, and Oceania) and ethnicity. Risk factors included in the calculation tool are age, sex, weight (kilograms), height (centimeters), previous fracture, parent fractured hip, current tobacco smoking, exposure to glucocorticoids, rheumatoid arthritis, secondary osteoporosis, alcohol intake of three or more units per day, and BMD (g/cm²) or, alternatively, *T*-score based on the NHANES III female reference data (Kanis, 2007).

The International Osteoporosis Foundation, the BHOF, the American Society for Bone and Mineral Research, and the International Society for Clinical Densitometry all endorse the use of FRAX (van den Bergh et al., 2010). The BHOF recommends using FRAX for postmenopausal women and men aged 50 years and older who are not on treatment, who have not had spine or hip fractures, and who have *T*-scores between –1.0 and –2.5 SD (LeBoff et al., 2022; van den Bergh et al., 2010). If the FRAX 10-year probability exceeds 20% for major osteoporotic fractures or 3% risk for hip fracture, BHOF guidelines recommend initiating drug treatment (LeBoff et al., 2022).

Increasing baseline FRAX 10-year probability was consistently associated with increased rates of incident fractures in a large cohort of adults with HIV (Battalora et al., 2014). Although FRAX may underestimate fracture risk in PWH, the EACS recommends FRAX screening in all persons aged 40 years and older (EACS, 2021).

DUAL-ENERGY X-RAY ABSORPTIOMETRY

BMD measurements are widely obtained using DXA scan. Relevant measurement locations include the hip, spine, and forearm. DXA is a two-dimensional system in which the size of the specimen is directly proportional to the estimate of area density. Overestimation of BMD values obtained from larger patients is a concern (Amorosa & Tebas, 2006a). Of greater concern is that DXA unfortunately has not been validated for fractures among PWH. Furthermore, fewer data exist on younger adults except in those taking TDF for pre-exposure prophylaxis. Additional concerns are the application of WHO definitions for osteoporosis and osteopenia to populations and skeletal sites other than those serving as the basis for the DXA correlations on which these bone abnormality definitions are described (Amorosa & Tebas, 2006b).

DXA is noninvasive and convenient, but it does not assess bone condition, bone structure, or bone quality, a factor directly linked to load-bearing strength (Ofotokun et al., 2011). It has been suggested that DXA may underestimate fracture risk in PWH (Ofotokun et al., 2011). In 2007, researchers demonstrated that approximately 50% of postmenopausal women experiencing a fracture did not meet the clinical definition of osteoporosis based on DXA values (Nguyen et al., 2007).

OTHER BMD MEASUREMENT TOOLS

Other BMD measurement tools exist and assist in the prediction of fragility fracture risk but have inherent limitations. Quantitative CT scanning (QCT) detects volumetric density and in some studies has been shown to detect a higher occurrence of osteoporosis and osteopenia (Pitukcheewanont et al., 2005). However, QCT is more expensive than DXA, requires a higher radiation dose, and is mainly used in research settings (Amorosa & Tebas, 2006a). Other tools, including quantitative ultrasound and analysis of biochemical and hormonal markers, may prove increasingly useful in the future.

Trabecular bone score (TBS) is a novel measurement of bone microarchitecture from DXA images. A high TBS value is associated with better bone structure, whereas low TBS values indicate worse bone structure (Silva et al., 2014). TBS is a proven OF predictor, even after adjusting for BMD, and is now included as an independent risk factor in the FRAX algorithm for fracture risk prediction (McCloskey et al., 2016).

Predictors of BMD and TBS were evaluated in a prospective, cross-sectional cohort study of virologically suppressed people with HIV, chronic hepatitis C (HCV), HIV/HCV coinfection, and uninfected controls. In a linear regression, despite both infections being associated with decreased BMD, only HCV, but not HIV, was associated with lower TBS score. Also, HIV/HCV-coinfected participants had lower TBS scores than HIV-monoinfected, HCV-monoinfected, and uninfected participants. Neither the use of TDF nor HCV viremia nor the severity of HCV liver disease was associated with lower TBS (Bedimo et al., 2018). This suggests that microstructural abnormalities underlie some of the higher fracture risk in HCV infection in PWH and the general population. In a recent study, despite significant differences in changes in BMD between the two drugs, there were no differences in TBS changes after initiation of TDF or ABC.

TREATMENT

Treatment of PWH with low BMD and associated complications should consider multiple factors. These include patient profile, patient age, risk factor reduction, potential for drug–drug interactions, underlying hepatic or renal disease, and likelihood of medication adherence.

IDENTIFY AND TREAT SECONDARY CAUSES OF LOW BONE MINERAL DENSITY

For persons with abnormal DXA scans (T-scores of 1 or less) or with a history of a fragility fracture, clinicians should evaluate and address secondary causes of osteoporosis. If low bone mass is identified on DXA or there is a history of a pathological fracture, laboratory evaluation for secondary causes of low BMD should be performed to identify appropriate next steps in treatment. Basic initial testing should include evaluation of serum creatinine, calcium, alkaline phosphatase, 25-hydroxy vitamin D, phosphorus, thyroid-secreting hormone, albumin, alanine aminotransferase (ALT), and a CBC (Camacho et al., 2020). Based initial test results and on a patients personal and family history, additional testing may be indicated. Intact parathyroid (PTH) and a 24-hour urine calcium may be considered in those with identified calcium abnormalities or a history or renal stones. Serum protein electrophoresis with immunofixation may be considered in patients with fragility fractures to assess for multiple myeloma. Bone turnover markers may be considered in those with suspected rapid loss of bone but are not currently recommended to screen for or diagnosis osteoporosis in clinical practice. Assessment of serum testosterone, particularly in men with HIV, can be an important test considering the high prevalence of hypogonadism in PWH.

BEHAVIORAL AND LIFESTYLE ADVICE

Several lifestyle factors including being sedentary and cigarette smoking are associated with low BMD and/or fractures in the general population. Modification of diet to optimize calcium and vitamin D intake, increasing weight-bearing exercise, and smoking cessation are prudent in general but especially among persons at increased risk of low BMD or fractures. Exercise, physical therapy, vision assessments, and environmental assessments have been shown to reduce fall risk (Tricco et al., 2017), while data to support increased physical activity to reduce fractures are less clear. In addition, because excess alcohol consumption (>3 units/d) and substance dependency are associated with fracture risk, strategies to limit or abstain from alcohol consumption should be discussed with patients.

SPECIFIC TREATMENTS FOR BONE LOSS

VITAMIN D AND CALCIUM REPLACEMENT

Vitamin D deficiency is common among PWH and may contribute to low BMD and fractures. Although there are no standardized guidelines for vitamin D and calcium repletion or supplementation, the IOM (2011) published a report providing dietary recommendations for calcium and vitamin D. It suggests 1,000 mg/d of calcium for most adults aged 19–50 years and for men up to age 71 years. No more than 1,200 mg/d of calcium is suggested for women aged older than 50 years and for men and women aged 71 years and older (IOM, 2011).

Specific to PWH, a study in 2014 (ACTG A5280) evaluated the effect of high-dose vitamin D_3 (4,000 IU/d) plus calcium supplementation (1,000 mg/d calcium carbonate) on BMD in 142 PWH (90% male, 33 years; BMI of 24.4 kg/m²; CD4 $^+$ T-cell count, 341 cells/mm³; HIV-1 RNA level, 4.5 $\log_{10}$ copies/mL; and mean 25(OH) vitamin D of 23 ng/mL) with DXA scanning done at baseline and then at week-48 after initiating ART with EFV/FTC/TDF. Supplementation with vitamin D/calcium mitigated loss of BMD particularly at the total hip (Overton, et al., 2014). The effect of vitamin D supplementation has subsequently been corroborated by others. Most notably, Havens and colleagues (2018b) reported on a randomized control trial of high-dose vitamin D. In this study of 214 young PWH (median age 22 years), 50,000 units of vitamin D monthly was associated with a significant increase in lumbar spine BMD (1.2% increase vs. no change in the placebo arm). No effect was seen on hip BMD. The group receiving vitamin D also experienced a significant decline in PTH and bone turnover markers and an increase in serum vitamin D levels.

Assuming minimal sun exposure in geographic regions of the United States and Canada, the IOM suggests 600 IU/d of vitamin D for most persons aged 1–70 years and 800 IUs for persons aged 71 years or older (IOM, 2011). These recommendations are not specific for PWH. However, it may be reasonable to monitor 25-hydroxy vitamin D levels in this population and recommend supplementation in situations of ART initiation and continued therapy if vitamin D levels are low (Overton et al., 2014; Yin et al., 2012a).

TESTOSTERONE REPLACEMENT

Testosterone deficiency is relatively common in men with HIV, especially in the aging population, and it is associated with a decrease in BMD. A recent publication identified the BMD benefits of testosterone supplementation in a cohort of men living with and without HIV (Grant et al., 2019). Testosterone use was more frequently reported in HIV-positive men compared to HIV-negative men (4% vs. 2%, $P < 0.001$). In the overall study population, testosterone use was associated with significantly higher BMD at both the lumbar spine and hip when compared to men not receiving testosterone. Clinicians should assess the risks and benefits of testosterone replacement in PWH with low BMD and low serum testosterone levels.

BISPHOSPHONATES

Currently, there are no specific guidelines for the treatment of BMD disorders among PWH. As noted earlier, diagnosis and management of bone disease among PWH generally follows guidance from the non-HIV population. The BHOF currently recommends pharmacologic treatment of postmenopausal women and men aged 50 and older with hip or vertebral fractures or a T-score of –2.5 or less at the femoral neck or spine after evaluation to exclude secondary causes (NOF, 2014). In addition, patients with a T-score between –1.0 and –2.5 at the femoral neck or spine and 10-year probability fracture by FRAX of 3% or greater at the hip and of 20% or greater for any osteoporosis-related fracture should be considered for treatment (LeBoff et al., 2022).

The class of drugs referred to as bisphosphonates inhibit osteoclast resorption and have can reduce vertebral and nonvertebral fractures by 25%–50% in HIV-negative individuals. These agents are indicated for prevention and treatment of osteoporosis and other bone diseases, including Paget's disease.

The effectiveness of these antiresorptive therapies in PWH has been evaluated in numerous placebo controlled RCTs. Five older studies evaluated patients with *T*-scores not within the osteoporotic range (Bolland et al., 2007; Guaraldi et al., 2004; Huang et al., 2009; McComsey et al., 2007; Mondy et al., 2005). Another trial included patients with *T*-scores of less than –2.5 (Rozenberg et al., 2012). Resulting data showed significant increases in BMD at the lumbar spine in all six studies and a large increase at the hip in three (Bolland et al., 2007; Huang et al., 2009; McComsey et al., 2007). The 2-year treatment trials (Bolland et al., 2007; Rozenberg et al., 2012) demonstrated the greatest change in BMD. Notably, an increase in BMD was detected in the placebo groups that were also given calcium and vitamin D.

Researchers evaluated the use of the intravenous bisphosphonate, zoledronic acid, to mitigate bone loss associated with ART (Hoy et al., 2018). This study included participants on TDF and low BMD and randomly assigned them to a switch from TDF or administration of a single dose of zoledronic acid or placebo. This drug was found to be safe and well-tolerated and was associated with a greater increase in BMD at the hip and lumbar spine (4.6% vs. 2.6% and 7.4% vs. 2.9%, respectively).

Long-term data have been published confirming the beneficial effect of bisphosphonates among PWH. Bolland and colleagues reported data on BMD on 25 men with HIV 11 years after receiving two doses of IV zoledronate. Their BMD remained significantly higher at the lumbar spine (3.7% higher), total hip (3/7% higher), and femoral neck (5.0% higher) compared to those given placebo. Bone turnover markers remained lower in the treatment arm as well suggesting that the effect of the bisphosphonate was mediated through reduced bone turnover (Bolland et al., 2019).

These data were corroborated by another RCT of zoledronate versus placebo that followed 63 PWH with bone loss for three years after treatment. The participants who received a single dose of zoledronate had an 11% increase in BMD at the lumbar spine at three years compared to a 4.3% loss in the placebo arm. More modest differences were seen in the femoral neck and total hip, but these changes did not reach statistical significance (Ofotokun et al., 2020).

A pediatric study evaluated the use of alendronate in perinatally infected children and adolescents with low BMD for age. Fifty-two participants (aged 11–24 years) were randomly assigned to weekly alendronate or placebo for 2 years. The therapy was well-tolerated with similar AEs in both groups and no cases of osteonecrosis or non-healing fractures. The group who received alendronate experienced 20% BMD gains in the lumbar spine at 1-year versus 7% in the placebo arm, with similar differences in the whole-body BMD (Jacobson et al., 2020).

Taken as a whole, these data suggest that bisphosphonates are safe and effective for use in PWH. It is this author's opinion that HIV providers should be more aggressive with the use of bisphosphonates in this high-risk population.

Adverse effects of bisphosphonates include osteonecrosis of the jaw (< 1 case per 100,000 py of exposure) and subtrochanteric fractures or atypical femoral shaft fractures (uncommon in patients with < 5 years of treatment) (Yin, 2012b). Thus, only patients with appropriate indication for treatment should be administered bisphosphonates, and the FDA recommends stopping treatment after 5 years (Yin, 2012b).

OTHER MEDICAL THERAPIES

Treatment options for low BMD typically include antiresorptive agents, which include bisphosphonates, estrogen-related therapies, denosumab (a RANKL inhibitor), and calcitonin, and anabolic agents, which include teriparatide (a recombinant parathyroid hormone (PTH) analogue), abaloparatide (a PTH-related protein analog), and romosozumab (a monoclonal antibody directed against sclerostin). The benefits of osteoporosis treatment have been best studied in postmenopausal women, and data in PWH to inform treatment with specific agents is also lacking. Currently FDA-approved treatment options specifically for men include alendronate, risedronate, zolendronic acid, teriparatide, and denosumab. Initial treatment with bisphosphonates or denosumab is recommended for patients with osteoporosis or osteopenia with high risk for fracture by the American College of Endocrinology (Camacho et al., 2020) and American College of Physicians (ACP) (Qaseem et al., 2020). The ACP recommends treatment for 5 years, during which time repeat bone density measure may not be helpful.

Anabolic agents can increase new bone formation, while romosozumab additionally inhibits bone resorption. Anabolic agents may be considered for patients with treatment failure (i.e., fracture or loss of BMD with initial therapy), corticosteroid-induced osteoporosis, or severe osteoporosis, which is defined as a *T*-score < –2.5 plus two or more vertebral fractures. Antiresorptive therapy should be initiated following discontinuation of denosumab, teriparatide, abaoloparatide, or romosozumab (LeBoff et al., 2022).

Combination therapy may be considered in patients with very low BMD (*T*-score < –3.0) or recent fractures. Combination of anabolics (e.g., teriparatide) and a potent antiresorptive (e.g., denosumab) may be considered in high-risk patients, although combining antiresorptive agents at the same time is not recommended.

ROLE OF ANTIRETROVIRAL THERAPY SELECTION AND SWITCHING

Because TDF is associated with greater initial loss of BMD compared to other antiretrovirals, the US Department of Health and Human Services (DHHS) HIV adult treatment guidelines recommend the avoidance of TDF in patients with osteoporosis (DHHS, 2022). Tenofovir alafenamide (TAF), a prodrug of tenofovir, is associated with less BMD loss compared to TDF in both initial and ART switch settings, and it may mitigate the BMD effect of TDF (Mills et al., 2016; Sax et al., 2014). There are limited data on the efficacy of ART switch strategies. HIV clinicians should generally consider avoiding TDF or ritonavir-boosted protease inhibitors in patients at risk for bone loss. Some older short-term studies found that switching virologically suppressed patients to abacavir or raltegravir resulted in improvement in BMD compared to TDF (Haskelberg et al., 2012; Yin et al., 2012a). For many PWH, TAF would be the preferred nucleoside analogue to use instead of TDF.

For management of osteopenia/osteoporosis, the DHHS guidelines recommend to consider changing the ART regimen (e.g., switching from TDF to TAF, and/or from lopinavir/ritonavir (LPV/r) to (rilpivirine) RPV or an unboosted integrase (INSTI) whenever possible) and supplement with vitamin D3 to raise serum 25-OH-vitamin D concentrations to >30 ng/mL. There is no clear benefit to administering daily supplemental vitamin D3 doses that are >4,000 IU. If patients are receiving a daily dose of vitamin D3 that is >4,000 IU, consider monitoring levels of 25-OH-vitamin D.

The field of metabolic bone disease in PWH remains a critical area of research—especially as this populations of patients successfully aged into the seventh and eighth decades of life and beyond. Additional data from clinical trials and observational cohorts are needed to identify the best preventive, screening, and treatment strategies for osteoporosis and fragility fractures for PWH.

REFERENCES

Agidigbi TS, Kim C. Reactive oxygen species in osteoclast differentiation and possible pharmaceutical targets of ROS-mediated osteoclast diseases. *Int J Mol Sci.* 2019:20:3576. http//:doi:10.3390/ijms2014357

Amorosa V, Tebas P. Bone disease and HIV infection. *Clin Infect Dis.* 2006a;42(1):108–114.

Amorosa V, Tebas P. Reply to Rojo and Ramos and to Vignolo et al. *Clin Infect Dis.* 2006b;43(1):113–114.

Anastos K, Lu D, Shi O, et al. The association of bone mineral density with HIV infection and antiretroviral treatment in women. *Antivir Ther.* 2007;12:1049–1058.

Battalora L, Armon C, Palella F, et al. Incident bone fracture and mortality in a large HIV cohort outpatient study, 2000-2017, USA. *Arch Osteoporos.* 2021;16(1):117. http://doi:10.1007/211657-21-00949-y

Battalora L, Buchacz K, Armon C, et al. Low bone mineral density is associated with increased risk of incident fracture in HIV-infected adults. *Antivir Ther.* 2016;21(1):45–54.

Battalora LA, Young B, Overton ET. Bones, fractures, antiretroviral therapy and HIV. *Curr Infect Dis Rep.* February 2014;16(2):393.

Bedimo R, Adams-Huet B, Poindexter J, et al. The differential effects of human immunodeficiency virus and hepatitis C virus on bone microarchitecture and fracture risk. *Clin Infect Dis.* 2018;66(9):1442–1447.

Bedimo R, Maalouf NM, Zhang S, et al. Osteoporotic fracture risk associated with cumulative exposure to tenofovir and other antiretroviral agents. *AIDS.* April 24, 2012;26(7):825–831.

Bedimo RJ, Drechsler H, Jain M, et al. The RADAR study: week 48 safety and efficacy of RALtegravir combined with boosted DARunavir compared to tenofovir/emtricitabine combined with boosted darunavir in antiretroviral-naive patients. Impact on bone health. *PLoS One.* 2014;9:e106221.

Bedimo R, Cutrell J, Zhang S, et al. Mechanisms of bone disease in HIV and hepatitis C virus: impact of bone turnover, tenofovir exposure, sex steroids and severity of liver disease. *AIDS.* 2016;30:601–608.

Berry SD, Samelson EJ, Pencina MJ, et al. Repeat bone mineral density screening and prediction of hip and major osteoporotic fracture. *JAMA.* 2013;310(12):1256–1262.

Bolland MJ, Grey AB, Horne AM, et al. Annual zoledronate increases bone density in highly active antiretroviral therapy-treated human immunodeficiency virus-infected men: a randomized controlled trial. *J Clin Endocrinol Metab.* 2007;92(4):1283–1288.

Bolland MJ, Horne AM, Briggs SE, et al. Effects of intravenous zoledronate on bone turnover and bone density persist for at least 11 years in HIV-infected men. *J Bone Miner Res.* 2019; 34:1248–1253.

Brown TT, Hoy J, Borderi M, et al. Recommendations for evaluation and management of bone disease in HIV. *Clin Infect Dis.* 2015;60:1242–1251.

Brown TT, McComsey GA, King MS, et al. Loss of bone mineral density after antiretroviral therapy initiation, independent of antiretroviral regimen. *J AIDS.* 2009; 51:554–561.

Brown TT, Qaqish RB. Antiretroviral therapy and the prevalence of osteopenia and osteoporosis: a meta-analytic review. *AIDS.* November 14, 2006;20(17):2165–2174.

Brown TT, Moser C, Currier JS, et al. Changes in bone mineral density after initiation of antiretroviral treatment with tenofovir disoproxil fumarate/emtricitabine plus atazanavir/ritonavir, darunavir/ritonavir, or raltegravir. *J Infect Dis.* 2015;212(8):1241–1249.

Camacho PM, Petak SM. American Association of Clinical Endocrinologists/American College of Endocrinology clinical practice guidelines for the diagnosis and treatment of postmenopausal osteoporosis—2020 update. *Endocr Pract.* 2020;26(Suppl 1):1–46.

Chang CJ, Chan YL, Pramukti I, et al. People with HIV infection had lower bone mineral density and increased fracture risk: a metaanalysis. *Arch Osteoporos.* 2021;16(1):47.

Cotter AG, Vrouenraets SM, Brady JJ, et al. Impact of switching from zidovudine to tenofovir disoproxil fumarate on bone mineral density and markers of bone metabolism in virologically suppressed HIV-1 infected patients; a substudy of the PREPARE study. *J Clin Endocrinol Metab.* 2013;98:1659–1666.

Dave JA, Cohen K, Micklesfield LK, et al. Antiretroviral therapy, especially efavirenz, is associated with low bone mineral density in HIV-infected South Africans. *PLoS One.* 2015;10(12):e0144286.

Department of Health and Human Services, US (DHHS). Panel on Antiretroviral Guidelines for Adults and Adolescents. Guidelines for the use of antiretroviral agents in adults and adolescents with HIV. Department of Health and Human Services. https://clinicalinfo.hiv.gov/en/guidelines/adult-and-adolescent-arv. Published 2022. Accessed September 29, 2022.

Dong HV, Cortes YI, Shiau S, Yin MT. Osteoporosis and fractures in HIV/hepatitis C virus coinfection: a systematic review and meta-analysis. *AIDS.* 2014;28:2119–2131.

El-Maouche D, Mehta SH, Sutcliffe C, et al. Controlled HIV viral replication, not liver disease severity associated with low bone mineral density in HIV/HCV co-infection. *J Hepatology.* 2011;55:770–776.

Ensrud KE, Lui LY, Crandall CJ, et al. Repeat bone mineral density screening measurement and fracture prediction in older men: a prospective cohort study. *J Clin Endocrinol Metab.* 2022;107(9):e3877–e3886.

Escota GV, Patel P, Brooks JT, et al. Short communication: the Veterans Aging Cohort Study Index is an effective tool to assess baseline frailty status in a contemporary cohort of HIV-infected persons. *AIDS Res Hum Retroviruses.* 2015;31(3):313–317. http://doi:10.1089/aid.2014.0225

Escota GV, Mondy K, Bush T, et al. High prevalence of low bone mineral density and substantial bone loss over 4 years among HIV-infected persons in the era of modern antiretroviral therapy. *AIDS Res Hum Retrov.* 2016;32(1):59–67.

European AIDS Clinical Society (EACS). Guidelines version 11.0. https://eacs.sanfordguide.com/. Published October 2021. Accessed September 29, 2022.

Goh SSL, Lai PSM, Tan ATB, Ponnampalavanar S. Reduced bone mineral density in human immunodeficiency virus-infected individuals: a meta-analysis of its prevalence and risk factors. *Osteoporos Int.* March 2018;29(3):595–613.

Gonciulea A, Wang R, Althoff KN, et al. Proteinuria is associated with increased risk of fragility fracture in men with or at risk of HIV infection. *J Acquir Immune Defic Syndr.* 2019;81(3):e85–e91.

Gourlay ML, Fine JP, Preisser JS; Study of Osteoporotic Fractures Research Group. Bone-density testing interval and transition to osteoporosis in older women. *N Engl J Med.* 2012 19;366(3):225–233.

Grant PM, Kitch D, McComsey GA, et al. Long-term bone mineral density changes in antiretroviral-treated HIV-infected individuals. *J Infect Dis.* 2016;214(4):607–611. PMID:27330053.

Grant PM, Li X, Jacobson LP, et al. Effect of testosterone use on bone mineral density in HIV-infected men. *AIDS Res Hum Retroviruses.* 2019;35(1):75–80.

Guaraldi G, Orlando G, Madeddu G, et al. Alendronate reduces bone resorption in HIV-associated osteopenia/osteoporosis. *HIV Clin Trials.* 2004;5(5):269–277.

Guo F, Song X, Li Y, et al. Longitudinal change in bone mineral density among Chinese individuals with HIV after initiation of antiretroviral therapy. *Osteoporos Int.* 2021;32(2):321–332.

Hansen AB, Gerstoft J, Kronborg G, et al. Incidence of low and high-energy fractures in persons with and without HIV infection: a Danish population-based cohort study. *AIDS.* 2012;26(3):285–293. PMID:22095195

Haskelberg H, Cordery DV, Amin J, et al. HLA alleles association with changes in bone mineral density in HIV-1-infected adults changing treatment to tenofovir–emtricitabine or abacavir–lamivudine. *PLoS One.* 2014;9(3):e93333.

Haskelberg H, Hoy JF, Amin J, et al. Changes in bone turnover and bone loss in HIV-infected patients changing treatment to tenofovir–emtricitabine or abacavir–lamivudine. *PLoS One.* 2012;7(6):e38377.

Havens PL, Stephensen CB, Van Loan MD; Adolescent Medicine Trials Network for HIV/AIDS Interventions (ATN) 109 Study Team. Vitamin D3 supplementation increases spine bone mineral density in adolescents and young adults with human immunodeficiency virus infection being treated with tenofovir disoproxil fumarate: a randomized, placebo-controlled trial. *Clin Infect Dis.* 2018a;66(2):220–228. PMID:29020329.

Havens PL, Long D, Schuster GU; Adolescent Medicine Trials Network for HIV/AIDS Interventions (ATN) 117 and 109 Study Teams. Tenofovir disoproxil fumarate appears to disrupt the relationship of vitamin D and parathyroid hormone. *Antivir Ther.* 2018b;66(2):220–228. http://doi:10.3851/IMP3269. [Epub ahead of print] PMID:30260797.

Hileman CO, Labbato DE, Storer NJ, et al. Is bone loss linked to chronic inflammation in antiretroviral-naïve HIV-infected adults? A 48-week matched cohort study. *AIDS.* 2014;28(12):1759–1767.

Hoy J, Grund B, Roediger M, et al.; INSIGHT START Bone Mineral Density Substudy Group. Effects of immediate versus deferred initiation of antiretroviral therapy on bone mineral density: a substudy of the INSIGHT Strategic Timing of Antiretroviral Therapy (START) study. [Abstract ADRLH-62]. Paper presented at the 15th European AIDS Conference and 17th International Workshop on Co-morbidities and Adverse Drug Reactions in HIV. Barcelona, Spain; October 21–24, 2015.

Hoy JF, Richardson R, Ebeling PR; ZEST Study Investigators. Zoledronic acid is superior to tenofovir disoproxil fumarate-switching for low bone mineral density in adults with HIV. *AIDS.* 2018;32(14):1967–1975. PMID:29927785.

Huang J, Meixner L, Fernandez S, et al. A double-blinded, randomized controlled trial of zoledronate therapy for HIV-associated osteopenia and osteoporosis. *AIDS.* 2009;23(1):51–57.

INSIGHT START Study Group. Initiation of antiretroviral therapy in early asymptomatic HIV infection. *N Engl J Med.* 2015;373:795–807.

Institute of Medicine (IOM). *Dietary reference intakes for calcium and vitamin D.* Washington, DC: National Academies Press; 2011. http://iom.nationalacademies.org/~/media/Files/Report%20Files/2010/Dietary-Reference-Intakes-for-Calcium-and-Vitamin-D/Vitamin%20D%20and%20Calcium%202010%20Report%20Brief.pdf. Accessed September 29, 2022.

Jacobson DL, Lindsey JC, Gordon C, et al. Alendronate improves bone mineral density in children and adolescents perinatally infected with human immunodeficiency virus with low bone mineral density for age. *Clin Infect Dis.* 2020;71:1281–1288.

Jespersen NA, Axelsen F, Dollerup J, et al. The burden of non-communicable diseases and mortality in people living with HIV (PLHIV) in the pre-, early- and late-HAART era. *HIV Med.* 2021;22(6):478–490.

Kanis JA, on behalf of the World Health Organization Scientific Group. *Assessment of osteoporosis at the primary health-care level. Technical report.* World Health Organization Collaborating Centre for Metabolic Bone Diseases. University of Sheffield, UK; 2007. https://www.shef.ac.uk/FRAX/pdfs/WHO_Technical_Report.pdf). Accessed September 29, 2022.

Kim JH, Noh J, Kim W, et al. Trends of age-related non-communicable diseases in people living with HIV and comparison with uninfected controls: A nationwide population-based study in South Korea. *HIV Med.* 2021;22(9):824–833.

Kuller LH, Tracy R, Belloso W, et al. Inflammatory and coagulation biomarkers and mortality in patients with HIV infection. *PLoS Med.* 2008;5:e203.

LaFleur J, Bress A, Crook J, et al. Renal and bone outcomes among HIV-infected patients exposed to EFV/TDF/FTC compared to other TDF-containing antiretroviral regimens: findings from the Veterans Health Administration (VHA) ID Week. New Orleans, LA; 2016.

Lafleur J, Cheng Y, Crook J, et al. *Regional variations in rates of osteopenia, osteoporosis, fractures, and bone mineral density screening in male US veterans.* American Society for Bone and Mineral Research Annual Meeting. Atlanta, GA; 2016.

Lawson-Ayayi S, Cazanave C, Kpozehouen A, et al. Chronic viral hepatitis is associated with low bone mineral density in HIV-infected patients, ANRS CO 3 Aquitaine Cohort. *J Acquir Immune Defic Syndr.* 2013;62:430–435.

LeBoff MS, Greenspan SL, Insogna KL, et al. The clinician's guide to prevention and treatment of osteoporosis. *Osteoporos Int.* April 28, 2022. http://doi:10.1007/s00198-021-05900-y. Epub ahead of print. Erratum in: *Osteoporos Int.* July 28, 2022.

LeBoff MS, Chou SH, Ratliff KA, et al. Supplemental vitamin D and incident fractures in midlife and older adults. *N Engl J Med.* 2022:387(4):299–309.

LeFevre ML, LeFevre NM. Vitamin D screening and supplementation in community-dwelling adults: common questions and answers. *Am Fam Physician.* 2018;97(4):254–260.

Liu Z, Xiao Y, Torresilla C, et al. Implication of different HIV-1 genes in the modulation of autophagy. *Viruses.* 2017;9:389. http://doi:10.3390/v9120389

Lo Re V 3rd, Guaraldi G, Leonard MB, et al. Viral hepatitis is associated with reduced bone mineral density in HIV-infected women but not men. *AIDS.* 2009;23:2191–2198.

Lo Re V 3rd, Volk J, Newcomb CW, et al. Risk of hip fracture associated with hepatitis C virus infection and hepatitis C/human immunodeficiency virus coinfection. *Hepatology.* 2012;56:1688–1698.

Llop M, Sifuentes WA, Bañón S, et al. Increased prevalence of asymptomatic vertebral fractures in HIV-infected patients over 50 years of age. *Arch Osteoporos.* 2018;13(1):56.

Maalouf NM, Zhang S, Drechsler H, et al. Hepatitis C co-infection and severity of liver disease as risk factor for osteoporotic fractures among HIV-infected patients. *J Bone Miner Res.* 2013;28(12):2577–2583.

Martin A, Bloch M, Amin J, et al. Simplification of antiretroviral therapy with tenofovir-emtricitabine or abacavir-lamivudine: a randomized, 96-week trial. *Clin Infect Dis.* 2009;49:1591–601.

McCloskey EV, Oden A, Harvey NC, et al. A meta-analysis of travecular bone score in fracture risk prediction and its relationship to FRAX. *J Bone Miner Res.* 2016;31(5):940–948.

McComsey GA, Kendall MA, Tebas P, et al. Alendronate with calcium and vitamin D supplementation is safe and effective for the treatment of decreased bone mineral density in HIV. *AIDS*. 2007;21(18):2473–2482.

McComsey GA, Kitch D, Daar ES, et al. Bone mineral density and fractures in antiretroviral-naive persons randomized to receive abacavir–lamivudine or tenofovir disoproxil fumarate–emtricitabine along with efavirenz or atazanavir–ritonavir: Aids Clinical Trials Group A5224s, a substudy of ACTG A5202. *J Infect Dis*. June 15, 2011;203(12):1791–1801.

McComsey GA, Tebas P, Shane E, et al. Bone disease in HIV infection: a practical review and recommendations for HIV care providers. *Clin Infect Dis*. 2010;51(8):937–946.

Mills A, Arribas JR, Andrade-Villanueva J, et al. Switching from tenofovir disoproxil fumarate to tenofovir alafenamide in antiretroviral regimens for virologically suppressed adults with HIV-1 infection: a randomised, active-controlled, multicentre, open-label, phase 3, non-inferiority study. *Lancet Infect Dis*. 2016;16(1):43–52.

Mondy K, Powderly WG, Claxton SA, et al. Alendronate, vitamin D, and calcium for the treatment of osteopenia/osteoporosis associated with HIV infection. *J AIDS*. 2005;38(4):426–431.

Moran CA, Weitzmann MN, Ofotokun I. The protease inhibitors and HIV-associated bone loss. *Curr Opin HIV AIDS*. 2016;11(3):333–342.

National Osteoporosis Foundation. *Clinician's guide to prevention and treatment of osteoporosis*. Washington, DC: National Osteoporosis Foundation; 2014.

Negredo E, Bonjoch A, Gómez-Mateu M, et al. Time of progression to osteopenia/osteoporosis in chronically HIV-infected patients: screening DXA scan. *PLoS One*. 2012;7(10):e46031.

Nguyen ND, Eisman JA, Center JR, Nguyen TV. Risk factors for fracture in nonosteoporotic men and women. *J Clin Endocrinol Metab*. 2007;92(3):955–962.

Ofotokun I, Weitzmann MN. HIV and bone metabolism. *Discov Med*. 2011;11(60):385–393.

Ofotokun I, Collins LF, Titanji K, et al. Antiretroviral therapy-induced bone loss is durably suppressed by a single dose of zoledronic acid in treatment-naïve persons with HIV infection: a phase IIB trial. *Clin Infect Dis*. 2020;71(7):1655–1663. http://doi:10.1093/cid/ciz1027. Online ahead of print.

Orwoll ES, Klein RF. Osteoporosis in men. *Endocr Rev*. 1995;16(1):87–116.

Overton ET, Chan ES, Brown TT, et al. Vitamin D and calcium attenuate bone loss with antiretroviral therapy initiation: a randomized trial. *Ann Intern Med*. 2015;162(12):815–824. PMID:26075752.

Pitukcheewanont P, Safani D, Church J, et al. Bone measures in HIV-1 infected children and adolescents: disparity between quantitative computed tomography and dual-energy X-ray absorptiometry measurements. *Osteoporosis Int*. 2005;16(11):1393–1396.

Pramukti I, Lindayani L, Chen YC, et al. Bone fracture among people living with HIV: a systematic review and meta-regression of prevalence, incidence, and risk factors. *PLoS One*. 2020;15:6:e0233501.

Premaor MO, Compston JE. The hidden burden of fractures in people living with HIV. *JBMR Plus*. 2018;2(5):247–256. PMID: 30283906.

Qaseem A, Forciea MA, McLean RM, et al. Treatment of low bone density or osteoporosis to prevent fractures in men and women: a clinical practice guideline update from the American College of Physicians. *Ann Intern Med*. 2017;166(11):818–839.

Raffi F, Babiker AG, Richert L, et al. Ritonavir-boosted darunavir combined with raltegravir or tenofovir-emtricitabine in antiretroviral-naive adults infected with HIV-1: 96 week results from the NEAT001/ANRS143 randomised non-inferiority trial. *Lancet*. 2014;384:1942–1951.

Raynaud-Messina B, Bracq L, Dupont M, et al. Bone degradation machinery of osteoclasts: an HIV-1 target that contributes to bone loss. *Proc Natl Acad Sci U S A*. 2018;115(11):E2556–E2565.

Rozenberg S, Lanoy E, Bentata M, et al. Effect of alendronate on HIV-associated osteoporosis: a randomized, double-blind, placebo-controlled, 96-week trial (ANRS 120). *AIDS Res Hum Retroviruses*. 2012;28(9):972–980.

Rukuni R, Rehman AM, Mukwasi-Kahari C, et al. Effect of HIV infection on growth and bone density in peripubertal children in the era of antiretroviral therapy: a cross-sectional study in Zimbabwe. *Lancet Child Adolesc Health*. 2021;5(8):569–581.

Sandler NG, Wand H, Roque A, et al. Plasma levels of soluble CD14 independently predict mortality in HIV infection. *J Infect Dis*. 2011;203:780–790.

Sax PE, Zolopa A, Brar I, et al. Tenofovir alafenamide vs. tenofovir disoproxil fumarate in single tablet regimens for initial HIV-1 therapy: a randomized phase 2 study. *J AIDS*. 2014;67(1):52–58.

Sharma A, Hoover DR, Shi Q, et al. Human immunodeficiency virus (HIV) and menopause are independently associated with lower bone mineral density: results from the Women's Interagency HIV Study. *Clin Infect Dis*. 2022;75(1):65–72.

Sharma A, Ma Y, Tien PC, et al. HIV infection is associated with abnormal bone microarchitecture: measurement of trabecular bone score in the Women's Interagency HIV Study. *J AIDS*. August 1, 2018;78(4):441–449.

Sharma A, Shi Q, Hoover DR, et al. Frailty predicts fractures among women with and at-risk for HIV: results from the Women's Interagency HIV Study. *AIDS*. 2019;33:455–463.

Silva BC, Leslie WD, Resch H, et al. Trabecular bone score: a noninvasive analytical method based upon the DXA image. *J Bone Miner Res*. 2014;28(3):518–530.

Starup-Linde J, Rosendahl SB, Storgaard M, Langdahl B. Management of osteoporosis in patients living with HIV-A systematic review and meta-analysis. *J Acquir Immune Defic Syndr*. 2020;83(1):1–8.

Stellbrink HJ, Orkin C, Arribas JR, et al. Comparison of changes in bone density and turnover with abacavir-lamivudine versus tenofovir-emtricitabine in HIV-infected adults: 48-week results from the ASSERT study. *Clin Infect Dis*. 2010;51:963–972.

Tenorio AR, Zheng Y, Bosch RJ, et al. Soluble markers of inflammation and coagulation but not T-cell activation predict non-AIDS-defining morbid events during suppressive antiretroviral treatment. *J Infect Dis*. 2014;210:1248–1259.

Thompson MA, Horberg MA, Agwu AL, et al. Primary care guidance for persons with human immunodeficiency virus: 2020 update by the HIV Medicine Association of the Infectious Diseases Society of America. *Clin Infect Dis*. 2021;73(11):e3572–e3605.

Tinago W, Cotter AG, Sabin CA, et al. Predictors of longitudinal change in bone mineral density in a cohort of HIV-positive and negative patients. *AIDS*. 2017;31:643–652.

Titanji K. Beyond antibodies: B cells and the OPG/RANK-RANKL pathway in health, non-HIV disease and HIV-induced bone loss. *Front Immunol*. 2017;8:1851.

Triant VA, Brown TT, Lee H, et al. Fracture prevalence among human immunodeficiency virus (HIV)-infected versus non-HIV-infected patients in a large US healthcare system. *J Clin Endocrinol Metab*. September 2008;93(9):3499–3504.

Tricco AC, Thomas SM, Veroniki AA, et al. Comparisons of interventions for preventing falls in older adults: a systematic review and meta-analysis. *JAMA*. 2017;7;318(17):1687–1699.

US Preventive Services Task Force; Krist AH, Davidson KW, et al. Screening for vitamin D deficiency in adults: US Preventive Services Task Force Recommendation Statement. *JAMA*. 2021;325(14):1436–1442.

US Preventive Services Task Force; Grossman DC, Curry SJ, et al. Vitamin D, calcium, or combined supplementation for the primary prevention of fractures in community-dwelling adults: US Preventive Services Task Force Recommendation Statement. *JAMA*. 2018;17;319(15):1592–1599.

van den Bergh JP, van Geel TA, Lems WF, et al. Assessment of individual fracture risk: FRAX and beyond. *Curr Osteoporosis Rep*. 2010;8(3):131–137.

van Vonderen MG, Lips P, van Agtmael MA, et al. First line zidovudine/lamivudine/lopinavir/ritonavir leads to greater bone loss compared to nevirapine/lopinavir/ritonavir. *AIDS*. 2009;23(11):1367–1376.

Womack JA, Goulet JL, Gibert C, et al. Increased risk of fragility fractures among HIV infected compared to uninfected male veterans. *PLoS One.* 2011;6(2):e17217.

Woolf AD, Pfleger B. Burden of major musculoskeletal conditions. *Bull World Health Organ.* 2003;81(9):646–656.

World Health Organization (WHO). WHO manual of diagnostic imaging. http://apps.who.int/iris/bitstream/10665/42457/1/9241545550_eng.pdf. Published 2002. Accessed September 29, 2022.

WHO. WHO technical report series 843: assessment of fracture risk and its application to screening for postmenopausal osteoporosis. Report of a WHO study group. *World Health Organ Tech Rep Ser.* 1994;843:1–129.

WHO. Metabolic Bone Disease Group. FRAX tool. http://www.shef.ac.uk/FRAX. Published 2008. Accessed September 29, 2022.

Yin MT, Kendall MA, Wu X, et al. Fractures after antiretroviral initiation. *AIDS.* 2012b;26:2175–2184.

Yin MT, Overton ET. Increasing clarity on bone loss associated with antiretroviral initiation. *J Infect Dis.* 2011;203(12):1705–1707.

Yin MT, Shi Q, Hoover DR, et al. Fracture incidence in HIV-infected women: results from the Women's Interagency HIV Study. *AIDS.* November 13, 2010;24(17):2679–2686.

Yin MT, Zhang CA, McMahon DJ, et al. Higher rates of bone loss in postmenopausal HIV-infected women: a longitudinal study. *J Clin Endocrinol Metab.* February 2012a;97(2):554–562.

Young B, Dao CN, Buchacz K, et al. Increased rates of bone fracture among HIV-infected persons in the HIV Outpatient Study (HOPS) compared with the US general population, 2000–2006. *Clin Infect Dis.* 2011;52(8):1061–1068.

Zhang T, Wilson IB, Zullo AR, et al. Hip fracture rates in nursing home residents with and without HIV. *J Am Med Dir Assoc.* 2022;23(3):517–518.

42.

IMMUNE RECONSTITUTION INFLAMMATORY SYNDROME (IRIS)

Dagan Coppock

CHAPTER GOAL

Upon completion of this chapter, the reader should be able to:

- Understand the epidemiology of IRIS and its associated opportunistic infections.

- Recognize the timing considerations regarding opportunistic infection treatment and antiretroviral therapy initiation as related to the risk for IRIS.

- Understand the management approaches to IRIS, based upon its presentation and the underlying opportunistic infection.

LEARNING OBJECTIVE

Review the current status of research and clinical recommendations regarding IRIS.

WHAT'S NEW?

- Clinical trial data suggest that the use of integrase strand transfer inhibitor (INSTI)-based antiretroviral therapy (ART) regimens, compared to non-INSTI-based regimens, do not increase the risk for IRIS.

KEY POINTS

- IRIS is associated with either worsening of a recognized infection (paradoxical IRIS) or an unrecognized infection (unmasking IRIS), which occurs in the setting of improved immunologic function.

- Most people presenting with IRIS should be maintained on ART, along with treatment for the associated infection.

INTRODUCTION

The hallmark of HIV pathogenesis is the gradual destruction of the cell-mediated immune system over a period of many years, as evidenced by a progressive and profound decline in CD4 $^+$ T lymphocytes. This decline leads to increased susceptibility to opportunistic infections (OIs), malignancies, and the development of acquired immunodeficiency syndrome (AIDS). Antiretroviral therapy (ART) can suppress HIV replication, and it allows for the regeneration of the immune system. Even people with advanced AIDS have a marked improvement in both quantity and quality of their immune system after starting ART. In a subset of those initiating ART, the harmonious, gradual reconstitution of the immune system does not occur; rather, there is a rapid immunologic recovery with an abrupt transition to a pathologic inflammatory state often causing clinical deterioration. Opportunistic and other infections, previously unrecognized or tolerated by the failing immune system, suddenly become the targets of this overzealous immunologic recovery. In this inflammatory state, people can clinically worsen despite an otherwise excellent response to ART, as evidenced by a decreased viral load and increased CD4 $^+$ T-cell counts. This paradoxical inflammatory response has been termed IRIS (French et al., 2004), which is used an umbrella term encompassing two clinical entities: (1) paradoxical IRIS, an exacerbation of a known OI, and (2) unmasking IRIS, a flare of an undiagnosed (subclinical) OI.

INCIDENCE AND ASSOCIATED OPPORTUNISTIC INFECTIONS

The incidence of IRIS is dependent on the population being studied. It occurs more frequently in persons with specific OIs, a higher viral load, and more significant immunosuppression (Müller et al., 2010). The HIV Outpatient Study—an eight-city, US-wide, prospective cohort study—evaluated 2,610 persons with 370 cases of IRIS (occurring in 276 people) who initiated or resumed ART and, during the next 6 months, demonstrated a decline in plasma HIV RNA viral load of at least 0.5 $\log_{10}$ copies/mL or an increase of at least 50% in CD4 $^+$ T-cell count per microliter; it reported that the incidence of IRIS was 10.6%. The most common IRIS-defining diagnoses were candidiasis (23%), cytomegalovirus (CMV) infection (3.5%), disseminated *Mycobacterium avium* intracellular (3.2%), *Pneumocystis* pneumonia (2.7%), *Varicella zoster* (2.4%), Kaposi's sarcoma (KS) (2.4%), non-Hodgkin's lymphoma (2.2%), and *Mycobacterium tuberculosis* (0.3%). IRIS was independently associated with CD4 $^+$ T-cell counts of less than 50 cells/mL versus at least 200 cells/mL (odds ratio (OR) 5.0) and a viral load of at least 5.0 $\log_{10}$ copies/mL versus less than 4.0 $\log_{10}$ copies/mL (OR 2.3) (Novak et al. 2012). In contrast, a study from the University of Washington HIV Cohort demonstrated a higher rate of IRIS in people with KS (29%), with no evident cases in people with CMV disease or *Candida* esophagitis. In this study, the highest IRIS-associated morbidity was in cases of visceral KS. The differences in clinical characteristics between these two studies may reflect population and geographic variability.

IRIS AND ANTIRETROVIRAL THERAPY

In addition to the potential demographic factors that might affect the presentation of IRIS, the choice of ART regimen may also play a role. The AIDS Clinical Trial Group (ACTG) reported the incidence and associations with IRIS in ACTG 5202, which was a phase 3b, randomized clinical trial conducted in the United States that compared the safety, tolerability, and efficacy of four commonly used, once-daily, initial ART regimens. Two dual nucleoside/nucleotide reverse transcriptase inhibitor fixed-dose combinations (tenofovir disoproxil fumarate/emtricitabine or abacavir/lamivudine) were compared when used in combination with either the nonnucleoside reverse transcriptase inhibitor (NNRTI) efavirenz or a ritonavir-boosted protease inhibitor, atazanavir/ritonavir. Among 1,848 eligible participants who initiated in this study, IRIS events occurred in 52 participants by week 48, with 4 participants having two events. Incidence rates were 6.05 (95% confidence interval (CI): 4.57–8.00) and 3.30 (95% CI: 2.51–4.33) cases/100 person-years (py) through 24 and 48 weeks, respectively. IRIS occurred 1–298 days after the initiation of ART, with 75% of cases occurring within 67 days, and 3 cases after 24 weeks. IRIS events included the following associated OIs or other clinical diagnoses: *Mycobacterium avium* complex (MAC) ($n = 11$); *Varicella zoster* virus ($n = 11$); herpes simplex virus ($n = 8$); KS ($n = 5$); HCV, tuberculosis (TB), and *Pneumocystis jirovecii* pneumonia (PCP) ($n = 4$ each); toxoplasmosis and cryptococcosis ($n = 2$ each); and CMV-associated colitis, progressive multifocal leukoencephalopathy (PML), *Mycobacterium kansasii*, eosinophilic folliculitis, and swollen lymph node ($n = 1$ each). The most commonly reported symptoms were fever and pain. There were no deaths from IRIS in this cohort. Among participants with IRIS, the median baseline HIV RNA was 4.9 $\log_{10}$ copies/mL, and the median CD4$^+$ T-cell count was 49 cells/mm^3. Fifty percent had prior AIDS-related illnesses. In univariate Cox proportional hazards models, an increased risk of IRIS was associated with baseline prior AIDS-related illness, higher HIV RNA level, lower CD4$^+$ T-cell count and percentage, lower CD8$^+$ T-cell count and higher percentage, and lower CD4$^+$:CD8$^+$ T-cell ratio (all $p \leq 0.01$). No significant association was observed with sex, age, or race/ethnicity ($p > 0.19$). Of note, IRIS events were more common with abacavir/lamivudine relative to tenofovir/emtricitabine for participants with low CD4$^+$ T-cell counts. This finding may reflect the more rapid CD4$^+$ T-cell increases observed with abacavir/lamivudine regimens (Fischl et al., 2010).

Early observational data raised concerns regarding INSTI-based regimens and their associations with IRIS; however, subsequent clinical trial data do not bear out these findings. In a retrospective cohort trial, 2,287 persons with CD4$^+$ T-cell counts below 200/mm^3 were evaluated by ART regimen. Cohorts consisted of participants receiving either INSTI-based or non-INSTI-based ART regimens. The odds ratio for developing IRIS was 1.99 (1.09–3.47) ($P = 0.04$) for the INSTI-based group (Dutertre et al., 2017). However, a clinical trial that evaluated standard two-nucleoside reverse transcriptase inhibitor/one-nonnucleoside reverse transcriptase inhibitor therapy compared with standard therapy intensified with raltegravir demonstrated no difference in the occurrence of IRIS between the two groups (86 (9.5%) with standard ART versus 89 (9.9%) participants with raltegravir-intensified ART, $p = 0.79$) (Kityo et al., 2019). In a clinical trial that compared efavirenz-based therapy with dolutegravir-based therapy, there were two reported cases of IRIS (one associated with KS, one associated with pulmonary tuberculosis) in the efavirenz group, while there were no reported cases in the dolutegravir group (NAMSAL, 2019). In summary, though INSTIs do lead to a more rapid reduction in viral load, available trials do not support the concern that they induce IRIS more than non-INSTI-based regimens.

ETIOLOGY AND PATHOGENESIS

Recovery of pathogen-specific T-cell responses and an increased production of proinflammatory chemokines and cytokines produced by the innate immune response after commencing ART may contribute to the immunopathogenesis of IRIS. Higher T-cell responses to nonstructural antigens of HCV in enzyme-linked immunosorbent spot assays and higher serum levels of antibodies to a mixture of virus proteins were demonstrated in people with HIV (PWH) and HCV coinfection who experienced an increase in serum liver enzyme levels after commencing ART (Cameron et al., 2011). People who develop TB IRIS have lower plasma levels of the chemokine CCL2 before commencing ART (Oliver et al., 2010).

The identification of biomarkers could be used to diagnose IRIS in the future and predict which persons might be at risk. A cohort of 45 HIV-1-infected, treatment-naive persons with baseline CD4$^+$ T-cell counts of 100 cells/μL or less who were started on ART, suppressed HIV RNA to less than 50 copies/mL, and seen every 1–3 months for 1 year were retrospectively evaluated for suspected or confirmed IRIS. Pre-ART levels of both D-dimer and the inflammatory biomarker C-reactive protein (CRP) were higher in IRIS cases versus controls (Porter et al., 2010). In another study, individuals with elevated baseline levels of CRP and the fibrosis biomarker hyaluronic acid were more likely to progress to AIDS, develop IRIS, or die within the first month after starting ART (Boulware et al., 2011). Large prospective studies to elucidate the predictive and diagnostic values of IRIS biomarkers are needed.

GUIDELINES FOR ART INITIATION

Current guidelines recommend the early initiation of ART with the exception of select clinical scenarios. US Department of Health and Human Services (USDHHS) guidelines recommend early initiation of ART despite the presence of OIs. However, there are exceptions for which a delay may be warranted (USDHHS, 2022). Notably, for cryptococcal meningitis, the initiation of ART is typically delayed until an individual receives 4–6 weeks of antifungal therapy (USDHHS, 2022). For tuberculous meningitis, the USDHHS guidelines recommend initiation within 2 to 8 weeks of initiating tuberculosis treatment, while the Infectious Diseases Society of America guidelines recommend a delay of 8 weeks for all individuals (Nahid, 2016). For pulmonary TB, both guidelines stratify initiation based on CD4 count (Nahid et al., 2016; USDHHS, 2022). ART can be initiated within 2 weeks of starting TB treatment for persons with a CD4$^+$ T-cell count less than 50 cells/mm^3, and between 2 and 8 weeks for persons with a CD4$^+$ T-cell count greater than 50 cells/mm^3. The evidence supporting these guidelines, as well as for other OIs, is discussed below.

ART INITIATION AND THE RISK OF NON-TUBERCULOSIS-ASSOCIATED IRIS

The timing of ART initiation and its association with OI-specific IRIS remains a concern for clinicians. In the ACTG 5164 study, 282 participants with an acute OI and a baseline median CD4$^+$ T-cell count of 29 cells/mm^3 were prospectively randomly assigned to immediate (< 14 days) versus delayed (>28 days) initiation of ART. In this study, which included participants diagnosed with PCP (63%), cryptococcal meningitis (12%), and bacterial infections (12%), earlier initiation of ART resulted in less progression to AIDS and/or death and no increase in adverse events or loss of virologic response compared to deferred ART. Participants with or on treatment for TB were excluded. Rates of IRIS in this study were low (7%) and did not differ by timing of ART (Zolopa et al., 2009). IRIS was reported in 23 cases and confirmed in 20: 8 participants in the immediate arm and 12 in the deferred arm. There was no evidence of an association of IRIS with the entry OI/bacterial infection: 13 (65%) IRIS cases were in participants with PCP who comprised 63% of the study population. IRIS developed a median of 33 days (interquartile range 26–72 days) after initiation of ART. There was no significant difference in the frequency of IRIS between participants who received corticosteroids during the treatment of their OI and those who did not receive corticosteroids: 9/150 (6%) versus 11/112 (9.8%), respectively (p = 0.35).

In contrast to the above study, early initiation of ART has been demonstrated in clinical trials focusing on cryptococcal meningitis. In a trial of patients treated for cryptococcal meningitis with fluconazole, ART initiation within 72 hours was associated with a higher rate of mortality compared to those who waited for at least 10 weeks

(Makadzange et al., 2010). A clinical trial conducted in Botswana compared the early (with 7 days) and late (after 28 days) ART initiation in patients being treated for cryptococcal meningitis (Bisson et al., 2013). There was no difference in mortality between the two study arms. However, the incidence of IRIS was higher in patients in the early initiation arm. Benefits to delayed initiation were also seen in a study conducted in Uganda and South Africa (Boulware et al., 2014). In this study patients were randomly assigned to receive ART within 48 hours of assignment or 4 weeks after assignment, and 177 patients underwent assignment after a median of 8 days of amphotericin. The 26-week mortality with early ART initiation was significantly higher than with delayed ART initiation (45% versus 30%; hazard ratio for death 1.73; P = 0.03). Based on the above findings, the USDHHS currently recommends delaying ART initiation by 4 to 6 weeks after starting antifungal treatment.

IRIS related to JC polyoma virus infection remains a clinical challenge as ART initiation and immune reconstitution is the only available treatment. Prior to ART, JC virus infection can lead to PML in people with advanced HIV infection. However, approximately 15% of individuals experience an exacerbation of PML after ART is commenced (Martin-Blondel et al., 2011). A review of 54 cases of PML IRIS evaluated the mortality of persons as stratified by steroid use. Of the 12 persons receiving steroids and 42 persons not receiving steroids, 5 and 14 died, respectively, suggesting a high mortality of PML IRIS, regardless of steroid use (Tan et al., 2009).

In people coinfected with HIV and viral hepatitis, IRIS is a frequent concern. Up to 25% of PWH and HBV or HCV coinfection experience a flare of hepatitis and/or elevation of serum liver enzyme levels after commencing ART (Cameron et al., 2011; Crane et al., 2009). Hepatitis flares in PWH and HBV coinfection are associated with a higher plasma HBV DNA level before ART (Crane et al., 2009), suggesting that pathogen load is an important determinant of disease. Even when ART with activity against HBV is selected for treatment, HBV IRIS can still occur, complicating the differential of a hepatitis flare (Crane et al., 2008). In recent years, the use of direct-acting antivirals (DAAs) for treating HCV has further complicated the differential. The use of DAAs has been associated with HBV reactivation (Bersoff-Matcha et al., 2017). This has led to changes in guidelines regarding the timing of ART initiation in people with viral hepatitis. For people who are both coinfected with HIV/HCV and have active HBV infection, USDHHS (2022) guidelines now recommend first initiating ART with activity against HBV prior to the initiation of DAAs.

TUBERCULOSIS IRIS AND ART INITIATION

For individuals with HIV and TB coinfection, unmasking and paradoxical IRIS can lead to two distinct clinical scenarios. In the context of TB, unmasking IRIS is the development of overt TB in people who initially screened negative for this infection, typically seen within the first 60 days following ART initiation (Dheda et al., 2004; Shelburne et al., 2006). It is thought to be due to an increase in circulating memory T-cells that were sequestered in lymphatic tissue prior to therapy. Alternatively, paradoxical IRIS involves worsening of signs and symptoms of TB in individuals with a known history of TB after they have been started on ART.

The HIV-CAUSAL Collaboration demonstrated that the incidence of TB decreased after ART initiation but not among persons aged older than 50 years or those with a CD4$^+$ T-cell count of less than 50 cells/mm^3. Despite an overall decrease in TB incidence, the increased rate during 3 months of ART suggests unmasking IRIS. This is a multinational cohort study among PWH from high-income countries. Among 65,121 individuals, 712 developed TB during 28 months of median follow-up (incidence, 3.0 cases per 1,000 py). The hazard ratio (HR) for TB for ART versus no ART was 0.56 (95% CI: 0.44–0.72) overall, 1.04 (95% CI: 0.64–1.68) for individuals aged older than 50 years, and 1.46 (95% CI: 0.70–3.04) for people with a CD4$^+$ T-cell count of less than 50 cells/mm^3. Compared with people who had not started ART, HRs differed by time since ART initiation: 1.36 (95% CI: 0.98–1.89) for initiation less than 3 months previously and 0.44 (95% CI: 0.34–0.58) for initiation 3 months or more previously. Compared with people who had not initiated ART, HRs less than 3 months after ART initiation were 0.67 (95% CI: 0.38–1.18), 1.51 (95% CI: 0.98–2.31), and 3.20 (95% CI: 1.34–7.60) for people aged younger than 35 years, 35–50 years, and older than 50 years, respectively, and 2.30 (95% CI: 1.03–5.14) for people with a CD4$^+$ T-cell counts of less than 50 cells/mm^3 (HIV-CAUSAL Collaboration, 2012).

In a South African cohort of 498 persons with advanced HIV, symptomatic individuals were screened for TB by chest X-ray and/or sputum examination. People who screened positive were initiated on anti-TB therapy prior to starting ART. Individuals who screened negative and went on to develop unmasking IRIS were found to have significantly elevated levels of interferon-γ (IFN-γ) and CRP at baseline prior to ART compared to non-IRIS, non-TB controls. These results suggest the presence of subclinical TB infection despite negative screening that was done prior to the initiation of ART (Haddow et al., 2009). Persons who exhibit paradoxical IRIS have been reported to have elevated tuberculin-specific effector memory CD4$^+$ T-cells prior to initiation of ART. Following the commencement of ART, increased levels of Th1-associated cytokines, IFN-γ, and tumor necrosis factor-α most likely contribute to the overwhelming inflammatory reaction to the TB antigen present (Bourgarit et al., 2009). PWH with *latent TB* (defined as >5 mm skin test induration or positive IFN-γ release assay) are at increased risk for progression to active TB compared to the HIV-negative population, which underscores the need to identify and treat people with latent disease. Active TB in PWH requires immediate treatment. However, optimal timing of ART has yet to be established. Potential for multiple adverse drug reactions, drug–drug interactions, and IRIS reactions has led to increased difficulty in defining the proper timing of ART.

TIMING OF ART WITH TB IRIS

In recent years, there has been debate on the timing of ART initiation relative to the initiation of TB treatment in known coinfected people. However, based on a number of trials, as discussed here, current USDHHS guidelines recommend an early, integrative approach to ART and TB treatment initiation.

In the SAPiT trial, there were no differences in rates of AIDS or death between people who started ART within 4 weeks after initiating TB treatment and those who started ART at 8–12 weeks (i.e., within 4 weeks after completing the intensive phase of TB treatment) (Abdool Karim, 2010). However, in people with baseline CD4$^+$ T-cell counts of less than 50 cells/mm^3, the rate of AIDS or death was lower in the earlier therapy group than in the later therapy group (8.5 vs. 26.3 cases per 100 py, a strong trend favoring the earlier treatment arm ($p = 0.06$)). For all people, regardless of CD4$^+$ T-cell count, earlier therapy was associated with a higher incidence of IRIS and of adverse events that required a switch in antiretroviral drugs compared to those who started therapy later. In this study, two deaths were attributed to IRIS.

In the CAMELIA study, people who had CD4$^+$ T-cell counts of less than 200 cells/mm^3 were randomly assigned to initiate ART at 2 or 8 weeks after initiation of TB treatment (Blanc et al., 2011). Study participants had a median CD4$^+$ T-cell count of 25 cells/mm^3 and high rates of disseminated TB disease. ART initiated at 2 weeks resulted in a 38% reduction in mortality ($p = 0.006$) compared with that of therapy initiated at 8 weeks. A significant reduction in mortality was seen in people with CD4$^+$ T-cell counts of 50 cells/mm^3 or less and in people with CD4$^+$ T-cell counts of 51–200 cells/mm^3. Overall, six deaths were associated with TB IRIS.

The ACTG 5221 (STRIDE) trial, a multinational study, randomly assigned ART-naive individuals with confirmed or probable TB and CD4$^+$ T-cell counts of less than 250 cells/mm^3 to earlier (< 2 weeks) or later (8–12 weeks) ART (Havlir et al., 2011). At study entry, the participants' median CD4$^+$ T-cell count was 77 cells/mm^3. The rates of mortality and AIDS diagnoses were not different between the earlier and later arms, although higher rates of IRIS were seen in the earlier arm. However, a significant reduction in AIDS or death was seen in the subset of people with CD4$^+$ T-cell counts of less than 50 cells/mm^3 who were randomly assigned to the earlier ART arm ($p = 0.02$).

Though the above studies focus on pulmonary TB, central nervous system TB is seen as a unique entity. A clinical trial conducted in Vietnam explored outcomes in HIV-associated TB meningitis (Torok et al., 2018). For the study population, individuals were randomly assigned to ART immediately or 2 months after the initiation of tuberculosis treatment. The investigators found that immediate ART did not improve outcomes. Further, there were significantly more grade 4 adverse events in the immediate initiation ART.

Given the previously discussed data, USDHHS guidelines recommend that, for patients with pulmonary TB, ART should be initiated within 2 weeks of starting tuberculosis treatment when an individual's CD4$^+$ T-cell count is less than 50 cells/mm^3 and by 8–12 weeks for all others. This reflects the observation that earlier ART initiation in TB-infected people improves mortality. However, for individuals with central nervous system TB, ART should be delayed for 8 weeks.

TREATMENT OF IRIS

When IRIS occurs, regardless of the OI, ART should be continued (USDHHS, 2022). Otherwise, the underlying OI should be treated as soon as possible. Although nonsteroidal anti-inflammatory drugs and corticosteroids are commonly used in clinical practice, the dosage and timing have not been well established in the medical literature. Regarding pulmonary TB-associated IRIS, a double-blind, placebo-controlled, randomized clinical trial, including those receiving both ART and anti-TB therapy and experiencing paradoxical IRIS, evaluated a tapering course of prednisone over 4 weeks. Individuals on steroid therapy had a significantly decreased length of hospitalization and marked improvement of symptoms related to IRIS, suggesting a potential role for steroids in the management of paradoxical IRIS (Meintjes et al., 2010). Though pulmonary TB-associated IRIS is typically self-limited, corticosteroids may be used to manage significant symptoms (USDHHS, 2022). However, for central nervous system TB, corticosteroids should be given adjunctively at the time of diagnosis based upon available clinical trial data (Girgis et al., 1991; Schoeman et al., 1997; Thwaites et al., 2004).

In other forms of IRIS, such as MAC, surgical drainage of necrotic lymphadenitis may be of benefit. In people with cryptococcal meningitis IRIS, CSF drainage may provide relief of increased intracranial pressure. While the data to support the use of corticosteroids in cryptococcal meningitis IRIS are sparse, Infectious Disease Society of America guidelines recommend considering their use in the setting of CNS inflammation and increased intracranial pressure (Perfect, 2010). Corticosteroid or other anti-inflammatory therapies may also be effective for treating some forms of IRIS, such as PML-associated IRIS (Martin-Blondel et al., 2011). However, in the previously described ACTG 5164 study, 63% of participants reported having *Pneumocystis* pneumonia as an OI. There was no significant difference in the frequency of IRIS between participants who received corticosteroids during the treatment and those who did not receive corticosteroids: 9/150 (6%) versus 11/112 (9.8%), respectively ($p = 0.35$).

In summary, in unmasking IRIS, management should focus on the diagnosis and treatment of the underlying OI. In paradoxical IRIS, treatment for the OI should be continued and alternate diagnoses should be excluded to ensure the individual is receiving the appropriate treatment. IRIS is typically managed supportively. ART should only be interrupted in severe, life-threatening situations where IRIS is unresponsive to supportive care. In certain conditions, corticosteroids may be used adjunctively to manage IRIS-related symptoms.

REFERENCES

Abdool Karim SS. Timing of initiation of antiretroviral drugs during tuberculosis therapy. *N Engl J Med*. February 5, 2010;362(8):697–706.

Bersoff-Matcha SJ, Cao K, et al. Hepatitis B virus reactivation associated with direct-acting antiviral therapy for chronic hepatitis C virus: a review of cases reported to the US Food and Drug Administration adverse event reporting system. *Ann Intern Med*. 2017;166(11):792–798.

Bisson GP, Molefi M, Bellamy S, et al. Early versus delayed antiretroviral therapy and cerebrospinal fluid fungal clearance in adults with HIV and cryptococcal meningitis. *Clin Infect Dis*. 2013;56(8):1165–1173.

Blanc FX, Sok T, Laureillard D, et al. Earlier versus later start of antiretroviral therapy in HIV-infected adults with tuberculosis. *N Engl J Med*. October 20, 2011;365(16):1471–1481.

Boulware DR, Hullsiek KH, Puronen CE, et al.; INSIGHT Study Group. Higher levels of CRP, D-dimer, IL-6, and hyaluronic acid before initiation of antiretroviral therapy (ART) are associated with increased risk of AIDS or death. *J Infect Dis*. June 1, 2011;203(11):1637–1646.

Boulware DR, Meya DB, Muzoora C, et al. Timing of antiretroviral therapy after diagnosis of cryptococcal meningitis. *NEJM*. 2014;370(26):2487–2498.

Bourgarit A, Carcelain G, Samri A, et al. TB-associated immune restoration syndrome in HIV-1-infected patients involves tuberculin-specific CD4 Th1 cells and can be predicted by KIR-negative gamma delta T cells. [Abstract 772]. Paper presented at the 16th Conference on Retroviruses and Opportunistic Infections. Montréal, Canada; February 8–11, 2009.

Cameron BA, Emerson CR, Workman C, et al. Alterations in immune function are associated with liver enzyme elevation in HIV and HCV co-infection after commencement of combination antiretroviral therapy. *J Clin Immunol*. 2011;31:1079–1083.

Crane M, Oliver B, Matthews G, et al. Immunopathogenesis of hepatic flare in HIV/hepatitis B virus (HBV)-coinfected individuals after the initiation of HBV-active antiretroviral therapy. *J Infect Dis*. 2009;199:974–981.

Crane M, Matthews G, Lewin SR. Hepatitis virus immune restoration disease of the liver. *Curr Opin HIV AIDS*. 2008;3(4):446–452.

Dheda K, Lampe FC, Johnson MA, et al. Outcome of HIV-associated tuberculosis in the era of highly active antiretroviral therapy. *J Infect Dis*. 2004;190(9):1670.

Dutertre M, Cuzin L, Demonchy E, et al. Initiation of antiretroviral therapy containing integrase inhibitors increases the risk of IRIS requiring hospitalization. *JAIDS*. 2017;76(1):e23–e26.

Fischl M, Mollan K, Pahwa S, et al. IRIS among US subjects starting ART in AIDS Clinical Trials Group Study A5202. [Abstract 791]. Paper presented at the 15th Conference on Retroviruses and Opportunistic infections. San Francisco, CA; February 16–19, 2010.

French MA, Price P, Stone SF. Immune restoration disease after antiretroviral therapy. *AIDS*. 2004;18:1615–1627.

Girgis NI, Farid Z, Kilpatrick ME, et al. Dexamethasone adjunctive treatment for tuberculous meningitis. *Pediatr Infect Dis J*. 1991;10(3):179.

Haddow L, Borrow P, Dibben O, et al. Cytokine profiles predict unmasking TB immune reconstitution inflammatory syndrome and are associated with unmasking and paradoxical presentations of TB immune reconstitution inflammatory syndrome. [Abstract 773]. Paper presented at the 16th Conference on Retroviruses and Opportunistic Infections. Montréal, Canada; February 8–11, 2009.

Havlir DV, Kendall MA, Ive P, et al. Timing of antiretroviral therapy for HIV-1 infection and tuberculosis. *N Engl J Med*. October 20, 2011;365(16):1482–1491.

HIV-CAUSAL Collaboration. Impact of antiretroviral therapy on tuberculosis incidence among HIV-positive patients in high-income countries. *Clin Infect Dis*. May 2012;54(9):1364–1372.

Kityo C, Szubert AJ, Siika A, et al. Raltegravir-intensified initial antiretroviral therapy in advanced HIV disease in Africa: a randomized controlled trial. *PLoS Medicine*. 2019;15(12):e1002706.

Makadzange AT, Ndhlovu CE, Takarinda K, et al. Early versus delayed initiation of antiretroviral therapy for concurrent HIV infection and cryptococcal meningitis in sub-Saharan Africa. *Clin Infect Dis.* 2010;50:1532–1538.

Martin-Blondel G, Delobel P, Blancher A, et al. Pathogenesis of the immune reconstitution inflammatory syndrome affecting the central nervous system in patients infected with HIV. *Brain.* 2011;134:928–946.

Meintjes G, Wilkinson RJ, Morroni C, et al. Randomized placebo-controlled trial of prednisone for paradoxical tuberculosis-associated immune reconstitution inflammatory syndrome. *AIDS.* September 24, 2010;24(15):2381–2390.

Müller M, Wandel S, Colebunders R, et al. Immune reconstitution inflammatory syndrome in patients starting antiretroviral therapy for HIV infection: a systematic review and meta-analysis. *Lancet Infect Dis.* 2010;10:251–261.

Nahid P, Dorman SE, Alipanah N, et. al. Official American Thoracic Society/Centers for Disease Control and Prevention/Infectious Diseases Society of America clinical practice guidelines: treatment of drug-susceptible tuberculosis. *Clin. Infect Dis.* 2016;63(7)e147–e195.

NAMSAL ANRS 12313 Study Group. Dultegravir-based or low-dose efavirenz-based regimen for the treatment of HIV-1. *NEJM.* 2019;381(9):816–826.

Novak RM, Richardson JT, Buchacz K, et al.; HIV Outpatient Study (HOPS) Investigators. Immune reconstitution inflammatory syndrome: incidence and implications for mortality. *AIDS.* March 27, 2012;26(6):721–730.

Oliver BG, Elliott JH, Price P, et al. Mediators of innate and adaptive immune responses differentially affect immune restoration disease associated with *Mycobacterium tuberculosis* in HIV patients beginning antiretroviral therapy. *J Infect Dis.* 2010;202:1728–1737.

Perfect JR. Clinical practice guidelines for the management of cryptococcal disease: 2010 update by the Infectious Diseases Society of America. *Clin Infect Dis.* 2010;50(3):291–322.

Porter BO, Ouedraogo GL, Hodge JN, et al. d-Dimer and CRP levels are elevated prior to antiretroviral treatment in patients who develop IRIS. *Clin Immunol.* July 2010;136(1):42–50.

Schoeman JF, Van Zyl LE, Laubscher JA, et al. Effect of corticosteroids on intracranial pressure, computed tomographic findings, and clinical outcome in young children with tuberculous meningitis. *Pediatrics.* 1997;99(2):226.

Shelburne SA, Montes M, Hamill RJ. Immune reconstitution inflammatory syndrome: more answers, more questions. *J Antimicrob Chemother.* 2006;57(2):167.

Tan K, Roda R, Ostrow L, et al. PML-IRIS in patients with HIV infection: clinical manifestations and treatment with steroids. *Neurology.* 2009;72(17):1458–1464.

Thwaites GE, Nguyen DB, Nguyen HD, et al. Dexamethasone for the treatment of tuberculous meningitis in adolescents and adults. *NEJM.* 2004;351(17):1741–1751.

Török ME, Yen NT, Chau TT, et al. Timing of initiation of antiretroviral therapy in human immunodeficiency virus (HIV)—associated tuberculous meningitis. *Clin Infect Dis.* June 2011;52(11):1374–1383.

US Department of Health and Human Services (USDHHS). Guidelines for the use of antiretroviral agents in adults and adolescents living with HIV. https://clinicalinfo.hiv.gov/en/guidelines. Published 2022. Accessed August 15, 2022.

Zolopa AR, Anderson J, Komarow L, et al. Early antiretroviral therapy reduces AIDS progression/death in individuals with acute opportunistic infections: a multicenter randomized strategy trial. *PLoS One.* 2009;4(5):e5575.

43.

HIV HEALTH CARE PROGRAMS AND INSURANCE COVERAGE IN THE U.S. HEALTH CARE SYSTEM

Leslie McGorman and Bruce J. Packett II

LEARNING OBJECTIVE

Upon completion of this chapter, the reader should be able to:

- Broadly understand the US health care system and coverage landscape as they relate to the provision of HIV care, treatment, and prevention, as well as associated medical coding and billing for reimbursement.

WHAT'S NEW?

There have been a number of short-term changes made to the health care system in response to COVID-19 and as part of the federal government's Public Health Emergency declaration. Many of those changes have served to enhance access for PWH and those at risk, including expanded telehealth access, "continuous coverage" Medicaid, and enhanced marketplace subsidy assistance (DHHS, n.d.). However, while efforts to increase access to health care coverage increased, HIV testing has seen a significant decline since the onset of the pandemic, and some PWH have fallen out of care (CDC, 2022). Between February 2020 and April 2022, Medicaid/Children's Health Insurance Program (CHIP) enrollment increased by nearly 24 percent (17 million people) (Corallo & Moreno, 2022). As with any potential change in coverage eligibility, HIV care providers can help prepare clients by linking them with community resources or a local Ryan White provider. Additionally, President Biden signed into law the Inflation Reduction Act in 2022, which includes a provision to extend American Rescue Plan health insurance premium subsidies aimed at ensuring people are able to keep affordable marketplace plans. These subsidies will be in effect for at least 3 more years.

The thirtieth anniversary of the Ryan White Comprehensive AIDS Resources Emergency (CARE) Act was commemorated on August 18, 2020. The CARE Act has been reauthorized four times since it was initially signed into law and aims to accommodate new and emerging needs of PWH as well as address ongoing disparities in access to care to improve HIV-related health outcomes. Congress appropriated additional funding for the total Ryan White Program in fiscal years 2020 and 2021, though some parts have not seen notable increases in several years.

Since 2019, several states have enacted measures allowing pharmacists to independently initiate pre-exposure prophylaxis or postexposure prophylaxis in a pharmacy setting. Requirements on whether or when a pharmacist must link a patient to a physician provider varies by state. Still other states allow for collaborative practice agreements between a pharmacist and physician or their respective public health department. Such changes are intended to help end the HIV epidemic by effectively expanding the HIV prevention workforce. In 2021, the first long-acting antiretroviral (LAI) therapy regimen (cabotegravir and rilpivirine, administered via injections monthly or every 2 months) was approved for the treatment of HIV. Later that year, long-acting cabotegravir (administered as injections every 2 months) was approved for HIV prevention. The long-acting nature of these therapies could considerably shift the nature of HIV prevention and treatment, particularly regarding care engagement and retention for some patients. However, accessibility has largely depended on how the patient receives health care coverage. Specifically, coverage across the private insurance market, Medicaid, Medicare, and state AIDS Drug Assistance Programs (ADAPs) vary and often include prior authorization requirements or other utilization management techniques.

In 2022, the US Supreme Court effectively overturned the landmark *Roe v. Wade* decision by allowing states to determine the parameters of legal abortion care. It is unknown how this ruling could impact HIV care, although it does allow for increased political reach into provider autonomy as it relates to reproductive health care. HIV health care providers must be aware of changing laws and how they may impact one's ability to provide care and/or protect patient privacy.

In 2022, the federal government announced its formal support for the Undetectable = Untransmittable (U = U) message. While there has long been scientific consensus that PWH who are on treatment and have an undetectable viral load cannot sexually transmit HIV, only certain departments within the government had adopted the message, thereby limiting the reach of U = U. Now, the Biden Administration has committed to utilizing U = U as a national mantra to guide HIV treatment and prevention efforts.

- It has been more than 12 years since passage of the landmark Patient Protection and Affordable Care Act (also called the Affordable Care Act (ACA)), and more than 8 years since implementation of the Health Insurance Marketplace, which greatly expanded the availability of health coverage for PWH in the United States.US. However, serious challenges such as affordability and access to treatment still remain and are especially evident in the 12 states that have chosen not to expand their Medicaid coverage. The ACA required all US citizens to have some form of health coverage, although the nature of that coverage varied widely. Subsequently, the passage of the Tax Cuts and Jobs Act of 2017 repealed the ACA's "individual mandate" to purchase insurance. As a result, individuals who were unable to afford insurance may have been heavily impacted by chronic lack of access to health coverage.

- The COVID-19 pandemic significantly undermined health insurance coverage, as broad surges in unemployment caused many to lose employer-sponsored insurance and disrupted access to care. While some of those issues have been corrected by the Biden Administration and the Inflation Reduction Act, we must expect that many of the variables around health care access—particularly for those with low incomes—will be dependent upon the particular policies and politics of the sitting administration at a given point in time. Congress has yet to pass legislation that would result in a long-term stabilization of the insurance market.

INTRODUCTION

HIV health care services in the United States have historically been covered by an assortment of federal, state, and local programs, such as Medicare, Medicaid, the Ryan White HIV/AIDS Program, and state and local health department–funded and/or administered programs. HIV/AIDS service organizations, local community-based organizations, federally qualified health centers, and grants from other sources also provide services for people living with HIV (PWH) who are underinsured or uninsured or meet a certain income threshold. These programs collectively constitute the long-standing pathways to insurance coverage, care, and access to HIV-related treatment and prevention for people living with and at risk for HIV. Some programs also provide access to HIV medications, including patient assistance programs, co-pay relief, and medications for co-occurring conditions common among PWH. The system of HIV care and prevention is a patchwork largely dependent upon government funding and political will.

AFFORDABLE CARE ACT

The ACA was signed into law by President Obama and was designed to reform health care coverage in the United States

(Levy, 2015). It represents the broadest reform to US health care system since the 1960s. When the ACA was enacted in 2010, approximately 46.5 million nonelderly Americans had no health insurance. The number dropped rapidly and reached an historic low of 27 million in 2016. The trend reversed during the Trump presidency owing to barriers erected by the administration, and approximately 1 million people became uninsured between 2017 and 2018 (KFF, 2020b). However, because of the Biden Administration's aggressive tactics to increase enrollment, by the end of 2021, 35 million people enrolled in coverage and the rate of uninsured people reached an all-time low (DHHS, 2022).

Passage of the ACA also directly affected provision of HIV care. Reforms which had a significant impact on PWH include:

1. Prohibiting discrimination by insurers against individuals with pre-existing conditions.

2. Requiring that all US citizens obtain health insurance coverage (this was subsequently effectively repealed, as noted above).

3. Expanding the Medicaid program to cover all individuals under 138% of the federal poverty level (FPL) (this was made optional for states by a 2012 Supreme Court ruling, see below).

4. Creating individual and small-group insurance markets ("exchanges") in each state. Along with the addition of federal tax credits for qualified individuals, these mechanisms have enabled low-income individuals to purchase more affordable insurance.

Ongoing public policy maneuvers, however, have brought about diverse changes in availability and affordability of private insurance coverage for PWH in many cases, depending on state of residence.

The constitutionality of various aspects of the ACA has been repeatedly challenged, even up to the US Supreme Court. The most momentous of these was a 2012 decision effectively making Medicaid expansion an optional, state-by-state decision. As of 2022, 38 states and the District of Columbia have chosen to adopt Medicaid expansion in some form. The remaining 12, to date, have declined. Four of these states are located outside of the US South, and the remaining eight are southern. As of 2021, Texas had 766,000 uninsured citizens who will qualify for coverage if the state expands Medicaid eligibility. Florida has the second largest uninsured population with 425,000 (Gee & Rapfogel, 2021). In its annual HIV Prevention Progress Report, the CDC for the first time listed "persons residing in the southern United States" as a specific population at increased risk of acquiring HIV, along with people of color, men who have sex with men, and various other groups (CDC, 2019).

Importantly, Medicaid remains the largest source of coverage for PWH in the United States, covering 42% of the population with HIV (KFF, 2019). In states that reject Medicaid expansion, individuals who are not below the poverty line but cannot afford commercial insurance remain uninsured. Low-income adults who do not qualify for Medicaid through other qualifying categories (e.g., are not disabled, elderly, caring for children, or pregnant) are thus left without access to any affordable health coverage options whatsoever. The lack of universal Medicaid expansion at present, coupled with significant flexibility provided to state lawmakers and insurers in the state insurance markets, has left PWH in each state with insurance coverage options of widely varying value. Although the Ryan White HIV/AIDS Program (see below) is a safety net program designed to "wrap around" other forms of health coverage, it is also affected by what each state can offer to its residents living with HIV (see section on "Medicaid" below, for additional details).

In 2018, Centers for Medicare and Medicaid Services (CMS) issued a final rule to increase the maximum use of ACA-noncompliant "short-term" insurance policies from 3 months to 364 days, thus facilitating uptake of these policies by people who wanted or needed to buy their insurance as inexpensively as possible. Often referred to as "junk insurance," these policies usually do not cover prescription drugs, maternity care, or care for people with pre-existing medical conditions. Purchasers are often not fully aware of their very limited utility at the time of purchase. While the Biden Administration has sought to expand accessibility of quality plans, as of 2022, it has not yet reversed this rule.

PRIVATE INSURANCE

Private health insurance in the United States is typically offered by private, for-profit, or nonprofit companies to various markets. In 2008, employment-based health insurance was the primary source of coverage for American workers (Rho and & Schmitt, 2010), offered as benefits or in the form of other compensation to employees by their employer. Individual insurance plans were less common before the ACA.

Some common forms of private insurance are indemnity plans, preferred provider plans, and health maintenance organizations. With indemnity plans, individuals can generally choose any health care provider and have a portion of the fees paid by the insurance. With preferred provider plans, individuals must choose from a defined network of clinicians, but the clinicians are generally employed by different groups. With health maintenance plans, individuals receive care from one or a small number of clinician groups hired by the insurer.

Reimbursement to clinicians varies widely with private insurance policies, with lower rates generally paid by managed care organizations. The provider networks within insurance plans can also affect reimbursement levels, as can plan benefits, co-pays, and cost-sharing mechanisms. Coverage of particular medications and treatments varies widely under private insurance plans.

STATE INSURANCE EXCHANGES

One of the most significant accomplishments of the ACA was the creation of marketplaces for individual and small-group insurance plans in each state (Center for Consumer Information & Oversight, 2022) Each state insurance exchange is simply a market forum where private insurance companies offer various qualified health plans to residents of that state. Individuals can access the marketplace online, by phone, or in person through assistants. Potential customers also use the marketplace to determine their eligibility for Medicaid or CHIP benefits (HealthCare.gov, Medicaid and CHIP coverage).

The ACA also makes tax credit subsidies available to some low- and medium-income individuals to purchase insurance through the state exchanges. Tax credits of gradated amounts are available to those with income levels between 133% and 400% FPL, and they are taken as up-front subsidies to the plan premium (HealthCare.gov, Premium tax credit glossary). For 2021 and 2022, the American Rescue Plan temporarily expanded eligibility for premium tax credits by eliminating the 400% FPL ceiling (IRS, 2022).

Plans offered within the markets vary widely in cost as well as coverage and benefit design. However, all are required to provide essential health benefits as a part of the insurance package including services within the following ten categories: ambulatory patient services; emergency services; hospitalizations; maternity and newborn care; mental health and substance use disorder services (including behavioral health treatment); prescription drugs; rehabilitative and habilitative services and devices; laboratory services; preventive and wellness services and chronic disease management; and pediatric services (including oral and vision care) (HealthCare.gov, Essential health benefits glossary). In addition, all state exchange plans are required to include a minimum percentage of all the Essential Community Providers (ECPs) in a geographic area in their provider networks. ECPs are providers that serve predominately low-income, medically underserved individuals. This includes Ryan White HIV/AIDS Program providers.

MEDICAID

Medicaid has long been the nation's public health insurance program for people with low-income status, limited resources, and disability. Originally, the program covered only certain populations, such as the medically disabled and pregnant persons, infants, and children living in poverty. Medicaid covers inpatient, ambulatory care, and skilled nursing care. It also covers prescription medications except for persons who also have Medicare coverage ("dual eligibles"). Coverage levels, eligibility criteria, and program benefits vary widely from state to state (Medicaid.gov, Benefits). Medicaid is financed jointly by the federal government and states. It is administered by state governments in accordance with certain basic federal eligibility and benefit standards (Medicaid.gov, Financing). At the federal level, the Medicaid program is run by the Centers for Medicare and Medicaid Services (CMS) under the US Department of Health and Human Services. Medicaid is the third largest domestic program in the federal budget, after Social Security and Medicare (Rudowitz &

Snyder, 2015). The federal government matches state spending for eligible beneficiaries without limit. The federal share for "traditional Medicaid"—children, parents and non-ACA expansion adults, the elderly, and people with disabilities—is based on a formula and the state's per capita income relative to other states. The design of Medicaid dictates that the government will pay a larger share of program costs in poorer states. The federal share (FMAO) varies by state and can be anywhere from 56% to 78% (2022) or higher. The ACA sought to expand the program's coverage to include all citizens below 138% FPL regardless of other categorizations (Rudowitz et al., 2021). However, as discussed earlier, this was not accepted by all states. Some states have partially expanded their Medicaid program in a variety of ways, and others have declined expansion altogether, largely for political reasons. The approximately 2.2 million eligible individuals in those states in the "coverage gap" are left with few options (KFF, 2022b). In 2022, Congress attempted to address this issue through the reconciliation process, but it did not make it into the final package. The premium tax credits described previously were also intended to help reach some of these individuals by giving them access to insurance plans of very low cost.

In 2021, 41 states reported that they used capitated managed care models to deliver Medicaid services to mitigate Medicaid budgetary costs through reductions of benefits, limitations to drug formularies, and other efforts (KFF, 2022a). Some others also offer managed care-type programs to particular populations in an effort to reduce costs. Managed care organizations (MCOs) contract directly with the state to provide services and benefits in a variety of capacities (KFF, Medicaid Managed Care Market Tracker). Some MCOs are operated by a parent firm that also participates in the private insurance market. Traditional Medicaid programs offer provider reimbursement through fee-for-service rates that are determined by the state. MCOs make agreements for provider reimbursement based on monthly capitation rates.

MEDICARE

Medicare is the federal health insurance program for people older than age 65 years and for those younger than 65 with permanent disabilities. The Medicare program is also administered by CMS. About one-quarter of PWH receive medical care through Medicare (KFF, 2016).

Medicare eligibility is tied to work history and contributions to Medicare through employment-based withholding. The number of PWH who use Medicare has increased because of longevity attributable to effective antiretroviral therapy and effective treatment of multiple chronic health conditions. Medicare covers HIV testing for beneficiaries.

Since Medicare Part D was launched in 2006, Medicare has provided prescription drug coverage under the Medicare Part D drug benefit. Most Medicare-eligible individuals can decide whether to participate through enrollment in one of several prescription drug plans that are marketed as stand-alone coverage or to rely on managed care plans ("Medicare Advantage"). When Medicare Part D was launched, Congress identified six

types of prescription drugs as "protected classes" and required that they be covered by Part D plans. Antiretroviral drugs were one of the protected classes, as well as cancer drugs, mental health treatments, and other medications that also require uninterrupted use, although that designation was under threat during the Trump administration. These protected classes were exempted from any prior authorization, step therapy or other "utilization management" techniques that would interrupt or delay patients' access to these drugs.

Medicare Part D also includes an "exceptions and appeals" process that can be used to request coverage of drugs not covered by the plan. Individual Part D plans differ widely in terms of premiums and other cost-sharing requirements. Specifically, Medicare Part D includes a sequence of cost-sharing requirements, including an initial deductible and subsequent "out-of-pocket" costs. Most Part D plans also have a coverage gap (also referred to as the Part D "donut hole") in which, after a certain amount of the costs have been paid through the coverage plan, any additional costs become the responsibility of the individual (Medicare.gov, Costs in the coverage gap; National Council on Aging, Tools & Training for Professionals; 2022) until the costs reach the catastrophic coverage threshold (Medicare.gov, Catastrophic coverage). At that point, nearly all costs are then covered by Medicare. The ACA closed this gap in 2020, although beneficiaries may still incur costs based on other factors.

Medicare reimbursement rates are similar to those of private insurance. Clinicians who accept Medicare reimbursement are subject to federal audits of their charts to check billed amounts against services documented.

RYAN WHITE HIV/AIDS PROGRAM

The Ryan White HIV/AIDS Program is a federal program designed specifically to ensure provision of care, treatment, and supportive services for PWH in the United States. First enacted in 1990, it is administered by the Health Resources and Services Administration under the US Department of Health and Human Services (HRSA, HIV/AIDS Bureau, Ryan White HIV/AIDS Program: about the Program).

Fundamentally, the Ryan White Program provides a "safety net" for health care services to PWH who have no other source of health coverage or are confronted with coverage limits. The program is designed to "wrap around" other forms of coverage and is—from a legal perspective—the "payer of last resort." This designation means that if an individual is eligible for any other program, they must access that coverage and benefits before accessing the Ryan White Program (HRSA, 2018).

As the third largest source of federal funding for HIV care in the United States after Medicare and Medicaid, the Ryan White Program is estimated to reach over 561,000 PWH each year (HRSA, 2021). Funding for the Ryan White Program is subject to Congressional appropriation each year. In addition to federal funding, some states and localities also provide funding to their Ryan White programs through state matching funds requirements.

Part A of the Ryan White Program provides funding to Eligible Metropolitan Areas and Transitional Grant Areas hardest hit by the HIV/AIDS epidemic for a wide range of services and efforts.

Part B provides funding to states and territories (HRSA, 2022). A vitally important component is the ADAP, which is specifically funded through allocations to the states under Part B along with state funding contributions. Each state's ADAP program provides HIV-related prescription drugs to low-income individuals with limited or no prescription drug coverage (KFF, 2020a). Many states also use ADAP funding to purchase health insurance and/or pay insurance premiums, copayments, or deductibles for PWH. All ADAP programs participate in the federal 340B Program, enabling them to purchase drugs at or below the statutorily defined 340B ceiling price.

Part C of the Ryan White Program funds providers and medical clinics to deliver comprehensive medical care and treatment to PWH who have no other source for care (HRSA, 2022). Part C also funds early intervention services, ambulatory care, and primary health care services for PWH in underserved or rural communities and communities of color. Finally, Part C also provides planning grants and capacity grants to support organizations in the delivery of high-quality, effective HIV care.

Part D of the Ryan White Program grants support services for women, infants, children, and youth (HRSA, 2022).

Part F provides funding for a variety of initiatives, including the Special Projects of National Significance, AIDS Education & Training Centers, dental programs, and the Minority AIDS Initiative (HRSA, 2022).

The benefits available through the ACA, together with support provided by Medicaid expansion in the majority of states, are now in place to provide some supports to PWH that were not available when the Ryan White CARE Act was created in 1990. Simultaneously, however, the number of PWH has increased over those decades and the proportion of PWH needing services provided by these programs is climbing.

In the 30 + years since the Ryan White Program was founded, organizations have learned how to make these programs dovetail to best meet the needs of PWH in a country without universal health care. The early passage and development of the Ryan White CARE Act set a critical precedent for the delivery of functional, HIV-focused services. This prototype, designed in close collaboration with the people it serves, subsequently influenced the ACA and Medicare expansion as these programs were similarly designed in consultation with program users. The Kaiser Family Foundation has asserted that "the Ryan White Program remains a critical component of the nation's response to HIV in the ACA era" (KFF, 2020a).

NETWORKS OF CARE

For HIV providers, inclusion in networks of care for health programs is of great importance. Most patients' health coverage limits them to: (1) seeing only certain providers who are "in network"; (2) being charged substantially higher fees for seeing "out of network" providers; or (3) being declined services by providers not included in the network.

The ACA requires that all plans in the state exchanges include a minimum percentage of all the ECPs in a geographic area in their provider network. As indicated previously, ECPs are providers that serve predominately low-income, medically underserved individuals. This includes Ryan White HIV/AIDS Program providers.

Reimbursement rates and schedules for providers who are part of the network are set by or negotiated with health coverage issuers and entities.

PROVIDER REIMBURSEMENT

Reimbursement for medical encounters and procedures depends heavily on thorough and accurate documentation of the medical visit, diagnosis, treatment, and services as recorded and submitted through coding claims. The level of complexity and severity of the medical encounter—and thus the level of reimbursement owed—is defined by the nature of the problem(s), the number of problems at issue, the amount of time spent with the patient, and other factors. Careful documentation of these factors is required to ensure adequate and appropriate reimbursement and is also generally considered a best practice to accurately communicate a provider's clinical decision-making. Other factors that are essential to document are the specific elements of the medical history, the physical examination, and medical decision-making. Documenting time spent on prevention services (e.g., counseling the patient about consistent condom use and disclosure to partners) and on promoting other behavioral changes (e.g., tobacco cessation, and weight loss) is also essential for accurate reimbursement of these services.

CODING

Standardized coding systems are used in the United States to process billing claims to private and public insurers. The two principal systems used for coding medical information in the United States are the International Classification of Diseases (ICD) and the Current Procedural Terminology (CPT) codes that make up the Healthcare Common Procedure Coding System (HCPCS). In general, CPT/HCPCS codes identify the services rendered, whereas ICD codes focus more on the diagnosis. CPT codes are created, maintained, and trademarked by the American Medical Association (AMA, 2022).

The HCPCS was created by CMS. It is based on CPT codes but provides for two levels of coding. Level I consists of AMA's CPT codes and provides for medical services and procedures furnished by clinicians. Level I codes are numeric. Level II codes are alphanumeric and apply primarily to medical devices and non-clinician services, such as ambulatory care, immunizations, diagnostic procedures, family counseling, and services provided by other health professionals (e.g., clinical nurses, psychologists, and pharmacists) (CMS, 2023).

Medicaid and Medicare services are reimbursed by CMS on the basis of the HCPCS codes for clinician activities.

The ICD is the international standard diagnostic classification for all epidemiological, health, and clinical usage. It is a coding and classification system of diseases, symptoms, injuries, and abnormal findings. It also documents the social circumstances and external causes of injury or diseases, as classified by the World Health Organization (WHO) (WHO, 2022).

In the context of reimbursement, ICD codes are used in conjunction with CPT codes to classify vital records and health condition codes associated with outpatient, inpatient, medical office utilization, and hospital charges.

REFERENCES

American Medical Association (AMA). CPT coding resources. https://www.ama-assn.org/practice-management/cpt/need-coding-resources. Published 2022. Accessed September 15, 2022.

Center for Consumer Information & Oversight. State-based exchanges. https://www.cms.gov/cciio/resources/fact-sheets-and-faqs/state-marketplaces.html. Published 2022. Accessed September 14, 2022.

Centers for Disease Control and Prevention (CDC). HIV prevention progress report, 2019. https://www.cdc.gov/hiv/pdf/policies/progressreports/cdc-hiv-preventionprogressreport.pdf. Published 2019. Accessed September 14, 2022.

CDC. HIV testing dropped sharply among key groups during first year of COVID-19 pandemic. https://www.cdc.gov/media/releases/2022/p0623-HIV-testing.html. June 23, 2022. Accessed September 15, 2022.

CDC. International classification of diseases, tenth revision, clinical modification (ICD-10-CM). National Center for Health Statistics. https://www.cdc.gov/nchs/icd/icd-10-cm.htm. n.d. Accessed September 14, 2022.

Centers for Medicare and Medicaid Services (CMS). List of CPT/HCPCS Codes. https://www.cms.gov/search/cms?keys=HCPCS+codes+. Published 3/16/2023. Accessed March 17, 2023.

Corallo B, Moreno S. Analysis of recent national trends in Medicaid and CHIP enrollment. KFF. https://www.kff.org/coronavirus-covid-19/issue-brief/analysis-of-recent-national-trends-in-medicaid-and-chip-enrollment/#:~:text=Data%20show%20that%20Medicaid%2FCHIP,64.5%25%20(Figure%202). September 12, 2022. Accessed September 15, 2022.

Department of Health and Human Services, US (DHHS). New reports show record 35 million people enrolled in coverage related to the Affordable Care Act, with historic 21 million people enrolled in Medicaid Expansion coverage. https://www.hhs.gov/about/news/2022/04/29/new-reports-show-record-35-million-people-enrolled-in-coverage-related-to-the-affordable-care-act.html#:~:text=media%40hhs.gov-,New%20Reports%20Show%20Record%2035%20Million%20People%20Enrolled%20in%20Coverage,Enrolled%20in%20Medicaid%20Expansion%20Coverage. Published April 29, 2022. Accessed September 15, 2022.

DHHS. Public health emergency declaration. https://www.phe.gov/Preparedness/legal/Pages/phedeclaration.aspx. n.d. Accessed September 15, 2022.

Gee E, Rapfogel N. Closing the Medicaid coverage gap would save 7,000 lives each year. Center for American Progress. https://www.americanprogress.org/article/closing-medicaid-coverage-gap-save-7000-lives-year/. Published September 10, 2021. Accessed September 15, 2022.

HealthCare.gov. Essential health benefits glossary. https://www.healthcare.gov/glossary/essential-health-benefits. n.d. Accessed September 14, 2022.

HealthCare.gov. https://www.healthcare.gov/medicaid-chip/getting-medicaid-chip/. n.d. Accessed September 14, 2022.

HealthCare.gov. Premium tax credit glossary. https://www.healthcare.gov/glossary/premium-tax-credit/. n.d. Accessed September 14, 2022.

Health Resources and Service Administration (HRSA). Eligible individuals & allowable uses of funds. https://ryanwhite.hrsa.gov/sites/default/files/ryanwhite/grants/service-category-pcn-16-02-final.pdf. Published 2018. Accessed September 14, 2022.

HRSA. HIV/AIDS Bureau, Ryan White HIV/AIDS Program: about the Program. https://ryanwhite.hrsa.gov/about. n.d. Accessed September 14, 2022.

HRSA. HIV/AIDS Bureau, Ryan White HIV/AIDS Program: Program parts & initiatives. https://ryanwhite.hrsa.gov/about/parts-and-initiatives. Published 2022. Accessed September 15, 2022.

HRSA. Ryan White HIV/AIDS Program annual client-level data report. Ryan White HIV/AIDS Program services report 2020. https://ryanwhite.hrsa.gov/sites/default/files/ryanwhite/about-program/RWHAP-annual-client-level-data-report-2020.pdf. Published December 2021. Accessed September 15, 2022.

HRSA. Ryan White HIV/AIDS Program. Coronavirus disease 2019 (COVID-19) frequently asked questions. https://hab.hrsa.gov/coronavirus/frequently-asked-questions. n.d. Accessed September 14, 2022.

Internal Revenue Service (IRS). The Premium Tax Credit—the basics. https://www.irs.gov/affordable-care-act/individuals-and-families/the-premium-tax-credit-the-basics. Published 2022. Accessed September 15, 2022.

Kaiser Family Foundation (KFF). 10 things to know about managed care. https://www.kff.org/medicaid/issue-brief/10-things-to-know-about-medicaid-managed-care/. February 23, 2022a. Accessed September 14, 2022.

KFF. AIDS drug assistance programs (ADAPs). http://kff.org/hivaids/fact-sheet/aids-drug-assistance-programs/. Published August 16, 2017. Accessed September 14, 2022.

KFF. Key facts about the uninsured population. https://www.kff.org/uninsured/issue-brief/key-facts-about-the-uninsured-population/. Published November 6, 2020b. Accessed September 14, 2022.

KFF. Medicaid and HIV. https://www.kff.org/hivaids/fact-sheet/medicaid-and-hiv/. Published October 1, 2019. Accessed September 14, 2022.

KFF. Medicaid managed care market tracker. https://www.kff.org/statedata/collection/medicaid-managed-care-tracker/. n.d. Accessed September 14, 2022.

KFF. Status of state Medicaid expansion decisions: interactive map. https://www.kff.org/medicaid/issue-brief/status-of-state-medicaid-expansion-decisions-interactive-map/. July 21, 2022b. Accessed September 15, 2022.

KFF. Medicare and HIV. https://www.kff.org/hivaids/fact-sheet/medicare-and-hiv/. October 14, 2016. Accessed September 14, 2022.

KFF. The Ryan White HIV/AIDS Program: the basics. https://www.kff.org/hivaids/fact-sheet/the-ryan-white-hivaids-program-the-basics/. October 22, 2020a. Accessed September 15, 2022.

Levy M. Patient Protection and Affordable Care Act (PPACA). *Encyclopedia Britannica*. https://www.britannica.com/topic/Patient-Protection-and-Affordable-Care-Act. Published June 26, 2015. Accessed September 15, 2022.

Medicaid.gov. Benefits. https://www.medicaid.gov/chip/benefits/index.html. n.d. Accessed September 15, 2022.

Medicaid.gov. Financing. https://www.medicaid.gov/chip/financing/index.html. n.d. Accessed September 15, 2022.

Medicare.gov. Catastrophic coverage. https://www.medicare.gov/drug-coverage-part-d/costs-for-medicare-drug-coverage/catastrophic-coverage. n.d. Accessed September 15, 2022.

Medicare.gov. Costs in the coverage gap. https://www.medicare.gov/drug-coverage-part-d/costs-for-medicare-drug-coverage/costs-in-the-coverage-gap. n.d. Accessed September 15, 2022.

National Council on Aging. Tools & training for professionals; donut hole: who pays what in Part D." https://www.ncoa.org/article/donut-hole-part-d. Published 2022. Accessed September 15, 2022.

Rho, HJ, Schmitt J. Health-insurance coverage rates for US workers, 1979–2008. https://cepr.net/documents/publications/hc-coverage-2010-03.pdf. Published March 2010. Accessed September 15, 2022.

Rudowitz R, Snyder L. Medicaid financing: how does it work and what are the implications? Kaiser Family Foundation. http://kff.org/medicaid/issue-brief/medicaid-financing-how-does-it-work-and-what-are-the-implications/. Published May 20, 2015. Accessed September 15, 2022.

Rudowitz R, Williams E, Hinton, E, Garfield R. Medicaid financing: the basics. Kaiser Family Foundation. https://www.kff.org/report-section/medicaid-financing-the-basics-issue-brief/. Published May 7, 2021. Accessed September 15, 2022.

The Henry J. Kaiser Family Foundation. The Ryan White HIV/AIDS Program: the basics. http://files.kff.org/attachment/fact-sheet-pdf-the-ryan-white-program. Published February 2017. Accessed September 15, 2022.

World Health Organization (WHO). ICD-11 2022 release. Better health with better information. https://www.who.int/news/item/11-02-2022-icd-11-2022-release. Published 2022. Accessed September 15, 2022.

44.

LEGAL ISSUES

Jarrett K. Sell

CHAPTER GOALS

- Demonstrate knowledge about legal issues surrounding HIV health care and communicate more effectively, professionally, and sensitively with patients and their families.

ROUTINE HIV TESTING (WITH CONSENT)

LEARNING OBJECTIVE

- Discuss the Centers for Disease Control and Prevention's (CDC) recommendations for routine HIV testing in various health care settings.

WHAT'S NEW?

- Before and during the COVID-19 pandemic in the United States, from 2019 to 2020, new HIV diagnoses reported to the CDC decreased by 17%.

- In the United States, from 2010–2019, Black men who have sex with men (MSM) with HIV were less likely (83%) than White MSM (90%) to know their status.%). The lowest percentages of known, diagnosed HIV were among 13–24-year-old (55%) and 25–34-year-old (71%) MSM.

- The US Preventive Services Task Force (USPSTF) recommends that clinicians screen for HIV infection in all adolescents and adults aged 15 to 65 years. Younger adolescents and older adults who are at increased risk of infection should also be screened.

KEY POINTS

- It is estimated that overall, 15% of people who do not know they have HIV account for 40% of transmissions to new HIV-negative persons.

- The CDC recommends that all people aged 13–65 receive an HIV test at least once as part of routine healthcare. Persons identified as at high risk for HIV infection should be retested at least annually.

- Routine testing delinks pre-and posttest counseling from testing.

- Both in routine and emergency care settings, many opportunities for routine HIV testing are missed.

An estimated 1.2 million people in the United States have HIV, including about 161,800 people who are unaware of their status. Nearly 40% of new HIV infections are transmitted by people who do not know they have the virus (CDC, 2006). Approximately half of unaware MSM and people who inject drugs who reported not having been tested in the past year reported not being offered HIV testing by any clinician despite having seen one. In the United States from 2010–2019, fewer Black MSM with HIV (83%) than White MSM (90%) knew their status, and the lowest percentages of diagnosed HIV were among 13–24-year-old (55%) and 25–34-year-old (71%) MSM (Pitasi et al., 2021).

A Morbidity and Mortality Weekly Report (MMWR) from the CDC in June 2018 evaluated a sample of 333 healthcare-seeking, heterosexual adults at increased risk for acquiring HIV: 194 (58%) reported not receiving an HIV test offer at a recent medical visit, and men (vs. women) had a significantly lower prevalence of provider-initiated HIV test offers (32% vs. 48%). Recent HIV testing was higher among recipients of provider-initiated offers compared with nonrecipients (71% vs. 16%). Provider-initiated HIV test offers are an important strategy for increasing HIV testing among heterosexual populations, especially men. However, despite the 2006 CDC recommendation for routine opt-out HIV testing, the percentage of ambulatory care visits at which an HIV test is performed only increased from 0.76% in 2009 to 2.41% in 2014, with HIV testing more often performed during visits for preventive care (Hoover et al., 2020).

A meta-analysis of 11 independent studies showed that the prevalence of high-risk sexual behavior is reduced substantially after people become aware that they have HIV (Marks et al., 2006). Estimated transmission is 3.5 times higher among persons who are unaware of their status, which contributes disproportionately to the number of new HIV infections each year in the United States, than among persons who are aware of their status (Marks et al., 2006). Modeling data showed that an estimated 49% of transmissions were from the 20% of persons living with HIV (PWH) unaware of their status (Hall et al., 2012).

A study in South Carolina found that among persons identified as late testers (persons who received an AIDS diagnosis within 1 year of HIV diagnosis), approximately three-fourths had visited a South Carolina healthcare facility prior to their HIV diagnosis. In addition, most of the late testers had made multiple visits, and most of their visits occurred 1 year or more before diagnosis of HIV. According to the report, the majority of diagnoses for these previous visits probably would not have prompted HIV testing under a risk-based testing strategy (CDC, 2006). The CDC published revised recommendations concerning routine HIV testing in healthcare settings in September 2006. The major recommendations are as follows:

- For patients in all healthcare settings.

- HIV screening is recommended for patients in all healthcare settings after patients are notified that testing will be performed unless patients decline (opt-out screening).

- Persons at high risk for HIV should be screened for HIV at least annually.

- Separate written consent for HIV testing should not be required; general consent for medical care should be considered sufficient to encompass consent for HIV testing.

- Prevention counseling should *not* be required as part of HIV diagnostic testing or HIV screening programs in healthcare settings.

- For pregnant women.

- HIV screening should be included in the routine panel of prenatal screening tests for all pregnant women.

- Repeat screening in the third trimester is recommended in certain jurisdictions with elevated rates of HIV among pregnant women.

Although the CDC recommends that prevention counseling should not be required with HIV diagnostic testing in healthcare settings, the elements of informed consent include some of the information communicated during pretest counseling. Also, risk assessment is needed to identify patients at high risk for HIV who should be screened at least annually. The CDC (2006) recommendations define informed consent as follows:

> A process of communication between patient and provider, through which an informed patient can choose whether to undergo HIV testing or decline to do so. Elements of informed consent typically include providing oral or written information regarding HIV, the risks and benefits of testing, the implications of HIV test results, how test results will be communicated, and the opportunity to ask questions.

Routine testing means that HIV testing is offered to all patients. Testing requires informed consent, but that consent can be included in the general consent to care agreements. Patients can choose to "opt out" of routine testing if they do not want to be tested. Opt-out testing in a 2022 systemic review and meta-analysis demonstrated a 12% higher uptake in HIV testing than opt-in testing (Soh et al., 2022).

The CDC recommends providers in clinical settings should offer HIV screening at least annually to all sexually active MSM. Additionally, HIV testing is recommended for all persons being evaluated for sexually transmitted infections (STIs) who are not already aware of their HIV status. Clinicians can also consider the potential benefits of more frequent HIV screening (e.g., every 3 or 6 months) for some asymptomatic sexually active MSM based on their individual risk factors, local HIV epidemiology, and local policies (DiNenno et al., 2017). The CDC also noted that additional research is needed to establish the individual- or community-level factors that might increase the risk for HIV acquisition for MSM and merit more frequent HIV screening. For MSM who are prescribed pre-exposure prophylaxis (PrEP), HIV testing every 3 months and immediate testing whenever signs and symptoms of acute HIV infection are reported is indicated (DiNenno et al., 2017).

The USPSTF recommended in 2019 that clinicians screen for HIV infection in all pregnant persons, including those who present in labor or at delivery whose HIV status is unknown (grade A recommendation) and all adolescents and adults aged 15 to 65 years. Younger adolescents and older adults who are at increased risk of infection should also be screened (grade A recommendation). The USPSTF Recommendation Summary found convincing evidence that identification and early treatment of HIV infection is of substantial benefit in reducing the risk of AIDS-related events or death. The USPSTF found convincing evidence that the use of antiretroviral therapy (ART) is of substantial benefit in decreasing the risk of HIV transmission to uninfected sex partners. The USPSTF also found convincing evidence that identification and treatment of pregnant women living with HIV infection is of substantial benefit in reducing the rate of mother-to-child transmission. The overall magnitude of the benefit of screening for HIV infection in adolescents, adults, and pregnant women is substantial (USPSTF, 2019) (Table 44.1).

Laws governing consent for HIV testing are state specific. Although all states require consent for an HIV test, most states that had required explicit written consent prior to the 2006 CDC revised HIV testing recommendations have changed their laws (Neff & Goldschmidt, 2011). Current state HIV testing laws are compiled by the CDC at https://www.cdc.gov/hiv/policies/law/states/testing.html.

Additional challenges in implementing routine HIV testing include cost of testing, follow-up notification of positive results in emergency departments and in-patient settings, and adoption of rapid testing. The COVID-19 pandemic also likely impacted routine HIV testing, as from 2019 to 2020 new HIV diagnoses reported to the CDC decreased by 17% (DiNenno et al., 2022). Future testing strategies may benefit from design that particularly vulnerable or marginalized populations. Transgender women, for example, who are disproportionately affected by HIV, were more likely to be tested if they had a usual source of health care and comfort with a health care provider (Lee et al., 2022). Targeted home HIV testing (Hecht et al., 2021) or community-based interventions, as seen in the community-led HIV self-testing study in Malawi that showed higher testing rates among adolescents in the community-led testing arm (84.6%) when compared to the standard of care arm (67.1%) (Indravudh et al., 2021), may also be strategies for increasing routine testing and HIV identification.

Table 44.1 US PREVENTATIVE SERVICES TASK FORCE HIV SCREENING RECOMMENDATIONS

POPULATION	RECOMMENDATION	GRADE
Pregnant persons	The USPSTF recommends that clinicians screen for HIV infection in all pregnant persons, including those who present in labor or at delivery whose HIV status is unknown.	A
Adolescents and adults aged 15–65 year	The USPSTF recommends that clinicians screen for HIV infection in adolescents and adults aged 15–65 years. Younger adolescents and older adults who are at increased risk of infection should also be screened. See the Clinical Considerations section for more information about assessment of risk, screening intervals, and rescreening in pregnancy.	A

SOURCE: The US Preventative Services Task Force. https://uspreventiveservicestaskforce.org/uspstf/recommendation/human-immunodeficiency-virus-hiv-infection-screening. Published 2019. Accessed August 30, 2022.

REFERENCES/RECOMMENDED READING

American Medical Association (AMA). AMA code of medical ethics opinion 8.1—routine universal screening for HIV. https://www.ama-assn.org/delivering-care/ethics/routine-universal-screening-hiv. Published 2022. Accessed August 25, 2022.

Centers for Disease Control and Prevention (CDC). Revised recommendations for HIV testing of adults, adolescents, and pregnant women in health-care settings. *MMWR Morbid Mortal Wkly Rep.* 2006;55(RR14):1–17.

Cossarini F, Hanna DB, Ginsberg MS, et al. Missed opportunities for HIV prevention: individuals who HIV seroconverted despite accessing healthcare. *AIDS Behav.* November 2018;22(11):3519–3524.

Dailey AF, Hoots BE, Hall HI, et al. Vital signs: human immunodeficiency virus testing and diagnosis delays—United States. *MMWR Morb Mortal Rep.* 2017; 66(47):1300–1306.

Diepstra KL, Cunningham T, Rhodes AG, et al. Prevalence and predictors of provider-initiated HIV test offers among heterosexual persons at increased risk for acquiring HIV infection—Virginia, 2016. *MMWR Morb Mortal Wkly Rep.* June 29, 2018;67(25):714–717.

DiNenno EA, Prejean J, Irwin K, et al. Recommendations for HIV screening of gay, bisexual, and other men who have sex with men—United States, 2017. *MMWR Morb Mortal Wkly Rep.* August 11, 2017; 66(31):830–832.

DiNenno EA, Delaney KP, Pitasi MA, et al. HIV testing before and during the COVID-19 pandemic—United States, 2019–2020. *MMWR Morb Mortal Wkly Rep.* 2022;71:820–824.

Lee K, Trujillo L, Olansky E, et al. Factors associated with use of HIV prevention and health care among transgender women—seven urban areas, 2019–2020. *MMWR Morb Mortal Wkly Rep.* 2022;71:673–679.

Hall HI, Holtgrave D, Maulsby C. HIV transmission rates from persons living with HIV who are aware and unaware of their infection. *AIDS.* 2012;26:893–896.

Hecht J, Sanchez T, Sullivan PS, DiNenno EA, Cramer N, Delaney KP. Increasing access to HIV testing through direct-to-consumer HIV self-test distribution—United States, March 31, 2020–March 30, 2021. *MMWR Morb Mortal Wkly Rep.* 2021;70:1322–1325.

Hoover KW, Huang YA, Tanner ML, et al. HIV testing trends at visits to physician offices, community health centers, and emergency departments—United States, 2009–2017. *MMWR Morb Mortal Wkly Rep.* 2020;69:776–780.

Indravudh PP, Fielding K, Kumwenda MK, et al. Effect of community-led delivery of HIV self-testing on HIV testing and antiretroviral therapy initiation in Malawi: a cluster-randomised trial. *PLoS Med.* May 11, 2021;18(5):e1003608.

Marks G, Crepaz N, Janssen RS. Estimating sexual transmission of HIV from persons aware and unaware that they are infected with the virus in the USA. *AIDS.* 2006;20:1447–1450.

Neff S, Goldschmidt R. Centers for Disease Control and Prevention 2006 human immunodeficiency virus testing recommendations and state testing laws. *JAMA.* 2011;305(17):1767–1768.

Pitasi MA, Beer L, Cha S, et al. Vital signs: HIV infection, diagnosis, treatment, and prevention among gay, bisexual, and other men who have sex with men—United States, 2010–2019. *MMWR Morb Mortal Wkly Rep.* 2021;70:1669–1675.

Soh QR, Oh LYJ, Chow EPF, et al. HIV testing uptake according to opt-in, opt-out or risk-based testing approaches: a systematic review and meta-analysis. *Curr HIV/AIDS Rep.* July 13, 2022;19(5):375–383.

US Preventive Services Task Force. Screening for HIV infection: US Preventive Services Task Force recommendation statement. *JAMA.* 2019;321(23):2326–2336.

Wejnert C, Prejean J, Hoots B, et al. Prevalence of missed opportunities for HIV testing among persons unaware of their infection. *JAMA.* 2018;319(24):2555–2557.

HIV TESTING WITHOUT CONSENT

LEARNING OBJECTIVE

- Discuss the circumstances under which it is allowable to test a patient for HIV without consent, including reference to applicable legal regulations.

WHAT'S NEW?

- The information on HIV testing without consent has remained consistent during the past few years.

KEY POINTS

- Many states allow HIV testing without consent in limited situations, such as emergency situations or when a healthcare worker or public safety officer has had a potential exposure to HIV.

- Some states require HIV testing of convicted sex offenders, and some states allow testing of persons charged with a crime capable of transmitting HIV, such as rape.

Although all states require consent for HIV testing (Halpern, 2005), there are situations in which it is possible to obtain an HIV test without the consent of the person to be tested. In some cases, HIV testing without consent may be standard practice. For example, in New York, newborn infants are tested without parental consent if their mother did not consent to HIV testing during pregnancy. Some states require HIV testing of convicted sexual offenders (e.g., Revised Code of Washington RCW 70.24.340).

A minority of states provide explicit exceptions for consent for HIV testing in emergency medical situations (Halpern, 2005). Some states allow for testing of source patients when there has been a potential exposure to HIV in a healthcare setting or when a public safety officer has had potential exposure. California and several other states allow for HIV testing of persons accused of a criminal act capable of transmitting HIV. California requires a court hearing showing there is probable cause to believe that the accused committed the offense and that blood, semen, or another bodily fluid capable of transmitting HIV (as identified in State Department of Health Services regulations) has been transferred from the accused to the victim (California Penal Code 1524.1(b)(3)(A)). A major challenge with testing without consent is getting the required court order (if required) from the appropriate authority so that testing and initiation of postexposure prophylaxis can take place in a timely manner (see Chapter 4). A survey showed that intensivists' decisions to pursue testing without consent, a not uncommon situation, are associated with their personal ethics and often erroneous perceptions of state laws but not with the laws themselves (Halpern et al., 2007). Because laws and regulations vary by state, the clinician is responsible for knowing the appropriate rules in the state in which they practice. Consultation with the local public health officer is advised whenever HIV testing without consent is believed to be necessary.

REFERENCES/RECOMMENDED READING

Halpern SD. HIV testing without consent in critically ill patients. *JAMA.* 2005;294(6):734–737.
Halpern SD, Metkus TS, Fuchs BD, et al. Nonconsented human immunodeficiency virus testing among critically ill patients: intensivists' practices and the influence of state laws. *Arch Intern Med.* 2007;167(21):2323–2328.

DISEASE REPORTING SYSTEM

LEARNING OBJECTIVE

- Discuss the system of disease reporting in the United States and identify reportable conditions related to HIV care.

WHAT'S NEW?

- The CDC and many states have implemented molecular surveillance, based on resistance testing data, to rapidly identify cluster outbreaks of community HIV transmission.

KEY POINTS

- All state and local departments of health use name-based HIV diagnosis and AIDS reporting to track HIV.

HIV/AIDS SURVEILLANCE

Since HIV/AIDS was first recognized as a disease, most state and city departments of health have used the reporting of AIDS cases to track the incidence and prevalence of HIV infections and HIV-related complications. Data on AIDS cases are reported in a standardized format to the CDC by all 50 states, the District of Columbia, and US dependencies and possessions.

The rationale frequently cited for using HIV rather than AIDS case surveillance is that it allows for a more thorough and accurate characterization of the populations in which HIV has been newly diagnosed and helps in the prioritization of prevention services (CDC, 2005; Holtgrave, 2004). Significant changes in HIV transmission and behavior can be achieved by appropriate programs. For example, aggressive efforts to increase the proportion of pregnant women with HIV who have been tested prior to delivery and potentially accept antiretroviral prophylaxis to prevent maternal–fetal transmission have been credited with the steep decline in mother-to-child HIV transmission (Wortley et al., 2001). Lab-based reporting of CD4 counts and HIV RNA for surveillance has become a helpful tool to assess the HIV care continuum, which includes diagnosis, engagement, linkage, retention in care, and viral suppression (Lubelchek et al., 2015; Wiewel et al., 2015).

In 2005, the CDC recommended that name-based HIV reporting be implemented using the same approach that is used for nationwide AIDS surveillance. All states successfully implemented confidential name-based HIV reporting by April 2008.

HIV MOLECULAR SURVEILLANCE

Name-based HIV case surveillance data can identify patterns in diagnosis rates, but in high-incident areas, recent, rapid transmission may not be identifiable amidst large numbers of cases. Partner-notification services staff interview persons with HIV to collect information about their partners; but not all index cases are interviewed, and partners nay not be known or located. However, analysis of HIV-1 genetic sequence data, which is known as molecular surveillance, can identify transmission clusters, enabling high-impact prevention efforts for social networks at high risk of HIV transmission (Oster et al., 2018). Molecular clusters are identified through analysis of HIV molecular sequence data generated from HIV-drug-resistance testing. This is also referred to as cluster response. Cluster response uses data routinely reported to health departments to identify communities where HIV may be spreading quickly. This information can then be used to identify gaps in prevention and care services and ensure that services reach the populations that need them the most (CDC, 2023). The technology in use by the CDC and provided to local health departments is

HIV-TRACE (TRAnsmission Cluster Engine), which is a platform that has been used extensively for rapid inference of transmission networks from large sets of pathogen genetic sequences to identify potential transmission links and to describe putative transmission cluster. HIV-TRACE identifies groups of putative transmission partners and assembles these partners in transmission clusters but cannot determine transmission directionality (Kosakovsky Pond et al., 2018).

As emphasized in the CDC draft document:

> Although some tools, such as Secure HIV-TRACE and MicrobeTrace, generate network diagrams of clusters based on genetic distance data, there are important limitations to drawing inferences from these data at an individual level. Although two persons infected with highly similar HIV strains could be directly linked through transmission, other transmission relationships could be consistent with this sequence similarity: both could have been infected from a third source, or they could be connected indirectly through a transmission chain including one or more intermediaries. Because of this scientific uncertainty, the potential for the misuse and misinterpretation of these data presents a concern. Moreover, presence of or patterns of linkages can be affected by timing of diagnoses and drug resistance testing. Although analysis of molecular data to identify growing transmission clusters can identify important opportunities for individual- and cluster-level public health interventions, inferences about specific transmission linkages or indirect inferences about sexual or other risk behaviors should not be used to guide services or follow-up at the individual level. Because of the potential for misinterpretation of these diagrams, it is not recommended to disseminate genetic network diagrams beyond the group of staff involved in the analysis of sequence data. (HIV Cluster Guidance Working Group, 2018)

The National Alliance of State and Territorial AIDS Directors (NASTAD, 2018) notes that:

> Emerging data-use and data-sharing activities raise questions about data privacy and confidentiality protections and the ethical uses and sharing of personally identifiable data. The fact that HIV surveillance data is, by and large, collected without explicit patient consent for enumerated data uses triggers additional ethical considerations for how health departments use and share this data. Data-sharing protections and limitations are important not only to inform emerging public health data-sharing activities, but also to restrict data sharing for non-public health purposes, such as criminal HIV exposure and transmission prosecutions.

NASTAD focused this analysis on 10 states (Illinois, Iowa, Louisiana, Massachusetts, Michigan, North Carolina, Tennessee, Virginia, Wisconsin, and Utah). Community engagement is an important component of this rapidly evolving surveillance methodology (NASTAD, 2018).

ANONYMOUS AND CONFIDENTIAL HIV TESTING

Although most studies have not shown a decrease in HIV testing in states that have adopted name-based reporting, data indicate that some people prefer anonymous HIV testing to name-based confidential testing (Charlebois et al., 2005). Many people are understandably reluctant to have their name entered in a database of PWH. Although the states have established elaborate precautions to prevent breaches of security, the risk of disclosure of HIV status can be intimidating. Therefore, in many areas, individuals can choose to be tested for HIV either anonymously (without giving any identifying information) or confidentially (with the HIV test result linked to identifying information, such as patient name).

In states that require HIV case reporting, only confidential testing results must be reported to public health authorities. Test results from anonymous testing are not reportable. However, they do provide the clinician with an important opportunity for educating and counseling patients about reducing high-risk behaviors and seeking HIV treatments, at which point they would be captured in systems linking HIV viral load and CD4 testing to the reporting database.

REPORTABLE HIV-RELATED DISEASES

Most states require reporting of conditions that commonly occur or are associated with HIV, including syphilis and other STIs, tuberculosis, hepatitis (A, B, or C), histoplasmosis, and HIV-related opportunistic infections. Certain microbiologic diagnoses that are made by culture or serology are reported directly by the laboratory to the appropriate state or local health authority.

THE CLINICIAN'S ROLE

Healthcare providers should know which illnesses and complications must be reported to their state health departments and the time frame within which reporting is required. They should understand that reporting of notifiable conditions is dependent on the jurisdiction, that a legal obligation is imposed upon practitioners by those states, and that sanctions (e.g., fines) can be imposed upon practitioners for failure to report (CDC, 2023).

REFERENCES/RECOMMENDED READING

Boyle BA, Bradley T, Bradley H, et al. Health Insurance Portability and Accountability Act of 1996: new national medical privacy standards. *AIDS Read*. 2003; 13:261–262, 265–266

Centers for Disease Control and Prevention (CDC). HIV cluster and outbreak detection and response. https://www.cdc.gov/hiv/programresources/guidance/cluster-outbreak/index.html. Published 2023. Accessed March 17, 2023.

CDC. Trends in HIV/AIDS diagnosis-33 States, 2001–2004. *MMWR Morb Mortal Wkly Rep.* 2005; 54(45):1149–1153.

Charlebois ED, Maiorana A, McLaughlin M, et al. Potential deterrent effect of name-based HIV infection surveillance. *J Acquir Immune Defic Syndr.* 2005;39(2):219–227.

HIV Cluster Guidance Working Group. Detecting and responding to HIV transmission clusters: a guide for health departments (draft). https://www.cdc.gov/hiv/pdf/funding/announcements/ps18-1802/CDC-HIV-PS18-1802-AttachmentE-Detecting-Investigating-and-Responding-to-HIV-Transmission-Clusters.pdf. Published 2018. Accessed August 25, 2022.

Holtgrave DR. Estimation of annual HIV transmission rates in the United States, 1978–-2000. *J Acquir Defic Syndr.* 2004;35(1):89–92.

Kosakovsky Pond SL, Weaver S, Leigh Brown AJ, et al. HIV-TRACE (TRAnsmission Cluster Engine): a tool for large scale molecular epidemiology of HIV-1 and other rapidly evolving pathogens. *Mol Biol Evol.* 2018;35(7):1812–1819.

Lubelchek RJ, Finnegan KJ, Hotton AL, et al. Assessing the use of HIV surveillance data to help gauge patient retention-in-care. *J AIDS.* 2015;69:S25–S30.

NASTAD. HIV data privacy and confidentiality legal & ethical considerations for health department data sharing. https://nastad.org/resources/hiv-data-privacy-and-confidentiality-legal-ethical-considerations-health-department-data. Published June 2018. Accessed August 25, 2022.

Oster AM, France AM, Panneer N, et al. Identifying clusters of recent and rapid HIV transmission through analysis of molecular surveillance data. *J Acquir Immune Defic Syndr.* 2018;79(5):543–550.

Wiewel E, Braunstein SL, Xiaet Q, et al. Monitoring outcomes for newly diagnosed and prevalent HIV cases using a care continuum created with New York City surveillance data. *J AIDS.* 2015;68:217–226.

Wortley PM, Lindegren ML, Fleming PL. Successful implementation of perinatal HIV prevention guidelines: a multistate surveillance evaluation. *MMWR Morbid Mortal Wkly Rep.* 2001;50(RR-6):17–28.

PARTNER NOTIFICATION AND PREVENTION FOR HIV-POSITIVE PATIENTS

LEARNING OBJECTIVE

.• Describe the requirements for partner-notification practices in HIV.

WHAT'S NEW?

• A recent analysis of partner service data submitted to the CDC from 2013 to 2017 found that 97.2% of partners were notified of their potential HIV exposure. However, only 52.3% of partners were tested for HIV, with 23.8% of tested partners being diagnosed with HIV.

KEY POINTS

• Many states require healthcare providers to discuss partner-notification options with PWH. The federal 1996 Ryan White CARE Act requires all states to adopt laws requiring notification of spouses of PWH.

• Many PWH do not disclose their HIV status to their partners out of fear of rejection, loss of financial support, and/or abuse. Their partners then remain unaware of their potential HIV exposure.

• Partner-notification programs typically allow PWH to anonymously inform their sexual and needle-sharing partners that they may have been exposed to HIV.

PARTNER-NOTIFICATION LEGAL REQUIREMENTS

In many states, healthcare providers are required to discuss partner-notification options with PWH. This is not only a legal requirement, carrying the possibility of civil and/or legal sanctions for violation of partner-notification laws, but also an ethical issue. Amendments to the federal Ryan White CARE Act in 1996 require states to take "administrative or legislative action to require that a good faith effort" is made to notify spouses of their potential exposure to HIV. This action must be taken by states in order to be eligible for CARE Act funds (Webber, 2004).

States can be categorized into three groups based on their rules and regulations for partner-notification programs: (1) states that require healthcare providers to give the contact's name to the local health officer, and the public health official then notifies the contact; (2) states that give the healthcare provider the choice of notifying either the local health officer or the contacts named by the source patient directly; and (3) states that make such disclosures to a state agency discretionary or optional (Lin & Liang, 2005). Healthcare providers should seek advice from local public health departments and their own attorneys to specifically understand their legal responsibilities.

THE CLINICIAN'S ROLE

Preventing harm not only to the patient but also to others should be the goal of every clinician. The CDC has recommended an increased emphasis on prevention efforts in the primary care of PWH (Box 44.1).

In general, PWH should be given the option of directly informing their sexual or needle-sharing contacts. A study of MSM found that knowledge of HIV status resulted in a significant decrease in behaviors capable of transmitting HIV;

Box 44.1 **METHODS FOR HEALTH CARE PROVIDERS TO HELP REDUCE HIV INFECTION**

• HIV testing and linkage to care

• HIV medications

• Access to condoms

• Prevention programs for PWH and their partners

• Prevention programs for people at high risk for HIV

• Substance use treatment and access to sterile needles and syringes

• STI screening and treatment

however, the behavioral changes were not permanent (Colfax et al., 2002).

Many PWH do not disclose their HIV status to their partners, fearing that they would be threatened, harmed, or abandoned. Non-disclosers, however, are not more likely than disclosers to use condoms or other disease prevention measures (Stein et al., 1998; Wolitski et al., 1998). When individuals are reluctant to disclose their HIV status to their partners themselves, partner-notification programs can assist (CDC, 2008).

PARTNER-NOTIFICATION PROGRAMS

Partner-notification programs are designed to allow PWH to inform their sexual and needle-sharing partners that they may have been exposed to HIV. For PWH who opt not to inform their partners themselves, these programs typically provide counselors who will inform the at-risk persons of possible HIV exposure without revealing the identity of the PWH who may have exposed them.

Partner-notification programs maximize the opportunity for persons to become aware of their HIV exposure and to access HIV testing and counseling. Partner notification may prevent an at-risk individual from acquiring HIV or, if they already have HIV, allow them to receive appropriate treatment and learn how to prevent the transmission of HIV to others.

Data looking at the effectiveness of partner notification, includes a 2013 Cochrane review of partner-notification strategies in people with a STI, including HIV, that was not able to identify a single optimal method of partner notification (Ferreira et al., 2013). A recent analysis of partner service data submitted to the CDC from 2013 to 2017 found that 97.2% of partners were notified of their potential HIV exposure (Song et al., 2022). However, only 52.3% of partners were tested for HIV, with 23.8% of tested partners being diagnosed with HIV. This 2022 study highlights the importance of and gaps in efforts to provide partner notification.

REFERENCES/RECOMMENDED READING

Centers for Disease Control and Prevention (CDC). Factsheet. Proven HIV prevention methods. https//www.cdc.gov/nchhstp/newsroom/docs/factsheets/methods-508.pdf. Published 2016. Accessed September 15, 2022.

CDC. Recommendations for partner services programs for HIV infection, syphilis, gonorrhea, and chlamydial infection. *MMWR Recomm Rep.* 2008;57(Rr-9):1–83.

Colfax GN, Buchbinder SP, Cornelisse PGA, et al. Sexual risk behaviors and implications for secondary HIV transmission during and after HIV seroconversion. *AIDS.* 2002;16:1529–1535.

Ferreira A, Young T, Mathews C, et al. Strategies for partner notification for sexually transmitted infections, including HIV. *Cochrane Database Syst Rev.* October 3, 2013;2013(10):CD002843.

Lin L, Liang BA. HIV and health law: striking the balance between legal mandates and medical ethics. *Virtual Mentor AMA J Ethics.* 2005;7(10).

Song W, Mulatu MS, Rao S, et al. Factors associated with partner notification, testing, and positivity in HIV partner services programs in the United States, 2013 to 2017. *Sex Transm Dis.* March 1, 2022;49(3):197–203

Stein MD, Freedberg KA, Sullivan LM, et al. Sexual ethics: disclosure of HIV-positive status to partners. *Arch Intern Med.* 1998;158:253–257.

Webber DW. Self-incrimination, partner notification, and the criminal law: negatives for the CDC's "prevention for positives" initiative. *AIDS Public Policy J.* 2004;19:54–66.

Wejnert C, Prejean J, Hoots B, et al. Prevalence of missed opportunities for HIV testing among persons unaware of their infection. *JAMA.* 2018;319(24):2555–2557.

ISSUES IN DISCLOSURE

LEARNING OBJECTIVE

- Discuss the healthcare provider's legal responsibilities to PWH who do not disclose their HIV status to sexual and needle-sharing partners.

WHAT'S NEW?

- Information regarding disclosure issues has remained consistent during the past several years.

KEY POINTS

- The obligation of healthcare providers to maintain patient confidentiality may be overridden to protect the public health or individuals who are endangered by PWH.

- Healthcare providers should consult an attorney or their state laws and regulations before making any such disclosures.

- Healthcare providers may have a "duty to warn" if there is an ongoing exposure to potential HIV transmission. Conversely, there may be criminal actions brought against patients based on information provided to local health departments about ongoing behaviors endangering the public health.

Information disclosed by a patient to a healthcare provider during the course of the provider–patient relationship is considered confidential. This confidentiality is essential for full and free disclosure of information so that effective counseling and therapy can be provided. In general, unless required by the law to do so, a healthcare provider is ethically barred from revealing confidential communications or information without the patient's consent.

The obligation to maintain patient confidence is not without limits, however, and it may be overridden by exceptions that are ethically and legally justified. Such justification may occur when a patient threatens to inflict bodily harm to another person or to self and there is a reasonable probability that the patient may carry out the threat, and when reports are required by law, such as with communicable diseases and gunshot and knife wounds. California established a physician's duty to warn third parties if there is an imminent threat of serious harm to a known third party (Tarasoff, 1976). Subsequent to the *Tarasoff* case, many other states have adopted this duty-to-warn requirement and even expanded it to unknown third parties. However, it is still not clear whether the duty to warn as identified in the *Tarasoff* case would apply to a sexual or needle-sharing partner of a PWH who had not disclosed their HIV status.

It is important to differentiate "permissive" disclosures allowed under state laws, usually to local public health officers, from "mandatory" disclosures as required by law. A mandatory disclosure is one that a healthcare provider must make, such as disclosure of reportable diseases or suspected child abuse. In a permissive disclosure, local regulations allow a healthcare provider to discuss a specific patient with local public health officials (e.g., to seek their assistance in modifying a patient's behavior).

It is within this legal and ethical framework that providers should consider their obligations when they are aware that a PWH is endangering others by engaging in acts that may lead to transmission of HIV. American Medical Association (AMA) guidelines issued in 1992 and updated in 1994, while recognizing a physician's obligation to protect the patient's confidentiality whenever possible, acknowledge that there are exceptions to this confidentiality:

> When necessary to protect the public health or when necessary to protect individuals, including healthcare workers, who are endangered by persons infected with HIV. If a physician knows that a seropositive individual is endangering a third party, the physician should, within the constraints of the law: (1) attempt to persuade the infected patient to cease endangering the third party; (2) if persuasion fails, notify authorities; and (3) if the authorities take no action, notify the endangered third party.

Given the legal implications of divulging a person's HIV status, healthcare providers should consult an attorney or become familiar with state laws and regulations before making any such disclosures.

PERINATAL/ADOLESCENT HIV DISCLOSURE

Complex disclosure challenges may arise during the peri/neonatal period. Local, regional, and national laws should be consulted in determining disclosure and privacy laws, as they apply to the peri/neonatal period. Likewise, disclosure of HIV status to young children or adolescents is a difficult challenge. HIV-status disclosure to children is quite low in Sub-Saharan Africa. This may be due to several factors, including parents'/caregivers' fear of the child disclosing status to others, a lack of knowledge on how to make the disclosure, and the assessment of whether the child can cope with the psychological impact of diagnosis (Doat et al., 2019).

The World Health Organization (WHO) recommends disclosing HIV status between 6 and 12 years, and the American Academy of Pediatrics recommends that children are informed at "school age." The WHO guidance notes that health care workers are often without the support of definitive, evidence-based policies and guidelines on when, how, and under what conditions children should be informed about their own or their caregivers' HIV status (Krauss et al., 2011).

Disclosure to Children of their Own HIV Status

Key conclusions of the WHO Guideline on HIV disclosure counseling for children up to 12 years of age:

- There is evidence of health benefit (e.g., reduced risk of death) and little evidence of psychological or emotional harm from disclosure of HIV status to children with HIV. Immediate emotional reactions dissipate with time and respond to program interventions.

- Disclosure of diagnosis, as described by published researchers and by practitioners, is not an isolated event but rather a step in the process of adjustment by the child, caregivers, and the community to an illness and the life challenges that it poses.

Disclosure to Children of their Parent's or Caregivers' HIV Status

- There is evidence of benefit to health for children (regardless of their HIV status) of caregivers with HIV if the caregiver discloses to them.

- The concerns of some caregivers that disclosure leads to increased behavioral problems in children and decreases the quality of the relationship are not supported by children's reports about their reactions to disclosure of their caregivers' HIV status. Even by parents' reports, anticipating and preparing for the understandable initial emotional reactions can improve the child's responses, and responses improve with time. Health care workers are often without the support of definitive, evidence-based policies and guidelines on when, how, and under what conditions children should be informed about their own or their caregivers' HIV status.

- There appears to be no harm to caregivers when they disclose their status to their children or wards.

Considering that virally suppressed people do not transmit HIV and that interrupting the transmission cycle is critical to ending the HIV epidemic, Budhwani and colleagues examined the relationship between age of disclosure and viral load suppression by evaluating data from a pediatric HIV clinic in the southern United States. Records from cases of perinatal transmission seen between 2008 and 2018 were analyzed (N = 61). The preliminary findings suggest that disclosing HIV-status between 10 and 12 years of age may promote viral suppression through medication adherence (Budhwani et al., 2020).

REFERENCES/RECOMMENDED READING

Budhwani H, Mills L, Marefka LEB, et al. Preliminary study on HIV status disclosure to perinatal infected children: retrospective analysis of administrative records from a pediatric HIV clinic in the southern United States. *BMC Res Notes*. 2020;13:253.

Doat AR, Negarandeh R, Hasanpour M. Disclosure of HIV status to children in Sub-Saharan Africa: a systematic review. *Medicina (Kaunas)*. 2019;55(8):433.

Downs L. The duty to protect a patient's right to confidentiality: Tarasoff, HIV, and confusion. *J Forensic Psychol Pract*. 2015;15(2): 160–170.

HIV.gov. HIV disclosure policies and procedures. https://www.hiv.gov/hiv-basics/living-well-with-hiv/your-legal-rights/limits-on-confidentiality. Published 2017. Accessed August 25, 2022.

Krauss B, Letteney S, de Baets A, Murugi J, Okero FA. *Guideline on HIV disclosure counselling for children up to 12 years of age*. Geneva: World Health Organization; 2011. https://apps.who.int/iris/bitstream/handle/10665/44777/9789241502863_eng.pdf;jsessionid=27A6CA8DA056F1823129425B95692717?sequence=1. Accessed August 25, 2022.

Lin L, Liang BA. HIV and health law: striking the balance between legal mandates and medical ethics. *Virtual Mentor Am Med Assoc J Ethics*. 2005;7(10).

Obermeyer CM, Baijal P, Pegurri E. Facilitating HIV disclosure across diverse settings: a review. *Am J Pub Health*. 2011;101(6):1011–1023.

Richardson R, Golden S, Hanssens C. Ending & defending against HIV criminalization—a manual for advocates: vol. 1. State and federal laws and prosecutions, 2nd ed. http://www.hivlawandpolicy.org/sites/www.hivlawandpolicy.org/files/HIV%20Crim%20Manual%20%28updated%205.4.15%29.pdf. Published 2015. Accessed August 25, 2022.

Simoni JM, Davis ML, Drossman JA, et al. Mothers with HIV/AIDS and their children: disclosure and guardianship issues. *Women Health*. 2000;31:39–54.

Tarasoff v. Regents of U. of California, 131 Cal. Rptr. 14, 551 P.2d 334 (1976).

Webber DW. Self-incrimination, partner notification, and the criminal law: negatives for the CDC's "prevention for positives" initiative. *AIDS Public Policy J*. 2004;19:54–66.

HIV CRIMINALIZATION

LEARNING OBJECTIVE

- Describe the scope, risks, and intentions of HIV criminalization laws that criminalize willful or knowing exposure of another person to HIV.

WHAT'S NEW?

- States continue to modify their HIV criminalization statutes in keeping with advancements in treatment and prevention) in the past few years.

- A national study of MSM in 2017 that found that Black MSM in states with HIV criminalization laws were more likely to report community discrimination against and intolerance toward PWH than Black MSM in states without such laws.

KEY POINTS

- HIV criminalization laws were enacted early in the HIV epidemic to limit the intentional spread of HIV, but these laws continue to be re-examined within the context of current scientific advancements in HIV care and the potential harms to PWH.

- Stigma and discrimination continue to be major challenges to the comprehensive response necessary to address the HIV public health crisis.

In an attempt to limit the spread of HIV, many states enacted laws that criminalize willful or knowing exposure of another person to HIV (Gostin, 1989). During the early years of the HIV epidemic, many states implemented HIV-specific criminal exposure laws (statutes and regulations). Initial funding in 1990 of the Ryan White Comprehensive AIDS Resources Emergency Act was contingent on states having criminal laws to prosecute individuals who knowingly exposed others to HIV (Mermin et al., 2021). Some of these state laws criminalize behaviors that cannot transmit HIV and apply regardless of actual transmission.

As of 2021, 35 states have laws that criminalize HIV exposure. The laws for the 50 states and the District of Columbia were assessed and categorized by the CDC into four categories.

1. HIV-specific laws that criminalize or control behaviors that can potentially expose another person to HIV.

2. Sexually transmitted disease (STI) and communicable, contagious, infectious disease (STI/communicable/infectious disease-specific) laws that criminalize or control behaviors that can potentially expose another person to STIs/communicable/infectious diseases. This might include HIV.

3. Sentence enhancement laws specific to HIV or STIs that do not criminalize a behavior but increase the sentence length when a person with HIV commits certain crimes.

4. No specific criminalization laws.

Some statutes do not require proof of intent to harm—only proof that the person knew that they had HIV, and, despite that knowledge, failed to inform at-risk contacts or use appropriate precautions (e.g., safer sex or clean needles) to prevent contacts from transmission. These laws have also been applied to PWH who solicited sex for money, a prisoner who bit a prison guard, and individuals who spat on another person. Although these statutes have been challenged on the alleged grounds of unconstitutional vagueness or violations of free speech or free association, most have been upheld. In addition to these laws, prosecutors have brought other criminal charges against PWH who unreasonably risk transmission of HIV through such acts as attempted murder, assault, and reckless endangerment (Gostin, 1989; Webber, 2004). These cases highlight the tension between public health and criminal justice approaches toward disclosure and HIV transmission (Csete, 2011; Obermeyer et al., 2011).

An analysis by CDC and US Department of Justice researchers found that, through 2011, a total of 67 laws explicitly focused on PWH had been enacted in 33 states. These laws vary as to what behaviors are criminalized or result in additional penalties. Many states have laws that require persons who are aware that they have HIV to disclose their status to sexual partners and/or needle-sharing partners. Some state laws criminalize one or more behaviors that, as noted by Lehman and colleagues (2014) pose low or negligible risk for HIV transmission. pose low or negligible risk for HIV transmission. The majority of laws were passed before studies showed that ART reduces HIV transmission risk, and most laws do not account for HIV prevention measures that reduce transmission risk, such as condom use, ART, and PrEP. Punishing people for behavior that is either consensual or poses no risk of HIV transmission only serves to further stigmatize already marginalized communities while missing opportunities for prevention education. The potential stigma associated with HIV criminalization laws was seen in a national study of MSM in 2017 that found that Black MSM in states with HIV criminalization laws were more likely to report community discrimination against PWH than Black MSM in states without such laws (aPR 1.14; 95% CI: 1.02–1.29; P = 0.02) and intolerance toward MSM (aPR 2.02; 95% CI: 1.43–2.86; P < 0.001) (Baugher et al., 2021).

National organizations and the federal government have recognized the need to update HIV criminalization laws to be consistent with current science and need for personal protection of PWH. The American Academy of HIV Medicine (AAHIVM), and its members are "opposed to laws that distinguish HIV disease from other comparable diseases or that create disproportionate penalties for disclosure, exposure, or transmission of HIV disease beyond normal public health ordinances." The AAHIVM "supports nonpunitive prevention approaches to HIV centered on current scientific understanding and evidence-based research." The HIV Medicine Association (HIVMA) also "strongly oppose laws that criminalize transmission or non-disclosure of HIV status and other infectious diseases because of the harmful affect these laws have on individual and public health." The Sero Project is a network of PWH and their allies fighting for freedom from stigma and injustice. The Sero Project is particularly focused on ending inappropriate criminal prosecutions of PWH, including for nondisclosure of their HIV status and potential or perceived HIV exposure or HIV transmission. In the United States, The National HIV/AIDS Strategy was updated in 2021 and identifies goals for 2022–2025, which includes Goal 3.1.1:

> Strengthen enforcement of civil rights laws (including language access services and disability rights), promote reform of state HIV criminalization laws, and assist states in protecting people with HIV from violence, retaliation, and discrimination associated with HIV status, homophobia, transphobia, xenophobia, racism, substance use, and sexism.

The CDC notes that since 2014, at least five states have modernized their HIV criminal laws. Changes include removing HIV prevention issues from the criminal code and including them under disease control regulations, requiring intent to transmit, actual HIV transmission, or providing defenses for taking measures to prevent transmission such as viral suppression or being noninfectious, condom use, and partner PrEP use.

Advances in effective ART and PrEP have called into question the necessity of some of the HIV criminalization laws, which were enacted early in the HIV epidemic when treatment and prevention options were not as advanced. Additionally, a 2017 study showed no association between HIV nor AIDS diagnosis rate and HIV criminalization laws across states, highlighting the limited efficacy of these laws in improving HIV prevention or detection (Sweeney et al., 2017).

REFERENCES/RECOMMENDED READING

Adam BD, Corriveau P, Elliott R, et al. HIV disclosure as practice and public policy. *Crit Public Health*. 2015;25(4):386–397.

American Academy of HIV Medicine. HIV criminalization. https://aahivm.org/hiv-criminalization/. n.d. Accessed August 25, 2022.

American Academy of HIV Medicine. Public policy platform. aahivm.org/wp-content/uploads/2019/06/policy-platform-updated-6.3.19.pdf. Updated June 3, 2019. Accessed August 25, 2022.

Baugher AR, Whiteman A, Jeffries WL 4th, et al. Black men who have sex with men living in states with HIV criminalization laws report high stigma, 23 U.S. cities, 2017. *AIDS*. August 1, 2021;35(10):1637–1645.

Centers for Disease Control and Prevention (CDC). HIV and STD criminal laws. https://www.cdc.gov/hiv/policies/law/states/exposure.html. Published 2022. Accessed August 25, 2022.

Center for HIV Law and Policy. HIV criminalization in the United States, CHLP. https://www.hivlawandpolicy.org/resources/map-hiv-criminalization-united-states-chlp-updated-2022. Updated 2022. Accessed August 25, 2022.

Center for HIV Law and Policy. State HIV laws HIV-specific criminal laws, state guidelines for health care workers with HIV, youth access to STI and HIV testing and treatment, HIV testing. http://www.hivlawandpolicy.org/state-hiv-laws. n.d. Accessed August 25, 2022.

Csete J, Kaplan K, Hayashi K, et al. Compulsory drug detention center experiences among a community-based sample of injection drug users in Bangkok, Thailand. *BMC Int Health Hum Rights*. 2011;11:12. doi:10.1186/1472-698X-11-12.

Francis LP, Francis JG. Criminalizing health-related behaviors dangerous to others? Disease transmission, transmission-facilitation, and the importance of trust. *Criminal Law Philosophy*. 2012;6:47–63.

Haire B, Kaldor J. HIV transmission law in the age of treatment-as-prevention. *J Med Ethics*. 2015;41:982–986.

HIVMA HIV Criminalization Reform and Advocacy. https://www.hivma.org/policy--advocacy/hiv-criminalization-reform-and-advocacy/. Published 2018. Accessed August 25, 2022.

Lehman JS, Carr MH, Nichol AJ, et al. Prevalence and public health implications of state laws that criminalize potential HIV exposure in the United States. *AIDS Behav*. 2014;18(6):997–1006.

Mermin J, Valentine SS, McCray E. HIV criminalisation laws and ending the US HIV epidemic. *Lancet HIV*. 2021;8(1):e4–e6.

Mykhalovskiy E. The public health implications of HIV criminalization: past, current, and future research directions. *Crit Public Health*. 2015;25(4):373–385.

Sero Project. HIV criminalization resources. http://www.seroproject.com/resources. Published 2022. Accessed August 25, 2022.

Sweeney P, Gray SC, Purcell DW, et al. Association of HIV diagnosis rates and laws criminalizing HIV exposure in the United States. *AIDS*. 2017;31(10):1483–1488.

The White House. National HIV/AIDS strategy for the United States 2022–2025. Washington, DC. https://hivgov-prod-v3.s3.amazon aws.com/s3fs-public/NHAS-2022-2025.pdf. Published 2021. Accessed August 25, 2022.

TREATING MINORS

LEARNING OBJECTIVE

- Describe legal issues related to treatment of minors with HIV.

WHAT'S NEW?

- Information regarding treatment of minors has remained consistent during the past several years.

KEY POINTS

- Medical treatment of minors (persons younger than age 18 years) must generally be authorized by a parent or legal guardian, with specific exceptions that vary across states.

- This area of law is often complex and variable. Healthcare providers unsure of their state laws and regulations should seek legal advice before treating minors for HIV.

The medical care of a *minor*—defined in most states as a person younger than age 18 years—must generally be authorized by his or her parent or legal guardian. This usually means that a parent or guardian of a minor is required to give informed consent on behalf of the minor for most medical decisions. However, there are exceptions to this rule, and certain minors can consent to certain types of medical care without the authority of a parent or legal guardian.

CONSENT FOR STI SERVICES AND MEDICAL TREATMENT

All 50 states and the District of Columbia explicitly allow minors to consent to STI services, although 11 states require that a minor be of a certain age (generally ages 12–14 years) before being allowed to consent. Thirty-two states explicitly include HIV testing and treatment in the package of STI services to which minors may consent.

MEDICAL TREATMENT

Most states have laws that authorize minors to consent to certain types of medical treatment, such as care for pregnancy; contraception and abortion care; treatment for contagious diseases, STIs, rape, sexual assault, mental health, and drug or alcohol abuse; and HIV testing. In many states, absent exceptional circumstances, a minor is not able to consent to HIV treatment, and consent must be obtained from the parent or legal guardian (e.g., see New York State Public Health Law 2504).

EXCEPTIONS

Almost all states have laws that authorize minors who have attained a certain status to make the majority of their own healthcare decisions. These may include minors who are married (or divorced), on active duty with the US Armed Forces, emancipated by a court order, or self-sufficient such that they have attained a designated age and live away from home and manage their own financial affairs.

LAWS RELATED TO INFORMING PARENTS

Eighteen states allow healthcare providers to inform a minor's parents that he, she, or they is seeking or receiving STI services. With the exception of one state (Iowa requires parental notification in the case of a positive HIV test), no state requires that providers notify parents (Guttmacher Institute, 2007; Ho et al., 2005). In some states, healthcare providers are prohibited from telling the minor's parent(s) or legal guardian about any test-related medical care unless the minor authorizes it (e.g., see New York State Public Health Law 2780.5).

SEEKING LEGAL ADVICE

Healthcare providers should be aware that this area of the law is very complex, highly variable by state, and rife with legal risks and exposure if an incorrect decision regarding treatment is made. Therefore, it is highly advisable that healthcare providers who are unsure of the law in their state consult a lawyer before providing HIV testing or treatment to a minor. Healthcare providers must be acutely aware of the importance of consulting and obtaining the informed consent of a parent or legal guardian of the minor when required by law.

REFERENCES/RECOMMENDED READING

Center for HIV Law and Policy. State HIV laws HIV-specific criminal laws, state guidelines for health care workers with HIV, youth access to STI and HIV testing and treatment, HIV testing. http://www.hivlawandpolicy.org/state-hiv-laws. n.d. Accessed August 25, 2022.

CDC. State laws that enable a minor to provide informed consent to receive HIV and STD services. https://www.cdc.gov/hiv/polic ies/law/states/minors.html. Published 2022. Accessed August 25, 2022.

Guttmacher Institute. Minors' access to STD services. State laws and policies. http://www.guttmacher.org/statecenter/spibs/spib_MASS. pdf. Published September 1, 2020. Accessed August 25, 2022.

Ho WW, Brandfield J, Retkin R, et al. Complexities in HIV consent in adolescents. *Clin Pediatr (Phil)*. 2005; 44:473–478.

Kaiser Foundation. Minors' authority to consent to STI services. http://kff.org/hivaids/state-indicator/minors-right-to-consent. Published 2022. Accessed August 25, 2022.

ADVANCE PLANNING

LEARNING OBJECTIVE

Discuss the use of durable power of attorney, advance directives, and physician orders for life-sustaining treatment for PWH.

WHAT'S NEW?

A physician order for life-sustaining treatment (POLST) form is becoming more commonly implemented as a part of advance care planning in many states.

People newly diagnosed with HIV (or any potentially life-threatening illness) face a myriad of legal concerns that affect almost every facet of their lives. At times, this may seem overwhelming to patient and provider alike. However, legal planning can greatly benefit PWH and their families. Providers can play an important role in informing patients of the benefits of planning ahead.

All providers should advise their patients to investigate and prepare three essential tools of effective legal planning:

1. A durable power of attorney for medical decision-making.

2. An advance directive ("living will").

3. A will.

DURABLE POWER OF ATTORNEY

A durable power of attorney makes legal provision for someone to make decisions in a patient's stead if he or she is no longer able to do so. Patients should consider two such documents to best protect their legal interests: one for healthcare decisions and one for legal and financial decisions. A patient may choose a single person to fill both roles, but the responsibilities are different. A durable power of attorney for financial issues may cover any and all financial concerns or may stipulate only specific tasks, such as paying standard household expenses or filing tax returns (NOLO, Estate Planning). A durable power of attorney for healthcare may cover any and all medical decisions or may stipulate only specific decisions can be made, such as consenting to or refusing any medical treatment. These documents are particularly important for couples who are not legally married, including gay and lesbian couples, because without a durable power of attorney, hospitals and courts usually defer to the closest biological relative to make medical decisions.

A power of attorney may take effect immediately when a patient signs it, or it may become effective only at a time or circumstance that the patient designates—for example, upon the patient's incapacity or other disability that hinders medical or financial decision-making (NOLO, Estate Planning). Patients must state in the document that a power of attorney is durable, or it will automatically end if the patient becomes incapacitated. In all cases, a power of attorney ends when the patient dies. Patients may choose to revoke the power of attorney at any time. If married patients grant power of attorney to a spouse, in some states (e.g., California, Illinois, and Texas), the power terminates if the couple divorces (NOLO, Estate Planning). Patients should consult an attorney in drafting a durable power of attorney to ensure that it is drawn up correctly.

ADVANCE DIRECTIVE

An advance directive is a document in which patients provide specific instructions about the kind of healthcare they do or do not want in the event that they have an incapacity that makes them unable to make or communicate medical decisions. These instructions are commonly referred to as a "living will." However, there is an important distinction: living wills generally are limited to cases of terminal illness, whereas advance directives may apply to any situation in which a patient is incapacitated, even temporarily. This distinction is especially compelling regarding PWH, who may experience AIDS-related dementia or other complications that may impair rational decision-making, but they may subsequently have improved executive function as a result of ART. Patients should know that an advance directive "may be the most convincing evidence of your wishes you can create" (American Association of Retired Persons, 1995). However, in a large national study of PWH, fewer than half reported having advance directives. The most important factor associated with having an advance directive was whether their practitioner had discussed end-of-life issues (Wenger et al., 2001). the HIV population ages, these discussions should routinely be part of intake medical visits and reviewed periodically.

Advance directives are valid in every US state and the District of Columbia, but the specifics of the law vary from state to state. Therefore, patients who spend significant time in more than one state or who move to another state should have directives adjusted to follow each state's guidelines (Caring Connections, n.d.). In creating an advance directive, the patient should consult an expert and should attempt to answer three important questions:

- What are my goals for treatment? Among other things, patients should consider their values relative to independence, their environment, and their religious beliefs.

- How specific should I be? No directive can cover all eventualities, but it is suggested that patients address anything that is especially important to them.

- How can I make sure that healthcare providers will follow my advance directive?

Most states give healthcare providers the right to refuse to honor directives on grounds of conscience. In such cases, healthcare providers generally are obligated to refer patients to other healthcare providers who will honor the directive. It is important to ask patients about their wishes. Generally, patients need both a durable power of attorney and an advance directive. In essence, the advance directive expresses a patient's specific wishes, and the durable power of attorney grants someone the authority to execute those wishes or to make healthcare decisions that could not be anticipated by the advance directive.

A 2001 study by Stein and Bonuck found that gay men and lesbians were more likely than the general population to have executed advance directives. However, given the importance of these documents to PWH, and because fewer than half of those studied had executed formal directives, healthcare providers are urged to assume a larger role in educating patients about advance care planning. Another study in 2000 affirmed previous results that intervention in an outpatient setting significantly increased the likelihood that PWH would execute advance care planning (Ho et al., 2000). A 2019 study of 154 PWH in Los Angeles and New Orleans found that only 26.0% of older adults had an advance directive, and 30.5% had a healthcare proxy (Nguyen et al., 2019).

Although the focus of advance care planning is usually on the healthcare and legal value of the process, another study showed that advance care planning also increased patients' sense of control and strengthened their relationships with their loved ones (Martin et al., 1999). However, more than 75% of all respondents in the Stein and Bonuck study (2001) said that their healthcare provider had never asked who should make medical decisions if patients were unable to do so themselves. Healthcare providers are encouraged to discuss these issues with patients.

PHYSICIAN ORDER FOR LIFE-SUSTAINING TREATMENT

A POLST form is becoming more commonly implemented as a part of advance care planning in many states. This form should be done with a healthcare provider, and it specifies medical treatments that a patient may or may not want in the event of a medical emergency or life-threatening event. In many cases it can complement the advanced directive and may be more appropriate for persons with a serious illness or advanced frailty near the end of life.

WILL

A will determines what happens to a person's property after his or her death. Despite considerable attention to wills in the popular press, do not assume that your patients have one—half of all Americans die without one (NOLO, Wills). Without a will, the courts will distribute a person's assets according to state laws. Wills are particularly important for people with minor children because, without a will, the state will decide the children's guardianship (NOLO, Estate planning). Wills are also important in situations in which persons are not legally married to their partner (e.g., common law marriage and unmarried gay and lesbian couples) because, without a will, survivors may inherit nothing and, worse, may lose personal property, because they cannot prove ownership (FindLaw, 2021).

Many people mistakenly believe that they do not need wills because they do not have large estates. In truth, everyone needs a will to ensure that their wishes are followed when their assets are distributed. Handwritten, unwitnessed wills (called *holographic wills*) are valid in approximately 25 states, but formal wills are preferable. A valid, legal will must include the following elements:

- It must be typewritten, or computer generated (except holographic wills, described previously).

- The document must expressly state that it is a "Will."

- The person making the will must date and sign it.

- The will must be signed by at least two or, in some states, three witnesses who will not inherit anything under the terms of the will.

Healthcare providers should be aware that legal planning is vital for all patients but especially for PWH. By focusing on the documents discussed previously (durable power of attorney, advance directives, POLST form, and wills) and by obtaining appropriate legal advice, the planning should not be difficult or confusing.

REFERENCES/RECOMMENDED READING

AARP. Advance directive forms. https://www.aarp.org/caregiving/financial-legal/free-printable-advance-directives/. Published March 18, 2013. Accessed August 25, 2022.

American Bar Association. Health care advance directives. https://www.americanbar.org/groups/public_education/resources/law_issues_for_consumers/directive_review/. Accessed August 25, 2022.

American Medical Association (AMA). Advance directives code of medical ethics opinion 5.2. https://www.ama-assn.org/delivering-care/ethics/advance-directives. Published November 2016. Accessed August 25, 2022.

Caring Connections. Advance care planning. www.caringinfo.org/i4a/pages/index.cfm?pageid=3278. n.d. Accessed August 30, 2022.

Centers for Disease Control and Prevention (CDC). HIV cluster and outbreak detection and response. https://www.cdc.gov/hiv/programresources/guidance/cluster-outbreak/index.html. Published 2023. Accessed March 17, 2023.

FindLaw. State laws: living wills. http://estate.findlaw.com/estate-planning/living-wills/estate-planning-law-state-living-wills.html. Published 2022. Accessed August 25, 2022.

FindLaw. Unmarried couples and property—basics. https//www.findlaw.com/family/living-together/unmarried-couples-and-property-basics.html. Published 2021. Accessed August 30, 2022.

Gostin LO. Public health strategies for confronting AIDS. Legislative and regulatory policy in the United States. *JAMA*. 1989;261(11):1621–1630.

HIV Cluster Guidance Working Group. Detecting and responding to HIV transmission clusters: a guide for health departments (draft). https://www.cdc.gov/hiv/pdf/funding/announcements/ps18-1802/CDC-HIV-PS18-1802-AttachmentE-Detecting-Investigating-and-Responding-to-HIV-Transmission-Clusters.pdf. Published 2018. Accessed August 25, 2022.

Ho VW, Thiel EC, Rubin HR, et al. The effect of advance care planning on completion of advance directives and patient satisfaction in people with HIV/AIDS. *AIDS Care*. 2000;12:97–108.

Martin DK, Thiel EC, Singer PC. A new model of advanced care planning: observations from people with HIV. *Arch Intern Med*. 1999;159(1):86–92.

Massachusetts Medical Society. Health care proxies and end of life care. http://www.massmed.org/Patient-Care/Health-Topics/Health-Care-Proxies-and-End-of-Life-Care/Health-Care-Prox ies-and-End-of-Life-Care/#.X16L4T-SmUk. n.d. Accessed August 25, 2022.

NASTAD. HIV data privacy and confidentiality legal & ethical considerations for health department data sharing. https://nastad.org/resources/hiv-data-privacy-and-confidentiality-legal-ethical-considerations-health-department-data. Published June 2018. Accessed August 25, 2022.

New York State Department of Health. Choosing your health care agent. https://www.health.ny.gov/professionals/patients/health_care_proxy/. Revised January 2020. Accessed August 25, 2022.

Nguyen AL, Seal D, Bruce O, et al. Caregiving preferences and advance care planning among older adults living with HIV. *AIDS Care.* February 2019;31(2):243–249.

NOLO. Estate planning: an overview. https://www.nolo.com/legal-encyclopedia/estate-planning-an-overview. n.d. Accessed August 25, 2022.

NOLO. Wills. https://www.nolo.com/legal-encyclopedia/wills. n.d. Accessed August 25, 2022.

Stein GL, Bonuck KA. Attitudes on end-of-life care and advance care planning in the lesbian and gay community. *J Palliat Med.* 2001;4(2):173–190.

Wenger NS, Kanouse DE, Collins RL, et al. End-of-life discussions and preferences among persons with HIV. *JAMA.* 2001; 285: 2880–2887.

Wolitski RJ Rietmeijer CA, Goldbaum GM, et al. HIV serostatus disclosure among gay men and bisexual men in four American citieis: general patterns and relation to sexual practices. *AIDS Care.* 1998;10(5):599–610.

ACKNOWLEDGMENTS

The author would like to acknowledge the contribution of Jeffrey Schouten to previous editions of this chapter.

INDEX